MOFFET'S
Pediatric Infectious Diseases
A Problem-Oriented Approach
FOURTH EDITION

D1408172

In Part One of formal scientific method, which is the statement of the problem, the main skill is in stating absolutely no more than you are positive you know. It is much better to enter a statement "Solve Problem: Why doesn't cycle work?" which sounds dumb but is correct, than it is to entery a statement "Solve Problem: What is wrong with the electrical system?" when you don't absolutely know the trouble is in the electrical system. What you should state is "Solve Problem: What is wrong with the cycle?" and then you should state as the first entry of Part Two: "Hypothesis Number One; The trouble is in the electrical system." You think of as many hypotheses as you can, then you design experiments to test them to see which are true and which are false. This careful approach to the beginning questions keeps you from taking a major wrong turn which might cause you weeks of extra work or can even hang you up completely. Scientific questions often have a surface appearance of dumbness for this reason. They are asked in order to prevent dumb mistakes later on.

ROBERT M. PIRSIG
Zen and the Art of Motorcycle Maintenance.
New York, William Morrow & Co., Inc., 1974

MOFFET'S
Pediatric Infectious Diseases
A Problem-Oriented Approach

FOURTH EDITION

Randall G. Fisher, MD
Associate Professor of Pediatrics
Eastern Virginia Medical School
Director, Pediatric Infectious Diseases Division
Children's Specialty Group, PLLC
Children's Hospital of the King's Daughters
Norfolk, VA

Thomas G. Boyce, MD, MPH
Assistant Professor of Pediatrics
Mayo Clinic College of Medicine
Division of Pediatric Infectious Diseases
Mayo Clinic
Rochester, MN

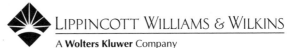
LIPPINCOTT WILLIAMS & WILKINS
A **Wolters Kluwer** Company
Philadelphia · Baltimore · New York · London
Buenos Aires · Hong Kong · Sydney · Tokyo

Acquisitions Editor: Anne M. Sydor
Developmental Editor: Kerry B. Barrett
Marketing Manager: Kathy Neely
Project Editor: Bridgett Dougherty
Compositor: Maryland Composition, Inc.
Printer: Edwards Brothers, Inc.

Third Edition 1989, JB Lippincott Co.
Second Edition 1981, JB Lippincott Co.
First Edition 1975, JB Lippincott Co.

Printed in the USA

Library of Congress Cataloging-in-Publication Data
Fisher, Randall G.
  Moffet's pediatric infectious diseases : a problem-oriented approach.-4th ed. / Randall G.
Fisher, Thomas G. Boyce.
    p. ; cm.
  Rev. ed. of: Pediatric infectious diseases / Hugh L. Moffet. 3rd ed. c1989.
  Includes bibliographical references and index.
  ISBN 0-7817-2943-2
  1. Communicable diseases in children. I. Title: Pediatric infectious diseases. II. Boyce,
Thomas G. III. Moffet, Hugh L., 1932- IV. Moffet, Hugh L., 1932- Pediatric infectious
diseases. V. Title.
  [DNLM: 1. Communicable Diseases—Child.   WC 100 F535m 2004]
RJ401.M63 2004
618.92'9—dc22
                                                              2004015194

Care has been taken to confirm the accuracy of the information presented and to describe
generally accepted practices. However, the authors, editors, and publisher are not responsible
for errors or omissions or for any consequences from application of the information in this
book and make no warranty, expressed or implied, with respect to the currency, completeness,
or accuracy of the contents of the publication. Application of this information in a particular
situation remains the professional responsibility of the practitioner.

The authors, editors, and publisher have exerted every effort to ensure that drug selection
and dosage set forth in this text are in accordance with current recommendations and practice
at the time of publication. However, in view of ongoing research, changes in government
regulations, and the constant flow of information relating to drug therapy and drug reactions,
the reader is urged to check the package insert for each drug for any change in indications and
dosage and for added warnings and precautions. This is particularly important when the
recommended agent is a new or infrequently employed drug.

Some drugs and medical devices presented in this publication have Food and Drug
Administration (FDA) clearance for limited use in restricted research settings. It is the
responsibility of the health care provider to ascertain the FDA status of each drug or device
planned for use in their clinical practice.

                                                        00 01 02 03 04 05

To my wife, Melody;
my sons, Garrett and Grayson;
and my parents, Garth and Jerry.
RGF

To my wife, Sharon;
my children, Natalie, Timothy, and Margaret;
and my parents, George and Gloria.
TGB

Foreword

Up until 1940, pediatricians distinguished themselves from all other medical practitioners by their expertise in child development and infectious diseases. In the 1930s, the discovery and development of chemotherapeutics was like a tornado in the study and treatment of bacterial diseases. Drs. Avery and MacLeod's work showing that the heritable property of virulence from one infectious strain of pneumococcus could be transferred to a noninfectious bacterium paved the way for the discovery of DNA. At this same time, Robert Austrian was about to publish his seminal work on antibodies particularly in relation to streptococcal infections.

With most of the new work related to antibacterial drugs, a few imaginative pediatricians focused their work on detailed descriptions and better cataloguing of infectious diseases, with the aim of improved integration of clinical pediatrics and the basic sciences. One of the leaders in this new endeavor was Hugh Moffet, who first published his widely read and easily understood textbook in 1975. In the decades that followed, new issues emerged, including increasing resistance of bacteria to the new antibiotics, increasing appreciation of the role of viruses in childhood infections, and the development of new vaccines. These concepts were incorporated into subsequent editions of Dr. Moffet's textbook. More recently, the explosion of information about HIV infection, other emerging infectious diseases, and opportunistic infections in immunocompromised hosts has resulted in a revolution in the practice of pediatric infectious diseases.

Drs. Fisher and Boyce, astute pediatricians and educators in the tradition of Dr. Moffet, have undertaken to bring this outstanding book up to date. They have successfully incorporated the deluge of new material. The reader will also find that they have maintained Dr. Moffet's learned, thoughtful, and delightfully expressed approach.

Lewis A. Barness, M.D.
Professor of Pediatrics
University of South Florida College of Medicine
Tampa, Florida

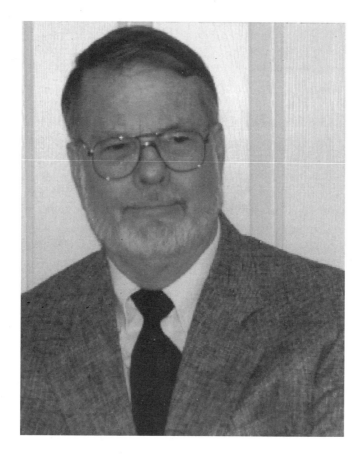

Hugh L. Moffet, MD

Preface

We are humbled at being allowed to tread, however clumsily, in the giant footsteps of Dr. Hugh L. Moffet, who wrote the first three editions of this exceptional textbook (in longhand on yellow legal pads, no less!). Those who have not attempted it themselves cannot comprehend the magnitude of that feat.

The genesis of the 4th edition, which you now hold, makes a rather interesting story. I was asked, by a graduating 3rd-year resident about to embark on private general pediatric practice, which infectious diseases textbook would be best for her to keep in her office. I didn't hesitate for even a fraction of a second to recommend Dr. Moffet's book, but I informed her that it was now slightly outdated; I advised her to await the next edition. She asked me when it would be published. As I had no idea, I called the publishing company to inquire. I was chagrined to learn that there were no plans for a 4th edition of the book. Dr. Moffet, I was informed, was retiring, and grinding out another edition of the book was not how he wanted to spend his retirement.

I was shell-shocked. My copy of the third edition was dog-eared. Its cover was half off. It was underlined here and there and had my chicken-scratchings in its margins. I had practiced general pediatrics for three years prior to taking on an infectious diseases fellowship, and Dr. Moffet's book had been a godsend. I determined right then and there that the book mustn't die on the vine, even if I had to do the 4th edition myself!

The rest, goes the cliché, is history.

In this revision and update, we have tried our best to preserve all the things we loved so much about the first three editions: the problem-oriented focus, the clear-headed thought processes, the logical progression of evaluation and workup, and the scientific integrity of the original author. Neither Dr. Boyce nor I was blessed with Dr. Moffet's singular talent. My prose tends to be too ornate, too intricate, and my conclusions about current literature too non-committal; Dr. Boyce's style, just the opposite: too brisk, too concise, too matter-of-fact. Between the two of us, though, these qualities even out somewhat, and the result is almost (and I emphasize *almost*) like vintage Dr. Moffet.

The number of things that have changed since the 3rd edition was published in 1989 is mind-boggling. As an example, in his Hepatitis chapter, Dr. Moffet lists hepatitis A, hepatitis B, and "non-A, non-B." There is no mention of *Chlamydia pneumoniae* in the Middle Respiratory Syndromes chapter because the organism had not yet been discovered. The explosion of information about HIV infection and AIDS began in earnest after the 3rd edition was published and continues, unabated, to the present day. Now, in addition to classic print journals, we have electronic pages, web-based journals, etc. No one could possibly stay entirely current and actually have time left over in which to see patients.

There is not room in any one-volume textbook for everything. Thus, in addition to a general updating, we have made some substantive changes to the 3rd edition. HIV and AIDS have been pulled out of the chapter on infectious mononucleosis and made into a separate chapter. Dr. Moffet's outstanding Chemotherapy chapter has been removed. It was our belief that antibiotics and antibiotic therapy change frequently, and there are now several excellent handbooks (such as Nelson's Pocket Book of Pediatric Antimicrobial Therapy) devoted to keeping up with these changes. As these handbooks are published more frequently than are textbooks like this one, we thought we would leave this subject to them. We have added a chapter on congenital immune deficiency syndromes, in response to the large number of questions we get asked about "how many infections is too many?" Interestingly, Dr. Moffet included a chapter called "Frequent Infections" in the first edition of this book. Some of Dr. Moffet's book was so close to perfect that we hesitated to change even a word. The first chapter, in particular, in which he outlines ideas about an overall approach to patient care, is ingenious. We changed very little. This chapter, for me at least, bears repeated thoughtful perusal.

Writing a textbook is one of those things that seems like a good idea at the time....This has been a tremendous, exhausting, yet ultimately rewarding experience for both of us. We have both continued to see patients throughout. While this has made progress slower than we would have liked, it is hoped that maintaining frequent patient contact brings a certain focus and perspective to the book that ultimately is worth it. We hope you enjoy this book as much as we enjoyed Dr. Moffet's earlier editions. We hope you refer to it again and again, dog-earing the pages as we have done to prior editions. Most of all, we hope you adopt Dr. Moffet's clear, structured approach to the practice of medicine and that this process will help you to unravel the complex, tangled knots that you will encounter in your practice of medicine.

Randall G. Fisher
Norfolk, Virginia

The idea for a 4th edition of this textbook was entirely Dr. Fisher's. Arriving at Vanderbilt in 1996 to begin my pediatric infectious diseases fellowship, I met a second-year fellow whose problem-oriented approach to patient care was remarkably similar to that of my mentor during my pediatric residency at the University of Wisconsin-Madison. The fellow was Randall Fisher and my mentor, of course, was Dr. Hugh L. Moffet. When Dr. Fisher suggested that we take on the task of a new edition, I declined, citing the lack of time for such a huge undertaking. Dr. Fisher pushed on and wrote much of the book himself, just as Dr. Moffet had done for three editions. Realizing I had missed an opportunity to be involved in such a worthwhile endeavor, I contacted Dr.

Fisher who graciously allowed me to assist with the book's completion.

Dr. Moffet was an outstanding clinician and an unparalleled teacher. His office was right around the corner from the pediatric ward. As did many residents before me, countless times I knocked on his door, and he always welcomed the visit with enthusiasm. As he adjusted the volume of the classical music station, he would roll up his sleeves and take notes on his yellow legal pad as we presented the history of a complex patient. He then helped us create a list of problems, based on anatomic diagnoses. Laboratory testing was always with a particular diagnosis in mind. Armed with an article from his extensive files, we were ready to apply the problem-oriented method to patient care. He used the same technique on the hospital wards, coming methodically but precisely to the diagnosis time and again, and all the while making us feel as if we had actually made the diagnosis ourselves. Dr. Fisher and I sincerely hope that the 4th edition of this book enables another generation of pediatricians to apply Dr. Moffet's approach to patient care.

Thomas G. Boyce
Rochester, Minnesota

Note: Both authors are happy to accept comments, suggestions, and constructive criticisms. Dr. Fisher may be contacted at fisherrg@chkd.com and Dr. Boyce may be contacted at boyce.thomas@mayo.edu.

Acknowledgments

We have been blessed to associate with and train under some of the best physicians in the world. Their wisdom and knowledge has contributed greatly to the book. We would like specifically to thank Drs. Peter F. Wright, Kathryn M. Edwards, William C. Gruber, Terence S. Dermody, James E. Crowe Jr, Gregory J. Wilson, Mark R. Denison, and Paul W. Spearman, who taught us, by example, how to be pediatric infectious diseases subspecialists during our fellowship training at Vanderbilt University. We would also like to thank Drs. Samuel L. Katz, Ross E. McKinney Jr, M. Bruce Edmonson, and Kathleen H. Rhodes, from whom we have gleaned a tremendous amount of knowledge. In addition, we would like to thank Barbara Campbell, Cynthia Hooker, and Inez Halverson, who have provided outstanding secretarial support for this project. This edition of the book could not have reached the presses without the hard work and vision of our editors Tim Hiscock, Kerry Barrett, and Anne Sydor.

Physicians who have reviewed portions of the manuscript and made substantive suggestions include Ross E. McKinney Jr, Judith V. Williams, Christopher K. Foley, Santa J. Johnston, Kenji M. Cunnion, Donald W. Lewis, W. Charles Huskins, Nancy K. Henry, Armando G. Correa, Philip R. Fischer, Bruce Z. Morgenstern, and Anthony A. Stans.

A beautiful illustration of the anatomy of bone infection was kindly provided by Dr. E. Stephen Buescher. Several photographs of dermatologic conditions were provided by Dr. Judith V. Williams.

Contents

CHAPTER 1

The Diagnosis and Management of Infectious Diseases

This chapter is intended as an introduction to some theoretical concepts about infectious diseases. It may be skimmed by physicians who are familiar with these concepts. It should not be omitted simply because it deals predominantly with generalizations, because many of these concepts can be extremely useful.

■ SPECIAL PROBLEMS OF CHILDREN

Children have a special susceptibility to or an increased severity of infections for a number of reasons.

1. *First exposure.* Exposure to an agent for the first time (e.g., to parainfluenza or influenza virus) often produces fever and a rather severe illness. A reexposure, such as may occur in an older child or an adult, is more likely to produce a mild illness, modified by the serum antibodies from the first infection, primarily immunoglobulin G (IgG), and by the antibodies in respiratory secretions, predominantly immunoglobulin A (IgA), as described in the section on the common cold (Chapter 2). Young children are also less likely to have cross-reacting antibodies from a previous infection with an antigenically related organism.
2. *Small passages.* The smaller passages of children (e.g., the bronchi, the larynx, and the eustachian tubes) are more easily obstructed by edema or secretions.
3. *Young cells.* There is considerable laboratory evidence that rapid growth rates such as those seen in fetal tissue make these cells more susceptible to infection with most viral agents (e.g., Coxsackie B viruses infect newborn but not adult mice). It may be that the special susceptibility of newborn humans to some viruses, such as Coxsackie B or herpes simplex, is related to the rapid growth rate of the infant's cells.

Decreased interferon production may be observed in young cells in cell cultures and in newborn animals, but the relation of this fact to the increased severity of viral infection in newborn animals is unproved.

4. *Immature immunologic defenses.* The fetus does not usually synthesize immunoglobulin M antibodies unless exposed to maternal infection. The newborn infant can synthesize IgM antibodies in response to infection but has no antibodies of the immunoglobulin M (IgM) type transmitted through the placenta from the maternal circulation. The importance of serum factors such as IgM in protecting the newborn from infection is not clearly established, but such factors probably would be helpful in providing opsonins to aid phagocytosis. Other immature immunologic functions in the newborn period include decreased complement activity, decreased neutrophil chemotaxis, and less effective cell-mediated immunity.

■ CLINICAL APPROACH TO INFECTIOUS DISEASES

The study of infectious diseases is different from the study of microbiology. Microbiology concentrates on the study of microorganisms, whereas the discipline of infectious diseases concerns itself with the study of patients. In clinical medicine, knowledge about microorganisms is only part of what is necessary to analyze the observations made of a patient with an infection.

Two Approaches

There are two approaches to infectious diseases: the etiologic agent approach and the anatomic syndrome approach (Fig. 1-1). Traditionally, the student's introduction to infectious diseases is in terms of the particular agent involved. The student learns to identify the characteristics of the infecting orga-

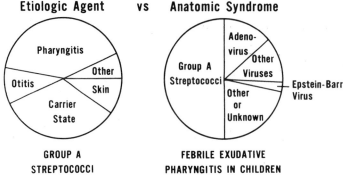

■ **FIGURE 1-1** Two approaches to infectious diseases: Anatomic syndrome versus etiologic agent.

nism and the diseases it may cause. However, patients cannot be easily categorized on the basis of etiologic agents, so that when clinical experience begins, the student must shift viewpoints to that of the clinician and think in terms of anatomic syndromes.[1,2] This is an important step in developing skill in clinical diagnosis. Syndromes can be defined in purely empirical and mutually exclusive terms, and a patient's illness often can be classified into a single anatomic syndrome.

These two approaches to infectious diseases can be illustrated by the example of group A streptococci and exudative pharyngitis (see Fig. 1-1). In the etiologic agent approach, the various kinds of illnesses that can be caused by Group A streptococci are considered. In the anatomic syndrome approach, a broad, general clinical pattern of the syndrome is defined (e.g., febrile exudative pharyngitis). After that, the various microorganisms that can cause this syndrome are evaluated.

It is important to make the anatomic syndrome diagnosis before trying to determine the specific etiologic diagnosis. This order of priority helps the clinician avoid overlooking reasonable possibilities. Although it is not customary to say, "influenza-like illness, possibly due to influenza virus," this sequence of phrasing a diagnosis helps remind the clinician that other viruses can produce an illness very similar to that produced by influenza virus. It is also an example of the two-step approach to diagnosis: first a descriptive syndrome diagnosis and second a probable etiologic diagnosis.

Agent versus Syndrome

The word "measles" can refer to either the disease or the virus. Similarly, the words "pertussis,"

"chickenpox," and "influenza" can refer to the syndrome or to the agent. However, many infectious diseases have been recognized that are best regarded as syndromes and that can be caused by a number of different agents. For example, a rubella-like illness can be caused by rubella virus or by other infectious agents. It is best to reserve the use of simple terms such as "rubella" or "measles" for cases in which the etiologic diagnosis is not in doubt; otherwise, terms that describe the syndrome, such as "rubella-like illness" should be used. Confusion does not arise if the agents are referred to by their taxonomic names, i.e., "rubella virus," "influenza virus," "*Bordetella pertussis*," or "varicella-zoster virus."

Normal versus Immunocompromised Child

When evaluating a child with a possible infectious problem, the approach may differ depending upon whether the child has a normal or a compromised immune system. The immunocompromising condition may be known, such as a child receiving chemotherapy for a malignancy, or suspected, such as a child with a history of severe, recurrent infections. Susceptibility to infection will vary depending on the nature and severity of the specific immunologic defect. In general, immunocompromised children require prompt and more aggressive therapy. These exigencies may appropriately lead the clinician to institute empiric therapy more readily. Coexisting infectious processes are also more likely in the immune compromised host. Finally, duration of therapy may also need to be lengthened.

Spectrum of Severity

There is a spectrum of severity of clinical illnesses caused by a single etiologic agent (Fig. 1-2). Most diseases are first recognized in their most severe form at autopsy. After the clinical patterns of illness in these fatal cases have been studied, a form of illness of moderate severity can often be diagnosed before death. After techniques have been developed for serologic diagnosis or for isolation of the agent, asymptomatic forms of the disease can be recognized.

The existence of various degrees of severity of any disease must be recognized when making generalizations about it. The physician should not consider diseases in terms of an average of all degrees of severity, because there are important clinical differences in the prognosis for different severities. The clinician must recognize that more vigorous therapy is needed for the severe form than for the milder form of an illness caused by the same agent.

The classic or severe form of a disease often is correctly diagnosed by a nurse, an observant family member, or a school teacher.[3] This form should not present any diagnostic difficulty to a physician who has seen the disease, but much more knowledge and skill is needed to diagnose moderate or atypical forms of a disease. Recognition of the mild or asymptomatic forms of an infection usually requires the use of laboratory tests. It is prudent to remember the old adage that atypical presentations of common illnesses are more frequent than classic presentations of rare illnesses.

■ THE DIAGNOSTIC PROCESS

Clinical diagnosis is an intellectual process the physician goes through in analyzing a patient's disease. It is a judgment that begins the moment a patient is first seen and the physician begins to reason from the general nature of the patient's signs and symptoms to the specific possible illnesses. It ends when the diagnosis cannot be further refined.

■ STEPS IN DIAGNOSIS

History and Physical Examination

The first history obtained is usually only an approximation and varies in quality according to the patient's ability to give information, the doctor's ability to elicit the necessary information, and the time available.

The experienced clinician forms hypotheses, also called tentative diagnoses or problems, early in the history taking and directs the questions toward testing these hypotheses.[4,5] One deliberately keeps the hypotheses broad and allows the history and questioning to shape them. This avoids the tendency to jump to diagnostic conclusions while still keeping the discussion within reasonable limits.

The important details of the physical examination can be completed in a brief period of time and should be complete relative to the disease suspected. Some parts of the examination should be repeated when indicated by the clinical situation.

In both the history and the physical examination, the critical information necessary to the final diagnosis of a complicated illness may not be obtained until the second or third evaluation of the important key features.

Working (Presumptive) Diagnoses

The clinician should always have presumptive (working) diagnoses on which to base laboratory studies and therapy. The presumptive diagnoses should be made early in the evaluation and are based on the history and physical examination, and, in some cases, on the initial laboratory studies.

Types of Diagnoses

Several kinds of presumptive diagnoses can be made for most illnesses,[6] as in the following list. Two have been described earlier as part of the two steps in the diagnostic process. A third type is often an emergency or urgent physiologic diagnosis and in pediatrics may be made on an urgent basis before the anatomic or syndrome diagnosis has been clarified.

1. *Anatomic:* describing the anatomic area involved (e.g., pharyngitis, pneumonia, or non-purulent

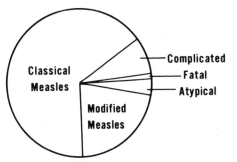

■ **FIGURE 1-2** Spectrum of severity of illness caused by a single etiologic agent such as measles virus.

meningitis); also called syndrome diagnoses. These diagnoses should be empirical and descriptive and should be easily agreed upon by reviewers of the data available.

2. *Etiologic:* indicating the cause of physiologic or anatomic disturbance (e.g., *Shigella*, meningococcus, or respiratory syncytial virus). The etiologic diagnosis should be given as the single most probable etiology, along with a list of the other reasonable possibilities, with comments about each possibility.

3. *Physiologic:* indicating the disturbances in physiology involved (e.g., respiratory acidosis, congestive heart failure, or endotoxic shock). Therapy directed at a physiologic disturbance is often possible as an immediate measure without knowledge of the etiologic agent involved. The physiologic diagnosis can often be expressed quantitatively (e.g., respiratory acidosis with a blood pH of 7.2 and P_{CO_2} of 50 torr).

Physiologic diagnoses should not be confused with theories of pathogenesis. Physiologic diagnoses can be defined operationally by empirical observations, as in shock, cerebral edema, or respiratory acidosis. Theories of pathogenesis cannot be defined by direct observation (e.g., antigen–antibody reaction, latent infection, viremia, and collagen disease).

Progressive Focusing on the Diagnosis

Anatomic syndromes should be defined precisely yet should be broad enough to include all possibilities.[5,7] After the anatomic syndrome is diagnosed, clinicians can gradually eliminate etiologic agents until they finally focus on the correct possibility. The principal problem in diagnosis is to consider that correct one. Attempting to make etiologic diagnoses before syndrome diagnoses is like trying to spear a fish. However, when the concept of anatomic syndromes is used, it is like casting a net, catching all the possible causes, then excluding those inconsistent with the data and gradually selecting the most likely.

Overlap of Categories

Patients' illnesses, especially early in their course, are difficult to categorize into a single syndrome. The diagnosis is gray, not black or white; mixed-up, not pure. This situation is best managed early

in the formulation of the patients' diagnoses or problem lists by being a "splitter" rather than a "lumper" and listing several separate problems rather than combining them. This is described further in a later section.

Pattern Diagnosis versus Physiologic Approach

The most frequent approach to diagnosis in practice is pattern diagnosis.[3,8] This involves recognizing and combining clinical features. Fever, red throat, and exudate would be combined as the syndrome or pattern of febrile exudative pharyngitis. The physician then takes the statistical probabilities in terms of age, sex, exposure, and other variables and arrives at a presumptive etiologic diagnosis for that patient, pending the results of the throat culture. Thus, multiple features make an anatomic pattern. The probable causes of that pattern make a probable etiologic diagnosis.

The physiologic approach to clinical diagnosis is most useful when the clinical pattern is unfamiliar to the physician. Such a situation may occur frequently, when the physician has had little clinical experience, or less often, when the experienced clinician encounters an unusual case. In unusual cases, the frequencies of various etiologies for a given pattern are of little value. The physician must then reason from the anatomic location and the physiologic disturbance and has little basis for discriminating among etiologic probabilities. In such cases, nonspecific laboratory studies are of little value. Specific tests, such as biopsy or computed tomography or direct culture of the involved area may be necessary if the illness is severe enough to justify such a study.

Algorithms

Rational approaches to the evaluation of certain clinical syndromes have been developed into algorithms. Overreliance on algorithms, particularly when the rationale behind their development has not been studied and internalized, stunts the diagnostic acumen of physicians in training. Emphasis should be placed on understanding disease processes rather than tracing algorithmic lines. Occasionally, the experienced clinician may find an algorithmic approach to an uncommon illness to be time- and resource-saving.

Presumptive and Final Etiologic Diagnoses

The broader the anatomic diagnosis and the more specific the etiologic possibilities it includes, the more likely it is to include the correct etiologic diagnosis. Like the detective in a mystery story who always has a working hypothesis for the identity of the criminal, the clinician needs to have a presumptive etiologic diagnosis as a guide to practical action for logical therapy.[3] If the physician has no presumptive etiologic diagnosis, there is no basis for rational specific therapy. The anatomic syndrome diagnosis rarely needs to be changed, because it is descriptive, and all skilled observers should agree on the descriptive formulation. However, the presumptive etiologic diagnoses may have to be changed when new information is obtained, because presumptive etiologic diagnoses are almost always practical and pragmatic.

The final etiologic diagnosis can be defined as the best diagnosis that can be made when all information, including laboratory data, is complete. The final diagnosis may be made late in the patient's illness. It need not always be made on the basis of laboratory tests but may be made by the course of the patient's illness or at a postmortem examination.

Fort Bragg fever, also called pretibial fever because the patients had fever and a rash on the lower legs, was recognized clinically in Fort Bragg, North Carolina, in 1942. The final etiologic diagnosis for this illness was not made until 10 years later, when *Leptospira autumnalis*, a spirochete, was identified in a soldier's blood after it had undergone 625 serial passages in guinea pigs.[9] Paired sera saved from these patients showed a rise in antibody titer when tested with this leptospira as the antigen. This example illustrates the value of paired sera in making a final laboratory diagnosis and shows how long a final diagnosis can be delayed.

Conclusive Etiologic Diagnoses

These conclusive diagnoses are not as frequent as laypersons might think. For the majority of patients with infectious diseases, a probable etiologic diagnosis is made rather than a conclusive one. However, a conclusive etiologic diagnosis is important because it allows the physician to:

- tailor immediate patient care;
- stop further unnecessary studies;
- adjust therapy more specifically;
- give a more accurate prognosis;

- learn more about a disease process;
- initiate preventive care, when necessary;
- ascertain which specific agents are common and severe enough to warrant vaccines; and
- recognize potential epidemics

A conclusive etiologic diagnosis allows discontinuance of laboratory studies and may provide guidance for specific antibiotic therapy. It may also reassure the patient or relatives, because it excludes more serious etiologies.

Every conclusive diagnosis increases the physician's knowledge, whereas unconfirmed diagnoses do not. For the scientific education of the physician, one conclusive diagnosis is worth a thousand equivocal, doubtful, unconfirmed diagnoses. The physician should use all methods available to establish the clinical diagnosis, provided that it is in the patient's best interest to do so. For the physician to benefit from a final diagnosis obtained later, it is essential to have accurate written observations of the early symptoms and signs so that they can be evaluated and analyzed.

Scientific analysis of therapy should be based on the results in patients with the best etiologic diagnosis possible. For conditions of unknown etiology, such as Kawasaki disease, the case definition must be as specific as possible in order to avoid including patients with other diagnoses.

A conclusive etiologic diagnosis is often desirable for public health reasons. For example, measles and diphtheria are of great public health importance, and confirmation by the most conclusive laboratory methods available is exceedingly important in justifying the massive preventive measures usually needed.

Laboratory Role

In the field of infectious diseases, the physician should rarely base decisions about a particular patient solely on laboratory studies. Rather, laboratory studies should be used to indicate whether the clinical diagnosis and the therapeutic decisions based on the clinical diagnosis were correct. Thus, laboratory results should be a control mechanism for retrospective interpretation of the patient's illness and a guide to the education of the physician for the treatment of future similar patients. Laboratory results may influence the physician to modify or change the diagnosis in a specific patient, but they should rarely be the first clues to the final diagnosis. A common error is to make a diagnosis based upon a laboratory test that is not consistent with the patient's clinical presentation, or, worse yet, based upon a laboratory test that was not indicated. The positive predictive value of a test is related not only to its sensitivity, but also to the prevalence of a disease in a population. When a test that is not indicated is obtained, as, for example, a Mantoux tuberculin test performed as a condition for school entrance in a child without any risk factors for disease, almost all the positive results are false positives. Similarly, serologic tests for Lyme disease drawn on patients who live in the Southeast and have a nonspecific exanthem are more likely to mislead than to inform the diagnostic process.

Sometimes the phrase "laboratory diagnosis" is used in contrast to the phrase "clinical diagnosis," as if a laboratory could make a judgment. This contrast is better made using the terms "presumptive diagnosis" and "final diagnosis," each of which is a human opinion that can be modified by laboratory data.

Definitions

Several types of definitions are recognized.

1. Dictionary definitions give a synonym or the literal meaning of the word. For example, the dictionary definition of laryngitis is "inflammation of the larynx." However, dictionary definitions often describe a set of circumstances that cannot be observed directly, such as the histologic appearance, but rather are deduced from other observations.
2. Operational definitions are definitions in which an observer does some sensory operation, such as looking, feeling, smelling, or listening, and the observation made defines the term.[10] For example, one operational definition of laryngitis is "what a patient has when the clinician observes the patient to have a barking cough, hoarseness, or loss of voice." A better operational definition of a barking cough might be "Go listen to that patient coughing in Room 16. That cough is a barking cough."
3. Circular definitions can best be described by examples:
   a. If a streptococcal infection is defined by recovery of group A streptococci from the throat culture by the bacteriology laboratory, then the throat culture is essential to the diagnosis of the infection.
   b. If a streptococcal infection is defined as a rise in titer to either antistreptolysin O, antistreptokinase, or antihyaluronidase, then all patients with streptococcal infections will have a rise in titer to one of these three antibodies.
   c. If the diagnosis of subacute bacterial endocarditis were limited to those patients who have positive blood cultures, then an analysis of cases with this diagnosis would reveal that 100% of patients with this diagnosis had a positive blood culture.

In the examples above, a streptococcal infection might be defined either by recovery of the organism or by demonstration of an antibody rise, but the test of such arbitrary definitions is their usefulness. In this case, an antibody rise against group A streptococcus is likely only if antibiotic therapy is not given, so this is not a useful way of making the diagnosis. Likewise, if one indiscriminately obtains throat cultures on every patient who comes to the office, a fair proportion of positive cultures will represent colonization rather than infection. The physician must be wary of circular definitions, particularly when they are used in the medical literature to make sweeping generalizations about a condition.

Classifications

Classifications are designed to be useful and are not intrinsically meaningful aside from their practical utility. Most laypeople have extremely simple views of medical diagnosis and do not discriminate between varieties of pneumonia, for example. Some clinicians use few diagnoses and tend to combine a number of clinically different pictures into the same general category. This process is sometimes called "lumping," but it is really oversimplification. However, the best clinicians discriminate as precisely as possible in the classification of types of pneumonia. As an analogy, in the English language, there is only one word for snow, because all snow is about the same to English-speaking people in their experience. However, the Alaskan natives are said to have many different words for snow, describing the varieties that they can distinguish, all of which are important to them. The most useful guide to the value of fine distinctions is whether such shades of differences have any utility in the experience of the physician using them.

The difference between lumping and splitting can be illustrated by several examples. Aseptic meningitis syndrome usually has a benign viral etiology. Acute encephalitis, on the other hand, usually has a serious prognosis and seldom has a specific etiology determined. The distinction between aseptic meningitis and acute encephalitis syndromes is very useful clinically, but the distinction is obscured by lumping the two together under the rubric "meningoencephalitis." Similarly, the use of the term "upper respiratory infection" or "URI" to include streptococcal pharyngitis and influenza-like illness is another example of a lumping oversimplification. It is certainly clinically useful to distinguish the benign common cold syndrome from the potentially serious streptococcal pharyngitis.

The terms "lumping" and "splitting" are also sometimes used in the context of how vigorously a clinician attempts to make all the patient's symptoms fit into a single clinical diagnosis. It is often preached at the pediatric bedside that pediatric patients only have one disease. In general, it is true that children's symptoms are most often related to a single underlying cause; however, it should be remembered that the presence of one disease does not necessarily exclude other diseases. In fact, in some cases, such as severe influenza virus infections, the presence of one disease (influenza) actually predisposes the patient to the development of another (bacterial superinfection).

Problem-Oriented Records

In the problem-oriented method, working diagnoses are called problems, and great emphasis is placed on the changing formulation of problems as additional information is obtained.[11-14] The problem-oriented system emphasizes the importance of stating the problem only in terms of what is reasonably certain and of avoiding working diagnoses that cannot be demonstrated by the available evidence. This concept is illustrated by the quotation from *Zen and the Art of Motorcycle Maintenance* on the front page of this book.

The Problem List

This list is a key part of the problem-oriented method. It has two main functions. The first is its use as an index or table of contents, for easier following of a problem through the mass of data. The second is that of forcing the physician to follow a rigid rule of accuracy in the wording of the patient's problem or working diagnosis. The problem name should be objective and descriptive and one that any clinician with the same data would accept.

Speculation in the problem list is banned by not allowing the use of "rule out" or "probable" in modifying the problem name. Therefore, the problem should not be put on the problem list too early (although it can be named tentatively in the assessment). After more data are obtained (hours in an acute illness, a day or two for more chronic illness), the problem can be put on the permanent problem list. As even more information is obtained, the problem name is refined, using arrows and dates.

A major purpose of this book is to provide operational definitions of infectious syndromes of children so the clinician can recognize the pattern and make a problem-oriented syndrome diagnosis. The second step of making an etiologic finding can then proceed using the probabilities and confirmatory laboratory tests also described in this book.

Flow Sheets

The problem-oriented method encourages the use of flow sheets. The flow sheet for purulent meningitis is an example of a rapid flow sheet (see Fig. 9-1). A flow sheet may be devised for following a patient with any acute, chronic, or recurrent illness. The best flow sheet is often the one improvised and individualized for a particular patient's needs.

Overdiagnosis

Physicians usually assume that their patients have a disease. However, some patients are overdiagnosed and may have what has been called "nondisease."[15] Patients may also be suffering from illnesses that do not have an organic etiology, but rather are manifestations of psychologic difficulties. Overdiagnosing can be avoided if anatomic syndrome diagnoses are maintained as exact descriptions of the problem, if absence of physiologic disturbance is always noted, and if "no organic basis" is kept in the list of possible etiologic diagnoses.

■ THE MANAGEMENT OF INFECTIONS

Diagnosis versus Management

It is useful to distinguish diagnostic problems from management problems. Although both problems may be present in various degrees, one is usually more prominent in any particular patient. If the etiologic diagnosis is not certain, most of the physician's effort is directed toward defining a working anatomic diagnosis and trying to determine the etiologic agent. When the patient has a physiologic diagnosis or an anatomic syndrome diagnosis, symptomatic and supportive treatment can be given. The patient still has a diagnostic problem until the etiologic diagnosis is reasonably certain. The first sentence of an oral presentation of a patient with an undiagnosed problem should state this fact. For example, "John is a 10-year-old boy with fever and arthralgia of undiagnosed cause."

In contrast, if the patient has a known etiologic diagnosis, the emphasis is on management and therapy. When the patient's problem and etiologic diagnosis are known, the evidence should be stated immediately in the presentation. For example, "Mary is a four-year-old girl with the problem of management of her staphylococcal empyema, a diagnosis based (at this moment) on finding clusters of gram-positive cocci in pus removed at thoracentesis."

Management versus Treatment

Treatment is too often regarded as giving drugs or performing operative procedures. Management is a broader term and should remind the physician of the importance of dealing with the patient's anxieties and following the course of the illness in order to anticipate complications and to alleviate the total impact of the illness.[16,17]

Management of Feelings

The anxiety of the parent and the interrelations of the child, parents, and the physician are important in dealing with infectious diseases, as in all illnesses. It is extremely important for the clinician to discuss the problems thoroughly with the family and the child if possible. Poor communication is especially likely if the patient's background is different from the physician's.[18] The clinician should provide individualized personal care with explanation of the symptoms to the patient, as well as instruction, encouragement, and support. In serious or chronic illnesses, ancillary support for the patient and the patient's family may also be appropriate. Failure to give the parents an adequate explanation is a significant reason for their failure to follow the physician's instructions.[19] Nurses are usually very helpful in interpreting problems and in giving instructions to the patient.

Anticipatory Diagnosis

As the clinician develops experience, there should be a trend toward earlier diagnosis of severe dis-

eases because of an increasing familiarity with the expected complications.[20–22] It is more important for the physician to recognize the early stages of a potentially dangerous disease than to recognize the advanced illness. Early diagnosis is essential for the primary care physician, but the earlier it is, the more difficult it is.[23] It is much more important to think of and prevent a life-threatening or permanently damaging complication than to allow the disease to progress under observation to a more dangerous but easily recognizable stage.[20] For example, orbital cellulitis should be recognized early and treated extremely vigorously to prevent the complication of cavernous sinus thrombosis. At the present stage of medicine, it is more important for the physician to know how to recognize orbital cellulitis than to know how to recognize cavernous sinus thrombosis, because the orbital cellulitis should usually not progress to cavernous sinus thrombosis under a physician's care.

Complications

Complications may make the diagnosis more difficult by overshadowing the usual findings of the primary disease. As soon as presumptive diagnoses are made, the known complications of the diagnoses should be mentally noted, and the signs and symptoms of these potential complications should be looked for frequently. This early recognition of complications is an essential part of management.

Follow-up of Outpatient Infections

As a general rule, the physician should arrange a specific follow-up visit or telephone call rather than leave this to the parents' discretion,[22] especially for young children with febrile illnesses, because many parents are not experienced in recognizing signs that the physician would recognize as serious.

Preventable Death

A review of the records of preventable deaths usually indicates that the principal error is failure to recognize the severity of the patient's illness. This error may be made by the patient or the parents simply because they have had no medical experience and do not know the signs of serious disease. It would be a useful public health practice to teach laypersons some of the danger signs of serious infectious illnesses, particularly in infants. This kind of educational effort is at least as valuable a preventive medicine procedure as teaching people the value of routine physical examinations and screening laboratory tests.

Occasionally, death occurs because the physician failed to recognize the severity of the patient's illness. Such a death might be prevented by knowledge of the clinical manifestations of expected complications and carefully specified follow-up arrangements for young infants.[21] The physician should also know the unusual or atypical course of an illness that has been diagnosed and should think of the unusual or atypical course.

Pessimist's List

Once the physician has made presumptive diagnoses, a list of the possible serious complications, a "pessimist's list," should be made. The physician should try to think of what diagnostic possibilities might be overlooked. The physician should think beyond the probable in order to be prepared for the unlikely and should plan for what to do if the worst occurs. This attitude should not lead the physician to undertake unnecessary diagnostic studies or treatments but should make one alert to the possibility of something other than what appears to be obvious.

Recognizing Alternatives

The clinician should have a complete understanding of the alternatives in the management of an illness. Problems of diagnosis usually involve a list of the various other possibilities (the differential diagnosis or assessment) and the procedures that follow logically from the list (the plan).

In problems of management, the clinician should consider all of the acceptable available alternatives. Errors can be made when the physician does not have a clear understanding of the alternatives and their consequences. It is more likely that an error will be made by failing to recognize a possible alternative than by choosing the wrong one. The physician should carefully consider all logical methods of treatment rather than try to follow a routine or regimen.

New Data

When a physician begins to believe a diagnostic hypothesis, conflicting data are sometimes ignored or misinterpreted. Newly acquired information may be used to confirm an existing hypothesis when, in fact, the information should be disregarded, used to reject the hypothesis, or used as the basis for a new hypothesis. The physician may exaggerate the importance of findings that fit with a preconceived idea.[24] The clinician should not block out new data that would change the current scientific consensus about a disease. This openness to scientific change has been called a "high tolerance for uncertainty"[23] and applies both to concepts about a disease and to a particular patient's problem.

The failure to believe new facts that would alter a decision has been called "defensive avoidance," as shown by calm inertia or denial in the face of new data that suggest that the current plan is a failure.[23] Working diagnoses should not be considered etiologic diagnoses. Clinicians should not become "invested" in a particular diagnosis or treatment plan; patient care must be patien rather than clinician-centered. Contingency plans are helpful and easier if complications are anticipated. It is a bad plan that permits no modification.

Redundant Predictors

When a patient has several of the classic predictors of a disease, the clinician may feel confident of the diagnosis. This confidence, however, may be unjustified if the signs and symptoms relied upon usually occur together, even in other disease states. For example, a physician may mistakenly make a clinical diagnosis of streptococcal pharyngitis based on the presence of fever, sore throat, painful swallowing, and a red throat on physical examination. It should be remembered that the latter three predictors are not independent. They usually occur together. Their presence does not increase the probability of the diagnosis of streptococcal pharyngitis proportionately. In contrast, a recent diagnosis of streptococcal pharyngitis in a sibling of the patient is an independent predictor, and increases the likelihood of the diagnosis in the patient.

Temporal Association versus Cause and Effect

When diagnostic uncertainty exists, a therapeutic trial of medication is often used to determine if the patient's condition improves. However, changes in disease states that coincide with administration of a drug may be due to chance variation or to the natural history of the disease process. For instance, children with the common cold often improve within one or two days of being given an antibiotic; this is due to the fact that by the time a child has been sick with a common cold long enough to see a physician, he is usually within 1 or 2 days of the natural end of the illness. Physicians must be wary about jumping to cause-and-effect conclusions based upon chance associations. Additionally, parents can be rather tenacious in beliefs that are based upon temporal associations.

Overgeneralization

Early in a physician's career, there is a natural tendency to extrapolate clinical experiences into generalizations about disease processes. This is particularly true when the clinician has cared for someone with a relatively uncommon disease. Because it is easier for the mind to recall diseases and syndromes when they are linked to actual patient experiences, one's own clinical happenstance takes mental precedence over medical teachings learned in classrooms, from textbooks, or from medical journal articles. If the patient in question had a classic form of the disease, this process is relatively harmless. However, personal clinical experiences must be placed in an appropriate context. One patient usually does not represent the whole. Obviously, the more patients with a particular disease the clinician has seen, the more closely the group of patients is likely to approximate a "typical" case.

Experienced physicians are also prone to this phenomenon, especially if one of their patients had a terrible complication of a common disease, or if the diagnosis of a catastrophic illness was missed because of a fairly benign presentation. Although the tendency is natural, clinicians must not take a "that's never going to happen to me again" approach to the care of patients with common, self-limited illnesses, because this leads to many unnecessary and potentially dangerous laboratory and imaging studies.

Decision Options

At any given time, there is a variety of possible decision options available to the physician. These can be described in the following general and medical terms:

1. *Disregard the situation.* Reassure the patient that the symptoms are not significant *but advise a return visit* or telephone call if new symptoms develop.

2. *Wait and observe.* Read, get consultation, do laboratory tests.
3. *Define the situation on the basis of present information.* Make a diagnosis.
4. *Manipulate the situation.* Give medication or operate.

It is useful for the clinician to review these four logical possibilities frequently to be sure that all of them are being considered in an individual case.

Occupational Rituals

Medicine has evolved rituals that function to maximize correct decisions and reduce the tensions that might arise from judgments made with incomplete knowledge.[25] Teaching rounds, work rounds, grand rounds, and morbidity and mortality conferences are, in part, designed to socialize the process of decision making and provide a structure for dealing with uncertainties. It may help the clinician to recognize that some of these conventions are rituals that were designed because it is not always easy to know what to do.

■ ANALYSIS OF LABORATORY DATA

There are several kinds of laboratory methods to aid in the etiologic diagnosis of infectious diseases: histology, culture (isolation of the agent), serology (demonstration of a significant antibody response to the agent), antigen detection, polymerase chain reaction (PCR), and skin tests.

Histologic Methods

Gram staining is the most useful histologic method and should always be done immediately on all purulent specimens. Occasionally, histologic observations are either pathognomonic, as in the Negri bodies in rabies, or highly specific, such as the intranuclear inclusions in cytomegalovirus infections. Fluorescent antibody and immune electron-microscopic methods have added the specificity of the antigen-antibody reaction to histologic methods and have made them increasingly valuable.[26]

Culture

This is the most frequently used laboratory procedure in infectious diseases. The first stage of this process is technically called the detection, recovery, or isolation of the agent. Bacteria or fungi may be detected by observing a colony on a plate or turbidity in a broth. Detection of a virus may be by cytopathic effect in cell culture, by interference, by hemadsorption, or by death or disease in an experimental animal.

The second stage in culturing is identification. Preliminary identification is based on general characteristics that allow the technologist to predict the final result according to probabilities based on past observations. Final identification of microorganisms is usually based on biochemical or serologic reactions; for example, by neutralization of the cytopathic effect by a type-specific antiserum (viruses) or by agglutination reaction with high dilutions of a specific antiserum (bacteria and fungi). Final identification may also be made by the use of fluorescent antibodies that attach to specific viral or bacterial antigens.

Detection and preliminary identification may be compared with procedures for final identification, which often require sending the isolate to a reference laboratory.

Serologic Methods (Antibody Detection)

These methods usually are based on the demonstration of a rise in the specific antibody titer between acute and convalescent sera. Antibody levels are measured in serum that is serially diluted with buffered saline (for example, 1 part serum to 1 part saline would be called 1:2 or "one to two"; the next dilution would be 1:4, and so on). The "titer" is the dilution at which antibody can still be detected. Serologic methods are especially useful in diseases in which the infectious agent may also be isolated in a carrier state or in a recurrence of latent infection, as well as in acute disease. Other infectious agents may be difficult or even dangerous to cultivate in the laboratory; serologic methods may be helpful in the diagnosis of these pathogens as well.

When an infectious agent is recovered from a patient without an increase in the antibody concentration against that agent, the implication is that the host has not responded to the agent. Therefore, the term "infection" is sometimes reserved for the limited sense of a significant (usually fourfold) antibody titer rise measured in serum obtained early in the illness and during convalescence.

Detection of specific IgM antibody has also been recognized as a method of proving recent infection on the basis of a single serum specimen. This is not necessarily a viable method for all types of infection;

Epstein-Barr virus, for example, may induce some IgM in asymptomatic reactivation of latent infection. Other diseases, such as cat scratch disease, are sometimes diagnosed based on only one sample by the intensity of the antibody response. In this case it has been determined that past infection rarely produces antibody titers higher than a certain cutoff level; therefore, antibody titers above that level may be assumed to represent acute infection.

Antigen Detection

Microbial antigens can be detected by a variety of methods, including direct and indirect fluorescent-antibody staining, coagglutination, counterimmunoelectrophoresis, latex agglutination, precipitin reactions, and enzyme-linked immunosorbent assays (ELISAs). Use of antigen detection methods, particularly latex agglutination tests, was once standard in the evaluation of many bacterial infections but has recently come under fire for being unreliable and for confusing the clinical situation more frequently than clarifying it.[26]

Polymerase Chain Reaction

Polymerase chain reaction (PCR) is a molecular diagnostic technique that uses primer, nucelotides, and enzymes in order to amplify DNA or RNA in clinical samples. Because this technique builds nucleic acids in logarithmic fashion (i.e., one copy becomes two copies, two copies become four copies, and so on), it is a sensitive method for detecting the presence of even very small numbers of pathogenic organisms, even after the organisms are no longer viable. It is a relatively complicated procedure and is prone to false positive results due to contamination. Laboratories that perform PCR on a regular basis are more reliable. PCR has become clinically very useful, especially in cases of herpes encephalitis, obviating the need for brain biopsy to secure the diagnosis.[27] It can also be helpful in the diagnosis of enteroviral infections and parvovirus B19 infections, among others.[28]

Skin Tests

Intradermal injection of an antigen can be used to detect delayed hypersensitivity, as in the tuberculin test. Delayed hypersensitivity usually indicates past infection with the microorganism and provides supportive evidence that the present illness may be caused by that agent. The value of skin tests is limited, however, because at the time the patient is first seen, the infection may be too early for a positive test. Alternatively, the patient may be anergic and immunologically unable to respond with a positive skin test. Skin tests for some agents (e.g., histoplasmosis) tend to stay positive for years after infection, and so may not be helpful in making the diagnosis of active infection.

Etiologic Association

The etiologic association of a particular syndrome with a specific infection is usually based on a statistical correlation, because infection, as demonstrated by an antibody titer rise, may occur coincidentally with an illness. For example, a streptococcal antibody titer rise would implicate the streptococcus as the cause of a concurrent febrile pharyngitis, but would not implicate it for a concurrent diarrheal illness.

Laboratory evidence of infection is therefore not necessarily proof of an etiologic relationship. The laboratory can only report what organism was detected. Even when the organism is recovered from the blood or other normally sterile site, the clinician must establish the significance of the laboratory result by following certain conventions for determining whether the individual illness is caused by the organism detected. These conventions are based on fundamental principles or assumptions of a general nature, such as Koch's postulates, stated in 1891. Interpretation of cultures becomes even more problematic when they are obtained from sites that are not normally sterile, such as an endotracheal tube in a mechanically ventilated patient.

The evolution of theories and standards for determining causation in infectious disease from Koch, Huebner, and Henle has been elegantly described and illustrated in a monograph by Alfred Evans.[29]

Associations versus Diagnosis

Etiologic association is a theoretical research problem for the medical scientist. It should not be confused with diagnosis, which is a practice problem for the clinician.

The problem of association is to determine whether a particular agent *ever* causes a particular naturally occurring illness. The establishment of such a causal relationship requires the set of conditions reviewed by Evans.[29] Experimental infections

can demonstrate that it is possible for the agent to cause the disease. Observations of outbreaks, or the statistical study of an agent in an illness compared with normal controls, can demonstrate that the agent is a probable cause of the naturally occurring illness. The clinician trying to make an etiologic diagnosis is often limited by practical circumstances. Sometimes, no laboratory tests are used. Sometimes, the clinician accepts the agent isolated as the probable cause of the illness. Sometimes, equivocal antibody results must be taken as the best diagnostic data available. Thus, the clinician may not often be able to reach a conclusive etiologic diagnosis, but the anatomic, physiologic, and presumptive diagnoses should always be made.

Possibilities and Probabilities

The clinician should learn to distinguish between probabilities and possibilities. Experimental infections can demonstrate that a given agent is a possible cause of a given syndrome. Epidemiologic observations of naturally occurring illnesses indicate what particular agents are the most probable cause of a syndrome. The probable cause of a syndrome depends on many variables, such as age, sex, exposures, season, and socioeconomic status. Until a final diagnosis can be made, the physician usually diagnoses the most probable of the possible agents; this diagnosis is based on epidemiologic, not experimental, studies.

Coincidental Infection

Sometimes, recovery of a virus from throat or rectal swabbing is only a coincidence. If asymptomatic infection or prolonged excretion of a virus is frequent, the statistical association of the virus with a particular syndrome is difficult. Some syndromes may be believed to be caused by a particular virus because the syndrome is rare, but recovery of the virus is frequent. Furthermore, a statistical difference between the recovery rate in normal and sick individuals may reflect an *effect* of the disease rather than its cause. Thus, the scientific criteria for etiologic association always require demonstration that the agent is a statistical cause of the naturally occurring disease and also observations of outbreaks or experimental human or animal infections.

■ REFERENCES

1. Evans AS. Clinical syndromes in adults caused by respiratory infection. Med Clin North Am 1967;51:803–18.

2. Horstman DM. Clinical virology. Am J Med 1965;38: 651–68.

3. Price RB, Vlahcevic ZR. Logical principles in differential diagnosis. Ann Intern Med 1971;75:89–5.

4. Barrows HS, Bennett K. The diagnostic (problem solving) skill of the neurologist. Arch Neurol 1972;26:273–7.

5. Kassirer JP, Garry GA. Clinical problem solving: a behavioral analysis. Ann Intern Med 1978;89:245–55.

6. Lipkin M, Almy TP, Kirkham FT Jr. The formulation of diagnosis and treatment. N Engl J Med 1966;275: 1049–2.

7. Blois MS. Clinical judgment and computers. N Engl J Med 1980;303:192–7.

8. Bolinger RE, Ahlers P. The science of "pattern recognition." JAMA 1975;233:1289–90.

9. Gochenour WS Jr, Smadel JE, Jackson EB, et al. Leptospiral etiology of Fort Bragg fever. Public Health Rep 1952;67: 811–3.

10. Hayakawa SI. Language in Thought and Action. 2nd ed. New York: Harcourt, Brace, and World, 1964.

11. Weed LA. Medical Records, Medical Education, and Patient Care: The Problem-Oriented Record as a Basic Tool. Cleveland: Case Western Reserve University Press, 1969.

12. Hurst JW. How to implement the Weed system (in order to improve patient care, education, and research by improving medical records). Arch Intern Med 1971;128:456–62.

13. Goldfinger SE. The problem-oriented record: a critique from a believer. N Engl J Med 1973;288:606–8.

14. Walker HK. The problem-oriented medical system. JAMA 1976;236:2397–8.

15. Meador CK. The art and science of non-disease. N Engl J Med 1965;272:92–5.

16. Tumulty PA. What is a clinician and what does he do? N Engl J Med 1970;283:20–4.

17. Carey WB, Sibinga MS. Avoiding pediatric pathogenesis in the management of acute minor illness. Pediatrics 1972;49: 553–62.

18. Kennell JH, Soroker E, Thomas P, et al. What parents of rheumatic fever patients don't understand about the disease and its prophylactic management. Pediatrics 1969;43: 160–7.

19. Francis V, Korsch BM, Morris MJ. Gaps in doctor-patient communication: patients' response to medical advice. Ann NY Acad Sci 1957;67:430–8.

20. Hodgkin K. Towards Earlier Diagnosis. 3rd ed. New York: Churchill Livingstone, 1975:1–15.

21. Stanton AN, McWeeny PM, Jay AL, et al. Management of acute illness in infants before admission to hospital. Br Med J 1980;1:897–9.

22. Dykes MHM. The physician: the key to the clinical application of scientific information (commentary). JAMA 1977; 237:239–41.

23. Janis IL, Mann L. Decision Making: A Psychological Analysis of Conflict, Choice, and Commitment. New York: Free Press, 1977.

24. Sox HC, Blatt MA, Higgins MC, et al. Probability: quantifying uncertainty. In: Blatt MA, Higgins MC, Marton KI, et al., eds. Medical Decision Making. Boston: Butterworth-Heineman, 1988:27–66.

25. Bosk CL. Occupational rituals in patient management. N Engl J Med 1980;303:71–6.

26. Perkins MD, Mirrett S, Reller LB. Rapid bacterial antigen detection is not clinically useful. J Clin Microbiol 1995;33: 1486–91.

27. Tang YW, Mitchell PS, Espy MJ, et al. Molecular diagnosis of herpes simplex virus infections in the central nervous system. J Clin Microbiol 1999;37:2127–36.

28. Markham AF. The polymerase chain reaction: a tool for molecular medicine. Br Med J 1996;94:148–52.

29. Evans AS. Causation and disease: the Henle-Koch postulates revisited. Yale J Biol Med 1976;49:175–95.

CHAPTER 2

Nose and Throat Syndromes

■ DEFINITIONS AND CLASSIFICATIONS

"Upper respiratory infection," often abbreviated URI, is a collective term. It has the same kind of meaning as "lower respiratory infection," i.e., it includes several anatomic syndromes. URI has become a lay term like "strep throat" or "flu."

The term "URI" is an oversimplification. The clinical skill of a physician is related to the ability to make specific diagnoses, which are based on discrimination and distinction between shades of differences, not on oversimplifications. In general, the best diagnosticians have a large number of possible anatomic syndromes to consider. The use of the collective term URI when a more specific diagnosis is possible implies unnecessarily superficial thinking.

In a study of emergency room visits, the diagnostic terms "common cold" and "rhinitis" were rarely used by the physicians, whereas the term URI was common.[1] Perhaps this was because the patient really had a more severe syndrome, sometimes referred to as the "uncommon cold," which may include acute bronchitis or some other diagnosis the vague term URI covers.[1]

Two syndromes are often misdiagnosed as upper respiratory infections. The first is a systemic syndrome, manifested by relatively high fever and general symptoms such as headache and fever, but with a normal physical examination. It is useful to classify such illnesses in diagnostic terms that emphasize the fever, such as "fever without localizing signs," as described in Chapter 10. This term is much more descriptive than "viral syndrome," an unsophisticated phrase that usually implies fever but is vague, assumes the etiology, and lacks an anatomic component.

The second misdiagnosed syndrome is distinguished by prominent respiratory symptoms (i.e., cough and sore throat) with a moderate to high fever or with generalized weakness. It is useful to classify such illnesses as influenza-like, as described in Chapter 7. Unfortunately, these distinctions between upper respiratory illnesses, systemic febrile illnesses, and influenza-like illnesses are not widely accepted, and medical communications continue to be hampered by the lumping of a variety of separable syndromes into the category of URI or "viral syndrome."

This chapter includes the common cold syndrome, purulent rhintis, and pharyngitis (see Box 2-1). Other respiratory syndromes are discussed in Chapters 7 and 8. Dental infections, gingivitis, stomatitis, and tongue infections are discussed in Chapter 4.

■ COMMON COLD SYNDROME

The common cold syndrome was defined in adults as a self-limited illness, with watery nasal discharge, nasal stuffiness, occasionally a scratchy throat, sneezing, chills, burning eyes and nasal mem-

---

BOX 2-1 ■ Classification of Upper Respiratory Infections

Anatomic Upper Respiratory Infections
- Common cold syndrome
  Sneezing
  Watery nasal discharge, often thickening and becoming yellow or green late in the course of the illness
  Nasal obstruction
  No significant fever
- Purulent rhinitis (rare)
  Foul-smelling, thick nasal discharge, with fever and/or excoriation near the nostril
- Pharyngitis
  Objective evidence of pharyngeal inflammation (i.e., red throat and/or exudate)
  Usually sore throat or fever

Misdiagnosed as Upper Respiratory Infections
- "Bronchitis"
- Influenza-like illness
- Fever without localizing signs

branes, and mild muscle aches. Cough may be present but is usually not prominent. Significant fever, defined as an oral temperature of 102°F (38.9°C) or higher, is unusual, especially in the older child. Common cold syndrome may reasonably be considered a rhinosinusitis. The lining of the sinuses is contiguous with the nasal mucosa and typically becomes inflamed during the course of a common cold.[2]

Possible Etiologies

Rhinoviruses

The most frequent cause of the common cold syndrome in adults and probably in teenagers is infection with one of the approximately 100 serotypes of rhinovirus. Reinfection with the same serotype can occur but is usually less symptomatic.[3] Unlike most other human viruses, rhinoviruses are temperature sensitive. They grow best at 33°C, about the temperature of the nasal mucosa, and growth is inhibited gradually at increasing temperatures. In vitro, most rhinoviruses do not grow well at 37°C, which is the reason they do not usually cause lower respiratory infection. It has been reported, however, that certain rhinoviruses can and do cause lower respiratory infection in some individuals,[4] and also that infection of the upper respiratory tract with a rhinovirus commonly induces wheezing in patients with asthma.[5]

Inoculation of susceptible volunteers with a rhinovirus results in an illness that begins about the first day after inoculation and lasts about 7 days. The virus continues to be recoverable from the nasopharynx for about 1–2 weeks. More than 90% of adult volunteers had nasal discharge, nasal obstruction, and inflamed nasal mucosa, and about 50% had sneezing and cough. About 10–30% of adults with the common cold syndrome will have a rhinovirus detected when proper cultures are done.

Coronaviruses

At least two serotypes of these viruses are causes of the common cold syndrome. Experimental infection in adult volunteers produced an illness similar to that caused by rhinoviruses. The incubation period is about 24 hours longer, and the duration of illness is generally 2–3 days shorter. Headache was reported by 85% of volunteers infected with coronavirus 229E versus about half of those infected with rhinovirus.[6] These viruses are difficult to detect in the laboratory.[7] They have been estimated to cause about 10% of adult upper respiratory infections. They are named for their appearance in electron micrographs as spheres with crownlike, petal-shaped projections. Coronavirus colds are most frequent in young children and gradually decrease in frequency throughout life.[8] Reinfection can occur. Wheezing is frequently present.[7]

Other Viruses

Summer "colds" are often mild infections with enteroviruses, which do not particularly cause diarrhea but do cause fevers, often with mild rhinitis or cough.

Mycoplasmas

Mycoplasma pneumoniae infection, as detected by monitoring of infants and young children, typically is asymptomatic.[9] When symptomatic, there can be mild rhinitis and cough, reasonably classified as a "common cold syndrome." More severe illness associated with *M. pneumoniae* infection is discussed in Chapter 7.

Modified Viral Infection (Reinfection)

In adults, many illnesses diagnosed as the common cold are probably modified infection caused by viruses that produce a mild illness on reinfection and a more severe disease on primary infection. The most common of these is respiratory syncytial virus, which circulates in epidemics yearly, and to which human adult volunteers can be productively infected repeatedly.[10,11] Influenza and the parainfluenza viruses can also cause this phenomenon. Adenoviruses and enteroviruses (Coxsackie and echoviruses) are also occasionally recovered from adults with illnesses resembling the common cold.

Prodrome of a More Serious Infection

Some serious infections, such as bronchiolitis, pneumonia, or meningitis may begin with symptoms resembling those of the common cold. In the case of bronchiolitis, the cold symptoms are part of the natural course of the disease. As for meningitis, the common cold syndrome may, in fact, be a risk factor for its development, due to disruption of the nasal mucosal barrier.[12]

Allergic Rhinitis

This condition closely resembles the common cold syndrome of infectious etiology. It can occur as early as the first month of life, especially if the baby is allergic to cow's milk,[13] but is rare in infancy. Mouth breathing, nasal rubbing, recurrent episodes of nasal bleeding, family or personal history of asthma or atopic dermatitis, seasonal episodes, and nasal eosinophilia support the diagnosis of allergic rhinitis.[14,15]

Nonallergic Rhinitis with Eosinophilia Syndrome (NARES)

Children 6–12 years of age may also have this syndrome, although it is usually associated with adults.[16] The syndrome is characterized by perennial rhinitis, negative allergy skin tests, normal serum immunoglobulin E (IgE), and nasal eosinophilia. It is a vasomotor rhinitis, with pale, boggy, edematous nasal mucosa, and usually responds to topical corticosteroids.

Nasal Polyps

Multiple and bilateral nasal polyps can be the presenting manifestation of cystic fibrosis, whether or not the obstruction or rhinorrhea respond to antiallergic therapy.[17]

Diagnostic Plan

Usually, no diagnostic studies are necessary or useful for the evaluation of a patient with the common cold syndrome.

Treatment

Antibiotics

Studies in college students, military recruits, and children have repeatedly documented the lack of efficacy of antibiotics in the treatment of the common cold.[18–20] A Cochrane database review of prospective placebo-controlled trials concluded that antibiotic treatment of the common cold produces no clinical benefit.[21] This is an expected outcome because bacteria do not cause the disease. Common cold is only occasionally complicated by secondary bacterial infection, and prophylaxis against this unusual occurrence is not effective.[22] Worse, the overuse of antibiotics in clinical pediatrics is a major contributing factor for the emergence of antimicrobial resistance in bacteria. Multiple studies have identified recent antibiotic use as a risk factor for invasive disease with resistant pneumococci.[23] Parental desire for antibiotics is not an indication for

their use in this benign, self-limited illness. Unfortunately, surveys show that although almost all physicians understand this concept, about half of them routinely prescribe antibiotics anyway.[24]

Cough Medications

Cough is not in itself an indication for cough suppression. Antitussive medicines are usually not necessary in the common cold but may be helpful for selective cases if the cough is not useful to raise sputum, interferes significantly with sleep, or precipitates vomiting. Severe or protracted coughing should make the physician rethink the diagnosis of common cold syndrome. Asthma is particularly underdiagnosed in this setting, as common cold can trigger an exacerbation of reactive airways disease (see Chapter 7). When needed, dextromethorphan is almost as potent an antitussive as codeine, but it is not addictive. Studies proving the antitussive effect of dextromethorphan in children are lacking. Parents should be educated about the fact that most of the combination cough medications that are available over-the-counter contain other drugs not necessary for treatment of the cough, which can produce significant side effects. Nonsensical combinations are also marketed, such as guaifenesin (thins mucus to make it easier to expectorate) and dextromethorphan (stops the cough that would expel the thinned mucus). Generally, stopping a cough requires a larger dose of dextromethorphan (0.5–1.0 mg/kg) than is recommended on the bottle. Attempting to achieve this dosage in combination syrups is likely to lead to overdosage of one of the other ingredients. Physicians should recommend the simplest formulations available if they choose to medicate cough at all.

Decongestants

Nose drops, nasal sprays, and oral decongestants may provide temporary relief of nasal obstruction. However, excessive use of nose drops can produce sensitization or rebound vasodilation (rhinitis medicamentosa). Several prospective, placebo-controlled studies of antihistamine-decongestant combinations in children have shown no measurable efficacy.[25,26] The younger the child, the less likely these medicines are to be effective. No study has ever shown clinical improvement in a child less than age 3 years with the use of these medications. Despite this, physicians continue to recommend over-the-counter antihistamine-decongestant medications, which have the potential to produce frightening and even life-threatening side effects.[27]

Expectorants

Drugs such as guaifenesin are intended to reduce the viscosity of sputum. They are unnecessary in the treatment of the uncomplicated common cold. Even in acute bronchitis their value is not clearly established. They may be of some benefit in the treatment of chronic bronchitis in adults. Toxic effects of iodides include acne and goiter. Iodides are contraindicated during pregnancy and breastfeeding, because they can produce goiter in the infant.

Antihistamines

The symptoms of the common cold are caused by virus replication and by the host immune response to the virus, not by histamine release. However, some patients can get partial relief from nasal congestion by the drying effects of antihistamines, a nonspecific side effect of these medications. A metaanalysis of all the prospective, placebo-controlled trials of antihistamines in common cold syndrome concluded "the primary literature offers little support for the use of antihistamines in the common cold."[28] Antihistamines may also produce sedation, decreased bladder tone, and rare severe reactions. If the cough is productive of sputum, the drying effect of antihistamines is undesirable.

Vitamin C

At present, the efficacy of vitamin C is not proved. It has been most highly touted as a preventive, rather than a treatment. A review in the *British Journal of Nutrition* of the six largest vitamin C supplementation studies (studies that used dosages of 1 g/day or greater) showed no reduction in the incidence of common cold in recipients of vitamin C.[29] This analysis included over 5,000 episodes. The relative risk of contracting a cold while on high-dose vitamin C was seen to be 0.99 (95% confidence interval 0.93–1.04). Adverse effects of high-dose vitamin C, other than stomach upset, are uncommon. The urine is acidified, however, which can lead to increased excretion of oxalic acid (a metabolic byproduct of ascorbic acid); this, in turn, can cause urinary tract calculi in predisposed individuals. Other than cost, perhaps the most important disadvantage is that this therapy may encourage people to use excessive doses of other, nonwater-soluble vitamins, some of which are exceedingly toxic.

Zinc Gluconate

A prospective study in adults with community-acquired common cold syndrome showed that subjects who received zinc gluconate lozenges every 2 hours for the duration of their colds recovered 3 days sooner, had half as many days with cough, one third fewer days of hoarseness and headache, two days less nasal drainage, and one third the duration of sore throat as compared with subjects in the placebo group.[30] There was no difference in resolution of fever, muscle aches, scratchy throat, or sneezing. Side effect profiles were impressive, with 20% of subjects experiencing nausea and 80% complaining of bad-taste reactions. The mechanism of action of zinc is unknown. An attempt to translate the adult experience into a pediatric population was unsuccessful.[31] No benefits of zinc gluconate have yet been demonstrated in childhood. The side effects, however, were preserved.

Other Therapies

Various other therapies have been tried, including anticholinergic nasal sprays, mast cell stabilizers, steroids, and new anti-viral agents active against enteroviruses including the rhinoviruses. Table 2-1 is a summary of these trials, along with the zinc trial mentioned above. The most effective therapy with the lowest side effect profile is probably nasal irrigation with warm salt water, but this has not been well studied. Commercial saline nasal sprays may not be entirely innocuous; most contain benzalkonium chloride, which is toxic to white blood cells in vitro.

Prevention

Vaccines

The need for rhinovirus vaccines, if indeed one exists, is based primarily on the frequency, rather than the severity, of rhinovirus infections. The large number of serotypes of rhinovirus, coupled with the fact that not all colds are due to rhinovirus infection, make a "common cold vaccine" impractical.

Avoid Exposure

Avoidance of exposure is not a practical measure within a family, although handwashing and not

TABLE 2-1. TRIALS OF TREATMENTS FOR THE COMMON COLD SYNDROME

DRUG	DOSING	DESIGN	RESULTS	SIDE EFFECTS	COMMENTS	REF.
Zinc	13 mg q 2hr	PRDBPCT[a]	Duration of cold sxs	Nausea 20%; bad taste 80%	High price to pay?	1
Ipatropium bromide	1–2 sprays per nostril qid	PRDBPCT	↓Nasal d/c (30%)	Bloody mucus (12%), dryness	Saline spray helped, too	2
Pirodavir (antiviral)	2 mg i.n. 6 times/d for 5 days	PRDBPCT	↓virus shedding; no sx relief	Dryness, bloody mucus, bad taste	Fancy drug without efficacy	3
Clemastine fumarate	1.34 mg po q 12 hr for 4 days	PRDBPCT	↓Runny nose, ↓sneezing on days 2–4	Dryness		4
Na Cromogly-cate	20 mg powder or 5.2 mg spray q 2hr for 2 days, then qid for 5 days	PRDBPCT	↓Duration; ↓severity on last several days	None		5
Prednisone	20 mg tid for 5 days	PRDBPCT	No effect; ↑virus titers	Negligible	Worthless and potentially dangerous	6
Antihista-mines	Many trials	Many designs	Little or no benefit	Dryness, sedation	More side effects than effects	

Note: None of these trials was performed in children.
[a]Prospective, randomized, double-blind, placebo-controlled trial.
Source: [1]Mossad SB, et al. Ann Intern Med 1996;125:81–88; [2]Hayden FG, et al. Ann Inten Med 1996;125:89–97; [3]Hayden FG, et al. Antimicrob Agents Chemother 1995;39:290–294; [4]Gwaltney JM, et al. Clin Infect Dis 1996;22:656–662; [5]Aberg N, et al. Clin Exper Allergy 1996;26:1045–1050; [6]Gustafson LM, et al. J Aller Clin Immunol 1996;97:1009–1014.

sharing glassware, silverware, etc. may be helpful. Attack rates for rhinovirus infection within a family are high but irregular.

Rhinoviruses can be transmitted by self-inocula-tion of the nose or conjunctivae with the fingers.[32] As nonenveloped, hard protein-shelled viruses, they can survive on environmental surfaces and fomites for prolonged periods. These viruses can be spread by large aerosol particles[33] but not usually by droplet nuclei, which implies that the virus is not likely to be spread beyond 6 feet by air. An instructional program on handwashing and germs decreased the incidence of respiratory infections in a day-care setting.[34]

■ PURULENT RHINITIS AND NASAL ABSCESS

Purulent rhinitis is an objective diagnosis that im-plies the presence of thick nasal discharge, usually yellow to green in color. This diagnosis does not imply the presence of bacterial infection. Even if exudate has been cleaned off, the nostrils usually appear crusted. Fever may be present but is usually not greater than 102°F (38.9°C). Excoriation around the nostril may be present.

This diagnostic classification should be used as a preliminary descriptive diagnosis only when there are no findings to suggest sinusitis or otitis. Most children for whom purulent rhinitis is the only find-ing are younger than 5 years. Purulent or febrile rhinitis usually has been specifically excluded from studies of antibiotic value in uncomplicated upper respiratory infections.

It is not unusual for nasal discharge to change from watery early in the course of a common cold to more viscous and yellow to green 4–7 days after the onset. This is part of the natural history of the common cold syndrome. The mucus changes color because of the influx of lymphocytes, which are there to lyse infected cells and clear the infection. Thus, the appearance of thickened and possibly col-ored nasal discharge is a good sign, usually her-alding recovery from the cold within 3–4 days. The child usually feels quite well by this time. Parents and physicians alike seem to believe that green mucus is tantamount to a bacterial infection that must be treated with antibiotics, but no study has ever shown a correlation between the color of nasal secretions and the presence of bacteria. Despite this fact, in one study 97% of physicians admitted to routinely prescribing antibiotics for "purulent rhinitis" of any duration.[24]

Sometimes, however, persistent purulent rhinitis is caused by bacterial infection of the sinuses. Often, it is the nasal mucosa or adenoidal lymphoid tissue that is the source of the pus. Bacterial sinusitis can be a reasonable diagnosis in cases when the nasal discharge persists for 10–14 days without improvement (See section on sinusitis, Chapter 5.)

Possible Etiologies

Group A Beta-hemolytic Streptococcus

This organism typically produces a thin, slightly bloody discharge. If there is a slow-healing excoriation about the nostril, Group A beta-hemolytic streptococcus is a likely etiology.[35]

Streptococcus pneumoniae

With this organism, also called the pneumococcus, the discharge is usually green and thick. If the discharge is protracted, or signs of sinusitis are present (fever, facial pain, periorbital swelling), the patient may respond to a course of therapy with amoxicillin.

Sinusitis

This diagnosis should be considered in any patient with purulent nasal discharge and is discussed in detail in Chapter 5.

Uncommon Causes

A foreign body should be considered in young children, especially if the discharge is unilateral and/or foul smelling. Nasal diphtheria is a rare cause of purulent rhinitis. A membrane is sometimes seen, and slight bleeding is often present. Allergic rhinitis is unlikely to produce a purulent discharge. Viral infections, such as those with adenoviruses, might produce purulent discharge, but this has not been documented. Purulent rhinitis without sinusitis caused by other bacteria, such as *H. influenzae* or *Staphylococcus aureus*, is difficult to document, because recovery of such normal flora on culture may be coincidental.

Diagnostic Plan

The nose should be examined carefully to exclude the presence of a foreign body. Occasionally, culture of the discharge to exclude Group A streptococcal infection may be indicated. Radiologic studies such as sinus x-rays or computed tomographic scans are usually not helpful.

Treatment

Many physicians use antibiotics to treat purulent rhinitis. Only a small prospective study of purulent rhinitis has been done, which indicated no benefit of cephalexin over placebo, with about 35 children in each group.[36] In a carefully controlled study of minor respiratory infections of children, true purulent rhinitis was observed as a complication in only 5 of about 670 patients.[37] Thickening and discoloration of mucus near the end of a common cold occurs with much greater regularity. In general, observation without treatment is indicated for patients with green nasal discharge unless the presence of Group A streptococci (which can be confirmed by culture) or a concomitant diagnosis of sinusitis is strongly suspected.

Complications

Acute purulent otitis media or sinusitis may occur as a complication of purulent rhinitis. The frequency of these complications is unknown, because no prospective study of purulent rhinitis has been done.

Nasal Septal Abscess or Hematoma

A history of a nasal furuncle or minor trauma is sometimes present in these cases.[38] Dental infections can be a source.[39] The swelling is usually bilateral and appears to arise medially. Fever and nasal obstruction are present, but the nasal discharge is usually serous rather than purulent.

Needle aspiration for confirmation and culture and surgical drainage are indicated.[40]

A nasal septal hematoma can be associated with bacteria without an abscess.[41] Hematomas can become infected and produce purulent drainage. The hematoma should be evacuated as an urgent procedure to prevent erosion of the nasal septal cartilage.

■ PHARYNGITIS

The terms "tonsillitis," "tonsillopharyngitis," and "pharyngitis" are often used interchangeably. In this section, the more general term "pharyngitis" is used for brevity, as the tonsils may have been removed. Pharyngitis is best defined by objective evidence of inflammation of the pharynx, such as exudate, ulceration, or definite erythema. Redness of the throat may occur as part of the general redness of all mucous membranes in a patient with fever. Therefore, a diagnosis of pharyngitis is not justified when the pharynx is no redder than the rest of the oral mucosa or if there is only slight injection of the pharynx.

The symptom of sore throat should be distinguished from the clinical diagnosis of pharyngitis, which should be based on the evidence of definite signs on physical examination. "Sore throat" often refers to tracheal irritation, as can often be demonstrated by asking the patient to point to the location of the soreness. In tracheitis, the patient usually points to the trachea in the midline with one finger. In pharyngitis, the patient typically points with one hand, using the thumb and forefinger to point to the tonsillar nodes.

Diagnostic Approach

It is important to get a thorough look at the pharynx with a good light using whatever restraint is necessary. The pharyngeal examination can be one of the more unpleasant parts of the physical examination, and there seems to be a tendency to rationalize a cursory look. Exudate, which usually resembles a thin layer of milk or cream on the surface, should be distinguished from cryptic debris, which is shiny, yellow-tinted, hard, and smooth and forms a cast of the tonsillar crypts. A cast of debris can be carefully picked out of the crypts, but this is not advisable. Submucosal spherical white areas may be seen, which give the tonsils the appearance of raw ground beef—red with white spheres mixed throughout. These white submucosal areas are not exudate but probably are nodules of lymphoid hyperplasia.

The palate, buccal mucosa, gums, and tongue should be examined for erythema or ulcers. The size and tenderness of the anterior (tonsillar) and posterior cervical nodes should be noted. Careful examination should be done for generalized lymphadenopathy, splenomegaly, liver tenderness, and edema of the eyelids or upper malar area, all of which suggest infectious mononucleosis. Absence of a heart murmur or dependent edema should be noted for their relevance to rheumatic fever and glomerulonephritis. Vital signs, including blood pressure, should be recorded. Poor quality of the heart sounds raises the question of diphtheritic myocarditis.

Anatomic Classification

Exudative Pharyngitis

The definition of exudative pharyngitis is the presence of a white or gray scum on the surface of the tonsils or pharynx. This scum resembles milk and is readily wiped off without producing bleeding. White material seen in the tonsillar crypts is usually cryptic debris, not exudate.

Ulcerative Pharyngitis

The criterion for ulcerative pharyngitis is the presence of circular or oval shallow ulcers on the soft palate, tonsillar area, or posterior pharynx. Herpangina is an older term still used for this syndrome, discussed later.

Membranous Pharyngitis

This is defined by the presence of a membrane (also called a pseudomembrane) on the tonsils, palate, or other part of the pharynx. It is defined as a gray-white layer of materials that can be peeled from the pharynx, usually leaving the surface underneath bleeding. Membranous pharyngitis is rare. In the United States, the cause is rarely diphtheria, which typically occurs in unimmunized children. Instead, most cases are due to infectious mononucleosis, particularly in teenagers and young adults.

Uvulitis

Uvulitis is uncommon. It can be associated with serious disease or can be an isolated finding. Several patterns have been recognized.[42–44] Uvulitis can occur in conjunction with streptococcal or other severe pharyngitis. In this case, the uvula is very red and swollen, as are the tonsils and the rest of the pharynx.

Uvulitis can also represent an extension of the acute inflammatory process of epiglottitis, so laryngeal or obstructive signs should be noted. A lateral soft-tissue roentgenogram of the neck might be indicated, as described in the section on epiglottitis. Isolated uvulitis has also been reported to occur with bacteremia due to *Haemophilus influenzae* type b (Hib) without epiglottitis. Since the advent of the conjugated Hib vaccine, epiglottitis and bacteremia due to this agent have become vanishingly rare in the United States. Prior to the routine use of this vaccine, Hib bacteremia occurred primarily in younger patients and produced high fever and toxicity. Uvulitis due to Group A streptococcal infection, in contrast, is more common in school-age children, and does not cause respiratory distress or high fever.

Other causes of uvulitis include acute uvular edema.[44] This can be an allergic reaction, so that the uvula is more swollen than red. Antihistamines have been recommended to shorten the course of this type of uvulitis.

Throat Culture

The most important and practical decision about pharyngitis is whether it is caused by the Group A streptococcus (*S. pyogenes*). The throat culture is a useful guide in this decision, but the clinician should make the final judgment as to its significance. Culturing for bacteria other than beta-hemolytic streptococci is unnecessary and usually more expensive.

The value of the throat culture has been clearly established by controlled clinical studies done in physicians' offices during the 1950s. Valuable studies were done by Breese, Stillerman, and others, who demonstrated that throat cultures are extremely useful for the prevention of rheumatic fever and therefore can be regarded as the gold standard for office practice. Rapid methods for the detection of Group A streptococcal antigen are discussed later.

The standard method for throat cultures, which has been best studied and is in longest use, is swabbing the symptomatic patient's throat, inoculating a sheep blood-agar plate, and streaking it with a flamed wire loop to separate the colonies.[45] Breese, Stillerman, and others have found this method sufficiently sensitive to identify those outpatients who needed antibiotic therapy to prevent complications. The principal variables involved with this method include use of clinical judgment to decide which patients to culture and which plates with few or questionable beta-hemolytic colonies to ignore. The more carefully one attends to the first question, the easier the second question is to answer. Indiscriminate testing of patients who lack objective evidence of pharyngitis leads to a decreased percentage of positive tests, and, more crucially, to an increased number of false-positive test results.[46] For this reason, the practice of allowing patients to have a "throat culture only" outpatient visit, during which the patient is not seen by a physician, is discouraged.

The standard throat culture method outlined above has been practical and accurate to the degree that acute rheumatic fever is virtually never observed by those physicians in private practice who use it as a guide to the diagnosis and treatment of streptococcal pharyngitis.

Etiologic Classification

For practical purposes, pharyngitis can be classified as streptococcal or nonstreptococcal on the basis of a conventional throat culture for beta-hemolytic streptococci. "Group A streptococci" and "beta-hemolytic streptococci" are two phrases that, although not synonymous, will be used interchangeably in this chapter, because beta-hemolytic streptococci that cause pharyngitis are almost always Group A.

The throat culture is primarily useful to exclude the diagnosis of streptococcal pharyngitis.[47] The recovery of beta-streptococci on throat culture does not prove a streptococcal infection; *infection* is usually defined by a streptococcal antibody titer rise (which may be partially inhibited by early antibiotic therapy). Although Group A streptococci may not always be the cause of the pharyngitis when found in the throat, their recovery from the throat is infrequent enough using office culture methods that a positive throat culture in a patient with pharyngitis is both a convenient and a practical basis for defining streptococcal pharyngitis. The carrier rate depends on many variables, discussed later in this section.

Frequency of Streptococcal Pharyngitis

Streptococcal pharyngitis is a common disease in children. In one study of school-age children, beta-hemolytic streptococcus was the most frequent cause of moderate to severe pharyngitis and the most common cause of fever greater than 101°F (38.4°C).[48] The frequency of beta-hemolytic streptococci as a cause of pharyngitis is closely related to age. In children less than 3 years of age, severe exudative pharyngitis was usually not streptoccocal in one study.[49] The exact reason why Group A streptococcal pharyngitis is not common in infants and young children is not well understood. Children less than 3 years of age who have school-age siblings may be at higher risk. Certainly they should have throat cultures if they have suggestive symptoms and older siblings or adults in the family have compatible illnesses or positive throat cultures. Clinical experience suggests that young children have a somewhat different pattern of illness, with fewer symptoms referable to the throat. It is not uncommon for a young child to not complain of throat pain at all, but rather to have headache, abdominal pain, fever, nausea and vomiting, or some combination of these symptoms. Streptococcal pharyngitis is certainly not unheard of in young children. One study of children with pharyngitis indicated that 17% of those less than 1 year, 19% of those 1–2 years, and 35% of those 2–3 years of age had Group A streptococci recovered.[50] Young adults without exposure to children, and older adults also do not frequently contract Group A streptococcal pharyngitis. However, a study of adults presenting to an emergency room with pharyngitis indicated that it is worthwhile to culture those patients with fever or exudates.[51]

Laboratory Methods

Throat Culture

Swabbing the tonsillar area for inoculation of a sheep blood-agar plate is the practical specific method for recognition of streptococcal pharyngitis. Nasal cultures need not be done and are much less sensitive than are throat cultures for the detection of Group A streptococci if the patient has pharyngitis. Viral culture of the throat is not a practical method for early diagnosis of viral pharyngitis. Viral agents causing pharyngitis are more likely to be recovered from a swab of the deep nasopharynx. Occasionally, viral throat cultures will have educational value for late confirmation of a clinical diagnosis.

Antistreptolysin O Titer

Serologic methods are also of no practical value in determining whether pharyngitis is streptococcal or not. A rise in antistreptolysin O (ASO) titer takes 3–6 weeks or longer, and waiting that long without antibiotic therapy increases the risk of acute rheumatic fever. Antibiotic therapy tends to prevent a rise in ASO titer, but if a rise occurs in spite of antibiotic therapy, this can be taken as accurate evidence of a streptococcal pharyngitis. Sometimes it is asserted that failure to develop an antibody titer rise is evidence that a patient was a streptococcal carrier and that the pharyngitis had some other cause. However, carriers should not be defined in this way, because the ASO titer is suppressed by antibiotic therapy, and more so by early treatment and larger doses (Fig. 2-1).[52–54]

The ASO titer may be useful to demonstrate that a recent unrecognized and untreated streptococcal

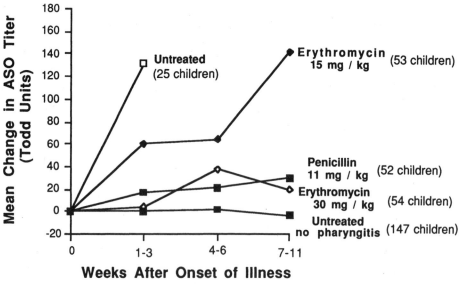

■ **FIGURE 2-1** Effect of various treatments on mean rise in ASO titer in children with moderate or severe group A streptococcal pharyngitis. (Redrawn from Moffet HL et al: Antimicrobial Agents and Chemotherapy-1963. © 1964, American Society for Microbiology)

infection has occurred in a patient with suspected acute rheumatic fever, as discussed in Chapter 18. However, it is neither necessary nor advisable to use ASO titers to follow the antibody response of patients with streptococcal pharyngitis who are adequately treated with antibiotics.

Antigen Detection Methods

Group A streptococcal antigen tests that detect the presence of streptococci in throat swabs are now widely available and are being used with increasing frequency in the routine evaluation of children with pharyngitis.

The most relevant problem of these rapid antigen tests is whether the sensitivity is sufficient. Studies show that most commercially available antigen detection kits have a sensitivity of about 90% compared with conventional throat culture techniques, especially if cultures with fewer than 10 colonies are considered negative.[55] However, many children with fewer than ten colonies of Group A streptococci on throat cultures will have a rise in their titer of antistreptococcal antibodies if untreated. This has led many clinicians to back up rapid antigen detection methods with conventional culture. Children with positive antigen tests are treated, and those with negative tests are not treated unless their throat culture becomes positive. Newer rapid antigen tests that utilize an optical immunoassay (OIA) may actually be more sensitive than traditional culture,[56] but are not yet widely available (in this study Todd-Hewitt broth culture was used as the gold standard). In a recent study, polymerase chain reaction was as sensitive as culture and much more so than antigen testing.[57] However, this test takes longer than rapid antigen testing and is not yet widely available.

The consequences of having rapidly available results in the office are important. The patient (or patient's family) is often interested in obtaining a rapid diagnosis so that therapy can begin as soon as possible. There is also a psychological benefit from obtaining a diagnosis on the day of the visit. Enthusiasm for these tests needs to be tempered by remembering that (1) streptococcal pharyngitis is a self-limited disease, in which the symptoms are modulated somewhat but not eliminated by antibiotic therapy, (2) there is no increased risk of non-suppurative complications by delaying therapy until the throat culture results are available, and (3) early institution of therapy against Group A strepto-

coccus may ameliorate the patient's antibody response, which may predispose to more frequent reinfection.[58]

The gold standard against which all these rapid antigen tests are measured is the usual office procedure of using a sheep blood-agar plate streaked on the surface and cultured in ordinary incubator temperature without CO_2 or anaerobic conditions. False-negative cultures may be obtained when throats are too gingerly or rapidly swabbed, or when the patient has had a recent dose of an antibiotic.

Nonspecific Laboratory Methods

These studies are of little value in the etiologic diagnosis of pharyngitis. Throat smears are of no value in making an etiologic diagnosis of any type of pharyngitis, and are likely to be misleading in the diagnosis of diphtheria because "diphtheroids" are frequently seen. Owing to an effective vaccine, diphtheria has become so rare that there are few technicians, bacteriologists, or pathologists who see it often enough to maintain competence in reading smears for corynebacteria. The interpretation of smears for diphtheria is frequently false positive.

White blood cell counts are often equivocal and are of no specific value in ruling in or out the diagnosis of streptococcal disease. The presence of lymphocytosis or atypical lymphocytes may aid in the diagnosis of infectious mononucleosis. High white blood cell counts may occur in viral, as well as in Group A streptococcal, pharyngitis.

C-reactive protein or other measures of inflammation are of no value in distinguishing streptococcal from viral pharyngitis.[59]

Reasons to Do Throat Cultures

Throat cultures for streptococci are recommended, especially for school-age and preschool children, when the following conditions are present:

1. Pharyngitis without hoarseness or significant cough, especially with fever
2. Febrile cervical adenitis
3. Illnesses with definite fever but no apparent focus of infection, especially if headache, abdominal pain, vomiting without diarrhea, or a scarlatiniform rash are present
4. Symptomatic family contacts of patients with streptococcal pharyngitis.[60] Asymptomatic family contacts should not be cultured.

TABLE 2-2. FINAL CLINICAL DIAGNOSES IN 230 CONSECUTIVE ADMISSIONS TO A CHILDRENS' HOME INFIRMARY OF SCHOOL-AGE CHILDREN WITH AN ORAL TEMPERATURE OF 101°F OR HIGHER

CLINICAL DIAGNOSIS	NUMBER	% WITH + TC[c] FOR GAS[d]
Pharyngitis	128	79
Otitis media	18	28
FWLS[a]	59	19
LRI[b]	13	8
Other	12	0
Total	230	

[a]Fever without localizing signs.
[b]Lower respiratory infections.
[c]Throat culture
[d]Group A streptococcus
Source: Moffet HL, Cramblett HG, Smith A. Group A streptococcal infections in a children's home; II. Clinical and epidemiologic patterns of illness. Pediatrics 1964;33:11–17.

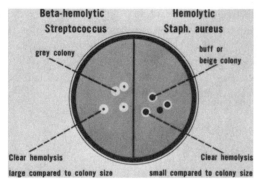

■ **FIGURE 2-2** Comparison of size of hemolysis zone produced by beta-hemolytic streptococci with that produced by hemolytic *S. aureus.*

As shown in Table 2-2, both otitis media and fever without localizing signs are associated with Group A streptococci significantly more frequently than they are seen in a normal control group. The office throat culture is a simple and inexpensive way to detect concurrent streptococcal pharyngitis. In patients with obvious acute otitis media that requires treatment with antibiotics (see Chapter 5), throat culture may be omitted because the antibiotics that treat otitis media also treat streptococcal pharyngitis.

Methods for Throat Culture

Personnel charged with obtaining throat cultures must be trained in the proper technique in order to derive useful information. A single cotton-tipped swab is used to swab the patient's tonsillar area. Refrigerating the swab overnight or retaining it at room temperature for several hours does not significantly reduce the accuracy of the method.[61] "False-negative" results where two consecutive cultures reveal one positive and one negative result are usually found in patients with small numbers of colonies and probably have little if any clinical significance.[48,52]

Anaerobic incubation or incubation in CO_2 may yield a slightly greater frequency of positive cultures for Group A streptococci.[62] However, the simpler, practical methods described above have been sufficiently sensitive for prevention of rheumatic fever by detecting streptococcal pharyngitis in office practice.[45] Selective media for Group A streptococci are available, but their increased sensitivity has not been proved necessary in office practice.

As mentioned above, after inoculation onto a sheep blood-agar plate, the culture should be streaked with a flamed wire loop. Beta-hemolysis can often be recognized after 12–16 hours of incubation at 37°C. The area of hemolysis is large compared with the colony size (Fig. 2-2). The plate should be reexamined for beta-hemolytic colonies after an additional 24 hours at room temperature, since this will detect approximately 10% of the additional positive cultures. Non-Group A beta-hemolytic streptococci are not inhibited by a bacitracin disk placed on the plate at the time of inoculation (Fig. 2-3).

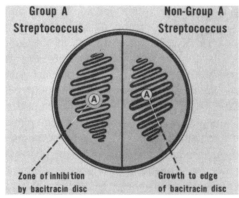

■ **FIGURE 2-3** Group A streptococci are inhibited by bacitracin, but other groups of streptococci are not.

Although there are more sensitive methods for the recovery of Group A streptococci, the above method is sensitive enough for practice purposes and avoids identifying small numbers of Group A streptococci in well individuals. The simple surface streaking method has a long history of successful discrimination between normal children and those at risk for acute rheumatic fever.[45]

Non-Group A Streptococcal Pharyngitis

The fact that beta-hemolytic streptococci other than Group A can cause streptococcal pharyngitis has been well established for at least 25 years. The primary basis of this evidence is food-borne outbreaks, where one of the non-Group A streptococci has contaminated food, particularly milk, and resulted in an outbreak of pharyngitis. Such outbreaks have confirmed that Group C or Group G streptococci can cause pharyngitis.[63] Of course, outbreaks of Group A streptococcal infection due to contaminated foodstuffs have also been reported, usually when food was contaminated by someone with active Group A streptococcal pharyngitis.[64] One outbreak of food-borne Group A streptococcal pharyngitis secondary to foodstuff contaminated by a cook with an infected hand wound has been reported.[65]

Group B streptococci also have a statistical relation with pharyngitis.[66] Because Groups C, G, and B can also be normal pharyngeal flora, it is still not known whether it is important to look for these organisms in nonoutbreak situations, or whether penicillin therapy should be given when they are recovered from the throat. A reasonable solution is that if on throat culture a patient with pharyngitis has streptococci that are not bacitracin sensitive, a recheck of the patient's symptoms should be done; if the patient is still sick, one could consider using penicillin, which may afford some symptomatic relief. However, it should be emphasized that there is no risk of acute rheumatic fever after non-Group A streptococcal pharyngitis.

Interpretation of Throat Culture

Carrier Rates

Interpretation of positive throat cultures is occasionally complicated by the fact that the isolation of Group A streptococci from the throat does not necessarily imply infection. The frequency of Group A streptococcal carriage in normal children has varied from study to study and is a function of the sensitivity of the culture method and the relative certainty of the patient's being "normal."[45] In a private practice, where the certainty that an individual was "normal" was great, Group A streptococci were recovered from 3–5% of children.[45,67] In a study in a children's home in which children were under close supervision, about 8% of normal children with nonpharyngeal disease had positive cultures with more than 10 colonies of Group A streptococci (see Table 2-2).[48] In surveys of schoolchildren, in which many have had a recent unreported illness, the recovery rate of Group A streptococci has usually been about 10–40% but has been as high as an average of 30% of "normal" (nonsick) individuals.[45]

The high carrier rates found in surveys of schoolchildren is best explained by use of excessively sensitive methods for recovery of Group A streptococci, use of multiple cultures, failure to assess the normality of the children by history and physical examination, and detection of a high convalescent carrier rate in a lower socioeconomic group that often did not seek medical care for illness.[45] The lower carrier rates of about 5–10% or less by Breese, Moffet, McCracken, and others reflect use of a single culture and careful screening to exclude convalescent individuals.[45,48,68]

Numbers of Colonies

In general, there is a correlation between the number of colonies of Group A streptococci found on throat culture and the clinical and laboratory findings of the patient. That is, the fewer the colonies on the culture plate, the less likely the patient is to have had recent or severe clinical pharyngitis, a typable Group A streptococcus, or an ASO titer rise. However, some patients with a severe pharyngitis do have fewer than 10 colonies; in one series, 33% of patients with fewer than 10 colonies had an ASO titer rise.[69] Another study revealed that 82 (29%) of 279 children with fewer than 10 colonies of beta-hemolytic streptococci had a typable organism, and one third of these 82 children had an ASO titer rise (Table 2-3). Thus, about 10% of children with fewer than 10 colonies will have both a typable Group A streptococcus and an ASO titer rise. Yet another study gave even a higher estimate: about half of patients with 10 or fewer colonies had a rise in ASO or anti-DNAse B titer.[53]

Sometimes there may be only two or three colonies of beta-hemolytic organisms and the organism

TABLE 2-3. TYPABILITY AND ASO TITER RISE AS A FUNCTION OF NUMBER OF COLONIES OF BETA-HEMOLYTIC STREPTOCOCCI IN UNTREATED CHILDREN STUDIED AT CHILDREN'S MEMORIAL HOSPITAL, CHICAGO, 1956–1968

	NUMBER OF COLONIES	TOTAL PATIENTS	PATIENTS WITH ASO TITER RISE (%)
Group A typable	<10	82	27 (33)
	>10	343	176 (51)
Group A nontypable	<10	125	30 (24)
	>10	338	143 (42)
Not Group A	<10	72	13 (18)
	>10	39	130 (30)

(Siegal AC, Johnson E, Loeffen M, Yarashus D; unpublished data.)

cannot be isolated on subculture to test bacitracin sensitivity. A repeat culture may clarify the situation and often reveals no Group A streptococci.[70] In this situation, withholding of antibiotics is usually reasonable.

■ STREPTOCOCCAL PHARYNGITIS

Objective evidence of pharyngitis and a throat culture positive for beta-hemolytic streptococci is the most practical basis for the presumptive diagnosis of streptococcal pharyngitis.

Importance

Nonsuppurative Complications

Streptococcal pharyngitis is important because a few untreated patients develop acute rheumatic fever and some patients with acute rheumatic fever suffer permanent damage to the heart valves. Thus, the most important reason for treating streptococcal pharyngitis is to prevent rheumatic fever and rheumatic heart disease. Relief of symptoms can usually be obtained with acetaminophen and gargling with warm water. Early therapy with antibiotics also provides a slightly more rapid improvement in symptoms, but antibiotic treatment need not be regarded as an urgent way to relieve symptoms.

Another nonsuppurative complication of streptococcal pharyngitis is acute glomerulonephritis. This complication is not prevented by treatment of the pharyngitis with antibiotics. These two complications are immunologically mediated, not caused by direct extension of infection.

Two interesting but rare nonsuppurative complications that have been associated with Group A streptococcus infection are: (1) poststreptococcal reactive arthritis (PSRA) and (2) pediatric autoimmune neuropsychiatric disorders associated with streptococcal infections (PANDAS). Patients with PSRA develop asymmetric, nonmigratory arthritis primarily involving the large joints, one to several weeks after streptococcal pharyngitis. Other features of acute rheumatic fever are absent.[71] Although usually not associated with long-term sequelae, about 5% of patients with PSRA have subsequently developed carditis, prompting some experts to recommend penicillin prophylaxis for up to 1 year in these patients.[72]

The theory behind the second of these syndromes, PANDAS, is that in some patients, streptococcal infection triggers exacerbation of extant obsessive-compulsive disorders (OCD) or tic disorders. This is believed to be mediated through the same mechanism that causes Sydenham's chorea.[73] Children prone to this usually have a known OCD or tic disorder, but sometimes latent OCD is uncovered by streptococcal infection. Treatment of the infection typically results in resolution of symptoms. The link between Group A streptococcus infection of the pharynx and OCD or tic disorder in these patients is not yet firmly established. Therefore, although the authors of original study[73] believe that patients with severe or frequent symptoms may require prophylactic treatment, there does not yet seem to be a clear indication for long-term antistreptococcal prophylaxis. The questions concerning PANDAS, its possible link to streptococcal infection, and the role of antibiotic therapy in this syndrome remain to be answered by prospective clinical trials.

Although the cause of Kawasaki disease is not known, up to 25% of patients with Kawasaki disease have a preceding Group A streptococcus infection.[74] At the least, there can be some overlap in the clinical symptomatology of streptococcal infection (especially with toxin-producing strains) and Kawasaki disease. Clinicians should certainly not exclude the possibility of Kawasaki disease in the patient with concomitant or recent streptococcal pharyngitis.[75] (See Chapter 11 on rash syndromes.)

Suppurative Complications

Direct purulent extensions of streptococcal pharyngitis include:

1. Otitis media (discussed in Chapter 5)
2. Sinusitis or mastoiditis (discussed in Chapter 5)
3. Peritonsillar cellulitis or abscess, which should be considered when one tonsil is larger and pushed toward the midline, with or without lateral deviation of the uvula. An abscess is difficult to distinguish clinically from cellulitis. Peritonsillar infections are discussed later in this chapter
4. Retropharyngeal abscess, an uncommon syndrome that typically produces difficulty swallowing and may be confused with epiglottitis (discussed in Chapter 6).

Clinical Diagnosis

Presumptive Diagnosis

The presumptive clinical diagnosis of streptococcal pharyngitis can be based on probability using epidemiologic and historical factors and observations from the physical examination. The following findings increase the probability that the pharyngitis is streptococcal:

1. Scarlatiniform rash
2. Fever greater than 101°F (38.4°C), definite exudate, and definite pharyngeal edema
3. Tender tonsillar nodes, palatal petechiae, and edema of the uvula
4. Frontal headache, abdominal pain, vomiting (especially in younger patients)
5. Age 5–16 years
6. Exposure to a sibling or other contact with known streptococcal pharyngitis
7. High frequency of streptococcal pharyngitis in the community at the time the patient is seen.

Conversely, the following findings decrease the likelihood that the pharyngitis is due to Group A streptococci:

1. Concurrent common cold-like symptoms, including runny nose, nasal stuffiness, hoarseness, or cough
2. Conjunctivitis
3. Absence of fever
3. Nonspecific (i.e., nonscarlatiniform) rash
4. Hepatomegaly or splenomegaly.

The above features assist the clinician in deciding whether to test for streptococcal pharyngitis; they are neither sufficiently sensitive nor specific to enable an accurate diagnosis without confirmation by throat culture.

Natural History of Streptococcal Pharyngitis

If a school-age child is seen very early in the course of streptococcal pharyngitis, tonsillar exudate may not yet be present (see Fig. 2-4). If the child is seen late in the course, the fever and redness of the pharynx may be gone, and only old exudate may remain. The clinical diagnosis becomes much less accurate after a day or two of illness.

Using clinical features to make the presumptive diagnosis of streptococcal pharyngitis, the physician can often decide to begin antibiotic treatment on the basis of a positive rapid streptococcal antigen test. Opting for conventional throat culture and awaiting its results is appropriate. Patients with negative rapid streptococcal antigen tests should almost never be treated with antibiotics pending results of conventional throat culture. Treatment of patients who have negative rapid antigen tests occasionally leads to confusing and expensive complications; a series of inappropriate laboratory tests may further alter the natural history and obscure a diagnosis that would have otherwise become apparent. One of the authors was recently consulted on a patient who, after being treated inappropriately for streptococcal pharyngitis despite a negative rapid antigen test, developed a moderately severe rash that was mistaken for Rocky Mountain spotted fever (RMSF) at an emergency treatment facility. An inappropriate serologic test for RMSF was ordered, which directed the physicians even further from the actual diagnosis, which was acute Epstein-Barr virus infection (see Chapter 3).

Treatment can be delayed 24 hours while awaiting throat culture results without any greater risk of either suppurative or nonsuppurative complica-

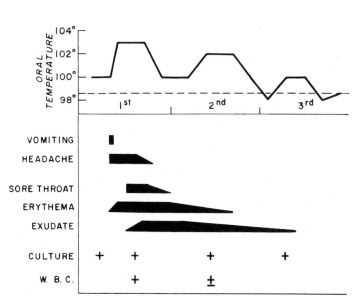

■ **FIGURE 2-4** Average course of streptococcal pharyngitis in school-age children over the first 3 days of illness, based on illnesses observed by Dr. Moffet twice a day during a 3-year period. Symptomatic therapy (aspirin, gargling) was given the first day, and antibiotics were begun on the second day. (Moffet HL et al: Pediatrics 1964;33:11–17)

tions. In fact, treatment may be delayed by several days without increasing the risk of acute rheumatic fever.[76] Therefore, the decision to treat presumptively should be based on: (1) unavailability of a rapid antigen test, and (2) a high likelihood that waiting for culture results will lead to an untreated child.

Treatment

Purpose

Antibiotic therapy is traditionally regarded as having the primary goal of prevention of suppurative and nonsuppurative complications. As was shown in military recruits in the 1950s, acute rheumatic fever can be reduced in frequency to about 0.02% in antibiotic-treated patients compared with about 2–3% in untreated controls.[77] Patients who developed rheumatic fever despite antibiotic therapy still had streptococci present in their throats after treatment.[78] Therefore, in many subsequent studies, eradication of the organism from the throat was equated with the adequacy of various antibiotic regimens.

During the 1950s and 1960s, treatment of streptococcal pharyngitis was intended to prevent rheumatic fever. It was recognized that fever and sore throat did improve, as could be shown statistically.[79] However, one frequently heard the statement that therapy did not change the natural history of streptococcal pharyngitis very much, and this concept became incorrectly altered to mean treatment did not change symptoms at all.

These studies have now been repeated in children.[58,80–82] It is not surprising to see that children, like recruits, do have statistically significant reduction of symptoms in the first 48–72 hours of penicillin treatment when compared with placebo or no treatment. However, it should be noted that those studies generally withheld antipyretics or other symptomatic therapy. Treatment of streptococcal pharyngitis also decreases the communicability of the infection to others. More than 80% of children will become culture negative for Group A streptococcus within 24 hours of the initiation of appropriate antibiotic therapy and, thus, may return to school or daycare thereafter.[83]

American Heart Association Recommendations

A committee of the American Heart Association (AHA) has made recommendations for the treatment of streptococcal pharyngitis based primarily on efficacy in eliminating organisms from the throat, as well as on efficacy in preventing acute rheumatic fever.[72] The AHA continues to recommend 10 days of oral penicillin V as the drug of choice for acute streptococcal pharyngitis. Several studies have suggested that shorter courses of oral cephalosporins are equally effective at eradicating the organism from the pharynx,[84,85] but studies proving protection against subsequent rheumatic fever are lacking, and these antimicrobial agents are considerably more expensive than penicillin. Group A streptococcus remains exquisitely sensitive to penicillin, and no penicillin-resistant Group A streptococcus strains have yet been detected.

Recommended Doses

The dose recommended by the AHA since 1984 has been oral penicillin V 125 mg or 250 mg three or four times a day for a full 10 days for adults or children.[72] Studies have demonstrated, however, equal eradication rates with the same total daily dose of penicillin V but given in divided doses twice a day, and compliance is likely to be better.[86] Some people feel that because, on a twice-a-day schedule, one missed dose makes the therapy effectively a once-a-day regimen, prescribing the medication three times a day provides an extra measure of safety. For intramuscular (one injection) benzathine penicillin, the dose is 1.2 million units for adults and 600,000 units for children less than 60 lbs. For children, 900,000 units of benzathine penicillin combined with 300,000 units of procaine is satisfactory. Intramuscular penicillin has the advantage that compliance with the regimen is assured. However, there are several disadvantages to this regimen. First is that the eradication rate of IM penicillin therapy is lower than most people think it is (approximately 79%).[87] Second, the administration of IM penicillin carries the risk of Hoigne's syndrome if it is inadvertently administered intravenously. Because IM penicillin is opaque and viscous, a moderate amount of blood may be drawn up into the syringe and not be detectable to the person administering the drug.[88] Hoigne's syndrome is a very dramatic, albeit harmless, reaction in which the patient may fall or flop down to the floor and make erratic body movements that resemble those of a fish out of water. Psychosis and true seizures may occur.[89] In the majority of cases the patient recovers spontaneously. Patients who have experienced Hoigne's syndrome are likely to be labeled "penicillin-allergic," although the syndrome is a nonallergic reaction to procaine; these patients may safely be administered penicillin or penicillin derivatives when they are needed. If IM penicillin is inadvertently administered into an artery, worse complications may occur, including distal tissue necrosis.[88]

Penicillin-allergic patients may be treated with erythromycin estolate at 30 to 40 mg/kg/day or erythromycin ethyl succinate at 40 mg/kg/day in divided doses two to four times per day for 10 days.

Carriers

The 1995 recommendations are liberal about not treating carriers: "Chronic streptococcal carriers usually do not need to be identified or treated with antibiotics. However, a difficult diagnostic problem arises when symptomatic upper respiratory tract viral infections develop in carriers. Because it is impossible to distinguish carriers from infected individuals, a single course of appropriate antibiotic therapy should be administered to any patient with pharyngitis and evidence of Group A streptococcus" infection.[72] Streptococcal carriers are not at risk for rheumatic fever, and are definitively not like "typhoid Mary." That is to say, carriers are not regarded as important reservoirs for the spread of streptococcal infection.

If, in some special circumstances, it is decided to eradicate the carrier state, clindamycin alone or rifampin plus penicillin can be used. In one study, clindamycin 20 mg/kg/day divided TID for 10 days eradicated carriage in 24 (92%) of 26 patients; by comparison, IM penicillin plus rifampin (20 mg/kg/day divided BID for 4 days) was effective in only 12 (55%) of 22 patients.[90]

Duration

The usual recommendation of 10 days of oral therapy is based on studies of eradication of the streptococcus, since no study has been done to determine the attack rate of rheumatic fever if shorter courses of penicillin are used.[91] It is assumed, and rationally so, that eradication of the organism is a reasonable surrogate for the prevention of rheumatic fever. In one study, one million units of oral penicillin twice a day for 5 days failed to eradicate the organism in about 40% of men, compared with a failure rate that approximated zero when the same total dose was given for 10 days. There was persistence of the carrier state in 70–80% of untreated controls. Thus, the longer therapy of 10 days is the conventional recommendation.

Antibiotics other than Penicillin

Sulfonamides should not be used for the treatment of streptococcal pharyngitis. In one study, the frequency of acute rheumatic fever after therapy of streptococcal pharyngitis with sulfadize was about 5%, not significantly different from that of an untreated control group of 264 individuals, of whom 11 (4%) developed rheumatic fever.[92] Trimethoprim-sulfamethoxazole (TMP-SMX) will not eradicate infection. As many as 20% of Group A streptococci are resistant to tetracycline, so it should not be used for therapy of streptococcal pharyngitis.[93] In the United States, an increasing percentage of Group A streptococcal isolates are resistant to erythromycin,[94] which is likely a consequence of increasing macrolide use.[95] Any of the oral cephalosporins is effective at eradicating Group A streptococcal infections of the throat, and some of them have a better eradication rate than that of penicillin, but they are more expensive, have a higher side effect profile, and have not been clinically proven to be otherwise advantageous. A single large-scale trial in children comparing a 10-day course of oral penicillin with a 5-day course of other antimicrobials in the treatment of culture-confirmed streptococcal pharyngitis has been published.[96] In this trial, 4,782 children were randomized, in a 1:2 ratio, to receive either 10 days of penicillin or 5 days of a different antimicrobial agent (amoxicillin/clavulanate, ceftibuten, cefuroxime axetil, loracarbef, clarithromycin, or erythromycin). Patients were followed for 12 months thereafter. Clinical response and acute eradication rates were similar. Of the 4,782 subjects enrolled, acute rheumatic fever (ARF) developed in only three, all of whom were in one of the 5-day treatment groups.[96] This difference was not statistically significant; however, because of the low baseline incidence of ARF, even a study of this size is insufficiently powered to detect a difference between the two groups.

Amoxicillin, though frequently used, has no microbiologic benefit over penicillin and is more expensive. Practitioners used to say they preferred amoxicillin because it could be given three times a day versus the four times a day regimen of penicillin; with studies showing successful eradication of Group A streptococci with thrice- and even twice-a-day penicillin therapy, that particular argument in favor of amoxicillin is no longer relevant. The last remaining point of discussion seems to be that amoxicillin is more palatable, and thus more likely to be taken. As no drug is effective if it is not ingested, amoxicillin may be considered in cases where the child is likely to be averse to taking penicillin. Ampicillin is also not better than penicillin,

and has the disadvantages of more frequent side effects, including diarrhea and rash. If used empirically, or when the culture is negative for Group A streptococci, the cause of the pharyngitis may be Epstein-Barr virus. In that case, ampicillin (and, to a lesser extent, amoxicillin) may cause an extensive maculopapular rash.

Recurrences

Clinical recurrences are best defined as pharyngitis and a positive culture within 30 days of starting therapy. Recurrence of the same type is usually not possible to distinguish from a new infection with a new type, because typing is not readily available. Bacteriologic recurrences are best defined as a positive follow-up culture within 30 days without clinical disease. This could also be called treatment failure but is not known to be associated with an increased risk of acute rheumatic fever if the treatment was appropriate.

Clinical or bacteriologic recurrences are relatively frequent (5–15%) after oral antibiotic therapy, depending on the dose and type of antibiotics used. Even intramuscular benzathine penicillin has a significant recurrence rate (about 20% of the same serotype). A "false" recurrence (recovery of a non-Group A streptococci) can be recognized by testing for bacitracin resistance. Ordinarily, reculture after therapy is not advisable except in patients with a history of rheumatic fever or rheumatic heart disease. However, some authorities recommend a follow-up culture as a precaution if the patient is given oral therapy and is judged unlikely to take the full course of antibiotics. There is no reason to obtain routine follow-up throat cultures except in patients not likely to comply with oral therapy.

Clinical recurrences should probably be treated with clindamycin or an oral cephalosporin, either of which is more effective than oral or intramuscular penicillin in such circumstances.[97] Erythromycin, once an effective second choice, is a less desirable choice because an increasing percentage of streptococcal isolates are erythromycin resistant.

Causes of Streptococcal Recurrences

1. *Nonadherence.* Because the symptoms of the disease are likely to disappear before 10 days passes, with or without antibiotic therapy, and because adherence to an antibiotic regimen when fully recovered from an illness is difficult, failure to complete the entire 10-day course of

oral antibiotic therapy is fairly common. Nonadherence with the 10-day penicillin regimen is certainly a cause of bacteriologic treatment failures. It has not been shown, however, that nonadherence is a cause of streptococcal recurrences.[98]

2. *Typability.* Several studies have shown a recurrence rate of about 20% if the original isolate was typable and about 10% if it was not.[98]

3. *Presence of beta-lactamase-producing anaerobic bacteria.* Cultures of tonsils removed at tonsillectomy have indicated that beta-lactamase-producing anaerobes, especially *Bacteroides* species, can often be grown.[99] It has been shown by a number of studies that antibiotics such as erythromycin, and clindamycin are more effective than beta-lactam antibiotics at eradicating Group A streptococci and in the treatment of a clinical recurrence of streptococcal pharyngitis. Beta-lactamase producing bacteria were more frequently recovered from children who fail penicillin therapy for Group A streptococci than in patients who did not fail therapy.[100] Further confirmation of this theory that beta-lactamase producers might be important was derived from a study of the clinical efficacy of penicillin, erythromycin, and clindamycin. Although such studies have not yet involved large numbers, it does appear that patients treated with clindamycin are more likely to have the Group A streptococci eradicated than are patients treated with erythromycin, who, in turn, are more likely to have the beta-streptococci eliminated than are patients treated with penicillin.[101] Some of this effect may be due to the fact that clindamycin achieves much higher tissue levels than do beta-lactam antibiotics. Given the side-effect profile of clindamycin, as well as the uncertain clinical significance of this phenomenon, penicillin remains the drug of choice for an initial episode of Group A streptococcal pharyngitis.

4. *Penicillin-tolerant Group A streptococci.* One of the theoretical explanations for recurrent Group A streptococcal infections after treatment with penicillin is that penicillin only inhibits, but does not kill, some strains of the organism. This theory is well established for Group B streptococci, where it applies to perhaps 5% of such isolates. In a study of the applicability of this theory to recurrent Group A streptococcal infections, there appeared to be an increased frequency of penicillin-tolerant streptococci in the recurrent cases.[102] However, further studies of the possible role of penicillin-tolerant Group A streptococci have not indicated that this is a clinically significant factor.[103] In addition, tolerance to penicillin among Group A streptococcus isolates is rare. Therefore, the possible role of tolerance as a cause of recurrences is not established.[104]

5. *Presence of penicillin-resistant staphylococci.* In the laboratory, penicillinase-producing *Staphylococcus aureus* protect Group A streptococci from the effects of penicillin.[105] This observation led to the hypothesis that the same effect might occur in patients with streptococcal pharyngitis, leading to recurrences. However, the bacteriologic recurrence rate does not appear to correlate with the presence of penicillinase-producing *S. aureus* in the throat.[99,106] Therapy with a penicillinase-resistant antibiotic such as nafcillin or cephalexin results in less frequent recurrences than does penicillin treatment, but the difference is not statistically significant.[99,106] Thus, treatment with the more expensive penicillinase-resistant penicillin is not indicated.

6. *Reinfection with the same serotype from the patient's toothbrush.* There are no clinical studies to show that this is a factor in recurrences. However, one study did show that toothbrushes may harbor the offending Group A streptococci for up to 15 days after the patient has been treated for streptococcal pharyngitis.[107]

Culture of Contacts

Other family members may also have a positive culture, but these contacts are unlikely to have been a source of recurrent infection. Speculation about the role of contacts in recurrent streptococcal pharyngitis has led some clinicians to culture even family pets. One study showed that culturing pets residing in the household is unlikely to yield a positive culture; no group A beta-hemolytic streptococci were recovered from any body site in a total of 230 dogs and cats.[108] The evidence favors regrowth of the patient's original serotype for one of the reasons above; only testimonial anecdotes support contacts as a source of reinfection.

Management of Recurrences

1. Make sure that recurrences are truly streptococcal **infections**, and that you are not just culturing Group A streptococcus from a carrier with a series of viral pharyngitides. Clinical features

of illness that suggest viral infection, i.e., cough, hoarseness, runny nose, indolent onset, etc. can be helpful. It may also be useful to obtain a throat culture on the patient when he is entirely asymptomatic to verify the carrier status.

2. Confirm that recurrences are caused by Group A streptococci by sending the isolate to a laboratory that can identify Group A by agglutination methods.

3. On the second or third clinical recurrence, use clindamycin instead of oral or intramuscular penicillin.

4. Give the patient with multiple recurrences a prophylaxis regimen similar to that used for prevention of acute rheumatic fever for approximately 3 months.[109] During this period, if the patient takes the medication as instructed, the physician can reassure the parents, based on a large body of controlled studies of rheumatic fever prevention, that the child is not at risk for rheumatic fever. Episodes of pharyngitis that occur during penicillin prophylaxis are likely to be viral in origin.

5. Consider a tonsillectomy for selected patients who have recurrent streptococcal pharyngitis. This may be, in the long run, less expensive than multiple courses of antibiotics and treatment visits, although the physician should take into consideration the size of the tonsils and the severity of the illness.

6. Have the patient dispose of his or her toothbrush and buy a new one sometime just before therapy is completed. Although there is no evidence that this will change the recurrence rate, the fact that many toothbrushes still harbor the same isolate as the one that caused the pharyngitis suggests that it may be helpful.[107]

Tonsillectomy

A prospective study has been done of the effect of tonsillectomy on severe recurrent pharyngitis with documented fever or cervical adenopathy or exudate or a positive culture for Group A streptococci.[110] After tonsillectomy (with or without adenoidectomy), there were moderately but significantly fewer throat infections than in children without tonsillectomy (who also had fewer infections than before admission to the control group). Some patients with frequent tonsillitis before tonsillectomy become patients with frequent pharyngitis after tonsillectomy.

Prevention

History of Rheumatic Fever

Daily oral penicillin or monthly benzathine penicillin injection is effective in the prevention of streptococcal infections. This type of prophylaxis is used almost exclusively for patients who have probably had rheumatic fever,[111] but it has been used in situations where there is a high risk of infection, such as military camps.

Management of Exposed Family Contacts

Family contacts should generally not be cultured unless they develop signs and symptoms suggestive of streptococcal pharyngitis. If there is a history of rheumatic fever in the family, parents and siblings should be cultured 2–3 days after the index patient has begun to receive antibiotic therapy, and should be treated if the culture is positive, even in the absence of symptoms.[112] Alternatively, reliable families, even with a history of rheumatic fever, may be cultured only when they develop symptoms.[113]

Severe PANDAS

Some children with frequent or severe PANDAS (discussed earlier) have been managed with antibiotic prophylaxis identical to that given to patients with a history of acute rheumatic fever, although with unproven benefit. Other therapies, such as immune globulin, remain investigational. These patients should be managed by an infectious diseases specialist in concert with a pediatric neurologist.

Axioms

The diagnosis and management of streptococcal pharyngitis is complex and controversial. There are conflicting studies regarding laboratory detection as well as practical guides to treatment. Axioms for the practitioner are provided in Box 2.

■ PERITONSILLAR CELLULITIS OR ABSCESS

Peritonsillar abscess can be defined as a collection of pus lateral to the tonsil that pushes the tonsil toward the midline. These abscesses are usually the result of severe tonsillitis. Peritonsillar cellulitis also displaces the tonsil medially but consists of edema and engorged mucosa without pus formation. The distinction between peritonsillar cellulitis and abscess can be difficult to make. Placing a needle into the swollen area and aspirating for pus is the traditional way of distinguishing the two; in recent years, investigators have studied intraoral sonography and computed tomographic scans as alternative methods. Computed tomography (CT) scans differentiate the two conditions with ease;[114] intraoral sonography, when tolerated, is also useful in this regard.[115] It is not entirely clear, however, that either of these methods yields results superior to those obtained by the old-fashioned methods. A review of 43 consecutive cases of clinically diagnosed peritonsillar abscess in children ages 7–8 years showed positive aspirate results in 76%; in 87% of these patients the abscess resolved; 6% each required two aspirations and immediate tonsillec-

tomy.[116] If the disease is detected early enough, neither biopsy nor surgical drainage is necessary.

Both of these entities are more frequent in teenagers and adults, perhaps a result of intense focal antigen-antibody reaction after years of making various streptococcal antibodies. In one study, the age range was 11–73 years, with half being 25 years or younger.[117]

Clinical Diagnosis

Usually, there is fever and painful swallowing. The patient may speak in a muffled "hot potato" voice. There may be ear pain and trismus on the affected side.[118] Trismus and painful swallowing result from inflammation abutting the muscles of mastication. Toxicity or neck swelling raises the question of extension down the neck. Age less than 12 years and trismus are more frequent in cellulitis; age 13 or older, dysphagia, and drooling are more common in abscess.[119]

Bacteria

Group A, non-Group A, alpha-hemolytic, and Group D streptococci are frequent.[119] The most common aerobic isolates are *Streptococcus pyogenes* (Group A streptococcus), *Streptococcus milleri* group, and viridans Streptococci.[120] Anaerobes may be more frequent than aerobes, especially in older adolescents and adults. *Fusobacterium* spp. and *Prevotella* spp. are most frequent, followed by *Actinomyces*, *Peptostreptococcus*, and others. Many patients have mixed infections. Mouth organisms like *Eikenella corrodens* are sometimes seen.[121] *H. influenzae* and *S. aureus* are not common.[122,123] Throat cultures are often negative, but cultures of the tonsillar needle aspirate may grow GAS or many of the above bacteria.[124]

Treatment

For ambulatory patients early in the course of the infection, oral clindamycin or amoxicillin/clavulanate is a rational choice. For hospitalized children, intravenous clindamycin is effective against streptococci, staphylococci, and almost all throat anaerobic bacteria. Ticarcillin/clavulanate or ampicillin/sulbactam are reasonable alternatives. One study showed that all but one isolate in a series of 53 abscesses contained bacteria that were sensitive to either penicillin or metronidazole, and recommended the combination of the two.[125] There is no consensus, however, on the optimal treatment for patients with peritonsillar abscess. Herzon published an exhaustive review of the management of peritonsillar abscess that used a cohort study of 123 patients, a national survey of management practices of otolaryngologists, and a meta-analysis in order to devise guidelines.[126] The conclusions were that: (1) needle aspiration should be used as the initial surgical drainage procedure for all patients who do not have indications for abscess tonsillectomy, and (2) antibiotic regimens for these patients should include penicillin. Intravenous penicillin has been used for years, but no direct comparative trials of penicillin to clindamycin have been performed. In one small, prospective trial, intramuscular procaine penicillin was as effective as ampicillin/sulbactam at effecting a cure. All patients underwent peroral drainage.[127] High doses of penicillin are needed to achieve good tonsillar tissue concentrations.[123]

Complications

Fatal necrotizing fasciitis of the neck has been reported in adults after late treatment.[128] Rarely, mediastinitis or other deep neck space infections may occur.[129] Lemierre's disease, also known as postanginal sepsis, is a rare condition associated with *Fusobacterium necrophorum* infection of the deep tissues of the neck in which intermittent bacteremia and septic embolization occur secondary to infection of the jugular vein (discussed later).[130]

Tonsillectomy

The need for tonsillectomy during the acute phase of the illness, or after recovery to prevent recurrences is the subject of some debate. Many otolaryngologists do routine tonsillectomy for all patients with peritonsillar abscess, because of a reported 15% recurrence rate. It turns out that in the United States, the recurrence rate is only 10%, which is significantly different from the rest of the world ($p > 0.02$).[126] A large abscess compromising the airway may require urgent drainage. Approximately 30% of patients will have a relative indication for immediate, or "quinsy" tonsillectomy.[126] If a tonsillectomy is to be performed, prospective data show that performing it immediately is technically simpler, associated with fewer working days lost (in adult patients), and less intraoperative blood loss.[131]

The majority of patients are not that sick, and really have peritonsillar cellulitis, which responds to intravenous antibiotics. In one review, only one of 41 patients who had needle drainage had a recurrent peritonsillitis.[132] Another study comparing in-

cision and drainage with needle aspiration found the advantages of needle aspiration alone outweighed its acceptably low failure rate.[133]

■ NONSTREPTOCOCCAL PHARYNGITIS

Nonstreptococcal pharyngitis can be defined as objective evidence of pharyngitis and a throat culture negative for beta-hemolytic streptococci. Ulcerative pharyngitis and membranous pharyngitis are special anatomic types of pharyngitis and are discussed in later sections.

It is a very common error to recover a microorganism from the throat of a patient with pharyngitis and say it is the cause. Many case reports of unusual causes of pharyngitis represent coincidental recovery of the agent. Recovery is less likely to be coincidental if there is bacteremia. However, statistical studies comparing normal controls and patients with pharyngitis are necessary to prove an association, as discussed in Chapter 1. Even experimental production of pharyngitis by inoculation of an agent may not be confirmed by epidemiologic studies, as exemplified by *M. hominis*, discussed below.

"Sore throat" is not pharyngitis and may be caused by trauma, allergy, and tracheal irritation from respiratory viruses, smoking, or inhalation of other irritants.[134] This section deals with definitive pharyngitis, as determined by objective observations on physical examination.

Possible Etiologies

Adenoviruses

These viruses are the most frequent cause of nonstreptococcal pharyngitis in young children (Box 3).[135–137] There are more than thirty respiratory serotypes of this virus, but most infections are caused by types 1–7.

Nasal obstruction or discharge and cough are often present. Conjunctivitis is sometimes seen. In some patients, a small pulmonary infiltrate, with or without evidence of pneumonia on physical examination, may be seen. Mild to moderate abdominal pain, with some loose stools, is occasionally present, as is otitis media (Fig. 2-5). A rash, usually lasting fewer than 3 days, may be observed. The rash is usually maculopapular but may rarely be petechial.

The tonsils frequently have flecks of superficial exudate or white spherical areas beneath their mucosal surfaces but occasionally have a necrotic-appearing exudate resembling that seen with infec-

BOX 2-3 ■ Causes of Nonstreptococcal Pharyngitis

Common
Adenovirus (especially in preschoolers)
EBV (especially in teenagers)
Herpes simplex type 1

Less Common
Enteroviruses
Influenza virus (in epidemics)
Respiratory syncytial virus (in epidemics)
Pharyngitis as part of a systemic disease (such as Kawasaki disease)
Measles
Parainfluenza virus
Meningococcus
Mumps
Arcanobacterium hemolyticum

Rare
Diphtheria
Anaerobes
Yersiniosis
Mycoplasma pneumoniae
Corynebacterium ulcerans, C. pseudodiphtheriticum
Non-Group A streptococci

Special Exposures
Herpes simplex type 2
Tularemia
H. ducreyi
Gonococcus

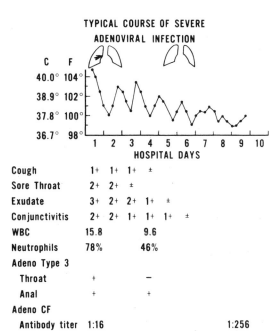

TYPICAL COURSE OF SEVERE ADENOVIRAL INFECTION

Cough	1+	1+	1+	±				
Sore Throat	2+	2+	±					
Exudate	3+	2+	2+	1+	±			
Conjunctivitis	2+	2+	1+	1+	1+	±		
WBC	15.8			9.6				
Neutrophils	78%			46%				
Adeno Type 3								
Throat	+			−				
Anal	+			+				
Adeno CF								
Antibody titer	1:16						1:256	

■ **FIGURE 2-5** Adenovirus pharyngitis is usually associated with conjunctivitis. Minimal pneumonia, otitis media, mild diarrhea, febrile convulsion, or leukocytosis with a predominance of neutrophils can be present.

tious mononucleosis. Typically in these cases the child is less than 5 years of age.

Adenovirus also causes a very specific syndrome known as pharyngoconjunctival fever.[138] Patients present with abrupt onset of pharyngitis, mild to moderate conjunctivitis, and fever. The pharyngitis is exudative in about a third of patients. Eye complaints are less than might be expected based on the appearance of the palpebral conjunctivae, which usually have a granular appearance. In severe cases, the appearance mimics subconjunctival hemorrhage. Fever to greater than 39°C (102.2°F) occurs in 50% of patients, and is accompanied by headache. The febrile episodes last from 4 to 7 days, and total duration of illness may approach 14 days.[138]

Herpes Simplex

Although more commonly associated with gingivostomatitis in toddlers, primary infection with herpes simplex type 1 may produce a sore throat with redness and sometimes a tonsillar exudate.[139] Typical ulcerations or bleeding may not appear until a day or two after the onset and may not be observed at all if the patient is not reexamined after the first visit (Fig. 2-6). Many teenagers reach college without neutralizing antibodies to this herpesvirus.[140]

Herpes simplex type 2 can cause exudative pharyngitis as well as ulcerative pharyngitis in individuals with oral-genital contact.[141,142]

Coxsackie and Echoviruses

These viruses typically produce ulcerative pharyngitis but are sometimes recovered from patients without vesicular or ulcerative lesions.[136,143] They may produce ulcerative lesions in the context of hand, foot, and mouth disease (see Chapter 11). Coxsackie B virus sometimes produces a definite pharyngitis along with several days of high fever. Exudate is uncommon in this situation.[144] Echovirus is sometimes associated with a definite pharyngitis.[145]

Parainfluenza Viruses

Usually, these viruses produce only a mild pharyngitis associated with a more prominent cough and

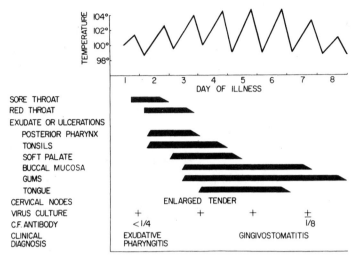

■ FIGURE 2-6 Typical course of ulcerative pharyngitis caused by herpes simplex virus. (Moffet HL, et al: J Pediatr 1968;73:51–60)

bronchitis. The frequency with which parainfluenza viruses are associated with pharyngitis is not clear, because most studies have combined patients with rhinitis, bronchitis, and pharyngitis.

Influenza Virus

This virus may produce pharyngeal erythema, but usually there is an additional Group A streptococcal infection if tonsillar exudate is present.[146] The sore throat observed with influenza virus infection is usually tracheal as opposed to pharyngeal.[147] The complaint of sore throat is usually out of proportion to the objective evidence seen on physical examination.

Respiratory Syncytial Virus

Although not usually thought of as a virus that causes pharyngitis, a review of 20 years of outpatient respiratory syncytial virus infection found that almost 70% of patients infected with this virus had pharyngitis on physical examination.[148] It is possible that some or all of these children had redness of the pharynx secondary to irritation from cough. Cough, wheezing, and tachypnea are usually more prominent clinical signs.

Epstein-Barr Virus

After 10 years of age, heterophile-positive infectious mononucleosis is a common cause of severe exudative pharyngitis, as discussed later in this chapter and in Chapter 3. The heterophile test is often false negative before the age of 10 years. Nonstreptococ-

cal febrile exudative pharyngitis was associated with a positive heterophile antibody test in only 3 (3%) of 93 younger children with nonstreptococcal pharyngitis in one study,[136] although some of these children may have had Epstein-Barr Virus (EBV) infections. EBV infection causing pharyngitis may be less common in children less than 10 years of age, although an insufficient amount of study has been performed in this age group. Acute EBV infection may be diagnosed by EBV serology at any age.

Mycoplasmas

Mycoplasma hominis is capable of causing exudative pharyngitis when experimentally inoculated into adult volunteers.[149] *Mycoplasma pneumoniae* may cause a mild pharyngitis in younger children, and a more pronounced pharyngitis in older children and young adults, usually associated with headache and cough.

Tularemia

Oropharyngeal tularemia is a very rare cause of nonstreptococcal pharyngitis. The pharyngitis and cervical adenopathy resemble those of streptococcal pharyngitis.[150,151] Alternatively, patients may have a membrane indistinguishable from that of diphtheria.

Gonococcus

"Sore throat" is a frequent symptom of gonorrhea in individuals with oral-genital contact, but exudative pharyngitis is not common. The frequency of *Neisseria gonorrheae* as a cause of pharyngitis has not been established by studies that exclude other causes, so that recovery of gonococcus from the throat may be coincidental to the pharyngitis, just as the presence of Group A streptococcus can be coincidental.[152]

Chancroid (*Haemophilus ducreyi* infection) also can be added to the list of causes of pharyngitis in persons with an orogenital exposure history.[153]

Anaerobes

Because anaerobes are normal inhabitants of the oropharynx, it is more difficult to prove a causative association between their isolation and the presence of pharyngitis. *Bacteroides melaninogenicus* is probably a relatively rare cause of pharyngitis.[154] It may produce a beta-lactamase that interferes with the penicillin therapy of streptococcal pharyngitis, as previously described. *Fusobacterium* species can be a rare cause of severe exudative pharyngitis with cellulitis of the neck and septic emboli.[155]

Diphtheria

Corynebacterium diphtheriae infection has become rare because of immunization, but should always be considered a possible cause of nonstreptococcal exudative pharyngitis. Early in the illness, the typical pseudomembrane may not be present. Usually, however, diphtheria produces a pseudomembrane on the soft palate, uvula, tonsil, or posterior pharynx. If such a membrane is present, the diagnosis should be "membranous pharyngitis," thus greatly limiting the etiologic possibilities, as described later in this chapter.

Arcanobacterium hemolyticum

Arcanobacterium hemolyticum has been reported to cause pharyngitis, occasionally with a scarlet fever-like rash in teenagers and young adults.[156] It is recovered more frequently from patients with acute pharyngitis than it is from controls. It has also been demonstrated that patients mount an antibody response to this organism following an episode of pharyngitis from which it was recovered.[157] In longitudinal studies, *Arcanobacterium hemolyticum* is isolated from approximately 2–3% of patients with acute pharyngitis.[158] Despite its resemblance to streptococcal pharyngitis, illness caused by *A. hemolyticum* is self-limited, and nonsuppurative complications do not occur.

Mumps

This virus occasionally produces pharyngitis.[159] However, the clinical diagnosis is usually based on minimal erythema. Pharyngitis may also be assumed to be present because the parotid or submandibular swelling is mistaken for cervical adenitis.

Measles

In classic measles, oral mucous membrane erythema may be prominent. In this case, the physician should recognize that the pharyngeal redness is of the same degree as that seen in all of the oral mucosa and that significant conjunctivitis and prominent cough are also present.

Other Microorganisms

Candida albicans is sometimes recovered from older children with severe pharyngitis, but it is probably coincidental.

Staphylococcus aureus, *Streptococcus pneumoniae*, fusiform bacteria, and spirochetes are agents that have not been proven to be causes of pharyngitis but are often coincidentally recovered from patients.

Chlamydia trachomatis has been implicated in pharyngitis by serologic studies performed in adults,[160] but these reports lacked important clinical details. This agent is probably not a cause of pharyngitis.[161]

In milk-borne yersiniosis involving all age groups, only adults were noted to have fever and pharyngitis with a throat culture positive for *Yersinia enterocolitica*.[162,163]

Noninfectious Causes

Rarely, lymphoma in teenagers presents as an exudative pharyngitis.[117]

Diagnostic Plan and Treatment

If the throat culture is negative for beta-hemolytic streptococci, few further diagnostic studies are useful except in special clinical circumstances. A slide test for infectious mononucleosis may be indicated for older children, or EBV serology for younger ones with suspicion of EBV infection. Viral cultures (e.g., for adenovirus) are occasionally of interest, especially in the immunocompromised host. Patients with risk factors for other agents, i.e., ingestion of undercooked meat (tularemia), history of orogenital contact (gonorrhea), should be evaluated for those specific diseases. This entails notifying the microbiology laboratory so that specimens are plated on proper media. Conventional throat cultures for Group A streptococcus will not detect the gonococcus. Tularemia is diagnosed by serology, as culturing the organism is hazardous to laboratory personnel.

No specific treatment is of value for nonstreptococcal pharyngitis except as noted earlier. In general, observation and the avoidance of unnecessary antibiotics are all that is necessary.

Postanginal Sepsis (Lemierre's Syndrome)

Rarely, pharyngitis is complicated by extension of the infection into the adjacent veins, with septic thrombophlebitis beginning in the tonsillar vein. This postanginal sepsis (also called Lemierre's syndrome) can occur in normal children (especially teenagers) as well as in immunocompromised children .[130, 155, 164, 165] Lemierre's syndrome is classically associated with *Fusobacterium necrophorum*, although other anaerobes that are part of the normal flora, such as *Bacteroides* or *Eikenella* are occasionally reported.

Physical findings include severe pharyngitis, tender tonsillar nodes, and tenderness and swelling along the lateral aspect of the sternocleidomastoid muscle (over the internal jugular vein).[164] The septic portion of the disease may follow the pharyngitis by 4–8 days. Therefore, in many cases, the pharyngitis may have resolved before the patient seeks medical care.[165] Septic pulmonary emboli may occur, as can septic embolization to abdominal organs, muscles, or joints. The knees and hips are the most commonly infected joints.[165] Ampicillin-sulbactam is reasonable empiric antibiotic therapy pending blood culture results, as *Eikenella* species are uniformly resistant to clindamycin.[166] Metronidazole retains good activity against most penicillin-resistant anaerobes, and may be added. All *Fusobacterium* species are sensitive to penicillin, and intravenous penicillin G is the drug of choice once the bacterium has been isolated and definitively identified.

Recurrences of Nonstreptococcal Pharyngitis

A frustrating problem to family and physician, recurrent nonstreptococcal pharyngitis remains a puzzle, primarily because of the difficulty of identifying an infectious cause or a host defect. Is this something we can now name as a syndrome (i.e.,

recurrent nonstreptococcal pharyngitis) with the causes yet to be found?

An increasingly recognized cause of pharyngitis, although it usually presents as fevers of uncertain etiology, is the syndrome known as periodic fever, adenitis, pharyngitis, and apthous stomatitis (PFAPA).[167] Not all of the features need to be present to make the diagnosis. The most consistent feature is a fever that is truly "periodic," i.e., comes and goes at a fixed interval, usually 28 days. Most patients have some degree of pharyngitis and adenitis, and may wrongly be treated as if they have recurrent streptococcal infection, especially if cultures are not routinely obtained. Fevers are usually high and the symptoms last 4 to 5 days and then spontaneously disappear. The etiology of this syndrome is still not known; information about treatment, prognosis, and differential diagnosis are contained in Chapter 10 on fever syndromes.

■ ULCERATIVE PHARYNGITIS AND HERPANGINA

Ulcerative pharyngitis is defined by ulcerations or vesicular lesions on the soft palate, anterior tonsillar fauces, or posterior pharynx. If glossitis or gingivostomatitis is present, the patient probably has herpetic gingivostomatitis (see Chapter 4). Thus, the diagnosis of ulcerative pharyngitis implies absence of erythematous, swollen, or bleeding gums and buccal mucosa.

"Herpangina" is a term first used in 1920 to describe pharyngitis with small vesicular lesions in the posterior pharynx. This term is still frequently used and now usually refers to any kind of vesicular or ulcerative pharyngitis.[168] Herpangina occurs almost exclusively in the summer or fall when Coxsackie and echoviruses are prevalent. Nodular pharyngitis without vesicles has been called acute lymphonodular pharyngitis,[169] and has been attributed to Coxsackie A virus. When ulcerative or vesicular stomatitis occurs with a vesicular or papular rash on the hands and/or feet, it is called hand, foot, and mouth disease (classically due to Coxsackie A16), and is discussed further in Chapter 11.

Possible Etiologies

Coxsackie A Virus

Because this virus grows poorly in cell culture, mouse inoculation is required to recover it. Coxsackie A virus is probably the most common cause of ulcerative pharyngitis.[170] Lesions begin shortly after the onset of fever, and may be papular at first, but quickly become vesicular and then ulcerative. By the time patients come to medical attention the lesions are usually ulcerative. There are often only a few lesions, from one to about 15, and they are small, 1–2 mm in diameter with surrounding erythema. The most common site is the anterior tonsillar pillar, but ulcers may occur anywhere in the mouth. Sometimes so-called hand, foot, and mouth syndrome really involves only the mouth; occasionally the rash on the hands and feet is seen without concomitant oral lesions. This syndrome is in general mild and self-limited, and lasts for 4–6 days. As the rash resolves, there is often fine desquamation of the papular lesions.

Herpes Simplex

In these cases, the ulcerations on the soft palate or pharynx are usually larger (3–8 mm in diameter) than those produced by Coxsackie A virus. If mouth or circular lip ulcers are also present, the cause is probably herpes simplex virus (Fig. 2-7). In one study of university students, ulcerative pharyngitis was the usual presentation of herpes simplex virus (HSV) infection, and only one-fourth of them also had anterior lesions of the mouth or lips.[171] Reactivation of HSV1 usually produces lip lesions ("cold sores") at any age. A history of genital exposure is probably more helpful in the diagnosis of HSV2 pharyngitis than is the actual appearance of the throat.

Other Causes

Coxsackie B viruses and echoviruses can also produce an ulcerative or vesicular pharyngitis that is indistinguishable from that caused by Coxsackie A virus.[169,172] There is some evidence that Coxsackie B virus infection is becoming more common in recent years.[173] Other enteroviruses, including poliovirus, can produce similar lesions, and this enanthem has been noted in both sporadic and epidemic poliomyelitis.[174] *Corynebacterium ulcerans* is a rare cause of ulcerative pharyngitis.[175] The disease is a zoonosis, and is seen in patients with animal contact or a history of consumption of contaminated raw milk. Primary syphilis can produce an ulcer of the tonsil, usually without fever, and with an appearance "suspicious" of a primary chancre.[176,177]

Diagnostic Plan

Antigen Detection

Often, the diagnosis of herpetic stomatitis is a clinical one, but herpes simplex antigen can be detected with a slide agglutination test,[178] or the virus can be cultured readily from active lesions when the diagnosis is in doubt. Virus isolation from any herpesvirus group-induced disease is maximized by sampling fresh (not crusted) lesions, and by rapid, cold transport and quick tissue culture inoculation. Polymerase chain reaction (PCR) can also be used to detect HSV DNA with high sensitivity and specificity.[179]

Virus Culture

Ulcerative pharyngitis is typically caused by a virus. Throat cultures for Group A streptococci can be obtained when there are signs and symptoms suggestive of a coexisting streptococcal infection. Cultures for virus may be of educational value but are rarely practical. Sometimes they give retrospective reassurance to the patient. Coxsackie A virus, the usual cause of ulcerative pharyngitis, is unlikely to be recovered unless suckling mice are injected

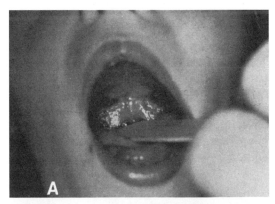

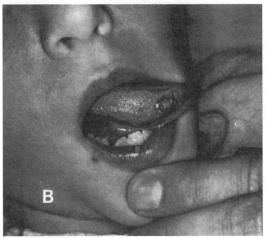

■ **FIGURE 2-7** Circular ulcers on the palate, lip, and tongue of a child with herpes simplex virus infection.

with the specimen, and this is both too expensive and too impractical to justify its use in the diagnosis of pharyngitis. Enteroviral PCR can be performed on throat swabs, but this technology is not yet widely available and offers little clinical benefit for this self-limited illness.[180]

Serum Antibodies

Serologic diagnosis is not practical for Coxsackie or echovirus infection. Paired sera could be obtained in an attempt to demonstrate herpes simplex virus infection, but this is seldom clinically useful.

Treatment

For the most part, symptomatic therapy is all that is required. Investigational antienteroviral agents may eventually be commercially available, but will probably not be indicated for these self-limited infections. Treatment of HSV pharyngitis is discussed under therapy for HSV gingivostomatitis in Chapter 4.

■ MEMBRANOUS PHARYNGITIS

Membranous pharyngitis can be defined as a definite membrane over the tonsils, pharynx, soft palate, or uvula. Bleeding is typical when the membrane is peeled off, as can be done with a swab or tongue blade. "Membrane" is used here as a synonym for "pseudomembrane" for convenience. In reality, there is a fundamental difference, in that pseudomembranes do not have a true epithelial layer.

Possible Etiologies

Infectious Mononucleosis

A membranous pharyngitis in the United States today is most likely to be caused by infectious mononucleosis, discussed in Chapter 3.

Diphtheria

Even though the disease is rare in the United States, diphtheria should be regarded as the presumptive cause of membranous pharyngitis in an unimmunized individual. There is a substantial group of parents who are now withholding vaccinations for their children either for religious or sociopolitical reasons. In addition, diphtheria has become common in the former Soviet Union, so the diagnosis should be suspected in patients with membranous pharyngitis and an appropriate travel history.

The incubation period is 2–5 days.[181] Typically the membrane is gray to black, depending upon how much blood it contains. It bleeds easily. It usually begins on the tonsils and spreads toward the uvula.[181] If the membrane extends over the soft palate and uvula, diphtheria is a much more likely diagnosis than infectious mononucleosis (Fig. 2-8).

Additional findings that suggest diphtheria include cervical adenitis with severe swelling of the neck (bullneck diphtheria); tachycardia, hypotension, or arrhythmia, which suggest myocarditis (this complication may occur as early as 3–5 days after the onset of illness); and proteinuria, secondary to the effect of the toxin on the kidneys. Palatal paralysis, which reflects a local effect of the toxin, may

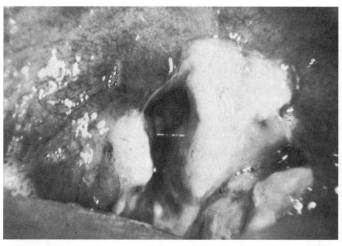

■ **FIGURE 2-8** Diphtheritic membrane on the soft palate and uvula. (Kallick CA et al.: Ill Med J 1970;137:505–512)

also occur in the first week of illness. Involvement of the nose, with a visible membrane or bleeding, or involvement of the larynx or trachea, resulting in croupy cough or stridor, occasionally coexists with the membranous pharyngitis.

Myocarditis may result in cardiogenic shock or congestive heart failure.[182,183] Occasionally, the development of electrocardiographic findings consistent with myocarditis is the best evidence available for the diagnosis of diphtheria when cultures have been negative. Late complications include most frequently a reversible polyneuritis, which involves the motor nerves and is usually symmetric.[184] Cutaneous diphtheria is manifested by a scaling rash or by ulcers with clearly demarcated edges. Most isolates are nontoxigenic.

Other Causes

Membranelike exudate has been described rarely in presumed viral or streptococcal pharyngitis. The exudate that forms after an adenotonsillectomy may resemble a membrane. *Arcanobacterium hemolyticum* has been reported to produce infections strongly mimicking diphtheria.[185] Rarely, other corynbacterium species (such as *C. pseudodiphtheriticum* or *C. ulcerans*) cause the clinical syndrome known as diphtheria. Oropharyngeal tularemia is a rare cause of membranous pharyngitis that can be indistinguishable from that of diphtheria.[186]

Diagnostic Plan

Tests for Infectious Mononucleosis

A slide test or serology for EBV infection should be done immediately, although they may not become positive until later. The peripheral blood should be examined for atypical lymphocytes. In the vaccinated child with no history of travel to an area of diphtheria endemicity, infectious mononucleosis is the likely cause.

Immunization History

Written evidence of recent adequate immunization against diphtheria does not exclude the diagnosis but makes it much less likely. It should be remembered that because the vaccine is a toxoid, it does not protect against nontoxigenic strains, which can cause infection but usually produce a disease that is not as severe. Prognosis for the patient with diphtheria is better if he or she is fully immunized.[187]

Throat Smear

Diphtheroids are species of *Corynebacterium* other than *Corynebacterium diphtheriae* that can be found in the throat of normal persons, so the diagnosis of diphtheria should not be based on a stain of a throat smear. Even the presence of typical-appearing organisms is not diagnostic of diphtheria. Fluorescent antibody methods may be useful if the antiserum is specific and proper controls are done. Considerable confusion may result if cross-reactions are reported as weakly positive, such as may occur with many other throat organisms found in patients without diphtheria.

Throat Culture

The diphtheria bacillus can be recognized by the appearance of its colonies on special media (tellurite or Tinsdale), but these media are often not immediately available. Fortunately, the organism also grows satisfactorily on sheep blood agar or chocolate agar plates. The toxigenicity of a diphtheria bacillus can be determined by several tests, which must be done in a reference laboratory. The essential test of virulence is the production of toxin.

Public Health Importance

The laboratory confirmation of a clinically suspected case of diphtheria is of great public health importance. Respiratory diphtheria is now rare in the United States, with only 49 cases reported from 1980 through 1999. However, toxigenic *C. diphtheriae* is occasionally isolated from cutaneous lesions, particularly in certain Native American communities. Cutaneous diphtheria can serve as both a reservoir and a source, and may be more important than is oropharyngeal carriage as a factor in some outbreaks.[188] One case of diphtheria usually leads to vigorous public health measures to prevent further spread. Many contacts are cultured and given diphtheria toxoid boosters. If there is clinical suspicion of early disease, antitoxin (horse serum) is given, and this is frequently associated with serum sickness. Therefore, bacteriologic confirmation of the first suspected cases is very important.

Outbreaks of respiratory diphtheria occurred in 1970 in Austin and San Antonio, Texas; Miami, Florida; and Chicago.[189] Cutaneous diphtheria was a reservoir for respiratory diphtheria in the Seattle, Washington area in the late 1970s.[190] The single most important factor in the public health problem posed by diphtheria is that approximately 50–60%

of adults in the United States are not up-to-date on their booster immunizations.[191] Immunity to diphtheria wanes, and boosters are required every 10 years.

In the acute situation, public health officials will not proceed with measures necessary to control an outbreak unless there is bacteriologic confirmation of suspected cases. "Epidemic" is the word that appears to be necessary in order to mobilize people to get booster immunizations.

Treatment

Airway

Patients with a pharyngeal membrane should have laryngoscopy or bronchoscopy with the physician ready to provide an airway, if needed.[192] Orotracheal intubation is one way of securing an emergency airway. However, tracheotomy will usually be advisable after intubation.

Antitoxin

If the clinical diagnosis is diphtheria, administration of antitoxin should never be delayed while awaiting laboratory confirmation. Antitoxin is able to neutralize free toxin and toxin that is adherent to cells, but cannot reverse the effects of toxin that has already entered cells. Therefore, both morbidity and mortality of diphtheria are related to the length of the delay in receiving antitoxin. In severe cases, antitoxin may need to be given intravenously, because of the delayed onset of action when given intramuscularly.[193] A test for allergy to the product, as described in the package circular, should be done before use, because it is a horse serum product.

Other Therapy

Some authorities recommend digoxin if congestive heart failure occurs, but it must be given cautiously.[189] Antibiotic therapy has minimal effect on the clinical progression and should never be used as a substitute for antitoxin. However, antibiotics decrease communicability. The disease is usually not communicable 48 hours after antibiotics are given. Oral erythromycin or intramuscular procaine penicillin G are given for 14 days. In a study in Thailand, corticosteroids failed to prevent or modify myocarditis or neuritis.[194]

Management of Contacts

With the assistance of public health authorities, household contacts of a patient with a clinical suspi-

cion of diphtheria should be examined and cultured without awaiting final laboratory confirmation of the index patient's culture. Contacts with signs suggestive of diphtheria should be treated with diphtheria antitoxin and parenteral penicillin (or erythromycin if they are penicillin allergic). All contacts of a patient with probable diphtheria, regardless of immunization status, should be treated with oral erythromycin for 7 days or intramuscular benzathine penicillin (1.2 million units for adults; 600,000 units for children less than 6 years of age), immunized with diphtheria toxoid, and undergo daily surveillance for clinical evidence of diphtheria or for the diphtheria organism, which presumably is present.[195] Cultures should be obtained at 1 day and 2 weeks after treatment. If surveillance is not possible, the unimmunized household contacts should also be given diphtheria antitoxin.[195]

All individuals with positive cultures should be isolated (see section on isolation, below). Even if asymptomatic, they should be treated with antitoxin because of the significant risk of serious disease, particularly myocarditis. Antitoxin should not be withheld while awaiting culture results if the diagnosis of diphtheria is strongly suspected on clinical grounds, regardless of immunization history. In a 1978 survey of children in Chicago, only 75% of those less than 10 years of age who had received three diphtheria toxoid vaccinations had protective levels of antibodies in their serum.[196]

Isolation Procedures

Droplet precautions are recommended for patients and carriers with pharyngeal diphtheria until at least two cultures of nose and throat are negative. Patients with cutaneous diphtheria require contact precautions. All medical personnel caring for patients with diphtheria should be up-to-date on diphtheria booster immunizations. Cultures of medical care personnel are neither necessary nor recommended. Diphtheria toxoid boosters are usually given to adequately immunized adults only at 10-year intervals. However, when an outbreak is present in a community with a large unimmunized population, diphtheria toxoid is usually given on a mass basis without individualization.

■ REFERENCES

1. Moffet HL. Common infections in ambulatory patients. Ann Intern Med 1978;89(Part 2):743–5.
2. Gwaltney JM Jr, Phillips CD, Miller RD, et al. Computed

tomographic study of the common cold. N Engl J Med 1994;330:25–30.

3. Fox JP, Cooney MK, Hall CE, et al. Rhinovirus in Seattle families, 1975-1979. Am J Epidemiol 1985;122:830–46.

4. McMillan JA, Weiner LB, Higgins AM, et al. Rhinovirus infection associated with severe illness among pediatric patients. Pediatr Infect Dis J 1993;12:321–5.

5. Rakes GP, Arruda E, Ingram JM, et al. Rhinovirus and respiratory syncytial virus in wheezing children requiring emergency care. IgE and eosinophil analyses. Am J Respir Crit Care Med 1999;159:785–90.

6. Bradburne AF, Bynoe ML, Tyrrell DAJ. Effects of a "new" human respiratory virus in volunteers. Br Med J 1967;3: 767–9.

7. Isaacs D, Flowers D, Clarke JR, et al. Epidemiology of coronavirus respiratory infections. Arch Dis Child 1983; 58:500–3.

8. McIntosh K, Chao RK, Krause HE, et al. Coronavirus infection in acute lower respiratory tract disease of infants. J Infect Dis 1974;130:502–7.

9. Fernald GW, Collier AM, Clyde WA, Jr. Respiratory infections due to *Mycoplasma pneumoniae* in infants and children. Pediatrics 1975;55:327–35.

10. Hall CB, Walsh EE, Long CE, Schnabel KC. Immunity to and frequency of reinfection with respiratory syncytial virus. J Infect Dis 1991;163:693–8.

11. Johnson KM, Bloom HH, Mufson MA, et al. Natural reinfection of adults by respiratory syncytial virus: possible relation to mild upper respiratory disease. N Engl J Med 1962;267:68–72.

12. Krasinski K, Nelson JD, Butler S, et al. Possible association of mycoplasma and viral respiratory infections with bacterial meningitis. Am J Epidemiol 1987;125:499–508.

13. Ingall M, Glaser J, Meltzer RS, et al. Allergic rhinitis in early infancy: review of the literature and report of a case in a newborn. Pediatrics 1965:36:108–12.

14. Miller RE, Paradise JL, Firday GA, et al. The nasal smear for eosinophils. Am J Dis Child 1982;136:1009—11.

15. Fagin J, Friedman R, Fireman P. Allergic rhinitis. Pediatr Clin North Am 1981;28:797–806.

16. Rupp GH, Friedman RA. Eosinophilic nonallergic rhinitis in children. Pediatrics 1982;70:437–9.

17. Stern RC, Boat TF, Wood RE, et al. Treatment and prognosis of nasal polyps in cystic fibrosis. Am J Dis Child 1982;136:1067–70.

18. Cronk GO, Naumann DE, McDermott H, et al. A controlled study of the effect of oral penicillin G in the treatment of nonspecific upper respiratory infections. Am J Med 1954;16:804–9.

19. Soyka LF, Robinson DS, Lachant N, et al. The misuse of antibiotics for the treatment of upper respiratory tract infections in children. Pediatrics 1975;55:552–6.

20. Taylor B, Abbott GE, Kerr MM, et al. Amoxicillin and co-trimoxazole in presumed viral respiratory infection in childhood: placebo-controlled trial. Br Med J 1977;2: 552–4.

21. Arroll B, Kenealy T. Antibiotics for the common cold. Cochrane Database Syst Rev 2000;2:CD000247.

22. Gadomski AM. Potential interventions for preventing pneumonia among young children: lack of effect of antibiotic treatment for upper respiratory infections. Pediatr Infect Dis J 1993;12:115–20.

23. Dowell SF, Schwartz B. Resistant pneumococci: protecting patients through judicious use of antibiotics. Am Fam Physician 1997;55:1647–54.

24. Watson RL, Dowell SF, Jayaraman M, et al. Antimicrobial use for pediatric upper respiratory infections: reported practice, actual practice, and parent beliefs. Pediatrics 1999;104:1251–57.

25. Clemens CJ, Taylor JA, Almquist JR, et al. Is an antihistamine-decongestant combination effective in temporarily relieving symptoms of the common cold in preschool children? J Pediatr 1997;130:463–6.

26. Hutton N, Wilson MH, Melliti ED, et al. Effectiveness of an antihistamine-decongestant combination for young children with the common cold: a randomized, controlled clinical trial. J Pediatr 1991;118:125–30.

27. Joseph MM, King WD. Dystonic reaction following recommended use of a cold syrup. Ann Emerg Med 1995;26: 749–51.

28. Luks D, Anderson MR. Antihistamines and the common cold. A review and critique of the literature. J Gen Int Med 1996;11:240–4.

29. Hamila H. Vitamin C intake and susceptibility to the common cold. Br J Nutr 1997;77:59–72.

30. Mossad SB, Macknin ML, Medendore SV, et al. Zinc gluconate lozenges for treating the common cold: a randomized, double-blind, placebo-controlled study. Ann Intern Med 1996;125:81–8.

31. Macknin ML, Piedmonte M, Calendine C, et al. Zinc gluconate lozenges for treating the common cold in children: a randomized, controlled trial. JAMA. 1998;279:1962–7.

32. Hendley JO, Wenzel RP, Gwaltney JM Jr. Transmission of rhinovirus colds by self-inoculation. N Engl J Med 1973; 288:1361–4.

33. Dick EC, Jennings LC, Mink KA, et al. Aerosol transmission of rhinovirus colds. J Infect Dis 1987;156:442–8.

34. Niffenegger JP. Proper handwashing promotes wellness in child care. J Pediatr Health Care 1997;11:26–31.

35. Hays GC, Mullard JE. Can nasal bacteria be predicted from clinical findings? Pediatrics 1972;49:596–9.

36. Todd JK, Todd N, Damato J, et al. Bacteriology and treatment of purulent nasopharyngitis: a double-blind, placebo-controlled evaluation. Pediatr Infect Dis J 1984;3: 226–32.

37. Townsend EH Jr, Radebaugh JF. Treatment of complications of respiratory illness in pediatric practice. N Engl J Med 1962;267:854–8.

38. Eavey RD, Malekzakeh M, Wright HT Jr. Bacterial meningitis secondary to abscess of the nasal septum. Pediatrics 1977;60:102–4.

39. Da Silva M, Helman J, Eliacher I, et al. Nasal septal abscess of dental origin. Arch Otolaryngol 1982;108:380–81.

40. Ambrus PS, Eavey RD, Baker AS, et al. Management of nasal septal abscess. Laryngoscope 1981;91:575–82.

41. Olsen KD, Carpenter RJ III, Kern EB. Nasal septal trauma in children. Pediatrics 1979;64:32–5.

42. Wynder SG, Lampe RM, Shoemaker ME. Uvulitis and *Haemophilus influenzae* b bacteremia. Pediatr Emerg Care 1986;2:23–35.

43. Li KI, Kiernan S, Wald ER, Reilly JS. Isolated uvulitis due to *Haemophilus influenzae* type b. Pediatrics 19847;74: 1054–7.

44. Reddy CR, Margolin SJ. Acute uvular edema. Am J Dis Child 1983;137:1204-5.

45. Breese BB, Hall CB. Beta-Hemolytic Streptoccocal Disease. Boston: Houghton Mifflin, 1978.

46. Bisno AL, Gerber MA, Gwaltney JM Jr, et al. Practice guidelines for the diagnosis and management of Group A streptococcal pharyngitis. Infectious Diseases Society of America. Clin Infect Dis 2002;35:113–25.

47. Wannamaker LW. Perplexity and precision in the diagnosis of streptococcal pharyngitis. Am J Dis Child 1972;124: 352–8.

48. Moffet HL, Cramblett HG, Smith A. Group A streptococcal infection in a children's home. II: clinical and epidemiologic patterns of illness. Pediatrics 1964;33:11–17.

49. Alpert JJ, Pickering MR, Warren RJ. Failure to isolate streptococci from children under the age of 3 years with exudative tonsillitis. Pediatrics 1966;38:663–6.

50. Schwartz RH, Hayden GF, Wientzen R. Children less than three-years-old with pharyngitis: are Group A streptococci really that uncommon? Clin Pediatr 1986;25:185–8.

51. Heckerling PS, Harris AA. Streptococcal pharyngitis in an adult emergency room population. J Fam Pract 1985;21: 302–7.

52. Kaplan EL, Top FH Jr, Dudding BA, et al. Diagnosis of streptococcal pharyngitis: differentiation of active infection from the carrier state in the symptomatic child. J Infect Dis 1971;123:490–501.

53. Moffet HL, Cramblett HG, Black JP, et al. Erythromycin estolate and phenoxymethly penicillin in the treatment of streptococcal pharyngitis. Antimicrob Agents Chemother 1964;1963:759–764.

54. Gerber MA, Randolph MR, Chanatry J, et al. Antigen detection test for streptococcal pharyngitis: evaluation of sensitivity with respect to true infections. J Pediatr 1986;108: 654–8.

55. Kellogg JA, Manzella JP. Detection of Group A streptococci in the laboratory or physician's office. JAMA 1986;255: 2638–42.

56. Gerber MA, Tanz RR, Kabat W, et al. Optical immunoassay for group A beta-hemolytic streptococcal pharyngitis. An office-based, multicenter investigation. JAMA 1997;277: 899–903.

57. Uhl JR, Adamson SC, Vetter EA, et al. Comparison of LightCycler PCR, rapid antigen immunoassay, and culture for detection of group A streptococci from throat swabs. J Clin Microbiol 2003;41:242–9.

58. Pinchichero ME, Disney FA, Talney WB, et al. Adverse and beneficial effects of immediate treatment of group A beta-hemolytic streptococcal pharyngitis with penicillin. Pediatr Infect Dis J 1987;6:635–43.

59. Moffet HL, Siegel AC, Doyle HK. Nonstreptococcal pharyngitis. J Pediatr 1968;73:51–60.

60. Honikman LH, Massell BF. Guidelines for the selective use of throat cultures in the diagnosis of streptococcal respiratory infection. Pediatrics 1971;48:573–82.

61. Moffet HL, Cramblett HG, Black JP. Group A streptococcal infections in a children's home. I: evaluation of practical bacteriologic methods. Pediatrics 1964;33:5–10.

62. Randolph MF, Redys JJ, Cope JB. Evaluation of aerobic and anaerobic methods for recovery of streptococci from throat cultures. J Pediatr 1984;104:897–9.

63. Benjamin JT, Perriello VA Jr. Pharyngitis due to group C hemolytic streptococci in children. J Pediatr 1976;89: 254–6.

64. Gallo G, Berzero R, Cattai N, et al. An outbreak of group A food-borne streptococcal pharyngitis. Eur J Epidemiol 1992;8:292–7.

65. Farley TA, Wilson SA, Mahoney F, et al. Direct inoculation of food as the cause of an outbreak of group A streptococcal pharyngitis. J Infect Dis 1993;167:1232–5.

66. Chretien JH, McGinniss CG, Thompson J, et al. Group B beta-hemolytic streptococci causing pharyngitis. J Clin Microbiol 1979;10:263–6.

67. Breese BB, Disney FA, Talpey W. The nature of a small group pediatric practice. II: the incidence of beta hemolytic streptococcal illness in a private pediatric practice. Pediatrics 1966;38:277–85.

68. Ginsburg CM, McCracken GH Jr, Crow SD, et al. Seroepidemiology of the Group-A streptococcal carriage state in a private pediatric practice. Am J Dis Child 1985;139: 614–17.

69. Kaplan EL, Top FH Jr, Dudding BA, et al. diagnosis of streptococcal pharyngitis: differentiation of active infection from the carrier state in the symptomatic child. J Infect Dis 1971;123:490–501.

70. Margileth AM, Mella GW, Zilvetti EE. Streptococci in children's respiratory infections: diagnosis and treatment. Clin Pediatr 1971;10:69–77.

71. Ahmed S, Ayoub EM, Scornik JC, et al. Poststreptococcal reactive arthritis: clinical characteristics and association with HLA-DR alleles. Arthritis Rheum 1998;41:1096–102.

72. Dajani A, Taubert K, Ferrieri P, et al. Treatment of acute streptococcal pharyngitis and prevention of rheumatic fever: a statement for health professionals. Pediatrics 1995; 96:758–64.

73. Swedo SE, Leonard HL, Garvey M, et al. Pediatric autoimmune neuropsychiatric disorders associated with streptococcal infections: clinical description of the first 50 cases. Am J Psychiatry 1998;155:264–71.

74. Dhillon R, Newton L, Rudd PT, et al. Management of Kawasaki disease in the British Isles. Arch Dis Child 1993; 69:637–8.

75. Hoare S, Abinun M, Cant AJ. Overlap between Kawasaki disease and group A streptococcal infection [letter]. Pediatr Infect Dis J 1997;16:633–64.

76. Cantanzareo FJ, Stetson CA, Morris AJ, et al. The role of the streptococcus in the pathogenesis of rheumatic fever. Am J Med 1954;17:749–59.

77. Mortimer EA Jr, Rammelkamp CH Jr. Prophylaxis of rheumatic fever. Circulation 1956;14:1144–52.

78. Cantanzareo FA, Rammelkamp CH Jr, Chamovitz R. Prevention of rheumatic fever by treatment of streptococcal infections. II: factors responsible for failures. N Engl J Med 1958;259:51–7.

79. Denny FW, Wannamaker LW, Hahn EO. Comparative effects of penicillin, aureomycin and terramycin on streptococcal tonsillitis and pharyngitis. Pediatrics 1953;11: 7–14.

80. Nelson JD. The effect of penicillin therapy on the symptoms and signs of streptococcal pharyngitis. Pediatr Infect Dis J 1984;3:10–3.

81. Hall CB, Breese BB. Does penicillin make Johnny's strep throat better? Pediatr Infect Dis J 1984;3:7–9.

82. Denny FW. Effect of treatment on streptococcal pharyngitis: Is the issue really settled? Pediatr Infect Dis J 1985;4:352–4.

83. Snellman LW, Stang HJ, Stang JM, et al. Duration of positive throat cultures for group A streptococci after initiation of antibiotic therapy. Pediatrics 1993;91:1166–70.

84. Pichichero ME, Goodch WM 3rd. Comparison of cefdinir and penicillin V in the treatment of pediatric streptococcal tonsillopharyngitis. Pediatr Infect Dis J 2000;19:S171–3.

85. Milatovic D, Adam D, Hamilton H, et al. Cefprozil versus penicillin V in treatment of streptococcal tonsillopharyngitis. Antimicrob Agents Chemother 1993;37:1620–3.

86. Krober MS, Weir MR, Themilis NJ, et al. Optimal dosing interval for penicillin treatment of streptococcal pharyngitis. Clin Pediatr 1990;29:646–8.

87. Feldman S, Bisno AL, Lott L, et al. Efficacy of benzathine penicillin G in group A streptococcal pharyngitis: reevaluation. J Pediatr 1987;110:783–7.

88. Weir MR. Intravascular injuries from intramuscular penicillin. Clin Pediatr 1988;27:85–90.

89. Silber TJ, D'Angelo L. Psychosis and seizures following the injection of penicillin G procaine: Hoigne's syndrome. Am J Dis Child 1985;139:335–7.

90. Tanz RR, Poncher JR, Corydon KE, et al. Clindamycin treatment of chronic pharyngeal carriage of group A streptococci. J Pediatr 1991;119:123–8.

91. Schwartz RH, Wientzen RL Jr, Pedreira F, et al. Penicillin V for group A streptococcal pharyngotonsillitis. A randomized trial of seven vs ten days' therapy. JAMA 1981;246:1790–5.

92. Morris AJ, Chamovitz R, Cantanzaro FJ, et al. Prevention of rheumatic fever by treatment of streptococcal infections: effect of sulfadiazine. JAMA 1956;160:114–6.

93. McCormack RG, Kaye D, Hood FW. Resistance of group A streptococci to tetracycline. N Engl J Med 1962;267:323–26.

94. Martin JM, Green M, Barbadora KA, Wald ER. Erythromycin-resistant group A streptococci in school children in Pittsburgh. N Engl J Med 2002;346:1200–6.

95. Bergman M, Huikko S, Pihlajamaki M, et al. Effect of macrolide consumption on erythromycin resistance in *streptococcus pyogenes* in Finland in 1997–2001. Clin Infect Dis 2004;38:1251–6.

96. Adam D, Scholz H, Helmerking M. Short-course antibiotic treatment of 4782 culture-proven cases of group A streptococcal tonsillopharyngitis and incidence of poststreptococcal sequelae. J Infect Dis 2000;182:509–16.

97. Breese BB, Disney FA, Talpey WB, et al. Beta-hemolytic streptococcal infection: comparison of penicillin and lincomycin in the treatment of recurrent infections or the carrier state. Am J Dis Child 1969;117:147–52.

98. Rosenstein BJ, Markowitz M, Goldstein E, et al. Factors involved in treatment failures following oral penicillin therapy of streptococcal pharyngitis. J Pediatr 1968;73:513–20.

99. Brook I. Role of anaerobic beta-lactamase-producing bacteria in upper respiratory tract infections. Pediatr Infect Dis J 1987;6:310–6.

100. Brook I. Role of beta-lactamase-producing bacteria in the failure of penicillin to eradicate group A streptococci. Pediatr Infect Dis J 1985;4:491–5.

101. Brook I, Hirokawa R. Treatment of patients with a history of recurrent tonsillitis due to group A streptococci. Clin Pediatr 1985;24:331–6.

102. Kim KS, Kaplan EL. Association of penicillin tolerance with failure to eradicate group A streptococci from patients with pharyngitis. J Pediatr 1985;107:681–4.

103. Feldman S, Bisno AL, Lott L, et al. Efficacy of benzathine penicillin G in group A streptococcal pharyngitis: reevaluation. J Pediatr 1987;110:783–7.

104. Dagan R, Ferne M, Sheinis M, et al. An epidemic of penicillin-tolerant group A streptococcal pharyngitis in children in a closed community: mass treatment with erythromycin. J Infect Dis 1987;156:514–6.

105. Simon HJ, Sadai W. Staphylococcal antagonism to penicillin-G therapy of hemolytic streptococcal pharyngeal infection: effect of oxacillin. Pediatrics 1963;31:463–9.

106. Stillerman M, Isenberg HG, Moody M. Streptococcal pharyngitis therapy: comparison of cephalexin, phenoxymethyl penicillin, and ampicillin. Am J Dis Child 1972;123:457–61.

107. Brook I, Gober AE. Persistence of group A beta-hemolytic streptococci in toothbrushes and removable orthodontic appliances following treatment of pharyngotonsillitis. Arch Otolaryngol Head Neck Surg 1998;124:993–5.

108. Wilson KS, Maroney SA, Gander RM. The family pet as an unlikely source of group A beta-hemolytic streptococcal infection in humans. Pediatr Infect Dis J 1995;14:372–5.

109. Breese BB, Denny FW, Dillon HC, et al. Consensus: difficult management problems in children with streptococcal pharyngitis. Pediatr Infect Dis J 1985;4:10–3.

110. Hendley JO. Tonsillectomy: justified but not mandated in special patients (editorial). N Engl J Med 1984;310:717–8.

111. Feinstein AR, Spagnuola M, Jonas S, et al. Prophylaxis of recurrent rheumatic fever: therapeutic-continuous oral penicillin vs. monthly injections. JAMA 1968;206:565–8.

112. Mortimer EA Jr, Boxerbaum B. Diagnosis and treatment: group A streptococcal infections. Pediatrics 1965;36:930–2.

113. Shulman ST, Amren DP, Bisno AL, et al. Prevention of rheumatic fever. Circulation 1984;70:1118A–22A.

114. Patel KS, Ahmad S, O'Leary G, et al. The role of computed tomography in the management of peritonsillar abscess. Otolaryngol Head Neck Surg 1992;107:727–32.

115. Buckley AR, Moss EH, Blokmanis A. Diagnosis of peritonsillar abscess: value of intraoral sonography. AJR Am J Roentgenol 1994;162:961–4.

116. Weinberg E, Brodsky L, Stanievich J, et al. Needle aspiration of peritonsillar abscess in children. Arch Otolaryngol—Head and Neck Surg 1993;119:169–72.

117. Schechter GL, Sly DE, Roper AL, et al. Changing face of treatment of peritonsillar abscess. Laryngoscope 1982;92:657–9.

118. McCurdy JA Jr. Peritonsillar abscess. Arch Otolaryngol 1977;103:414–18.

119. Shoemaker M, Lampe RM, Weir MR. Peritonsillitis: abscess or cellulitis? Pediatr Infect Dis J 1986;5:435–9.

120. Jousimies-Somer H, Savolainen S, Matkie A, et al. Bacteriologic findings in peritonsillar abscesses in young adults. Clin Infect Dis 1993;16Suppl A:S212–18.

121. Knudsen TD, Simko EJ. Eikenella corrodens: an unexpected pathogen causing a persistent peritonsillar abscess. Ear Nose Throat J 1995;74:114–17.

122. Sugita R, Kawamura S, Ichikawa G, et al. Microorganisms isolated from peritonsillar abscess and indicated chemotherapy. Arch Otolaryngol 1982;108:655–8.

123. Maisel RH. Peritonsillar abscess: tonsil antibiotic levels in patients treated by acute abscess surgery. Laryngoscope 1982;92:80–7.

124. Gray WC. Throat culture in impending peritonsillar abscess. South Med J 1984;77:1545–7.

125. Prior A, Montgomery P, Mitchelmore I, et al. The microbiology and antibiotic treatment of peritonsillar abscesses. Clin Otolaryngol Allied Sci 1995;20:219–23.

126. Herzon FS, Harris P. Peritonsillar abscess: Incidence, current management practices, and a proposal for treatment guidelines. Laryngoscope 1995;105(8 Part 3 S74):1–17.

127. Yilmaz T, Unal OF, Figen G, et al. A comparison of procaine penicillin with sulbactam-ampicillin in the treatment of peritonsillar abscess. Eur Arch Otorhinolaryngol 1998; 255:163–5.

128. Wenig BL, Shikowitz MJ, Abramson AL. Necrotizing fasciitis as a lethal complication of peritonsillar abscess. Laryngoscope 1984;94:1576–9.

129. Nielsen TR, Clement F, Andeasson HK. Mediastinitis—a rare complication of a peritonsillar abscess. J Otolaryngol Otol 1996;110:175–6.

130. Moreno S, Garcia Altozano J, Pinilla B, et al. Lemierre's disease: postanginal bacteremia and pulmonary involvement caused by *Fusobacterium necrophorum*. Rev Infect Dis 1989;11:319–24.

131. Fagan JJ, Wormald PJ. Quinsy tonsillectomy or interval tonsillectomy—a prospective, randomized trial. South Afr Med J 1994;84:689–90.

132. Fried MP, Forrest JO. Peritonsillitis. Arch Otolaryngol 1981;107:283–6.

133. Spires JR, Owens JJ, Woodson GE, et al. Treatment of peritonsillar abscess: a prospective study of aspiration vs. incision and drainage. Arch Otolaryngol Head Neck Surg 1987;113:984–6.

134. Schwartz RH, Wientzen RL, Grundfast KM. Sore throats in adolescents. Pediatr Infect Dis J 1982;1:443–7.

135. Glezen WP, Clyde WA, Senior RJ, et al. Group A streptococci, mycoplasmas, and viruses associated with acute pharyngitis. JAMA 1967;202:455–60.

136. Moffet HL, Siegel AC, Doyle HK. Non-streptococcal pharyngitis. J Pediatr 1968;73:51–60.

137. Ruuskanen O, Sarkkinen H, Meurman O, et al. Rapid diagnosis of adenoviral tonsillitis: a prospective clinical study. J Pediatr 1984;104:725–8.

138. Giladi N, Herman J. Pharyngoconjunctival fever. Arch Dis Child 1984;59:1182–3.

139. Evans AS, Dick EC. Acute pharyngitis and tonsillitis in University of Wisconsin students. JAMA 1964;190: 699–708.

140. Glezen WP, Fernald GW, Lohr JA. Acute respiratory disease of university students with special reference to the etiologic role of Herpesvirus hominis. Am J Epidemiol 1975;101:111–21.

141. Young EJ, Vainrub B, Musher DM, et al. Acute pharyngotonsillitis cause by herpesvirus type 2. JAMA 1978;239: 1885–6.

142. Chang T-W. Herpetic angina following orogenital exposure. J Am Vener Dis Assoc 1975;1:163–4.

143. Cramblett HG, Moffet HL, Black JP, et al. Coxsackie virus infections. J Pediatr 1964;64:406–14.

144. Moffet HL, Cramblett HG, Smith A. Group A streptococcal infections in a children's home. II: clinical and epidemiologic patterns of illness. Pediatrics 1964;33:11–17.

145. Anonymous. Echovirus type 9 outbreak—New York. MMWR 1978;28:392–4.

146. Moffet HL, Cramblett HG, Middleton GK, et al. Outbreak of influenza B in a children's home. JAMA 1962;182: 834–8.

147. Schultz I, Gendelfinger B, Rosenbaum M, et al. Comparison of clinical manifestations of respiratory illnesses due to Asian strain influenza, adenovirus and unknown cause. J Lab Clin Med 1960;55:497–509.

148. Fisher RG, Gruber WC, Edwards KM, et al. Twenty years of outpatient respiratory syncytial virus infection: a framework for vaccine efficacy trials. Pediatrics 1999;e7:2.

149. Mufson MA, Ludwig WM, Purcell RH, et al. Exudative pharyngitis following experimental Mycoplasma hominis type 1 infection. JAMA 1965;192:1146–52.

150. Jacobs RF, Condrey YM, Yamauchi T. Tularemia in adults and children: a changing presentation. Pediatrics 1985;46: 818–22.

151. Tyson HK. Tularemia: an unappreciated cause of exudative pharyngitis. Pediatrics 1976;58:864–6.

152. Wallin J, Siegel MS. Pharyngeal Neisseria gonorrhoeae: Colonizer or pathogen? Br Med J 1979;1:1462–3.

153. Kinghorn GR, Hafiz S, McEntegart MG. Oropharyngeal *Haemophilus ducreyi* infection. Br Med J 1983;287:650.

154. Brook I, Gober AE. *Bacteroides melaningogenicus*: its recovery from tonsils of children with acute tonsillitis. Arch Otolaryngol 1983;109:818–20.

155. Vogel LC, Boyer KM. Metastatic complications of *Fusobacterium necrophorum* sepsis. Am J Dis Child 1980;134: 356–8.

156. Miller RA, Brancato F, Holmes KK. *Corynebacterium haemolyticum* as a cause of pharyngitis and scarlatiniform rash in young adults. Ann Intern Med 1986;105:867–72.

157. Nyman M, Alugupalli KR, Stromberg S, et al. Antibody response to *Arcanobacterium haemolyticum* infection in humans. J Infect Dis 1997;175:1515–8.

158. Mackenzie A, Fuitte LA, Chan FT, et al. Incidence and pathogenicity of *Arcanobacterium haemolyticum* during a 2-year study in Ottawa. Clin Infect Dis 1995;21:177–81.

159. Person DA, Smith TF, Herrmann EC Jr. Experiences in laboratory diagnosis of mumps virus infections in routine medical practice. Mayo Clin Proc 1971;46:544–8.

160. Komaroff AL, Aronson MD, Pass TM, et al. Viral and bacterial organisms associated with pharyngitis in a school-aged population. J Pediatr 1986;109:747–52.

161. Neinstein LS, Inderlied C. Low prevalence of *Chlamydia trachomatis* in the oropharynx of adolescents. Pediatr Infect Dis J 1986;5:660–2.

162. Rose FB, Camp CJ, Antes EJ. Family outbreak of fatal *Yersinia enterocolitica* pharyngitis. Am J Med 1987;82:636–7.

163. Tacket CO, Davis BR, Carter GP, et al. *Yersinia enterocolitica* pharyngitis. Ann Intern Med 1983;99:40–2.

164. Irigoyen MM, Katz M, Larsen JG. Postanginal sepsis in adolescence. Pediatr Infect Dis J 1983;2:248–50.

165. Leugers CM, Clover R. Lemierre syndrome: post-anginal sepsis. J Am Board Fam Pract 1995;8:384–91.

166. Celikel TH, Muthuswamy PP. Septic pulmonary emboli

secondary to internal jugular vein phlebitis (postanginal sepsis) caused by *Eikenella corrodens*. Am Rev Resp Dis1984;130:510–3.

167. Thomas KT, Feder HM, Lawton AR, et al. Periodic fever syndrome in children. J Pediatr 1999;135;15–21.

168. Cherry JD, Jahn CL. Herpangina: the etiologic spectrum. Pediatrics 1965;36:632–4.

169. Steigman AJ, Lipton MM, Braspennickx H. Acute lymphonodular pharngitis: a newly described condition due to Coxsackie A virus. J Pediatr 1962;61:331–6.

170. Parrott RH, Wolf SI, Nudelman J, et al. Clinical and laboratory differentiation between herpangina and infectious (herpetic) gingivostomatitis. Pediatrics 1954;14:122–9.

171. Glezen WP, Fernald GW, Lohr JA. Acute respiratory disease of university students with special reference to the etiologic role of Herpesvirus hominis. Am J Epidemiol 1975;101:111–21.

172. Suzaki N, Ishikawa K, Horiuchi T, et al. Age-related symptomatology of echo 11 virus infections in children. Pediatrics 1980;65:284–6.

173. Nakayama T, Urano T, Osano M, et al. Outbreak of herpangina associated with Coxsackie virus B3 infection. Pediatr Infect Dis J 1989;8:495–8.

174. Zahorsky J. Herpangina: a specific infectious disease. Arch Pediatr 1924;41:181–4.

175. Liesky BA, Goldberger AC, Tompkins LS, et al. Infections caused by nondiphtheria corynebacteria. Rev Infect Dis 1982;4:1220–35.

176. Viers WA. Primary syphilis of the tonsil: presentation of four cases. Laryngoscope 1981;91:1507–11.

177. Fiumara NJ, Walker EA. Primary syphilis of the tonsil. Arch Otolaryngol 1982;108:43–44.

178. Cohen PR. Tests for detecting herpes simplex virus and varicella-zoster virus infections. Dermatol Clin 1994;12: 51–68.

179. Espy MJ, Uhl JR, Mitchell PS, et al. Diagnosis of herpes simplex virus infection in the clinical laboratory by LightCycler PCR. J Clin Microbiol 2000;38:795–9.

180. Kuan MM. Detection and rapid differentiation of human enteroviruses following genomic amplification. J Clin Microbiol 1997;35:2598–601.

181. Hodes H. Diphtheria. Pediatr Clin North Am 1979;26: 445–59.

182. Morgan BC. Cardiac complications of diphtheria. Pediatrics 1963;32:549–57.

183. Tahernia AC. Electrocardiographic abnormalities and serum transaminase levels in diphtheritic myocarditis. J Pediatr 1969;75:1008–14.

184. Dietze WE, Sudderth JF. Post-diphtheria polyneuritis: 3 case reports. Laryngoscope 1972;82:765–80.

185. Green SL, LaPeter KS. Pseudodiphtheritic membranous pharyngitis caused by *Corynebacterium hemolyticum*. JAMA 1981;245:2330–1.

186. Luotonen J, Syrjala H, Jokinene K, et al. Tularemia in otolaryngologic practice. An analysis of 127 cases. Arch Otolaryngol—Head Neck Surg 1986;42:77–80.

187. Doege TC, Heath CW, Sherman II. Diphtheria in the United States: 1959–1960. Pediatrics 1962;30:194–205.

188. Bowler CJ, Mandal BK, Schlecht B, et al. Diphtheria: the continuing hazard. Arch. Dis Child 1988;63:194–5.

189. McClosky RV, Eller JJ, Green M, et al. The 1970 epidemic of diphtheria in San Antonio. Ann Intern Med 1972;75: 495–502.

190. Bader M, Pedersen AHB, Spearman J, et al. An unusual case of cutaneous diphtheria. JAMA 1978;240:1382–3.

191. Popovic T, Wharton M, Wenger JD, et al. Are we ready for diphtheria? A report from the Diphtheria Diagnostic Workshop, Atlanta, 11 and 12 July 1994. J Infect Dis 1995; 171:765–7.

192. Dobie RA, Tobey DN. Clinical features of diphtheria in the respiratory tract. JAMA 1979;242:2197–2201.

193. Tasman A, Minkenhof JE, Vink HH, et al. Importance of intravenous injection of diphtheria antiserum. Lancet 1958;1:1299–304.

194. Thisyakorn U, Wongvanich J, Kumpeng V. Failure of corticosteroid therapy to prevent diphtheritic myocarditis or neuritis. Pediatr Infect Dis J 1984;3:126–8.

195. Public Health Service Advisory Committee on Immunization Practices. Diphtheria antitoxin for case contacts. MMWR 1977;26:402–7.

196. Nelson LA, Peri BA, Rieger CHL, et al. Immunity to diphtheria in an urban population. Pediatrics 1978;61:703–10.

CHAPTER 3

Infectious Mononucleosis and Mononucleosis-like Syndromes

■ CLASSIC INFECTIOUS MONONUCLEOSIS

Definitions and Classifications

Terminology is a problem in infectious mononucleosis (IM) and related syndromes, and historical usage needs to be integrated with practical and meaningful definitions. Clinical IM was classified by Hoagland in 1960 as having pharyngeal (very common), typhoidal (fever only), and icteric forms. The last two forms are now readily recognized if Epstein-Barr virus (EBV) serology is done in patients with acute hepatitis and in febrile patients with atypical lymphocytes on blood smear. The classification used in this book is outlined in Table 3-1. Classic IM is defined as meeting all three criteria of clinical, hematologic, and serologic features.

The clinical features of classic IM (or "mono") typically include at least three of the following: exudative pharyngitis, generalized lymphadenopathy, splenomegaly, malar facial swelling, and easy fatigability. The hematologic feature is the presence in the peripheral blood smear of at least 5% atypical lymphocytes (Fig. 3-1). The serologic feature is a slide test positive for IM antibodies (agglutinins for sheep or horse erythrocytes). This book uses "heterophile antibody" to mean the current customary usage; namely, the sheep or horse erythrocyte-agglutinating antibody that is absorbed by guinea pig antigen but not by beef antigen. Perhaps Paul and Bunnell's original speculation was correct that the agent of IM (EBV) has a cross-reacting antigen that usually stimulates humans (except many young children) to produce such a heterophile antibody.[1]

Primary EBV infection can now be demonstrated by antibody titers. However, "EBV infection" and "infectious mononucleosis" should not be used as synonyms: EBV infection often does not result in classic IM, and mono-like illness can have causes other than EBV infection. This distinction in terminology is analogous to distinguishing between mumps virus infection and parotitis. EBV is a possible etiology of many syndromes that are not like IM, as discussed in chapters on other syndromes. Heterophile-negative IM is discussed in the section on mono-like syndromes.

Clinical Diagnosis

Pharyngitis

Febrile exudative pharyngitis is the most frequent clinical picture of IM.[2–9] It often is severe and may resemble the membranous pharyngitis of diphtheria. Concurrent Group A streptococcal pharyngitis is no more common than in normal controls.[6] However, a throat culture to exclude concurrent streptococcal pharyngitis is reasonable in this situation, as the pharyngitis of Group A streptococcus and that of EBV infection are clinically indistinguishable. A certain number of streptococcal carriers will be falsely identified as having streptococcal pharyngitis when this approach is taken. Therefore, if the diagnosis of IM is clinically obvious the pharyngitis can be attributed to EBV infection, and the throat culture omitted. Petechiae on the hard palate are an occasional feature of both streptococcal and EBV pharyngitis.

Lymphadenopathy

Most patients with IM have generalized adenopathy. Enlargement of the anterior cervical (tonsillar) nodes is of little diagnostic value, since it may accompany tonsillitis from any cause. Posterior cervical adenopathy is much more suggestive of IM.[5]

Splenomegaly

Most patients with classic IM have splenomegaly, a sign that may make the physician suspect IM. Athletic teenagers often have well-developed

TABLE 3-1. LOGICAL COMBINATIONS OF THREE FEATURES OF INFECTIOUS MONONUCLEOSIS-LIKE SYNDROMES

DIAGNOSTIC CLASSIFICATION	CLINICAL	HEMATOLOGIC	SEROLOGIC
Classical IM	+	+	+
IM without atypical lymphocytosis	+	0	+
Asymptomatic IM	0	+ or 0	+
Heterophile-negative IM	+	+	0
Pharyngitis, lymphadenopathy, splenomegaly	+	0	0
Atypical lymphocytosis	0	+	0

abdominal musculature that impairs palpation, but typically they have splenic enlargement by percussion.

Edema around Eyes

Edema of the upper eyelid, and especially edema of the upper cheek just below the eye, is an extremely useful, if often overlooked, finding that is present in about one third of adolescents or young adults with IM (Figure 3-2).[5] This feature was first described by Hoagland and is sometimes called "Hoagland's sign."

Jaundice

About 5% of young adults with IM have jaundice. In one series of children under 16, serum aminotransferase levels were elevated in about 40% during the acute illness.[7] When unusually high alkaline phosphatase levels are found in nongrowing teenagers or young adults with minimal and dispropor-

tionately low bilirubin levels, IM should be suspected.[8]

Mild Abdominal Pain

The enlarged liver or spleen may produce mild upper abdominal pain and tenderness on palpation.

Rash

A maculopapular rash has been noted in about 10% of children[3] but was noted in 40% of patients in one large series.[9] If the patient has been given ampicillin (a poor choice for any pharyngitis), a rash occurs in 70–100% and usually is confluent and extensive and may be frightening. In bygone days, the appearance of a rash in patients with IM upon exposure to ampicillin was used as a diagnostic test. The rash may also occur in patients with IM due to cytomegalovirus (CMV) infection, as well as in patients with acute lymphocytic leukemia.[10] Rash may also occur upon treatment with other antibiot-

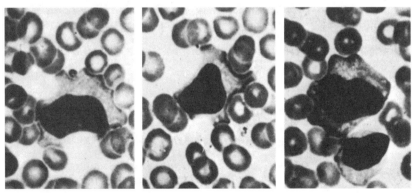

■ **FIGURE 3-1** Dented or scalloped cytoplasm of atypical lymphocytes. This finding is readily recognized by even an inexperienced observer and is very suggestive of infectious mononucleosis. (Photo from Dr. I. Davidsohn)

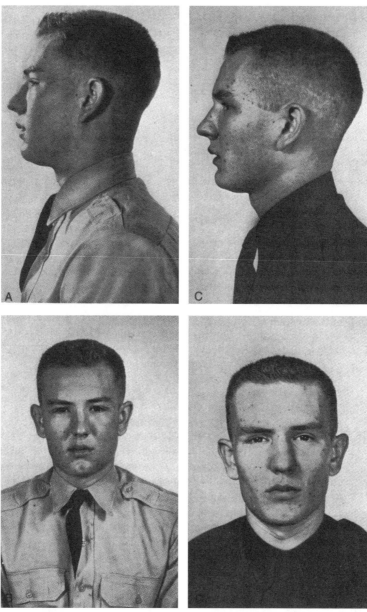

■ **FIGURE 3-2** Eye swelling during infectious mononucleosis. (*A* and *B*) during illness; (*C* and *D*) after recovery. (Copyright 1958 CIBA Pharmaceutical Company, Division of CIBA-GEIGY Corporation. Reproduced with permission from *Clinical Symposia*. All rights reserved.)

ics, including amoxicillin and cephalexin.[11] The mechanism by which antibiotic-associated rash is produced in patients with IM is not understood.

Easy Fatigability

Most children who are old enough to articulate this symptom will volunteer it or acknowledge it on questioning.

Laboratory Approach

Atypical Lymphocytosis

An increase in the number of lymphocytes with atypical forms is usually found in IM. Atypical lymphocytosis can be observed in association with many viral diseases (Box 3–1), some nonviral diseases (toxoplasmosis, babesiosis, malaria, tsutsugamushi scrub

---

BOX 3-1 ■ Causes of Lymphocytosis

Atypical lymphocytosis
Common
Epstein-Barr virus
Cytomegalovirus
Uncommon
Hepatitis A virus[a]
Respiratory syncytial virus[a],[15]
HIV (Acute retroviral syndrome)[b]
Rare
Toxoplasmosis[a]
Babesiosis[a]
Malaria[c]
Drug-hypersensitivity syndromes
Toxin exposure
Malignancies (especially non-Hodgkin's
    lymphoma)

Typical lymphocytosis
Pertussis
Acute infectious lymphocytosis[16]

[a]Usually does not cause an atypical lymphocytosis.
[b]Frequently causes atypical lymphocytosis.
[c]Almost always associated with some degree of atypical lymphocytosis.

---

typhus), poisoning, toxin exposure, radiation, malignancies, drug reactions, and allergies.[4],[12] Some authorities emphasize that the atypical lymphocytes of IM can often be distinguished from those of other diseases, but few laboratory technologists can make this distinction accurately. Thus, the finding of atypical lymphocytes is not specific, but it is useful to stimulate a search for more specific diagnostic information, especially if more than 10% of the lymphocytes are atypical. Some laboratories report a small percentage of atypical lymphocytes in many patients who do not have IM. This finding is usually of no significance. Patients with IM commonly also have a "shift" toward the lymphocyte lineage, in that greater than 50% of the white blood cells are lymphocytic. Experienced observers use many features of staining and morphology to recognize atypical lymphocytes. For the physician who does not examine smears often, the presence of denting or scalloping of lymphocytes by erythrocytes is a useful finding (Fig. 3-1). Dented cytoplasm is also seen in the atypical lymphocytes of the mono-like syndrome caused by cytomegalovirus.

Pertussis is classically associated with a lymphocytosis, but the lymphocytes are not atypical and the clinical presentation does not resemble IM (see

Chapter 7). Rarely, other infections may be associated with extremely high white blood cell counts with a lymphocytic predominance. This pattern has been termed acute infectious lymphocytosis. Typically, the etiologic agent is not discovered. Cases attributable to viral[13] and even parasitic[14] infections have been described. Atypical lymphocytes are not observed. As the lymphocytosis resolves, a transient eosinophilia sometimes develops.

Serologic Diagnosis

The traditional serologic test for heterophile antibody is a tube dilution test using sheep erythrocytes as antigen, but cumbersome tube tests are no longer necessary. Several slide tests using horse or sheep erythrocytes are simple and rapid screening tests for the antibody and can easily be repeated in a week or so if the initial test is negative but the diagnosis is still suspected. When the person reading the test is experienced in the practice, slide screening tests (such as Monospot®), have a high degree of specificity for IM; that is, false-positive results are uncommon.[17],[18] A small percentage of normal individuals, however, will have persistently false-positive slide tests.

The principal limitation of these tests is their low sensitivity. A negative slide screening test in no way eliminates the diagnosis of IM. The negative predictive value of the slide test was found to be 82% in one recent study involving 299 children and adolescents with clinically and serologically defined IM.[19] Another study showed that 271 (82%) of 329 patients with clinical IM who eventually had positive heterophile antibody tests required more than one sample before a positive result was obtained.[20] Finally, in a small cohort, no correlation could be found between severity of disease and the percent positive by heterophile antibody testing.[21] This implies that even patients who are very sick with EBV-induced IM may test falsely negative by heterophile antibody testing methods. Clinical practice backs up the experience reported in these studies; we have seen hospitalized patients with EBV-induced IM who had 2 or even 3 negative Monospot® tests. In these patients, the diagnosis can be made by testing for specific antibody production with EBV serology. Those with CMV-induced IM are also negative by heterophile antibody tests, so inclusion of CMV titers is often helpful in evaluation of patients with clinically suspect IM but negative slide screening tests.

Interpreting EBV serologic results is simpler if you use this seemingly silly but useful analogy and think of EBV as a peanut M&M. The candy coating is the viral capsid antigen (VCA). Since the candy is the first thing you taste when eating a peanut M&M, this reminds you that antibodies, both immunoglobulin M (IgM) and immunoglobulin G (IgG), to VCA are the first antibodies the immune system makes after EBV infection. The next layer is the chocolate, which represents EBV early antigen (EA). Antibody to EA, therefore, is made second. Finally, the peanut symbolizes the Epstein-Barr nuclear antigen (EBNA). Antibody to EBNA arises last. IgG antibody to VCA and antibody to EBNA persist for life, but antibody to early antigen wanes, usually within 6–9 months (Table 3-2). Stretching the analogy slightly further, remembering that chocolate melts makes it easy to recall that antibody to EA goes away over time.

Duration of Positivity

The most useful specific antibody for diagnosing primary EBV infection is the IgM EBV capsid antibody (Table 3-2). This appears within one month and becomes negative by three months in 80% of patients. As noted above, antibody to EA disappears within 9 months in most patients, but can persist for several years. There is no clinical significance to this phenomenon. The heterophile antibody test may remain positive in 75% of patients for up to one year.

Age Frequency

A positive heterophile slide test occurs most frequently in the 10- to 29-year-old group.[9,22] In one series of 575 cases of heterophile-positive IM in Georgia, less than 1% were 4 years of age or younger, only 5% were less than 10 years of age, and only 3% were 30 years of age or older.[9] This is not to suggest, however, that EBV infection does not occur in young children, but rather that it may be harder to diagnose. It is not known why young children do not reliably produce heterophile antibodies in response to EBV infection. These patients can be diagnosed, however, by specific EBV serology. In the study cited above, all patients, including those less than 2 years of age, mounted a measurable serologic response to the viral capsid antigen, although Monospot® testing was often negative.

In summary, the majority of children less than 10 years of age who have EBV infections are asymptomatic or have illnesses that do not resemble classic IM.[23,24] However, if a young child does appear to have classic IM, specific EBV antibody tests, in addition to a test for heterophile antibody, should be done. Some will be rapid slide test positive; one study showed that 35% of children ages 2 and 3

TABLE 3-2. ANTIBODIES USUALLY INCLUDED IN AN EBV-ANTIBODY PANEL (EBV SEROLOGY), AND THEIR INTERPRETATION

ANTIBODY AND TYPE	ANTIGEN TO WHICH THE ANTIBODY IS DIRECTED	COMMENTS
VCA IgM antibody	Viral capsid antigen (VCA)	Arises quickly; gone by 4 months; absence does not rule out acute EBV infection
VCA IgG antibody	VCA	Peaks at 3 weeks; remains for life
EA antibody	EBV early antigen	Arises slightly later than antibody to VCA; usually wanes and becomes undetectable by 6–9 months; in some patients may persist for several years, but this is of no clinical significance
EBNA antibody	Epstein-Barr nuclear antigen	Arises more than 1 month after infection; remains for life. Occasionally, EBNA responses are mounted late or not at all

years were positive, versus 80% of children between the ages of 4 and 11 years.[25]

Contagion

Initial lytic replication of EBV probably takes place in mucosal epithelial cells of the oropharynx. From there the virus infects and then immortalizes B cells, in which it establishes latency. It has been shown to be periodically shed from the oropharynx. Several recent investigations suggest that replication in B cells must occasionally be lytic; using polymerase chain reaction (PCR), EBV DNA can be found in the serum of at least 20% of patients with EBV-induced IM.[26,27] Studies have also identified not only EBV genome, but also replication-competent EBV particles in the urine of patients with IM,[28] although there is no epidemiologic evidence supporting transmission of the virus through urine.

The spread of the disease by saliva was deduced by Hoagland as early as 1960 from West Point cadets.[29] He noted lack of spread among roommates, and an incubation period of 5–7 weeks based on histories of brief episodes of intimate kissing. He also noted an incubation period of 21 days after blood transfusions.

Outbreaks have been reported, documented by EBV-specific serology.[30] However, outbreaks reported on the basis of slide tests may well be pseudo-outbreaks related to improper performance and interpretation of the tests.[31] Studies of families have indicated that about one-fourth of susceptible members will develop infection as evidenced by seroconversion, but that the younger children will usually not develop clinical disease.[32] EBV has been recovered from the pharynx 9 days before onset of symptoms and can persist for as long as 6 months.[32,33] It has also been shown that asymptomatic shedding of EBV in saliva can and does occur intermittently throughout life after EBV infection. At any point in time, between 6 and 20% of adults have measurable amounts of EBV in their saliva.[34] Many factors, including stress and intercurrent illness, have been implicated in the periodic asymptomatic reactivation of EBV replication.

Treatment and Prevention

Rest is usually the only treatment necessary. Most patients have significant fatigue, so rest is not difficult to enforce. Corticosteroid therapy for 6–10 days has been advocated for severe cases, such as those with potential airway obstruction. Corticosteroids are effective in reducing fever and other symptoms,[35] but it is doubtful that such potent therapy is justified for symptomatic relief in a self-limiting illness, and therapy may even prolong recovery.

In vitro, acyclovir inhibits lytic replication of EBV. Acyclovir given intravenously (10 mg/kg) every 8 hours for 7 days was statistically more effective than placebo, but only when six measures of improvement were combined.[36] Liver enzymes were not improved in the treated group. Another study looked at using prednisolone and acyclovir in uncomplicated IM. Oropharyngeal EBV shedding was significantly decreased in the treatment group, but no effect was observed on duration of illness, sore throat, weight loss, or other symptomatic parameters.[37] The lack of effect of acyclovir is intuitive, because the clinical manifestations of EBV infection are primarily due to the host immune response, not to viral replication.

Recently, ranitidine was investigated as a potential treatment for IM in a randomized, prospective clinical trial. No statistically significant differences could be found between the treatment and placebo groups.[38]

■ COMPLICATIONS OF INFECTIOUS MONONUCLEOSIS AND EPSTEIN-BARR VIRUS INFECTION

Complications typically associated with the clinical syndrome of IM, and those associated with EBV infection (not necessarily in the context of symptomatic IM) will be discussed separately. Complications listed as local and hematologic, such as peritonsillar abscess, partial airway obstruction, and acute hemolytic anemia, most often occur in patients who have clinically typical IM, but many of the other complications of EBV infection occur in patients who do not have typical mono-like illnesses.

Complications of Infectious Mononucleosis

Spontaneous rupture of the spleen can occur, especially during the first two weeks of the illness when the spleen is enlarging, but this complication is rare in childhood. Later rupture is presumed to be related to trauma to the still-enlarged spleen.[39] Return to nonathletic classroom activities can be based on the patient's strength and fatigability.

Return to competitive athletics after the patient feels well enough cannot easily be based on time alone, since recommendations have ranged from 3 weeks to 6 months. A normal spleen size is a more reasonable guide than use of an arbitrary time. This usually can be determined by a plain abdominal film.[39] Before especially traumatic body-contact sports, ultrasonic confirmation of a normal spleen size is sometimes advisable if the x-ray is equivocal.

Airway obstruction secondary to tonsillar and pharyngeal lymphoid hypertrophy and edema can occur. The teenager may be anxious and may avoid lying down because of difficulty swallowing secretions. Usually, airway obstruction can be anticipated and treated with corticosteroids, which often produces dramatic relief secondary to shrinking of the hypertrophied lymphoid tissue. Tracheal intubation and tracheotomy have been required in some patients.

Pneumonia with nodules or pleural effusion appears to be very rare, but concurrent mycoplasmal pneumonia may be more common and more severe than is generally expected and may account for some of the pneumonia attributed to IM.

Neurologic complications, such as aseptic meningitis, encephalitis, myelitis, peripheral nerve paralysis, or Guillain-Barré syndrome are usually self-limited and reversible. However, EBV-induced encephalitis may be severe, and a recent retrospective study of cases of EBV encephalitis suggests that outcomes may not be universally good.[40] EBV has been recovered from the spinal fluid. Occasionally, the neurologic involvement is the first or predominant finding, so serologic tests for EBV should be done routinely in such illness whenever the etiology is not known. The more specific serologic tests should always be done, especially for young children, who may not have a positive heterophile test. Seizures may occur in children with a convulsive disorder as a result of increased clearance of phenytoin. Hallucinations or acute visual distortions have been described as a complication and called "Alice in Wonderland syndrome" because of the shrinking or enlarging perceptions.[41]

Clinical hepatitis is found in about 5% of cases and subclinical hepatitis in 20–40%. Acute liver failure has been reported, as well as unexplained death.

Hematologic complications include hemolytic anemia with a positive direct Coombs test; fortunately, this complication is rare. Severe neutropenia is much more common, but usually does not lead to superinfection with bacteria or fungi. Thrombocytopenia is also not rare, and occasionally pancytopenia with capillary leak syndrome (with expanded plasma volume, pulmonary edema, and ascites) has been reported.

Acute renal failure as a result of severe rhabdomyolysis has been reported. Nephrotic syndrome has also been seen,[42] as has interstitial nephritis.[43] Concurrent genital ulceration of the labia has been reported in the absence of herpes simplex infection. Cardiac complications include complete heart block, severe myocarditis, and pericarditis.

Complications of EBV Infection

Numerous complications have been reported during EBV infection, some of which may be coincidental occurrences (Box 3–2). Sometimes, the EBV infection is manifested as a classic IM illness, but in younger children, there occasionally are no clinical findings or atypical lymphocytes to lead the clinician to suspect EBV. The malignancies associated with EBV, such as Burkitt's lymphoma and nasopharyngeal carcinoma, are not listed, as their presentation is not acute, nor do they resemble an infectious disease. Chronic or recurrent clinical IM or fatigue attributed to IM is discussed later.

EBV is associated with lymphoproliferative disease in patients with congenital or acquired immunodeficiency, and it is the most common cause of post-transplant lymphoproliferative disease (PTLD). These patients have impaired T-cell immunity and are unable to control the proliferation of EBV-infected B cells. Although they may present with symptoms of IM, more commonly they present with localized or disseminated lymphoproliferation involving the lymph nodes, liver, lung, kidney, bone marrow, central nervous sytem, or small intestine. The diagnosis requires demonstration of EBV genome in biopsy material.

Diagnosis

In some reported cases, there were no atypical lymphocytes to provide a clue to the diagnosis of EBV infection, as in the reference listed for migraine and chorea. However, these cryptic EBV complications are included on the list for completeness.

In general, when children do not have atypical lymphocytosis with EBV infections, they also do not have the clinical features of classic IM.[96] Thus children manifest at least two distinct patterns of

BOX 3-2 ■ Complications Associated with EBV Infection

Local

Peritonsillar abscess; postanginal sepsis[44,45]
Partial airway obstruction[46]
Splenic rupture[29]
Liver failure[47]
Mediastinal lymphadenopathy[48]
Sinusitis, orbital cellulitis[49]
Hematemesis, melena[50]
Membranous laryngitis[51]

Hematologic

Hemolytic anemia,[52] cryoglobulinemia[53]
Thrombocytopenia[54]
Agranulocytosis; pancytopenia[55,56]
Hemophagocytic syndrome[57]
Angioimmunoblastic lymphadenopathy[58]
X-linked lymphoproliferative syndrome[59,60]
Post-transplant lymphoproliferative disease[61]
Aplastic anemia[62]

Neurologic or Behavioral

Encephalitis[63]
Polyneuritis[64,65]
Ataxia, paralysis, cerebellitis[64,66]
Hallucinations; psychosis[41,67]
Depression; anxiety[68]
Seizures secondary to increased phenytoin clearance[69]
Migraine; chorea[70]
Lumbosacral radiculoplexopathy[71]
Aphonia[72] (palsy of the recurrent laryngeal nerve)
Cranial neuritis[73]
Retrobulbar neuritis[74]
Opsoclonus-myoclonus[75]

Other

Deafness[76]
Myocarditis[77,78]
Pancreatitis[79]
Renal failure; rhabdomyolysis[80,81]
Mycoplasmal pneumonia[82]
Cold-induced acrocyanosis or urticaria[83,84]
Genital ulceration[85,86]
Inappropriate secretion of antidiuretic hormone[87]
Migratory polyarthritis[88]
Pleural effusion[89]
Erythema multiforme[90]
Pneumonia[91]
Gianotti-Crosti syndrome[92]
Gall bladder hydrops[93]
Precipitation of hereditary angioedema[94]
Acute aqueductal stenosis[95]

EBV infection—the classic clinical IM pattern with atypical lymphocytes and an asymptomatic or atypical form without lymphocytosis. An earlier study from Israel also clearly described some young children who had atypical lymphocytes with nonspecific symptoms and negative heterophile tests.[97]

When the diseases and disorders listed as complications are encountered as diagnostic problems, the most useful test is for IgM antibody to EBV capsid antigen, which is usually included in any EBV antibody panel.

Treatment

Corticosteroid treatment is often used, especially for more severe complications, but should be individualized. For a teenager with partial respiratory obstruction, a burst of prednisone beginning with 60 mg and tapering over 10 days can be used.[98] For hemolytic anemia or an ongoing problem, a moderate daily dose (40 mg for a teenager) can be continued and then tapered when sufficient improvement occurs.

■ MONO-LIKE ILLNESS

There are three logical combinations of the clinical or hematologic features of heterophile-negative mono-like syndromes: the clinical features, the hematologic features, or both (see Table 3.1). Atypical lymphocytosis has been discussed earlier. If only the rapid slide serology test is negative, the pattern is usually called heterophile-negative mono-like illness (Box 3–3).

Heterophile-Negative Mono-like Illness

EBV Infection

This virus is the most frequent cause of heterophile-negative IM syndrome.[99–101] The heterophile antibody may not be produced because of the young age of the patient, or it may be missed because of the timing of the serum collection. Dual infections with EBV and other herpesviruses can occur.[102]

CMV Infection

This virus is another common cause of heterophile-negative IM, accounting for 30 (70%) of 43 patients in one study.[101] Fever, atypical lymphocytosis, splenomegaly, and occasionally hepatic involvement can be caused by this virus whether acquired by blood transfusion or by other routes, particularly

---

BOX 3-3 ■ Causes of Mono-like Syndrome with Negative Heterophile Antibody Tests

With atypical lymphocytosis
EBV
Cytomegalovirus
Acute toxoplasmosis
Hepatitis A
HHV-6
Acute HIV infection

Without atypical lymphocytosis
EBV
Cytomegalovirus
Acute toxoplasmosis
Coxsackie virus
Adenovirus
Herpes simplex virus
Rubella
Drugs (e.g., phenytoin, sulfa)
Malignancies

---

saliva. Pharyngitis is less common in CMV than it is in EBV mononucleosis. Cough is often present.[100] CMV infection is more likely to resemble classic EBV-induced IM in young children than it is in teenagers or adults. Lymphadenopathy tends to be less pronounced than in children with EBV.[103]

CMV infection should be considered in individuals who develop fever and atypical lymphocytosis 2–3 weeks after transfusion, although this syndrome is becoming less common.

Although EBV infection is the most common cause of heterophile-negative IM overall, in adults[104] CMV seems to predominate. In a review of immunologically normal adults (mean age, 28 years) with CMV-induced IM, splenomegaly and adenopathy occurred in about one-third, tonsillitis in 6%, and mild elevation of serum transaminases in 90%.[105] About 26% had atypical lymphocytes on the peripheral blood smear.

In a report of 124 children from birth to 12 years with symptoms clinically compatible with IM, EBV was more common than CMV at all ages. However, 14 (70%) of the 20 CMV cases were diagnosed in children from birth to age four years, whereas in EBV IM, cases were fairly evenly distributed among the age groups.[106] In a comparison of cytomegalovirus mononucleosis from Brazil, exudative tonsillitis was seen in children but not in adults. The mean age of the children was 5 years, and their illnesses were typically mono-like.[107]

Acute Toxoplasmosis

This protozoan can cause fever, atypical lymphocytosis, generalized lymphadenopathy, splenomegaly, and myalgia.[108] Leukopenia or a rash may also be present. Often, there is a history of exposure to cats, undercooked meat such as venison or lamb, or goat's milk.

Hepatitis A

As discussed in Chapter 13, hepatitis A can occasionally present as a mono-like illness with fever, hepatosplenomegaly, elevated liver enzymes, generalized lymphadenopathy, and atypical lymphocytes.

Human Herpes Virus Type 6

Because human herpes virus type 6 (HHV-6) is a member of the same virus family, and causes similar pathologic changes in monocytes, as EBV, it is not surprising that HHV-6 has been recently described as the cause of a mononucleosis-like syndrome in young adults. The clinical features of this illness were indistinguishable from those of EBV or CMV infection, and patients developed a mild atypical lymphocytosis.[109] Caution must be taken in interpreting serologic tests for this virus, however, given the fact that EBV is a known polyclonal B-cell activator, and has been shown specifically to increase antibody titers against HHV-6.[110] EBV infection is not likely to stimulate the production of HHV-6 antibody without concurrently causing an antibody response to EBV.

Human Immunodeficiency Virus

It has been shown that the majority of patients who contract human immunodeficiency virus (HIV) infection have an acute HIV syndrome several weeks after acquisition of infection. This syndrome clinically resembles IM.[111] A fair number of these patients also have an atypical lymphocytosis. It is important to remember acute HIV syndrome in the differential diagnosis of heterophile-negative mono-like illness, especially in patients known to be sexually active. HIV infection is discussed in more detail in Chapter 20.

Mono-like Illness Without Atypical Lymphocytosis

This syndrome consists of the clinical manifestations of IM, such as febrile pharyngitis with lymphadenopathy or splenomegaly, without atypical lymphocytosis. Cervical lymphadenopathy is discussed in Chapter 6.

Cytomegalovirus can produce a mono-like syndrome without atypical lymphocytes.[112] Acute toxoplasmosis typically produces generalized lymphadenopathy and fever, but splenomegaly and pharyngitis are occasionally observed.

Coxsackievirus

These viruses have been associated with a syndrome of febrile pharyngitis, generalized lymphadenopathy, conjunctivitis, and *painful* liver or spleen enlargement.[113] A few patients had atypical lymphocytosis or a rash.

Other Infectious Causes

Adenovirus, herpes simplex, HHV-6, HIV, and other agents such as those causing nonstreptococcal pharyngitis can cause a mono-like illness. Rubella virus infection without a rash can produce this pattern.

Drugs

Phenytoin, sulfas, and other drugs can produce a heterophile-negative IM-like syndrome.

Malignancies

Lymphoma or other hematologic malignancy also can cause fever with splenomegaly or hepatosplenomegaly.

Diagnostic Plan

Serology

IgM antibody can be determined for specific agents such as cytomegalovirus, toxoplasma, and rubella. If IgM-specific antibodies are not available, paired sera can be evaluated for antibodies to EBV, CMV, toxoplasmosis, or other viruses. A definitive serologic result will eliminate concern over a possible lymphatic malignancy. Lymphoma or leukemia is a consideration when the adenopathy and splenomegaly persist after the initial febrile period.

Unfortunately, enzyme-linked immunosorbent assay (ELISA)/Western Blot will not always detect acute HIV infection because of the time required for the antibody response to develop. PCR testing is much more sensitive in this setting, but can occa-

sionally produce false positive results,[114] which can be a source of undue stress for patients. A judicious approach to this problem might be to consider the diagnosis of HIV infection in patients with a mononucleosis-like syndrome, but only order PCR testing when EBV and CMV serology is negative or when the patient has risk factors for HIV infection.

■ CHRONIC OR RECURRENT EBV INFECTION

Chronic active EBV (CABEV) infection is a very rare disorder that has been defined by the presence of the following three features: severe illness of more than six months' duration that begins as a primary EBV infection or that is associated with abnormal EBV antibody titers; histologic evidence of organ disease, such as pneumonitis, hepatitis, bone marrow hypoplasia, or uveitis; and demonstration of EBV antigens or EBV DNA in tissue. There are often extreme elevations of virus-specific antibody titers.[115] In contrast, chronic fatigue syndrome, which is not caused by EBV, is a different disorder in which patients may have slightly elevated antibody titers to EBV and other viruses.

The majority of patients suspected of chronic or recurrent EBV infection lack the clinical and laboratory parameters described above, but develop their illness immediately after a documented clinical episode of IM. In these cases, it is advisable to use "post-mononucleosis fatigue" as a diagnostic category. A fair number of teenagers develop prolonged easy fatigability after IM. Many of them fit the socioeconomic and psychological profile of patients who develop chronic fatigue syndrome (CFS), but the illness never gets severe enough to meet diagnostic criteria for CFS. If antibody titers fall to levels typically associated with past EBV infection, the diagnosis of chronic active EBV infection is effectively ruled out. The pathogenesis of post-mononucleosis fatigue is not understood.

There does appear to be a true syndrome of chronic active EBV infection, however. The most common symptoms are those associated with acute EBV infection, viz., pharyngitis, adenopathy, fever, headaches, and fatigue. Some patients also complain of myalgias, arthralgias, and depression. It is not known why the virus, which normally transforms B cells and establishes latency, would produce a chronic infection with ongoing viral replication in some people. Some investigators have found differences in the production of immediate early gene products thought to be important in the induction of latency.[116] Others believe that, epidemiologically at least, there appears to be a familial component.[117] Time and experience with this rare clinical entity may eventually provide an answer to this question. In the meantime, the diagnosis of CAEBV infection should be made with caution, and only when the diagnostic criteria outlined above are met. Patients suspected of having this very rare syndrome should be managed in concert with an infectious diseases specialist.

■ CHRONIC FATIGUE SYNDROME

In contrast, chronic fatigue syndrome is a different and much more common phenomenon sometimes seen in adolescents and young adults. There is no known infectious cause. Patients usually date the onset of their fatigue to the time of an acute illness in the distant past. The illness may have been a mono-like illness, sometimes even confirmed as due to EBV infection. However, patients with CFS are no more likely than healthy controls to have serologic or virologic evidence of recent EBV infection.[118]

Patients with CFS are often high-achievers who have difficulty resuming normal activities after a period of convalescence from the acute illness. As a result of inactivity, they become deconditioned, so that even mild exertion causes extreme fatigue. Psychosocial and psychosomatic aspects may also play a role in the genesis and perpetuation of the syndrome. There may even be an element of classical conditioning in the on-going syndrome; specifically, expectation of illness makes recovery difficult. CFS is a diagnosis of exclusion, and other causes of fatigue, such as anemia and hypothyroidism, should be ruled out. The diagnostic criteria are listed in Table 3-3. Management is supportive. The physician must often walk a fine line: terse dismissal of the illness as non-disease is counterproductive, but excessive laboratory testing and sympathy for the illness may exacerbate or perpetuate the syndrome. A program of gradually increasing physical activity is important to recovery; a physical therapist may be able to assist the physician in planning a program. Evaluation by a psychologist or psychiatrist can assist the patient in dealing with the depression and family stress that nearly always either accompanies or precipitates CFS in adolescents. Many of these teenagers were overcommitted to extracurricular activities before the development

of their fatigue and may need to prioritize which activities to resume. Homebound schooling should be avoided, and regular school attendance should be strongly encouraged.

TABLE 3-3. CENTERS FOR DISEASE CONTROL AND PREVENTION'S REVISED CASE DEFINITION OF CHRONIC FATIGUE SYNDROME[119]

Clinically evaluated, unexplained, persistent or relapsing fatigue for 6 months or longer that is:

- of new or definite onset
- not the result of ongoing exertion
- not substantially alleviated by rest

resulting in substantial reduction in previous levels of occupational, educational, social, or personal activities AND

The presence of at least four of the following symptoms:

- Impaired concentration or short-term memory
- Sore throat
- Tender cervical or axillary lymph nodes
- Muscle pain
- Arthralgia without swelling or redness
- Headaches of new type, pattern, or severity
- Nonrestorative sleep
- Postexertional malaise lasting more than 24 hours

■ REFERENCES

1. Paul JR, Bunnell WW. The presence of heterophile antibodies in infectious mononucleosis. Am J Med Sci 1932; 183:90–104. (Reprinted in Rev Infect Dis 1982;4: 1062–8.)
2. Shurin SB. Infectious mononucleosis. Pediatr Clin North Am 1979;26:315–26.
3. Chin TDY. Diagnosis of infectious mononucleosis. South Med J 1976;69:654–8.
4. Rapp CE Jr, Hewetson JF. Infectious mononucleosis and the Epstein-Barr virus. Am J Dis Child 1978;132:78–86.
5. Hoagland RJ. The clinical manifestations of infectious mononucleosis: a report of two hundred cases. Am J Med Sci 1960;240:21–8.
6. Chretien JH, Esswein JG. How frequent is bacterial superinfection of the pharynx in infectious mononucleosis? Observations on incidence, recognition, and management with antibiotics. Clin Pediatr 1976;15:424–7.
7. Baehner RL, Shuler SE. Infectious mononucleosis: clinical expressions, serologic findings, complications, prognosis. Clin Pediatr 1967;6:393–9.

8. Shuster F, Ognibene AJ. Dissociation of serum bilirubin and alkaline phosphatase in infectious mononucleosis JAMA 1969;209:267–8.

9. Heath CW Jr, Brodsky AL, Potolosky AI. Infectious mononucleosis in a general population. Am J Epidemiol 1972; 95:46–52.

10. Kerns DL. Ampicillin rash in childhood. Am J Dis Child 1973;125:187–90.

11. McCloskey GL, Massa MC. Cephalexin rash in infectious mononucleosis. Cutis 1997;59:251–4.

12. Lascari AD, Bapat VR. Syndromes of infectious mononucleosis. Clin Pediatr 1970;9:300–5.

13. Arnez M, Cizman M, Jazbec J, et al. Acute infectious lymphocytosis caused by coxsackievirus B2. Pediatr Infect Dis J 1996;15:1127–8.

14. Arribas JM, Fernandez GH, Escalera GI, et al. Acute infectious lymphocytosis associated with *Giardia lamblia* and *Blastocystis hominis* coinfection. An Esp Pediatr 2001;54: 518–20.

15. Naqvi SH, Dunkle LM. Atypical lymphocytosis in respiratory syncytial virus pneumonia. Pediatr Infect Dis 1986; 5:494.

16. Saulsbury FT. B cell proliferation in acute infectious lymphocytosis. Pediatr Infect Dis J 1987;6:1127–9.

17. Horwitz CA, Henle W, Henle G, et al. Spurious rapid infectious mononucleosis test results in non-infectious mononucleosis sera. Am J Clin Pathol 1982;78:48–53.

18. Horwitz CA, Henle W, Henle G, et al. Persistent falsely positive rapid tests for infectious mononucleosis. Am J Clin Pathol 1979;72:807–11.

19. Votava M, Bartosova D, Krchnakova A, et al. Diagnostic importance of heterophile antibodies and immunoglobulin IgA, IgE, IgM and low-avidity IgG against Epstein-Barr virus capsid antigen in children. Acta Virol 1996;40: 99–101.

20. Hrnjakovic-Cvjetkovic I, Jerant-Patic V, Cvjetkovic D, et al. Serologic diagnosis of infectious mononucleosis (Serbo-Croatian). Medicinski Pregled 1996;49:291–5.

21. Mach E, Bielec D, Szeniawska A, et al. Dynamics of the Paul Bunnel-Davidson test during infectious mononucleosis (Polish). Medycyna Doswiadczalna I Mikrobiologia 1993;45:379–83.

22. Vahlquist B, Edelund H, Tvetaras E. Infectious mononucleosis and pseudomononucleosis in childhood. Acta Pediatr Scand 1958;47:120–31.

23. Fleisher G, Henle W, Henle G, et al. Primary infection with Epstein-Barr virus in infants in the United States: clinical and serological observations. J Infect Dis 1979; 139:553–8.

24. Fleisher G, Lennette ET, Henle G, et al. Incidence of heterophil antibody responses in children with infectious mononucleosis. J Pediatr 1979;94:723–8.

25. Sumaya CV, Ench Y. Epstein-Barr virus infectious mononucleosis in children. II: heterophil antibody and viral-specific responses. Pediatrics 1985;75:1011–9.

26. Gan YJ, Sullivan JL, Sixbey JW. Detection of cell-free Epstein-Barr virus DNA in serum during acute infectious mononucleosis. J Infect Dis 1994;170:436–9.

27. Prang NS, Hornef MW, Jager M. et al. Lytic replication of EBV in the peripheral blood: analysis of viral gene expression in B lymphocytes during IM and in the normal carrier state. Blood 1997;89:1655–77.

28. Landau Z, Gross R, Sanilevich A, et al. Presence of infective Epstein-Barr virus in the urine of patients with infectious mononucleosis. J Med Virol 1994;44:229–33.

29. Hoaglund RJ. The incubation period of infectious mononucleosis. Am J Pub Health 1964;54:1699–705.

30. Ginsburg CM, Henle G, Henle W. An outbreak of infectious mononucleosis among the personnel of an outpatient clinic. Am J Epidemiol 1976;104:571–5.

31. Armstrong CW, Hackler RL, Miller GB Jr. Two pseudo-outbreaks of infectious mononucleosis. Pediatr Infect Dis 1986;5:325–7.

32. Fleisher GR, Pasquariello PS, Warren WS, et al. Intrafamilial transmission of Epstein-Barr virus infections. J Pediatr 1981;98:16–9.

33. Niederman JC, Miller G, Pearson HA, et al. Infectious mononucleosis: Epstein-Barr-virus shedding in saliva and the oropharynx. N Engl J Med 1976;294:1355–9.

34. Chang RS, Lewis JP, Abildgaard CF. Prevalence of oropharyngeal excretors of leukocyte-transforming agents among a human population. N Engl J Med 1973;289:1325–9.

35. Bender CE. The value of corticosteroids in the treatment of infectious mononucleosis. JAMA 1967;199:529–31.

36. Andersson J, Britton S, Ernberg I, et al. Effect of acyclovir on infectious mononucleosis: a double-blind, placebo-controlled study. J Infect Dis 1986;153:283–90.

37. Tynell E, Aurelius E, Brandell A, et al. Acyclovir and prednisolone treatment of acute infectious momucleosis: a multicenter, double-blind, placebo-controlled study. J Infect Dis 1996;174:324–31.

38. Vendelbo Johansen L, Lildholdt T, Bende M, et al. Infectious mononucleosis treated by an antihistamine: a comparison of the efficacy of ranitidine (Zantac) vs placebo in the treatment of infectious mononucleosis. Clin Otolaryngol 1997;22:123–5.

39. Maki DG, Reich RM. Infectious mononucleosis in the athlete: diagnosis, complications, and management. Am J Sports Med 1982;10:162–3.

40. Domachowski JB, Cunningham CK, Cummings DL, et al. Acute manifestations and neurologic sequelae of Epstein-Barr virus encephalitis in children. Pediatr Infect Dis J 1996;15:871–5.

41. Sanguineti G, Crovato F, De Marchi R, et al. "Alice in Wonderland" syndrome in a patient with infectious mononucleosis. J Infect Dis 1983;147:782.

42. Blowey DL. Nephrotic syndrome associated with EBV infection. Pediatr Nephrol 1996;10:507–8.

43. Lopez-Navidad A, Domingo P, Lopez-Talavera JC, et al. Epstein-Barr virus infection associated with interstitial nephritis and chronic fatigue. Scand J Infect Dis 1996;28: 185–7.

44. Dagan R, Powell KW. Postanginal sepsis following infectious mononucleosis. Arch Intern Med 1987;147:1581–3.

45. Portman M, Ingall D, Westenfelder G, et al. Peritonsillar abscess complicating infectious mononucleosis. J Pediatr 1984;104:742–4.

46. Alpert G, Fleisher GR. Complications of infection with Epstein-Barr virus during childhood: a study of children admitted to the hospital. Pediatr Infect Dis J 1984;3: 304–7.

47. Harries JT, Ferguson AW. Fatal infectious mononucleosis with liver failure in two sisters. Arch Dis Child 1968;43: 480–5.

48. Waterhouse BE, Lapidus PH. Infectious mononucleosis associated with a mass in the anterior mediastinum. N Engl J Med 1967;277:1137–9.

49. Givner LB, McGehee D, Taber LH, et al. Sinusitis, orbital cellulitis, and polymicrobial bacteremia in a patient with primary Epstein-Barr virus infection. Pediatr Infect Dis J 1984;3:254–6.

50. Koay CB, Norval C. An unusual presentation of an unusual complication of infectious mononucleosis: haematemesis and melaena. J Laryngol Otol 1995;109;335–6.

51. DiGirolama S. Anselmi M, Piccini A, et al. Aspecific membranous laryngitis after infectious mononucleosis. Int J Pediatr Otorhinolaryngol 1996;34:171–4.

52. Fekete AM, Kerpelman EJ. Acute hemolytic anemia complicating infectious mononucleosis. JAMA 1965;194:1326–7.

53. Witzke O, Kassubek J, Bonmann E, et al. Cryoglobulinemia: a complication of infectious disease. Clin Invest 1994;72:1048–50.

54. Andiman WA. Primary Epstein-Barr virus infection and thrombocytopenia during late infancy. J Pediatr 1976;89:435–8.

55. Neel EU. Infectious mononucleosis: death due to agranulocytosis and pneumonia. JAMA 1976;236:1493–4.

56. Koppes GM, Ratkin GA, Coltman CA. Pancytopenia and "capillary leak syndrome" with infectious mononucleosis. South Med J 1976;69:145–8.

57. Wilson ER, Malluh A, Stagno S, et al. Fatal Epstein-Barr virus-associated hemophagocytic syndrome. J Pediatr 1981;98:260–2.

58. Seigneurin JM, Mingat J, Lenoir GM, et al. Angioimmunoblastic lymphadenopathy after infectious mononucleosis. Br Med J 1981;282:1574–5.

59. Hamilton JK, Sullivan JL, Maurer HS, et al. X-linked lymphoproliferative syndrome registry report. J. Pediatr 1980;96:669–73.

60. Lederman HM, Yolken R, D'Souza BJ, et al. Chronic disseminated Epstein-Barr virus infection and humoral immunodeficiency: detection of viral antigen by ELISA inhibition assay. Pediatr Infect Dis J 1983;2:388–90.

61. Cohen JI. Epstein-Barr virus infection. N Engl J Med 2000;343:481–92.

62. Lazarus KH, Baehner RL. Aplastic anemia complicating infectious mononucleosis: a case report and review of the literature. Pediatrics 1981;67:907–10.

63. Halsted CC, Chang RS. Infectious mononucleosis and encephalitis: recovery of EB virus from spinal fluid. Pediatrics 1979;64:257–8.

64. Silverstein A, Steinberg G, Nathanson M. Nervous system involvement in infectious mononucleosis. Arch Neurol 1972;26:353–8.

65. Salazar A, Martinez H, Sotelo J. Ophthalmoplegic polyneuropathy associated with infectious mononucleosis. Ann Neurol 1983;13:219–20.

66. deFraiture DM, Sie TH, Boezeman EH, et al. Cerebellitis as an uncommon complication of infectious mononucleosis. Neth J Med 1997;51:79–82.

67. Rubin RL. Adolescent infectious mononucleosis with psychosis. J Clin Psychiatry 1978;39:63–5.

68. Hendler N, Leahy W. Psychiatric and neurologic sequelae of infectious mononucleosis. Am J Psychiatry 1978;135:842–4.

69. Leppik IE, Ramani V, Sawchuk RJ, et al. Increased clearance of phenytoin during infectious mononucleosis. N Engl J Med 1979;300:481–3.

70. Leavell R, Ray CG, Ferry PC, et al. Unusual acute neurologic presentations with Epstein-Barr virus infection. Arch Neurol 1986;43:186–8.

71. Sharma KR, Sriram S, Fries T, et al. Lumbosacral radiculoplexopathy as a manifestation of EBV infection. Neurology 1993;43:2550–4.

72. Parano E, Pavone L, Musumeci S, et al. Acute palsy of the recurrent laryngeal nerve complicating EBV infection. Neuropediatrics 1996;27:164–6.

73. Connolly M, Junker AK, Chan KW, et al. Cranial neuropathy, polyneuropathy and thrombocytopenia with EBV infection. Dev Med Child Neurol 1994;36:1010–5.

74. Anderson MD, Kennedy CA, Lewis AW, et al. Retrobulbar neuritis complicating acute EBV infection. Clin Infect Dis. 1994;18:799–801.

75. Sheth RD, Horwitz SJ, Aronoff S, et al. Opsoclonus myoclonus syndrome secondary to EBV infection. J Child Neurol 1995;10:297–9.

76. Williams LL, Lowery HW, Glaser R. Sudden hearing loss following infectious mononucleosis: possible effect of altered immunoregulation. Pediatrics 1985;75:1020–7.

77. Frischman W, Kraus ME, Zabkar J, et al. Infectious mononucleosis and fatal myocarditis. Chest 1977;72:535–8.

78. Hudgins JM. Infectious mononucleosis complicated by myocarditis and pericarditis. JAMA 1976;235:2626–7.

79. Koutras A. Epstein-Barr virus infection with pancreatitis, hepatitis and proctitis. Pediatr Infect Dis J 1983;2:312–3.

80. Lowery TA, Rutsky EA, Hartley MW, et al. Renal failure in infectious mononucleosis. South Med J 1976;69:1212–5.

81. Kantor RJ, Norden CW, Wein TP. Infectious mononucleosis associated with rhabdomyolysis and renal failure. South Med J 1978;71:346–7.

82. Dearth JC, Rhodes KH. Infectious mononucleosis complicated by severe Mycoplasma pneumoniae infection. Am J Dis Child 1980;134:744–6.

83. Dickerman JD, Howard P, Dopp S, et al. Infectious mononucleosis initially seen as cold-induced acrocyanosis: association with auto-anti-M and anti-I antibodies. Am J Dis Child 1980;134:159–60.

84. Mesko JW, We LYF. Infectious mononucleosis and cold urticaria (letter). JAMA. 1982;248:828.

85. Brown ZA, Stenchever MA. Genital ulceration and infectious mononucleosis: report of a case. Am J Obstet Gynecol 1977;127:673–4.

86. Portnoy J, Ahronheim GA, Ghibu F, et al. Recovery of Epstein-Barr virus from genital ulcers. N Engl J Med 1984;311:966–8.

87. Mouallem M, Friedman E, Rubinstein E, et al. Inappropriate antidiuretic hormone secretion with infectious mononucleosis (letter). N Engl J Med 1984;311:262.

88. Venuta A, Laudizi L, Micheli A, et al. [Migrant polyarthritis and EBV infection] (Italian). Pediatria Medica e Chirurgica 1997;19:135–6.

89. Takakura Y, Kobayashi Y, Takahashi Y, et al. [Infectious mononucleosis with pleural effusion.] (Japanese). Rinsho Ketsueki—Japanese J Clin Hematol 1996;37:719–24.

90. Hughes J, Burrows NP. Infectious mononucleosis presenting as erythema multiforme. Clin Exp Dermatol 1993;18:373–4.

91. Sriskandan S, Labrecque LG, Schofield J. Diffuse pneumonia associated with infectious mononucleosis: detection of Epstein-Barr virus in lung tissue by in situ hybridization. Clin Infect Dis 1996;22:578–9.

92. Schopf RE. [Gianotti-Crosti syndrome in EBV infection.] (German). Hautarzt 1995;46:714–6.

93. Dinulos J, Mirchell DK, Gerton J. et al. Hydrops of the gallbladder associaed with EBV infection: a report of two cases and review of the literature. Pediatr Infect Dis J 1994; 13:924–9.

94. Weidenbach H, Beckh KH, Lerch MM, et al. Precipitation of hereditary angioedema by infectious mononucleosis [letter]. Lancet 1993;342:934.

95. Cotton MF, Reiley T, Robinson CC, et al. Acute aqueductal stenosis in a patient with Epstein-Barr virus infectious mononucleosis. Pediatr Infect Dis J 1994;13:224–7.

96. Fleisher GR, Paradise JE, Lennette ET. Leukocyte response in childhood infectious mononucleosis. Am J Dis Child 1981;135:699–702.

97. Tamir D, Benderly A, Levy J, et al. Infectious mononucleosis and Epstein-Barr virus in childhood. Pediatrics 1974; 53:330–5.

98. Brandfronbrener A, Epstein A, Wu S, et al. Corticosteroid therapy in Epstein-Barr virus infection. Arch Intern Med 1986;146:337–9.

99. Evans AS. Infectious mononucleosis and related syndromes. Am J Med Sci 1978;276:325–39.

100. Klemola E, von Essen R, Henle G, et al. Infectious-mono-nucleosis-like disease with negative heterophile agglutination test: clinical features in relation to Epstein-Barr virus and cytomegalovirus antibodies. J Infect Dis 1970;121: 608–14.

101. Horwitz CA, Henle W, Henle G, et al. Heterophile-negative infectious mononucleosis and mononucleosis-like illnesses: laboratory confirmation of 43 cases. Am J Med 1977;63:947–57.

102. Lemon SM, Hutt LM, Huang YT, et al. Simultaneous infection with multiple herpesviruses. Am J Med 1979;66: 270–6.

103. Begovac J, Soldo I, Presecki V. Cytomegalovirus mononucleosis in children compared with the infection in adults and with Epstein-Barr virus mononucleosis. J Infect 1988; 17:121–5.

104. Horwitz CA, Henle W, Henle G. Diagnostic aspects of the cytomegalovirus mononucleosis syndrome in previously healthy persons. Postgrad Med 1979;66:153–8.

105. Cohen JI, Corey GR. Cytomegalovirus infection in the normal host. Medicine 1985;64:100–14.

106. Lajo A, Borque C, DellCastillo F, et al. Mononucleosis caused by Epstein-Barr virus and cytomegalovirus in children: comparative study of 124 cases. Pediatr Infect Dis J 1994;13:56–60.

107. Pannuti CS, Vilas Boas LS, Angelo MJO, et al. Cytomegalovirus mononucleosis in children and adults: differences in clinical presentation. Scand J Infect Dis 1985;17:153–6.

108. Kean BH, Kimball AC, Christensen WN. An epidemic of acute toxoplasmosis. JAMA. 1969;208:1002–4.

109. Steeper TA, Horwitz CA, Ablashi DV, et al. The spectrum of clinical and laboratory findings resulting from human herpes virus-6 (HHV-6) in patients with mononucleosis-like illnesses not resulting from Epstein-Barr virus or cytomegalovirus. Am J Clin Pathol 1990;93:776–83.

110. Linde A, Fridell E, Dahl H, et al. Effect of primary Epstein-Barr virus infection on human herpes virus-6, cytomegalovirus, and measles virus immunoglobulin G titers. J Clin Microbiol 1990;28:211–5.

111. Rosenberg ES, Caliendo AM, Walker BD. Acute HIV infection among patients tested for mononucleosis [letter]. N Engl J Med 1999;340:969.

112. Causey JQ. Spontaneous cytomegalovirus mononucleosis-like syndrome and aseptic meningitis. South Med J 1976; 69:1384–7.

113. Siegel W, Spencer FJ, Smith DJ, et al. Two new variants of infection with Coxsackie virus Group B, type 5, in young children: a syndrome of lymphadenopathy, pharyngitis, and hepatomegaly or splenomegaly, or both, or one of pneumonia. N Engl J Med 1963;268:1210–6.

114. Rich JD, Merriman NA, Mylonakis E, et al. Misdiagnosis of HIV infection by HIV-1 plasma viral load testing: a case series. Ann Intern Med 1999;130:37–9.

115. Straus SE. The chronic mononucleosis syndrome. J Infect Dis 1988;157:405–12.

116. Schwarzmann F, Jager M, Hornef M, et al. Epstein-Barr viral gene expression in B lymphocytes. Leuk Lymphoma 1998;30:123–9.

117. Joncas JH, Ghibu F, Blagdon M, et al. A familial syndrome of susceptibility to chronic active Epstein-Barr virus infection. Can Med Assn J 1984;130:280–4.

118. Sumaya CV. Serologic and virologic epidemiology of Epstein-Barr virus: relevance to chronic fatigue syndrome. Rev Infect Dis 1991; 13: S19–25.

119. Fukuda K, Straus SE, Hickie I,et al. The chronic fatigue syndrome: a comprehensive approach to its definition and study. International Chronic Fatigue Syndrome Study Group. Ann Intern Med 1994;121:953–9.

CHAPTER 4

Mouth and Salivary Gland Syndromes

■ GINGIVITIS, STOMATITIS, AND DENTAL INFECTIONS

Definitions

Inflammatory disease of the oral cavity should be diagnosed first in terms of the anatomic area involved, and then in terms of the probable etiology. Anatomic diagnoses commonly used include stomatitis (inflammation of the buccal mucosa), gingivitis (inflammation of the gums), gingivostomatitis, and glossitis (inflammation of the tongue). Inflammation of the lips is best called labiitis (Table 4.1).

Clinical Patterns

Recurrent Aphthous Stomatitis

Called "canker sores" by laypersons, these lesions usually appear as a superficial red ring with a shallow mucosal ulceration covered by a gray membrane (Figure 4-1). They involve the wet, moveable mucosa—typically the buccal mucosa, occasionally the ventral surface of the tongue, and less commonly the lips or gums. These lesions do not involve the attached gingiva or hard palate. In the most severe form, the lesion extends into the submucosa and is called periadenitis aphthae. The cause of aphthous stomatitis remains uncertain, but investigations suggest several associations. First, aphthous ulcers are associated with poor cytotoxic T lymphocyte function and/or neutropenia.[1] Second, some patients with recurrent aphthous stomatitis have poor regulation of the inflammatory cytokine cascade.[2]

Recurrent aphthous stomatitis in association with fever may be a clue to a syndrome of unknown cause called PFAPA (periodic fever, adenitis, pharyngitis, and aphthous stomatitis) (see Chapter 10).[3] Children with human immunodeficiency virus (HIV) infection can also be afflicted with refractory aphthous ulcers.[4] Children with cyclic neutropenia

TABLE 4-1. MOUTH AND DENTAL INFLAMMATORY DIESEASE

SYNDROME	POSSIBLE CAUSES
Buccal stomatitis	Apthous stomatitis (unknown cause? *Strep. sangits*) Behçet syndrome; Trauma
Gingivitis	Herpes simplex Enteroviruses (hand-foot-mouth syndrome)
Gingivostomatitis	Herpes simplex Stevens-Johnson syndrome *Candida albicans* Oral erythema multiforme
Necrotizing ulcerative gingivitis (Vincent's angina)	Periodontitis (poor hygiene; fusobacteria and spirochetes as secondary invaders)
Labiitis	Herpes simplex (ulcers or general edema)
Glossitis	Group A streptoccocci, *Staph. aureus, H. influenzae*, herpes simplex (ulcerative)
Gum abscess	Local normal oral flora; rarely, occult bacteremia (embolic)
Pulpitis	Normal local flora
Periapical abscess	Normal local flora
Uvulitis	Group A streptococci, *H. influenzae, Strep. pneumoniae*

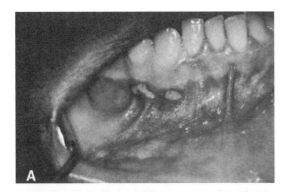

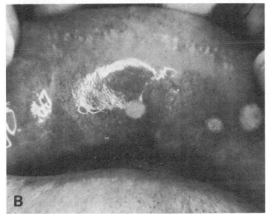

■ **FIGURE 4-1** Aphthous stomatitis. (**A**) Lesions of mucosa below the gingiva. (Photo from Dr. John Duffy) (**B**) Lesions of the upper lip. (Photo from Dr. Edward Graykowski)

or chronic granulomatous disease (CGD) may also present with recurrent aphthous ulcers.[5,6] Interestingly, most carriers of X-linked CGD have recurrent aphthous ulcers as well.[7] Rarely, recurrent aphthous stomatitis is a clue to the diagnosis of Behçet's disease, discussed below.

Whether infectious agents sometimes cause aphthous ulcers is not known. Most attempts at associating infectious agents with this disease have been fruitless. Physical and psychological stress precipitates attacks in susceptible people, probably by affecting the function of the immune system.[8]

Aphthous ulcers resolve without treatment. Pain relief may be afforded by treatment with over-the-counter products. Frequent or severe ulceration may respond to topical application of nonaqueous steroid sprays intended for intranasal use. The mucosa is simply wiped dry, and the ulcer is sprayed. This may be done twice a day and usually results in rapid resolution. Some patients with recurrent aphthous ulceration respond to a toothpaste that does not contain sodium lauryl sulfate.[9] Severe, re-

fractory, or widespread aphthous ulceration such as that seen in HIV disease is occasionally treated with thalidomide.[10] These patients should be in the care of an infectious diseases specialist.

Necrotizing Ulcerative Gingivitis

Formerly called "trench mouth" (because it was common in soldiers in the trenches in WWII) or "Vincent's angina," necrotizing ulcerative gingivitis (NUG) occurs at the gingival papillae between the teeth (Fig. 4-2, panel A).[11] The diagnostic triad of NUG is pain, interdental ulceration, and bleeding,

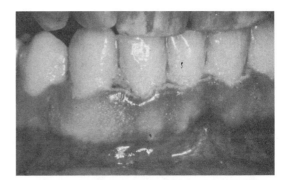

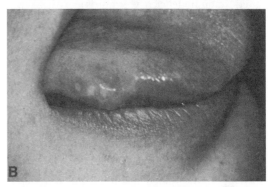

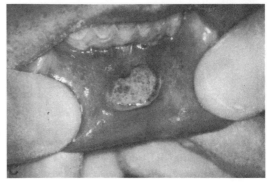

■ **FIGURE 4-2** (**A**) Necrotizing ulcerative gingivitis showing involvement of the papillae of the gums between the teeth. (**B**) Traumatic lesion of tongue. (**C**) Traumatic lesion of lower lip. (Photos from Dr. John Duffy)

and patients may also develop fetid breath and form a pseudomembrane.[12] NUG has been attributed to a synergistic infection with spirochetes, fusobacteria, or, in childhood especially, *Actinobacillus actinomycetemcomitans*.[13] All of these organisms are normal inhabitants of the mouth, so a causal association has been hard to prove. Molecular techniques have shown, however, that the spirochetes found in these lesions contain pathogen-specific determinants and that patients with NUG often have a serological response to these spirochetes, which would not be expected if they were not pathogenic.[14]

Most cases occur in adults, but the disease can be seen in adolescents or younger children. Although it occurs with higher frequency in people who live in crowded settings, it is not thought to be contagious.[15] Transmission by fomites or vectors has never been documented.[16] The lay diagnosis of "trench mouth" in a young child is likely to refer to herpes simplex gingivostomatitis.

In adults, risk factors for NUG include poor oral hygiene, unusual emotional stress, inadequate sleep, Caucasian race, age 18–21 years, and recent illness.[12] Severe juvenile NUG should raise the question of a defect in neutrophil locomotion. Acquired immunodeficiency syndrome (AIDS) patients also are at higher risk of NUG, and occasionally acute NUG is the presenting sign of HIV infection, at least in young adults.[17] In children with cancer, especially those with neutropenia, poor nutrition, and marginal oral hygiene, acute NUG can result in loss of teeth.[18]

Penicillin usually results in dramatic improvement.[19] Interestingly, the effectiveness of the antiparasitic drug metronidazole against anaerobes was discovered when it was used for trichomonal vaginitis and produced dramatic improvement in a patient with NUG.

Gum Abscess

This abscess may be seen before the eruption of teeth.[19] It is usually caused by normal mouth flora, but a case caused by the gonococcus has been reported.[20] It is also called a parulis or "gum boil."

Gingivitis or cystic, pink, nontender gingival masses about 1 cm in diameter have been described in patients with occult pneumococcal bacteremia (see Chapter 10).[21]

Glossitis

A swollen, painful tongue can be caused by acute bacterial infection of any type but in children is most likely to be due to Group A beta-hemolytic streptococcal, staphylococcal, or *Haemophilus influenzae* type b (Hib) infection.[22] The latter has become exceedingly rare since the institution of an effective H. flu type b vaccine. In patients with HIV infection or other severe immune suppression, herpes simplex virus can cause a syndrome known as herpetic geometric glossitis.[23] This clinical syndrome is marked by painful tongue fissures or furrows, and responds to intravenous acyclovir.

Glossitis has also been associated with systemic diseases, especially vitamin B12 deficiency and pernicious anemia.[24] Geometric tongue is a noninfectious condition seen in fair numbers of otherwise well children. The pattern on the tongue changes with time, and is not symptomatic. Coated tongue is a condition that can be seen in normal children during the course of acute infection with respiratory viruses. The cause of coated tongue is not well delineated. It goes away with resolution of the respiratory infection. The exception is "coated tongue" in patients with immune suppression[25]—this clinical scenario is likely to be a manifestation of thrush and should be treated (discussed later). Coated tongue is also a common finding in typhoid fever.

Pulpitis and Periapical Abscess

Infection of the pulp of a tooth is the most common cause of toothache.[19] Pain is severe, and is exacerbated by hot, cold, and percussion. Occasionally, facial cellulitis develops. The definitive treatment is incision and drainage, although antibiotics are usually also prescribed.[26]

Complications of Dental Infections

A periapical abscess of a mandibular tooth can drain to the outside of the lower gum as a sinus tract (parulis) or can spread medially to produce a neck space infection.[27] An abscess of a maxillary tooth can spread medially to form a submucosal abscess of the hard palate, or laterally to produce facial cellulitis.[27] Chronic proliferative periostitis (Garre's osteomyelitis) usually is a reaction to adjacent dental infection. It produces an "onion skin" appearance of the mandible on x-ray, and resembles Caffey's disease. Treatment of the dental problem is indicated, but systemic antibiotics are usually not required.[27]

Uvulitis

A red or swollen uvula may have several causes, discussed in the section on pharyngitis (Chapter 2).

Possible Etiologies

Herpes Simplex

This virus is the usual cause of acute gingivostomatitis in children. The primary infection typically occurs in the first 6 years of life. The illness is often associated with fever. There is often slight bleeding when the gums or buccal mucosa are touched. Glossitis may be present, with superficial circular ulceration of the tongue covered with a thin layer of white or gray exudate (see Fig. 2-7). Carefully moving the buccal mucosa out of the way with a tongue depressor will usually reveal ulcers on the gingivae. Lip involvement is not common in the first infection. The incubation period is about 7 days, with a range of 3–9 days.[28] The patient usually improves in 3–5 days and has recovered by 14 days. Outbreaks of acute gingivostomatitis caused by this virus have been observed in young children in nurseries or orphanages.[28]

Reactivation of latent herpes simplex virus (HSV) infection can also cause recurrent stomatitis, gingivostomatitis, or labiitis. Recurrences are usually extraoral, on or near the lips (see Fig. 11-9), unlike the primary infection, which is usually intraoral. The severity of recurrent illness is usually much less than that of the first episode. However, occasionally there is a recurrence of severe stomatitis with fever and mucosal bleeding. HSV is the most common trigger of erythema multiforme (EM) in children, in some cases leading to recurrent episodes of EM.[29,30] Recurrent labiitis or stomatitis caused by HSV can be precipitated by another illness, such as pneumococcal pneumonia, or meningococcal or *H. influenzae* meningitis. Occasionally, the labiitis or stomatitis precedes signs of the precipitating disease, so the child should be examined carefully for another disease if some clinical findings seem atypical or overly severe to be explained by herpetic stomatitis alone.

As mentioned above, HSV can also cause herpetic geometric glossitis in patients with immune deficiency states. It has been reported in one child after cardiac transplant, and in one child with acute myelogenous leukemia in addition to being seen in children with AIDS.[23]

HSV stomatitis may present a difficult diagnostic problem when a febrile child is seen early in the illness and the stomatitis has not yet appeared. When stomatitis occurs a day or two later, it is difficult to be certain that the gingivostomatitis does not represent a secondary reactivation of a latent infection by fever of some other cause. In one study, the fever sometimes preceded stomatitis by a day or two, and HSV was believed to be the cause of both the fever and of the later stomatitis.[31] However, in experimental infections in adults with other viruses, HSV was frequently recovered before the experimental illness, suggesting that HSV often is a coincidental isolate associated with another infectious process.[32]

Virus excretion in patients with recurrent herpes labialis is greater during episodes of the common cold or after oral trauma.[33] Patients with prodromal symptoms that lead them to expect a recurrence often have increased excretion of the virus in the absence of visible lesions.

Coxsackievirus

Stomatitis somewhat resembling aphthous stomatitis can be caused by Coxsackievirus A. However, the lesions of coxsackievirus infection are usually smaller and more erythematous and tend to be more predominantly located in the posterior oropharynx. The illness is called hand-foot-and-mouth syndrome when it is associated with a papular rash on the palms and soles, as described in Chapter 11. The disease sometimes presents with stomatitis alone.

Behçet's Syndrome

Aphthous stomatitis rarely is an indication that a child has Behçet syndrome.[34,35] This syndrome has been observed in children as young as 2 months of age and eventually may include arthritis, erythema nodosum, sterile cellulitis, perineal or genital ulcerations, and involvement of the eye, gastrointestinal tract, or neurologic system.[35] Corticosteroid therapy usually provides symptomatic relief.[36] Children with suspected or confirmed Behçet's syndrome should be managed in concert with a pediatric rheumatologist.

Candida albicans

Stomatitis produced by this yeast typically occurs in young infants and often involves the tongue as well as the buccal mucosa. When yeasts are found to be a cause of stomatitis after about 6 months of age, a defect of cell-mediated immunity should be suspected.[37] Chronic mucocutaneous candidiasis is discussed in Chapter 23.

Syphilis

The chancre of primary syphilis is a rare cause of an ulcer on the lip, buccal mucosa, or palate. Regional lymphadenopathy is usually present.[38]

Stevens-Johnson Syndrome

Severe gingivostomatitis is also rarely caused by Stevens-Johnson syndrome (discussed in Chapter 11). Typically, there is involvement of at least one other mucous membrane such as the conjunctiva or the urethra. This syndrome probably represents a hypersensitivity reaction. It is most commonly drug induced, but is occasionally secondary to an infectious process.[39]

Other Causes

Neutropenia from any cause should be excluded by a white blood count and differential study when ulcerative or necrotic lesions are seen on the gums.[11] Langerhans cell histiocytosis is a rare cause of necrotizing gingivitis.[40] Infectious mononucleosis is rarely associated with gingivitis or stomatitis.[11]

Trauma of the buccal mucosa or the gums can produce lesions resembling the ulcerations of stomatitis (Fig. 4-2). It is commonly secondary to chewing, operative procedures, or suctioning. Lichen planus can produce lesions in the buccal mucosa resembling those of aphthous stomatitis.

Vesicular stomatitis virus of cattle rarely produces infections in humans. Such infections occur in people who are exposed to cattle or who work with the virus in the laboratory.[41] The clinical manifestations include headache, fever, vomiting, and pharyngitis. Vesicular lesions occur on the gums, buccal mucosa, pharynx, and, rarely, lips or fingers.

In addition to glossitis, as mentioned above, stomatitis and mucosal ulcerations have long been recognized as signs of vitamin B12 deficiency. Oral changes may precede the development of anemia and macrocytosis.[42] Glossodynia is another prominent feature of the oral symptoms in patients with pernicious anemia.[24]

Diagnostic Plan

Gram stain and culture for *Candida albicans* may be indicated. Culture and PCR for HSV are usually positive in typical cases of acute gingivostomatitis.

The clinical features of this illness are familiar enough that most clinicians can make the diagnosis by history and physical examination alone. Chemotherapy-induced neutropenia is often associated with mucositis. If the mucositis is more severe or more prolonged than expected, concomitant HSV infection should be ruled out by PCR or culture.

Laboratory studies to rule out vitamin B12 deficiency and pernicious anemia may be indicated. Recurrent aphthous ulceration, especially in the presence of fever, should prompt evaluation of cyclic neutropenia and consideration of the diagnosis of PFAPA, as well as disorders of neutrophil function such as CGD. Patients with HIV infection who develop severe or recurrent aphthous stomatitis should be referred to a specialist in pediatric infectious diseases.

Treatment

Supportive Measures

In severe stomatitis, the affected child will often not eat solids well. Cold foods such as ice cream may be soothing. Bland oral fluids should be encouraged in order to prevent dehydration and provide nourishment. Drinking citrus juices may cause pain. It may be necessary to administer intravenous fluids to small children with high fever who refuse oral fluids.

Gentian violet stains linens and neither provides pain relief nor influences the course of the illness. Local anesthetic ointments such as viscous lidocaine or maximum-strength benzocaine applied to the mouth may provide some pain relief, but are usually not used because of reports of children injuring themselves by biting on anesthetized mucosa or lips. Rinsing with dilute bland mouthwashes or with weak bicarbonate solutions may be soothing. Antibiotics are not necessary. Periodontal disease should be treated by a dentist.

Specific Therapy

A controlled trial of topical acyclovir ointment demonstrated no clinical benefit over placebo in the treatment of recurrent HSV labialis.[43] More recently, a large trial of penciclovir cream showed a minimal benefit (median time to healing of lesions 4.8 days versus 5.5 days with placebo).[44] Oral antiviral agents provide similarly disappointing results when administered at the onset of symptoms in patients with recurrent HSV stomatitis.[45] In contrast, they are effective for treatment of primary infection. A double-blind, placebo-controlled trial showed benefit of acyclovir therapy for primary herpetic gingivostomatitis in a subset of children hospitalized for the disease.[46] Children had mild to moderate disease based on the number of lesions, and all presented to the hospital or doctor's office within 72 hours of the onset of the illness. In this group, 15 mg/kg of acyclovir, given 5 times a day for 7 days reduced the duration of oral lesions from 4–10 days, cut short the eating and drinking difficulty to 3 days rather than 6, and caused viral shedding to stop in 1 day versus 5 days in the placebo group.[46] Toddlers and young children admitted to the hospital for hydration therapy because of severe herpetic gingivostomatitis are often given intravenous acyclovir.

Penicillin is usually effective for necrotizing ulcerative gingivitis.

Oral candidiasis can be treated with nystatin, 200,000 units per dose. For refractory cases, a persistent source such as a pacifier, thumb sucking, or the nipple of the mother or bottle should be excluded. For areas with a thick coating of thrush, such as the tongue, the nystatin must often be brushed on with a cotton swab to be effective. Administering nystatin every 3 hours rather than every 6 hours may cure refractory cases.[47] Clotrimazole (troches for older children, topical or vaginal for application to the nipple and buccal mucosa) and emulsified miconazole suppositories or vaginal cream have also been advocated.[47] Cases that fail all of the above measures, or cases of thrush in immunocompromised hosts, are probably best treated with oral fluconazole.[48]

Prevention

Herpes simplex vaccines have been periodically reported to be effective. However, a double-blind study showed no difference between the effectiveness of a placebo and the vaccine, with both having about a 70% efficacy in preventing recurrent labial lesions.[49] This high rate of spontaneous improvement probably accounts for the reported success of past vaccines.

Long-term oral acyclovir greatly limits the number of recurrences of HSV infection in immunodeficient patients.[50] Oral or intravenous acyclovir is used to prevent reactivation of latent HSV during periods of maximum immunosuppression for patients with neutropenia following bone marrow transplant or chemotherapy.[51] Prophylactic acyclovir may also be considered for immunocompetent people with frequent recurrences of HSV stomatitis. In adults, 400 mg of oral acyclovir twice daily decreased the number of clinical episodes of HSV stomatitis by 53% compared with placebo.[52]

The prophylactic use of oral glutamine in children receiving cancer chemotherapy has been shown to decrease the severity and duration of mucositis.[53]

■ PAROTITIS AND SIALITIS

Painful enlargement of a salivary gland (sialitis) most commonly involves the parotid. Parotitis can be diagnosed when there is enlargement of the parotid gland accompanied by fever. A layperson may mistakenly believe that a child has "mumps," when in reality it is the anterior cervical (tonsillar) lymph nodes that are enlarged. The clinician should be able to distinguish cervical adenitis from parotitis by looking carefully at the anatomic location of the swelling. When the parotid gland is enlarged, the swelling is equally distributed above and below the angle of the jaw (except that edema sometimes lowers the center of the swelling somewhat). In contrast, when cervical nodes are enlarged, the center of the swelling is located below the jaw. Minimal parotid swelling can best be detected by inspection of the parotid area rather than by palpation.

Several other findings are helpful in recognizing parotitis. Parotid enlargement may occur rapidly if major ducts are obstructed. Parotitis is usually somewhat painful because of stretching of the capsule and is usually made worse by foods that stimulate production of saliva. A bacterial infection, such as a cervical abscess, is usually tender to palpation, whereas parotitis is usually not tender unless it is suppurative (which is rare outside of the neonatal period). In parotitis, the openings of Stensen's ducts, which are easily seen in the buccal mucosa, are often red and swollen and may exude pus if the condition is suppurative (Fig. 4-3).

Submandibular salivary gland enlargement should also be looked for in patients with exposure to mumps or with concurrent parotitis. Enlargement of this salivary gland is often mistaken for lymph node enlargement. Apparent enlargement of a single salivary gland sometimes turns out to be either a soft-tissue abscess not related to the gland or a lymph node.

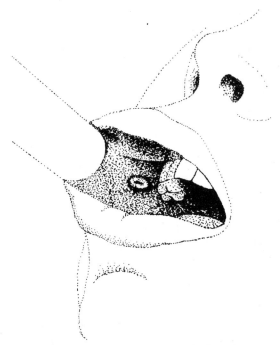

■ **FIGURE 4-3** Edematous Stensen's duct orifice, often present in parotitis of any cause.

Mumps versus Parotitis

The word "mumps" originally referred to the swelling seen in epidemic parotitis. Mumps virus is a common cause of parotitis, but parotitis may also be caused by other infectious and inflammatory conditions. In addition, parotitis occurs in only 30–40% of mumps virus infections. Therefore, the word "mumps" should not be used as a synonym for parotitis. The best problem-oriented diagnostic phrasing is "parotitis, probably caused by mumps virus." Outbreaks of parotitis, or cases of parotitis that can be related to exposure to another person with parotitis, are almost always caused by mumps virus (Box 4–1).

Infectious Causes

Mumps Virus Infection

In the past, this was by far the most common cause of parotitis. With routine use of measles-mumps-rubella (MMR) vaccine, mumps is now uncommon, with fewer than 400 U.S. cases reported annually. Classical mumps virus infection is painful parotitis, with enlargement of the parotid glands, and fever. Parotid swelling is unilateral at the onset and subsequently becomes bilateral in three-quarters of cases.

Edema of the openings of Stensen's ducts in the mouth can often be seen. The other salivary glands may also be enlarged. Edema of the neck or presternal area can occur in severe cases. Headache and vomiting may be severe. The incubation period is longer than that of the other common childhood diseases, averaging 21 days, so the exposure may have been forgotten.

Other Viruses

Parainfluenza virus is one of the most common causes of acute parotitis.[54] Other viruses that can cause parotitis include influenza virus, lymphocytic choriomeningitis virus, Coxsackie A and B viruses, echoviruses, and Epstein-Barr virus.[55,56]

Cat Scratch Disease

This bacterial disease can rarely cause inflammation of the lymph nodes within the parotid gland, producing a clinical syndrome closely resembling parotitis.[57]

Bacterial (Suppurative) Parotitis

The usual cause of bacterial parotitis is *Staphylococcus aureus*.[55] Occasionally *H. influenzae* causes suppurative parotitis.[58] Postoperative suppurative parotitis is rare in children.[59] In such cases, purulent material can often be expressed from the ducts. Suppurative parotitis can occur in the newborn period, especially in premature infants.[55,60] In these cases, gramnegative rods such as *Klebsiella* or *Pseudomonas* may be recovered.

Both immune compromised and immune competent hosts with *Salmonella* parotitis have been reported.[60] *Streptococcus pneumoniae* seems to be a more common cause among children with HIV infection.[61] This bacterium probably gets to the parotid gland via the bloodstream.

Other

Mycobacterium tuberculosis is a rare cause of parotid enlargement due to granulomatous parotitis.[62] Nontuberculous mycobacteria including *Mycobacterium avium* complex are also seen.[63] Mycobacteria may infect the gland itself, or the lymphoid tissue that resides within the parotid gland. Actinomycosis is a rare cause of parotitis;[64] it is usually associated with a more typical facial or cervical lesion.

BOX 4-1 ■ Causes of Parotitis

Acute

Nonsuppurative
Mumps virus
Parainfluenza viruses
Influenza viruses
Coxsackie viruses
Echovirus
Epstein-Barr virus
Cytomegalovirus
Lymphocytic choriomeningitis virus
Drugs
   iodides
   nitrofurantoin
   cimetidine

Suppurative
Staphylococcus aureus
Streptococcus pyogenes
Streptococcus pneumoniae[a]
Haemophilus species
Pseudomonas aeruginosa[b]
Escherichia coli[b]
Klebsiella species[b]
Proteus species[b]
Salmonella species[b]
Anaerobic bacteria
Peptostreptococci
Prevotella species
Fusobacteria
Actinomyces species

Recurrent
Juvenile recurrent parotitis
Sialithiasis
Sialectasis
Self-induced pneumoparotitis

Subacute or Chronic
Bartonella henselae (cat scratch)
Mycobacterium tuberculosis[c]
Mycobacterium avium intercellulare[c]
Mixed connective tissue disease
Masseter muscle hypertrophy

Sarcoidosis
Milkulicz's disease
Sjögren's syndrome
Mucoepidermoid carcinoma

[a]Higher incidence in children with HIV/AIDS.
[b]Especially seen in neonates.
[c]Causes granulomatous parotitis.

Noninfectious Causes

Reactive Follicular Hyperplasia

The parotid gland is the only salivary gland that contains lymphoid tissue within it. Reactive follicular hyperplasia may, therefore, cause a clinical syndrome indistinguishable from recurrent parotitis. This has been reported in otherwise well children,[65] but is very common in children infected with HIV. Children with HIV infection may also be more susceptible to suppurative and viral parotitis.

Salivary Gland Stones

Sialolithiasis is rare in children. The average age at presentation is about 10 years.[55] Stones may result in fever, suppurative parotitis, and trismus. Sometimes, they can be palpated, and they may be radiopaque, especially those in the submandibular duct.

Persistent or Recurrent Parotid Enlargement

The widespread lay belief that a second mumps virus infection is a common cause of recurrent parotitis is incorrect and is based on the lack of understanding that parotitis can have many causes. Parotitis has been observed in a few patients who had mumps virus antibody before the parotitis and subsequently developed a fourfold rise in titer to mumps virus.[66] However, viral cultures were not done, and it is difficult to exclude cross-reacting antibody to a parainfluenza virus. Parotitis with isolation of mumps virus in spite of past live mumps-virus vaccine has been documented.[67] A second episode of parotitis might result from a virus other than mumps, but several other possibilities should always be considered.

The syndrome of juvenile recurrent parotitis is

an under-appreciated cause of parotitis in children. In some series, it is the second most common salivary gland disease of childhood (after mumps), and it is probably the most common cause of recurrent parotitis in children.[68] This condition is characterized by periodic acute or subacute parotid swelling, usually accompanied by pain as well as fever and malaise. Between attacks the child is free of subjective symptoms. Typical onset is between 3 and 6 years of age.[69] Exacerbations occur every 3–4 months, but usually subside after puberty. Both sporadic and autosomal-dominant forms have been described.[70] Sialograms show multiple small sialectases. Ultrasound reveals hypoechoic heterogeneous areas and is more sensitive than sialograms in detecting changes over time.[71] Histologic findings include dilated interlobular ducts with surrounding infiltration.[68] Although various bacteria have been cultured from the saliva of such children, episodes resolve with or without antibiotics in 2–5 days.

Salivary stasis may occur in children, sometimes due to parotid duct narrowing (sialectasis), which presumably is secondary to past inflammation.[55,72] Drug hypersensitivity, such as from iodides or nitrofurantoin,[73] and rheumatoid mandibular joint swelling also can cause recurrent sialectasis.

A rare cause of persistent or recurrent parotid enlargement is Sjögren's syndrome, which occurs uncommonly in children.[74] Mikulicz's disease usually occurs in adults but has been observed in children and is usually associated with inadequate tears as well as lacrimal and salivary gland enlargement, often with a collagen disease such as systemic lupus erythematosus.[75] In adolescent girls, mixed connective-tissue disease is a rare cause of persistent parotid enlargement with intermittent fever and arthritis.[76] There is a single case report of Wegener's granulomatosis presenting as swelling of the major salivary glands.[77]

Pneumoparotitis is an unusual cause of (usually) bilateral parotid gland swelling.[78] It is caused by forcing air retrograde through Stensen's duct and actually inflating the parotid gland. It has been reported secondary to dental procedures and anesthesia ("anesthetic mumps"). Those who play wind instruments are also at higher risk. Several cases of children who autoinflated their parotid glands, either by blowing with great force against the palm of the hand or by performing a Valsalva maneuver against a closed mouth, have been reported.[78] In this situation, recurrent parotid swelling occurs. Patients are afebrile, and the parotid is not erythematous. Crepitus over the gland, and the production of air or frothy but clear saliva from Stensen's duct upon external pressure over the parotid are pathognomonic. Patients who repeatedly autoinflate the parotid glands should be referred for psychologic counseling.

Infantile cortical hyperostosis, which occurs in the first year of life, is occasionally mistaken for persistent mumps.[79] Sarcoidosis also is a rare cause of persistent parotid enlargement in children.[80] Neoplasms of the parotid gland are likewise rare. Unilateral hypertrophy of the masseter muscle is occasionally mistaken for parotid enlargement.

Mucoepidermoid carcinoma, the most common malignant salivary neoplasm in adults, is rarely found in teenagers.[81]

Complications of Mumps Virus Infection

The frequency of various complications of mumps has not been adequately studied in a prospective fashion. Some reported serious complications might in reality have been coincidental, because mumps was a frequent disease before the vaccine was available. The proven complications include the following:

1. *Orchitis* appears to occur in about 10–20% of adult men with mumps, although the frequency has been studied prospectively in very few outbreaks.[82,83] *Oophoritis* may occur as frequently as orchitis, but atrophy apparently does not occur, presumably because the ovary is not surrounded by an inelastic tunica albuginea, as is the testis.
2. *Deafness* appears to be exceedingly rare,[84,85] but there are no adequate data on its frequency.
3. *Aseptic meningitis syndrome* is common, but significant permanent neurologic sequelae are rare. The patient may have severe headache and transient delirium, but brain involvement (encephalitis) is rare (see Chapter 9).[86]
4. *Encephalitis*, defined as a severe and persistent disturbance of consciousness with cerebrospinal fluid lymphocytosis, is rare.[86] Death caused by mumps virus infection has rarely been documented by virus isolation with exclusion of other causes.
5. *Pancreatitis* is probably less frequent than is commonly believed. The serum amylase concentration may be elevated because of parotitis rather than pancreatitis.

Very rare complications, and reported complications that may have been coincidental, include the following:

1. *Endocardial fibroelastosis* (EF), long suspected of being associated with antecedent mumps virus infection because of studies showing positive mumps skin tests in infants with this disease, has now been shown by PCR to be definitely associated with mumps infection.[87] EF is a "vanishing" disease that used to be much more common. Of 29 infants who died of EF, more than 70% had evidence of mumps virus genome in myocardial samples by PCR testing. None of 65 control myocardial samples tested positive.[87]

2. *Hydrocephalus* secondary to aqueductal stenosis has been reported in experimental infections in rodents but has not been shown to occur in humans.

3. Other rare complications attributed to mumps virus include arthritis, thyroiditis, myocarditis, facial paralysis, transient psychosis, thrombocytopenic purpura, and transverse myelitis.[88–91] Diabetes mellitus in children has been suggested as a possible late sequela of mumps virus infection, but this is not proved.

Laboratory Studies

Virus Cultures

Mumps, parainfluenza, cytomegalovirus, and influenza viruses are relatively easily isolated in laboratories equipped for virus isolation.

Serum Antibodies

Enzyme immunoassay is available commercially and is the most sensitive test. Assays for both immunoglobulin M (IgM) and immunoglobulin G (IgG) are available. IgM antibodies peak about a week after the onset of illness. The diagnosis can also be made by documenting a fourfold or greater rise of IgG titers in specimens obtained 2 to 4 weeks apart.

Mumps Skin Test

This skin test antigen, once commercially and readily available, is unreliable and is no longer used.

Serum Amylase

In patients with parotitis, the serum amylase concentration is elevated. This may be a useful laboratory guide to help distinguish parotitis from cervical adenitis or other masses in the neck. However, amylase elevation is not specific for mumps parotitis. Fractionated amylase measurements are usually available, which separates parotid amylase from that of pancreatic origin.

Imaging Studies

In juvenile recurrent parotitis, ultrasound is the imaging study of first choice.[92] Sialograms may also be helpful, and, in some cases, at least transiently therapeutic. In chronic parotitis, computed tomography scanning may help to define the process.

Histopathology

In chronic or frequently recurrent parotitis of unknown etiology, biopsy may be indicated. Sometimes biopsy will aid in the diagnosis of chronic parotid infections with atypical mycobacteria or actinomyces species.[93]

Treatment

Parotitis

There is no specific treatment for viral parotitis, and symptomatic treatment is rarely needed. Bed rest to prevent complications is often advocated by laypersons who fear that orchitis may occur even in the prepubertal male. Bed rest is of no proven value, but complications that occur in patients allowed activity are usually blamed on the activity and on the person who allowed it.

Acute suppurative parotitis occurring in neonates or in postoperative children should be treated with broad-spectrum antibiotics that cover staphylococci and streptococci as well as gram-negative organisms and anaerobes. *Klebsiella*, *Salmonella*, and *Pseudomonas* are among the gram-negative pathogens isolated from babies with this condition. Strictly anaerobic cases, as well as mixed infections have been documented.[94] Antibiotic therapy can be tailored after the results of Gram stain and particularly culture are available. Material expressed from Stensen's duct is the best source of the infecting organism.

Recurrent suppurative parotitis should be treated with antistaphylococcal antibiotics. Frequent recurrences should prompt evaluation for possible stones or duct narrowing. There may be a familial disposition.

Although juvenile recurrent parotitis usually spontaneously resolves by puberty, the disease can cause frequent and troublesome symptoms. For this reason, some authors have advocated superficial parotidectomy.[95] Complete remission was achieved in eight of ten patients treated with surgery, partial remission in the other two, and no patient experienced facial nerve impairment. This option should be reserved only for patients with extreme forms of this condition.

Orchitis

In one controlled study of orchitis, steroids were of no value in relief of pain, swelling, or tenderness and apparently did not influence the extent of testicular atrophy seen 6 months after infection.[82] Aspirin or codeine and support of the scrotum usually provide some relief. Other causes of orchitis are discussed in Chapter 15.

Prevention

Live-attenuated mumps virus vaccine is safe and effective. Two doses of mumps vaccine (given as MMR), separated by at least 4 weeks, are routinely recommended for all children. The first dose of MMR should be given at 12 months of age. Persons exposed to mumps who have not previously been vaccinated can be given mumps vaccine in an attempt to produce vaccine-virus illness in advance of the wild-virus illness. However, the efficacy of this measure in preventing infection and complications from the current exposure has not been proved. The vaccine will provide protection against any subsequent exposures. Many adults are immune because of previous subclinical infection.

■ **REFERENCES**

1. Sun A, Chiang CP, Chiou PS, et al. Immunomodulation by levamisole in patients with recurrent aphthous ulceration or oral lichen planus. J Oral Pathol Med 1994;23:172–7.
2. Yamamoto T, Yoneda K, Ueda E, et al. Serum cytokines, interleukin-2 receptor, and soluble intercellular adhesion molecule-1 in oral disorders. Oral Surg Oral Med Oral Pathol 1994;78:727–35.
3. Thomas KT, Feder HM Jr, Lawton AR, et al. Periodic fever syndrome in children. J Pediatr 1999;135:15–21.
4. Greenspan D, Greenspan JS. HIV-related oral disease. Lancet 1996;348:729–33.
5. Rodenas JM, Ortego N, Herranz MT, et al. Cyclic neutropenia: a cause of recurrent apthous stomatitis not to be missed. Dermatology 1992;184:205–7.
6. Charon JA, Mergenhagen SE, Gallin JI. Gingivitis and oral ulceration in patients with neutrophil dysfunction. J Oral Pathol 1985;14:150–5.
7. Kragballe K, Borregaard N, Brandrup F, et al. Relation of monocyte and neutrophil oxidative metabolism to skin and oral lesions in carriers of chronic granulomatous disease. Clin Exp Immnol 1981;43:390–8.
8. McCartan BE, Lamey PJ, Wallace AM. Salivary cortisol and anxiety in recurrent aphthous stomatitis. J Oral Pathol Med 1996;25:357–9.
9. Herlofson BB, Barkvoll P. The effect of two toothpaste detergents on the frequency of recurrent aphthous ulcers. Acta Odontol Scand 1996;54:150–3.
10. Jacobson JM, Greenspan JS, Spritzler J, et al. Thalidomide for the treatment of oral aphthous ulcers in patients with human immunodeficiency virus infection. National Institute of Allergy and Infectious Diseases AIDS Clinical Trials Group. N Engl J Med 1997;336:1487–93.
11. Baer PN, Benjamin SD. Periodontal Disease in Children and Adolescents, Chapters 3 and 11. Philadelphia: J.B.Lippincott, 1974.
12. Horning GM, Cohen ME. Necrotizing ulcerative gingivitis, periodontitis, and stomatitis: clinical staging and predisposing factors. J Periodontol 1995;66:990–8.
13. Dougherty MA, Slots J. Periodontal disease in young individuals. J Calif Dent Assoc 1993;21:55–69.
14. Riviere GR, Wagoner MA, Baker-Zander SA, et al. Identification of spirochetes related to Treponema pallidum in necrotizing ulcerative gingivitis and chronic periodontitis. N Engl J Med 1991;325:539–43.
15. Stammers AF. Vincent's infection: observations and conclusions regarding the etiology and treatment of 1017 civilian cases. Br Dent J 1944;76:147–55.
16. Melnick SL, Roseman JM, Engel D, et al. Epidemiology of acute necrotizing ulcerative gingivitis. Epidemiol Rev 1988; 10:191–211.
17. Rowland RW, Escobar MR, Friedman RB, et al. Painful gingivitis may be an early sign of infection with the human immunodeficiency virus. Clin Infect Dis 1993;16:233–6.
18. Ryan ME, Hopkins K, Wilbur RB. Acute necrotizing ulcerative gingivitis in children with cancer. Am J Dis Child 1983; 137:592–4.
19. Summers GW. The diagnosis and management of dental infections. Pediatr Clin North Am 1976;9:717–28.
20. Urban M, Hervadda AR. Gonococcal gum abscess in a 10-week-old infant. Clin Pediatr 1977;16:193–4.
21. Burech DL, Koranyi K, Haynes RE, et al. Pneumococcal bacteremia associated with gingival lesions in infants. Am J Dis Child 1975;129:1283–4.
22. San Joaquin VH, Granum M, Surpure JS, et al. Acute glossitis and septicemia owing to Haemophilus influenzae type b. Am J Dis Child 1980;134:91.
23. Theriault A, Cohen PR. Herpetic geometric glossitis in a pediatric patient with acute myelogenous leukemia. Am J Clin Oncol 1997;20:567–8.
24. Schmitt RJ, Sheridan PJ, Rogers RS 3d. Pernicious anemia with associated glossodynia. J Am Dent Assoc 1988;117:838–40.
25. Nicolatou O, Theodoridou M, Mostrou G, et al. Oral lesions in children with perinatally acquired human immunodeficiency virus infection. J Oral Pathol Med 1999;28:49–53.

26. Chow AM, Roser SM, Brady FA. Orofacial odontogenic infections. Ann Intern Med 1978;88:392–402.

27. Wright JM, Taylor PP, Allen EP, et al. A review of the oral manifestations of infections in pediatric patients. Pediatr Infect Dis 1984;3:80–8.

28. Hale BD, Rendtorff FC, Walker LC, et al. Epidemic herpetic stomatitis in an orphanage nursery. JAMA 1963;183:1068–72.

29. Weston WL, Brice SL, Jester JD, et al. Herpes simplex virus in childhood erythema multiforme. Pediatrics 1992;89:32–4.

30. Weston WL, Morelli JG. Herpes simplex virus-associated erythema multiforme in prepubertal children. Arch Pediatr Adolesc Med 1997;151:1014–6.

31. Moffet HL, Sigel AC, Doyle HK. Non-streptococcal pharyngitis. J Pediatr 1968;73:51–61.

32. Lindgren KM, Douglas RG Jr, Cough RB. Significance of Herpesvirus hominis in respiratory secretions of man. N Engl J Med 1968;278:517–23.

33. Spruance SL. Pathogenesis of herpes simplex labialis: Excretion of virus in the oral cavity. J Clin Microbiol 1984;19:675–9.

34. Mundy TM, Miller JJ III. Behcet's disease presenting as chronic aphthous stomatitis in a child. Pediatrics 1978;62:205–8.

35. Ammann AJ, Johnson A, Fyfe GA, et al. Behcet's syndrome. J Pediatr 1985;107:41–3.

36. James DG. Behcet's syndrome [editorial]. N Engl J Med 1979;301:431–2.

37. Driezen S. Oral candidiasis. Am J Med 1984;77:28–33.

38. Goldberg MP. The oral mucosa in childhood. Pediatr Clin North Am 1978;25:239–62.

39. Roujeau JC, Stern RS. Severe adverse cutaneous reactions to drugs. N Engl J Med 1994;331:1272–85.

40. Quraishi MS, Blayeny AW, Walker D, et al. Langerhans cell histiocytosis: head and neck manifestations in children. Head Neck 1995;17:226–31.

41. Fields BN, Hawkins K. Human infection with the virus of vesicular stomatitis during an epizootic. N Engl J Med 1967;277:989–94.

42. Field EA, Speechley JA, Rugman FR, et al. Oral signs and symptoms in patients with undiagnosed vitamin B12 deficiency. J Oral Pathol Med 1995;24:468–70.

43. Spruance SL, Schnipper LE, Overall JC Jr, et al. Treatment of herpes simplex labialis with topical acyclovir in polyethylene glycol. J Infect Dis 1982;146:85–90.

44. Spruance SL, Rea TL, Thoming C, et al. Penciclovir cream for the treatment of herpes simplex labialis. A randomized, multicenter, double-blind, placebo-controlled trial. Topical Penciclovir Collaborative Study Group. JAMA 1997;277:1374–9.

45. Leigh IM. Management of non-genital herpes simplex virus infections in immunocompetent patients. Am J Med 1988;85(2A):34–8.

46. Amir J, Harel L, Smetana Z, et al. Treatment of herpes simplex gingivostomatitis with acyclovir in children: a randomised double blind placebo controlled study. Br Med J 1997;314:1800-3.

47. Hughes WT. Persistent thrush in young infants. Pediatr Infect Dis J 1987;6:1074–5.

48. Pons V, Greenspan D, Lozada-Nur F, et al. Oropharyngeal candidiasis in patients with AIDS: randomized comparison of fluconazole versus nystatin oral suspensions. Clin Infect Dis 1997;24:1204–7.

49. Allen WP, Rapp F. Concept review of genital herpes virus vaccines. J Infect Dis 1982;145:413–21.

50. Gallant JE, Moore RD, Chaisson RE. Prophylaxis for opportunistic infections in patients with HIV infection. Ann Intern Med 1994;120:932–44.

51. Shepp DH, Dandliker PS, Flournoy N, et al. Sequential intravenous and twice-daily oral acyclovir for extended prophylaxis of herpes simplex virus infection in marrow transplant patients. Transplantation 1987;43:654–8.

52. Rooney JF, Straus SE, Mannix ML, et al. Oral acyclovir to suppress frequently recurrent herpes labialis. A double-blind, placebo-controlled trial. Ann Intern Med 1993;118:268–72.

53. Anderson PM, Schroeder G, Skubitz KM. Oral glutamine reduces the duration and severity of stomatitis after cytotoxic cancer chemotherapy. Cancer 1998;83:1433–9.

54. Cullen SJ, Baublis JV. Parinfluenza type 3 parotitis in two immunodeficient children. J Pediatr 1980;96:437–8.

55. Myer C, Cotton RT. Salivary gland disease in children: a review. Part 1: Acquired non-neoplastic disease. Clin Pediatr (Phila) 1986;25:314–22.

56. Krilov LR, Swenson P. Acute parotitis associated with influenza A infection. J Infect Dis 1985;152:853.

57. Earle AS, Wolinsky E. Cat scratch disease with involvement of intraparotid lymph nodes. Case report. Plastic Reconst Surg 1978;61:917–9.

58. Fainstein V, Musher DM, Young EJ. Acute bilateral suppurative parotitis due to Haemophilus influenzae: report of two cases. Arch Intern Med 1979;139:712–3.

59. David RB, O'Connell EJ. Suppurative parotitis in children. Am J Dis Child 1970;119:332–5.

60. Grossenbacher R, Steiner D. Salmonella parotitis with abscess formation. Otolaryngol-Head Neck Surg 1992;106:98–100.

61. Stellbrink H-J, Albrecht H, Greten H. Pneumococcal parotitis and cervical lymph node abscesses in an HIV-infected patient. Clin Invest 1994;72:1037–40.

62. Rowe-Jones JM, Vowles R, Leighton SEJ, et al. Diffuse tuberculous parotitis. J Laryngol Otol 1992;106:1094–5.

63. Green PA, Fordham von Reyn C, Smith RP Jr. Mycobacterium avium complex parotid lymphadenitis: successful therapy with clarithromycin and ethambutol. Pediatr Infect Dis J 1993;12:615–7.

64. Hensher R, Bowerman J. Actinomycosis of the parotid gland. Br J Oral Maxillofac Surg 1985;23:128–34.

65. Otrakji CL, Carreno T, Tesini SS, et al. Reactive follicular hyperplasia of intraparotid lymphoid tissue presenting as a recurrent parotid enlargement. Pediatr Pathol 1992;12:737–41.

66. Biedel CW. Recurrent mumps parotitis following natural infection and immunization. Am J Dis Child 1978;132:678–80.

67. Westmore GA, Pickard BH, Stern H. Isolation of mumps from the inner ear after sudden deafness. Br Med J 1979;1:14–5.

68. Ericson S, Zetterlund B, Ohman J. Recurrent parotitis and sialectasis in childhood. Clinical, radiologic, immunologic, bacteriologic, and histologic study. Ann Otol Rhinol Laryngol 1991;100:527–35.

69. Cohen HA, Gross S, Nussinovitch M, et al. Recurrent parotitis. Arch Dis Child 1992;67:1036–7.

70. Reid E, Douglas F, Crow Y, et al. Autosomal dominant juvenile recurrent parotitis. J Med Gen 1998;35:417–9.

71. Shimizu M, Ussmuller J, Donath K, et al. Sonographic analysis of recurrent parotitis in children: a comparative study with sialographic findings. Oral Surg Oral Med Oral Pathol Oral Radiol Endodontics 1998;86:606–15.

72. Blatt IM. Chronic and recurrent inflammations about the salivary glands with special reference to children: a report of 25 cases. Laryngoscope 1966;76:917–33.

73. Pellinen TJ, Kalske J. Nitrofurantoin-induced parotitis. Br Med J 1982;285:344.

74. Chudwin DS, Daniels TE, Wara DW, et al. Spectrum of Sjogren syndrome in children. J Pediatr 1981;98:213–7.

75. Romero RW, Nesbitt LT Jr, Ichinose H. Mikulicz disease and subsequent lupus erythematosus development. JAMA 1977;237:2507–10.

76. Sanders DY, Huntley CC, Sharp GS. Mixed connective tissue disease in a child. J Pediatr 1973;83:642–5.

77. Ah-See KW, McLaren K, Maran AG. Wegener's granulomatosis presenting as major salivary gland enlargement. J Laryngol Otol 1996;110:691–3.

78. Goguen LA, April MM, Karmody CS, et al. Self-induced pneumoparotitis. Arch Otol-Head Neck Surg 1995;121:1426–9.

79. Cayler GC, Peterson CA. Infantile cortical hyperostosis: report of seventeen cases. Am J Dis Child 1956;91:119–25.

80. Cohen DL. Sicca syndrome: an unusual manifestation of sarcoidosis in childhood. Am J Dis Child 1983;137:289–90.

81. Conley J, Tinsley PP Jr. Treatment and prognosis of mucoepidermoid carcinoma in the pediatric age group. Arch Otolaryngol 1985;111:322–4.

82. Kocen RS, Critchley E. Mumps epididymo-orchitis and its treatment with cortisone. Br J Med 1961;2:20–4.

83. Philip RN, Reinhard KR, Lackman DB. Observations on a mumps epidemic in a "virgin" population. Am J Hyg 1959;69:91–111.

84. Smith MHD. Mumps virus vaccine [letter]. Pediatrics 1969;42:907–9.

85. Levitt LP, Rick TA, Kinde SW, et al. Central nervous system mumps. Neurology 1970;20:829–34.

86. Editorial: Mumps vaccine: More information needed. N Engl J Med 1968;278:275–6.

87. Ni J, Bowles NE, Kim YH, et al. Viral infection of the myocardium in endocardial fibroelastosis. Molecular evidence for the role of mumps virus as an etiologic agent. Circulation 1997;95:133–9.

88. Brown NJ, Richmond SJ. Fatal mumps myocarditis in an 8-month-old child. Br Med J 1980;2:355–6.

89. Gold HE, Boxerbaum B, Leslie HJ Jr. Mumps arthritis. Am J Dis Child 1968;116:547–8.

90. Eylan E, Zmuchy R, Sheba CH. Mumps virus and subacute thyroiditis: evidence of a causal association. Lancet 1957;1:1062–3.

91. Kolars CP, Spink WW. Thrombocytopenic purpura as a complication of mumps. JAMA 1958;168:2213–5.

92. Chitre VV, Premchandra DJ. Recurrent parotitis. Arch Dis Child 1997;77:359–63.

93. Wright GL, Smith RJH, Katz CD, et al. Benign parotid diseases of childhood. Laryngoscope 1985;95:915–9.

94. Brook I, Frazier EH, Thompson DH. Aerobic and anaerobic microbiology of acute suppurative parotitis. Laryngoscope 1991;101:170–2.

95. Sadeghi N, Black MJ, Frenkiel S. Parotidectomy for the treatment of chronic recurrent parotitis. J Otolaryngol 1996;25:305–7.

CHAPTER 5

Eye, Ear, and Sinus Syndromes

■ ACUTE OTITIS MEDIA

Otitis media is best considered a disease of eustachian tube dysfunction. The bacteria trapped in the middle ear represent the nasopharyngeal flora. Antibiotic treatment is aided by gradual and spontaneous improvement in eustachian tube function during the natural history of the disease. The physiology and mechanism of eustachian tube dysfunction and the frequency of various pathogens have been well reviewed.[1,2]

Ear Examination

Cleaning of the Ear Canal

The ear should be examined as thoroughly as possible before attempting to remove the earwax, because such attempts sometimes make adequate removal and visibility more difficult.

Suctioning is the most effective method of removing wax. A bent 14-gauge blunt needle attached by tubing to a trap and a suction machine is popular and is especially useful for sticky wax. Water irrigation is also useful if there is no perforation. It can be done using either an ear syringe or a water-jet machine of the type used for cleaning between teeth. The water-jet machine should be set at its lowest force because perforation can occur at the highest force. Tools such as a dull loop or a dewaxing speculum also can be used. Large cotton swabs are not helpful, but small nasopharyngeal swabs can be. Calcium alginate swabs are very flexible and can be bent into an effective and pliable loop. Wax solvents or hydrogen peroxide followed by water irrigation or suction have been found useful by some physicians. However, severe local reactions to commercial wax solvents have been reported. These reactions can be avoided by rinsing the ear canal with water after allowing the solvent a few minutes to work.

Appearance of the Tympanic Membranes

After the wax has been adequately removed, the tympanic membranes should be carefully examined. The eardrum is normally gray or pink, but can also be red, blue, or injected (prominent blood vessels). Tympanic membranes are often red in a crying infant or in a baby with fever from any cause. Comparing the degree of erythema with the other tympanic membrane may be helpful.

The drum normally appears thin and reflects the otoscope light. Diseased drums can appear dull or thick without light reflection. The drum has a normal position but can be bulging or retracted (atelectatic). Perforations, calcifications, whitish exudate, or bullae may be noted. Landmarks should be noted as an aid to description. The more complete the description, the easier it is to gauge improvement at the time of follow-up examination. A simple diagram of the eardrum can be sketched and labeled for the patient's record (Fig. 5-1).

Pneumatic Otoscopy

The mobility of the eardrum should be evaluated by applying pressure and suction, usually by means of a rubber bulb attached to the head of the otoscope by a rubber tube. For this technique to be effective, there must be an adequate air seal between the speculum and the ear canal.[1] Failure to perform an evaluation of the tympanic membrane's mobility is one of the most frequent mistakes in pediatric practice. Any examination of the middle ear that

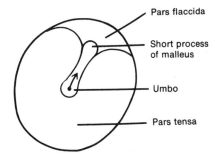

■ FIGURE 5-1 Diagram of landmarks of right tympanic membrane. Note that a line from the umbo to the short process points to the right, the side being examined.

does not include an assessment of mobility is incomplete. Incomplete examination often leads to incorrect diagnosis; in this case, it often leads to overdiagnosis of otitis media, an error that is to be strenuously avoided.

Failure of the eardrum to move with suction and pressure implies that the middle ear is full of fluid or is under negative pressure. A normal eardrum moves in and out easily with gentle pressure changes (Fig. 5-2A). If the drum only moves outward, it may be atelectatic (collapsed), as in the tympanogram shown in Figure 5-2C. Pneumatic otoscopy is a reasonably accurate way of detecting and observing the course of fluid in the middle ear. Rarely, an immobile drum is caused by a rigid or scarred membrane or an undetected perforation.

Tympanometry

In tympanometry, also called impedance audiometry, changes in the reflection of sound energy by the tympanic membrane are measured in the external ear canal in response to changes in ear-canal pressure (Figure 5-2).[3] As in pneumatic otoscopy, a pressure seal is required. This method has been especially useful in studying the development of middle-ear effusions and in screening young children for asymptomatic effusions, because large numbers of examinations are needed to make the equipment cost effective. Tympanometry is also being used to investigate the onset, diagnosis, and course of acute otitis media. As a more objective measure of the presence of middle ear fluid, tympanometry is also a good training tool for medical students, residents, physicians assistants, and nurse practitioners; the "student" can examine the middle ear using pneumatic otoscopy first, and then confirm the validity of his/her examination by tympanometry.

Acoustic Reflectometry

Middle-ear effusions can be detected by a simple acoustic otoscope and confirmed by myringotomy or tympanocentesis.[4]

Tympanocentesis

Since the 1970s, needle puncture of the tympanic membrane (tympanocentesis) has been used sporadically. It can be useful to derive statistical information about the frequency of various bacteria in middle-ear effusions. Tympanocentesis is also used

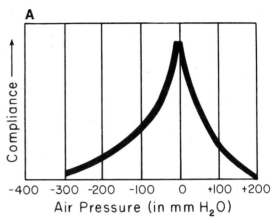

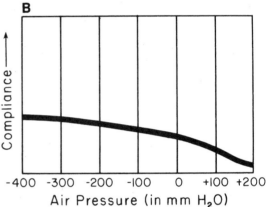

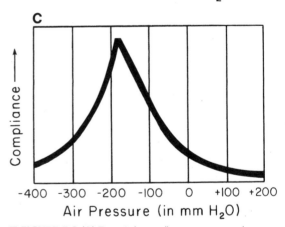

■ **FIGURE 5-2 (A)** Type A (normal) tympanogram demonstrating normal middle-ear pressure and compliance. **(B)** Type B tympanogram, as found with serous otitis or perforation, demonstrating reduced eardrum compliance and no point of peak compliance throughout the air pressure range. **(C)** Type C tympanogram demonstrating negative middle-ear pressure (retracted tympanic membrane). (Rees TS: Clin Pediatr 1976;15:368–73).

by some physicians in particular situations, as described later. The technique has been described for both aerobic and anaerobic collection of specimens.[5] In 6 (5%) of 122 children with bilateral acute otitis media, culture results revealed different pathogens from the two ears.[6] This is unlikely to be clinically significant, as many cases self-resolve without therapy, as discussed later. However, it may explain why on some occasions one side may respond poorly and the other well to treatment.

Criteria for tympanocentesis include: (1) a severely ill child who has developed otitis while receiving an antibiotic or who is still toxic after 48 to 72 hours of antibiotic therapy; (2) otitis in the sick-appearing newborn or in an immunocompromised child; (3) middle-ear effusion in a toxic infant without other signs of infection or in whom there is a suppurative complication without accessible culture material (i.e., brain abscess or cerebral venous sinus thrombosis); or, sometimes, (4) chronic middle-ear effusion with an acute exacerbation. In addition, continued clinical failure after changing antibiotics is a relative indication for tympanocentesis.

Predisposing Factors

Otitis media is generally more common in boys than in girls. Eskimos and Native Americans have a particularly high incidence. Patients with cleft palate, submucous cleft palate, Down syndrome, supine swallowing (bottle-propping), allergic rhinitis, environmental tobacco smoke exposure, or exclusive bottle feeding have a higher incidence of middle-ear infection. Most cases of acute otitis media are preceded by a viral respiratory infection.[7] All respiratory viruses can predispose to the development of otitis media.

Classic Clinical Findings

The classic clinical picture of otitis media is the sudden development of fever and otalgia in a patient with a respiratory infection, usually the common cold syndrome. Unfortunately, the classic findings are often absent. Fever is variably present. Small children are not able to complain of ear pain, but may tug at or dig into their ears. Ear tugging in and of itself (i.e., in the complete absence of other signs of disease) is not usually a sign of acute otitis media.[8] Young children may have nonspecific signs of illness, such as irritability, decreased appetite, or diarrhea.

Examination of the ear may reveal a red tympanic membrane that is tense or bulging or may show the presence of pus behind the thickened membrane. Insufflation shows decreased movement with both positive and negative pressure. The tympanic membrane may have blisters or bullae on it (bullous myringitis, discussed later). A gray bulging membrane may be found.[9] Very high fever (above 40°C) is rare.[10] The white blood cell count is of no predictive value.[11]

Classification

Otitis media can be classified on the basis of a number of variables. The onset and course can be acute, subacute, chronic, asymptomatic, or recurrent. Accurate classification on the basis of middle-ear fluid is possible only if fluid is examined directly; that is, only if there is spontaneous perforation with drainage or if tympanocentesis or myringotomy is performed. The middle-ear fluid may be purulent (cloudy, with many white blood cells), serous (clear and yellow like serum), or mucoid (sticky, with threads of mucus).

Problem-oriented diagnoses are not yet widely used to describe acute otitis media, but they are gaining in popularity. The frequency of antibiotic prescriptions for otitis media has hastened the development of resistance in *Streptococcus pneumoniae,* which has forced pediatricians to come to terms with the concept of problem-oriented diagnosis in otitis media in order to have a conceptual basis for a "watch and wait" approach to certain kinds of otitis media. It is, therefore, helpful to make problem-oriented descriptive diagnoses on the basis of the onset and course of the illness and the appearance and mobility of the tympanic membrane. If middle-ear fluid is obtained for examination, additional diagnostic descriptions can be given. A reasonable classification according to diagnoses that can usually be made is shown in Box 5-1.

The management of a patient with otitis media needs to be based on the specific subgroup diagnosis. The following are some examples of this approach:

1. *Fever with red, but mobile drums.* This category, sometimes loosely called "red ear," is probably the most frequent form of so-called acute otitis media reported in series published before 1970. However, those who believe that middle-ear fluid is required for the diagnosis do not regard red but mobile tympanic membranes as otitis media. This is probably the most reasonable po-

---

BOX 5-1 ■ Problem-orinted Classification of Otitis Media

Fever and red, mobile drums
Acute otitis media
Otitis media with effusion
Bullous myringitis
Recurrent otitis media
Draining ear
Acute otitis media with perforation versus otitis externa
Chronic otitis media without perforation
Chronic otitis media with perforation
Acute otitis media in a child with tympanostomy tubes
Chronically draining ear in a child with tympanostomy tubes
Asymptomatic middle-ear effusion

---

sition, because tympanic membranes can become transiently red with crying or fever. Most young children who are brought to the doctor's office and have a speculum placed into their external ear canal have *both* fever and crying. Inclusion of many febrile children with "red ears" in early studies of otitis media probably decreased the accuracy of these studies and led to some reports that a placebo was as effective as an antibiotic. The frequency of development of middle-ear fluid in these patients has not been adequately studied, but it is reasonable to suspect that large series that concluded antibiotics were no more effective than placebo probably included many such patients.

2. *Acute otitis media (AOM).* This diagnostic category corresponds to what has been called acute purulent otitis media. This is a disease with a sudden onset, ear pain, and usually some degree of fever. Patients are clearly suffering from a moderate to severe illness. The eardrum is usually red, the normal landmarks are obscured, and there is fluid behind the drum that can be appreciated visually or by poor mobility on insufflation. The exact consistency of fluid seen behind the inflamed tympanic membrane in this condition is not always easy to determine; it may be assumed that pus is there based on the presentation and course of this illness. This is the classification of otitis media that usually calls for antimicrobial therapy, as discussed later.

3. *Otitis media with effusion (OME).* This is the cur-

rent classification of a disease that used to be more frequently referred to as "serous otitis media." OME is a condition in which the patient has fluid behind the tympanic membrane, but has neither signs nor symptoms of acute illness. The patient may have some dullness or even some redness to the drum. Otalgia, if present at all, is mild. Older patients may complain of decreased hearing acuity or may say that they feel as if they should but cannot "pop their ears." OME may follow a course of AOM, or it may arise by itself. Some patients have bacteria recovered on tympanocentesis, but most do not. Many of these effusions will resolve spontaneously over the course of 1 to 3 months.

4. *Bullous myringitis.* This condition is characterized by the formation of blebs, vesicles, or bullae on the tympanic membrane, sometimes creating a cobblestone appearance. It tends to be quite painful, although some children do not seem to be bothered by it. It was originally linked to mycoplasmal infection, but has subsequently been shown to be simply a variant of AOM, as discussed later.

5. *Recurrent otitis media.* This is defined by recurrences of AOM with normal tympanic membranes between acute episodes.

6. *Draining ear.* This is a preliminary diagnosis that should eventually be resolved into either acute otitis externa, AOM with perforation, or chronic otitis media with perforation.

7. *Chronic middle-ear effusion.* If the effusion persists for more than 3 months, as it does in 5–10% of acute cases, it is defined as chronic. Myringotomy with aspiration is often the first step in surgical treatment. If the effusion reaccumulates, ventilation tubes may be necessary, as described later in this chapter. In general, the longer the middle-ear fluid is present, the more viscous it becomes, and thus the more difficult it is for it to drain spontaneously.

8. *Asymptomatic middle-ear effusion of unknown duration.* This problem-oriented diagnosis can be made when immobile, dull eardrums are noted on a routine examination. A good air seal is needed for the test. This condition is also called asymptomatic OME, although this term assumes that the fluid is serous rather than purulent or mucoid. Asymptomatic effusion can be a stage in the course of AOM. This particular condition should never prompt a course of antibiotics.

9. *Draining ear in a child with tympanostomy tubes.* It is appropriate to consider this as a separate category because the management is different from that of the child without tympanostomy tubes. As in a child without tympanostomy tubes, this should be classified as either acute or chronic drainage.

Possible Infectious Causes

Bacteria

In children with otitis media, the most frequent bacteria recovered from ear puncture are *S. pneumoniae* (pneumococcus), nontypable *Haemophilus influenzae,* and *Moraxella catarrhalis.* The frequency of the various organisms recovered by needle puncture or myringotomy is diagrammed in Figure 5-3.

Approximately 30% of middle-ear cultures show no growth. This sometimes is the result of a failure of the culture techniques to detect fastidious bacteria, small numbers of bacteria, bacteria no longer capable of replication because of antibiotic therapy, or microorganisms other than bacteria. Sometimes the patient's bacterial infection has been eradicated, although signs and symptoms of inflammation are still present. In other words, you may have cured the patient, but the patient may not know that he has been cured. It used to be thought that anaerobic bacteria accounted for much of this "no-growth" percentage,[12] but this is no longer believed to be the case. Aerobic pathogens can be found in middle-ear fluid by polymerase chain reaction (PCR) in a high percentage of "sterile" effusions.[13] It is still not clear whether this means these patients will benefit from antibiotic therapy. The 30% figure also suggests that in some cases, middle-ear fluid is sterile and not formed as a response to bacterial infection. It supports the concepts that (1) eustachian tube dys-

function is the basic mechanism of otitis media, and (2) not all cases of otitis media require therapy.

Gram-negative enteric bacteria and *S. aureus* were the bacteria most frequently recovered from the middle ear of premature or term neonates in some early studies and may have represented the nasopharyngeal flora of these infants,[14] as subsequent studies have indicated that these bacteria are uncommon in infections. Young infants occasionally have Group B streptococci recovered from the middle ear.[15] The recovery of *Neisseria* species or of *S. epidermidis,* which are not usually associated with disease, also suggests that some bacteria recovered from the middle ear are, in fact, normal flora of the nasopharynx that have reached the middle ear after eustachian tube dysfunction and are not the cause of the otitis media. In addition, inadequate disinfection of the ear canal before tympanocentesis may be a factor, as *S. epidermidis* and diphtheroids are especially likely contaminants from the external ear canal.[16] The possible contribution of these low-virulence organisms to the illness has not been adequately evaluated; they may be important in some cases. If a young infant (less than 2 months of age) has otitis media and appears toxic, hospitalization, tympanocentesis, lumbar puncture, blood culture, and intravenous antibiotics are indicated. AOM with low-grade fever in a well-appearing young infant can usually be treated with oral antibiotics provided that close follow-up can be ensured.

Viruses

It has now been well established that viruses can not only predispose to otitis media because of inflammation of the eustachian tubes, but they can also be etiologic agents of otitis media.[17,18] Respiratory syncytial virus, parainfluenza viruses, cox-

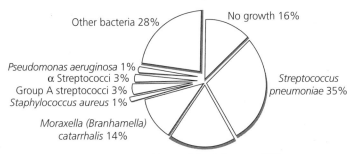

■ **FIGURE 5-3** Frequency of various microorganisms found by tympanocentesis in 2807 cases of acute otitis media. (Adapted from Bluestone CD, et al. Pediatr Infect Dis J 1992;11:S7–S11)

sackie viruses, and others have been recovered from middle-ear fluid by conventional cell culture.[19] Studies suggest that the concomitant presence of a viral pathogen and a bacterial pathogen in the middle-ear space signals a disease process that is more difficult to eradicate.[20] On occasion, a virus is the only pathogen recovered. Viral antigens and genetic material have also been found by ELISA and PCR. PCR positivity for viral antigens does not prove active infection, as dead or replication-incompetent viruses will still produce a positive PCR.

Any respiratory viral infection can serve as an inciting event for the development of AOM. It is often thought that RSV is the agent most likely to do so;[21] however, the most comprehensive study on this issue to date shows that the difference in the prevalence of otitis media in children with culture-proven respiratory syncytial virus infection versus the prevalence in infection with other respiratory viruses is small.[22]

Mycoplasma

Bullous myringitis occurs in some cases of experimental infection of human volunteers with *Mycoplasma pneumoniae*.[23] However, later studies emphasize the fact that *Mycoplasma* is a rare cause of otitis media, even in the presence of bullous myringitis.[24] In fact, when tympanocenteses are performed in patients with bullous myringitis, the breakdown of pathogens mirrors that in patients with AOM in the absence of bullae (i.e., *S. pneumoniae* is most common, followed by nontypable *H. influenzae*, and then by *M. catarrhalis*).[24] These findings suggest bullous myringitis is, in fact, nothing more than a variant of AOM. As such, it should be treated with the same antibiotics one would choose for uncomplicated AOM. The clinician should feel absolutely no compulsion to add erythromycin or to use an erythromycin-containing antibiotic or a newer macrolide in the treatment of patients with bullous myringitis.

Chlamydia

Chlamydia trachomatis appears to be a cause of some recurrent middle-ear effusions, as discussed later. Special culture techniques and PCR revealed the presence of *C. pneumoniae* in a small percentage of both acute and refractory cases of otitis media. In most cases it was not the sole pathogen recovered.[25]

Noninfectious Etiologies

Hemorrhagic or bullous myringitis can result from trauma.

Treatment

Many cooperative studies of antibiotics have been done, and excellent reviews are available.[26,27] It is important to distinguish the subgroup of otitis media to which a particular management applies.

No Antibiotic Treatment

Physicians in some European countries have adopted a strategy of watchful waiting (or as one author phrased it, "masterful inactivity"[28]) for most cases of AOM. Analgesics are given. Several published studies show a remarkable success rate using this strategy.[28,29] Physicians in the United States have been reluctant to adopt this concept because of concerns about mastoiditis, persistent effusions, spontaneous perforation, and other complications.[26,27] However, the rapid emergence of penicillin-resistant *S. pneumoniae* in most areas of the United States has necessitated a rethinking of our routine antibiotic approach to the care of patients with otitis media. In the late 1980s, papers that urged pediatricians to withhold therapy for a subset of children with otitis media began to emerge.[30,31] It has been well recognized for years that a high percentage of cases labeled "otitis media" will resolve without antibiotic therapy.

Recent recommendations from the American Academy of Pediatrics have emphasized a selective approach to the treatment of otitis media.[32] Patients with OME (mild redness of the tympanic membrane, low-grade to no fever, a serous fluid collection behind the drum, and no toxicity) are best observed without antibiotic therapy. Analgesia, preferably with acetaminophen with or without topical analgesics, may be prescribed if needed. Patients with "red ear" should never be administered antibiotic therapy.

Acute Otitis Media

Patients with true AOM (i.e., bright red, bulging tympanic membranes; moderate to high fever; severe otalgia; or toxicity) are clear candidates for antibiotic therapy. Therapy should be directed at the pathogens most likely to require therapy (see next paragraph).

Virgil Howie's early studies of the bacterial etiology of otitis media using placebo therapy and serial tympanocenteses reveal that the spontaneous resolution rate of otitis media is, to a large extent, determined by the specific pathogen.[33] His data show that of 25 children who had "nonpathogens" (most of which were probably *M. catarrhalis*) at the time of the first tympanocentesis, 7 (28%) had no exudate at 2- to 7-day follow-up. Thirteen (52%) of the 25 had a persistently positive culture. *H. influenzae* was somewhat less likely to spontaneously resolve: of 21 initial isolates, 3 (14%) had no exudate and 12 (57%) remained culture positive by the repeat tympanocentesis. In contrast, of 45 children with isolates of *S. pneumoniae*, only 2 (4%) had no exudate, and 36 (82%) were still culture positive at follow-up tympanocentesis.[33] Persistence of viable bacteria after failed treatment also varies by pathogen, being highest in *S. pneumoniae* infections.[34] In this study, only 5% of cultures of AOM treatment failures yielded *M. catarrhalis*, despite the fact that almost 90% of the *M. catarrhalis* isolates were beta-lactamase producers.[34] Experience and subsequent clinical research have proved this fact: AOM caused by *S. pneumoniae* is the least likely to resolve on its own. Group A streptococcal otitis also has a low spontaneous resolution rate. If there were a way of knowing which pathogen the patient was harboring, antibiotic therapy could almost certainly be safely withheld for most patients with *H. influenzae* and almost all patients with *M. catarrhalis* ear infections. The fact that suppurative complications of otitis media such as mastoiditis are almost never caused by *M. catarrhalis* further underscores the low pathogenic potential of this organism in otitis media.

It is difficult to establish the exact etiologic agent in any one case of AOM; nasopharyngeal cultures do not reflect the pathogen infecting the middle-ear space and are therefore not recommended. Because there is no way, short of obtaining middle-ear fluid for culture, of knowing with certainty what pathogen is inhabiting the middle ear of a patient, and because suppurative complications are potentially devastating, antibiotic therapy against AOM should, first and foremost, be directed against the pneumococcus. In doing this, some activity against beta-lactamase-producing *H. influenzae* and *M. catarrhalis* will be lost, but the trade-off is reasonable, given the fact that most patients with these other pathogens will undergo spontaneous resolution of their disease, even if they have true AOM at the onset. Studies of inflammatory mediators in serum

have shown that the body's response to the pneumococcus differs markedly from its response to other pathogens of otitis media.[35] These serologic findings have a clinical correlate: patients with pneumococcal otitis media are, in general, sicker than those with AOM due to *H. influenzae* or *M. catarrhalis*. Specifically, children with *S. pneumoniae* AOM are more likely to have a temperature of greater than 38.5°C and to have red and bulging tympanic membranes.[36,36a] The difference is more pronounced in children less than 24 months of age, in whom the findings of fever and a red, bulging tympanic membrane have a sensitivity of almost 60%, and absence of these findings has a specificity of 98% for otitis media caused by *S. pneumoniae*. Pneumococcal otitis media, therefore, can almost be looked on as a separate disease from otitis caused by other bacteria. One editorial suggested that physicians should think only about pneumococcus when planning therapy for AOM.[37]

Amoxicillin is still the best drug for initial treatment of AOM, despite increasing penicillin resistance in *S. pneumoniae* isolates, mainly because of its excellent penetration into the middle-ear space and its slow elimination.[38,39] "Resistance" is not absolute, but is related to the concentration of drug needed to inhibit the growth of a bacterial isolate (MIC). Once the MIC is exceeded, bacterial killing will take place. The rationale behind high-dose amoxicillin therapy is to achieve middle-ear fluid levels that exceed the MIC of the organism. If there is a high prevalence (greater than about 25%) of penicillin-resistant *S. pneumoniae* in your area, it is prudent to begin therapy with an amoxicillin dose of approximately 80–90 mg/kg/day, as opposed to the more traditional dosing of 40–45 mg/kg/day. In areas of low prevalence, low- or intermediate-dose amoxicillin can be started, with a follow-up visit in 48–72 hours. Early studies showed that lack of clinical improvement in the first 2–3 days predicted clinical failure of the antibiotic regimen; later studies correlated the clinical response with early eradication of the infecting organisms.[40] Changing therapy early in the course of disease is preferable to treating with an ineffective antibiotic for a full 10 days. The most commonly used second-line agent is amoxicillin-clavulanic acid. A new formulation of this antibiotic that contains these agents in a 14:1 ratio and allows for a high-dose regimen without excessive rates of diarrhea has improved tolerability. A child with no improvement after consecutive 3-day courses of two different antibiotics should probably undergo tympanocentesis. This has the benefit of draining the pus, which may be therapeutic, in addition to enabling a sample to be obtained for culture and sensitivity testing.

A patient with unilateral AOM and ipsilateral conjunctivitis has otitis-conjunctivitis syndrome. Patients with this syndrome are more likely to have *H. influenzae* as the causative agent of their AOM. Because of the high likelihood of beta-lactamase production by *H. influenzae* isolates, patients with otitis-conjunctivitis syndrome should be treated with a drug that is beta-lactamase stable. Trimethoprim-sulfamethoxazole (FMP-SMX), amoxicillin-clavulanate, a second- or third-generation cephalosporin, or a macrolide would be appropriate. Cost concerns favor a trial of TMP-SMX. No systematic comparison of these alternatives in this situation has been performed.

Several acceptable alternative initial therapies are available for penicillin-allergic patients. Cefpodoxime, cefuroxime, and cefprozil have been tested and found to be reasonably effective in the treatment of AOM. Cefdinir is a similar drug that has the advantage of being more palatable. Caution must be used when prescribing cephalosporins to patients with true penicillin allergy, as there is a small (<5%) incidence of cross-sensitivity. Cefaclor suspension should not be used. This antibiotic is unstable in suspension; one of the breakdown products causes a rash to occur in some patients. Developing a rash while taking cefaclor suspension, therefore, does not prove cephalosporin allergy. In any case, cefaclor is a poor choice as empiric therapy for AOM because its activity against *S. pneumoniae* is unacceptably low. Loracarbef, ceftibuten, and cefixime also have relatively poor activity against *S. pneumoniae*. Clindamycin has activity against most strains of the pneumococcus, but no activity against *H. influenzae* or *M. catarrhalis*, and its use should probably be reserved for cases in which *S. pneumoniae* has been cultured from middle ear fluid. The combination of erythromycin ethylsuccinate and sulfisoxazole suffers from the fact that these two drugs are antagonistic. The newer macrolides (azithromycin and clarithromycin) are popular but offer no particular advantage over other agents. Pneumococcal resistance against these agents appears to be on the rise.

Persistent middle ear effusion

Effusion is still present in about 50% of children 10 days after treatment,[41] especially those younger than 24 months.[42] With time, the effusion resolves: 90% are resolved within 3 months. After that time, few cases resolve.[43]

It used to be common practice to have a 2-week follow-up visit for all children with AOM. Because the natural history of the disease is that at least half of the children will not have a normal ear examination at that visit, it is prudent to delay the follow-up visit to approximately 4 weeks in children whose symptoms have resolved. As mentioned earlier, children who still have ongoing moderate to severe symptoms should be seen sooner than 2 weeks, preferably at 2 to 3 days. Children with continued effusion, but without symptoms at 4-week follow-up are best managed by watchful waiting and follow-up evaluation. TMP-SMX for 14 days failed to promote resolution of effusion in a controlled study.[41]

Persistence of middle-ear fluid after acute otitis media occurs more commonly in white children under 2 years of age and can cause transiently impaired hearing, although long-term follow-up reveals normal hearing and normal speech and language development in most.[44] When an episode of AOM results in persistence of middle ear fluid for 3 months, as described in the preceding section, and the tympanic membrane remains immobile, consultation with an ear specialist is advisable. A short course of oral steroids in concert with antimicrobial therapy has been advocated as a last resort before referral to an otolaryngologist,[45] but not all studies have shown a beneficial effect.[46] Recent guidelines recommend against their use.[46a]

Bullous myringitis

As discussed previously, this condition should be considered a variant of AOM, and treated appropriately. If there are associated middle or lower respiratory findings, it may be reasonable to consider therapy with a macrolide, although data about the efficacy of this approach are lacking.

Asymptomatic effusion

OME can be asymptomatic in early infancy and may be detected only by routine examination at well-child visits.[47] Fifty percent of effusions in young infants resolve in one month, but about 15% will remain unresolved after 3 months. Therapy of this primarily benign condition with TMP-SMX for 4 weeks significantly increases the frequency of resolution compared with placebo, but the therapy itself is not benign. A 2-week course of amoxicillin also hastens resolution. In the era of antimicrobial resistance, an approach of no antibiotic therapy and monthly follow-up seems wise, especially in the absence of risk factors for severe or disseminated infection (extreme young age, prematurity, or immunodeficiency states). Antihistamine-decongestant combinations offer no additional benefit.[48]

Neonatal otitis media

Examination of the ear in the newborn requires relatively deeper penetration with the speculum and pulling of the pinna down and posteriorly in order to straighten the canal.[49] In the first 3 months of life, hospitalized infants, especially those in intensive care units, may have *S. aureus* or enteric gram-negative bacilli recovered on tympanocentesis,[50] whereas infants this age seen as outpatients are likely to have the conventional pathogens.[51]

It has been suggested that amniotic fluid viscosity is a relevant variable in resorption of middle-ear fluid in the first 48 hours of life and may be relevant to the pathogenesis of later middle-ear effusions and infections in young infants.[52] The eustachian tube is more horizontal, and the tensor veli palatini muscle, the contraction of which opens the tube, does not have mature function in the young infant. In fact, innervation and function of this muscle usually is not complete until about the age of 6 years. This helps to explain why recurrent otitis media becomes a relatively rare disease in children over the age of 6.

Other Treatment

Oral decongestants and antihistamines were of no value for AOM or for chronic effusion in two controlled studies.[21,48] In the third study, antihistamines for AOM were associated with a longer duration of middle ear effusion.[52a] In many children, antihistamines produce sedation, masking the neurologic symptoms of rare complications such as meningitis or brain abscess. However, antihistamines may be helpful in recurrent OME in children with documented allergic problems. The use of nonsedating antihistamines in children with this condition has not been evaluated.

Allergies and upper respiratory infections appear to disrupt eustachian tube function. Prevention of otitis media by symptomatic treatment of allergies has not been demonstrated. The incidence of AOM are decreased in children given influenza vaccination[53] and also in children who were treated with respiratory syncytial virus-enriched IVIG for the prevention of RSV disease.[54]

Myringotomy

Incision of the tympanic membrane may be useful for relief of pain but does not appear to significantly alter the clinical course or prognosis of the illness.[22] It rarely has been used in the treatment of AOM since the 1970s and usually need not be considered unless medical therapy fails. Myringotomy should only be performed by physicians experienced with the procedure. In selected cases, tympanocentesis can be done to relieve pressure. More frequently, tympanocentesis is performed to obtain fluid for culture in refractory cases. The recovery and speciation of pathogens is very helpful because antibiotic susceptibility testing can be performed and the results used to guide antimicrobial decisions.

Some physicians are now using a laser device to puncture the tympanic membrane, principally for relief of pressure, in cases of severe or refractory AOM. The true utility of the procedure awaits further study; it shows some potential in reducing the unnecessary use of antibiotic therapy.

Analgesics

Acetaminophen or ibuprofen may be used for relief of ear pain. On rare occasions, a dose or two of codeine may be indicated for severe pain. Topical application of Auralgan, containing dehydrated glycerin, antipyrine, and benzocaine, may be of some value in pain relief and may soften earwax for easier removal. This preparation is especially useful in the first two or three days of therapy for a full-blown case of AOM, in which pain can be intense.

Duration of Therapy and Follow-Up

Reexamination, as mentioned earlier, should be done in 48–72 hours in severe or unresponsive cases. It can be postponed to 4 weeks for others. Older children (greater than age 3 or 4) may not require a formal follow-up examination at all: if the child says he is feeling better, the condition is almost always resolved. Keep in mind that even at a 4-week follow-up visit, some fluid may still be present, although it may be sterile.

The optimal duration of therapy has undergone some intensive investigation over the past few years.[55] Antibiotics with long half-lives, such as azithromycin, have been recommended to be given for only 5 days. This recommendation is based on the fact that a 5-day course provides almost 10 days of antimicrobial coverage given the disappearance of the active drug from the tissues. More recently, recommendations have been published that children at low risk for suppurative complications, (such as children greater than 4 years old, children without a history of frequent or severe AOM, and children without severe disease at the time of diagnosis) can be treated for 5–7 days with conventional antibiotics.[32] Children less than 5 years old, those with frequent AOM or a history of severe AOM or AOM with complications, and patients with high fever or who are ill appearing at the time of diagnosis should continue to receive a full 10-day course of antibiotic therapy.

Studies have shown that one intramuscular injection of ceftriaxone is as effective as a 10-day course of amoxicillin-clavulanate for the initial treatment of AOM.[56] For treatment of previously unresponsive cases, three consecutive days of therapy is superior to a single injection.[57] However, the use of ceftriaxone for treatment of otitis media should not be routine. A single dose of intramuscular ceftriaxone has been shown to increase penicillin resistance among the pneumococci colonizing the nasopharynx.[58] Although some refractory cases of AOM due to multiply resistant organisms will respond to a 3-consecutive-day schedule of intramuscular ceftriaxone,[32] this approach to therapy is painful and inconvenient. Sometimes it can allow a patient to avoid ear surgery, and in those cases it seems to be the lesser of two evils.

Draining Ears

A new discharge from the external ear canal can be caused by perforated AOM or acute otitis externa. Ear drainage is an expected finding in the child with tympanostomy tubes and AOM. A chronically draining ear can be caused by chronic otitis media with perforation, with the draining pus producing secondary otitis externa. A chronically draining ear is seldom attributable to otitis externa alone. Chronic drainage may also be a sign of mastoiditis.

■ OTITIS EXTERNA

Acute Otitis Externa

Otitis externa is defined as redness, itching, or edema of the external ear canal, with or without exudate. The ear canal is usually very painful, the pain perhaps aggravated by chewing. Typically, pain is produced by moving the pinna and by insertion of the speculum into the external ear. Fever is uncommon. There may be erythema and edema around the external auditory canal, so that the physician may at first suspect mastoiditis or parotitis. "Swimmer's ear" is an otitis externa apparently initiated or exacerbated by water in the ear.

Chronic Otitis Externa

This condition is usually secondary to chronic drainage from a perforated eardrum.

Malignant otitis externa

Occurring predominately in adults, especially diabetics, malignant otitis has been observed rarely in newborn infants, and in children with diabetes mellitus or other immunocompromising conditions.[59,60] It is characterized by progressive, invasive external-ear infection, typically caused by *Pseudomonas aeruginosa*. It is likely that the child will be in poor general health. The disease may invade the bone of the mastoid, mandible, or skull, with cranial nerve paralysis or even death.[61] Technetium bone scan may be helpful in the early diagnosis of osteomyelitis associated with malignant otitis externa.[61] A 4-week course of parenteral antibiotics active against *Pseudomonas* has been advised, with surgical drainage only if no clinical response is obtained with antibiotics.[62] Both an aminoglycoside and an antipseudomonal penicillin should be used, at least for the first week. Patients who get through this illness may be beset with late complications including sensorineural hearing loss,[63] stenosis of the external canal, or necrosis of the tympanic membrane.[64]

Mechanisms

Otitis externa is usually related to water in the ear canal. This may be caused by excessive exposure to water, such as in swimming (especially under water) or heated whirlpool baths, or by a contaminated infant bath sponge or failure to dry the ear after exposure to water. The external ear canal protects itself with a layer of cerumen, which normally removes contaminants by trapping and moving them slowly toward the outlet of the canal, where they can be removed by gentle swabbing. Anything that damages this layer can predispose to external otitis, including excessive or vigorous cerumen removal with a cotton-tipped swab. Parents should be instructed that it is neither necessary nor advisable to put cotton-tipped swabs into the external ear canal. Problems of earwax build-up in the external canal are also sometimes related to attempts at wax removal. Inexperienced people may actually be pushing the earwax closer to the tympanic membrane, where it can collect. Once the wax dries, it is harder for it to move toward the outlet as it should. This can also macerate the epithelium of the canal and predispose to otitis externa.

Otitis externa is more common in the summer. This is presumably because more people are swimming in the summertime; however, some experts believe that excessive humidity of the hot summer air may be a cause, as well.

Etiologies

The principal differential diagnostic problem in a draining ear is distinguishing otitis externa from otitis media with perforation and drainage obscuring the eardrum. The problem is complicated by the fact that a chronically draining ear secondary to otitis media may predispose to subsequent otitis externa. A history of recent swimming or of past otitis media is helpful. Physical examination including manipulation of the canal is also helpful. Patients with rupture of the tympanic membrane (TM) from otitis media will often have a history of severe ear pain with rather sudden resolution, as rupture of the TM often brings relief of pressure pain. They may also have had fever prior to the rupture of the TM. In contrast, patients with otitis externa usually have increasing symptomatology, without a history of relief. Fever is uncommon. Movement of the tragus is sharply painful.

Suctioning of the drainage may allow the clinician to see the perforation of the TM. Perforations may also alter the results of tympanometry, as it measures the volume of air communicating with the external auditory canal.

P. aeruginosa is the organism most often recovered in acute otitis externa, whereas *S. pneumoniae, H. influenzae,* or beta-hemolytic streptococci are more common in AOM with rupture. In addition to *Pseudomonas, Proteus* species, *Escherichia coli,* or anaerobes may be recovered from a chronically draining ear. *Candida, Aspergillus,* or other fungi can cause otitis externa, especially in hot, damp climates.[62]

Allergic otitis externa is not unusual and may result from eardrops or chronic eczematoid otitis externa. Other diseases, such as Langerhans cell his-tiocytosis and Wegener's granulomatosis, are rare causes of draining ears.

Laboratory Approach

Gram Stain

In a chronically draining ear, a Gram stain may reveal more than one kind of gram-negative rod. If only one grows out in culture, the other may be an anaerobe.

Culture

Patients with external ear drainage secondary to otitis externa need not have cultures performed. Patients with chronic otitis media with drainage through a perforated TM or myringotomy tube should have cultures done on the pus. Swabbing pus that is already present in the canal usually yields a mixture of aerobes and anaerobes, most of which are commensals and do not provide any useful information. If the area can be cleaned first, fresh pus is occasionally recoverable. An ENT specialist is able to suction pus from the PE tube orifice or from a perforation, and thus get a more useful specimen. If a culture is obtained within 24 to 48 hours in perforated otitis media, it may provide useful information even without disinfection of the ear canal.[65] This is a practical office procedure for any office set up to do throat cultures for beta-hemolytic streptococci, although *H. influenzae* will not be recovered unless the swab is smeared on a chocolate agar plate and incubated in a candle jar.

Often, the culture shows no growth or yields only a skin contaminant. However, if pneumococci, *H. influenzae,* or beta-hemolytic streptococci are recovered, the culture is useful and indicates drainage from a recently perforated otitis media. Recovery of *P. aeruginosa, S. aureus,* or an enteric gram-negative rod suggests exudate from otitis externa or a chronically infected, perforated otitis media. Pseudomonads, however, are frequently commensal; their recovery must be interpreted in clinical context.

Treatment of Otitis Externa

Antibacterial Eardrops

Dilute (0.25%) acetic acid can be effective against *P. aeruginosa* and is inexpensive. A 1:1 mixture of household vinegar (dilute acetic acid) and rubbing (isopropyl) alcohol adds the drying effect of alcohol and may also be used. Cortisporin (polymixin B-bacitracin-neomycin-hydrocortisone) suspension can be used without much irritation of the middle ear if the drainage is from a perforation. The clear Cortisporin solution has a theoretical advantage of allowing the canal to be better visualized, but is more acidic than the suspension and often is poorly tolerated because of burning or stinging.[62] Ophthalmic solutions of Cortisporin or gentamicin may be tried even if Cortisporin suspension is not tolerated.[62] Hydrocortisone-acetic acid (VoSoL-HC) appeared to be as effective as Cortisporin solution in the treatment of otitis externa.[66] Otic Domeboro solution (2% acetic acid in modified Burrow's solution) is another effective local agent that is applied every 3 or 4 hours. It will relieve pain and reduce edema. Umbilical tape or commercially available ear wicks can be used if there is edema of the canal. If the edema is marked, topical agents are unlikely to reach their intended sites. In this situation, referral to an ENT specialist for daily suctioning of debris and wick placement is often necessary.

Prophylactic use of an antifungal, antibacterial medication (VoSoL) appeared to prevent swimmer's ear in a controlled study of campers.[67] Otic Domeboro left in for 5 minutes is also effective when given on arising, after swimming, and at bedtime.[62] A hair dryer may be helpful, but the use of cotton swabs to dry the ear is not recommended,[62] as trauma to the canal facilitates the development of otitis externa (OE). Ear hoods are of no value.

Analgesia

Dry heat may be helpful for pain. A few doses of acetaminophen, ibuprofen, or even codeine may sometimes be necessary.

■ CHRONIC AND RECURRENT OTITIS MEDIA

Definitions

Recurrent otitis media

Recurrent AOM has been defined as more than three episodes of AOM within 6 months.[68] The middle ear is normal, without effusions, between episodes.

Chronic otitis media

Called chronic serous otitis in the past, this pattern is usually defined as a middle-ear effusion that has been present for at least 3 months.[68] Persistent structural changes, such as a persistent eardrum perforation, imply past otitis but not necessarily chronic infection. Management of these problems remains difficult for most physicians, and only an introductory discussion of the principles will be given. Some sort of eustachian tube dysfunction is the principal predisposing factor.

Chronic Draining Ear

The diagnosis of chronic draining ear can be made on the basis of a reliable history. Typically, there is a chronic suppurative otitis media (CSOM) with a perforation. Perforations that occur at the margin are a special problem, because they are often associated with cholesteatomas, discussed later in this section. Chronic draining ear may also be a sign of mastoiditis. CSOM in the child with tympanostomy tubes is a particularly common problem, occurring in 5% to 10% of tube insertions.[69]

Recurrent Draining Ear

Recurrent draining ear should be the working diagnosis when an ear discharge is present intermittently. The diagnosis of otitis externa can be made if a perforation can be excluded, as discussed earlier in the chapter.

Persistent Middle-Ear Effusion

When an episode of otitis media results in persistence of middle-ear fluid for 3 months, as described in the preceding section, and the tympanic membrane remains immobile, consultation with an ear specialist is advisable.[70,71] Persistence of middle-ear fluid after AOM is more common in white children under age 2.[72]

Terms that imply knowledge about the character of the middle-ear fluid (such as serous otitis) or the mechanism of pathogenesis (such as secretory otitis) should be reserved for cases in which the physician is certain they are correct. Otherwise, the term otitis media with effusion (OME) should be used.

Rarely, the drum appears purple or blue as a result of bloody fluid.[73] Trauma can also cause this clinical picture.

Bone conduction (sound heard through the mastoid) is better than air conduction (sound heard through the external auditory canal). Sound from a tuning fork placed on the top of the skull is lateralized to the ear with the greater impairment of hearing.

If the ear is punctured for examination of the fluid early in the course of the illness, the fluid is usually thin and yellow (serous); later in the course, the fluid becomes more viscid and adhesive (glue-like), and the eardrum may appear retracted. Some authorities believe that production of fluid of these two consistencies is caused by different mechanisms rather than by differences in duration of illness,[74] but this remains unproved.

A spinal fluid leak into the middle ear is a rare cause of unilateral middle-ear fluid and can result from head trauma or without any recognized injury.[75]

Possible Mechanisms

Eustachian Tube Dysfunction

For all practical purposes, all children from birth to age 4 or 5 can be considered to have some degree of eustachian tube dysfunction, as the innervation of the tensor veli palatini muscle is not complete. A subset of children has very poor function: obstruction, reflux, and failure to clear middle-ear fluid are the most common dysfunctions. For example, cleft palate is invariably associated with OME secondary to eustachian tube dysfunction.[76]

Other Mechanisms

Risk of recurrent or chronic middle-ear infections may also occur or be increased by mechanisms independent of eustachian tube dysfunction. Defects of mucociliary action[77] or of protective immunologic mechanisms of the middle ear may also be involved in infection in the absence of true obstruction. The clearing of the middle-ear fluid of bacteria in *H. influenzae* or *S. pneumoniae* infection is closely related to whether a specific antibody can be found in the fluid.[78] Therefore, some children with immunoglobulin deficiencies have frequent otitis media (see chapter 23). Exposure to environmental tobacco smoke and day-care attendance both increase the risk of AOM. Breast-feeding is protective against AOM, probably because of the transfer of secretory IgA as well as a more upright feeding position in comparison to bottle-fed infants.[79]

Allergy

Hypersecretion of mucus on an allergic basis is another possible explanation of middle-ear fluid for-

mation without obstruction.[80] Obstruction of the eustachian tube by edema of lymphoid hypertrophy secondary to allergy has also been postulated.[81]

Disordered Mucous Production or Primary Ciliary Dyskinesia

Patients with cystic fibrosis are at risk of frequent otitis media. Ciliary dysmotility as a predisposing factor in frequent AOM is discussed in the section on primary ciliary dyskinesia, later in this Chapter (and in Chapter 23).

Infectious Causes

Recurrent Otitis

The bacteria in recurrent AOM are the same as those in a single first episode, except that in children who have undergone multiple courses of antibiotic therapy, the causative agents tend to become increasingly resistant over time.[82] Second episodes are more often new infections with a different pathogen than they are recrudescences of the old pathogen.

Chronic Otitis Media

Typically, these patients have had several courses of different antibiotics, so the nasopharyngeal flora and the middle-ear fluid often contain resistant bacteria. *P. aeruginosa* was recovered frequently on tympanocentesis in one study of 36 children with chronic otitis media.[83] Another study found *H. influenzae* most frequently in serous effusions (62%) and *S. epidermidis* (42%) in mucoid effusions.[84] *S. aureus*, viridans group streptococci, *S. pneumoniae*, enteric gram-negative rods, and anaerobes were also frequent. Bacteria have been recovered from tympanocenteses in the absence of middle-ear effusions in a carefully done study.[74]

Chronic suppurative otitis (CSOM) that has been treated with numerous courses of conventional antibiotics often is caused by penicillin-resistant *S. pneumoniae*. Many samples are culture negative.

When faced with a child with chronic draining ears despite multiple courses of antibiotics, the clinician should make sure the child does not have mastoiditis. An ENT specialist should examine the patient, and careful cultures should be obtained. Intravenous clindamycin and gentamicin should provide adequate antibiotic coverage pending the results of culture. Topical antibiotic drops may be simultaneously administered.

Viral or Mycoplasmal Infections

Viruses are certainly a cause of AOM, as described earlier. Viral or mycoplasmal infections have been proposed as a possible cause of OME, but there is little evidence to support this notion. Viral cultures of serous ear fluid rarely reveal a virus.[85] Outbreaks of some viruses have, however, been temporally associated with an increased frequency of OME.[85]

Chlamydia

Recurrent otitis media occurs twice as frequently in infants born to women who had chlamydia in the cervix.[86]

Other

Although *M. tuberculosis* is a rare cause of chronic otitis media, it is important to identify.[87] A chronically draining TM is usually found, often with associated hearing loss and sometimes with unilateral facial palsy.[88] Nontuberculosis mycobacteria and fungi are also occasional causes of CSOM and require specific culture mediator detection.

Treatment and Prevention

Culture of the ear drainage is sometimes helpful as a guide to antibiotic therapy in chronic otitis media. If there is a permanently perforated eardrum, the organisms often enter the middle ear from the outside, and enteric bacteria or *S. aureus* may be found. Systemic antibiotic therapy is often indicated for CSOM, but the perforation should be repaired if possible. Occasionally, the discharge is a primary foreign-body response to a tympanostomy tube. In this case, removal of the tube will usually result in abatement of the discharge.

A study comparing topical ofloxacin otic solution to oral amoxicillin-clavulanate for the child with tympanostomy tubes and AOM showed no significant difference in the cure rate.[89] Topical ofloxacin has good activity against *Pseudomonas* and is thus usually effective for cases of CSOM in children with tympanostomy tubes as well. Rarely, intravenous antipseudomonal agents are required.[69]

Chemoprophylaxis

In the recent past, children with frequent episodes of AOM were often given chemoprophylaxis to pre-vent the development of new episodes. Ampicillin was shown to be effective for prophylaxis of native Alaskan children with frequent purulent otitis media.[90] Chemoprophylaxis with sulfisoxazole was more effective than placebo in a study of New York children with frequent otitis media.[91] However, in this era of increasing antibiotic resistance among the organisms that cause otitis media, some experts question the wisdom of initiating chemoprophylaxis under any circumstances. In essence, chemoprophylaxis is designed to provide a continuous low concentration of antibiotic in the middle-ear space, a condition that, at least in theory, maximizes the chances of developing antibiotic resistance. There are no prospective trials evaluating whether chemoprophylaxis actually produces more antimicrobial resistance, but the setting is certainly ideal. Thus maximizing treatment by episode, and referring the most refractory patients for myringotomy tube placement is often a better option than chemoprophylaxis.

Vaccine Prophylaxis

The use of the polysaccharide pneumococcal vaccine has not proved efficacious[92] in the prevention of recurrent otitis media, except perhaps in asthmatic children.[93] However, the protein-conjugate pneumococcal vaccine is immunogenic in both otitis-free and otitis-prone children.[94] The vaccine also decreases, albeit modestly, the incidence of otitis media in vaccine recipients.[94a] All of the major serotypes of the pneumococcus that cause otitis media are in the conjugate vaccine, and presumably good antibody titers to these pathogens should be helpful in the host defense against otitis media. In some studies vaccination against influenza virus has been shown to decrease the incidence of AOM in children by approximately 30%.[95] However, a repeat randomized controlled trial failed to demonstrate a reduction in AOM in children give a inactivated influenza vaccine.[95a]

Other Therapy

Antihistamines and nasal decongestants are of unproved value, either alone or in combination.[96] An antihistamine was no better than placebo in one study of treatment and prevention of OME.[97] There is not much evidence supporting the pathogenic role of allergies in OME; therefore, most experts do not recommend referral to an allergist, even for those who seem allergy prone. Obviously, allergen avoidance pays other dividends to these patients.

Cigarette smoke exposure should be minimized. If possible, day-care attendance should be kept to a minimum, and children should be enrolled in small day-care centers if available. Breast-feeding should be encouraged. There is no scientific evidence to support claims that alternative therapies, such as chiropractic manipulation, homeopathy, or naturopathic remedies, provide any benefit to patients with frequent otitis media.[32,46a] Two studies from the same group showed that children who chew xylitol-containing gum have a reduced incidence of otitis media,[98,99] unfortunately, the age group that has the highest incidence of recurrent otitis media is too young to obtain these benefits.

Stopping the practice of allowing the baby to suck from a bottle while supine (bottle-propping) may eliminate many situations of recurrent otitis media.[100]

Complications

Hearing Impairment

Serial audiometric examinations of patients with AOM indicate some temporary hearing loss in the majority and persistent hearing loss in about 12%.[101] Because of the correlation between the appearance of the eardrum and hearing loss, audiometry should be considered at 6 and 12 months after a protracted episode of middle-ear space disease,[102] as such hearing impairment could potentially result in substantial learning and speech acquisition delays if not recognized.[103]

Extension of Infection

Brain abscess, meningitis, and lateral sinus thrombosis are rare sequelae of otitis media because the use of antibiotics has become widespread.[104] Mastoiditis (discussed later) is much more common than any of the preceding complications. The occurrence of infection in contiguous spaces other than the mastoid is rare, even in countries that do not routinely prescribe antibiotic therapy for children with otitis media.[30]

Paralysis

Facial nerve paralysis or oculosympathetic nerve paralysis (constricted pupil with ptosis) is rare but has been reported.[105]

Vestibular Symptoms

Occasionally, children with otitis media present with balance problems secondary to involvement of the vestibular system.[106]

Cholesteatoma

An enlarging mass of stratified squamous epithelium, a cholesteatoma is dangerous because it is invasive and can erode bone. It can begin with an invagination or perforation of the tympanic membrane. It usually is related to chronic adhesive middle-ear infection.[107] Adhesive OM refers to a condition caused by healing of chronic inflammation in the middle ear that leads to proliferation of fibrous tissue in the mucosal lining and impairment of ossicular movement. Rarely, a cholesteatoma is congenital[108] or the result of implantation of tympanostomy tubes.[109] On otoscopic examination, a cholesteatoma appears as white, shiny, greasy debris behind the tympanic membrane, often accompanied by foul-smelling discharge. It cannot be cured by antibiotics but must be removed surgically before it becomes infected and allows infection to spread to bone or brain. Cholesteatoma is usually a silent, painless disease.

Otitic Hydrocephalus

Bulging of the anterior fontanelle may be a complication of severe bilateral otitis media.[110] It can be secondary to increased intracranial pressure with spontaneous recovery, or less commonly, a result of lateral sinus thrombosis.

Referral to an Otolaryngologist

Referral for ear infection is indicated under the following conditions:[111–114]

1. For myringotomy for unusually severe pain, concurrent intracranial suppuration, or a suspected unusual pathogen in an immunosuppressed child. Myringotomy may also be indicated for children with persistence of acute symptomatic otitis media that progresses or fails to improve at all after reasonable first- and second-line therapy. In this case, myringotomy is not performed simply to allay symptoms, but to provide material for culture and antibiotic sensitivities. The timing of referral for this procedure may depend somewhat on the prevalence and severity of antibiotic-resistant pneumococcal

isolates in a practitioner's patient population. In general, there is a higher percentage of resistant organisms among patients with frequent otitis media, a history of recent broad-spectrum antimicrobial use, and day-care attendance. Even children who have never had even a single course of antibiotics may harbor drug-resistant organisms if they attend a day care or reside with siblings with recent antibiotic use.[115] Simple myringotomy in the office is usually not sufficient to facilitate adequate drainage of an effusion that persists after an ordinary episode of AOM.[116]

2. For tympanostomy tube placement for persistent (more than 3 or 4 months) middle-ear effusion, or for recurrent otitis media (four or more episodes in 6 months or 6 or more episodes in 12 months) when all other measures have failed. Tympanostomy tube placement should be performed at a time that will maximize its benefit. For example, it is often possible to avoid tympanostomy tube placement near the end of the respiratory virus season, when frequent recurrent AOM is likely to resolve anyway. Similarly, because the peak age of AOM is 6 to 24 months, if the child is approaching his or her second birthday, the frequency of middle ear infections is likely to decrease even without tube placement. Parents should clearly understand that improvement from the procedure is temporary (usually 6 to 9 months). Tympanostomy tubes have been associated with the long-term development of tympanosclerosis,[117] which can impair tympanic membrane mobility.

3. For mastoidectomy for simple chronic mastoiditis with draining purulent otitis media that fails to stop after 1 to 2 weeks of appropriate intravenous antibiotics[118] and for acute suppurative mastoiditis with postauricular swelling (see next section).

Studies on the value of adenoidectomy in the prevention of eustachian tube obstruction and recurrent otitis media have reached conflicting results; however, it is now generally believed that recurrent AOM in and of itself is not an appropriate indication for adenoidectomy.

■ MASTOIDITIS

Mastoiditis refers to infection of the mastoid air spaces and/or the bones that surround them. The mastoid air cells communicate with the middle ear, and their mucous membrane is contiguous with that of the middle ear. All purulent middle-ear infections, therefore, probably involve the mastoid air spaces to some degree. The clinical syndrome known as acute mastoiditis is a more severe involvement of those air spaces or bone in the infectious process. Pressure can build up in the middle-ear space when the tympanic membrane is intact and the eustachian tube is completely obstructed; this probably participates in the pathogenesis of acute mastoiditis.

Acute mastoiditis is an uncommon but not rare complication of otitis media. Although accurate numbers are not kept, acute mastoiditis is probably on the rise in the last few years.[119] This slightly increased incidence is likely not due to, as some have speculated, the decreased use of antibiotics in otitis media, but rather to the rise in resistant organisms due to the overuse of antibiotic therapy.[120] Mastoiditis occurred in 4 cases out of 6800 in a Dutch study of otitis media in which antibiotics were never given at the time of presentation but were reserved for patients who failed a trial of "tincture of time" plus pain medications. All patients had mild cases of mastoiditis that responded to oral antibiotic therapy no more intensive that what we use to treat uncomplicated otitis media in the United States.[30]

Acute mastoiditis should be suspected when otitis media is complicated by mastoid pain, tenderness, erythema, or swelling behind the ear. Often, there has been recent perforation of the tympanic membrane; drainage may or may not be ongoing at the time of examination. The ear typically is pushed forward and down by the postauricular swelling in children less than 1 year of age, whereas older children have a pneumatized mastoid process, and the ear lobe is elevated.[121] Radiographs typically reveal clouding or one or both mastoids and may show destruction and coalescence of mastoid air cells (osteitis). Mastoiditis may be considered an abscess; antibiotic therapy may help contain or localize infection, but surgical drainage is often required.

Chronic mastoiditis typically occurs in children with a chronic draining ear, who may have no physical signs of mastoid disease.

Computed Tomography Scans

Where there is clinical evidence suggesting intracranial complications, a cholesteatoma, or chronic mastoiditis producing a chronically draining ear, a computed tomography (CT) scan is usually helpful.[122,123]

Differential Diagnosis

Otitis externa may produce sufficient redness around the ear canal to resemble mastoiditis, but the tenderness is centered in the canal, not over the mastoid area. In otitis externa, there is often pain when the auricle is gently manipulated, whereas this does not usually occur with mastoiditis. A furuncle within the ear canal can produce swelling and tenderness, but is usually not associated with fever or "toxicity." Parotitis may push the ear out and can be mistaken for mastoiditis. Cellulitis or a wound infection behind the ear usually has a visible site of injury on careful examination.

Possible Etiologies

In acute mastoiditis, pneumococci, other streptococci, and *S. aureus* appear to be the most common causes.[121] *H. influenzae* and the bacteria found in chronic mastoiditis are less likely. *M. catarrhalis* is almost never seen.

In chronic mastoiditis or in acute mastoiditis complicating chronic otitis that has been treated with many courses of antibiotics, anaerobic bacteria, enteric bacteria, and *P. aeruginosa* are more likely.[124] In the last few years, we have seen several cases of acute mastoiditis caused by multiply drug-resistant *S. pneumoniae* in patients with frequent otitis media and numerous courses of broad-spectrum antibiotics.

Rarely, mycobacteria such as *M. tuberculosis* or *M. avium-intracellulare* will produce an acute or chronic mastoiditis in an immunocompetent child.[125]

Some patients with acute suppurative mastoiditis and cultures reported to be sterile may in reality have been infected with anaerobic upper-respiratory flora such as *Fusobacterium*.[126]

Treatment

For acute mastoiditis, a myringotomy should be done if the ear is not already draining adequately. Intravenous antibiotics (such as a third-generation cephalosporin) that cover the most likely pathogens should be given and adjusted in accordance with culture results. Antibiotic therapy should be continued for a minimum of 3 weeks; in cases with extensive bony involvement, 6 weeks is sometimes required. In one study, the mastoid radiograph played no part in the decision to operate, which was based on the presence of a subperiostial abscess,[127] manifested clinically by postauricular fluctuance. Some children in that study who had postauricular swelling thought to be small abscesses were managed with antibiotics alone or incision and drainage after needle aspiration. A few children thought to have acute disease were found at operation to have unrecognized chronic mastoid disease, including one cholesteatoma.

The authors of another study of acute mastoiditis recommended that children without a neurologic complication or subperiosteal abscess be treated with myringotomy and intravenous antibiotics and that the need for mastoidectomy be reassessed in those who fail to respond in 24 to 48 hours.[128]

In a chronically draining ear that fails to respond to two or more courses of oral antibiotics, a CT scan may indicate a chronic coalescent mastoiditis, which will usually improve after mastoidectomy. Antibiotic therapy should cover anaerobes and *P. aeruginosa*; for example, intravenous clindamycin and gentamicin, or the combination of ceftazidime or ticarcillin and gentamicin can be given until culture results are known. Many microbiology laboratories will not culture surface ear drainage for anaerobes. Ear drainage should be gram stained and, in chronic disease, stained for acid-fast organisms.

Complications

Unrecognized mastoiditis can extend to the brain or meninges, producing brain abscess or meningitis.[123,128,129] Even in the antibiotic era, complications of mastoiditis can occur: Goldstein et al. noted that 18 (25%) of 72 children with mastoiditis required total mastoidectomy for subperiosteal or Bezold's abscess (an abscess of the deep neck spaces), or cholesteatoma; complete or partial facial paralysis occurred in 31%; petrositis requiring mastoidectomy was found in 6%; and labyrinthitis was diagnosed in 7%.[130] Lateral sinus thrombosis is a rare complication.

■ SINUSITIS

Definitions

Sinusitis in children is a complex and controversial subject.[131–133] Dr. Ellen Wald proposed what is perhaps the most useful operational definition in her extensive studies of sinusitis in childhood; sinusitis may be reasonably diagnosed when children have symptoms of a common cold that last longer than 10 days without any improvement. This will be discussed in more detail later. Any sort of operational definition is better than the consensus definition from a symposium on sinusitis, which was "an inflammation of the mucosal lining of the paranasal sinuses." Sinusitis can be classified as acute if < 4 weeks in duration, subacute when 1–3 months in duration, and chronic if it lasts greater than 3 months.

Acute purulent sinusitis can be defined as pus in a sinus, as seen coming from an orifice of a sinus or found at aspiration of the sinus. Radiologic sinusitis can be defined as mucosal thickening, air-fluid interfaces, or complete sinus opacification. Sinus pain is pain in the area of a sinus, particularly under the maxillary or frontal bones. Other sinus symptoms include nasal discharge and obstruction, malodorous breath, and daytime cough. The problem-oriented diagnosis of sinusitis symptoms can be used when sinus roentgenograms are not done and the sinus openings cannot be directly observed. The particular sinuses involved should be stated.

Experimental Studies

Sinus pain has been well studied by experiments in adults using stimulation by an electric probe, heat and cold, or sinus pressure.[134] In the classic studies of sinus pain by McAuliffe and associates in 1943, it was found that the most pain-sensitive area is the mucosa covering the nasal openings (ostia) of the paranasal sinuses (Fig. 5-4). Although pain may be referred to the sinus cavity, the mucosal cavity within the sinus is relatively insensitive to pain.[134]

These investigators used a wire insulated by varnish to its tip to produce the faradic current stimulation. The same electric stimulus that was felt as 1+ pain on the tongue was felt as 4+ to 6+ pain on the nasal turbinates and 6+ to 9+ pain when applied to the sinus ostia. However, the same stimulus produced only 1+ to 2+ pain when applied to the mucosa in the frontal or maxillary sinus cavity.[134] The stimulus to the opening of the sinus cavity produced pain that was referred to a site other than the opening, namely, the cavity of the sinus. The pain was described as diffuse, deep, aching, nonpulsatile, and sustained. Pain in the back of the head or the neck never resulted from stimulation of the nasal mucosa. These investigators concluded that headaches not associated with turbinate engorgement or inflammation and not reduced by nasal vasoconstriction or nasal anesthesia are not caused by disease of the nasal or perinasal structures.[134]

Sinus pain and sinus symptoms are probably many times more frequent than true bacterial sinusitis. This is probably because of the common practice of diagnosing sinusitis when nasal symptoms are present and pain is referred to the sinuses. This fact may partially explain why somewhere between 30% and 65% of episodes of "sinusitis" resolve without therapy. It stands to reason that many cases self-diagnosed as sinusitis are really inflammation localized primarily to the nasal mucosa and might

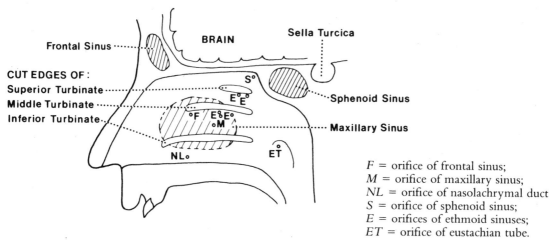

F = orifice of frontal sinus;
M = orifice of maxillary sinus;
NL = orifice of nasolachrymal duct
S = orifice of sphenoid sinus;
E = orifices of ethmoid sinuses;
ET = orifice of eustachian tube.

■ **FIGURE 5-4** Orifices of paranasal sinuses, nasolacrimal duct, and eustachian tube.

be more accurately called sinus pain or sinus symptoms.

Age Factors

The age distribution of sinusitis in children depends on the age at which the sinuses develop and are large enough to form a cavity that can be obstructed.[135] Development of the maxillary and ethmoid sinuses begins in utero, but these sinuses are not usually well enough developed to be clinically relevant until about the age of 2 years. The frontal and sphenoid sinuses are identifiable and can become clinically important by about 6 years of age, although most patients with clinical infections of these sinuses are at least age 10. In general, the younger the child, the less frequent the complaint of sinus pain, an observation that has been attributed to their relatively large ostia, which are less likely to be under pressure.

Predisposing Factors

Sinusitis follows retention of secretions, which may have several contributing factors: first, obstruction of the sinus ostia; second, decrease in number or function of cilia; third, a change in the production or the viscosity of the secretions. The most common predisposing factor is a recent viral upper respiratory infection; bacterial sinusitis complicates 0.5–5% of episodes of the common cold.[136] Mechanical obstruction can be caused by nasal mucosal swelling from viral infection, swimming, trauma, foreign bodies, polyps, or a deviated nasal septum.[131] Nasotracheal intubation may also lead to obstruction and the development of sinusitis in intensive care unit patients.[137] Ciliary function is abnormal in patients with primary ciliary dyskinesia (with or without situs inversus [Kartagener's syndrome]).[138] Viral infections, especially influenza or parainfluenza virus infection, can rapidly immobilize cilia, even in normal hosts.[131] Cigarette or cigar smoking also leads to inactivation of cilia on respiratory epithelial cells and exposure to environmental tabacco smoke alters nasal mycociliary clearance.[138a] Mucous secretions are abnormally viscous in patients with cystic fibrosis[139] and become abnormally copious in patients with respiratory viral infections. Patients with chronic rhinitis due to allergy and patients with asthma are prone to the development of sinusitis.[140,141] Occasionally,

---

> ### BOX 5-2 ■ Possible Predisposing Factors for Recurrent or Persistent Sinusitis
>
> Allergy
> Primary ciliary dyskinesia
> Wegener's granulomatosis
> Nonbacterial infection (i.e., fungal sinusitis—see text)
> Nasotracheal intubation
> Nasogasmic tube
> Cystic fibrosis
> Angiofibroma of nasopharynx
> Immunocompromised status
> Dental infection
> Cyanotic congenital heart disease

patients with deficiencies in immune function, especially humoral immune deficiencies, will have chronic or recurrent sinusitis.[142] Although this has not been well studied in children, one study of adult patients with HIV/AIDS showed a 54% prevalence of self-diagnosed sinusitis. Patients also self-reported that their sinonasal disease severity was significantly higher than that of mouth or throat disease, ear disease, or neck and salivary gland disease.[143] Finally, cyanotic congenital heart disease is frequently complicated by sinusitis (Box 5-2).

Association with Other Diseases

Purulent otitis media occurs with purulent sinusitis. Bronchiectasis is often secondary to or associated with sinusitis.

Cystic fibrosis should be considered in patients with chronic sinusitis or nasal polyposis.[139] Wegener's granulomatosis is a rare disease that may present as a clinical triad of chronic sinusitis, nodular or cavitary pulmonary lesions with hemoptysis, and hematuria.[144] Angiofibroma of the posterior nasopharynx typically occurs in adolescent boys and may produce refractory sinusitis because of obstruction.[145]

Midline granuloma is an extremely rare disease associated with sinusitis. Fungal sinusitis should be considered in immunocompromised individuals, but also occurs in healthy persons.[142] The prevalence of fungal sinusitis increases with the duration of the symptoms. Mucormycosis is fortunately a rare disease that should be considered when severe necrotizing rhinitis is observed in patients with diabetes mellitus or malignancy.

Primary Ciliary Dyskinesia (PCD)

Primary ciliary dyskinesia (PCD) is the term for diseases that are characterized by various ultrastructural aberrations in the dynein arms or radial spokes of the cilia of the respiratory epithelium of the nose, bronchi, and middle ear.[138] Also, the tails of spermatozoa are usually immotile because of absent dynein arms. Mucociliary clearance is defective because of the resultant inadequacy of ciliary motion. Acute sinusitis and otitis media are frequent, and eventually bronchiectasis occurs.[146,147] Children with PCD also often have chronic rhinitis, nasal polyps, absent or underdeveloped sinuses, chronic bronchitis, and recurrent pneumonia. The diagnosis can be made by electron microscopy of biopsies taken from the nasal mucosa.

A subgroup of PCD, Kartagener's syndrome, was described early because of its associated dextrocardia.[148] The syndrome is a triad of sinusitis, bronchiectasis, and situs inversus and is usually suspected if the chest x-ray is properly labeled as to left and right sides. In about half of patients with PCD, the heart rotates normally to the left during embryonic development, whereas the other half (those with Kartagener's syndrome) have dextrocardia.[149]

Acute Purulent Sinusitis

Acute purulent sinusitis, as mentioned earlier, is best defined as pus in a sinus cavity. This can be a relatively certain diagnosis if pus is seen to appear at a meatus immediately after the area is wiped or if pus is obtained by cannulation or puncture of a sinus.[131,132] Tenderness to pressure over a sinus and opaque transillumination, which are suggestive of sinusitis in adults, are not helpful in young children, although children may have pain on percussion.[135] This physical examination finding is part of the most clear-cut pattern of sinusitis in school-age children or adolescents, which is marked by leukocytosis, purulent nasal discharge, and sinus pain. Radiographically, there may be air-fluid levels visible in a sinus, but sometimes plain films are normal. The microbiology typically reflects the normal flora of the nasopharynx in children.

In younger children, sinusitis usually presents differently than in older children, often as a protracted common cold.[150] Fatigue, malodorous breath, nasal discharge that persists without improvement for 10 days, daytime and nighttime cough (probably by a respiratory reflex mechanism), and brief morning periorbital swelling have all been correlated with purulent sinusitis documented by sinus aspiration.[151]

In teenagers and adults, nasal allergy can mimic sinusitis and may respond to immunotherapy.

Other Patterns of Sinusitis

Subacute or chronic sinusitis is more likely to be related to an underlying disease. Anaerobes have predominated in studies of chronic sinusitis, but the usual respiratory flora may be found.[152] These patients are more likely to have pathogens that are resistant to standard antimicrobials. Studies in adults with chronic sinusitis have indicated a high incidence of fungal pathogens.[153] Fungal infections of the sinus produce a long-standing, indolent disease course. Allergic inflammation, especially in sinusitis induced by *Aspergillus* species, may predominate. Other black molds (dematiaceous fungi) are also commonly found. Although these molds are noninvasive, patients often develop problems secondary to pressure phenomena and may present, for example, with proptosis complicating the course of a chronic sinusitis.[154] The diagnostic criteria for allergic fungal sinusitis are as follows: radiographically confirmed sinusitis; presence of thick, black allergic mucini within a sinus, demonstration of fungal hyphae in the allergic mucini, absence of fungal invasion; and absence of immune compromise.[154a]

Diagnostic Approach

Clinical Diagnosis

Most children with acute, uncomplicated sinusitis may be diagnosed by history and physical examination alone, without resorting to either laboratory tests or diagnostic radiology. The criteria discussed earlier, namely persistent nasal drainage in association with a cold that lasts at least 10 days and is not improving, is a reasonable operative definition of sinusitis. However, it should be realized that this definition results in overdiagnosis of bacterial sinusitis. In both adults and children with uncomplicated colds, about 20–30% will still have symptoms of cough or nasal discharge after 10 days of illness.[136,155]

Radiography

The reliability of radiographic findings has recently been clarified. At one time, it was believed that many children had radiologic evidence of sinusitis even in the complete absence of symptoms. This belief was based on reviews of films obtained in children with head injuries. However, newer studies of patients who were carefully selected on the basis of the absence of symptoms indicated that radiographic abnormalities of the maxillary sinuses were rare and that children who had abnormal sinuses but who were thought to be "normal" really had respiratory complaints. In children older than one year, abnormal maxillary sinus radiographs are rare and generally indicate inflammatory disease.[156] Whether this disease requires therapy is another matter.

Certain radiographic views are good at showing sinusitis in certain sinuses: for example, the antero-posterior view demonstrates the ethmoid sinuses, whereas the lateral view shows the frontal and sphenoid sinuses. Visualizing the maxillary sinuses requires a Waters's view. Air-fluid interfaces and complete opacification are fairly obvious x-ray signs of sinusitis; mucosal thickening is less specific, but in the right clinical situation can still be helpful. The sinus mucosae should not be thicker than 5 mm in adults or adolescents, nor should they be thicker than 4 mm in children. An abnormal Waters's view x-ray coupled with clinical signs and symptoms of sinusitis correlates with positive culture on sinus aspiration 86% of the time.[157]

Computed tomography is an even more sensitive way to view sinus disease at any age. Unfortunately, however, it has been demonstrated that during the course of an uncomplicated common cold, most people have abnormalities of their sinuses by CT scan.[158] Thus, this imaging modality may be overly sensitive for use in the diagnosis of sinus disease and should be reserved for patients who fail to respond to therapy or who have historical or physical examination findings suggestive of suppurative complications of their sinus disease. A recent study in adults with chronic sinusitis showed no correlation between findings on CT scan and severity of clinical symptoms.[159] One final reason for discouraging the use of CT scans is their expense and inconvenience.

Clinical study shows that ultrasonic examination of the sinuses is not as sensitive as either roentgenography or MRI imaging, but may be useful for follow-up imaging in some cases.[160]

Cultures

Sinus aspiration can be done in selected situations by an otolaryngologist in the outpatient setting.[135,150] Quantitative culture of the aspirate aids in its interpretation. This is the gold standard that has helped define sinusitis syndromes.

Indications for maxillary sinus puncture include immunosuppression, life-threatening complications, and rarely, relief of severe pain. Culture in acute sinusitis yields the usual normal upper respiratory flora of children, with a predominance of *S. pneumoniae, H. influenzae,* and *M. catarrhalis.*[135] In chronic sinusitis, anaerobes are frequently found and may predominate.[152] As mentioned earlier, various types of fungi are also occasional causes of chronic sinusitis in children. Culture of the nasal surface correlates poorly with puncture cultures and is not recommended, although culture of pus from a sinus ostium after it has been wiped may be of some value.[135]

Children with cystic fibrosis are likely to have *P. aeruginosa* and anaerobes, as well as the usual respiratory flora, on maxillary sinus aspiration.[161]

Differential Diagnosis

The clinical diagnosis of sinusitis in childhood is fairly uncomplicated. However, there are other disease states that mimic sinusitis that must be eliminated (see Box 5-3), especially when making the diagnosis without radiologic guidance.

Treatment

Antibiotics

The first consideration is whether antibiotic therapy is indicated.[132] A placebo was almost as effective as amoxicillin in one study.[162] This result may be partially due to the fact that the study may have included people with "sinus pain" rather than a true sinus infection. There is little standardization in the

---

BOX 5-3 ■ Differential Diagnosis of Sinusitis

1. **Chronic or copious nasal discharge**
   Nasal foreign body
   Allergic rhinitis
   Rhinitis medicamentosa
2. **Persistent cough**
   Cough-variant asthma
   Cystic fibrosis
   Pertussis
   Atypical pneumonia
   Gastroesophageal reflux

diagnosis of sinusitis, especially in children. This problem has led to a lack of consensus in the approach to treatment. Careful studies of sinusitis in children suggest that improvement occurs relatively rapidly; within 48 hours, most children feel significantly better, defervesce, and have decreased cough.[152]

In an early study, antibiotic treatment of patients who met the clinical diagnostic criteria resulted in quicker resolution of symptoms than did treatment with placebo.[151] An attempt to replicate that study in 188 children with 10–28 days of "sinus symptoms" failed to demonstrate benefit over placebo using either amoxicillin or amoxicillin/clavulanic acid.[163] When bacterial maxillary sinusitis is present, therapy directed at the normal upper respiratory flora is effective.[152] Amoxicillin remains the drug of first choice, even in the era of antibiotic resistance, because high levels can be achieved in the sinuses. Amoxicillin-clavulanate offers the additional benefit of predictable coverage against beta-lactamase producing organisms such as *H. influenzae* and *M. catarrhalis*; its benefits must be weighed against its increased cost and side effects when compared with amoxicillin. Although studies in adult patients suggest that azithromycin[164] and clarithromycin[165] may both be fairly effective in the treatment of sinusitis, studies in children are lacking. Immunocytochemical study of the mucosal epithelia of adults and children with sinusitis (with and without cystic fibrosis) suggests that the pathophysiology of sinus infection in children may differ from that of adults,[166] which makes extrapolation of adult studies that much more hazardous. Clarithromycin is somewhat weak against nontypable *H. influenzae,* and neither clarithromycin nor azithromycin is consistently active in vitro against penicillin-resistant *S. pneumoniae.*

Traditionally, it was believed that a long course of therapy was necessary. Adults were generally treated for 21 days. Most experts are now treating adults with shorter courses, and for children a 10- to 14-day course is adequate. Longer therapy may be appropriate in certain situations (e.g., when a patient is improving greatly but is not completely well at the end of a 2-week course). Children with chronic sinusitis may require 3 to 4 weeks of continuous antibiotic therapy. Those who fail to respond to this course of antibiotics should probably be referred to an otolaryngologist for evaluation, sinus puncture, and culture.

Adjunctive Therapy

Decongestants

Oral decongestants and antihistamines have not been demonstrated to be effective. Topical application of vasoconstrictive drugs may have some initial benefit, at least in symptom relief. However, in addition to shrinking the nasal mucosa, they also tend to induce ciliary stasis. These medicines should be used judiciously because overuse causes rhinitis medicamentosa (rebound vasodilatation), worsening the patient's condition.

Normal Saline and Hypertonic Saline Nose Sprays

Although there is probably no harm in using over-the-counter normal saline nose drops or sprays, they have never been demonstrated to be effective as adjunctive therapy for children with sinusitis. In vitro, the benzalkonium chloride used as a preservative causes leukocyte inactivity and death. Studies attempting to find a clinical correlate of this phenomenon are ongoing. Nose drops may be used (in infants and toddlers) to loosen up mucus so it can be more effectively removed by bulb suctioning. Hypertonic saline, however, demonstrated no benefits and was associated with burning in 32% of recipients in a recent double-blinded, randomized trial.[167]

Other Therapy

Both intranasal corticosteroids and oral leukotriene receptor antagonists have been used for patients with sinusitis. Although some patients may benefit from these adjunctive therapies, their use should not be routine.

Sinus Puncture and Aspiration

Persistence of a nasal discharge in an otherwise asymptomatic child at the end of a 2-week course of antibiotics is not sufficient grounds for performing a sinus aspiration.[132] If there is clinical and radiologic evidence of persistent sinusitis after several 2-week courses of appropriate antimicrobials, aspiration of the maxillary sinus and irrigation is advisable. The Proetz irrigation procedure done by an otolaryngologist may also help frontal and ethmoid sinusitis.[132]

Antral puncture of the maxillary sinus by an otolaryngologist may be appropriate if chronic maxillary sinusitis does not resolve after one or two irrigations.[132] Some otolaryngologists do not lavage the sinuses in younger children but do the antrostomy when medical measures have failed, as both lavage and antrostomy require a general anesthetic.[168]

Complications

Extension of Infection

Acute frontal sinusitis may be associated with brain abscess, epidural abscess, or meningitis.[131,169] Orbital cellulitis (discussed in the next section) is an important complication of ethmoid or maxillary sinusitis.[170,171] Other complications include frontal osteomyelitis (Pott's puffy tumor), orbital abscess,[172] optic neuritis,[173] bacterial carotid aneurysms,[174] and cavernous or lateral sinus thrombosis (Box 5-4).[175] A recent review of suppurative complications of sinusitis in adults at one hospital showed that, of patients with established complications, 23% had epidural abscess, 18% each had subdural empyema and meningitis, 14% had cerebral abscess, and 9% had superior sagittal sinus thrombosis, cavernous sinus thrombosis, and osteomyelitis.[176] Antibiotic therapy for those infections should include coverage for anaerobes; for example, a third-generation cephalosporin plus metronidazole, or ticarcillin-clavulanate plus gentamicin.

Reactive or Parainfectious Meningitis

Acute sinusitis or mastoiditis is occasionally associated with a spinal fluid pleocytosis with a negative culture. The white cell count may sometimes be greater than 1000/mcL, but the glucose concentration is typically normal. This can be called "reactive meningitis" and is usually secondary to infection near the meninges that is not producing a true bacterial meningitis, as discussed in Chapter 9. The treatment for this kind of reactive meningitis should be vigorous and should consist of intravenous antibiotics like those recommended for central nervous system extensions of sinus infections, unless blood cultures or well-obtained sinus cultures reveal an organism that should be treated differently. The patient should be evaluated for possible brain abscess (see Chapter 9), although early in the acute stages of the illness any brain involvement may not be detectable by CT.

■ ORBITAL CELLULITIS

It is customary to make a distinction between periorbital cellulitis and orbital cellulitis.[177-180] Orbital cellulitis implies inflammation behind the orbital septum, as indicated by proptosis and limitation of eye motion. Fever and leukocytosis are usually present. Periorbital cellulitis (often called preseptal cellulitis) does not have the more serious findings of orbital cellulitis and is defined by redness and edema of the eyelids and periorbital area. Usually, it is unilateral. It has many possible causes, including severe conjunctivitis, local trauma, impetigo, insect bites, or infection with *H. influenzae*, *S. aureus*, or Group A streptococci.[177] It can be secondary to bacteremia, particularly with *H. influenzae*, without any apparent focus.[179] Facial swelling caused by maxillary or ethmoid sinusitis can be confused with periorbital cellulitis.

Cellulitis of the cheek area should be referred to as facial or buccal cellulitis. This disease (discussed in Chapter 6), once quite common, was often associated with *H. influenzae* bacteremia in infants and young children. It has, fortunately, become a rarity in the era of conjugate *Hib* vaccine use.

Mechanisms

Orbital cellulitis is usually an extension of an infection from a paranasal sinus or an injury near the eye. Sinusitis, usually ethmoid sinusitis in young children, is the usual source of the infection. A traumatic wound near the eye is an occasional source. It is useful to distinguish these two sources, because gram-negative enteric bacteria or *S. aureus* are more likely from traumatic cellulitis, whereas orbital cellulitis secondary to ethmoid sinusitis is usually caused by upper respiratory tract pathogens. Rarely, orbital cellulitis is an extension of a pustule or stye near the eye or of a dental abscess. In children 10 years of age and older, frontal sinusitis is a more likely cause of orbital cellulitis than is ethmoid sinus infection.

The orbital veins connect with facial veins without valves, so skin infections near the nose can be a source of orbital cellulitis. There are no lymphatics in the periorbital space, and edema tends to appear primarily in the upper eyelid, where the most loose tissue and potential space is present.

Orbital cellulitis secondary to frontal sinusitis requires aggressive therapy such as open drainage because of the proximity of the sinus to the brain.

Clinical Diagnosis

Redness and swelling of the periorbital area along with fever are sufficient for a presumptive diagnosis of periorbital cellulitis. Other common findings include headache and purulent nasal discharge. If there is proptosis, limitation of eye motion, eye pain, or decreased vision (Fig. 5-5), the diagnosis should be orbital cellulitis. Early proptosis may be subtle; tilting the child's head down and looking down on the head from the apex may reveal proptosis not evident from face-to-face examination. Loss of retinal vein pulsation indicates thrombosis, but often the fundus cannot be adequately examined because of the severe swelling of the eyelids. Bilateral proptosis is uncommon and suggests cavernous sinus thrombosis. Papilledema is usually not present but sometimes is observed if the eyelids can be separated enough to examine the fundi. The severity and toxicity of the illness may be made milder by preceding oral antibiotics. A spectrum of severity can be observed, ranging from periorbital inflammatory edema to cavernous sinus thrombosis (Fig. 5-6). A CT scan of the orbit may suggest an abscess, but operative drainage often is not necessary, especially if the onset is acute and not delayed by prior antibiotic therapy.

Laboratory Approach

Typically, there is a marked leukocytosis. Pus present in the eye or nose may be cultured, but the results cannot be considered as conclusive as a positive blood culture. Unfortunately, blood cultures are often negative. In one series of 59 cases, cultures were positive in only 6 (10%).[181] If the patient has a subperiosteal abscess, Gram stain and culture of material removed at surgery has the best chance of providing direct etiologic confirmation. Ethmoid sinus aspirate, if required for patient well-being, is also definitive.

Aspiration of subcutaneous fluid for Gram stain

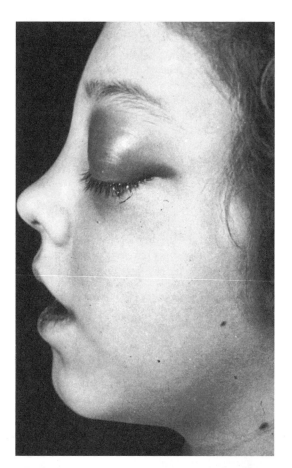

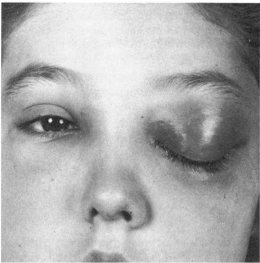

■ **FIGURE 5-5** Orbital cellulitis. Beta-hemolytic streptococci were recovered from pus obtained by operative drainage of the ethmoid sinus.

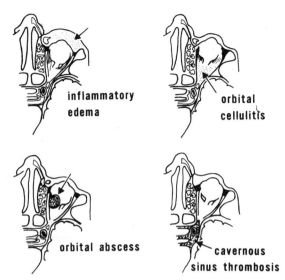

■ **FIGURE 5-6** Spectrum of severity of infection involving the orbit, from inflammatory edema to cavernous sinus thrombosis. (Chandler JR et al: Laryngoscope 1970;80:1414)

and culture is useful in cellulitis in many locations, but obtaining this kind of sample near the eye is a very precise procedure that requires the child to be completely restrained and preferably anesthetized.

Differential Diagnosis

Purulent Conjunctivitis

If severe enough, conjunctivitis (particularly gonococcal) may produce enough surrounding edema and erythema to cause periorbital cellulitis.

Adenoviral Conjunctivitis

In young children (5 months to about 2 years of age), adenovirus infection of the conjunctiva produces much more adnexal inflammation than it does in adults. Conjunctivitis due to this virus can produce a clinical picture difficult to distinguish from periorbital cellulitis. A series of 80 children referred to ophthalmology consultation for either periorbital or orbital cellulitis included 13 patients with adenovirus types 8 or 19. These cases occurred between December and March. A distinguishing feature on physical examination was the presence of a whitish membrane on the palpebral conjunctivae; this was seen in 12 of the patients on the initial examination, and the 13th developed it within 3 days.[182] A history of exposure to a playmate or a family member with recent ocular infection may

be helpful. The presence of preauricular nodes and follicular versus nonfollicular nature of the conjunctivitis did not prove to be helpful in distinguishing adenoviral conjunctivitis from periorbital cellulitis in this series of patients. As adenoviral culture of the eye takes about a week to become positive, culture is helpful only as a confirmatory test and for epidemiologic purposes. Rapid diagnosis is possible through PCR;[183] this test, if it is available, should be considered in infants and toddlers with the clinical picture described earlier.

Viral Infections Near the Eye

Herpes simplex can produce cellulitis in the area of the pustules, which may occur near the eye (Fig. 5-7). Secondary bacterial infection is often suspected because of the intense inflammatory reaction to the virus. Herpes simplex virus infections of the eye may be associated with gingivostomatitis.

Other Infectious Causes

Clostridial myonecrosis of the eyelid after trauma near the eye has been reported.[184]

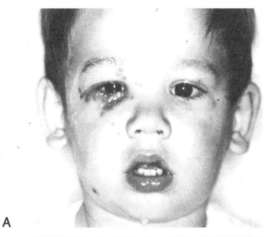

A

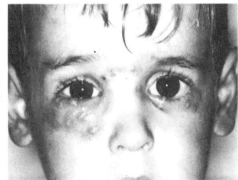

B

■ **FIGURE 5-7** Herpes simplex virus infection near the eye. Diagnosis was confirmed by virus isolations.

Idiopathic Orbital Inflammatory Pseudotumor

Inflammatory pseudotumors, when they occur in childhood, are almost always asymptomatic lung lesions found when chest x-rays are obtained for other reasons.[185] Extrapulmonary tumors are usually in the abdomen or pelvis, but they rarely may occur in the orbit. The tumor is nonmalignant and of unknown etiology. When it occurs in the orbit, it produces early-morning swelling, chemosis, conjunctival injection, proptosis, a palpable superior orbital mass, and limitation of eye movement.[186] Because biopsy often shows eosinophilic infiltration, a parasitic etiology might be considered. Papilledema or iritis develops in about one-third of children.

The edema responds to corticosteroids. However, because steroid therapy may allow bacterial orbital cellulitis to worsen, the diagnosis of pseudotumor requiring corticosteroids should be made with great caution.

Other Causes

Rhabdomyosarcoma is the most common primary malignancy of the eye in children. Sarcoidosis can produce supraorbital swelling.[187] Idiopathic orbital myositis can produce limited adduction, pain, and a swollen eyelid. These patients are neither febrile nor ill-appearing.[188] Retinoblastoma can present with a picture that closely resembles orbital cellulitis.[189] Of two reported cases of malignant lymphoma complicated by hemophagocytosis that resembled orbital cellulitis, one was in a 16-year-old female.[190] Rarely, other neoplasms such as Burkitt's lymphoma, leukemia, or Langerhans cell histiocytosis (Letterer-Siwe disease) can present with an orbital cellulitis-like picture. Finally, infarction of a facial bone, with resultant fever and proptosis, has been reported in patients with hemoglobinopathies.[191] Dysthyroid exophthalmia should be readily distinguishable from orbital cellulitis.

Possible Etiologies

The reported series of cases in orbital cellulitis have not included enough positive blood cultures to give reliable information about the frequency of various bacterial causes. It is clear, however, that the introduction of universal immunization against *H. influenzae* type b (Hib) has changed the microbiology of this disease. A retrospective report from a tertiary care children's hospital reported that only 1 of 70 cases of peri- and orbital cellulitis had a blood culture positive for Hib. This occurred in a child who was unvaccinated. They report no new cases of periorbital cellulitis and *H. influenzae* bacteremia in the 10 years from 1988 to 1998.[181] In a separate series of 133 blood cultures obtained from patients with orbital cellulitis, only two were positive for Hib. Of 101 patients discharged after July of 1987, none had a positive culture for Hib.[192] These reports are in contrast to earlier series, in which *H. influenzae* type b was the most frequently recovered bacterium in cases with positive blood cultures.

S. aureus is the most common cause when periorbital cellulitis develops following trauma or an insect bite. It is less frequently recovered from blood culture when the patient has ethmoid sinusitis as the source of infection and has not had previous antibiotic therapy. Pneumococci or beta-hemolytic streptococci are occasional causes.[180]

Gram-negative enteric bacteria or *P. aeruginosa* may also cause orbital cellulitis secondary to contaminated wounds. The frequency of *P. aeruginosa* is increased in patients with AIDS.[193] In one series of eight adult patients with AIDS and orbital cellulitis, *Aspergillus fumigatus* was the most common pathogen. This series also included two patients with *P. aeruginosa*.[194] There are no published series of orbital infections in children with HIV/AIDS. *P. aeruginosa* is a rare cause of orbital cellulitis secondary to conjunctivitis in very young infants.[195]

Fungal orbital abscesses are rare, but can occur, typically in patients with diabetic ketoacidosis. *Aspergillus* and the agents of mucormycosis are the most common pathogens. "Orbital apex syndrome," marked by paralysis of all the ocular muscles, may occur. Therapy includes intravenous amphotericin B and surgical debridement.

The larvae of *Echinococcus granulosis* can cause hydatid cysts of the orbit that may mimic orbital abscess. Patients present with noninflammatory proptosis and dull orbital pain.

Diagnostic Approach

Pus should be Gram stained and cultured, whether found in a wound near the eye, exuding from the conjunctivae, or present as a nasal or posterior pharyngeal discharge. Culture of the blood is positive in some cases and is therefore a useful procedure.

CT scan of the orbit may be useful to define an orbital abscess or subperiosteal abscess that may require operative drainage. CT should include narrow cuts of the frontal lobes. A preliminary report suggests that standardized orbital ultrasound may be more sensitive than CT scan in picking up subperiosteal abscesses.[196]

The use of lumbar puncture in the evaluation of children with orbital cellulitis has been on the rise; one retrospective study showed that 62% of patients underwent the procedure from 1985–1991, whereas only 14% had a spinal tap as part of the initial workup during the years 1979–1984.[197] Despite the increase in the number of lumbar punctures, the yield was no greater; in fact, only 2 (1%) of 214 patients had meningitis, and the diagnosis was strongly suspected in both prior to the procedure. In general, lumbar puncture is not indicated unless the patient either has signs or symptoms suggestive of intracranial complication, or meets other criteria for the performance of a lumbar puncture (e.g., very young with high fever, immunocompromised host).

Treatment

Hospitalization

Because of the severity of complications and the need for intravenous antibiotics, hospitalization is indicated in all patients with clinical findings suggestive of orbital cellulitis.

Antibiotic Therapy

Intravenous ceftriaxone, cefotaxime, or cefepime would be a logical empiric antibiotic if the source is sinusitis, because the usual pathogens are susceptible. Nafcillin or some other penicillinase-resistant penicillin should be included if the patient is less than 3 months old, if the Gram stain of the pus shows staphylococci, or if the infection is secondary to a wound and no satisfactory material is available for Gram stain. Gentamicin and nafcillin should be used initially if there has been a grossly contaminated penetrating wound. Anaerobic coverage should be added if the source was chronically infected sinuses or a dental abscess.

Duration of antibiotic therapy must be individualized. Usually, periorbital cellulitis is treated with IV antibiotics until redness and swelling is significantly decreased, then oral antibiotics are given for an additional 7 to 10 days. Patients with orbital involvement are usually given parenteral antibiotics for 1 to 2 weeks and continued on oral antibiotics with close outpatient follow-up to complete a 3- to 4-week total course of therapy, depending on the patient's clinical response.[170,197a]

Adjunctive Therapies and Measures

Patients need to have serial visual examinations. These may be performed at the bedside. It is helpful, if possible, to have all the examinations administered by the same person, to minimize interobserver variability. CT scan should be repeated if the patient is slow to improve on standard therapy, or if physical findings or clinical course suggest the development of a complication. If sinusitis is present, as it is in up to 96% of patients with orbital cellulitis and 81% of patients with periorbital cellulitis,[192] nasal vasoconstrictor sprays may be of value to shrink nasal mucosa and allow drainage through the meatus. Cocaine is sometimes used by local application by otolaryngologists, who should be consulted. Potent vasoconstrictors given by nasal spray are sometimes judiciously used.

For all cases of orbital cellulitis, early consultation with a pediatric ophthalmologist is strongly recommended.

Operative Drainage

Pus may be present behind or adjacent to the globe or in the subperiosteal area contiguous with the ethmoid sinus. Operative drainage by an ophthalmologist may be necessary if there is no response to adequate antibiotic therapy, particularly if visual acuity is decreased.[198]

Not all patients with CT findings of orbital abscess need to have operative drainage, as a trial of antibiotic therapy may produce resolution, especially if it is started early in the illness.[199] Periosteal abscesses are more prone to nonsurgical resolution than are true "orbital abscesses," in which the entire orbit is filled with pus. Pressure phenomena from the abscess can compromise vision; in such cases early drainage is advisable to spare visual acuity. Other relative indications for surgical drainage include age greater than 9 years, presence of frontal sinusitis, suspicion of anaerobic infection (presence of gas within the abscess space on CT), evidence of chronic sinusitis, optic nerve or retinal compromise, and infection of dental origin.[199]

Complications

Complications have been rare since the availability of antibiotics. Compression or stretching of the optic nerve may produce loss of vision. Exposure keratitis can occur if the proptotic eye is not protected.

Suppurative complications include meningitis, estimated to occur in about 2% of patients, cavernous sinus thrombosis and brain abscesses, which occur in about 1% apiece, and the more common local abscesses (subperiosteal abscesses occur in about 7% of patients). Cavernous sinus thrombosis usually is secondary to staphylococcal furuncles near the nose.[200] Eye involvement is typically bilateral, and retinal veins appear engorged. Pus in the anterior chamber (hypopyon) is a rare complication.[201]

Loss of vision to one degree or another occurs in approximately 1% of patients with orbital cellulitis. Primary or secondary optic neuritis can occur but is rare.

Usual Course

Typically, the cellulitis responds to appropriate therapy with lessened toxicity, a gradual decrease in fever, and a darkening of the skin color from pink or red to a darker red to purple. Swelling below the opposite eye may be expected to occur with improvement, as this subcutaneous tissue easily becomes edematous.

Progression from unilateral to bilateral eye involvement, with continued or worsening signs of toxicity, suggests the development of cavernous sinus thrombosis and requires immediate evaluation with magnetic resonance venography (MRV).

■ EYE INFECTIONS

Classification

Eye infections are classified by anatomic location.[202–204] Minor pustular infections involving the lids are common in children. Penetrating eye injuries and infections secondary to injury or foreign bodies are also relatively common. Corneal infection (keratitis) is relatively uncommon in children, as is chronic infection of the lid margins (blepharitis).[202]

Pustules and conjunctivitis can be managed by pediatricians and family practitioners, but the other eye infections discussed later in this section usually mandate consultation with an ophthalmologist. These more difficult infections are mentioned so that the physician can be aware of them and recognize the general principles and terminology involved.

Pustules

It is useful to distinguish two types of hordeolum. The first, and more common, is an external hordeolum, which is a superficial staphylococcal infection of a gland of Zeis (sebaceous glands that extend along the base of the eyelashes). This type of hordeolum is popularly referred to as a sty. A sty is a self-limited infection; with or without therapy they invariably point and drain within several days. Warm compresses may speed this process. Incision may lessen pain but is not necessary. There is no indication for antibiotic therapy for the common sty.[205] An internal hordeolum, on the other hand, is an infection of a meibomian gland. These glands are located within the tarsus and seldom drain spontaneously. Symptoms are considerably worse than those of the common sty. Therapy for an internal hordeolum consists of oral antistaphylococcal antibiotics and warm compresses.

The lacrimal sac may become infected, particularly if partially obstructed. Infants and young children with nasolacrimal duct obstruction are prone to this condition. The sac is located nasally, below the inner canthus. Infection of the lacrimal sac is called dacryocystitis. It occurs in acute and chronic forms. The infection is usually staphylococcal or pneumococcal but may be caused by other bacteria. A review of 54 cases of acute and chronic dacryocystitis revealed that two-thirds of cases were the chronic, insidious form.[206] The average age of all patients was 20 months, with a range of 4 months to 5 years. Chronic dacryocystitis was usually successfully treated by outpatient nasolacrimal duct probing; patients with acute dacryocystitis were admitted to the hospital for intravenous antibiotics with or without surgical intervention. One case was complicated by orbital cellulitis. In almost all cases, nasolacrimal duct probing was ultimately required.[206]

S. epidermidis and *S. aureus* can be cultured so frequently from asymptomatic persons that they can be considered normal flora.[202,207] Therefore, the clinical presentation and Gram stain of an eye discharge are essential in the infants without bowel control, gram-negative enteric bacteria can occasionally be cultured from the eye, presumably carried there on the hands.

■ CONJUNCTIVITIS

Conjunctivitis can be defined as a definite redness of the conjunctivae, with hyperemia and congestion of the vessels and various severities of purulent exudate. Preauricular adenopathy may be present. When the redness involves only the palpebral conjunctivae, it may be very difficult to be sure that conjunctivitis is present because the redness may be the result of hyperemia of all mucous membranes and skin with flushing of the skin and oral mucosa. When the vessels of bulbar conjunctivae are congested and hyperemic, the diagnosis of conjunctivitis can be made with more certainty.

In most cases of conjunctivitis, the redness is more prominent away from the cornea. Redness that is intense near the cornea suggests keratitis or iridocyclitis (discussed later). These conditions are often accompanied by pain, whereas acute conjunctivitis is more often associated with itching, burning, or a foreign body sensation. Acute conjunctivitis never causes a decrease in visual acuity; change in vision should prompt a search for other eye diseases.

Classification

It is useful to distinguish several syndromes of conjunctivitis (Box 5-5).

Nonpurulent Conjunctivitis

The two most common causes of nonpurulent conjunctivitis are allergy and viral infection; sometimes they are difficult to differentiate. With either cause, purulent exudate is minimal and usually is present only in the morning or after sleeping. Stasis and drying of serous secretions may also produce the appearance of purulence on awakening from sleep. With viral conjunctivitis, itching is not usually prominent, and symptoms are usually unilateral at onset, although the other eye often becomes secondarily infected. Sometimes the lymphoid follicles enlarge, producing a pebbly appearance called follicular conjunctivitis; this also usually indicates a viral cause. Adenoviruses of various serotypes are the most common infectious cause of this pattern in children. Patients may present with mild photophobia, a foreign body sensation, watering, and redness. Subconjunctival hemorrhage is occasionally present. A grayish-pink, friable membrane that adheres to the palpebral conjunctiva is the most specific sign of adenoviral conjunctivitis.[182] The membrane may be removed with a cotton swab, which affords a great deal of symptomatic relief. However, it may reform several times over a 3- to 4-day period and may bleed slightly when removed. Patients

---

BOX 5-5 ■ Causes of Various Conjunctivitis Syndromes

Nonpurulent
Adnovirus (frequent)
Allergy (frequent)
Herpes simplex virus
Ultraviolet light
Kawasaki disease
Measles

Purulent
Mild
  H. influenzae (nontypable)
  H. aegyptius
  Moraxella spp., especially catarrhalis
  Gram-positive anaerobes (susceptible to common antibiotics)
  S. pyogenes

Severe
  N. gonorrheae
  N. meningitidis
  S. aureus
  S. pneumoniae
  H. influenzae (in children less than 5 years)

Follicular
Adenovirus
Nontrachomatis chlamydiae (C. pneumoniae, C. psittaci)

Oculoglandular
Tularemia (Francisella tularensis)
Sporotrichosis, tuberculosis, syphilis (rare)
B. henselae (cat-scratch bacillus)
Adenovirus

Neonatal
N. gonorrheae
C. trachomatis
S. pneumoniae
S. aureus
Haemophilus spp.
Herpes simplex virus (rare)
Chemical (secondary to eye prophylaxis)
Rarely, other species listed under purulent

Hemorrhagic conjunctivitis
Enterovirus type 70
Coxsackie virus type A24
Adenovirus type 11 (occasionally, other types)

Otitis-Conjunctivitis Syndrome
H. influenzae (nontypable)

Keratoconjunctivitis
Adenovirus (several types)

often have contact with another person with conjunctivitis. Occasionally, a common source is implicated, such as a swimming pool. Prodromal upper respiratory tract infection signs such as pharyngitis or rhinitis are frequently present. Adenoviral conjunctivitis is highly contagious. The incubation period is approximately 5 to 10 days, but may be as long as 21 days. The virus is shed for 7 to 12 days. Total duration of adenoviral conjunctivitis is usually from 2 to 4 weeks.[205] Good hand washing is important in limiting spread. It is impractical to exclude children from day care for this period of time, and antimicrobial therapy is obviously of no benefit. Occasionally, a diffuse, punctate keratitis forms that outlasts the conjunctivitis. Treatment is symptomatic, with cold compresses and acetaminophen. If keratitis is severe, ophthalmology consultation should be obtained.

Allergic conjunctivitis is also quite common, and presents with itching and tearing as the most prominent symptoms. Usually both eyes are involved and often there are concomitant symptoms of allergic rhinitis. The presence of eosinophils in conjunctival scrapings supports the diagnosis, but their absence does not exclude allergy.[208] Allergic conjunctivitis may respond to topical or systemic antihistamines. Reduction of exposure to known allergens or immunotherapy for those with other signs of allergies may also be helpful.

Purulent Conjunctivitis

In this form, purulent exudate (pus) is present to a greater degree and throughout the day, and edema of the eyelids may be present.[209] Bacterial conjunctivitis may be unilateral or bilateral. Chemosis may be prominent. Gonococcal conjunctivitis is marked by copious, thick secretions.

Bacterial conjunctivitis outside the neonatal period is a self-limited syndrome, with resolution in about 1–2 weeks, even without therapy.[210] Any kind of topical antibiotic ointment or drops will shorten the course somewhat. As there is no particular therapeutic benefit of one preparation over the others, caregivers may be allowed the choice of therapeutic agents. Sulfa-containing eyedrops carry a small but real risk of allergic reactions including anaphylaxis and Stevens-Johnson syndrome, and the drops sting on application. Neomycin- or other aminoglycoside-containing preparations may induce an allergic blepharoconjunctivitis that is much more severe than was the original disease. Very young children with bacterial conjunctivitis (who may not tolerate ocular application of antibiotics) may be treated with oral antibiotics, if treatment is deemed necessary.

Rarely, bacterial conjunctivitis may be severe, particularly in the immunocompromised child. This form can be sight- and even life-threatening and requires prompt attention and intravenous antibiotic therapy. Gram stain of conjunctival material may provide guidance as to the initial therapy, which can then be changed if the culture results so dictate. Gram-positive cocci on original Gram staining should be treated with topical erythromycin or ciprofloxacin and with intravenous nafcillin or cefuroxime. If the Gram stain shows gram-negative cocci, treatment should be started with topical erythromycin in concert with intravenous cefuroxime or ceftriaxone.

Follicular Conjunctivitis

Some cases of conjunctivitis, particularly those that preferentially involve the palpebral conjunctivae, are associated with a prominent follicular pattern. Adenovirus accounts for most, but not all, cases of this syndrome. Four of 15 samples from patients with chronic conjunctivitis with a follicular pattern were found by PCR to be caused by nontrachomatis species of chlamydia, such as *C. pneumoniae* or *C. psittaci*, versus none of 24 control samples.[211] There are no data on this infection in children, nor are there sufficient data to ascertain the frequency of nontrachomatis chlamydial species as the cause of follicular conjunctivitis. In the patients described in the preceding study, short courses of antibiotics were insufficient to eradicate the clinical problem.

Oculoglandular Syndrome

This syndrome is characterized by conjunctivitis and ipsilateral preauricular adenopathy. The conjunctivitis is often in the form of one or multiple granulomas of the palpebral conjunctiva. In an endemic area, cat scratch disease is the most common cause, and both the conjunctivitis and adenopathy are painless. Tularemia may also cause this syndrome, in which case both the node and the conjunctiva are usually very painful.[212] Patients with adenoviral conjunctivitis quite commonly have a palpable preauricular node. In contrast, bacterial conjunctivitis is not typically associated with adenopathy.

Neonatal Conjunctivitis

The term ophthalmia neonatorum is giving way to "conjunctivitis in the newborn" or "neonatal conjunctivitis." In the developed world, many cases are averted by the use of prophylaxis, discussed later. Although many etiologies are possible, the most important agents of neonatal conjunctivitis are *Chlamydia trachomatis* and *Neisseria gonorrheae*. *S. aureus* is another cause that must be considered. *C. trachomatis* conjunctivitis may begin at any time between birth and age 3 weeks, but generally these babies present at about a week of age. *N. gonorrheae* conjunctivitis usually presents earlier. The discharge associated with *N. gonorrheae* conjunctivitis typically is copious and mucopurulent and rapidly reaccumulates after removal. However, etiologic diagnoses in neonatal conjunctivitis cannot be made by historic and clinical findings.

Babies who present in the first weeks of life with conjunctivitis should be investigated for an etiologic diagnosis. Gram stain and culture of the exudate should be obtained. Cells should be scraped from the lower palpebral conjunctivae for chlamydial antigen testing (e.g., by EIA or DFA), chlamydial culture, and/or a nucleic acid amplification test (where available). If gram-negative diplococci are seen on Gram stain, the baby should be hospitalized with a diagnosis of probable gonococcal infection. An investigation for disseminated disease, including a careful physical examination, blood culture, and lumbar puncture with cerebrospinal fluid culture should be performed. Disseminated disease is found only in a small percentage of patients, but proper treatment is imperative. Treatment for gonococcal conjunctivitis in the newborn is with ceftriaxone 50 mg/kg (maximum dose 125 mg) IV or IM. A single dose is usually sufficient to eradicate disease, but patients are often given multiple doses while awaiting the results of blood and cerebrospinal fluid cultures. Frequent saline irrigation of the eyes is an adjunctive therapy that may be helpful in patients with thick exudates. Patients with chlamydial conjunctivitis should be treated with oral erythromycin, 50 mg/kg/day divided into four doses and administered for 14 days. Topical erythromycin therapy is inferior to oral therapy because oral therapy eradicates carriage of the organism. Limited experience with azithromycin suggests it may also be effective, but trials are lacking.

Neonates with either gonococcal or chlamydial conjunctivitis should be evaluated for the possibility of syphilis and HIV infection.

Conjunctivitis-Otitis Syndrome

The association of unilateral conjunctivitis with an ipsilateral otitis media is usually caused by nontypable *H. influenzae* infection.[213] Patients with this syndrome should be initially treated with a beta-lactamase stable oral antibiotic. Concomitant topical antibiotics are not necessary.

Conjunctivitis in Immunosuppressed Hosts

Many opportunistic bacteria can cause conjunctivitis; *P. aeruginosa* is especially prominent. Primary fungal conjunctivitis almost never occurs, even in severely compromised hosts.

Acute Hemorrhagic Conjunctivitis

Adenovirus conjunctivitis is sometimes complicated by subconjunctival hemorrhage. Enterovirus 70[214] and coxsackievirus A24[215] are occasional causes of this disease.

Keratoconjunctivitis

In this pattern, the cornea is also involved, as suggested by corneal pain, and confirmed by the observation of subepithelial infiltrates on the cornea seen on slit-lamp examination. A foreign body sensation is also a frequent complaint. Severe or persistent foreign body sensation should prompt the physician to perform fluorescein staining and to refer the patient for slit-lamp examination. These patients should also have a close examination of the palpebral conjunctivae, as a membrane there (such as is seen in adenoviral conjunctivitis) can also produce the same symptoms (see previous discussion).

Patients with keratoconjunctivitis usually have a mucoid rather than a purulent exudate, and lacrimation can be prominent. The redness of the conjunctivae may be worse centrally than it is in the periphery. This pattern is unusual in children, but can be seen in outbreaks of adenovirus types 8, 19, and 37, which have been well documented in the United States.[216] Herpes simplex virus infection can also produce this pattern. Fluorescein staining followed by slit-lamp examination may reveal a dendritic pattern on the cornea. Patients suspected of having herpes simplex virus keratitis should be referred to an ophthalmologist on an urgent basis, as this infection can also be sight threatening. Such patients may or may not have simultaneous periocular herpetic skin lesions.

Differential Diagnosis of Infective Conjunctivitis

Conjunctivitis Associated with Systemic Diseases

Several systemic diseases, infectious and noninfectious, are associated with conjunctival involvement. Toxic shock syndrome, whether caused by *S. aureus* or *S. pyogenes*, is usually accompanied by a diffuse conjunctival injection. Children with Kawasaki disease almost always have conjunctivitis, which is bilateral, nonpurulent, spares the limbus, and usually affects the bulbar conjunctiva to a greater extent than the palpebral conjunctiva. Patients with Stevens-Johnson syndrome usually have conjunctival injection.

Periorbital Edema

Edema of the lids and congestion of the conjunctival vessels is difficult to distinguish from conjunctivitis, but the conjunctival tissue between the vessels is not excessively red. Migratory palpebral erythema and edema has been described in adenoviral pharyngoconjunctival fever.[217] In periorbital or orbital cellulitis, discussed earlier in this chapter, both edema and congested conjunctival vessels are present. Infectious mononucleosis and trichinosis are causes of periorbital edema and should be considered. One of the authors has been consulted on a patient whose initial manifestation of Henoch-Schönlein purpura was periorbital edema.

Conjunctivitis Medicamentosa

Over-the-counter decongestant-containing eyedrops can lead to a fairly severe conjunctivitis. It usually occurs after 4 or more days of use, but can occur after as little as 8 hours.[218] In a series of 70 patients with this condition, conjunctival hyperemia was the most prominent pattern, seen in 50 patients.[218] Follicular conjunctivitis was seen in 17 cases, and an eczematoid blepharoconjunctivitis was seen in a very small number of patients (3 of 70). Treatment of this condition consists primarily of discontinuing the use of over-the-counter eyedrops. On average, conjunctivitis persisted for 4 weeks after stopping the eyedrops.

Dysversion of the Lateral Eyelashes

Recurrent red, watery, sore, and itchy eyes in children may be due to this condition, in which fine, long, flexible lateral eyelashes curve inward and rub on the conjunctiva and cornea, causing the symptoms of the syndrome. This condition can be diagnosed by close inspection of the lateral eyelashes. Treatment consists of manual repositioning of the eyelashes. Failure to recognize this fairly common condition may lead to unnecessary use of topical antibiotic preparations.[219]

Ptosis

A droopy eyelid may appear to be a swollen upper eyelid, but no inflammation is present.

Allergy

This is discussed in the section on nonpurulent conjunctivitis

Nasolacrimal Duct Obstruction (Obstructed Tear Duct, Dacryostenosis)

Nasolacrimal duct obstruction may be either congenital or acquired. Infants with nasolacrimal duct obstruction will present with what appears to be chronic or recurrent episodes of purulent conjunctivitis. The eyes will be especially full of secretions just after awakening, and the parent may report that the eye is "sealed shut." The difficulty in caring for these patients has always been in differentiating true conjunctival infection from the symptoms that occur completely as epiphenomena of the obstruction to the normal flow of tears. A study looking at conjunctival culture results from 158 children with nasolacrimal duct obstruction and 176 normal controls revealed that the number and types of organisms grown in culture were the same in each group. Additionally, the rate of spontaneous resolution of infection that did occur was not statistically different.[220] These results suggest that frequent culturing and topical antibiotic therapy are probably not necessary in the management of these patients.

Pediatricians have long recommended nasolacrimal duct massage, which is done by placing the tip of the fifth finger between the inner canthus of the eye and the bridge of the nose and gently rolling it downward and centrally for 5 minutes at a time several times a day. However, no studies document the efficacy of this therapy. Most cases spontaneously resolve with growth, although some require surgical probing. Patients who develop dacryocystitis almost always end up requiring surgical care.[206]

Neonatal Conjunctivitis Prophylaxis

Erythromycin 0.5% ointment, tetracycline 1% ointment, and silver nitrate 1% solution are all effective in preventing gonorrheal ophthalmia neonatorum. However, none effectively prevents chlamydial conjunctivitis.[222-224] None of the prophylactic regimens is 100% effective in preventing gonococcal infection, however, especially if there has been prolonged rupture of membranes or if the mother's disease is severe. A single trial showed that a 2.5% solution of povidone-iodine was a more effective prophylactic agent against *C. trachomatis* than either silver nitrate or erythromycin, and it was equally effective against *N. gonorrheae*.[224]

Nongonococcal, nonchlamydial neonatal conjunctivitis can also be prevented by these agents. A large, prospective, randomized trial of silver nitrate versus either erythromycin ointment or no prophylaxis showed that both preparations decreased the incidence of conjunctivitis in the first 2 months of life in babies born to mothers who were carefully screened to exclude the presence of *N. gonorrheae* infection. Overall, 107 (17%) of 630 neonates developed mild conjunctivitis, most within the first 2 weeks of life.[225] The authors concluded that parental choice of prophylaxis agent including no prophylaxis at all is reasonable if the mother has had good prenatal care and is carefully screened for sexually transmitted diseases during pregnancy.

■ KERATITIS

Keratitis (corneal inflammation) typically is unilateral and produces pain as well as a foreign body sensation. Aside from outbreaks of adenovirus keratoconjunctivitis (discussed previously), keratitis is an uncommon condition in childhood. Because infection of the cornea may lead to scarring, corneal rupture, and loss of vision, this condition is potentially urgent, and patients suspected of having keratitis should be referred to the care of an ophthalmologist as quickly as possible. Keratitis should be suspected when eye symptoms such as pain, lacrimation, and photophobia are severe.[226] Fluorescein staining in the pediatrician's office may reveal corneal ulcers.

Herpes simplex virus is the leading cause of keratitis in the developed world, but its incidence in childhood is low.[227] Damage to vision rarely occurs in primary keratitis in childhood, but some loss of vision may be difficult to prevent even with antiviral eyedrops.[209] The infection is usually unilateral. The virus typically produces a dendritic (branching) lesion, although sometimes the lesion is ameboid. The diagnosis can be strongly suspected on clinical grounds; scraped stromal specimens may be used for viral culture. Local therapy with a topical antiviral agent (usually trifluridine) is the treatment of choice. The use of topical steroids in the eye is dangerous because herpetic infection may be made more severe by steroids. Paradoxically, severe cases, especially those involving the stroma, may require the anti-inflammatory action of a topical steroid;[227,228] the management is complex and requires expert attention. Steroids, if used, are weaned as quickly as possible.[205] Steroids can also produce side effects of ocular hypertension and posterior subcapsular cataracts.[225] There is no benefit to the addition of oral acyclovir to the regimen.[229] Even after successful treatment, recurrence is seen in 30–50% of adult patients.[205]

Other viruses of the herpesvirus group also can produce keratitis, but do so less frequently than herpes simplex virus (HSV-1). Keratitis from varicella zoster virus (VZV) occurs during primary chickenpox on rare occasions.[230] VZV more commonly causes keratitis upon endogenous reactivation (zoster); the disease is known as herpes zoster ophthalmicus. As in most cases of zoster (shingles), waning cellular immunity is the harbinger of this condition; therefore it is seen in childhood mostly in the setting of immune deficiency syndromes. Dendritic lesions of the cornea may be seen, but they are usually slightly different from those of HSV and far less destructive. Dendritic keratitis mimicking that of HSV has also been reported from Epstein-Barr virus (EBV) infection. Cytomegalovirus (CMV) can cause keratitis; this infection is usually accompanied by retinitis and is seen in immune-suppressed patients. Measles virus, which commonly causes conjunctivitis, occasionally involves the cornea. In healthy, well-nourished children, it is transient and resolves without therapy. It can be devastating in children with vitamin A deficiency.

Bacterial keratitis can be acute and destructive. A scratched cornea or foreign body is a frequent predisposing factor, especially if bacterially contaminated eyedrops have been used. Contact lens wearers have an 80-fold increased risk of acquiring this disease.[231] The risk for patients who use extended wear lenses is three to eight times higher still.[232] A prospective trial has shown that it is primarily the wearing of contact lenses for extended periods of time (as opposed to the material used to make the contacts) that predisposes to infection.[233] *P. aeruginosa* is the most common pathogen in cases attributed to infection following overnight wear of soft contact lenses.[205] This pathogen can produce a very fulminant keratitis, with subsequent loss of the eye.[233] *S. aureus* and the pneumococcus are the most frequent causes of bacterially infected corneal ulcers not associated with soft contact lens wear.[234]

Rare bacterial causes include *Listeria,* many members of the Enterobacteriaceae family, atypical mycobacteria, *Nocardia,* anaerobes such as *Propionibacterium acnes, Peptostreptococcus,* and others. *Shigella* keratitis has been reported. It can be treated with topical neomycin-bacitracin-polymyxin or topical sulfa or gentamicin ophthalmic preparations.[235] Enterobacteriaciae such as *Serratia marcescens* infections are hard to prevent because the concentrations of antibacterials that would need to be in contact lens solutions to prevent their growth are toxic to the eye.[236]

Fungi can also be a cause of keratitis, especially after a corneal injury from a branch or a stick of wood. A variety of fungal species have been implicated. Most are soil saprophytes. Fungi with septate, branching hyphae such as *Aspergillus* species are common in hot, humid climes near the equator, whereas in the southern United States pigmented fungi such as *Curvularia* predominate, and in the northern United States and Canada, *Candida* species are the most frequent pathogens. Amebic keratitis can also occur from contact lens wear and tends to be severe. The rarity of corneal infections is a testament to the powerful antibacterial activity of tears and the resilience of an intact corneal epithelial layer. One study, which cultured contact lens cases of 101 lens wearers who used hydrogen peroxide as a disinfectant and only used commercial saline solutions, showed that 81% of the cases were contaminated. Seventy-seven percent were positive for bacterial pathogens, 24% for fungi, and 20% for protozoa. Acanthameba were found in 8%. All bacteria isolated produced catalase, which inactivates hydrogen peroxide.[237] Contact lens wearers should be encouraged to scrub their lens cases frequently, to wash them in very hot water, and to allow them to air dry between uses.

Laboratory evaluation of keratitis should include a direct microscopic examination and culture of a corneal scraping for fungi, as well as a Gram stain and bacterial culture. Culture yield may be increased by using BactoR2A low-nutrient agar.[238]

Dendritic or ameboid keratitis should be cultured for viruses, particularly HSV.

Bacterial keratitis is treated with local and systemic antibiotics after culture is obtained. Traditionally, two antimicrobials have been used, but monotherapy with fluoroquinolones has been popular since a topical preparation became available.[205] However, ciprofloxacin-resistant isolates of *P. aeruginosa* are beginning to be a problem.[239] Mycotic keratitis is usually treated with local application of amphotericin B solution. Steroids or antibacterial antibiotics may make fungal keratitis worse.

Congenital syphilis is a cause of interstitial stromal keratitis. Clinical manifestations usually begin sometime between the ages of 5 and 25 years. The condition begins as a peripheral corneal inflammation and progresses centrally. It is usually bilateral and may impair vision significantly.

Noninfectious causes include keratitis, ichthyosis, and deafness (KID) syndrome;[240] Cogan's syndrome, which is a vasculitic disorder of unknown etiology;[241] incontinentia pigmenti;[242] and tyrosinemia type II, in which tyrosine builds up in the cornea and induces an inflammatory reaction.[243] Abuse of topical anesthetic drops can also cause a ring keratitis.[244]

■ UVEITIS

Uveitis is inflammation of the uveal tract (iris, ciliary body, and choroid). It is usually classified as anterior (iridocyclitis) or posterior (chorioretinitis). Uveitis can be secondary to a number of causes including trauma, chemical irritation, pauciarticular rheumatoid arthritis, a nearby infectious process, or sarcoidosis.[245] In most cases, however, the cause cannot be found, and it is referred to as endogenous uveitis or uveitis of obscure etiology.

Iridocyclitis

Clinical Picture

Acute iridocyclitis may resemble conjunctivitis because of the redness of the conjunctiva, but iridocyclitis is usually associated with pain and is much more serious than conjunctivitis, being a true ophthalmologic emergency. It is distinguished from conjunctivitis by the photophobia and the prominent inflammation near the cornea. The individual blood vessels are not as well seen as in conjunctivitis, and they do not move with the conjunctivae. There may be a slight constriction of the affected pupil, which may be irregular. There is absence of purulent secretions, although tearing may be present. The iridocyclitis of juvenile rheumatoid arthritis (JRA) is insidious and may be entirely asymptomatic.

Etiologies

Many of the herpesviruses have been implicated. Herpes simplex virus usually produces iridocyclitis in association with corneal disease, discussed earlier. EBV produces a follicular conjunctivitis in a small percentage of children with infectious mononucleosis, and a subset of them may develop iridocyclitis. VZV rarely produces an anterior uveitis during primary chickenpox and can also produce the disease on reactivation, sometimes in the absence of typical zosteriform skin lesions.[246] HHV-6 infection has been implicated in the onset and reactivation of some cases of iridocyclitis associated with JRA.[247] Finally, CMV may cause an anterior uveitis, although it usually causes a chorioretinitis. The disease is usually asymptomatic and occurs in patients with advanced AIDS or other severe immune suppression.

Several ocular complications are seen in primary mumps virus infection. The most common of these is dacryoadenitis, but conjunctivitis, scleritis, keratitis, and iridocyclitis can also be seen.[248] Enteroviruses such as coxsackievirus A24 and enterovirus 71 cause a follicular conjunctivitis that is rarely associated with iridocyclitis. At least two large outbreaks of echovirus 11 that caused fairly severe uveitis in babies and toddlers have been reported from eastern Europe;[249] to date, similar outbreaks have not been seen in the United States. Kawasaki disease had uveitis as an early finding in 66% of cases in one series.[250]

Mycobacterium tuberculosis can infect any part of the eye; iridocyclitis due to *M. tuberculosis* has been reported in a 2-year-old girl who lived in a nonendemic area.[251]

Syphilis is a possible cause of chronic iridocyclitis. It may occur in conjunction with interstitial keratitis, which is a late finding of congenital syphilis, or it may arise during secondary syphilis. Any patient suspected of having syphilitic iridocyclitis should undergo lumbar puncture to rule out asymptomatic neurosyphilis. Leptospirosis and Rocky Mountain spotted fever are rare causes of acute uveitis, but typically there are more prominent manifestations of the disease.

Acute iridocyclitis can be produced by rheumatoid disease, although a chronic iritis with insidious onset is more frequent. The iritis can be detected late in the disease by recognition of irregular pupils, but regular slit-lamp examination is needed for early detection of clinically silent iritis in children with pauciarticular juvenile rheumatoid arthritis (JRA). Rarely, iridocyclitis may be the presenting symptom of undiagnosed JRA. Young girls with pauciarticular disease who are antinuclear antibody (ANA) positive are at particular risk. They should be screened every 3 to 4 months.[252] Other noninfectious causes include tubointerstitial nephritis with uveitis (TINU syndrome),[253] a disease of unknown etiology seen in adolescents; bilateral iridocyclitis with retinal capillaritis (BIRC),[254] another syndrome of questionable etiology seen mostly in teenagers; and sarcoidosis.[255] Iridocyclitis also has been reported as an adverse reaction to chronic ibuprofen use.[256]

Chorioretinitis

Chorioretinitis can be congential or acquired. Congenital chorioretinitis is usually suspected in newborn or young infants because of other associated defects, as described in Chapter 19. However, it is sometimes first detected by routine funduscopic examination. Acquired chorioretinitis is usually first recognized because of decreased vision or floating spots or specks.

Etiologies

Toxoplasmosis is probably the most frequent cause of congenital chorioretinitis and is discussed in Chapter 19. Cytomegalovirus is a rare cause of congenital chorioretinitis. Chorioretinitis recognized in infancy and childhood usually is secondary to congenital toxoplasmosis but can be an acquired disease.[257] Diagnosis can usually be made clinically. PCR of vitreous fluid can be a useful diagnostic test in patients with chorioretinitis in which the diagnosis is in doubt.[258] *Toxocara canis* infection, caused by ingestion of dog roundworm ova, is an occasional cause of acquired chorioretinitis. It typically is associated with eosinophilia.

Chorioretinitis is commonly found in patients with the syndrome of congenital varicella zoster infection. However, in utero primary varicella zoster virus infection sometimes causes unrecognized retinitis. For this reason, any patient who presents within the first year of life with zoster should be referred to an ophthalmologist for retinal examination.[259]

Rare infectious causes of acute chorioretinitis include tuberculosis, histoplasmosis and other granulomatous disease, amebiasis, coxsackie B4 virus,[260] and herpes simplex virus. Rarely, chorioretinitis complicates Epstein-Barr virus–induced infectious mononucleosis.[261] Secondary syphilis can also produce chorioretinitis, usually in immunosuppressed patients.[262] Lyme disease (*Borrelia burgdorferi* infection) can cause either bilateral or unilateral choioretinitis.[263] *Bartonella henselae* (the cat scratch bacillus) has been associated with a neuroretinitis and stellate pattern seen on the retina.[264] Optic nerve involvement is common, and a small percentage have residual visual loss after the acute illness has resolved.[265] No treatment benefit has been proven by controlled trial, but the combination of doxycycline and rifampin for 4 to 6 weeks produced quicker resolution than that seen in historical controls.[266]

Aicardi syndrome has a characteristic chorioretinopathy and neurological defects and can resemble the clinical appearance of severe congenital toxoplasmosis.[267] The infants are typically females, with infantile spasms, mental retardation, and vertebral anomalies. The etiology is unknown. Children with chronic granulomatous disease frequently have "punched out" retinal lesions with pigment clumping. Nine (24%) of 38 patients and 3 (8%) of 36 carriers were noted to have retinal pathology on slit-lamp examination.[268]

Cytomegalovirus chorioretinitis has been observed in immunosuppressed adults with renal allografts.[269] Disseminated cryptococcosis has also been described as a cause of chorioretinitis in severe immune suppression.[270]

Eye involvement occurs in about 50% of patients with subacute sclerosing panencephalitis. Usually the eye problems occur at the same time as other neurologic symptoms, but can precede them by weeks or even months.[271]

Treatment

A mydriatic such as 1% atropine is the emergency treatment for acute iridocyclitis pending identification of its cause. Local, or even systemic, corticosteroids may be indicated, but an ophthalmologist should be consulted. For recently detected ocular toxoplasmosis, steroids plus antiparasitic chemotherapy with pyrimethamine, sulfadiazine, and foli-

nic acid are indicated. A recent phase I trial showed that atovaquone was well tolerated in 17 patients with ocular toxoplasmosis. All patients showed signs of improvement within 1 to 3 weeks of starting therapy, and visual acuity improved from a mean of 20/200 to a mean of 20/25 during an average follow-up length of 10 months.[272] Further study will be needed, but this approach looks promising.

Complications

Acute iridocyclitis may become chronic and lead to posterior synechiae (adhesions), cataract formation, or glaucoma.

■ INTRAOCULAR INFECTIONS

Pus in the anterior chamber of the eye is called a hypopyon. It can be an extension of a bacterial infection within the eye, or it can be a sterile reaction to a corneal infection. Blood in the same area is called a hyphema and is usually a result of an injury to the eye.

Penetrating eye injuries carry a great risk of infection within the eye (endophthalmitis), and antibiotic prophylaxis is advisable. An 8-year-old boy with endophthalmitis secondary to an intraocular graphite pencil lead has been reported.[273] Nafcillin and gentamicin is a reasonable combination. An ophthalmologist should be consulted. Intravitreous or subscleral administration of antibiotics is often indicated, especially in severe or relapsing cases.

Endophthalmitis also occurs after eye surgery, although the incidence of postsurgical infection is low, 0.09% in one large series.[274] The microorganisms isolated from postoperative endophthalmitis do not differ much from those of posttraumatic infection; the incidence of gram-negative organisms and fungi may be slightly higher.[275,276] No direct comparison has been performed. *Propionibacterium acnes* is a fairly common cause of late-onset, insidious postoperative endophthalmitis.[277] Finally, *Bacillus cereus* deserves special mention as a cause of this infection. Usually associated with food poisoning, *B. cereus* is an uncommon but devastating pathogen in endophthalmitis.

Candidal endophthalmitis may occur in premature infants, usually in association with candidemia and disseminated candidal infection.[278] In adult patients, the incidence of endophthalmitis in patients with systemic candidal infection is considerably lower than it once was, presumably secondary to a trend toward rapid institution of antifungal therapy.[279] No thorough review of the incidence in neonatal intensive care units has been published, but experience suggests that the adult data are being mirrored in the premature babies. Amphotericin B is the drug of choice.

Ceftazidime penetrates aqueous humor well and is probably useful in penetrating eye injuries when gram-negative enteric bacilli, especially *Pseudomonas* species, are suspected.[280]

■ REFERENCES

1. Bluestone CD. Recent advances in the pathogenesis, diagnosis, and management of otitis media. Pediatr Clin North Am 1981;28:727–55.
2. Klein JO, Bluestone CD. Acute otitis media. Pediatr Infect Dis 1982;1:66–73.
3. Groothuis JR, Sell SHW, Wright PF, et al. Otitis media in infancy: tympanometric findings. Pediatrics 1979;63:435–42.
4. Lampe RM, Weir MR, Spier J, et al. Acoustic reflectometry in the detection of middle ear effusion. Pediatrics 1985;76:75–8.
5. Brooks I. A' practical technique for tympanocentesis for culturing aerobic and anaerobic bacteria. Pediatrics 1980;65:626–7.
6. Pelton SI, Teele DW, Shurin PA, et al. Disparate cultures of middle ear fluids: results from children with bilateral otitis media. Am J Dis Child 1980;134:951–3.
7. Henderson FW, Collier AM, Sanyal MA, et al. A longitudinal study of respiratory viruses and bacteria in the etiology of acute otitis media with effusion. N Engl J Med 1982;306:1377–83.
8. Baker RB. Is ear pulling associated with ear infection [letter]? Pediatrics 1992;90:1006–7.
9. Schwartz RH, Rodriguez WJ, Sait T. The gray bulging immobile eardrum. an important sign of acute otitis media. Pediatr Infect Dis 1983;2:173.
10. Schwartz RH, Rodriguez WJ, Brook I, et al. The febrile response in acute otitis media. JAMA 1981;245:2057–8.
11. Schwartz RH, Hayden GF, Rodriguez WJ, et al. Leukocyte counts in children with acute otitis media. Pediatr Emerg Care 1986;2:10–4.
12. Brook I. Otitis media in children: a prospective study of aerobic and anaerobic bacteriology. Laryngoscope 1979;89:992–7.
13. Liederman EM, Post JC, Aul JJ, et al. Analysis of adult otitis media: polymerase chain reaction versus culture for bacteria and viruses. Ann Otol Rhinol Laryngol 1998;107:10–6.
14. Tetzlaff TR, Ashworth C, Nelson JD. Otitis media in children less than 12 weeks of age. Pediatrics 1977;59:827–32.
15. Bonadio WA, Jeruc W, Anderson Y, Smith D. Systemic infection due to group B beta-hemolytic streptococcus in children. A review of 75 outpatient-evaluated cases during 13 years. Clin Pediatr 1992;31:230–3.
16. Riding KH, Bluestone CD, Michaels RH, et al. Microbiology of recurrent and chronic otitis media with effusion. J Pediatr 1978;93:729–43.
17. Shaw CB, Obermyer N, Wetmore SJ, et al. Incidence of adenovirus and respiratory syncytial virus in chronic otitis media with effusion using the polymerase chain reaction. Otolaryngol Head Neck Surg 1995;113:234–41.
18. Pitkaranta A, Virolaiinen A, Jerro J, et al. Detection of rhinovirus, respiratory syncytial virus and coronavirus infection in acute otitis media by reverse transcriptase polymerase chain reaction. Pediatrics 1998;102:291–5.
19. Chonmaitree T, Howie VM, Truant AL. Presence of respiratory viruses in middle ear fluids and nasal wash specimens from children with acute otitis media. Pediatrics 1986;77:698–702.
20. Patel JA, Reisner B, Vizirinia N, et al. Bacteriologic failure of amoxicillin-clavulanate in treatment of acute otitis media caused by nontypeable *Haemophilus influenzae*. J Pediatr 1995;126:799–806.
21. Heikkinen T, Thint M, Chonmaitree T. Prevalence of various respiratory viruses in the middle ear during acute otitis media. N Engl J Med 1998;340:260–4.
22. Fisher RG, Gruber WC, Edwards KM, et al. Twenty years of outpatient respiratory syncytial virus infection: a framework for vaccine efficacy trials. Pediatrics 1997;2:e7.
23. Rifkind D, Chanock R, Kravetz H, et al. Ear involvement (myringitis) and primary atypical pneumonia following inoculation of volunteers with Eaton agent. Am Rev Resp Dis 1962;85:479–89.
24. Roberts DB. The etiology of bullous myringitis and the role mycoplasmas in ear disease: a review. Pediatrics 1980;65:761–6.
25. Block SL, Hammerschlag MR, Hedrick J, et al. *Chlamydia pneumoniae* in acute otitis media. Pediatr Infect Dis J 1997;16:858–62.
26. Marchant CD, Shurin PA. Therapy of otitis media. Pediatr Clin North Am 1983;30:281–96.
27. McCracken GH. Antimicrobial therapy for acute otitis media. Pediatr Infect Dis 1984;3:383–6.
28. Fry J. Antibiotics in acute tonsillitis and acute otitis media. Br Med J 1958;2:883–7.
29. Van Buchem FL, Peters MF, van 't Hof MA. Acute otitis media: a new treatment strategy. Br Med J (Clin Res Ed) 1985;6:290:1033–7.
30. Dowell SF, Marcy SM, Phillips WR, et al. Otitis media—principles of judicious use of antimicrobial agents. Pediatrics 1998;101(suppl):S65–71.
31. Hirschmann JV. Methods for decreasing antibiotic use in otitis media. Lancet 1998;352:672.
32. American Academy of Pediatrics Subcommittee on Management of Acute Otitis Media. Diagnosis and Management of acute otitis media. Pediatrics 2004;113:145–65.
33. Howie VM. Natural history of otitis media. Ann Otol Rhinol Laryngol 1975;84(suppl 19):67–72.
34. Gehanno P, N'Guyen L, Derriennic M, et al. Pathogens isolated during treatment failures in otitis. Pediatr Infect Dis J 1998;17:885–90.
35. Heikinen T, Ghaffar F, Okorodudu AO, Chonmaitree T. Serum interleukin-6 in bacterial and non-bacterial acute otitis media. Pediatrics 1998;102:296–9.
36. Rodriguez WJ, Schwartz RH. *Streptococcus pneumoniae* causes otitis media with higher fever and more redness of tympanic membranes than *Haemophilus influenzae* or *Moraxella catarrhalis*. Pediatr Infect Dis J 1999;18:942–4.
36a. Palmu AA, Herva E, Savolainen H, et al. Association of

clinical signs and symptoms with bacterial findings in acute otitis media. Clin Infect Dis 2004;38:234–42.

37. Olson LC, Jackson MA. Only the pneumococcus. Pediatr Infect Dis J 1999;18:849–50.

38. Blumer JL. Pharmacokinetics and pharmacodynamics of new and old antimicrobial agents for acute otitis media. Pediatr Infect Dis J 1998;17:1070–5.

39. Harrison CJ. Using antibiotic concentrations in middle ear fluid to predict potential clinical efficacy. Pediatr Infect Dis J 1997;16(suppl):S12–16.

40. Dagan R, Leibovitz E, Greenberg D, et al. Early eradication of pathogens from middle ear fluid during antibiotic treatment of acute otitis media is associated with improved clinical outcome. Pediatr Infect Dis J 1998;17:776–82.

40a. Anne S, Reisman RE. Risk of administering cephalosporin antibiotics to patients with histories of penicillin allergy. Ann Allergy Asthma Immunol 1995;74:167–70.

41. Schwartz RH, Rodriguez WJ. Trimethoprim-sulfamethoxazole treatment of persistent otitis media with effusion. Pediatr Infect Dis 1982;1:333–5.

42. Shurin PA, Pelton SI, Donner A, et al. Persistence of middle ear effusion after acute otitis media in children. N Engl J Med 1979;300:1121–3.

43. Schwartz RH, Rodriguez WJ, Grundfast KM. Duration of middle ear effusion after acute otitis media. Pediatr Infect Dis 1984;3:204–7.

44. Roberts JE, Rosenfeld RM, Ziesel SA. Otitis media and speech and language: a meta-analysis of prospective studies. Pediatrics 2004;113:238–48.

45. Rosenfeld RM, Mandel EM, Bluestone CD. Systemic steroids for otitis media with effusion in children. Arch Otolaryngol 1991;117:984–9.

46. Lambert PR. Oral steroid therapy for chronic middle ear effusion: a double-blind crossover study. Otolaryngol Head Neck Surg 1986;95:193–9.

46a. Rosenfeld RM, Culpepper L, Doyle KJ, et al. Clinical practice guidelines: otitis media with effusion. Otolaryngol-Head Neck Surg 2004;130:595–118.

47. Marchant CD, Shurin PA, Turczyk VA, et al. Course and outcome of otitis media in early infancy: a prospective study. J Pediatr 1984;104:826–31.

48. Mandel EM, Rockette HE, Bluestone CD, et al. Efficacy of amoxicillin with and without decongestant-antihistamine for otitis media with effusion in children. N Engl J Med 1987;316:432–7.

49. Eavey RD, Stool SE, Peckham GJ, et al. How to examine the ear of the neonate. Clin Pediatr (Phila) 1976;15:338–41.

50. Berman SA, Balkany TJ, Simmons MA. Otitis media in the neonatal intensive care unit. Pediatrics 1978;62:198–201.

51. Shurin PA, Howie RM, Pelton SI, et al. Bacterial etiology of otitis media during the first six weeks of life. J Pediatr 1978;92:893–6.

52. Jaffe BF. Amniotic fluid microviscosity and middle ear effusion. Pediatrics 1980;65:362–3.

52a. Chonmaitree T, Saeed K, Uchida T, et al. A randomized, placebo-controlled trial of the effect of antihistamine or corticosteroid treatment in acute otitis media. J Pediatr 2003;143:377–85.

53. Clements DA, Langdon L, Bland C, Walter E. Influenza A vaccine decreases the incidence of otitis media in 6– to 30-month-old children in day care. Arch Pediatr Adol Med 1995;149:1113–7.

54. Simoes EA, Groothius Jr, Tristram DA, et al. Respiratory syncytial virus-enriched globulin for the prevention of acute otitis media in high risk children. J Pediatr 1996;129:214–9.

55. Cohen H, Levy C, Boucherat M, et al. A multicenter, randomized, double-blind trial of 5 versus 10 days of antibiotic therapy for acute otitis media in young children. J Pediatr 1998;133:634–9.

56. Varsano I, Volovitz B, Horev Z, et al. Intramuscular ceftriaxone compared with oral amoxicillin-clavulanate for treatment of acute otitis media in children. Eur J Pediatr 1997;156:858–63.

57. Leibovitz E, Piglansky L, Raiz S, et al. Bacteriologic and clinical efficacy of one day vs three day intramuscular ceftriaxone for treatment of nonresponsive acute otitis media in children. Pediatr Infect Dis J 2000;19:1040–5.

58. Heikkinen T, Saeed KA, McCormick DP, et al. A single intramuscular dose of ceftriaxone changes nasopharyngeal bacterial flora in children with acute otitis media. Acta Pediatr 2000;89:1316–21.

59. Coser PL, Stamm AEC, Lobo RC, et al. Malignant external otitis in infants. Laryngoscope 1980;90:312–6.

60. Merritt WT, Bass JW, Bruhn FW. Malignant external otitis in an adolescent with diabetes. J Pediatr 1980;96:872–3.

61. Hirsch B. Infections of the external ear. Am J Otolaryngol 1992;13:144–5.

62. Marcy SM. Infections of the external ear. Pediatr Infect Dis 1985;4:192–201.

63. Sobie S, Brodsky L, Stanievich JF. Necrotizing external otitis in children: report of two cases and review of the literature. Laryngoscope 1987;97:598–601.

64. Evans P, Hoffmann L. Malignant external otitis: a case report and review. Am Fam Physician 1994;49:427–31.

65. Schwartz RH, Rodriguez WJ. Draining ears in acute otitis media: reliability of culture. Laryngoscope 1980;90:1717–9.

66. Ordonez GE, Kime CE, Updegraff WR, et al. Effective treatment of acute, diffuse otitis externa. I: a controlled comparison of hydrocortisone-acetic acid, nonaqueous and hydrocortisone-neomycin-polymyxin B otic solutions. Curr Ther Res 1978;23(suppl):S13–14.

67. Heilig D, Heilig M, Glassman JM. Prophylactic use of a topical nonaqueous acetic acid medication for the prevention of otitis externa (swimmer's ear): a two-year study with follow up. Curr Ther Res 1979;26:862–73.

68. Riding KH, Bluestone CD, Michaels RH, et al. Microbiology of recurrent and chronic otitis media with effusion. J Pediatr 1978;93:739–43.

69. Sabella C. Management of otorrhea in infants and children. Pediatr Infect Dis J 2000;19:1007–8.

70. Greydanus DE, O'Connell EJ, McDonald TJ. Middle ear effusions: current concepts. Mayo Clin Proc 1977;52:497–503.

71. Bierman CW, Furukawa CT. Medical management of serous otitis in children. Pediatrics 1978;61:768–74.

72. Shurin PA, Pelton SI, Donner A, et al. Persistence of middle ear effusion after acute otitis media in children. N Engl J Med 1979;300:1121–3.

73. Paparella MM. Blue ear drum and its management. Ann Otol Rhinol Laryngol 1976;85(suppl):S293–5.

74. Fraser JG. Secretory otitis media in childhood. A survey of current understanding and management. Clin Pediatr (Phila) 1971;10:261–4.

75. Wolfowitz B. Spontaneous CSF otorrhea simulating serous otitis. Arch Otolaryngol 1979;105:496–9.

76. Paradise JL, Bluestone CD, Delder H. The universality of otitis media in 50 infants with cleft palate. Pediatrics 1969;44:35–42.

77. Lim DJ. Functional morphology of the lining membrane of the middle ear and eustachian tube: an overview. Ann Otol Rhinol Laryngol 1974;83(suppl):S5–26.

78. Sloyer JL Jr, Howie VM, Ploussard JH, et al. Immune response to acute otitis media: association between middle ear fluid antibody and the clearing of clinical infection. J Clin Microbiol 1976;4:306–8.

79. Paradise JL, Rockette HE, Colborn DK, et al. Otitis media in 2253 Pittsburgh-area infants: prevalence and risk factors during the first two years of life. Pediatrics 1997;99: 318–33.

80. Sade K. The biopathology of secretory otitis media. Ann Otol Rhinol Laryngol 1974;83(suppl):S59–71.

81. Dees SC, Kelkowitz D III. Secretory otitis media in allergic children. Am J Dis Child 1972;124:364–8.

82. Leibovitz E, Raiz S, Piglansky L, et al. Resistance pattern of middle ear fluid isolates in acute otitis media recently treated with antibiotics. Pediatr Infect Dis J 1998;17: 463–9.

83. Kenna MR, Bluestone CD. Microbiology of chronic suppurative otitis media in children. Pediatr Infect Dis 1986; 5:223–5.

84. Giebink GS, Mills EL, Huff JS, et al. The microbiology of serous and mucoid otitis media. Pediatrics 1979;63: 915–9.

85. Adlington P, Davis JR. Virus studies in secretory otitis media. J Laryngol 1969;83:161–73.

86. Schaefer C, Harrison FIR, Boyce WT, et al. Illnesses in infants born to women with *Chlamydia trachomatis* infection. Am J Dis Child 1985;139:127–33.

87. Skolnik PR, Nadol JB Jr, Baker AS. Tuberculosis of the middle ear: review of the literature with an instructive case report. Rev Infect Dis 1986;8:403–10.

88. Kirsch CM, Wehner JH, Jensen WA, et al. Tuberculous otitis media. South Med J 1995;88:363–6.

89. Goldblatt EL, Dohar J, Nozza RJ, et al. Topical ofloxacin versus systemic amoxicillin/clavulanate in purulent otorrhea in children with tympanostomy tubes. Int J Pediatr Otorhinolaryngol 1998;46:91–101.

90. Maynard JE, Fleshman JK, Tschopp CF. Otitis media in Alaskan Eskimo children: prospective evaluation of chemoprophylaxis. JAMA 1972;219:597–9.

91. Perrin JM, Charney E, MacWhinney JB Jr, et al. Sulfisoxazole as chemoprophylaxis for recurrent otitis media: a double blind crossover study in pediatric practice. N Engl J Med 1974;291:664–7.

92. Howie VM, Ploussard J, Sloyer JL, et al. Use of pneumococcal polysaccharide vaccine in preventing otitis media in infants: different results between racial groups. Pediatrics 1984;73:79–81.

93. Schuller DE. Prophylaxis of otitis media in asthmatic children. Pediatr Infect Dis 1983;2:280–3.

94. Barnett ED, Pelton SI, Cabral HJ, et al. Immune response to pneumococcal conjugate and polysaccharide vaccines in otitis-prone and otitis-free children. Clin Infect Dis 1999;29:191–2.

94a. Black S, Shinefield H, Fireman B, et al. Efficacy, safety and immunogenicity of heptavalent pneumococcal conjugate vaccine in children. Pediatr Infect Dis J 2000;19:187–95.

95. Heikkinen T, Ruuskanen O, Waris M, et al. Influenza vaccination in the prevention of acute otitis media in children. Am J Dis Child 1991;145:445–8.

95a. Hoberman A, Greenberg DP, Paradise JL, et al. Effectiveness of inactivated influenza vaccine in preventing acute otitis media in young children: a randomized controlled trial. JAMA 2003;290:1608–16.

96. Klein SW, Olson AL, Perrin J, et al. Prevention and treatment of serous otitis media with an oral antihistamine: a double blinded study in pediatric practice. Clin Pediatr (Phila) 1980;19:342–7.

97. Lampe RM, Weir MR. Erythromycin prophylaxis for recurrent otitis media. Clin Pediatr (Phila) 1986;25:510–5.

98. Uhari M, Kontiokari T, Koskela M, Niemela M. Xylitol chewing gum in prevention of acute otitis media: double blind randomised trial. Br Med J 1996;313:1180–4.

99. Uhari M, Kontiokari T, Niemela M. A novel use of xylitol sugar in preventing acute otitis media. Pediatrics 1998; 102:879–84.

100. Schwartz RH. Prevention of otitis media: a multitude of yellow brick roads. Pediatr Infect Dis 1982;1:3–7.

101. Olmsted RW, Alvarez MC, Moroney JD, et al. The pattern of hearing following acute otitis media. J Pediatr 1964; 65:252–5.

102. Swigart E, Stool SE. Hearing sensitivity and physical characteristics of the eardrum observed during otoscopic examination. Clin Pediatr (Phila) 1977;16:556–60.

103. FrielPatti S, FinitzoHieber T, Conti G, et al. Language delay in infants associated with middle ear disease and mild, fluctuating hearing impairment. Pediatr Infect Dis 1982;1:104–9.

104. Gower D, McGuirt WF. Intracranial complications of acute and chronic infectious ear disease: a problem still with us. Laryngoscope 1986;93:1028–33.

105. Kamitsuka M, Feldman K, Richardson M. Facial paralysis associated with otitis media. Pediatr Infect Dis 1985;4: 682–4.

106. Casselbrant ML, Furman JM, Rubenstein E, Mandel EM. Effect of otitis media on the vestibular system in children. Ann Otol Rhinol Laryngol 1995;104:620–4.

107. Bluestone CD, Cantekin EI, Berry QC, et al. Function of the eustachian tube related to surgical management of acquired aural cholesteatoma in children. Laryngoscope 1978;89:1155–63.

108. Curtis AW. Congenital middle ear cholesteatoma: two unusual cases and a review of the literature. Laryngoscope 1979;89:1159–65.

109. Schwartz RH, Linda RE. Iatrogenic implantation cholesteatoma: an unusual complication of tympanostomy tubes. J Pediatr 1979;94:432–3.

110. Catalana P. Otitic hydrocephalus. Pediatr Infect Dis 1985; 4:563–4.

111. Bluestone CD, Carder HM, Coffey JD, et al. Consensus: management of the child with a chronic draining ear. Pediatr Infect Dis 1985;4:607–12.

112. Bluestone CD. Surgical management of otitis media. Pediatr Infect Dis 1984;3:392–6.

113. Paradise JL, Rogers KD. On otitis media, child development, and tympanostomy tubes: new answers or old questions. Pediatrics 1986;77:88–92.

114. Gates GA. Otologic referral: indications and expectations. Pediatr Infect Dis 1986;5:1–5.

115. Zenni MK, Cheatham SH, Thompson JM, et al. *Streptococcus pneumoniae* colonization in the young child: association with otitis media and resistance to penicillin. J Pediatr 1995;127:533–7.

116. Schwartz RH, Rodriguez WJ, Schwartz DM. Office myringotomy for acute otitis media: its value in preventing middle ear infections. Laryngoscope 1981;91:1–4.

117. Riley DN, Herberger S, McBride G, Law K. Myringotomy and ventilation tube insertion: a ten-year follow-up. J Laryngol Otol 1997;111:257–61.

118. Kenna MA, Bluestone CD, Reilly JS, et al. Medical management of chronic suppurative otitis media without cholesteatoma in children. Laryngoscope 1986;96: 146–51.

119. Hoppe JE, Koster S, Bootz F, Niethammer D. Acute mastoiditis—relevant once again. Infection 1994;22: 178–82.

120. Antonelli PJ, Dhanani N, Giannoni CM, Kubilis PS. Impact of resistant pneumococcus on rates of acute mastoiditis. Otolaryngol-Head Neck Surg 1999;121:190–4.

121. Ginsburg CM, Rudoy R, Nelson JD. Acute mastoiditis in infants and children. Clin Pediatr (Phila) 1980;19: 549–53.

122. Mafee MF, Singleton EL, Valcassori GE, et al. Acute otomastoiditis and its complications: role of CT. Radiology 1985;155:391–7.

123. Venezio FR, Naidich TP, Shulman ST. Complications of mastoiditis with special emphasis on venous sinus thrombosis. J Pediatr 1982;101:509–13.

124. Brook I. Aerobic and anaerobic bacteriology of chronic mastoiditis in children. Am J Dis Child 1981;135:478–9.

125. Wardrop PA, Pillsbury HC. *Mycobacterium avium* acute mastoiditis. Arch Otolaryngol 1984;110:686–7.

126. Moloy PJ. Anaerobic mastoiditis: a report of two cases with complications. Laryngoscope 1982;92:1311–5.

127. Hawkins DB, Dru D, House JW, et al. Acute mastoiditis in children: a review of 54 cases. Laryngoscope 1983;93: 568–72.

128. Ogle JW, Lauer BA. Acute mastoiditis. Am J Dis Child 1986;140:1178–82.

129. Holt GR, Gates GA. Masked mastoiditis. Laryngoscope 1983;93:1034–7.

130. Goldstein NA, Casselbrant ML, Bluestone CD, Kurs-Lasky M. Intratemporal complications of acute otitis media in infants and children. Otolaryngol-Head Neck Surg 1998;119:444–54.

131. Wald ER, Pang D, Milmoe GJ, et al. Sinusitis and its complications in the pediatric patient. Pediatr Clin North Am 1981;28:777–96.

132. Bluestone CD. Medical and surgical therapy of sinusitis. Pediatr Infect Dis 1984;3(suppl):S13–18.

133. Siegel JD. Diagnosis and management of acute sinusitis in children. Pediatr Infect Dis 1987;6:95–9.

134. McAuliffe GW, Goodell H, Wolff HG. Experimental studies on headache: pain from the nasal and paranasal structures. Assoc Nerv Mental Dis Res Publ 1943;23:185–208.

135. Wald ER. Acute sinusitis in children. Pediatr Infect Dis 1983;2:61–8.

136. Wald ER, Guerra N, Byers C. Upper respiratory tract infections in young children; duration of and frequency of complications. Pediatrics 1991;87:129–33.

137. Kronberg FG, Goodwin WJ. Sinusitis in intensive care unit patients. Laryngoscope 1985;95:936–8.

138. Meeks M, Bush A. Primary ciliary dyskinesia (PCD). Pediatr Pulmonol 2000;29:307–16.

138a. Bascom R, Kesavanathan J, Fitzgerald TK, et al. Side-stream tobacco smoke exposure acutely alters human nasal mucociliary clearance. Environ Health Perspect 1995;103:1026–30.

139. Gharib P, Allen RP, Joos HA, et al. Paranasal sinuses in cystic fibrosis. Am J Dis Child 1964;108:488–502.

140. Shapiro GC. Role of allergy in sinusitis. Pediatr Infect Dis 1985;4:S55–9.

141. Lehrer JF, Ali M, Silver J, et al. Recognition and treatment of allergy in sinusitis and pharyngotonsillitis. Arch Otolaryngol 1981;107:543–6.

142. Morgan MA, Wilson WR, Neel HB, et al. Fungal sinusitis in healthy and immunocompromised individuals. Am J Clin Pathol 1984;82:597–601.

143. Porter JP, Patel AA, Dewey CM, Stewart MG. Prevalence of sinonasal symptoms in patients with HIV infection. Am J Rhinol 1999;13:203–8.

144. Hall SL, Miller LC, Duggan E, et al. Wegeners granulomatosis in pediatric patients. J Pediatr 1985;106:739–44.

145. Sessions RB, Zarin DP, Bryan RN. Juvenile nasopharyngeal angiofibroma. Am J Dis Child 1981;135:535–7.

146. Jahrsdoerfer R, Feldman PS, Rubel RW, et al. Otitis media and the immotile cilia syndrome. Laryngoscope 1979;89: 769–78.

147. Fischer TJ, McAdams JA, Entis GN, et al. Middle ear ciliary defect in Kartagener's syndrome. Pediatrics 1978; 62:443–5.

148. Woodring JH, Royer JM, McDonagh D. Kartagener's Syndrome. JAMA 1982;247:2814–6.

149. Eliasson R, Mossberg B, Camner P, et al. The immotile cilia syndrome: a congenital ciliary abnormality as an etiologic factor in chronic airway infections and male sterility. N Engl J Med 1977;297:1–6.

150. Wald ER. Diagnostic considerations. Pediatr Infect Dis 1985;4:S61–3.

151. Wald ER, Milmoe GJ, Bowen A, et al. Acute maxillary sinusitis in children. New Engl J Med 1981;304:749–54.

152. Brook I. Bacteriologic features of chronic sinusitis in children. JAMA 1981;246:967–9.

153. Ponikau JU, Sherris DA, Kern EB, et al. The diagnosis and incidence of fungal sinusitis. Mayo Clin Proc 1999; 74:877–84.

154. Carter KD, Graham SM, Carpenter KM. Ophthalmic manifestations of allergic fungal sinusitis. Am J Ophthalmol 1999;127:189–95.

154a. DeShazo RD, Chapin K, Swain RE. Fungal sinusitis. N Engl J Med 1997;337:245–9.

155. Gwaltney JM Jr, Hendley JO, Simon G, Jordan WS Jr. Rhinovirus infections in an industrial population. II. Characteristics of illness and antibody response. JAMA 1967;202:494–500.

156. Kovatch AL, Wald ER, Ledesma Medina J, et al. Maxillary sinus radiographs in children with nonrespiratory complaints. Pediatrics 1984;73:306–8.

157. Lebeda MD, Haller JR, Graham SM, Hoffmaan HT. Evalu-

ation of Maxillary Sinus aspiration in patients with fever of unknown origin. Laryngoscope 1995;105:683–5.

158. Gwaltney JM Jr. Computed tomographic study of the common cold. N Engl J Med 1994;330:25–30.

159. Stewart MG, Sicard MW, Piccirillo JF, Diaz-Marchan PJ. Severity staging in chronic sinusitis: are CT scan findings related to patient symptoms? Am J Rhinol 1999;13: 161–7.

160. Katz RM, Friedman S, Diament M, et al. A comparison of imaging techniques in patients with chronic sinusitis (x-ray, MRI, A-mode ultrasound). Allerg Proc 1995;16: 123–7.

161. Shapiro ED, Wald ER, Rodnan JB, et al. Bacteriology of the maxillary sinuses in patients with cystic fibrosis. J Infect Dis 1982;146:589–93.

162. Wald ER, Chiponis D, Ledesma Medina J. Comparative effectiveness of amoxicillin and amoxicillin-clavulanate potassium in acute paranasal sinus infections in children: a double blind, placebo controlled trial. Pediatrics 1986; 77:795–800.

163. Garbutt JM, Goldstein M, Gellman E, et al. A randomized, placebo-controlled trial of antimicrobial treatment for children with clinically diagnosed acute sinusitis. Pediatrics 2001;107:619–25.

164. Klapan I, Culig J, Oreskovic K, et al. Azithromycin versus amoxicillin/clavulanate in the treatment of acute sinusitis. Am J Otolaryngol 1999;20:7–11.

165. Lasko B, Lau CY, Saint-Pierre C, et al. Efficacy and safety of oral levofloxacin compared with clarithromycin in the treatment of acute sinusitis in adults: a multicentre, double-blind, randomized study. J Int Med Res 1998;26: 281–91.

166. Coltrera MD, Mathison SM, Goodpaster TA, Gown AM. Abnormal expression of the cystic fibrosis transmembrane regulator in chronic sinusitis in cystic fibrosis and non-cystic fibrosis patients. Ann Otol Rhinol Laryngol 1999;108:576–81.

167. Adam P, Stiffman M, Blake RL Jr. A clinical trial of hypertonic saline nasal spray in subjects with the common cold or rhinosinusitis. Arch Fam Med 1998;7:39–43.

168. Gross CW. Surgical management: an otolaryngologist's perspective. Pediatr Infect Dis 1985;4(suppl):S67–70.

169. Sable NS, Hengerer A, Powell KR. Acute frontal sinusitis with intracranial complications. Pediatr Infect Dis 1984; 3:58–61.

170. Givner LB. Periorbital versus orbital cellulitis. Pediatr Infect Dis J 2002;21:1157–8.

171. Brook I, Friedman EM, Rodriguez WJ, et al. Complications of sinusitis in children. Pediatrics 1980;66:568–72.

172. Harris GJ. Subperiosteal abscess of the orbit. Arch Ophthalmol 1983;101:751–7.

173. Sanborn GE, Kivlin JD, Stevens M. Optic neuritis secondary to sinus disease. Arch Otolaryngol 1984;110:816–9.

174. Rout D, Sharma A, Mohan PJ, et al. Bacterial aneurysms of the intracavernous carotid artery. J Neurosurg 1984; 60:1236–42.

175. Goldenberg RA. Lateral sinus thrombosis: medical or surgical treatment? Arch Otolaryngol 1985;111:56–8.

176. Gallagher RM, Gross CW, Phillips CD. Suppurative intracranial complications of sinusitis. Laryngoscope 1998; 108:1635–42.

177. Teele DW. Management of the child with a red and swollen eye. Pediatr Infect Dis 1983;2:258–62.

178. Jackson K, Baker SR. Clinical implications of orbital cellulitis. Laryngoscope 1986;96:568–74.

179. Shapiro ED, Wald ER, Brozanski BA. Periorbital cellulitis and paranasal sinusitis: reappraisal. Pediatr Infect Dis 1982;1:91–4.

180. Israele V, Nelson JD. Periorbital and orbital cellulitis. Pediatr Infect Dis J 1987;6:404–10.

181. Donahue SP, Schwartz G. Preseptal and orbital cellulitis in childhood: a changing microbiologic spectrum. Ophthalmol 1998;105:1902–5.

182. Ruttum MS, Ogawa G. Adenovirus conjunctivitis mimics preseptal and orbital cellulitis in young children. Pediatr Infect Dis J 1996;15:266–7.

183. Kinchington P, Turse S, Kowalski R, Gordon Y. Use of polymerase chain reaction for the detection of adenovirus in ocular swab specimens. Invest Ophthalmol Vis Sci 1994;35:4126–34.

184. Porter RC, Smith HG, Hutto JO, et al. Clostridial myonecrosis: an unusual presentation. Pediatr Infect Dis 1984;3:340–2.

185. Fisher RG, Wright PF, Johnson JE. Inflammatory pseudotumor presenting as fever of unknown origin. Clin Infect Dis 1995;21:1492–4.

186. Mottow LS, Jakobiec EA. Idiopathic inflammatory orbital pseudotumor in childhood. Arch Ophthalmol 1978;96: 1410–7.

187. Richtsmeier AJ Jr, Dray P, Costas C, et al. Sarcoidosis with supraorbital swelling. Am J Dis Child 1986;140: 189–90.

188. Slavin ML, Glaser JS. Idiopathic orbital myositis: report of six cases. Arch Ophthalmol 1982;100:1261–5.

189. Mullaney PB, Karcioglu ZA, Huaman AM, al-Mesfer S. Retinoblastoma associated orbital cellulitis. Br J Ophthalmol 1998;82:517–21.

190. Nakajima A, Abe T, Takagi T, et al. Two cases of malignant lymphoma complicated by hemophagocytosis resembling orbital cellulitis. Jap J Ophthalmol 1997;41: 186–91.

191. Seeler RA. Exophthalmos in hemoglobin SC disease. J Pediatr 1983;102:90–1.

192. Barone SR, Aiuto LT. Periorbital and orbital cellulitis in the *Haemophilus influenzae* vaccine era. J Pediatr Ophthalmol Strabismus 1997;34:293–6.

193. Nash E, Livingston P, Margo CE. Orbital cellulitis in the acquired immunodeficiency syndrome. Arch Ophthalmol 1997;115:677–9.

194. Kronish JW, Johnson TE, Gilberg SM, et al. Orbital infections in patients with human immunodeficiency virus infection. Ophthalmol 1996;103:1483–92.

195. Weiss IS. *Pseudomonas* orbital cellulitis. Am J Ophthalmol 1979;87:368–70.

196. Kaplan DM, Briscoe D, Gatot A, et al. The use of standardized orbital ultrasound in the diagnosis of sinus induced infections of the orbit in children: a preliminary report. Int J Pediatr Otorhinolaryngol 1999;48:155–62.

197. Ciarallo LR, Rowe PC. Lumbar puncture in children with periorbital and orbital cellulitis. J Pediatr 1993;122: 355–9.

197a. Starkey CR, Steele RW. Medical management of orbital cellulitis. Pediatr Infect Dis J 2001;20:1002–5.

198. Chandler JR, Langenbrunner DJ, Stevens ER. The pathogenesis of orbital complications in acute sinusitis. Laryngoscope 1970;80:1414–28.

199. Garcia GH, Harris GJ. Criteria for nonsurgical management of subperiosteal abscess of the orbit: analysis of outcomes 1988–1998. Ophthalmol 2000;107:1454–6.

200. Sofferman RA. Cavernous sinus thrombophlebitis secondary to sphenoid sinusitis. Laryngoscope 1983;93: 797–9.

201. GomezBarreto J, Nahmias AD. Hypopyon and orbital cellulitis associated with *Haemophilus influenzae* type b meningitis. Am J Dis Child 1977;131:215–7.

202. Siegel JD. Eye infections encountered by the pediatrician. Pediatr Infect Dis 1986;5:741–8.

203. Matoba A. Ocular viral infections. Pediatr Infect Dis 1984; 3:358–68.

204. Annable WL. Therapy for ocular infections. Pediatr Clin North Am 1983;30:389–96.

205. Baum J. Infections of the eye. Clin Infect Dis 1995;21: 479–88.

206. Campolattaro BN, Lueder GT, Tychsen L. Spectrum of pediatric dacrocystitis: medical and surgical management of 54 cases. J Pediatr Opthalmol Strabismus 1997;34: 143–53.

207. Gigliotti F, Williams WT, Hayden FG, et al. Etiology of acute conjunctivitis in children. J Pediatr 1981;98: 531–6.

208. Abelson MB, Madiwale N, Weston JH. Conjunctival eosinophils in allergic ocular disease. Arch Ophthalmol 1983;101:555–6.

209. Sandstrom KI, Bell TA, Chandler JW, et al. Microbial causes of neonatal conjunctivitis. J Pediatr 1984;105: 706–11.

210. Gigliotti F, Hendley JO, Morgan J, et al. Efficacy of topical antibiotic therapy in acute conjunctivitis in children. J Pediatr 1984;104:623–6.

211. Lietman T, Brooks D, Moncada J, et al. Chronic follicular conjunctivitis associated with *Chlamydia psittaci* or *Chlamydia pneumoniae*. Clin Infect Dis 1998;26:1335–40.

212. Halperin SA, Gast T, Ferrieri P. Oculoglandular syndrome caused by *Francisella tularensis*. Clin Pediatr (Phila) 1985;24:520–2.

213. Bodor FF, Marchant CD, Shurin PA, et al. Bacterial etiology of conjunctivitis-otitis media syndrome. Pediatrics 1985;76:26–8.

214. Patriarca PA, Onorato IM, Sklar VEF, et al. Acute hemorrhagic conjunctivitis: investigation of a large-scalle community outbreak in Dade County, Florida. JAMA 1983; 249:1283–9.

215. Christopher S, Theogaraj S, Godbole S, et al. An epidemic of acute hemorrhagic conjunctivitis due to coxsackievirus A24. J Infect Dis 1982;146:16–9.

216. Keenlyside RA, Hierholzer JC, D'Angelo LJ. Keratoconjunctivitis associated with adenovirus type 37: an extended outbreak in an ophthalmologist's office. J Infect Dis 1983;147:191–8.

217. Giladi N, Herman J. Pharyngoconjunctival fever. Arch Dis Child 1984;59:1182–3.

218. Soparkar CN, Wilhelmus KR, Koch DD, et al. Acute and chronic conjunctivitis due to over-the-counter ophthalmic decongestants. Arch Ophthalmol 1997;115:34–8.

219. Sadiz SA, Downes RN. Dysversion of lateral eyelashes in children: a new diagnosis. Eye 1996;10:473–5.

220. MacEwan CJ, Phillips MG, Young JD. Value of bacterial culturing in the course of congenital nasolacrimal duct (NLD) obstruction. J Pediatr Ophthalmol Strabismus 1994;31:246–50.

221. Laga M, Plummer FA, Piot P, et al. Prophylaxis of gonococcal and chlamydial ophthalmia neonatorum: a comparison of silver nitrate and tetracycline. N Engl J Med 1988;318:653–7.

222. Hammerschlag MR, Cummings C, Roblin PM, Williams TH, Delke I. Efficacy of neonatal ocular prophylaxis for the prevention of chlamydial and gonococcal conjunctivitis. N Engl J Med 1989;320:769–72.

223. Bell TA, Sandstrom KI, Gravett MG, et al. Comparison of ophthalmic silver nitrate solution and erythromycin ointment for prevention of natally acquired *Chlamydia trachomatis*. Sex Trans Dis 1987;14:195–200.

224. Isenberg SJ, Apt L, Wood M. A controlled trial of povidone-iodine as prophylaxis against ophthalmia neonatorum. N Engl J Med 1995;332:562–6.

225. Bell TA, Grayston JT, Krohn MA, Kronmal RA. Randomized trial of silver nitrate, erythromycin, and no eye prophylaxis for the prevention of conjunctivitis among newborns not at risk for gonococcal ophthalmitis. Pediatrics 1993;92:755–60.

226. Schaefer F, Bruttin O, Zografos L, Guex-Crosier Y. Bacterial keratitis: a prospective clinical and microbiological study. Br J Opthalmol 2001;85:842–7.

227. Poirier RH. Herpetic ocular infections of childhood. Arch Ophthalmol 1978;98:704–6.

228. Thomas CI, Purnell EW, Rosenthal MS. Treatment of herpetic keratitis with IUD and corticosteroids: report of 105 cases. Am J Ophthalmol 1965;60:204–17.

229. The Herpetic Eye Disease Study Group. A controlled trial of oral acyclovir for the prevention of stromal keratitis or iritis in patients with herpes simplex virus epithelial keratitis. Arch Ophthalmol 1997;115:703–12.

230. Power WJ, Hogan RN, Hu S, Foster CS. Primary varicella-zoster keratitis: diagnosis by polymerase chain reaction. Am J Ophthalmol 1997;123:252–4.

231. Dart JKG, Stapleton F, Minassian D. Contact lenses and other risk factors in microbial keratitis. Lancet 1991;338: 650–3.

232. Dart J. Extended-wear contact lenses, microbial keratitis, and public health. Lancet 1999;354:174–5.

233. Levy B, McNamara N, Corzine J, Abbott RL. Prospective trial of daily and extended wear disposable contact lenses. Cornea 1997;16:274–6.

234. Locatcher Khorazo D, Seegal BC. Microbiology of the Eye. St Louis: CV Mosby, 1972.

235. Tobias JD, Starke JR, Tosi MF. *Shigella* keratitis: a report of two cases and a review of the literature. Pediatr Infect Dis 1987;6:79–81.

236. Parment PA. The role of *Serratia marcescens* in soft contact lens associated ocular infections: a review. Acta Ophthalmol Scand 1997;75:67–71.

237. Gray TB, Cursons RT, Sherwan JF, Rose PR. Acanthamoeba, bacterial, and fungal contamination of contact lens storage cases. Br J Ophthalmol 1995;79:601–5.

238. Horgan SE, Matheson MM, McLoughlin-Borlace L, Dart JK. Use of a low nutrient culture medium for the identification of bacteria causing severe ocular infection. J Med Microbiol 1999;48:701–3.

239. Garg P, Sharma S, Rao GN. Ciprofloxacin-resistant *Pseudomonas* keratitis. Ophthalmol 1999;106(suppl): S319–23.

240. Kone-Paut I, Hesse S. Palix C, et al. Keratitis, ichthyosis, and deafness (KID) syndrome in half sibs. Pediatr Dermatol 1998;15:219–21.

241. Romain PL, Aretz HT. Weekly clinicopathological exercises: Case 6-1999: A 17 1/2-year-old girl with a thoracoabdominal aneurysm. N Engl J Med 1999;340:635–41.

242. Ferreira RC, Ferreira LC, Forstot L, King R. Corneal abnormalities associated with incontinentia pigmenti. Am J Ophthalmol 1997;123:549–51.

243. al-Hemidan AI, al-Hazzaa SA. Richner-Hanhart syndrome (tyrosinemia type II). Case report and literature review. Ophthalmol Genetics 1995;16:21–6.

244. Varga JH, Rubinfeld RS, Wolf TC, et al. Topical anesthetic abuse ring keratitis: report of four cases. Cornea 1997; 16:424–9.

245. Kataria S, Trevathan GE, Holland JE, et al. Ocular presentation of sarcoidosis in children. Clin Pediatr (Phila) 1983;22:793–7.

246. Yamamoto S, Tada R, Shimomura Y, et al. Detecting varicella-zoster virus DNA in iridocyclitis using polymerase chain reaction: a case of zoster sine herpete [letter]. Arch Opthalmol 1995;113:1358–9.

247. Wiersbitzky S, Ratzmann GW, Bruns R, Wiersbitzky H. Reactivation in children of juvenile chronic arthritis and chronic iridocyclitis associated with human herpesvirus-6 infection. Padiatrie und Grenzgebiete 1993;31:203–5.

248. Shah MA, Nair AU, Khubchandani RP, Kumta NB. Ocular complications following mumps [letter]. Indian Pediatr 1992;29:937–8.

249. Lashkevich VA, Umanskaia SV, Koroleva GA, et al. Outbreak of enteroviral uveitis in children in Omsk in 1987–1988. Voprosy Virusologii 1990;35:33–8.

250. Burns JC, Joffe L, Sargent RA, et al. Anterior uveitis associated with Kawasaki syndrome. Pediatr Infect Dis 1985; 4:258–61.

251. Gain P, Mosnier JF, Gravelet C, et al. Iris tuberculosis. A propos of a case diagnosed by iridectomy. J Francais Ophthalmol 1994;17:525–8.

252. Section on Rheumatology and Section on Ophthalmology. Guidelines for ophthalmic examinations in children with juvenile rheumatoid arthritis. Pediatrics 1993;92: 295–6.

253. Querfeld U, Baisch C, Soergel M, et al. Acute tubulointerstitial nephritis and uveitis (TINU syndrome) in childhood. Monatsschrift Kinderheilkunde 1991;139: 336–41.

254. Matsuo T, Matsuo N. Bilateral iridocyclitis with retinal capillaritis in juveniles. Ophthalmol 1997;104:939–44.

255. Ohara K, Okubo A, Sasaki H, Kamata K. Branch retinal vein occlusion in a child with ocular sarcoidosis. Am J Ophthalmol 1995;119:806–7.

256. Kaplan BH, Nevitt MP, Pach JM, Herman DC. Aseptic meningitis and iridocyclitis related to ibuprofen. Am J Ophthalmol 1994;117:119–20.

257. Ronday MJ, Luyendijk L, Baarsma GS, et al. Presumed acquired ocular toxoplasmosis. Arch Ophthalmol 1995; 113:1524–9.

258. Montoya JG, Parmley S, Liesenfeld O, et al. Use of the polymerase chain reaction for diagnosis of ocular toxoplasmosis. Ophthalmol 1999;106:1554–63.

259. Fisher RG, Edwards KM. Varicella-zoster. Pediatr Rev 1998;19:62–7.

260. Hirakata K, Oshima T, Azuma N. Chorioretinitis induced by coxsackievirus B4 infection. Am J Ophthalmol 1990; 109:225–7.

261. Kelly SP, Rosenthal AR, Nicholson KG, Woodward CG. Retinochoroiditis in acute Epstein-Barr virus infection. Br J Ophthalmol 1989;73:1002–3.

262. Radolf JD, Kaplan RP. Unusual manifestations of secondary syphilis and abnormal humoral immune response to Treponema pallidum antigens in a homosexual man with asymptomatic immunodeficiency virus infection. J Am Acad Dermatol 1988;18:423–8.

263. Niutta A, Barcaroli J, Palombi E. Monolateral chorioretinitis with multiple foci in one case of Lyme disease. Ann Ophthalmol 1993;25:257–61.

264. Ghauri RR, Lee AG. Optic disk edema with a macular star. Survey Ophthalmol 1998;43:270–4.

265. Kerkhoff FT, Ossewaarde JM, de Loos WS, Rothova A. Presumed ocular bartonellosis. Br J Ophthalmol 1999; 83:270–5.

266. Reed JB, Scales DK, Wong MT, et al. Bartonella henselae neuroretinitis in cat scratch disease. Diagnosis, management, and sequelae. Ophthalmol 1998;105:459–66.

267. Willis J, Rosman NP. The Aicardi syndrome versus congenital infection: diagnostic considerations. J Pediatr 1980;96:235–9.

268. Goldblatt D, Butcher J, Thrasher AJ, Russell-Eggistt I. Chorioretinal lesions in patients and carriers of chronic granulomatous disease. J Pediatr 1999;134:780–3.

269. Murray HW, Knox DL, Green WR, et al. Cytomegalovirus retinitis in adults: a manifestation of disseminated viral infection. Am J Med 1977;63:574–84.

270. Henderly DE, Liggett PE, Rao NA. Cryptococcal chorioretinitis and endophthalmitis. Retina 1987;7:75–9.

271. Zagami AS, Lethlean AK. Chorioretinitis as a possible very early manifestation of subacute sclerosing pancencephalitis. Aust New Zeal J Med 1991;21:350–2.

272. Pearson PA, Piracha AR, Sen HA, Jaffe GJ. Atovaquone for the treatment of toxoplasma retinochoroiditis in immunocompetent patients. Ophthalmol 1999;106: 148–53.

273. Hamanaka N, Ikeda T, Inokuchi N, et al. A case of intraocular foreign body due to graphite pencil lead complicated by endophthalmitis. Ophthalmol Surg Lasers 1999; 30:229–31.

274. Aaberg TM Jr, Flynn HW Jr, Schiffman J, Newton J. Nosocomial acute-onset postoperative endophthalmitis survey. A 10-year review of incidence and outcomes. Ophthalmol 1998;105:1004–10.

275. Kunimoto DY, Das T, Sharma S, et al. Microbiologic spectrum and susceptibility of isolates: part I. Postoperative endophthalmitis. Am J Ophthalmol 1999;128:240–2.

276. Kunimoto DY, Das T, Sharma S, et al. Microbiologic spectrum and susceptibility of isolates: part II. Posttraumatic endophthalmitis. Am J Ophthalmol 1999;128:242–4.

277. Clark WL, Kaiser PK, Flynn HW Jr, et al. Treatment strategies and visual acuity outcomes in chronic postoperative Propionibacterium acnes ophthalmitis. Ophthalmol 1999;106:1665–70.

278. Baley JE, Kliegman RM, Fanaroff AA. Disseminated fungal infections in very low-birth-weight infants: clinical manifestations and epidemiology. Pediatrics 1984;73:144–52.

279. Scherer WJ, Lee K. Implications of early systemic therapy on the incidence of endogenous fungal endophthalmitis. Ophthalmol 1997;104:1593–8.

280. Axelrod JL, Kochman RS, Horowitz MA, et al. Ceftazidime concentrations in human aqueous humor. Arch Ophthalmol 1984;102:923–5.

CHAPTER 6

Face and Neck Syndromes

■ CERVICAL ADENITIS AND ADENOPATHY

Cervical adenitis is defined as enlarged, tender lymph nodes in the neck. Unilateral acute cervical adenitis is usually caused by a pyogenic bacterium.[1] Involvement of the anterior cervical (tonsillar) nodes under the angle of the jaw suggests a tonsillar disease. The submandibular nodes may be involved. Enlargement of the posterior cervical nodes behind the sternocleidomastoid muscle is more likely to be associated with infectious mononucleosis.

The diagnosis should be cervical adenopathy if there is no erythema over the node and no tenderness. Many patients without such evidence of local inflammation have an infectious cause of the adenopathy, but many noninfectious diseases also result in cervical adenopathy.

Acute Unilateral Cervical Adenitis

A practical approach to cervical adenitis is to divide it into acute febrile unilateral cervical adenitis and all other forms. Acute unilateral cervical lymphadenitis can be empirically treated with oral antibiotics active against the two most likely etiologic agents, *Staphylococcus aureus* and Group A streptococci (such as dicloxacillin, cephalexin, or amoxicillin/clavulanate). Some improvement in clinical symptoms should take place within 48 hours, and ultimately most patients are cured, especially if they are seen early in the illness. However, a small proportion of patients will not respond, especially if the swelling appeared rapidly or is already large, and will continue to have an enlarging node. For such patients, oral antibiotic therapy on an outpatient basis usually does not produce a cure, and it is necessary to hospitalize them.

After hospitalization, an intravenous antibiotic such as nafcillin or clindamycin can be given for approximately 24–48 hours. During this time, the surrounding inflammatory process typically becomes less prominent, and the node will feel firmer and harder. Although the feeling of the node does not suggest that it is compressible or fluctuant, the tenseness of the node is probably caused by pus under pressure. Within the node is a variable area of liquefaction (Fig. 6-1) surrounded by an intensely inflammatory process with firmness secondary to infiltration of cells. Ultrasound may help define the process.

After about 24–48 hours of antibiotic therapy, it is often appropriate to do an incision and drainage of the lymph nodes, usually with a drain left in. The infecting organism may grow out of a culture of pus, as it may not be eliminated by antibiotic therapy, even if it is sensitive to the drug that was administered.

With this approach, most patients will have a short hospital stay and minimal complications. Once the fever is reduced by intravenous antibiotics, and after incision and drainage has been done and the drain removed in a day or so, healing usually occurs rapidly. The patient can then be discharged on oral antibiotics.

The management of other kinds of cervical adenitis is different and depends on whether the disease is chronic or subacute.

Infectious Etiologies

There is overlap between the causes of cervical adenitis and adenopathy, as the bacteria that can cause adenitis can also cause adenopathy, particularly if the findings are made milder by previous antibiotic therapy or by partial immunity of the patient. Thus Group A streptococci, one of the most frequent causes of cervical adenitis, is also a common cause of cervical adenopathy, which is usually bilateral. Infectious causes of cervical adenitis or adenopathy, in approximate order of frequency, are shown in Box 6–1.

Group A Streptococci and Staphylococcus Aureus

Determining whether Group A streptococci or staphylococci are the most common cause of acute

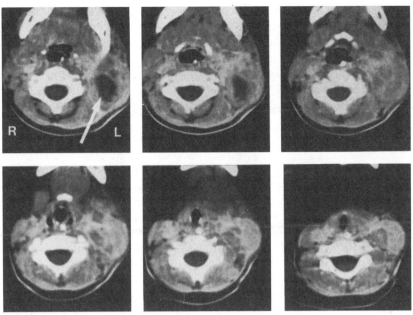

■ **FIGURE 6-1** Six cuts of a neck CT scan showing irregular liquefaction (arrow) and loculation in infected cervical lymph node. Liquid pus and semisolid material were obtained at incision and drainage, when the surgeon broke up the loculated septae. (CT scan from Dr. Richard Logan)

BOX 6-1 ■ Infectious Causes of Cervical Adenitis

Acute Cervical Adenitis
S. aureus
Group A streptococci
Other streptococci, including pneumococci
Anaerobic mouth flora, especially after dental
  work
Epstein-Barr virus (EBV)*
Cytomegalovirus (CMV)*
Adenovirus*
Enterovirus*
H. influenzae
Mycoplasma hominis (newborn)
Kawasaki disease

Chronic or Subacute Adenitis/Adenopathy
Nontuberculous mycobacteria
Bartonella henselae (cat scratch disease)
Human immunodeficiency virus (HIV)*
Tularemia
Fungi (histoplasmosis, coccidioidomycosis)
*M. tuberculosis**
Toxoplasmosis*
Actinomycosis/nocardiosis

*Commonly associated with bilateral cervical or generalized adenopathy

---

unilateral cervical lymphadenitis is fraught with difficulty. It is generally agreed that approximately 65–90% of all cases are due to one or the other. One series suggested that the incidence of Group A streptococcus and *S. aureus* was nearly identical.[2] In a series of children who had not received antibiotics, Group A streptococci were the most frequent cause of cervical adenitis, as demonstrated by culture of the organism by needle aspiration, incision and drainage of the fluctuant nodes, or rising antistreptolysin O titers.[3] In some cases, *S. aureus* was recovered from the node, by itself, or in concert with Group A streptococcus, and an antibody response to Group A streptococcus was demonstrated. Another series ranked beta-hemolytic streptococci second to *S. aureus* regardless of prior antibiotic therapy.[4] Throat culture is not necessarily predictive of the infecting organism; some patients have positive throat cultures for Group A streptococcus when the lymphadenitis is due to *S. aureus*; sometimes, beta-hemolytic streptococci are not recovered from the throat, even though the organism is recovered by needle aspiration of the node.[3,4] Published studies may underestimate the frequency of Group A streptococcus, as these children tend to recover after simple antibiotic therapy and thus not go on to drainage and culture.

S. aureus is more likely in patients who have had unsuccessful antibiotic therapy and require incision and drainage; in one series of 65 such patients *S. aureus* was four times more frequently recovered.[5] However, as noted earlier, one series found no relation between previous penicillin therapy and recovery of *S. aureus* on node aspiration.[4] Staphylococcal adenitis also may occur in young infants as a result of nursery colonization.[6]

Other Bacteria

Pneumococci, anaerobic bacteria, or gram-negative rods rarely produce cervical adenitis, especially in young infants.[4,6] Neonates may also develop a syndrome called "cellulitis-adenitis syndrome" secondary to Group B streptococci. This condition is more common in males.[7] Dental infections may be a predisposing factor for some unusual organisms, particularly anaerobes.[8] *Haemophilus influenzae* is a rare cause of cervical adenitis.

Infectious Mononucleosis

Cervical adenitis in older children and adolescents can be caused by Epstein-Barr virus (EBV). The tenderness is variable depending on the severity of the pharyngitis and often is associated with splenomegaly and generalized adenopathy (Chapter 3). EBV can be associated with a unilateral neck mass.[9]

Subacute Cervical Adenitis

Nontuberculous Mycobacteria

Most of these mycobacteria, previously called unclassified, anonymous, or atypical, have now been

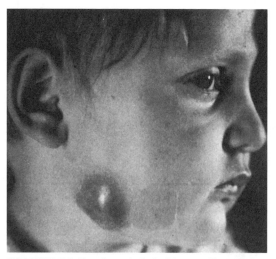

■ **FIGURE 6-2** Chronic cervical adenitis caused by *Mycobacterium scrofulaceum*. (Photo from Dr. Henry Rikkers)

assigned species names. Prior to 1978, the most common species recovered from cervical adenitis in children was *Mycobacterium scrofulaceum*, named for scrofula, an old term for tuberculous cervical adenitis (Fig. 6-2).[10,11] An abrupt shift to *M. avium intercellulare* complex took place in the late 1970s. The reason behind this epidemiologic change is not explained.[12]

Nontuberculous mycobacterial adenitis is a disease that affects predominantly children between the ages of 1 and 5. It is almost always unilateral and has a predilection for the anterior cervical nodes in the submandibular area near the angle of the jaw.[12] In two series, there was a slight female predominance.[13] Patients are otherwise healthy and present with painless lymph node swelling without significant fever or other systemic symptoms. Signs of local inflammation are scant. Over time, the nodes may develop a violaceous hue, but are usually neither bright red nor hot. Left untreated, many will progress to spontaneous rupture and develop a chronic draining sinus tract; the clinical course is variable, however, and the local progression of any one case is difficult to predict.[12] Disseminated disease does not occur in the immunocompetent host.

The histologic appearance of a biopsy specimen of the node depends somewhat on how old the lesion is when it is resected; they tend to progress from dimorphic granulomas to caseating granulomas and finally to calcified granulomas. Acid-fast bacilli can often be found in the smear of aspirated pus or biopsy section. In one large series, 88% of patients had a positive tuberculin skin test (TST) of from 6–15 mm; 9 of 13 "nonresponders" were positive if rechallenged with second-strength (250 TU) purified protein derivative (PPD).[12] This TST response, in contrast to that caused by BCG immunization, seems to last for years. In some cases, nontuberculous mycobacterial adenitis that occurred before the age of 5 years has been responsible for making a preemployment TST positive in adulthood.[12] Others have found the initial TST response less reliable; Hazra et al. reported that only 2 of 13 patients were TST positive at presentation.[13] Skin tests using representative atypical mycobacterial antigens can be compared with the reaction to a standard tuberculin test: in nontuberculous mycobacterial diseases, a larger area of induration is produced by an atypical antigen. Unfortunately, nontuberculous mycobacterial skin-test antigens have been recalled by the FDA because proof of reproducibility was lacking. Culture of a nontuberculous mycobacterium from a node is conclusive, but in one series, only about one-third of children with the diagnosis based on skin tests had a positive culture.[14]

Excisional biopsy of the node is the treatment of choice.[14] Whether chemotherapy prevents progression of disease is unknown. Reports of anecdotal success may reflect the natural history of this infection. The use of antimicrobials should be reserved for cases in which surgical excision carries considerable risk, or when surgical excision is incomplete (usually because of proximity of the facial nerve). The combination of clarithromycin (20–30 mg/kg/day) in two divided doses and ethambutol (15 mg/kg/day) as a single dose is a rational choice based on representative sensitivity patterns of atypical mycobacteria.[13] If the organism is obtained, therapy can be tailored to susceptibility testing done in a reference laboratory. A prolonged course of therapy may be necessary and should usually be undertaken with the assistance of an infectious diseases specialist.

Tuberculous Adenitis

This is rare in children born in the United States but should be considered in children from other countries or in those with a history of exposure to tuberculosis.[15] *Mycobacterium tuberculosis* is more likely to infect nodes behind the sternocleidomastoid muscle or deep in the neck just above the clavicle.[12] In the past, most patients with *M. tuberculosis* lymphadenitis usually had lung or mediastinal involvement as well, probably because of presentation later in the course of illness. However, a recent series of 60 patients with tuberculous cervical lymphadenitis reported abnormal chest x-ray findings in only 10 (16%).[16] In this series, the commonest age group affected was 11 to 20 years, constitutional symptoms were uncommon, and the TST was > 10 mm in 95% and > 15 mm in 84% of patients. Treatment is the same as for pulmonary tuberculosis (see Chapter 8).

Tularemia

Cervical adenitis can be caused by *Francisella tularensis,* spread by a tick bite or handling of infected tissue carcasses.[17,18] The node typically is unresponsive to antistaphylococcal antibiotics and becomes fluctuant and may ulcerate. There is usually a history of an acute illness characterized by fever, headache, abdominal pain, and malaise that antedates the development of the lymphadenopathy.

Careful physical examination may reveal a healing ulcer at the site of a tick bite on the scalp or concomitant inflammation of either the conjunctivae or the pharynx. Diagnosis is made by demonstrating an antibody response to *Francisella tularensis.* Classically, this requires a fourfold or greater increase in antibody titer of paired sera. However, because exposure to *F. tularensis* is uncommon, a presumptive diagnosis can also be made when a single antibody titer is 1:160 or greater. Antibodies may not be detected until the second or third week of illness. Culture is not recommended because of the risk of laboratory personnel acquiring inhalational disease.

Toxoplasmosis

The relative frequency of toxoplasmosis as a cause of cervical adenitis or adenopathy in the United States is not clearly established.[19] Probably, it is frequently undiagnosed because the patient improves and diagnostic studies are not done. In one outbreak, 25 (68%) of 37 patients were ill enough to seek medical attention, but the correct diagnosis was made in only 3 (12%).[20] The most common presenting symptoms were fever, lymphadenopathy, headache, and myalgia.

Exposure to cat feces or undercooked meat may signal a need to suspect the diagnosis. Toxoplasmosis should also be considered when atypical lymphocytosis is present with a negative heterophile test. It can be confirmed by demonstrating a fourfold rise in titer of immunoglobulin (IgG) to *Toxoplasma* antibodies or by the presence of IgM antibodies in a single specimen. However, the quality of available tests is highly variable; false-positive and, to a lesser extent, false-negative results have been a problem with some commercial kits.[21]

A highly sensitive polymerase chain reaction (PCR) that worked well in the diagnosis of both encephalitis and myocarditis due to *Toxoplasma gondii* failed to identify the organism in 8 of 9 lymph nodes with histologically proven toxoplasma infection.[22] The histopathologic findings, however, are highly characteristic and can be identified by experienced pathologists.[23] The cyst form of the parasite can sometimes be seen in histologic sections of excised lymph nodes.[24]

Cat Scratch Disease

The enlarged nodes are in the head and neck in about one-fourth of patients with cat scratch disease (CSD) (Fig. 6–3).[25] Cat scratches are found in some patients; a history of cat exposure is very common. Bacteremia with *Bartonella henselae*, the agent of CSD, is more common in kittens than in full-grown cats and in cats that spend part of their time outdoors than in those restricted to a home environment. Suppuration occurs in 10–25% of infected nodes.[25,26] Despite the fact that this disease was originally called cat scratch fever, systemic symptoms such as fever are relatively uncommon; about one-fourth may have temperature elevation to greater than 38.3°C (101°F), usually for less than a week. A rash, conjunctivitis, or parotid enlargement is noted in 3–5% of patients. The enlarged node is usually noticed about 2 weeks after the scratch but may occur as late as 7 weeks or as early as 3 days.[25] In certain locations (such as the southeastern United States), this condition is one of the most common causes of subacute lymphadenopathy in childhood. Cats can also transmit the infection by licking nonintact skin. Surgical removal or biopsy is unnecessary for diagnosis, but is sometimes performed for patient comfort .

The diagnosis is usually made serologically, with a single elevated titer of *B. henselae* IgG or IgM often considered diagnostic, although unfortunately, both false-negative and false-positive results are relatively common.[27] In our experience, some children with CSD have negative serology until relatively late in the disease; therefore, if suspicion of CSD is high, serologic titers should be repeated. If the diagnosis remains in doubt, definitive etiologic diagnosis can now be obtained by PCR of aspirated pus.[28] A small percentage of patients who appear to have an enlarged node as the sole manifestation of CSD can be demonstrated to have hepatic and splenic microabscesses by abdominal ultrasound.[29] This procedure should not, however, be used as a diagnostic test for CSD. The presence of asymptomatic hepatosplenic abscesses does not mandate therapy.

Actinomycosis

"Lumpy jaw" is the most characteristic pattern of actinomycosis in cattle, but it is a very rare disease in humans.[30] Usually, there is a firm, tender mass in the submandibular area, which often results in draining sinuses. Drainage from these sinuses may contain characteristic "sulfur granules."[30] The infection spreads locally without regard for potential spaces or fascial planes. Males outnumber females. Rarely, the disease extends to the mandible and produces osteomyelitis. Typically, the center of the mass becomes black and necrotic.

Nocardiosis

Cervicofacial nocardiosis in children can occur without any immune deficiency and typically presents as a pustule and regional submandibular adenopathy, either of which may produce chronic drainage.[31] The drainage may contain sulfur granules, mimicking actinomycosis. *Nocardia* are weakly acid-fast, and Kinyoun stain will sometimes differentiate the two diseases.[32]

Fungi

Histoplasmosis, blastomycosis, and coccidiodomycosis are occasionally causes of cervical adenitis in areas of the United States where these organisms are endemic.[33] Fungi are a special consideration in children with leukemia.[34]

Other Causes

Patients with acute HIV infection may present with a monolike illness, which often includes bilateral cervical adenopathy.[35] *Yersinia enterocolitica* is a rare cause of cervical adenitis.[36]

Lymphogranuloma venereum is also a rare cause of cervical lymphadenitis and is found in individuals with oral-genital contact.[37] Syphilis is a rare cause that can be excluded by a VDRL test.

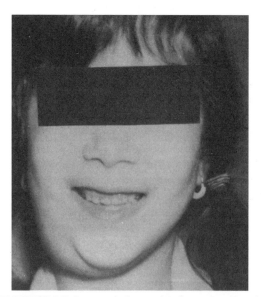

■ **FIGURE 6-3** Cat scratch disease showing regional lymph node enlargement. (Photo from Dr. Andrew Margileth)

Mycoplasma hominis is a possible cause of cervical adenitis in the newborn perod.[38] This infection is probably a result of aspiration of normal flora of the uterine cervix before or during delivery.

Kawasaki Disease

"Mucocutaneous lymph node syndrome" is a synonym for this cause of cervical lymphadenopathy; it is discussed in Chapter 11.

Noninfectious Causes

Congenital Neck Anomalies

Cystic hygroma, bronchial cleft cysts, or thyroglossal duct cysts can be mistaken for lymph nodes. These cysts may become infected and the masses mistaken for cervical adenopathy.

Sinus Histiocytosis

Also called Rosai-Dorfman disease, this is a cause of massive painless cervical lymphadenopathy with fever, leukocytosis, and hypergammaglobulinemia.[39,40] It is benign but may last for several years. The involved lymph nodes show dilated sinuses with numerous histiocytes. The cause is unknown.

Autoimmune Lymphoproliferative Syndrome

This disorder results when lymphocytes fail to undergo the normal process of apoptosis (programmed cell death).[41] It presents with subacute or chronic bilateral cervical (or sometimes generalized) lymphadenopathy. Hypergammaglobulinemia and splenomegaly are common features, as are various autoimmune phenomena, such as hemolytic anemia and thrombocytopenia.[42] Some patients' symptoms respond to corticosteroids. Severe hypersplenism may necessitate splenectomy.

Histiocytic Necrotizing Lymphadenitis (Kikuchi's Disease)

Originally described in Japan in 1972, this is an uncommonly recognized cause of cervical adenopathy in children, adolescents, and young adults.[43] Fever is common, and leukopenia is present in 20% of patients, often prompting concern of malignancy and biopsy of an enlarged node.[44] Although cases are initially often misdiagnosed as lymphoma, Kikuchi's disease can be distinguished from lymphoma histologically by virtue of its polymorphous appearance and its focal, circumscribed involvement of lymph nodes. Females are affected four times as frequently as males. Nodes are rarely greater than 2 cm in size and are not tender or fixed. The cause is unknown. Spontaneous resolution occurs in 1 to 6 months.[45]

Neoplasms

Non-Hodgkin's lymphoma or Hodgkin's disease are rare causes of cervical adenopathy in children. Eosinophilia may be present. Other clues include elevated serum uric acid and lactate dehydrogenase (LDH) and mediastinal lymphadenopathy on chest x-ray. Typically, the adenopathy is painless and without signs of inflammation. Lymph nodes with these characteristics that are large (> 4 cm) or rapidly expanding should undergo excisional biopsy to rule out malignant causes.

Drugs

Phenytoin can be a cause of cervical adenopathy.

Diagnostic Plan

A white blood cell count and differential study may reveal leukocytosis, which implies bacterial adenitis. Atypical lymphocytosis suggests infectious mononucleosis or, rarely, toxoplasmosis. A rapid slide serologic test for infectious mononucleosis antibodies should be done if the child is 5 years of age or older. Specific serologic tests for EBV may be helpful. Serologic evaluation for toxoplasmosis, coccidioidomycosis, HIV, or cytomegalovirus (CMV) may be selectively used.

A tuberculin test is usually indicated in a patient with cervical adenitis or adenopathy that does not respond to initial antibiotic therapy or whose adenopathy persists for longer than 2 weeks. Equivocal or even positive reactions may be the result of crossreactions from nontuberculous mycobacterial infection. A recent study reported 15 mm induration in 17 (59%) of 29 children with nontuberculous mycobacterial lymphadenitis.[46] Definitive diagnosis can usually be made by culture or DNA probe of material obtained by excisional biopsy.

The chest radiograph is occasionally abnormal in tuberculous cervical adenitis but is essentially always normal in adenitis due to nontuberculous mycobacteria. It may reveal mediastinal lymphadenopathy if cervical adenopathy is caused by a neoplasm or a fungal disease such as histoplasmosis.

For acute cervical adenitis, needle aspiration or incision and drainage, with Gram stain and culture of the pus, is often conclusive. Aspiration of fluctuant nodes should usually be performed if 48 hours of antimicrobial therapy has failed or if the infection is severe enough to require intravenous antibiotics and there is "aspiratable" material present. Anaerobic culture of pus may be useful.[47] Smear and culture of the pus for acid-fast organisms and for fungi should also be done. In subacute or chronic adenitis, surgical excision is preferred over incision and drainage.[13] Biopsy or excision of the node with histologic examination may reveal the caseating granulomatous lesions of mycobacteria or fungi, the noncaseating granulomas typical of CSD or tularemia, the "sulfur granules" of actinomycosis, or the eosinophilic histiocytes of toxoplasmosis.

CSD is often diagnosed on clinical grounds alone, especially if the kitten exposure history is strong or if a telltale papule can be found. This is especially true in areas with a high incidence of CSD, such as the southeastern United States. As mentioned earlier, serologic tests are widely available but lack sensitivity and specificity. Aspirated pus can be sent to a reference laboratory for PCR diagnosis of *B. henselae* infection.[28] Skin testing with cat-scratch disease antigen has fallen out of favor; antigen is no longer available.

Treatment

Local heat may be of value for symptomatic relief in mild cases. As the majority of cases are due to either Group A streptococci or *S. aureus*, initial treatment should be with an antimicrobial agent that covers both pathogens. Cephalexin, clindamycin, or amoxicillin-clavulanate would be appropriate. In some areas of the country, community-acquired strains of methicillin-resistant *S. aureus* are becoming common.[47a] Fortunately, these organisms are generally susceptible to clindamycin. Usually, the nodes will shrink soon after the antibiotic is started. If there is no improvement in 2 or 3 days, needle aspiration of the node should be considered, and antibiotic therapy should be changed as guided by Gram stain and culture. If there is still no decrease in nodal size in another 3 days, incision and drainage of the node will probably be necessary. When the mass becomes fluctuant, the abscess should be incised widely and the septae broken up.

If the tuberculin test is positive or nontuberculous mycobacteria is suspected clinically, the node should be excised surgically to prevent a chronic draining sinus from developing.

Antituberculous chemotherapy is indicated if *M. tuberculosis* is found. Although surgical excision was commonly advocated in the past, a recent series reported excellent outcomes in 60 cases of tuberculous cervical lymphadenopathy. In this series, excisional biopsy was performed in only four patients; the remainder received 6 months of combination chemotherapy only. Six months after completion of therapy, there were no local or systemic recurrences.[16]

Excision is sufficient for nontuberculous mycobacterial adenitis, but sometimes complete resection is impossible without compromising the facial nerve. In such cases, clarithromycin and ethambutol may be used pending susceptibility testing, as described above. Most cases of CSD adenitis resolve without specific antimicrobial therapy.

■ TORTICOLLIS

Torticollis (wryneck) can be divided into congenital and acquired categories. Congenital torticollis is almost never secondary to infection. This condition presents within the first few months of life and is often accompanied by a sternocleidomastoid "tumor."[48] Acquired torticollis may occur as a complication of cervical adenitis, peritonsillar infection, or retropharyngeal abscess.[49] In one survey, a head or neck inflammatory focus was found in 85% of children presenting with acute nontraumatic acquired torticollis.[50]

When it occurs after known trauma, it may be caused by atlantoaxial rotatory subluxation, best diagnosed by spiral computed tomography (CT) imaging.[51] This condition is important to diagnose because reduction becomes more difficult with time.[52]

Sandifer's syndrome is the occurrence of torticollis in association with hiatal hernia and severe gastroesophageal reflux. Surgical correction of the hernia corrects the torticollis.[53] Toddlers may present with head tilt resembling torticollis but without limitation of motion of the neck secondary to ocular muscle disorders.[54] An interesting case of a 6-year-old girl who presented with torticollis as the first manifestation of systemic onset juvenile rheumatoid arthritis has been reported.[55] A teenager with torticollis from osteomyelitis of the first rib has been described.[56]

Recurrent torticollis can be caused by recurrently infected congenital anomalies of the neck, such as branchial cleft cysts or a laryngeal pyriform sinus diverticulum.[57] CT can be useful in detecting such anomalies.

■ FACE AND NECK INFECTIONS

Cellulitis of the face and neck, suppurative thyroiditis, and retropharyngeal abscess are discussed in this section. Orbital cellulitis, which is usually related to sinusitis, is discussed in Chapter 5 and tonsillar complications of peritonsillar abscess and postanginal sepsis are discussed in Chapter 2.

Facial (Buccal) Cellulitis

"Facial" or "buccal" cellulitis refers to cellulitis of the cheeks. This is another disease that is currently seldom seen because of the efficacy of the conjugated H. influenzae type b vaccine.[57a] In the absence of a wound or maxillary sinusitis, it typically occurs in infants less than 2 years of age.[58] The cheek is usually swollen and faintly red and later sometimes becomes bluish-purple-red. The patient may be ill-appearing and have a high fever. Blood cultures are positive in from 55–86% of patients.[59] The condition can be bilateral, and small outbreaks were observed in the past.[60,61] Rarely, the infant with infectious facial cellulitis is afebrile but usually has a leukocytosis.

H. influenzae type b is the usual cause. Other serotypes of H. influenzae are not prone to cause this infection. The bluish-purple hue of the cheeks is not specific for H. influenzae, as it has also been observed with pneumococcal cellulitis.[62] Meningitis may complicate up to 9% of bacteremic buccal cellulitis.[63] Thus, lumbar puncture is indicated in the young child with buccal cellulitis thought to be due to H. influenzae type b. In the newborn period, or in the school-age child with a dental abscess, S. aureus is a possible cause. S. aureus is also seen in some children who have facial cellulitis secondary to a wound or other small portal of entry. Group B streptococcus can cause facial cellulitis in the first 3 months of life, usually as part of the cellulitis-adenitis syndrome mentioned earlier.[64]

Treatment

Ceftriaxone or cefotaxime are useful to treat facial cellulitis because they are effective against ampicillin-resistant H. influenzae and most strains of S. pneumoniae. Antistaphylococcal coverage should be added if the facial cellulitis stems from a dental abscess. Ampicillin-sulbactam is effective against ampicillin-resistant H. influenzae and has the advantage of being effective for rare anaerobes as well as many strains of S. aureus.

Unusual Causes

Acute wound infections usually can easily be related to a recent injury. However, some bacteria can cause a facial abscess that is chronic and indolent, with the original injury having been minor and forgotten. Nontuberculous mycobacteria such as M. chelonei can result in such a pattern.[65] Incision and drainage is typically needed. Such rapidly growing nontuberculous mycobacteria usually are resistant to conventional antituberculous drugs. Therapy depends on the particular species and should be discussed with an infectious diseases specialist.

Facial edema with induration is an uncommon complication of severe cystic acne.[66]

Other conditions resembling infectious facial cellulitis include trauma, insect bite, burn, atopic dermatitis, contact dermatitis, erythema infectiosum, and exposure to cold.[67] A special subset of cold panniculitis that occurs in the summertime is so-called popsicle panniculitis.[68]

Ludwig's Angina and Other Neck Space Infections

Definitions

Ludwig's angina is defined as indurated cellulitis of the submandibular or sublingual spaces.[69,70] It is rare and usually related to a dental infection, a laceration of the floor of the mouth, or mandibular fracture. A case related to tongue piercing has also been reported.[71]

Other neck infections can be classified by the anatomic compartments formed by the superficial cervical fascia and the three layers of deep cervical fascia.[72,73] Superficial fascial-space infections occur above the platysma muscle and rarely extend through the deep fascia but can extend into the axillary area.[72] The anterior cervical fascial space, enclosed by the superficial layer of the deep fascia, encloses the parotid and submandibular glands. The middle layer encloses the larynx, esophagus, and thyroid gland. The deep layer is located in front of the vertebra and extends from the base of the skull to the coccyx.[72] These various spaces and compartments have names and numbers, but for the clinician who is not an otolaryngologist, the areas are best named for the nearest familiar gland or anatomic landmark. Examples include the space within the carotid sheath, the submandibular space (Ludwig's angina), the lateral pharyngeal space (parapharyngeal abscess), the peritonsillar space (peritonsillar abscess), the buccal space, the retropharyngeal space (retropharyngeal or prevertebral abscess), and the parotid space.[72,74] Fortunately, deep neck infections are rare in children.

Diagnostic Studies

Computed tomography is an excellent way to define the extent of cervical infections and to distinguish phlegmon from abscess.[75]

Infecting Microorganisms

The usual bacteria involved in neck space infections are viridans streptococci, *S. aureus*, *S. epidermidis*, beta-hemolytic streptococci, and mouth anaerobes.[76] The prevalence of group A streptococcus as a cause of deep neck infections has dropped considerably in recent years, probably due to prompt antibiotic therapy of streptococcus pharyngitis; only 8 (7%) of 110 deep neck abscesses grew Group A streptococci in one review.[76]

Treatment

Neck space infections should be treated aggressively with antibiotics effective against anaerobes and *S. aureus*, such as ampicillin-sulbactam or clindamycin, with early surgical consultation for proper drainage.[77,78] An abscess that is small or not yet liquefied (so-called phlegmon) can sometimes be managed without surgical drainage.

Complications

The most common and devastating complication of Ludwig's angina is airway obstruction, which can occur quickly and without much warning. In one review of deep neck abscesses, 50% of patients with Ludwig's angina who were not given a tracheotomy at the time of presentation required emergency tracheotomy later.[76] The authors of that review advocate tracheotomy in all patients with this condition. In another survey, only 1 of 14 patients required tracheotomy; these authors believe that early surgical intervention coupled with aggressive antimicro-

bial therapy can reduce the rate of tracheotomy and mortality.[79] Ludwig's angina (submandibular-submental fascial cellulitis) can extend to produce a mediastinal abscess. Jugular thrombophlebitis with septic pulmonary emboli can occur (postanginal sepsis or Lemierre's syndrome,[80] discussed in Chapter 2). Necrotizing fasciitis can occur in the neck, as it can in any fascial area, and in these rare cases results in similar complications as well as in airway obstruction.[81]

Neck Abscesses

Cervical adenitis can produce a neck abscess and is discussed in the section on cervical adenitis. Torticollis is often secondary to cervical node infection and is also discussed in that section.

Congenital anomalies that can become infected include thyroglossal duct cysts and branchial cleft cysts or sinus tracts. The infected thyroglossal duct cyst is always below the level of the hyoid bone, at or very near the midline of the neck. Recurrent inflammation sometimes causes rupture with drainage through an external sinus tract.[82] Branchial cleft cysts or fistulae can be infected; these are usually located along the anterior border of the sternocleidomastoid muscle below the hyoid bone, although first branchial cleft fistulae can actually open into the external ear canal.[82] Branchial cleft cysts can also become abscesses and are treated by incision and drainage with operative removal of all remnant structures.

Most cystic hygromas are located behind the sternocleidomastoid muscle in the supraclavicular fossa and are soft and rounded and transilluminate well.[83] Now the approach is usually to dissect out the entire lesion.

Retropharyngeal Abscess

The incidence of retropharyngeal abscess, the most common of deep cervical space abscesses in childhood, has decreased greatly in the antibiotic era. Although uncommon, it is important to consider this condition because of the potential for severe and even life-threatening complications. Because it usually is the result of infection of the retropharyngeal lymph nodes, which regress at or before puberty, it is much more common in young children. One review of 65 cases of retropharyngeal abscess revealed that half the patients were younger than 3 years of age, and 71% were younger than 6 years.[84] It has, however, been noted to occur in older children and adults.[85] In adults it is more likely to be secondary to trauma, foreign bodies, or as a complication of dental infection.[86] In childhood it is usually secondary to severe adenotonsillar disease. The most common aerobes include alpha- and gamma-hemolytic streptococci, *S. aureus*, *Haemophilus* species, and Group A beta-hemolytic streptococci. Anaerobes most frequently isolated include *Bacteroides*, Peptostreptococci, and Fusobacteria. Infection is often polymicrobial.[87, 87a] Rarely, cervical vertebral infection such as tuberculosis presents as a cervical abscess.[88]

Diagnosis

Painful or difficult swallowing, drooling secretions, or regurgitation can occur. Meningismus may be present. Airway compromise and stridor may be relatively late signs in infants. Direct examination often reveals a posterior pharyngeal mass bulging forward. Inspiratory lateral roentgenograms of the soft tissues of the neck should reveal bulging of the retropharyngeal tissues into the pharynx.[89] Caution must be used in interpreting lateral neck x-rays taken during *expiration*; one report describes the appearance of retropharyngeal thickening and even deep neck space air pockets in infants whose *inspiratory* films were entirely normal.[90]

CT can be a valuable tool. Two studies that compared preoperative CT scan findings with surgical findings concluded that CT scanning had a sensitivity of 85–90% and a specificity of 87–88%.[91,92] Therefore, some experts recommend that all children who present with a disease compatible with deep neck abscess be initially treated with intravenous antibiotics, and that surgery be reserved for those who are either acutely ill at the time of presentation or who fail to respond to intravenous antibiotics.[93] Once the patient clinically requires surgery, however, it is best to obtain CT scanning prior to the surgical procedure. A cautionary tale about an infant who had multiple abscesses, one of which caused recurrent disease about 1 week after successful surgical drainage of the largest, has been reported.[94]

One small study concluded that measuring the distance from the internal carotid artery to the cervical vertebra by color Doppler ultrasonography detected retropharyngeal abscess in 5 cases and was negative in all 50 controls.[95] This procedure also allowed the investigators to monitor progress, without exposing patients to radiation, by doing serial ultrasonographic measurements. The true clinical utility of this procedure awaits further study.

Other causes of retropharyngeal masses include cystic hygroma, neuroblastoma or other neurogenic neoplasms, or an enlarged thyroid.[96] However, none of these would be likely to produce the fever, leukocytosis, or toxicity of an abscess.

Treatment

Tracheal intubation is needed to secure the airway in advanced cases. A retropharyngeal phlegmon without true abscess formation usually responds to parenteral antibiotic therapy alone. There is some evidence that early antibiotic therapy may prevent cellulitis from progressing to abscess. True abscesses are approached surgically; this can be done intraorally in most cases. The abscess is aspirated for culture and detection of pus and is incised and drained if pus in present.[89] Some otolaryngologists treat small abscesses (i.e., < 1–2 cm) conservatively and monitor with serial CT scans. Antibiotic therapy should cover the group A streptococcus, *S. aureus,* and anaerobes. Ampicillin-sulbactam or clindamycin would be reasonable choices.

Complications

The abscess can dissect into the mediastinum or burst into the pharynx, with resultant empyema or aspiration of pus.[97,98]

Suppurative Thyroiditis

Suppurative thyroiditis is rare in children.[99,100] This is thought to be secondary to the excellent blood and lymphatic supply of the thyroid, in addition to its protective capsule and high local iodine content. Injecting bacterial suspensions directly into the thyroid artery does not produce suppurative thyroiditis in dogs.[101] Nonsuppurative bacterial thyroiditis can occur in newborns.[102]

The disease is usually preceded by an upper respiratory tract infection. Patients then present with fever, cough, dysphagia, and a tender left anterior neck mass. The mass is usually nonfluctuant at first, but many progress to fluctuance. The left pole of the thyroid is involved in almost 90% of cases. This is because the pathogenesis of this condition in childhood almost always involves a pyriform sinus fistula, which occurs on the left. Therefore, patients who present with suppurative thyroiditis should undergo barium esophagogram to detect the abnormality. A thorough review of all pediatric cases in the literature showed that esophagograms were abnormal in 89% of children with suppurative thyroiditis.[103] In others, pyriform sinus fistulae were discovered by surgical exploration, even though esophagograms were normal (acute inflammation may temporarily close the sinus tract, producing a false negative test). Pyriform sinus fistulae must be surgically repaired or the condition will recur. Thyroglossal duct remnants also have been associated with the development of suppurative thyroiditis.

Early literature reports suggested that *S. aureus* and *S. pneumoniae* were common etiologic agents.[104] Review of all published cases shows, however, that most cases are caused by indigenous microflora of the oropharynx. Streptococcal species of one type or another have accounted for almost half of all cases. Following streptococcal species, *Bacteroides*, *Peptococcus*, *Staphylococcus*, Enterobacteriaciae, *Eikenella*, and *Haemophilus* species have been found, in approximately that order. About 40% of cultures grow more than one species of bacteria. Anaerobic bacteria are found in about one-third, sometimes alone, and sometimes in mixed infection. *S. pneumoniae* has not been reported as a pathogen of suppurative thyroiditis in childhood.

Psittacosis can produce thyroiditis. Fungi and mycobacteria can cause infectious thyroiditis, especially in immunocompromised hosts.[105] *Pneumocystis jiroveci* (previously *P. carinii*) is a pathogen of increasing importance in adults with severe immune compromise;[106] this agent has not yet been reported as a cause of thyroiditis in children.

The disease may be mistaken for cervical adenitis, but the mass may be seen to move with swallowing. Skillful physical examination should make the diagnosis obvious, except that the condition is rare enough that the clinician may not suspect it. Ultrasound is useful to differentiate this condition from malignancy.[107] CT scanning with and without contrast may also help to narrow the differential diagnosis.[108] Suppurative thyroiditis will enhance with contrast. Thyroid scans are abnormal in 100% of cases. Thyroid function tests have been normal in all pediatric cases outside the neonatal period. Nonsuppurative thyroiditis is a frequent initial misdiagnosis.[110]

Initial antibiotic agents should include coverage for anaerobic organisms. Ampicillin-sulbactam plus an aminoglycoside, penicillin plus clindamycin, or mevoppnem would seem to be logical antibiotic choices, but none of these has been adequately studied. Surgical drainage and repair of fistulous tracts are important facets of the management of this condition.

Esophagitis

Children with esophagitis are usually immunocompromised, and the causes are usually *Candida albicans*, herpes simplex virus (HSV), or cytomegalovirus (CMV). Newborn infants can have candidal esophagitis, producing frequent emesis.[111] Although candidal esophagitis can occur in normal persons who have received antibiotics,[112] this diagnosis in a host who is presumed to be immunologically normal should prompt evaluation for acquired or congenital immunodeficiency (Chapter 23). HSV esophagitis has been observed in normal children as an extension of oral herpes.[113]

The symptoms typically include difficult or painful swallowing and retrosternal pain. CMV may produce more systemic symptoms, such as nausea, vomiting, and fever. Candidal esophagitis can occur in the absence of thrush; between a fifth[114] and half[115] of all immunocompromised patients eventually proven to have candidal esophagitis have a normal oropharynx by physical examination. Radiologic examination with contrast medium appears to be sensitive and reveals ulcerations, abnormal motility, or plaques.[116] Alternatively, esophagoscopy with smear, biopsy, and culture can be done.

Esophagitis due to HSV is treated with acyclovir, and that due to CMV is treated with ganciclovir. Candidal esophagitis almost always responds to fluconazole. Refractory cases may be treated with itraconazole, voriconazole or intravenous amphotericin B, or caspofungia.[117]

■ REFERENCES

1. Marcy SM. Infections of lymph nodes of the head and neck. Pediatr Infect Dis 1983;2:397–405.
2. Yamauchi T, Ferrieri P, Anthony BG. The aetiology of acute cervical lymphadenitis in children: serological and bacteriological studies. J Med Microbiol 1980;13:37–43.
3. Dajini AS, Garcia RE, Wolinsky E. Etiology of cervical lymphadenitis in children. N Engl J Med 1963;268:1329–33.
4. Barton LL, Feigin RD. Childhood cervical lymphadenitis: a reappraisal. J Pediatr 1974;84:846–52.
5. Simo T, Hartley C, Rapado F, et al. Microbiology and antibiotic treatment of head and neck abscesses in children. Clin Otolaryngol Allied Sci 1998;23:164–8.
6. Boyce JM, Garner JS, Twenge JA, et al. Nosocomial staphylococcal cervical lymphadenitis in infants: report of an outbreak. Pediatrics 1976;57:854–60.

7. Baker CJ. Group B streptococcal cellulitis-adenitis in infants. Am J Dis Child 1982;136:631–3.

8. Bradford BJ, Plotkin SA. Cervical adenitis caused by anaerobic bacteria. J Pediatr 1976;88:1060.

9. Dudley JP. Epstein-Barr virus and a unilateral neck mass: its occurrence and diagnosis in a patient with no other signs of infection. Arch Otolaryngol 1982;108:253–4.

10. White MP, Bangash H, Goel KM, et al. Non-tuberculous mycobacterial lymphadenitis. Arch Dis Child 1986;61:368–71.

11. Schaad JB, Votteler TP, McCracken GR Jr, et al. Management of atypical mycobacterial lymphadenitis in childhood: a review based on 380 cases. J Pediatr 1979;95:356–60.

12. Wolinsky E. Mycobacterial lymphadenitis in children: a prospective study of 105 nontuberculous cases with long-term follow-up. Clin Infect Dis 1995;20:954–63.

13. Hazra R, Robson CD, Perrez-Atayde, Husson RN. Lymphadenitis due to nontubercuous mycobacteria in children: presentation and response to therapy. Clin Infect Dis 1999;28:123–9.

14. Altman RP, Margileth AM. Cervical lymphadenopathy from atypical mycobacteria: diagnosis and surgical treatment. J Pediatr Surg 1975;10:419–22.

15. Tomblin JL, Roberts FJ. Tuberculous cervical lymphadenitis. Can Med Assoc J 1979;121:324–30.

16. Jha BC, Dass A, Nagarkar NM, et al. Cervical tuberculous lymphadenopathy: changing clincial patterns and concepts in management. Postgrad Med J 2001;77:185–7.

17. Jacobs RF, Condrey YM, Yamauchi T. Tularemia in adults and children: a changing presentation. Pediatrics 1985;76:818–22.

18. Speert DP, Britt WJ, Kaplan EL. Tick-borne tularemia presenting as ulcerative lymphadenitis. Clin Pediatr 1979;18:239–41.

19. Rafaty FM. Cervical adenopathy secondary to toxoplasmosis. Arch Otolaryngol 1977;103:547–9.

20. Teutsch SM, Juranek DD, Sulzer A, et al. Epidemic toxoplasmosis associated with infected cats. N Engl J Med 1979;300:695–9.

21. Wilson M, Remington JS, Clavet C, et al. Evaluation of six commercial kits for detection of human immunoglobulin M antibodies to Toxoplasma gondii. J Clin Microbiol 1997;35:3112–5.

22. Weiss LM, Chen YY, Berry GJ, Strickler JG, et al. Infrequent detection of Toxoplasma gondii genome in toxoplasmic lymphadenitis: a polymerase chain reaction study. Human Pathol 1992;23:154–8.

23. Dorfman RF, Remington JS. Value of lymph node biopsy in the diagnosis of acute acquired toxoplasmosis. N Engl J Med 1973;289:878–91.

24. Aisner SC, Aisner J, Moravec C, et al. Acquired toxoplasmic lymphadenitis with demonstration of the cyst form. Am J Clin Pathol 1983;79:125–7.

25. Carithers HA. Cat-scratch disease. Am J Dis Child 1985;139:1124–33.

26. Margileth AM. Cat scratch disease: nonbacterial regional lymphadenitis: the study of 145 patients and a review of the literature. Pediatrics 1968;42:803–18.

27. Bergmans AM, Peeters MF, Schellekens JF, et al. Pitfalls and fallacies of cat scratch disease serology: evaluation of Bartonella henselae-based indirect fluorescence assay and enzyme-linked immunoassay. J Clin Microbiol 1997;35:1931–7.

28. Goral S, Anderson B, Hager C, Edwards KM. Detection of Rochalimaea henselae DNA by polymerase chain reaction from suppurative nodes of children with cat-scratch disease. Pediatr Infect Dis J 1994;13:994–7.

29. Estrada B, Silio M, Begue RE, Van Dyke RB. Unsuspected hepatosplenic involvement in patients hospitalized with cat-scratch disease. Pediatr Infect Dis J 1996;15:720–1.

30. del Rosario N, Rickman L. Cervicofacial actinomycosis. Arch Otolaryngol 1986;113:777–8.

31. Seidel SF, Younce DC, Hupp JR, Kaminski ZC. Cervicofacial nocardiosis: report of a case. J Oral Maxillofac Surg 1994;52:188–91.

32. Lampe RM, Baker CJ, Septimus EJ, et al. Cervicofacial nocardiosis in children. J Pediatr 1981;99:593–5.

33. Zinman HM, Read SE. Blastomycosis presenting as a neck abscess. Pediatr Infect Dis 1986;5:491–2.

34. Shenep JL, Kalwinsky DK, Feldman S, et al. Mycotic cervical lymphadenitis following oral mucositis in children with leukemia. J Pediatr 1985;106:243–6.

35. Kahn JO, Walker BD. Acute human immunodeficiency virus type 1 infection. N Engl J Med 1998;339:33–9.

36. Jaffe KM, Smith AL. Yersinia enterocolitica cervical lymphadenitis. J Pediatr 1980;97:937–9.

37. Thorsteinsson SB, Musher DM, Min KW, et al. Lymphogranuloma venereum: a cause of cervical lymphadenopathy. JAMA 1976;235:1882.

38. Powell DA, Miller K, Clyde WA Jr. Submandibular adenitis in a newborn caused by Mycoplasma hominis. Pediatrics 1979;63:798–9.

39. Rosai J, Dorfman RF. Sinus histiocytosis with massive lymphadenopathy: a pseudolymphomatous benign disorder. Cancer 1972;30:1174–88.

40. Buchino JJ, Byrd RP, Kmetz DR. Disseminated sinus histiocytosis with massive lymphadenopathy. Arch Pathol Lab Med 1982;106:13–6.

41. Infante AJ, Britton HA, DeNapoli T, et al. The clinical spectrum in a large kindred with autoimmune lymphoproliferative syndrome caused by a Fas mutation that impairs lymphocyte apoptosis. J Pediatr 1998;133:629–33.

42. Bleesing JJ, Straus SE, Fleisher TA. Autoimmune lymphoproliferative syndrome: a human disorder of abnormal lymphocyte survival. Pediatr Clin North Am 2000;47:1291–310.

43. Lerosey Y, Lecler-Scarella V, Francois A, Andriue Guitrancourt J. A pseudo-tumoral form of Kikuchi's disease in children: a case report and review of the literature. Int J Pediatr Otorhinolaryngol 1998;45:1–6.

44. Boyce TG, Moffet HL, Roh SK, Desouky SS. Kikuchi's disease (histiocytic necrotizing lymphadenitis). Arch Pediatr Adol Med 1994;148:427–8.

45. Ali MH, Horton LWL. Necrotizing lymphadenitis without granulocytic infiltration (Kikuchi's disease). J Clin Pathol 1985;38:1252–7.

46. Haimi-Cohen Y, Zeharia, Mimouni M, Soukhman M, Amir J. Skin indurations in response to tuberculin testing in patients with nontuberculous mycobacterial lymphadenitis. Clin Infect Dis 2001;33:1786–8.

47. Brook I. Aerobic and anaerobic bacteriology of cervical adenitis in children. Clin Pediatr (Phila) 1980;19:693–6.

47a. Sattler CA, Mason EO J, Kaplan SL. Prospective comparison of risk factors and demographic and clinical characteristics of community-acquired, methicillin-resistant versus methicillin-susceptible *Staphylococcus aureus* infection in children. Pediatr Infect Dis J 2002; 21:910–7.

48. Cheng JC, Tang SP, Chen TM. Sternocleidomastoid pseudotumor and congenital muscular torticollis in infants: a prospective study of 510 cases. J Pediatr 1999;134:712–6.

49. Harries PG. Retropharyngeal abscess and acute torticollis. J Laryngol Otol 1997;3:1183–5.

50. Bredencamp JK, Maceri DR. Inflammatory torticollis in children. Arch Otolaryngol Head Neck Surg 1990;116:310–3.

51. Nicholson P, Higgins T, Forgarty E, et al. Three-dimensional spiral CT scanning in children with acute torticollis. Int Orthoped 1999;23:47–50.

52. Schwarz N. The fate of missed atlanto-axial rotatory subluxation in children. Arch Ortho Trauma Surg 1998;117:288–9.

53. Tekou H, Akue B, Senah KC, et al. Sandifer's syndrome—a report of one case. W Afr J Med 1997;16:48–9.

54. Williams CR, O'Flynn E, Clarke NM, Morris RJ. Torticollis secondary to ocular pathology. J Bone Joint Surg(B) 1996;78:620–4.

55. Uziel Y, Rathaus V, Pomeranz A, et al. Torticollis as the sole initial presenting sign of systemic onset juvenile rheumatoid arthritis. J Rheumatol 1998;25:166–8.

56. Steinberg GG. Osteomyelitis of the rib presenting as painful torticollis. J Bone Joint Surg(A) 1979;61:614–5.

57. Makino SI, Tsuchida Y, Yoshioka H, et al. The endoscopic and surgical management of pyriform sinus fistulae in infants and children. J Pediatr Surg 1986;21:398–401.

57a. Fisher RG, Benjamin DK Jr. Facial cellulitis in childhood: a changing spectrum. South Med J 2002;95:672–4.

58. Chartrand SA, Harrison CJ. Buccal cellulitis reevaluated. Am J Dis Child 1986;140:891–3.

59. Rapkin RH, Bautista G. *Haemophilus influenzae* cellulitis. Am J Dis Child 1972;124:540–2.

60. Landwirth J. Bilateral cellulitis of the cheeks in an infant due to *Haemophilus influenzae*. Clin Pediatr (Phila) 1977;16:182–4.

61. Siddiqui WH, Reed TD. *Haemophilus influenzae* buccal cellulitis: five cases in eight weeks. J Pediatr 1977;91:687–8.

62. Thirumoorthi MC, Asmar BI, Dajani AS. Violaceous discoloration in pneumococcal cellulitis. Pediatrics 1978;62:492–3.

63. Baker RC, Bausher JC. Meningitis complicating acute bacteremic facial cellulitis. Pediatr Infect Dis 1986;5:421–3.

64. Hauger SB. Facial cellulitis: an early indicator of group B streptococcal bacteremia. Pediatrics 1981;67:376–7.

65. Hamrick HJ, Maddux DW, Lowry EK, et al. *Mycobacterium chelonei* facial abscess: case presentation and review of cutaneous infection due to Runyon Group IV organisms. Pediatr Infect Dis 1984;3:335–40.

66. Connelly MG, Winkelmann RK. Solid facial edema as a complication of acne vulgaris. Arch Dermatol 1985;121:87–90.

67. Lowe LB Jr. Cold panniculitis in children. Am J Dis Child 1968;115:709–13.

68. Epstein EH Jr, Oren ME. Popsicle panniculitis. N Engl J Med 1970;282:966–7.

69. Gross SJ, Nieburg PI. Ludwig's angina in childhood. Am J Dis Child 1977;131:291–2.

70. Finch RG, Snider GE Jr, Sprinkle PM. Ludwig's angina. JAMA 1980;243:1171–3.

71. Perkins CS, Meisner J, Harrison JM. A complication of tongue piercing. Br Dental J 1997;182:147–8.

72. Paonessa DF, Goldstein JC. Anatomy and physiology of head and neck infections (with emphasis on the fascia of the head and neck). Otolaryngol Clin North Am 1976;9:561–90.

73. Megran DW, Scheifele DW, Chow AW. Odontogenic infections. Pediatr Infect Dis 1984;3:257–65.

74. Schuit KE, Johnson JT. Infections of the head and neck. Pediatr Clin North Am 1981;28:965–71.

75. Nyberg DA, Jeffrey RB, Brant-Zawadzki M, et al. Computed tomography of cervical infections. J Comput Assist Tomogr 1985;9:288–96.

76. Har-El G, Aroesty JH, Shaha A, Lucente FE. Changing trends in deep neck abscess. A retrospective study of 110 patients. Oral Surg Oral Med Oral Pathol 1994;77:446–50.

77. Bartlett JG, Gorbach SL. Anaerobic infections of the head and neck. Otolaryngol Clin North Am 1976;9:655–78.

78. Levitt GW. Cervical fascia and deep neck infections. Otolaryngol Cln North Am 1976;9:703–16.

79. Juang YC, Cheng DL, Wang LS, et al. Ludwig's angina: an analysis of 14 cases. Scand J Infect Dis 1989;21:121–5.

80. Shannon GW, Ellis CV, Stepp WP. Oropharyngeal *Bacteroides melaninogenicus* infection with septicemia: Lemierre's syndrome. J Fam Pract 1983;16:159–66.

81. Gallia LJ, Johnson JT. Cervical necrotizing fasciitis. Otolaryngol Head Neck Surg 1981;89:935–7.

82. Myers EN, Cunningham MJ. Inflammatory presentations of congenital head and neck masses. Pediatr Infect Dis J 1988;7:S162–8.

83. Pounds LA. Neck masses of congenital origin. Pediatr Clin North Am 1981;28:841–4.

84. Thompson JW, Cohen SR, Reddix P. Retropharyngeal abscess in children. Laryngoscope 1988;98:589–92.

85. Barratt GE, Koopman CF Jr, Coulthard SW. Retropharyngeal abscess—a ten-year experience. Laryngoscope 1984;94:455–63.

86. Goldenberg D, Golz A, Joachims HZ. Retropharyngeal abscess: a clinical review. J Laryngol Otol 1997;111:546–60.

87. Brook I. Microbiology of retropharyngeal abscesses in children. Am J Dis Child 1987;141:202–4.

87a. Asmar BI. Bacteriology of retropharyngeal abscess in children. Pediatr Infect Dis J 1990;9:595–7.

88. Neumann JL, Schleuter DP. Retropharyngeal abscess as the presenting feature of tuberculosis of the cervical spine. Am Rev Resp Dis 1974;110:508–11.

89. Seid AB, Dunbar JS, Cotton RT. Retropharyngeal abscesses in children revisited. Laryngoscope 1979;89:1717–24.

90. Currarino G, Williams B. Air collection in the retropharyngeal soft tissues observed in lateral expiratory films of the neck in 9 infants. Pediatr Radiol 1993;23:186–8.

91. Stone ME, Walner DL, Koch BL, et al. Correlation between computed tomography and surgical findings in retropharyngeal inflammatory processes in children. Int J Pediatr Otorhinolaryngol 1999;49:121–5.

92. Lazor JB, Cunningham MJ, Eavey RD, Weber AL. Comparison of computed tomography and surgical findings in deep neck infections. Otolaryngol Head Neck Surg 1994;111:746–50.

93. Eliashar R, Sichel YV, Gomori JM, et al. Role of computed tomography scan in the diagnosis and treatment of deep neck infections in children [letter]. Laryngoscope 1999; 109:844.

94. Gaglani MJ, Edwards MS. Clinical indicators of childhood retropharyngeal abscess. Am J Emerg Med 1995;13: 333–6.

95. Chao HC, Chiu CH, Lin SJ, Lin TY. Color Doppler ultrasonography of retropharyngeal abscess. J Otolaryngol 1999; 28:138–41.

96. McCook TA, Felman AH. Retropharyngeal masses in infants and young children. Am J Dis Child 1979;133:41–3.

97. Ramilo J, Harris VJ, White H. Empyema as a complication of retropharyngeal and neck abscesses in children. Radiology 1978;126:743–6.

98. Murray PM, Finegold SM. Anaerobic mediastinitis. Rev Infect Dis 1984;6(suppl):S123–7.

99. Taylor WE Jr, Myer CM III, Hays LL, et al. Acute suppurative thyroiditis in children. Laryngoscope 1982;92: 1269–73.

100. Taguchi T, Okuno A, Fujita K, et al. Etiologic factors in acute suppurative thyroiditis. J Infect Dis 1982;146:447.

101. Womack WA, Cole WH. Thyroiditis. Surgery 1944;16: 770–81.

102. Nelson AJ. Neonatal suppurative thyroiditis. Pediatr Infect Dis 1983;2:243–4.

103. Rich EJ, Mendelman PM. Acute suppurative thyroiditis in pediatric patients. Pediatr Infect Dis J 1987;6:936–40.

104. Berger SA, Zonszein J, Villamena P, Mittman N. Infectious diseases of the thyroid gland. Rev Infect Dis 1983;5: 108–18.

105. Berger SA, Zonszein J, Villamena P, et al. Infectious diseases of the thyroid gland. Rev Infect Dis 1983;5:108–22.

106. Yu EH, Ko WC, Chuang YC, Wu TJ. Suppurative *Acinetobacter baumanii* thyroiditis with bacteremic pneumonia: case report and review. Clin Infect Dis 1998;27:1286–90.

107. Conrad C. Ultrasonography of the thyroid. Eur J Radiol 1985;5:218–20.

108. Vibhaker SD, Eckhauser C, Bellon EM. Computed tomography of the nasopharynx and neck. J Comp Tomogr 1983; 7:259–69.

110. Bussman YC, Song ML, Bell MJ, et al. Suppurative thyroiditis with gas formation due to mixed anaerobic infection. J Pediatr 1977;90:321–2.

111. Petru A, Azimi PH. Esophagitis associated with *Candida* infection in a neonate. Clin Pediatr 1984;23:179–81.

112. Hachiya KA, Kobayashi RH, Antonson DL. Candida esophagitis following antibiotic usage. Pediatr Infect Dis 1982; 1:168–70.

113. Ashenburg C, Rothstein FC, Dahms BB. Herpes esophagitis in the immunocompetent child. J Pediatr 1986;108:584–7.

114. Wilcox CM, Straub RF, Clark WS. Prospective evaluation of oropharyngeal findings in human immunodeficiency virus-infected patients with esophageal ulceration. Am J Gastroenterol 1995;90:1938–41.

115. Sheft DJ, Shrago G. Esophageal moniliasis: the spectrum of disease. JAMA 1970;213:1859–62.

116. Levine MS, Macones AJ Jr, Laufer I. *Candida* esophagitis: accuracy of radiographic diagnosis. Radiology 1985;154: 581–7.

117. Pappas PG, Rex JH, Sabel JD, et al. Guidelines for treatment of Candidiasis. Clin Infect Dis 2004;38:161–89.

CHAPTER 7

Middle Respiratory Syndromes

■ GENERAL CONCEPTS

The middle respiratory tract can be defined as the area from the top of the larynx to the bronchioles. Pharyngitis and other upper respiratory infections are discussed in Chapter 2. Pneumonia syndromes are discussed in Chapter 8, although the frequency and some of the physiologic problems of both pneumonia and middle respiratory syndromes are discussed in this section.

Respiratory physiology, respiratory insufficiency, and arterial blood gas analysis are discussed in simplified terms. More specialized textbooks should be consulted for further details.[1–3]

Symptoms in Pulmonary Disease

Tachypnea

Rapid breathing is often obvious, but counting and observing respirations is generally neglected. The child should be observed and examined without clothing covering the chest. If there is no cough or other physical sign of pulmonary disease accompanying the tachypnea, a metabolic acidosis (such as diabetic acidosis or acidosis from dehydration) should be suspected. In this case, the hyperventilation is a respiratory compensation for metabolic acidosis. If cough and other pulmonary signs are present, hypoxemia is the likely cause of the tachypnea. Fever in young children will often cause both tachypnea and tachycardia.

Acute Chest Pain

In children with respiratory disease, acute chest pain is usually increased by breathing (pleuritic) and indicates pleural disease, usually infection. Pain on coughing also implies pleuritic disease. In young children, pleural disease is manifested by splinting or unequal expansion.

Chest pain may be caused by pneumothorax or pneumomediastinum, which may be spontaneous or occur after mild trauma or coughing. Chest pain may also be related to anxiety, costochondritis, or strained intercostal muscles. Pulmonary embolism or infarction is exceedingly rare in children and should suggest a thrombotic disorder. Coxsackie B virus infection can cause fever and chest pain (pleurodynia).

Physical Signs in Pulmonary Disease

Anxiety

Facial expression and hyperactivity may imply anxiety, which in turn implies hypoxemia. Nasal flaring, retractions, and grunting also may be observed by simple inspection of the patient.

Splinting

Pain on inspiration can sometimes be inferred by observing protection of the involved side by holding it, not moving it as well, or by lying on it.

Names for Chest Signs

Rales are a fine crackling noise that may be simulated by rubbing the hair behind your ear between thumb and forefinger. They are also referred to as crackles and are more commonly inspiratory. They may be heard in pneumonia, bronchiolitis, atelectasis, and heart failure. End-inspiratory rales are typical of pneumonia. Rales that disappear after coughing are usually of no significance. Rhonchi are harsh upper airway noises that typically occur during both inspiration and expiration. Wheezes are high-pitched, whistling noises that occur most commonly during expiration and are produced by airflow through a partially obstructed airway. Polyphonic (musical) wheezes are typical of asthma, whereas those in other conditions (such as bronchomalacia) are often monophonic. Stridor is a high-pitched crowing sound that usually indicates large airway obstruction. If the obstruction is extrathoracic (from nose to midtrachea), the stridor is mostly inspiratory, as in croup; if the obstruction is intrathoracic, the stridor is usually expiratory. Stertor is the name given to loud noises that occur because of nasopharyngeal restriction, usually from mucus (similar to snoring). Dyspnea, or distress during breathing, is manifested in children by nasal flaring, suprasternal and infrasternal retractions, cyanosis, and a rapid respiratory rate.

Apnea Spells

Periods of not breathing (apnea) can have many causes. Apnea of less than 15 seconds is often a normal finding in infants, whereas apneic episodes longer than 15 seconds are usually abnormal. Certain infections can produce apnea,[4,5] especially pertussis, chlamydia, and respiratory syncytial virus (RSV) infection (Box 7-1). Lower respiratory tract infection was the fourth most common discharge diagnosis in a study of 130 infants admitted with a diagnosis of apparent life-threatening event (ALTE).[6] Among children with RSV infection, risk factors for apnea include young age, prematurity, hypercapnia, hypothermia, and atelectasis on chext x-ray.

Noninfectious causes in infants include seizures and gastroesophageal reflux.[7]

Classification

In middle and lower respiratory infections, a complete diagnosis ideally includes an anatomic diagnosis (such as "right middle lobe pneumonia"), an etiologic diagnosis (such as "probably pneumococcal"), and a physiologic diagnosis formulated as

quantitatively as possible (such as "respiratory acidosis, probably well compensated now"). Thus, respiratory syndromes can be classified on the basis of anatomic syndrome, etiologic agent, or physiologic problem.

Anatomic Syndrome

It is customary to use the diagnostic term that indicates the most severe illness if more than one anatomic area is involved. For example, if the patient has both bronchitis and pneumonia, usually only pneumonia is recorded. Furthermore, a multiple term such as laryngotracheobronchitis (LTB) has the disadvantage of vagueness and diffuseness. The diagnosis of "croup syndrome" or "laryngitis" more accurately identifies the site of the most dangerous involvement: the larynx. The anatomic diagnosis should localize the disease as specifically as possible. For example, "bilateral interstitial pneumonia" is much more meaningful than simply "pneumonia." In the following sections, the anatomic diagnoses are discussed, beginning with the larynx at the top of the tracheobronchial tree and descending to the small bronchioles (Box 7-2). Syndromes involving the alveoli and pleural space are discussed in Chapter 8.

Etiologic Classification

In the following sections, the etiologic diagnoses are discussed in terms of probabilities for each anatomic syndrome. A clinical prediction of the etiology of a patient's lower respiratory infection can be made on the basis of the anatomic area involved, the particular clinical manifestations of the illness,

---

BOX 7-1 ■ Causes of Apnea in Infancy

Infectious
Respiratory syncytial virus (RSV)
Pertussis
Chlamydial pneumonia
Rotavirus[8]
Epstein-Barr virus[9]
Pneumocystis jiroveci (formerly *carinii*) pneumonia
Other lower respiratory-tract infections

Noninfectious
Gastroesophageal reflux
Seizures
Prematurity
Others

BOX 7-2 ■ Classification of Middle Respiratory Syndromes

Cough only
Laryngitis
    Supraglottitis (epiglottitis)
    Croup
    Episodic croup ("spasmodic" croup)
    Purulent tracheobronchitis
Acute bronchitis
Pertussis-like illness
Influenza-like illness
Bronchiolitis
Asthmatic bronchitis
Asthma

past statistical studies of similar cases, and Gram staining of specimens to be cultured.

The general principles for the use of laboratory procedures and cultures for both pneumonia and middle respiratory infections are discussed at the beginning of chapter 8. Etiologic diagnoses are important and necessary for specific chemotherapy. However, in severe lower respiratory infections, the early diagnosis and treatment of physiologic disturbances may be lifesaving.

Physiologic Disturbances

The physician should identify and evaluate the degree of physiologic disturbances in all patients with significant respiratory problems (Table 7-1).

Frequency

In a study of consecutive visits by 1,570 ill children to a pediatric group's office in Rochester, New York, approximately one-fourth of all illnesses were respiratory infections.[10] In a study of visits to an emergency room during hours that physicians' offices were closed, children less than 18 years of age accounted for about 60% of the visits.[11] Of the 858 randomly selected visits for infections, about 24% were classified as upper respiratory, 12% as middle respiratory, 6% as lower respiratory, 23% as pararespiratory (such as otitis or sinusitis), and 35% other infections. Thus, middle respiratory (airway) syndromes were twice as common as lower respiratory syndromes (pneumonia).

Respiratory Insufficiency

Respiratory insufficiency can lead to acute respiratory failure, defined as hypoxemia, hypercarbia (respiratory acidosis) or both.[12] The clinician must be able to recognize the clinical signs that suggest impending respiratory failure.[13,14]

Respiratory Acidosis

Resulting from excess CO_2 (hypercarbia), respiratory acidosis is secondary to hypoventilation or a severe ventilation–perfusion mismatch. Signs of acute respiratory acidosis include sweating, anxious expression on the face, falling rates of respiration and pulse, and rising blood pressure. Cyanosis is a late sign. A widened QRS pattern on EKG also occurs later. Because acute CO_2 retention is typically the result of hypoventilation, it is usually best treated by mechanical ventilation unless the cause of the hypoventilation can be rapidly reversed.

Hypoxemia

This is defined as a low arterial pO_2, whereas hypoxia implies oxygen deficiency in the tissues. Hypoxemia is usually secondary to ventilation–perfusion imbalance, venous-to-arterial shunt, hypo-

TABLE 7-1. MIDDLE AND LOWER RESPIRATORY PHYSIOLOGIC PROBLEMS

PROBLEM	EXAMPLES
High airway obstruction	Croup; foreign body; purulent tracheobronchitis
Low airway obstruction	Bronchiolitis; asthma; foreign body
Respiratory muscle weakness	Any acute prolonged lower respiratory infection, especially in a premature or debilitated infant or in a patient with muscle disease
Impaired diffusion of oxygen (alveolar diffusion block)	Interstitial fibrosis
Restriction of lung expansion	Pneumothorax; pleural effusion; ascites; severe obesity
Perfusion–ventilation mismatching	Atelectasis; arteriovenous shunting; reduced pulmonary blood flow; shock, especially septic
Respiratory center depression	Drugs; head injury
Central hyperventilation	Meningitis; encephalitis
Acidotic hyperventilation	Diabetes

ventilation, or diffusion impairment. Signs of hypoxemia include tachypnea, cyanosis, restlessness, poor judgment, weakness, and confusion. In severe hypoxia, the muscle tone is poor, and the patient is often limp. Hypoxemia is best treated with oxygen, first with increased concentrations, then assisted ventilation if necessary. Spot or continuous monitoring of oxygen saturation provides a useful guide for the administration of oxygen.

Anticipation of Respiratory Insufficiency

The most serious error in the treatment of middle or lower respiratory infections is to fail to recognize how seriously ill the patient really is. Early recognition of respiratory insufficiency is difficult unless the physician is experienced and can make frequent clinical observations. Therefore, if there is doubt, the patient should be transferred to a location where intensive observation can be done and arterial blood gases measured frequently and accurately.

■ COUGH ONLY

Cough only is a useful preliminary diagnosis when cough is present without fever, rhonchi, rales, or dyspnea. By definition, it is an isolated symptom, without lower respiratory signs and without fever (rectal temperature 101°F = 38.4°C). Chronic cough can be defined as persistence of a cough for more than 3 weeks.[15] Except for psychological coughs,[16] this symptom usually reflects irritation of the tracheobronchial tree. This irritation may be caused by inhalants (such as cigarette smoke), local inflammation, or secretions entering the trachea from above (sinuses). Cough only is rarely caused by pulmonary parenchymal disease, as discussed later.

Causes and Diagnostic Approach

The possible causes of cough only are listed in Box 7-3. Asthma is a common cause of chronic cough in children.[17,18] Although there is much controversy about the diagnosis of cough-variant asthma, most experts agree that some children do display their asthma with cough alone. These children have abnormal pulmonary function tests and an abnormal response to methacholine challenge similar to those with classic asthma. Children with cough-variant ashthma often have a family or personal history of atopy. Cough is likely to be worse at night, to disrupt sleep, and to sound like the cough of a classic

BOX 7-3 ■ Possible Causes of Cough Only
Cough-variant asthma
Postinfectious (after bronchitis, influenza, pertussis, mycoplasmal infection)
Foreign body in larynx or bronchus
Rhinitis, sinusitis, or postnasal drip syndrome
Habit cough
Smoking (active or passive)
Irritation of the pleura, diaphragm, or pericardium
Irritation of the auricular branch of the vagus nerve (foreign body or wax in ear canal)
Elongated uvula
Tourette's syndrome
Gastroesophageal reflux
Vascular ring or vascular sling
Pollution or irritant exposure (environmental dust, cigarette smoke, etc.)

asthmatic.[19] Cough may also be exacerbated by exercise or exposure to cold air. Some of these patients will go on to develop classic wheezing asthma over time. Chronic cough is by no means synonymous with cough-variant asthma, however, and failure to respond to bronchodilator or anti-inflammatory therapy over the course of several weeks should lead the physician to consider other diagnostic possibilities.

Cystic fibrosis is a rare cause of cough only. Sweat chloride concentration should be measured in children who have nasal polyps, poor growth, or both in addition to cough. Radiologic evidence of pulmonary disease is usually present in patients with cough secondary to cystic fibrosis.

The quality of the cough may also be instructive. Seal-like or croupy cough suggests tracheomalacia. The cough of children with vascular rings may have a similar quality.

Subacute or chronic sinusitis may cause cough in the absence of either headache or fever, as discussed in Chapter 5. History may reveal that the cough began during an episode of the common cold syndrome. Thus it must be differentiated from postviral cough syndrome, which occurs in the absence of demonstrable sinus infection. Sinus serie x-rays or coronal computed tomography (CT) may be helpful when the diagnosis is seriously considered.[20]

Gastroesophageal reflux (GER) may cause a wet-sounding cough that occurs mostly when the infant or child is lying down. Paradoxically, it has been shown that thickening the formula with rice cereal actually increases the frequency of cough in infants with GER.[21]

Children may aspirate a foreign body, such as a peanut, which may lodge in any part of the airway. Typically, the child is 1 to 2 years old.[22] There may be a history of a foreign body in the mouth, usually a food, with an episode of falling or choking, followed by persistent cough, unilateral wheezing, and decreased air entry on the affected side.[23] Unfortunately, the actual aspiration event is often unwitnessed and may be followed by a clinically silent stage. The aspirated foreign body is often vegetable matter and is therefore radiolucent. This may rarely lead to a child presenting with a chronic intractable pneumonia.[24] Laryngoscopy or bronchoscopy is often necessary. If a foreign body is suspected, rigid rather than flexible bronchoscopy is preferred.[25]

A careful history and physical examination can establish the cause of cough in most cases. Chest x-ray is usually indicated. Children older than 6 years should undergo pulmonary function testing. Exercise challenge or methacholine challenge are usually not necessary. A history of possible exposures to tuberculosis should be taken and, if positive, tuberculin skin testing performed. In one series of children with chronic cough, a trial of therapy directed at the most likely cause established the diagnosis in 58% of cases.[26]

Barium swallow or endoscopy should be considered if the preceding studies are negative and the cough persists, especially in infants.[27]

Treatment

No specific therapy is needed in the absence of a specific etiology. Symptomatic therapy includes attempts to improve humidification and use of over-the-counter antihistamines to decrease postnasal drip.

Cough syrups are discussed in Chapter 2. They should be avoided in young children, as no cough suppressant has been studied for efficacy or safety in children less than 2 years of age.

■ LARYNGEAL SYNDROMES

Definitions

The manifestations of laryngitis may include stridor and voice changes such as hoarseness, a barking or brassy cough, or aphonia (usually due to refusal to speak). The child may indicate to the parent that the "throat" (laryngeal area) is sore.

In adults, laryngitis is recognized by hoarseness. In children, subglottic laryngitis is usually called croup. Inspiratory stridor is the most characteristic sign in laryngitis and is the hallmark of high respiratory obstruction of any cause (Table 7-2). Substernal inspiratory retraction is typically present in moderate to severe cases and also is a general sign of upper airway (extrathoracic) obstruction.

TABLE 7-2. FINDINGS IN LARYNGEAL SYNDROMES

	SUBGLOTTIC (VIRAL CROUP)	SUPRAGLOTTIC (EPIGLOTTITIS)	PURULENT TRACHEO-BRONCHITIS
Appearance	Usually not seriously ill	Seriously ill, drooling	Variable
Preferred position	Lying	Sitting	Variable
Barking cough	Typical	Rare	Possible
Hoarseness or aphonia	Variable	Typical	Uncommon
Red or edematous epiglottis	Absent	Typical	Absent
Inspiratory stridor or retraction	Present	Present	Variable
Expiratory wheezes	Absent	Absent	Often present
Fever	Variable	Usually high	Moderately high
Purulent secretions in trachea	Absent	Rare	Typical
Course	Gradual—days	Rapid—hours	Rapid atelectasis; airway needed

A child with laryngitis or any other upper airway obstruction has trouble getting air *into* the lungs, whereas the child with bronchiolitis, or other lower airway (intrathoracic) obstruction, has trouble getting air *out of* the lungs. In laryngitis, breath sounds are usually decreased throughout all lung fields, and this is usually described as poor air entry or exchange.

Classification

The literature contains a dizzying array of different diagnostic terms for the various conditions that affect the larynx and trachea. Laryngitis is a working diagnosis that is best used when the location of the laryngeal disease cannot be further identified. Laryngitis can be classified into subglottic or supraglottic laryngitis. Although it is useful to distinguish between supraglottic and subglottic laryngitis, this distinction is often difficult when the child is first seen. Laryngitis or croup syndrome is a useful preliminary descriptive diagnosis until more definitive information (such as a lateral roentgenogram of the neck) is available. "Croup syndrome" also has been used to emphasize the variety of possible causes and location of the laryngeal disease. In this section, "croup" is used to refer to subglottic laryngitis, presumably viral (Table 7-2). "Epiglottitis" is an imprecise term often used in place of the better "supraglottitis;" the latter term is superior because the epiglottis may be minimally involved in some cases in which most of the swelling is in the aryepiglottic folds. Spasmodic croup is also a poor name, due to the lack of evidence that laryngospasm plays an etiologic role in the condition. Preferred terms are as follows (with the usual terms in parentheses): croup, supraglottitis (epiglottitis), episodic croup (spasmodic croup), and suppurative tracheitis, laryngotracheitis, laryngotracheobronchitis, or laryngotracheobronchopneumonitis (bacterial tracheitis), depending on the extent of the bacterial superinfection.

Severe laryngitis, whether subglottic or supraglottic, is an extremely important pediatric emergency. It may be necessary to call an anesthesiologist or otorhinolaryngologist to perform tracheal intubation or tracheostomy. The primary care physician in training should learn to perform difficult intubations as well as emergency ventilation with a bag and mask. However, intubation may be impossible in some patients with supraglottitis (epiglottitis), so an operative airway procedure, such as tracheostomy or cricothyroid membrane puncture, may be needed.

Age and Frequency

Laryngitis in adults characteristically produces only hoarseness or loss of voice. However, when children have laryngitis, they may have a much more serious illness because the larynx is smaller. Edema in a child's larynx thus produces more obstruction of the airway than the same amount of edema in an adult. Another important factor is that young children are usually experiencing primary infection with a particular respiratory virus, whereas adults will have been previously infected. Primary infection with the parainfluenza viruses and respiratory syncytial virus tends to be more severe and to spread more widely in the respiratory tract. This is in contrast to second or later infections, in which these viruses tend to be restricted to the upper airway.

Hospitalization is needed for only a small percentage of patients with laryngitis seen in an office or outpatient clinic. Although only a few children hospitalized because of croup are likely to need intubation, the possibility of acute progression of the obstruction must always be remembered.

Viral croup tends to be seasonal, especially when caused by parainfluenza virus type 1, its most frequent etiologic agent. Peak time for admissions from croup in temperate climates is late fall, and the epidemic is more severe in odd-numbered years.[28] Parainfluenza type 3 can also produce severe croup in an endemic pattern. Summertime croup may be due to enteroviruses, adenovirus, or parainfluenza type 3.

Supraglottitis, in contrast, has no seasonal peak. This disease, almost always caused by *Haemophilus influenzae* type b bacteremia, has been virtually eradicated. The peak age frequency for croup is 1–3 years. Supraglottitis occurs in older children, with a peak between 3 and 6 years. Suppurative tracheobronchitis also tends to be a disease of preschool and school-age children.

Physiologic Principles

Laryngeal Edema

The major components in laryngeal obstruction in laryngitis are edema and spasm.

Laryngitis is a classic example of a respiratory infection in which the main problem is upper airway obstruction. Some children have severe enough respiratory obstruction so that if the obstruction is not relieved by an endotracheal tube or tracheotomy, death may occur.

Laryngospasm

Laryngospasm is a feared complication of supraglottitis. Manipulation of the posterior pharynx, such as gagging the patient with a tongue blade, may produce aspiration of secretions, laryngospasm, or both and lead to rapid obstruction of the airway. Examination of the posterior pharynx should not be attempted in the child with severe respiratory distress suspected to be caused by supraglottitis, especially if it involves restraining the child in the supine position. In an older child who can cooperate and in whom supraglottitis is thought to be unlikely, a skilled laryngoscopist can sometimes perform indirect laryngoscopy to exclude the diagnosis.[29] However, equipment and skills should be available for bag and mask ventilation and intubation if direct visual examination is attempted.

The principal cause of episodic croup ("spasmodic croup") is not, as the name suggests, laryngospasm, but rather acute edematous swelling of the subglottic tissues. What causes this process is not well understood. The appearance of the tissues is that of noninflammatory edema.

Purulent Secretions

Rarely, purulent secretions add to obstruction in the trachea and major bronchi. Suctioning is unnecessary in most forms of laryngitis and should usually be avoided, because trauma from the suctioning tube may make the spasm or edema worse.

Hypoxemia

The principal physiologic disturbance in croup is hypoxemia,[30] the mechanism of which is complex. It may be caused by a diffusion block from involvement of the lower airways with infection or by pulmonary edema secondary to high resistance. In any case, low arterial pO_2 is frequently present in croup.[30] CO_2 retention is unusual, and the pCO_2 is usually low because of hyperventilation. When the pCO_2 becomes normal or elevated, the ventilation may be inadequate, indicating a more serious situation (see Fig. 7-1). Except for a rising pCO_2, blood gases are not well correlated with the need for intubation.[31]

Clinical Appearance of Laryngeal Syndromes

Acute upper respiratory obstruction can be classified into several anatomic syndromes on the basis of the location of the obstruction and the clinical findings (Table 7-2). However, the syndromes often cannot be distinguished early in the course. Mild viral croup and episodic croup often may not be distinguishable.

Supraglottitis (Epiglottitis)

Obstruction by edema at and above the glottis (vocal cords) is characterized by pooling of secretions in the pharynx, with drooling. The position of comfort is sitting with the chin forward (Fig. 7-2).[32] Respirations may be slow and careful. Swelling of the entire neck is sometimes observed. The voice is absent (aphonia) or is hoarse, muffled, or guttural. The patient generally appears quite anxious. Onset of the disease is usually quite rapid, and, because this condition is usually accompanied by

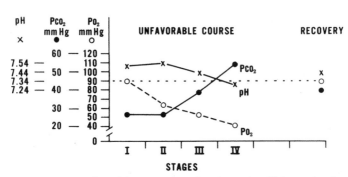

■ FIGURE 7-1 Unfavorable progression of respiratory insufficiency, showing progressive fall of arterial pO_2. PCO_2 elevation is a late finding.

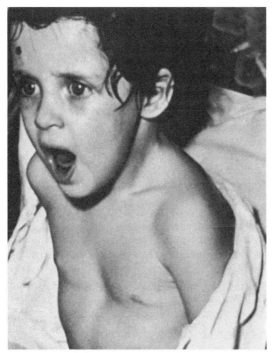

■ **FIGURE 7-2** Typical appearance in severe supraglottic obstruction. See text. (Fearon B: Pediatr Clin North Am 1962; 9:1095–1112)

bacteremia, high fever is seen. This syndrome is an urgent situation, because obstruction may occur suddenly. The epiglottis may be cherry red and spherical, but rarely it can be normal, with the edema localized to the aryepiglottic folds.

Croup

Obstruction by edema below the vocal cords is characterized by pooling of secretions below the vocal cords in the trachea or by edema in the conus elasticus, the loose alveolar tissue below the vocal cords. The position of comfort is usually a lying position, but the child may prefer lying on the back with the neck hyperextended over a pillow. Respiration is usually rapid. There is a brassy or barking cough, usually without hoarseness. Aphonia is uncommon. This form of laryngitis usually has a gradual onset and course, with fatigue as a major factor in respiratory insufficiency. There is sometimes a history of croup.

Purulent Tracheobronchitis

Also called bacterial tracheitis and pseudomembranous tracheitis, purulent tracheobronchitis should be considered as a separate entity, because the physiologic disturbance and treatment are different from those of the preceding two syndromes.[33–37] The condition resembles croup with minimal laryngeal manifestations. Often, a foreign body is suspected because of focal low-pitched inspiratory and expiratory wheezes.[35] It is characterized by pooling of purulent secretions in the trachea and major bronchi. Copious amounts of purulent secretions may be coughed up or suctioned. Laryngeal manifestations are minimal or variable, so that the severity of obstruction may not be recognized. Brassy cough and croupy stridor are usually not present, although viral tracheitis may be a predisposing factor.[36] However, coarse inspiratory and expiratory wheezes, and sometimes rales, can be heard with a stethoscope. Air trapping is common. The wheezing may be lateralized to one major bronchus, which is partially obstructed by purulent secretions, and this may raise the suspicion of a foreign body. Atelectasis is common in severe cases. Chest x-ray may reveal diffuse pulmonary involvement, and sometimes loose pseudomembranes can be seen. Lateral films more easily reveal the narrowing of the tracheal airway with shaggy borders due to thick, purulent secretions.

Acute respiratory insufficiency may occur because of acute obstruction at the trachea or several major bronchi. Nasotracheal intubation or bronchoscopy and suctioning may be lifesaving. A tracheostomy may be necessary to facilitate suctioning. It is important to diagnose this condition rapidly, as a delay in diagnosis leads to poorer outcome.

Episodic Croup (Spasmodic Croup)

This clinical pattern is characterized by sudden onset of croupy cough and inspiratory stridor that typically lasts less than a day or begins to improve in less than a day.[38] Recurrences are common. The syndrome usually develops in a child who was well or only minimally sick at the time he was placed to bed. The patient then awakens with a brassy cough, with or without inspiratory stridor. Fever is absent.

Laryngoscopic examination reveals that the symptoms are caused by the rapid accumulation of edema in the laryngeal tissues. Viral infections are usually implicated, but why some children develop this sudden edema is not well understood. This predisposition tends to run in families. Long-term follow-up studies reveal a higher incidence of asthma in patients with a history of episodic croup.

Rapid response to mist is usually seen. Sometimes, the drive to the hospital will be enough to completely eliminate the symptoms. It tends to recur, sometimes in the same night, and almost always on subsequent nights for 1 to 4 days. During the day the child will occur well or nearly so. Parents can expose the child to mist from the bathroom shower, or may be able to hold off a recurrence by adequately humidifying the child's bedroom. Mist need not be cool. Despite its initial sometimes frightening appearance, episodic croup is almost always benign.

Possible Etiologies

Viruses

Parainfluenza viruses are the most common viral cause of croup and appear to account for 30–40% of the laryngitis in children.[39] Extrapolations from epidemiologic studies suggest that parainfluenza viruses account for approximately 250,000 emergency room visits, 70,000 hospitalizations, and about $190 million in health care costs each year in the United States alone.[40] Parainfluenza viruses types 1 and 3 cause moderate to severe croup, whereas the course of croup secondary to parainfluenza virus type 2 is generally mild. RSV, influenza A and B, adenoviruses, and enteroviruses are occasional causes of croup syndrome, as is the newly discovered human metapupumovirus.[39] Croup caused by a virus usually has a gradual onset and gradual course, although croup secondary to influenza virus can be unusually severe.[41]

There is a fairly high rate of croup syndrome in children with measles infection. Several outbreaks of measles were reported among undervaccinated populations in the early 1990s; in one of these, 82 (19%) of 440 children diagnosed as having measles also had croup.[42]

Herpes simplex virus (HSV) has been identified as the cause of prolonged croup symptoms in patients with severe gingivostomatitis.[43] Epstein-Barr virus (EBV) was the cause in one 12-year-old who developed a pseudomembrane.[44]

Parainfluenza or influenza viruses appear to be rare causes of supraglottic laryngitis.[45]

A particularly recalcitrant cause of recurrent hoarseness, stridor, and sometimes respiratory obstruction is laryngeal papillomatosis, a condition caused by human papillomaviruses (usually serotype 6 or 11) that are acquired via passage through the birth canal. Multiple and sometimes frequent surgical procedures may be required to relieve obstructive symptoms.

Bacteria

H. influenzae supraglottitis may be an extreme medical emergency. It usually is characterized by the findings of supraglottic obstruction, with a red swollen epiglottis and a rapid course.[46,47] In a few cases of H. influenzae laryngitis, the subglottic area may be the major focus of the obstruction.

Other bacteria, particularly Groups A, B, or C beta-hemolytic streptococci, may rarely produce severe laryngitis.[48–50] Mycoplasma pneumoniae has been associated with croup in some patients. Diphtheria may produce a membranous obstruction in the larynx or trachea. This disease is now relatively rare but should still be considered, especially when exudative pharyngitis is present with croup in an unimmunized child. Staphylococcus aureus is the usual cause of purulent tracheobronchitis according to cultures of the purulent tracheal aspirates. Gram-negative enteric organisms are rarely implicated in purulent laryngotracheobronchitis.

Previous immunization with H. influenzae type b vaccine does not exclude the possibility of H. influenzae supraglottitis, but a child who has received the entire immunization series is highly unlikely to develop this disease. In addition, herd immunity from the widespread use of the vaccine has rendered the condition rare, even in unimmunized children.

Fungi

Inspiratory stridor in a young infant and supraglottitis in immunocompromised adults have been caused by Candida albicans.[51,52] One of us has managed a young child with recurrent croup caused by infection with Sporothrix shenkii, which was exacerbated by treatment with systemic corticosteroids.[52a]

Foreign Body

Aspiration of a foreign body into the larynx or esophagus by a small child can produce the croup syndrome, usually with subglottic obstruction.[53,54] The illness may closely resemble infectious croup, especially if fever develops because of pneumonia in the obstructed lung.

Gastroesophageal Reflux

Gastroesophageal reflux (GER) can be a cause of episodic croup. One retrospective study of 66 patients with recurrent croup episodes found that 47% of the patients had GER.[55] Because of its retrospective nature this study was likely subject to selection bias. However, the authors did demonstrate a "dose-response" relationship of sorts; children who were hospitalized three or more times for croup had a higher prevalence of GER.[55] These patients tended to be younger and to have a shorter interval between episodes of croup. No controls were evaluated. Another small study documented that eight of eight children with recurrent croup who underwent esophageal pH probe studies had GER. Six control subjects had normal pH probe studies.[56]

Allergy or Irritation

Allergic laryngeal edema can be severe and dangerous. Inhaled irritants can produce laryngeal spasm in individuals who are particularly susceptible. This may be one possible cause of episodic croup. Some cases appear to be precipitated by cold air (e.g., from an air conditioner). Aspiration of a small amount of gastric contents also appears to be an occasional cause of laryngeal irritation and a crouplike illness. Toxic inhalants can produce an episodic croup.[57] Hot beverages can cause thermal epiglottitis in infants.

Other Syndromes

Laryngitis may be suspected when upper airway obstruction results in inspiratory stridor. Retropharyngeal abscess can produce stridor and is discussed further in Chapter 6. Epilepsy can cause recurrent laryngospasm.[58] Hereditary angioedema can produce the rapid onset of symptoms of croup. This condition is related to C1 esterase inhibitor deficiency.[58a] Teenagers may present with acute upper airway obstruction due to vocal cord dysfunction. This condition is caused by paradoxical closure of the vocal cords and may present with stridor or wheezing. It is most common in adolescent females and responds to speech therapy and psychotherapy.[59]

Diagnostic Approach

Lateral Neck Radiograph

These radiographs, ordered for viewing the soft tissues rather than the cervical spine, are frequently used to determine the area of obstruction when the patient's condition is good (Figs. 7-3 and 7-4). Radiographs of the lateral neck require experience to interpret, and comparison with diagrams of this area may be helpful (Figs. 7-3 and 7-4). Anteroposterior views may show subglottic edema in supraglottic laryngitis, in addition to supraglottic edema.[60] A radiopaque foreign body can be excluded by these radiographs. A review of lateral neck radiographs by radiologists who did not know the diagnosis indicated that for subglottic laryngitis, the interpretation is very reliable except in severe cases with unreadable roentgenograms.[61] A newer

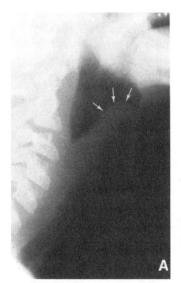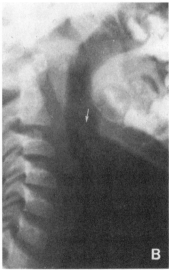

■ **FIGURE 7-3** Roentgenogram of lateral neck in epiglottis. (**A**) Epiglottitis; (**B**) normal. Compare with Figure 7-4. (Rapkin RH: J Pediatr 1972;80:96–98)

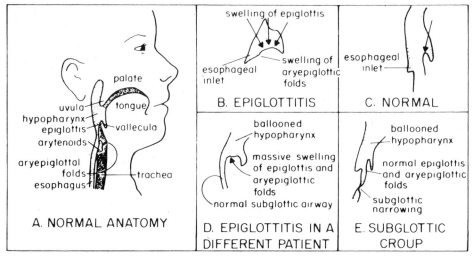

■ **FIGURE 7-4** Diagrams of lateral neck radiographs in laryngitis. (**A**) Normal anatomy; the esophagus is normally not visible on lateral neck roentgenograms because it does not contain air. (**B**) Roentgenogram in epiglottitis; as shown in Figure 7-3A. (**C**) Normal roentgenogram as shown in Figure 7-3B. (**D**) Roentgenogram in another case of epiglottitis. (**E**) Roentgenogram in subglottic laryngitis. (**D** and **E** from Poole CA, Altman D: Radiology 1963;80:798–805)

study compared the results of plain radiography with diagnosis made at microlaryngoscopy and bronchoscopy in 144 children with acute upper airway obstruction.[62] X-ray diagnosis was > 86% sensitive for diagnosing suppurative laryngotracheitis, foreign body, and innominate artery compression. The sensitivity of plain films in the diagnosis of laryngomalacia and tracheomalacia was 5% and 62%, respectively.[62] Another review indicated that poor-quality radiographs interfered with accurate radiologic interpretation.[63]

A child in severe respiratory distress should not be sent for a radiograph but should have a direct examination with operating room facilities, an anesthesiologist, and an otolaryngologist who can intubate or do endoscopy or tracheostomy. Even a mildly ill child should be accompanied by someone capable of providing an emergency airway or ventilation.

White Blood Cell Count and Differential

Sometimes, a white cell count and differential is used as a guide to whether antibiotics should be used; these studies usually are of no special value. No laboratory values were of use in distinguishing viral croup from purulent tracheobronchitis in one small study.[64]

Cultures

Throat culture for bacteria is of no value. Tracheal secretions recovered at the time of intubation should be cultured for *H. influenzae* and other bacteria, as well as for viruses. Blood culture may be of value in children with suspected supraglottitis, although the yield is low. Patients with croup need not undergo blood culturing. In a study of 249 highly febrile (temperature > 39°C) children between the ages of 3 and 36 months who had a clinical diagnosis of croup,[65] none had a positive culture.

Arterial Blood Gases

If the patient appears seriously ill and possibly in need of an airway soon, then restraint, such as for arterial puncture, should not be done. Capillary blood gases are most useful in a gradually progressive illness where the adequacy of air exchange may be difficult to assess but did not correlate with the need for endotracheal intubation in one study of croup and epiglottitis.[31]

Treatment of Suspected Supraglottitis

Although supraglottitis is rarely seen, its diagnosis and treatment are critical because it can be rapidly fatal. Therefore, a discussion of its treatment is first.

It is sometimes difficult for the clinician to distinguish between the two major kinds of laryngitis; a cautious approach is indicated. Hospitals should have their own written protocol for management of a child with suspected supraglottitis.[47,66,67] The following approach is based on the possibility that the child might have supraglottitis (Box 7-4).

Tracheal Intubation

In severe laryngeal obstruction, tracheal intubation may be needed.[68–73] It has been used successfully instead of tracheotomy in most cases of acute epiglottitis, but the risk of delayed or unsuccessful intubation is always present, especially if laryngeal edema is severe.

The principal value of this procedure is its immediate availability for emergency use. It appears to be preferable when experienced personnel are available for intubation. The major disadvantage is the occasional postintubation complication of subglottic stenosis, which is a greater problem than removal of the tube from a tracheostomy.

Tracheostomy

Routine elective tracheostomy was advocated in the early 1970s for patients with supraglottitis, because usually 20 or 30 minutes were necessary to mobilize personnel to do an urgent tracheotomy, and intubation was difficult.[68,74]

Antibiotics

Ceftriaxone (or its equivalent) is indicated for febrile, toxic patients. Antibiotics do not decrease the need for careful observation early in the course of severe laryngitis and have a lower priority than evaluation of the airway.

Treatment of Croup

The management of severe croup includes many of the same steps described previously for supraglottitis (Box 7-4). Other treatment possibilities for croup follow.

Nebulized Racemic Epinephrine

This is a mixture of equal parts of d and l (ordinary) epinephrine. Because d-epinephrine has relatively little activity, the equal parts mixture gets its activity almost entirely from the l-epinephrine (the form commonly available diluted 1:1000). Thus, the standard preparation of 2.25% racemic (d,l) epinephrine is physiologically equivalent to 1% epinephrine (USP). A small but well-designed study that assigned 16 children with severe croup to racemic epinephrine and 15 to l-epinephrine treatment demonstrated that l-epinephrine is at least as effective as racemic epinephrine.[75] L-epinephrine has the advantages of lower cost, more widespread availability, and potentially lower adverse event rate.

Epinephrine apparently produces relief of obstruction by local vasoconstriction, which shrinks the edematous mucosa. Epinephrine is widely used

---

BOX 7-4 ■ Summary of Priorities in Severe Laryngitis

1. Allow the child to assume a position of comfort while observing respirations and taking history. Offer oxygen by mask when available.
2. Obtain the proper size bag and face mask, oxygen supply, and intubating equipment.
3. Call an otolaryngologist and anesthesiologist (who should notify the operating room) if history and examination or if lateral neck film indicates supraglottic obstruction.
4. Ventilate with bag and mask (or mouth to mouth) if respiratory arrest occurs.
5. Accompany the child from the office to the hospital or from the emergency room to the radiology department, ward, or operating room, and be prepared to resuscitate and provide an airway.
6. Examine gently. If child is in distress, do not restrain. Use a light to examine pharynx, without gagging.
7. Avoid unessential manipulation, such as venipunctures or injections.
8. Request 0.3 mg/kg of dexamethasone, a mist tent, 4 mL of 1:8 racemic epinephrine, a respiratory therapist and respiratory equipment to deliver the racemic epinephrine.
9. Obtain a lateral film soft tissues of the neck, at the bedside if possible.
10. Use racemic epinephrine as part of oxygen therapy, if tolerated.
11. Use dexamethasone IM or IV if intubation attempt is anticipated.
12. Intubate in operating room or area with setup for tracheostomy if needed.

and appears to be helpful in laryngotracheitis, at least for several hours.[76] The usual dose is 2.5% racemic epinephrine or 1% l-epinephrine diluted 1:8 (0.5 ml of epinephrine in 3.5 ml distilled water) given by face mask without positive pressure.[77] One drawback of nebulized epinephrine has been the potential for rebound, wherein the patient transiently improves but then becomes quite suddenly worse when the therapy "wears off." Because of this concern, it was once widely believed that patients who received epinephrine in the emergency department needed to be admitted to the hospital. A prospective cohort study showed that patients with croup who received both epinephrine and dexamethasone and, at the end of a two-hour observation period, had neither stridor nor intercostal retractions at rest could be safely discharged home.[78] Of 82 patients treated in this way, only 6 required more therapy within the next 48 hours and only 2 required hospital admission.[78] Nebulized epinephrine is not without risk, however. A recent report tells of a young child who developed an acute myocardial infarction after receiving multiple doses of racemic epinephrine in the emergency department.[79]

Corticosteroids

Although some small, early studies showed no benefit from the administration of corticosteroids, there is now a substantial body of literature supporting their use. Steroid therapy should be reserved for patients with moderate to severe croup and used sparingly, if at all, in patients who present with classic episodic croup, who usually respond quite rapidly to nebulized saline. Patients with severe episodic croup, however, do respond to corticosteroids; thus, this treatment can be selectively employed. If the patient requires a prolonged course of therapy or increasing doses to control symptoms, referral to an ear, nose, and throat specialist for laryngoscopy should be made. Many studies have been criticized for failing to sort out episodic croup, but this criticism is not correct. Supraglottitis and purulent tracheobronchitis are readily excluded clinically, whereas patients with mild episodic croup rarely are hospitalized. Patients with severe episodic croup requiring hospitalization often cannot be adequately distinguished from patients with viral croup, as defined in this section. Thus, studies with adequate numbers and adequate controls that indicate benefit should not be discarded because of failure to make clinical diagnostic determinations that are difficult or impossible. The variations in severity should fall equally into placebo and treated groups if randomization is done correctly.

Studies show that corticosteroids are effective in croup whether they are administered intramuscularly, by nebulization, or by the oral route. A prospective, randomized, blinded study of 144 children with moderate to severe croup compared intramuscular dexamethasone or inhaled budesonide to placebo.[80] All patients were also given nebulized epinephrine. Hospitalization rates were 71% in the placebo group, 38% in the nebulized budesonide group, and 23% in the intramuscular dexamethasone group.[80] Oral dexamethasone at a dose of 0.15 mg/kg administered to patients with mild croup produced a measurable benefit: none of 50 patients who received the steroid treatment versus 8 (16%) of 50 who received placebo returned for further medical care during the same illness.[81] This study, however, failed to demonstrate a difference in the total duration of croup symptoms or the duration of symptoms of viral illness. This result is in agreement with the conclusions of a meta-analysis of 24 studies of corticosteroids in the management of croup, which demonstrated improved croup scores at 6 and 12 hours after steroid administration, but not at 24 hours.[82] The benefits of glucocorticoid treatment in laryngotracheitis, then, are transient but real; short-term improvement is often all that is needed to alleviate troublesome symptoms and avert hospitalization in this patient group.

Currently, 0.3 to 0.5 mg/kg of dexamethasone intramuscularly can be recommended in severe croup, especially when there will be a delay of 30 minutes or longer before receiving oxygen and mist in the hospital.

Epinephrine

Use of a trial of 0.01 ml/kg of the standard aqueous solution of 1:1000 epinephrine intramuscularly is reasonable when an *allergic* basis is strongly suspected, whether of episodic croup or supraglottic allergic edema.

Helium–Oxygen Mixtures

Because its density is less than nitrogen, helium, when mixed with oxygen, should facilitate oxygen passage through partially obstructed airways. However, its use is still investigational, and in one study in newborns with subglottic stenosis, the mixture resulted in hypoxemia.[83]

Complications

Pulmonary Edema

Laryngeal obstruction can produce pulmonary edema, manifested by extensive pulmonary infiltrates without cardiac enlargement.[84,85] The treatment includes positive end-expiratory pressure (PEEP), oxygen, morphine, and a diuretic such as furosemide.

Extralaryngeal Infection

Meningitis, pericarditis, and septic arthritis are extremely rare complications of *H. influenzae* epiglottitis.[46]

■ BRONCHITIS AND COUGHING SYNDROMES

Definitions

There exists no clear consensus on an operational definition of acute bronchitis in childhood. The dictionary definition, "inflammation of the bronchi," is clearly inconvenient for diagnostic purposes, as the bronchi cannot be visualized noninvasively. For many busy practitioners, the term *bronchitis* has been a "trash can" diagnosis, into which all children who are "too sick to have a common cold, but too well to have pneumonia" have been tossed. Physicians may also make the diagnosis of bronchitis to justify the administration of antimicrobial agents when they are expected by a child's parents,[86] although the diagnosis generally fails to provide an indication for antibiotic therapy. Acute bronchitis is probably best defined as cough with rhonchi or coarse crackles that clear with coughing and no evidence of pneumonia. The cough may be paroxysmal or nighttime. Tracheitis is often present. Fever is generally present but usually not significant. If marked lymphocytosis or a whoop is present, it is a pertussis-like illness (Table 7-3). If headache and weakness are prominent, the condition should be diagnosed as an influenza-like illness. If wheezing is present and persistent, the illness is usually diagnosed as asthmatic bronchitis (Table 7-4).

Bronchiolitis and asthmatic bronchitis are discussed in a later section on wheezing syndromes.

Classification

Acute bronchitis in children can be classified into subgroups and possible etiologies according to additional features (see Table 7-3). The table distin-

TABLE 7-3. CLASSIFICATION OF ACUTE COUGHING SYNDROMES

SUBGROUPS	CHARACTERISTIC FEATURES
Acute bronchitis	Cough, coarse rhonchi or wheezes Coarse crackles that clear on coughing Fever variable
Pertussis-like illness	Acute bronchitis, plus lymphocytosis and/or paroxysmal coughing spells with or without inspiratory whoop or post-tussive emesis
Influenza-like illness	Acute bronchitis, plus marked myalgia and/or headache, fever with chills, influenza epidemic in community
Other	Foreign body aspiration: toddler, focal wheezing Chlamydia: 1–6 months, usually afebrile, with or without, peripheral eosinophilia Measles: unvaccinated, conjunctivitis, possible lymphopenia Allergy: see asthmatic bronchitis and Table 7–4

guishing bronchiolitis, asthmatic bronchitis, and asthma (Table 7-4) should be used to complete the spectrum of syndromes.

Epidemiology and Pathology

The diagnosis of "bronchitis" is very common in pediatric practice. In one study of 5,489 outpatients with respiratory tract illnesses other than common cold, 40% were assigned the diagnosis of acute bronchitis.[87]

Clearly established predisposing factors include day-care attendance and passive smoking. Former premature babies with bronchopulmonary dysplasia often present with recurrent bronchitis. Some reports suggest that children with IgG subclass deficiencies are at higher risk for bronchitis, especially in recurrent or chronic form.[88,89] Measurement of IgG subclasses is not likely to be informative in children younger than 3 years.

TABLE 7-4. DIFFERENTIATION OF THREE WHEEZING SYNDROMES

	BRONCHIOLITIS	ASTHMATIC BRONCHITIS	ASTHMA
Usual age	< 2 years	1–4 years	> 4 years
Recurrences	Not yet	Sometimes	Repeated
Presumed location	Bronchioles	Small bronchi	All bronchi
Auscultatory Features	Coarse sounds, Wheezes, rhonchi	Wheezes, rhonchi	Musical wheezes
Usual etiology*	RSV, hMPV, AV, PIV, IV, EV	RV, AV, PIV, IV, EV, other respiratory viruses	Allergens, inhalants, or respiratory viruses

*In approximate decreasing order of frequency

RSV = respiratory syncytial virus, hMPV = human metapneumovirus, AV = adenovirus, PIV = parainfluenza viruses, RV = rhinoviruses, IV = influenza viruses, EV = enteroviruses

Because bronchitis is rarely fatal, little is known about the histopathology of this condition. One report examined the results of bronchial biopsy and bronchial wash specimens in nonatopic children with a history of chronic bronchitis.[90] Despite the fact that the specimens were collected at a time when the children had not had a recent acute infection, 87% of the specimens showed extensive respiratory epithelial damage. Lymphocytic infiltration, edema, increased protein content of mucus, and decreased mucociliary function were all demonstrated.[90]

Causes

Respiratory Viruses

The grand majority of cases are due to infection with a respiratory virus. Adenoviruses (especially types 4 and 7), influenza, parainfluenza, and RSV are the most common causes of acute bronchitis in childhood. Rhinovirus and some enteroviruses are also capable of causing acute bronchitis.[87] Adenoviruses have been reported to produce an illness indistinguishable from classical whooping cough, including the marked lymphocytosis[91]. However, subsequent reports concluded that the adenovirus may have been reactivated by *Bordetella pertussis* (which is very difficult to culture), and statistical evidence does not support a role for adenoviruses in pertussis-like illnesses.[92] Of the parainfluenza viruses, type 3 is a more common cause of bronchitis than either type 1 or type 2, in contradistinction to the relative frequencies seen in croup.

Measles virus infection always involves the bronchi. As discussed in Chapter 11 on rashes, coughing and fever are prominent before the eruption of the rash.

Mycoplasmas

Mycoplasma pneumoniae is an occasional cause of acute bronchitis, especially in school-age children.[91] Radiologic or clinical evidence of pneumonia is not detected, despite prominent cough and fever. Poor air exchange and even cyanosis may be present. Cold agglutinins are often positive in this disease, although the presence of IgM antibodies to *M. pneumoniae* is a more sensitive and specific test.

Chlamydia

C. trachomatis can cause cough and tachypnea in the infant 1 to 6 months of age along with a bilateral interstitial pneumonia and sometimes an eosinophilia.[93] It is discussed further in the section on pulmonary infiltrates with eosinophilia in Chapter 8.

There is conflicting information on the role of *C. pneumoniae* in acute bronchitis, largely because the diagnosis of *C. pneumoniae* infection is fraught with difficulty. Because it grows in cell culture only, it cannot be cultivated on typical agar plates used for isolating bacteria. It needs to be transported in proper media and kept cold. Direct antigen testing is fairly unreliable. Of late, reports on the use of polymerase chain reaction (PCR) in the detection of *C. pneumoniae* have been appearing, but further evaluation will be required. Serologic responses can be suggestive of recent infection; an IgM response appears in about 3 weeks and IgG at about 6 to

8 weeks. Grayston and colleagues suggest that a fourfold rise in antibody titer between acute and convalescent samples, or a single IgM titer of 1:16 or higher, or a single IgG titer of 1:512 or higher are reasonable criteria for proof of *C. pneumoniae* infection.[94]

A study of 365 adults with acute repiratory illnesses found that 9 (47%) of 19 with serologic evidence of *C. pneumoniae* infection had bronchospasm at the time of evaluation, and that there was a strong quantitative association of *C. pneumoniae* antibody titer and wheezing.[95] In contrast, a study that attempted to find *C. pneumoniae* in gargled water specimens of 193 children with respiratory infections was solidly unsuccessful;[96] indirect immunofluorescence was negative in all, enzyme immunosorbent assay was negative in all, and PCR detected *C. pneumoniae* in a total of 3 cases (1.6%). Of those three, all had subacute or chronic bronchitis-like symptoms, and in two the chest x-ray confirmed involvement of the pulmonary parenchyma.[96] Part of the problem may be that the nasopharynx, not the oropharynx, is the optimal site for isolation of the organism.

Passive Smoking

Infants exposed to smoking parents have twice the risk of an attack of bronchitis or pneumonia in the first year of life.[97]

Foreign Body

This was discussed in the preceding section on cough only.

Bacterial Infections

The possible bacterial etiologies of acute bronchitis in children have not been adequately studied. *B. pertussis* causes a bronchitic syndrome, usually in association with other features, as discussed later. In acute exacerbations in adults with chronic bronchitis, nontypable *H. influenzae* has been found more frequently than during remissions, and antibiotic therapy directed at *H. influenzae* usually is helpful.

Children may have bacterial bronchitis complicating sinusitis,[98] or more commonly, the symptoms of sinusitis may mimic those of bronchitis.

Bacteria, particularly *S. aureus,* can cause a purulent tracheobronchitis, which can be mistaken for laryngitis or a foreign body, as discussed in the section on laryngeal syndrome.

Chronic Bronchitis

In children, unlike adults, chronic bronchitis is not adequately defined.[98] Practitioner surveys revealed an absence of a widely accepted operational definition.[99] In addition to children with asthma or cystic fibrosis,[98,99] chronic bronchitis can be proved by endoscopy in children with IgG subclass abnormalities.[100]

Cast (Plastic) Bronchitis

In children with chronic bronchitis (usually secondary to asthma), large, branching bronchial casts may be expectorated or removed at bronchoscopy.[101] This condition was once thought to be extremely rare in childhood, and the diagnosis is still seldom established. A report from a pulmonologist from Spain who has personally seen and treated over 74 children with cast bronchitis, however, suggests that cast bronchitis may be more common than is generally appreciated.[102] Adults are often diagnosed with cast bronchitis when they expectorate casts after vigorous coughing. Young children swallow, rather than expectorate, whatever they bring up with coughing. Dr. Perez-Soler, therefore, performed early morning gastric aspirates to look for casts. He found casts ranging from 0.5–2.0 cm in length and 0.2–0.7 cm in diameter. They were composed of epithelial cells, varying numbers of inflammatory cells, and noncellular fibrinous material. Clinically, 90% of the patients were between 6 months and 3 years of age; the main symptoms were dyspnea and low-grade fever. Physical examination revealed diffuse wheezing, sometimes with rales. Sixty-five (88%) of the cases took more than 9 months to completely resolve.[102]

■ PERTUSSIS-LIKE ILLNESS

Typical Pertussis

An acute prolonged bronchitis plus either a marked lymphocytosis or a characteristic whoop can be defined as typical pertussis (see Table 7-3). The disease has historically been divided into three stages. The *catarrhal stage* lasts for little more than a week and is marked by common cold-like symptoms. The *paroxysmal stage* is named for the forceful coughing spells. This stage may last from a week to a month. Finally, a long *convalescent stage* leads to eventual recovery. Infants with classic pertussis usually have close contact with an adult with the disease. Pertussis in adults or children, however, often follows a less classic course[103] (resembling a refractory bronchitis, such as that seen with *C. pneumoniae* infection), so the exposure may be unknown. The clinical picture in infancy is characterized by a paroxysmal cough followed by an inspiratory whoop. Post-tussive emesis is another frequent symptom. Lymphocytosis (total white blood cell count above 15,000 with greater than 60% lymphocytes) is a helpful clue when present. Lymphocyte counts may be high enough to raise suspicion of leukemia. However, lymphocytosis is less common in infants less than 2 months of age.[104] Adenopathy and splenomegaly are not present, and eosinophilia may be frequent but masked by the lymphocytosis.[105]

Atypical Pertussis

In young infants infection with *B. pertussis* can occur without a whoop.[106] They may have mild disease or severe disease with vomiting following coughing. The diagnosis may be suspected only because of a known exposure to an older sibling or parent.

Cases of neonatal pertussis occurring within the first three weeks of life have been described.[107] All infants had extreme lymphocytosis, apneic spells, feeding difficulties, neurologic complications, and bronchopneumonia. Two of the infants had about a week of gradually increasing difficulty before hospitalization. In one study of infants less than 6 months of age, about half of 35 nonhospitalized infants did not have a whoop and were usually cultured because of exposure to a known case.[106] Pertussis is often misdiagnosed in infants as bronchiolitis or pneumonia.[108]

Older children, adolescents, or adults, many of whom have partial immunity because of either prior immunization, prior infection, or both, usually lack features of classic pertussis. Paroxysmal coughing is still fairly frequent, but the whoop is often absent.[109] Laboratory parameters such as lymphocytosis are entirely missing; one study of pertussis in adults seen in an emergency room setting found that both total white count and absolute lymphocyte count in patients with pertussis were indistinguishable from those of patients with other cough illnesses.[110] Seizures, apnea, and other central nervous system manifestations occasionally seen in babies with pertussis are absent in older patients.

Differential Diagnosis

Classic pertussis produces a readily diagnosable clinical syndrome. However, other pathogens can also cause pertussis-like syndromes. In a serologic study in children who coughed for greater than 7 days and had no evidence of *B. pertussis* infection, adenovirus was the most frequent pathogen found, followed by the parainfluenza viruses, *Mycoplasma pneumoniae*, and RSV.[111] Patients with adenovirus did not cough for as long a period as did those with pertussis, but more than 80% met the Centers for Disease Control and Prevention (CDC) diagnostic criteria (two weeks or more of cough, associated with paroxysms, inspiratory "whoop," or post-tussive emesis, without other obvious cause). Whooping occurred in 20% of children without a serologic diagnosis of pertussis, and post-tussive emesis was noted in greater than 50% of patients with a serologic diagnosis of adenovirus infection.[111] However, serologic evidence of adenovirus infection is not always reliable, and a serologic response may be occasioned by *B. pertussis* infection. An outbreak of pertussis-like illness secondary to *C. pneumoniae* has been reported from Japan.[112]

Diagnostic Approach

A chest roentgenogram is indicated in most patients with acute bronchitis, depending on the severity or duration of the illness and the age of the patient. A tuberculin skin test is indicated for children with acute bronchitis and a history of possible exposure to *Mycobacterium tuberculosis*.

Culture

If lymphocytosis is present or if pertussis is present in the community, culture for *B. pertussis* should be done. The organism is fastidious and difficult to grow in culture; the probability of isolating the organism is, in part, related to the manner in which the culture is obtained and handled. Yield is maximized by obtaining Bordet-Gengou plates from the microbiology laboratory *before* getting the specimen from the patient. A calcium alginate swab should be used and the posterior nasopharynx somewhat vigorously swabbed. The specimen is then plated on the agar at the bedside and transported to the laboratory by hand immediately thereafter. If direct bedside inoculation is not possible, Regan-Lowe transport medium should be used. Cultures are more likely to be positive if they are obtained within the first 3 weeks of the onset of illness. Sensitivity of properly performed culture or direct fluorescent antibody testing approaches 80% if done in the early stages of illness in patients who have not been on antibiotic therapy.[113] Atypical pertussis in adults or immunized children is usually culture negative but has been detected by serologic studies (see following).[114]

Fluorescent-Antibody Staining of Smear

Fluorescent-antibody methods are useful for rapid diagnosis from a nasal smear and complement the culture for *B. pertussis*.

Polymerase Chain Reaction

PCR diagnosis of pertussis is becoming more widely used; preliminary studies suggest that it is more sensitive than culture. In a study of patients undergoing nasopharyngeal swab testing for pertussis, 319 consecutive specimens were tested by culture, direct fluorescent antibody (DFA), and PCR. Cases were defined by the CDC clinical criteria plus either a positive DFA or PCR. The sensitivity of culture was 15%, DFA 52%, and PCR 93%.[115] A more recent study suggests that LightCycler PCR may be even more sensitive than conventional PCR.[115a]

Chlamydia Studies

Methods used in studies for *Chlamydia* are described in the section on pulmonary infiltrates with eosinophilia in Chapter 8.

Serum Antibodies

Natural infection with *B. pertussis* causes an increase in specific serum IgG, IgM, and IgA. Immunization produces boosted titers of IgG and IgM, but not of IgA. A serologic diagnosis is made by finding an agglutinizing titer rise of either IgA or IgG to *B. pertussis* components pertussis toxin (PT), filamentous hemagglutinin, pertactin, fimbriae, or sonicated whole organism. High antibody titers on a single sample can be diagnostic if age-specific norms are used. IgA antibodies against *B. pertussis* appear in the nasopharyngeal secretions during the second or third week of illness and persist for at least 3 months. One study of 525 cases and 321 controls showed that a single serum sample was not very helpful if it was drawn between the first and third week of the onset of coughing; in convalescent samples, drawn between 5 and 10 weeks after onset, detection of IgG directed at pertussis toxin was the best single test, with a sensitivity varying from 61% in infants to 74% in previously unvaccinated schoolchildren.[116]

Unfortunately, serologic diagnosis of pertussis is not widely used and therefore not readily available; it is performed in some reference laboratories.[113,114]

Treatment of Acute Bronchitis
Observation

Antibiotics are not indicated for most children with bronchitis. Cough syrups with expectorants or decongestants have no demonstrated value but may help some patients.

Asthmatic bronchitis is discussed in the section on bronchiolitis. Wheezing with bronchitis may respond well to therapies used for asthma.

Antibiotics

Amoxicillin is sometimes used to treat young children and infants because of the belief that *H. influenzae* may be an occasional cause of acute bronchitis in this age group. Erythromycin or one of the newer macrolides (clarithromycin or azithromycin) is a better choice, as they have some efficacy against *Chlamydia*, *Mycoplasma*, and *B. pertussis*.

Some children diagnosed with bronchitis probably have bacterial sinusitis as the cause of their cough, and these children may benefit from a course of antibiotics. In general, if cough is present for more than 2 weeks, observation alone for 5–7 days or a trial of anti-asthma medications is warranted. If the cough is present for less than 2 weeks and is not getting better, attempts at both anatomic and etiologic diagnosis should be made. This would include such studies as chest x-ray, coronal sinus CT, serology for *Mycoplasma* and *Chlamydia pneumoniae*, and a test for pertussis. Other studies, such as peak flow measurement, pulmonary function studies, and tuberculin skin testing, should also be considered.

Treatment of Pertussis

Erythromycin should be used if pertussis is suspected. The estolate form has been thought to be more active than the ethylsuccinate form; however, there are no compelling data to suggest that this is true.[117] It should be remembered that the pharmacokinetics and dosing recommendations of the two preparations are different. The estolate preparation can be dosed at 30 mg/kg/day divided BID or TID, wheras the ethylsuccinate form is dosed at 40 mg/kg/day divided QID.[118] On the basis of more frequent case reports, the estolate form was thought to be more likely to cause cholestatic jaundice. Population-based studies have shown that rates of this complication are similar with all forms of erythromycin.[119]

An open-label study of azithromycin showed that after a 5-day course, the organism was eradicated from the nasopharynx of all 34 patients when tested at 14 days.[120] The significance of this finding is uncertain because *B. pertussis* is difficult to culture even in the absense of prior therapy. More recently, a randomized trial compared both microbiologic and clinical cure rates in 153 patients (including 62 culture-positive cases) receiving either 7 days of clarithromycin or 14 days of erythromycin. In an intent-to-treat analysis, microbiologic eradication was documented in 89% of patients in each arm of the study. Clinical cure was documented in 94% of patients receiving clarithromycin and 89% of patients receiving erythromycin.[121]

Erythromycin is effective in eliminating the organism from the nasopharyngeal secretions and probably alters the course of the illness if given shortly after the paroxysmal stage has begun.[122] Bacterial relapse may occur if erythromycin is used for fewer than 14 days, but the significance of this with respect to contagion is not known. Recently, the use of erythromycin in newborns has been associated with an increased risk of hypertrophic pyloric stenosis.[123] The slightly increased risk of pyloric stenosis needs to be weighed against the risk of clinical pertussis, which can be severe in this age group. Whether other macrolides would have a similar effect is not known.

Early studies looking at the use of pertussis hyperimmune globulin showed no benefit but used relatively low doses. A randomized, double-blind, placebo-controlled trial of high-titer pertussis immune globulin in 73 children with clinical pertussis demonstrated a decrease in the duration of whoops from 21 days in the placebo group to 9 days in those receiving pertussis immune globulin.[124] Unfortunately, pertussis immunoglobin is not commercially available. Unfortunately, pertussis immunoglobin is not commercially available.

Salbutamol (albuterol), a beta-2 agonist, has seemed to be helpful in pertussis in a few small studies but has not been thoroughly studied and is not used much for therapy in the United States.

Corticosteroids are not well studied in humans but caused increased mortality in a mouse model; they are not advocated by many in the United States.

Hospitalization

Infants less than 12 months old with pertussis—and older children with severe pertussis—should be hospitalized. The patient should be put in a single-patient room with droplet precautions.[125] Monitoring for apnea should be done. Parenteral feeding may be advisable for very sick young infants.[108] Measuring capillary pCO_2 for hypercapnia may be helpful in severe cases. Recording the number of paroxysmal coughing attacks per 8- or 12-hour nursing shift can provide a guide to the progress of the illness and help in discharge planning.

Mist, Oxygen, and Suctioning

Mist is indicated to prevent drying of bronchial secretions if the relative humidity of the hospital room is low. In pertussis, suctioning of the oropharynx should be done after a coughing spell, particularly if sticky secretions are obtainable. Intubation or bronchoscopy to facilitate suctioning may be helpful in severely ill young infants. Oxygen can be delivered by tent or face mask, particularly if there are periods of cyanosis. In some severe cases, mechanical ventilation may be needed.

Complications of Pertussis

Apnea

Episodes of apnea and bradycardia are common in severe pertussis and may be related to a toxin produced by the organism, as these episodes may occur in the absence of paroxysmal coughing spells.[126,127] All complications of pertussis are more common in young infants; this is particularly true for apnea. Such a toxin might also explain other neurologic complications such as seizures and encephalopathy.[126,127]

Pneumonia

The initial pneumonia in pertussis is typically perihilar, often producing irregularity of the right heart border, the "shaggy heart." In severe cases, the pneumonia may progress, and other bacteria, such as *S. aureus* or *Pseudomonas aeruginosa,* may produce a secondary pneumonia. The degree of hypoxia often seems to be more severe than the radiologic picture would indicate. Dyspnea between paroxysms, tachypnea, and fever are not present in uncomplicated pertussis and suggest a secondary bacterial pneumonia (or a primary diagnosis other than pertussis).

Atelectasis

This is a frequent complication of pertussis and typically involves the right middle or right upper lobe.[128] Before modern respiratory therapy techniques were used, reexpansion took a month or two and sometimes as long as 10 or 11 months.[130,131] Now, bronchiectasis or change in pulmonary function is rare.

Encephalopathy

This is a rare complication of pertussis. It might occur because of hypoxemia but may also be due to the heat-stable pertussis toxin, which is histamine-sensitizing, lymphocyte-stimulating, and stimulating to the pancreatic islets.[127] Hypoglycemia may be a contributing factor.[105] A report of a 7-year-old unimmunized girl who developed encephalopathy with pertussis demonstrated a titer of antibody to filamentous hemagglutinin (FHA) in cerebrospinal fluid (CSF) that was 9-fold higher than that found in serum.[132] The CSF/serum ratio of albumin was normal. This suggests that the patient had antibody production within the CSF to a *B. pertussis* antigen other than pertussis toxin.[132] Convulsions during a severe illness occasionally occur, but long-term brain damage is rare.

In a surveillance study in the United States from 1979 to 1981, seizures were reported for 4% of 1,277 patients and encephalopathy was reported for 0.4% of patients, all younger than 1 year of age.[133] Current figures for seizures and encephalopathy are similar; the odd reports of encephalopathy in a school-age child[132] or cerebellar ataxia in adolescents[134] have begun to appear.

Long-term Lung Function

Adults with a history of pertussis during childhood have a small but measureable decrease in lung function compared with those who do not have a history of pertussis.[135]

Prevention of Pertussis

Exposed Contacts

Erythromycin is currently recommended for all exposed family contacts. Treatment of the index case eliminates the organism in 4 days but must be continued for 14 days to avoid bacteriologic relapse.[137] A recent prospective, placebo-controlled study of household contacts of patients with culture-proven pertussis showed that although erythromycin significantly decreased the number of culture-positive cough illnesses, the total number of cases of severe cough illnesses clinically compatible with pertussis was unchanged by prophylaxis.[138] It is probable that the decreased number of culture-positive cases would translate into a reduction in tertiary cases and community spread. Women with pertussis during labor did not transmit the infection to the nursing infant if both were given erythromycin.[139]

Pertussis vaccine, as a DTaP booster, is recommended for previously immunized children less than 7 years of age who are in contact with a known or suspected case of pertussis, unless a dose has been received within the past 3 years.[140]

Primary Immunization of Children

Pertussis immunization, given as DPT vaccine, is fairly reactogenic. Local pain, swelling, fever, febrile seizures, an unusual high-pitched cry, inconsolability, and hypotonic-hyporesponsive episodes have been temporally associated with its receipt. Because of this, and the public misconception that whole-cell pertussis vaccine was causally associated with encephalopathy, many people (and even entire countries) chose to risk natural pertussis rather than obtain the vaccine. A large outbreak of pertussis, associated with mortality, occurred in England in the late 1970s when pertussis vaccination was discontinued.[141]

Fortunately, immunogenic and protective acellular pertussis vaccines have been developed and are now the only pertussis vaccines used in the United States. Five acellular vaccines containing from two to five antigens are licensed for use in the United States. All have been shown to be immunogenic and protective. The incidence of side effects from acellular vaccines is considerably lower than that of whole-cell vaccines. Uncommonly, patients will experience swelling of an entire limb after a booster dose of acellular pertussis vaccine.[142] Complete recovery without permanent sequelae occurred in all patients. The incidence of this side effect does not seem to be related to the number of antigens contained in the vaccine. Routine pertussis vaccination is an immensely important public health measure, and unlike polio (wherein a chance at eradication exists), pertussis is an ever-present threat. Parents and caregivers should be educated about the improved safety and decreased reactogenicity of acellular pertussis vaccines, and every effort should be made to immunize all infants and children.

Booster Immunization of Adults

Immunity to pertussis, whether engendered by natural infection or by vaccination, is relatively short-lived. Most children who received the complete primary vaccine series are susceptible to pertussis infection by the time they reach the age of 12 years.[143] Pertussis causes anywhere from 12% to 28% of prolonged cough illnesses in adults.[144] Although adults usually experience atypical pertussis, the disease is still quite distressing and long-lived. Additionally, they serve as a reservoir for the bacterium and aid in spreading the infection to fully susceptible infants, who suffer more severe disease.[144a]

Two formulations of a cellular pertussis vaccine combined with dT for use in adolescents and adults are currently under review by the Food and Drug Administration (FDA). Acellular pertussis vaccines are well tolerated and immunogenic in adults. Only a small amount of antigen is necessary to boost antibody responses.[145] Some unusual reactions to the vaccine were seen in several trials; most notably, late or biphasic local reactions, occuring 5 to 7 days after vaccine receipt.[109] Unfortunately, only about 60% of the adult population is currently in compliance with the every-10-year booster dose of dT vaccine, and it is difficult to imagine that number escalating with the addition of the acellular pertussis component. Moreover, mathematical modeling of the epidemiology of pertussis predicts that an adult vaccination program would be unable to produce herd immunity, and thus might have only a marginal effect on the incidence of severe pertussis in young children.[146] The underlying epidemiologic principle is that it is difficult to produce significant herd immunity to an endemic disease using a vaccine that causes short-lived immunity. Selective immunization of adults with extensive child contact may prove to be equally effective and considerably less expensive.[147]

■ INFLUENZA-LIKE ILLNESS

Definitions

Influenza and *flu* are words that are often used by laypersons to refer to almost any gastrointestinal or respiratory illness. The physician may sometimes wish to use the patients' understanding of these words to communicate with them. However, for best communication among physicians, it is preferable to avoid the word *flu* and to use *influenza* only in the context of influenza virus infection or influenza-like illness, a phrase usually used to refer to the classic pattern of illness produced by the influenza virus.

Classic influenza-like illness is characterized by fever, cough, headache, sore throat often localized to the trachea, muscle aches, and weakness (Box 7-5). Onset is generally quite abrupt. Influenza virus illness occurs in the context of an epidemic or outbreak; sporadic cases are rare. Thus, epidemiologic clues are helpful in establishing a presumptive diagnosis of influenza. Fever is usually a prominent component of the illness, especially in young children; one study showed that the majority of young children with proven influenza virus infection had a fever of higher than 38.9°C.[148] In order for a respiratory illness without significant fever to be classified as influenza-like, myalgia should be prominent.

Physical examination usually reveals no remarkable respiratory signs to correspond with the respiratory symptoms. Dyspnea and fine crackles are not present in uncomplicated cases. Coarse crackles that clear with coughing may be heard. Influenza-like illnesses sometimes resemble bronchitis or laryngitis, but there is severe weakness or prostration that seems out of proportion to the rest of the illness.

Spectrum of Severity

The classic pattern of influenza-like illness is that of an acute illness of only a few days' duration, but the severity of the illness is variable. In severe cases, the temperature can be as high as 104°F to 105°F (40°C to 40.5°C) for 5 to 7 days, although school-age children usually do not appear critically ill at

---

BOX 7-5 ■ Typical Findings in Influenza Virus Infection

- Fever (> 101°F or 38.3°C), usually with sweating; occasionally with shivering
- Cough
- Headache
- Sore throat often localized to trachea; substernal pressure; "congestive feeling"; occasionally hoarseness
- Fatigue, weakness, excessive sleeping, or prostration
- Muscle pains; eye pain; dizziness
- Anorexia
- Significant respiratory signs, such as rales, are not common
- Abdominal signs and symptoms are uncommon, except in the very young

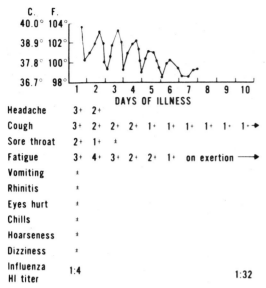

■ **FIGURE 7-5** Typical course of influenza virus infection in a child.

any point. In the mildest pattern, the patient does not have a high fever but has myalgia or weakness and hoarseness, nasal obstruction, or cough that may persist for several weeks (Fig. 7-5).

Influenza Virus Infection in Young Children

The presentation of influenza in infants and young children may differ from that seen in school-age children, teenagers, and adults. Children less than 6 months of age have a high incidence of influenza-related hospitalization.[149] Typically, it presents as an undifferentiated viral illness with fever.[148] The patient may appear moderately toxic and have clear rhinorrhea, irritability, and cough. Gastrointestinal symptoms are much more common in young children and may dominate the clinical picture. One study of 53 infants (< 12 months of age) found that diarrhea was a prominent symptom in 18 (34%).[150] Young children may also present with febrile seizures. Classic laryngotracheitis or croup syndrome is seen in young children with influenza, and its course tends to be more severe than that seen with parainfluenza viruses.[151]

Causes of Influenza-like Illnesses

Influenza Virus

Influenza virus is the usual cause of influenza-like illness in large outbreaks in civilians.[152–154] In school-age children, the clinical findings are usually classic, as closely observed in an outbreak involving 280 children in a children's home (see Box 7-5).[152] A large study showed that symptoms and signs that were more common in children than in adults were anorexia, abdominal pain, nausea and vomiting, cervical lymphadenopathy, and temperature greater than 38.9°C.[148] Symptoms that were more prominent in adults than in children were sneezing and sputum production.

Muscle pain and tenderness, particularly in the calf muscles, are not uncommon in children and are typically associated with elevated muscle enzyme concentrations (especially creatine phosphokinase) in the serum.[155,156] Myalgia may become so severe that the child will be unable or unwilling to walk. Most cases are caused by influenza B virus.[155] The onset of myositis is sometimes several days after that of the influenza-like illness and resolves without residual weakness over about a week.

Disease caused by influenza virus infection is more severe in children with underlying medical problems such as bronchopulmonary dysplasia, diabetes mellitus, congenital heart diseases, neuromuscular disorders, or neoplasms. Chronic respiratory disease such as bronchopulmonary dysplasia is the most common background medical problem seen in children hospitalized with influenza virus infection.[157]

Other Viruses

Adenoviruses are the second most frequent cause of influenza-like illness in military bases and also in civilians.[158,159] Parainfluenza viruses are a frequent cause of influenza-like illness.[160,161] Myalgia or weakness is usually not recognized by children, and headaches or general aches are not prominent in adults. Coxsackieviruses are an occasional cause of influenzalike illness.[162]

Other Infectious Agents

Mycoplasma pneumoniae may produce influenzalike illnesses without pneumonia.[163] Group A streptococcus should be considered a possible cause of influenza-like illness, because fever, headache, sore throat, and myalgia may occur in streptococcal pharyngitis. Summertime influenza-like illness should bring to mind the possibility of Rocky Mountain spotted fever. Several potential agents of bioterrorism (e.g., anthrax, plague, tularemia, and smallpox) can present initially as a severe influenza-like illness.

Laboratory Approach

Group A streptococcal infection should be excluded in children with an influenzalike illness if there is objective evidence of pharyngitis. Early streptococcal pharyngitis may resemble an influenza-like illness, and concurrent streptococcal pharyngitis may occur with illness caused by a virus.

Serum Antibodies

Influenza, parainfluenza, and adenovirus infection can be confirmed by demonstration of a rise in titer between a serum specimen obtained early in the illness and one obtained about 2 weeks later. A serologic study comparing the prevalence of specific IgA, IgM, and IgG and the kinetics of antibody production in patients with culture- or antigen-detection-proven influenza virus infection showed that: (1) the prevalence of IgA against influenza virus in controls was less than 4%, and (2) IgA, and the bulk of IgG was synthesized within the first week of illness. Therefore, a measurable titer of influenza-specific IgA on a single sample is highly suggestive of acute influenza virus infection.[164] Measurement of influenza-specific IgA, however, is not widely available. Antibody production to influenza virus can be measured either by ELISA or by hemagglutination-inhibition. Both methods are reasonably sensitive. Laboratory confirmation of such a virus infection is of retrospective interest primarily for severe illnesses. Serologic studies for these viruses are of special interest when influenzalike illnesses are first appearing in a community, because the presence of confirmed influenza virus infection may be useful in stimulating public health measures, such as immunization, throughout the state.

Viral Cultures

The viruses that can cause influenza-like illnesses grow readily in cell cultures. Viral cultures are also useful to confirm the presence of influenza virus in a community and to define the virus type.

In the first 3 or 4 days of symptomatic influenza virus infection, about 70–90% of children shed the virus, but by the fifth day of illness, this drops to about 20%.[165] The virus titer and frequency of recovery increase with severe illness.[152,165]

Rapid Antigen Detection Tests

Commercially available antigen detection kits for the diagnosis of influenza infection are widely available. Some kits detect influenza A only, whereas others detect both influenza A and B. The test is sensitive and fairly reliable if a good nasopharyngeal or oropharyngeal swab specimen is obtained. In general, nose washes provide better results than nasopharyngeal swab specimens, but either is acceptable. The test can be run in less than 30 minutes and is helpful when rapid diagnosis is desirable.

Multi-virus Rapid Tests

It is possible to screen for influenza virus infection and, at the same time, screen for RSV, respiratory adenoviruses, and the parainfluenza viruses using the fluorescent antibody method. This test, unlike the rapid antigen detection kits discussed previously, requires a nose wash specimen and is highly observer-dependent. Cells from the nose wash are fixed to a glass slide, then a mix of antibodies is allowed to react with the specimen. Antibodies thus attached to the viral antigens are then labeled with fluorescein-tagged antibodies. Skilled performance and observation are required. The test is only available at select institutions.

PCR

Influenza virus infections lack a viremic phase, and PCR examinations of serum are almost always negative.[166] However, PCR of respiratory secretions has been experimentally shown to correlate well (98% concordance) with standard rapid antigen detection tests.[167] The future of rapid diagnosis of severe acute respiratory tract disease will probably evolve along these lines. The ability to rapidly pinpoint the etiologic diagnosis of respiratory illnesses will be a great boon to the practicing physician.

Treatment of Influenza

Antibiotic therapy of an influenza-like illness is unnecessary unless concurrent group A streptococcal infection, otitis media, or pneumonia is present. Symptomatic therapy includes acetaminophen or NSAIDs (but not aspirin, which may increase the risk of Reye's syndrome) for headache and myalgia. Cough syrup is rarely necessary.

Amantadine hydrochloride has been shown to be of value in both prevention and treatment of influenza A virus infection in placebo-controlled, double-blind studies in adults and children.[168,169] Rimantadine is a drug of similar chemical composition and mode of action but with a much lower incidence of CNS side effects. Rimantadine is metabolized by the liver before being excreted renally; its dosage needs some adjustment for patients with renal failure. It can be given once a day, which makes it an attractive option. Rimantadine is approved for prophylaxis in children as young as 1 year of age. Although it is only approved for treatment of children age 13 years or older, many physicians use it for this purpose in younger children.[168]

Zanamivir and oseltamivir are neuraminidase inhibitors. Unlike amantadine and rimantadine, these compounds are active against both influenza A and influenza B isolates.[170] Zanamivir is delivered locally to the site of influenza virus replication by an inhalational device. The main side effect is bronchospasm, which may be severe, especially in patients with a previous history of ashthma.[171] The package insert contains a warning that zanamivir generally should not be given to patients with underlying airway disease. This drug is approved for treatment of influenza in persons 7 years and older; it has not yet been approved for prophylaxis.

Oseltamivir is a neuraminidase inhibitor that is taken by mouth. Inhibitory concentrations of the drug reach the lungs, and the drug has been shown to provide benefit to subjects with experimental influenza virus infections in clinical trials.[172] The principal side effect of oseltamivir is nausea and vomiting, which occurred in up to 14% of recipients as compared with 9% of placebo recipients.[172] This can usually be alleviated by taking the medication with food. Oseltamivir is approved for prophylaxis in children older than 12 years and for treatment in children over 12 months. None of the four antiviral agents has been demonstrated to be effective in preventing serious influenza-related complications.

Most children with influenza seen in the outpatient setting do not require specific antiviral therapy. However, for the child with influenza who is at high risk for complications, antiviral therapy should be considered. This includes children for whom the influenza vaccine is recommended. Antiviral therapy should also be considered for any child with influenza whose illness is severe enough to require hospitalization. No antiviral therapy is effective against influenza if started greater than 48 hours after the onset of symptoms.

Complications

Pneumonia or Bronchiolitis

Influenza-like illness caused by influenza virus or another virus is sometimes complicated by pneumonia or bronchiolitis.[153,157] This subject is discussed further in the sections on atypical pneumonia and fulminating pneumonia in Chapter 8.

Toxic Shock Syndrome

S. aureus can superinfect patients with influenza virus infection, and if it is a toxin-1 producing strain, the patient may develop hypotension, rash, and the other manifestations discussed in Chapter 10.[173,174]

Encephalopathy

Rarely, influenza virus infection is complicated by an acute encephalitis or encephalopathy.[175] It can occur during infection with influenza or as a postinfectious complication.[176]

Reye's syndrome is an acute encephalopathy and hepatopathy that has been associated with influenza virus infection and the intake of aspirin or aspirin-containing products. Reye's syndrome is discussed in more detail in Chapter 9.

Others

Other rare complications include renal failure from myoglobinuria,[177] Stevens-Johnson syndrome, and Guillain-Barré syndrome. Leukopenia may accompany influenza virus infection with some frequency; pancytopenia, anemia, and thrombocytopenia that developed concurrently with influenza virus infection and resolved spontaneously when the respiratory disease abated have been reported.[178] Chronic pulmonary disease such as pulmonary fibrosis or bronchiectasis can follow childhood influenza.[179] In a study of volunteers experimentally infected with wild influenza virus, increased bronchial reactivity occurred and persisted about 4 weeks.[180]

Prevention of Influenza

Chemoprophylaxis

Amantadine or rimantidine can be given daily to exposed susceptible children older than 12 months of age at risk for severe complications (the same group that should have received vaccine). Prophylaxis should be continued until such time as the influenza virus is no longer in the community, usually about 6–12 weeks.[168] Chemoprophylaxis can also be considered for immunodeficient patients who are unable to mount a suitable response to influenza vaccination.

Neither drug interferes with the immune response to influenza vaccine, which should have been given before the virus entered the community but may still be given afterward. These drugs have activity only against influenza A virus, for which they are between 70–90% effective at preventing symptomatic infection. They do not have activity against influenza B virus. Amantidine can increase the risk of seizures in those with a seizure disorder and is also associated with other neurologic side effects (such as nervousness, lightheadedness, and difficulty concentrating) in about 13% of patients. These side effects occur about half as frequently with rimantidine, which is more expensive.

Studies of the prevention of influenza infection by neuraminidase inhibitors have shown that they are 70–90% effective in prophylaxis.[170,181] They are active against both influenza A and B. Oseltamivir is approved for prophylaxis in children age 12 years or older and can be used in a similar fashion to that described for amantidine and rimantidine. Zanamivir is not approved for prophylaxis. The neuraminidase inhibitors do not impair immune responses to influenza vaccine.

Inactivated Influenza Vaccine

Children at risk for severe complications of influenza virus infection include those who have chronic cardiac or pulmonary disease, such as asthma, cystic fibrosis and bronchopulmonary dysplasia, those receiving long-term aspirin therapy, and those with poorly controlled metabolic, renal, or hematologic diseases. Children who are immunocompromised by disease or chemotherapy generally should be immunized at a time when they are likely to respond to inactivated-virus vaccines[168] if possible, but the vaccine should not be withheld because of concern regarding poor immune response.

Recommendations regarding dosages and preparations for children 6 months to 12 years of age are made each year, usually in the summer, and should be implemented before December.[168] As children serve as reservoirs of influenza virus in the community, many are now advocating influenza vaccination for all schoolchildren.[182] Concerns about inactivated influenza vaccine precipitating acute attacks in patients with asthma have been largely put to rest.[183] Although egg hypersensitivity has long been regarded as an absolute contraindication to influenza vaccination (as the vaccine virus is grown in embryonated eggs), a multicenter trial showed that the vaccine could be safely administered even to patients with reliable histories and demonstrated responses to oral egg challenge.[184] This group of investigators administered the vaccine to 83 patients with egg allergy and saw no adverse reactions, even in patients with positive vaccine skin prick tests. They gave one-tenth of the recommended vaccine dose first, followed by the remaining nine-tenths 30 minutes later.

Live-Attenuated Influenza Vaccine

A trivalent live-attenuated influenza vaccine that is administered by nasal spray (FluMist) has been FDA-approved for use in healthy persons ages 5 to 49 years old. Unfortunately, the vaccine is most efficacious in a group for which it is not approved (i.e., children with little prior experience with influenza).[185] Its superior efficacy in young children may relate to its ability to induce a mucosal immune response,[186] which has been shown to be poor in unprimed children receiving the inactivated vaccine.[187] Children younger than 5 years old are also the age group in which the convenience of a nasal spray vaccine would be most welcome.

The reason for the exclusion relates to a possible increased risk of asthma episodes in young children receiving the vaccine. In a large safety study, 14 (0.7%) of 2,032 children ages 1 to 4 years old developed an episode of asthma in the 6 weeks after vaccination with FluMist as compared with 2 (0.2%) of 1,025 placebo recipients in that age group ($P = 0.11$).[187a] Although this difference was not statistically significant at the 95% confidence level, the FDA decided that further study was needed before it could recommend use of the vaccine in children younger than 5. Studies regarding the safety and immunogenicity of this vaccine in young children and in immunocompromised patients are ongoing. Currently it is not recommended for these groups, but future studies may expand its indications.

■ BRONCHIOLITIS AND WHEEZING

The term *bronchiolitis* indicates inflammation of the bronchioles, although this cannot be observed directly. There is no clinical definition of bronchiolitis as a syndrome that is universally accepted; the one used in the 1975 edition of this text, based on a collaborative study, is given following.[188]

Three characteristics are typical features of bronchiolitis:

1. Acute generalized peripheral airway obstruction ("air trapping"), as recognized by tachypnea, decreased breath sounds, and low diaphragms on chest roentgenogram
2. Occurrence in the infant age group (less than one year of age), because their airways are smaller and contribute a larger fraction of airway resistance

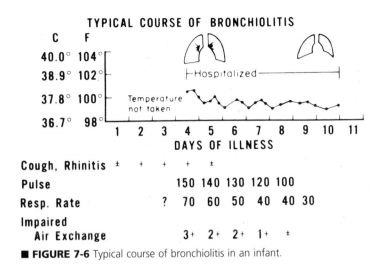

■ **FIGURE 7-6** Typical course of bronchiolitis in an infant.

3. Usually, no evidence of similar episodes in the past

A broader clinical definition of bronchiolitis can be given by describing the classic clinical pattern of illness requiring hospitalization see next section. Variations from the classic pattern may still be legitimately classified as bronchiolitis as a presumptive diagnosis pending further observations.

Classic Clinical Bronchiolitis

Typically, an infant in the first year of life has minor respiratory symptoms for a few days.[189] Then, the parents recognize increasing difficulty and rate of breathing (Fig. 7-6). When the infant is first examined, there is usually tachypnea, bilateral intercostal retractions, and poor air exchange (diminished breath sounds) in all lung fields. Wheezing is a prominent feature. After therapy with humidified oxygen, alveolar aeration may improve, as indicated by louder breath sounds. Coarse inspiratory and expiratory breath sounds, or coarse inspiratory crackles, may then be heard throughout the chest. In bronchiolitis, the crackles are coarse and are often heard through most of inspiration and sometimes during expiration, suggesting disease in the small air passages rather than in the alveoli. This contrasts with pneumonia, in which the crackles are fine and occur at the end of inspiration.

An inspiratory chest roentgenogram will almost always show low diaphragms (hyperinflation). Occasionally, the film shows intercostal lung bulging, areas of linear atelectasis, or small areas of interstitial pneumonia. Segmental or patchy pulmonary densities usually represent atelectasis. True consolidation is rarely seen.[190] The principal physiologic problem in bronchiolitis is obstruction of the lower respiratory passages, not fluid in the alveoli ("pneumonia"). If sparse pulmonary densities are seen, an appropriate problem-oriented diagnosis would be "bronchiolitis with patchy pneumonia." The severity of symptoms often waxes and wanes before there is evidence of clear improvement. Oxygen saturation as measured by pulse oximetry can also vary from moment to moment. Often, the ability of the infant to breast- or bottle-feed is the best index of disease severity and the most useful indication for hospitalization. Dyspnea lasts about 5 days (see Fig. 7-6).

In a population-based cohort of 280 children hospitalized for bronchiolitis from 1990–1999, the median age at the diagnosis was 4 months, and nearly two-thirds of the patients were male. Fourteen percent were born at before 36 weeks of gestation, 5% has congenital heart disease, 2% has bronchopulmonary dysplasia, and 12% had a prior diagnosis of reactive airways. Two-thirds of patients required supplemental oxygen, 27% were admitted to the intensive care unit, and 6% required mechanical ventilation. The mean hospital stay was 2.7 days (range 1–15 days).[190a]

Other Wheezing Syndromes

The following definitions were used in the 1975 edition of this book and still seem to be in fairly common usage in the United States.

Acute bronchial asthma, asthmatic bronchitis, and bronchiolitis all refer to illnesses with acute lower respiratory (peripheral airway) obstruction (see Table 7-4). The term *asthma* (or *bronchial asthma*) is usually reserved for recurrent episodes of wheezing that have an allergic, viral, or exercise-induced basis and typically respond to bronchodilators, inhaled corticosteroids, or both. This diagnosis can rarely be made with accuracy during the first episode in infants and usually is not used until the episodes recur and until responses to bronchodilators and antiinflammatory therapies are demonstrated.

The term *asthmatic bronchitis* can be used to describe the illness of a young child who has had several episodes of bronchitis with wheezing. Other terms in common use include *reactive airways disease* (RAD) and *reactive obstructive airways disease syndrome* (ROADS). Usually, the child is 1 to 4 years of age and may have no further evidence of asthma later in life. If recurrent episodes continue, the term *asthma* is used.

Bronchiolitis is usually the most appropriate diagnosis for the first episode of acute lower respiratory obstruction in an infant. Usually, the infant is younger than 1 year if it is the first episode. In two large population-based studies of bronchiolitis hospitalizations, 64–67% occurred in children less than 6 months of age.[191,192] Recovery of a virus is more likely in an infant with a first episode (bronchiolitis) than in one with a history of wheezing (asthmatic bronchitis).[193]

Physiologic Disturbances

Lower Respiratory Obstruction

One of the reasons that the young infant has more difficulty with respiratory tract obstruction may be the small size of the airways and their greater contribution to total airway resistance.[194,195] The principal mechanism of obstruction in bronchiolitis is presumed to be edema of the bronchioles, because improvement often occurs within a few days. Review of autopsy findings in acute bronchiolitis shows that the bronchioles are plugged with mucus and necrotic cell debris, but this probably is more characteristic of fatal cases.[196] Bronchospasm, as defined by improved air exchange after administration of bronchodilators, rarely can be documented. Secretions may be present in the bronchi, as evidenced by coarse crackles, but these are not a constant finding. Attempts to aspirate these secretions are usually unnecessary and may be harmful.

Immune Response and Disease Severity

A formalin-inactivated vaccine in the 1960s caused recipients to mount an antibody response, but exacerbated clinical disease when patients were infected with wild-type RSV.[197] Some investigators showed that these antibodies were nonneutralizing, which fueled speculation that passive antibodies worsened RSV disease.[198] Subsequent studies have conclusively proven that passive antibody to RSV is at least partially protective against severe disease, and that the higher the antibody titer the better.[199] Murine models suggest that enhanced illness was the result of selective activation of type 2 CD4+ lymphocytes, leading to altered cytokine (e.g., IL-4) and immunoglobulin (e.g., IgE) production.[200] Among infants with RSV infection, those manifesting bronchiolitis have significantly higher titers of RSV-specific IgE in nasopharyngeal secretions than those without bronchiolitis.[201] However, what determines whether the immune response to RSV infection is predominantly type 1 or type 2 remains unknown.

Hypoxemia

Because of the bronchiolar obstruction, there is uneven ventilation of various parts of the lung, resulting in ventilation-perfusion disparity ("mismatch") and therefore hypoxemia.[202] The arterial pCO_2 is usually normal in mild cases or may be low because of hyperventilation, as shown in Figure 7-1. In patients with more severe obstruction of the smaller airways, CO_2 retention also occurs but is rare except as a late finding.[202,203] Severe persistent obstruction can result in acute respiratory failure.

Causes of Bronchiolitis or Wheezing

The syndrome of bronchiolitis occurs every month of the year in the northern United States and should be regarded as having many possible etiologies.[204] It is useful to distinguish between epidemic bronchiolitis, which is usually caused by RSV, and sporadic bronchiolitis, which may have a number of possible causes.

Viral Infection

Respiratory syncytial virus is the most frequent viral cause of bronchiolitis throughout the world. These infections tend to be seasonal and typically are associated with outbreaks (Fig. 7-7). About 65% of in-

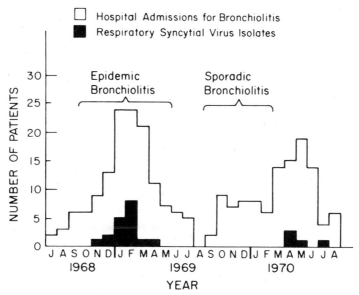

■ FIGURE 7-7 Sporadic and epidemic bronchiolitis. Note months in fall and early winter of 1969 when admissions to Children's Memorial Hospital for bronchiolitis were not associated with respiratory syncytial virus isolations (sporadic bronchiolitis).

fants experience RSV infection within the first 12 months of life; by age 2, almost all children have been infected at least once. RSV-positive bronchiolitis occurs primarily in infants less than 6 months of age, usually with less fever or leukocytosis than is observed with RSV-negative bronchiolitis.[189] Re-infection with RSV is extremely common; sometimes children are infected twice within a single RSV "season." Fortunately, disease with reinfection is usually less severe than that seen with primary infection.

Adenoviruses are an occasional cause of bronchiolitis.[205,206] Influenza virus, parainfluenza viruses, and rhinoviruses also can cause bronchiolitis.[207] In longitudinal studies of respiratory diseases in infants, a large proportion have no virus isolated. To some extent, this may be due to the technical difficulties of virus cultures. However, it also may indicate that other, unknown, viruses are important or that nonviral etiologies (allergy) are also frequently involved. This supposition was confirmed with the discovery of human metapneumovirus (hMPV), a paramyxovirus that causes a spectrum of illness very similar to that of RSV.[207a] In a study of over 600 outpatient visits from children under 5 years old with lower respiratory tract illness from 1976 to 2001, archived nasal wash specimens were tested for hMPV by reverse transcriptase

PCR.[207b] Overall, 12% of lower respiratory tract infections were found to be caused by hMPV infection. hMPV was associated with bronchiolitis (59%), croup (18%), asthma exacerbation (14%), and pneumonia (8%). In a prospective, population-based study of 675 hospitalizations for respiratory disease in children younger than 5 years old, RSV was responsible for 18%, parainfluenza 6%, hMPV 4%, and influenza 3%.[207c] Half of children hospitalized with hMPV infection received supplemental oxygen, and 15% required admission to the intensive care unit. All hMPV infections occurred from January to May, with a peak in March, which is slightly later than RSV season. The peak age of infection was 6 to 12 months of age, as compared with RSV infection, which peaks in the first 6 months of life.[207c]

Cytomegalovirus can produce bronchiolitis in immunocompromised children but has not been reported as a cause of bronchiolitis in normal children.[208]

Allergy

Many infants apparently have an allergic basis for their symptoms.[196,209] This is particularly true of sporadic bronchiolitis as opposed to epidemic bronchiolitis.

Both parainfluenza viruses and RSV stimulate

some children to produce significant amounts of virus-specific IgE antibody and histamine in nasal secretions.[207] Interestingly, it is these children who respond to the virus infection with wheezing, suggesting a role for immediate hypersensitivity reactions in both the initial illness and the recurrent wheezing or asthma that may occur later in many cases. Investigations have been unable, however, to link either total eosinophil count or the serum concentration of eosinophil cationic protein with the subsequent development of asthma.[210] It is likely that the pathogenesis of wheezing relates to a complex interplay of cytokines, chemokines, adhesion molecules, and other mediators of inflammation. The specifics of these responses are currently under investigation both in naturally infected humans and in experimental animal models.

Mycoplasma Infection

M. pneumoniae is an uncommon cause of bronchiolitis in infants.[204] It was recovered from about 50% of wheezing-associated respiratory illnesses in children 9 to 15 years of age but from only 3% of children less than 2 years of age who had a similar illness.

Cystic Fibrosis

This disease can cause an acute persistent episode of expiratory obstruction, often initially diagnosed as bronchiolitis (Fig. 7-8). Persistence of expiratory obstruction with low diaphragms for longer than 1 week in bronchiolitis should suggest the possibility of cystic fibrosis. Recurrent expiratory obstruction can also be caused by cystic fibrosis.

Others

Congestive heart failure may mimic bronchiolitis. In addition, bronchiolitis of unusual severity may be the first manifestation of previously undiagnosed congenital heart disease.

Course

Bronchiolitis has a spectrum of severity. The average illness lasts 3 to 7 days. The hospitalization rate is 1–2%[190,191,199] and the mortality rate is approximately 2.4 per 100,000 infants younger than 1 year of age.[211] Case-fatality rates are highest in patients with underlying severe cardiac or pulmonary disease. Although the rate of secondary bacterial infec-

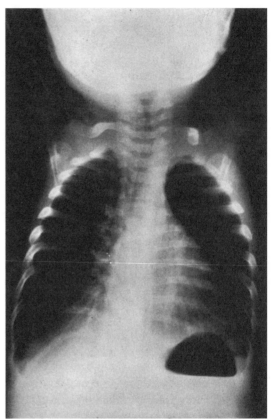

■ **FIGURE 7-8** Low diaphragms in a patient with bronchiolitis. This infant had respiratory syncytial virus isolated but had a progressively worsening course and died, with cystic fibrosis of the pancreas.

tion is low, patients with bronchiolitis may develop pneumonia, especially after cardiac or respiratory arrest and resuscitation.

The recent survival of more very low birthweight infants and more infants with bronchopulmonary dysplasia have added to the pool of infants with greater severity of bronchiolitis. Despite this, the incidence of death due to bronchiolitis has not increased over the past two decades.[211]

At first, rapid respiratory rates usually indicate good compensation by the patient. In severe cases, the respiratory rate may decrease as the infant becomes fatigued and may indicate impending respiratory failure. Infants who are weak or debilitated before the illness may become unable to ventilate adequately relatively early in the illness. In such infants, respiratory acidosis and cardiac arrest may occur, and measurement of arterial pO_2, pCO_2, and pH may be helpful to warn the physician of progressive respiratory failure and impending cardiac arrest.

Diagnostic Approach

Chest Roentgenogram

A chest film is useful to confirm low diaphragms and to exclude pneumonia and cardiomegaly (Fig. 7-8).

White Cell Count and Differential

In bronchiolitis, white cell counts are typically not helpful.

Cultures

Viral cultures may be available in some centers, but culture results do not influence the initial management.

Rapid Antigen Testing

Rapid antigen testing for RSV can be performed easily using a commercially available ELISA kit. It takes approximately 20 minutes to perform, but samples are usually batched. The test is almost always positive in children with RSV bronchiolitis because these patients typically shed large quantities of virus from the nasopharynx. Nasal washes are more reliable samples, but naspharyngeal swabbing is also acceptable.

When identification of other viruses is desirable, nasal washings can be tested using fluorescein-tagged antibodies, as described earlier.

RT-PCR

Although still experimental, RT-PCR techniques for the detection of respiratory viruses in children with bronchiolitis are under development. A study that enrolled 216 children with bronchiolitis showed a 97% correlation between RT-PCR results and results of virus isolation and immunofluorescence tests.[212] This technique is also able to distinguish between RSV-A and RSV-B.

Clinical Diagnosis

During the middle of an RSV epidemic, the majority of babies less than 6 months of age who present with classic clinical features of bronchiolitis are infected with RSV.

Treatment

Humidified Oxygen

Essentially all infants sick enough to be hospitalized with RSV infection have some degree of hypoxemia.

Therefore, humidified oxygen guided by O_2 saturation monitoring should be offered to all patients. Humidified oxygen is the only treatment consistently proven to provide benefit for patients with RSV bronchiolitis and is thus the mainstay of therapy. A level of 30–40% oxygen is usually sufficient to improve the hypoxemia and does not result in CO_2 retention.[202]

Mist Therapy

Use of mist has not been shown to be of value in bronchiolitis. In one small controlled study, mist therapy was associated with longer periods of cough and rhonchi but a lesser duration of anxiety in infants with pneumonitis and lower respiratory obstruction.[213] In asthma, mist therapy sometimes makes the child worse,[214] and occasionally an infant with bronchiolitis appears to improve after removal from mist, probably because of bronchospasm. Cool mist can produce hypothermia in a young infant.[215]

Epinephrine and Bronchodilators

In the distant past, a clinical trial of 0.01 ml/kg (up to 0.3 ml) of subcutaneous epinephrine (1:1000) was sometimes employed in an effort to help sort out bronchiolitis from allergic disease. This method was never particularly successful, although it sometimes produced rapid improvement in older infants with allergy-mediated disease. No data have shown that an early trial of epinephrine prevents hospitalization in patients who present to emergency departments with bronchiolitis. In addition, the use of nebulized epinephrine in infants hospitalized with bronchiolitis does not reduce the length of hospital stay.[215a] Therefore, a trial of epinephrine is no longer recommended for patients with clinical histories and physical examinations highly suggestive of bronchiolitis. It may be used in severely ill children in whom the diagnosis is not clear. Epinephrine should not be used if tachycardia is severe (consistently more than 200 per minute).

Bronchodilators such as albuterol are in wide use for the treatment of moderate to severe bronchiolitis. Chart review indicates that about 85% of children hospitalized for RSV bronchiolitis are prescribed bronchodilator therapy (RG Fisher, unpublished data), despite lack of convincing data for its usefulness. A meta-analysis of 20 randomized controlled trials reported modest short-term improvement in clinical scores, but no effect on oxygenation, rate of hospitalization, or duration of hospitalization.[216] Given the marginal benefit and the total annual cost of $37 million to provide inhaled bronchodilator therapy to infants with first-time bronchiolitis, routine use is not justified. Careful thought reveals that the idea of using bronchodilator therapy, extrapolated from response in patients with asthma, is probably wrongheaded from the start. The pathophysiology of wheezing in these babies differs from that of asthmatics. Young infants, who become sickest with RSV infection, lack both the amount of smooth muscle[217] and the beta-adrenergic receptors[218] they would need to derive a clinical response from bronchodilators. Moreover, the primary cause of airway narrowing is edema and mucous plugging, not bronchospasm.

Nevertheless, a clinical bias remains that some patients do respond to nebulized bronchodilator therapy, and because virtually no other therapeutic option exists, a trial of a bronchodilator is endorsed by most experts. However, if bronchodilators are used, careful pre- and posttherapeutic assessment should be employed and the therapy stopped if a clear benefit cannot be ascertained. Unfortunately, both clinical observation and published clinical research show that physicians tend to continue bronchodilators despite obvious indication of no benefit. One study showed that although 61% of patients with bronchiolitis who were initially started on bronchodilators had clear, chart-documented evidence of no response to therapy, 87% of them continued to receive nebulized albuterol throughout their hospital course.[219] Amazingly, 54% continued to receive albuterol as outpatients after hospital discharge. This approach to the treatment of bronchiolitis is wasteful of health care dollars and exposes the patient to the unnecessary risk of side effects or paradoxical worsening of lung function.[220]

Intravenous Bronchodilators

In severe, life-threatening cases, the physician can try aminophylline, but such potent agents should be avoided except in extreme cases. Theophylline blood-level measurements are essential when high doses are used. A retrospective study showed no value for theophylline in moderate bronchiolitis.[221] Another study of 15 infants with bronchiolitis (14 of whom had proven RSV infection) requiring mechanical ventilation and continuous positive airway pressure (CPAP) noted no adverse effects of aminophilline and general improvement in many measures of respiratory function.[222] As with aersolized bronchodilator therapy, this form of treatment should be discontinued if no response is seen.

Antibiotics

The incidence of secondary bacterial infection in bronchiolitis is very low. Hall and colleagues documented bacterial infection in only 7 (1.2%) of 565 cases;[223] Greenes and Harper found a positive blood culture in only 1 (0.2%) of 411 children aged 3 to 36 months, even though subjects were selected for the study because of the presence of high fever (> 39°C).[65] A separate study looked at secondary bacterial infections in very young infants (< 90 days) in whom evaluations for sepsis were likely to be undertaken: 165 (78%) of 211 consecutive babies with fever and bronchiolitis underwent some combination of blood, urine, and CSF cultures; not a single case of bacterial infection was found.[224] Secondary bacterial pneumonia is rare even if a definite pulmonary infiltrate is present. Unfortunately, antibiotics are often prescribed inappropriately in this setting.

Acute otitis media (AOM), on the other hand, is common in patients with RSV-induced bronchiolitis. In one study of 42 children with bronchiolitis, 36 (86%) had AOM at some time during the clinical course.[225] Middle-ear fluid cultures revealed a bacterial pathogen in all cases, and the proportion of cases due to *S. pneumoniae*, nontypable *H. influenzae*, and *Moraxella catarrhalis* mirrored that seen in all middle-ear fluid culture studies. RSV is also frequently found in the middle-ear fluid, but not usually as a solitary pathogen. Therapy of AOM in this setting need not differ from the usual approach.

Corticosteroids

It is suspected that much of the pathology in bronchiolitis is due to host response (inflammation) rather than to viral replication, so it would seem logical that antiinflammatory therapy would prove beneficial. Unfortunately, studies of heterogeneous patients have not shown any statistical difference between corticosteroid and placebo-treated groups, either in terms of benefit or adverse effects of corticosteroids.[188] Newer studies again confirm no short- or long-term benefit from either oral[226] or nebulized corticosteroids.[227] The latter study started therapy as early in the course as possible and continued it for 6 weeks, but still showed no benefit. Observation of some individual cases seems to indicate that corticosteroids influence favorably the course of life-threatening disease; however, without blinding and without controls, these cases amount to little more than anecdotes. Thus there is currently no scientific support for the use of corticosteroids in the treatment of bronchiolitis. Certainly they should not be used outside the direst circumstances.

Diuretics

In the very sick patient with bronchiolitis, one or more doses of a diuretic may be helpful if there is evidence of fluid overload.[98] Careful fluid management from the outset may allow the clinician to avoid diuretic use.

Inhaled Nitric Oxide

Nitric oxide exerts a bronchodilatory effect and has been used with varying success in the treatment of other respiratory diseases. One small prospective study of inhaled nitric oxide in infants with bronchiolitis was not promising; no apparent bronchodilatory effect and no measurable clinical benefit was demonstrated.[228]

Helium-Oxygen (Heliox)

The theory behind heliox is that oxygen as well as aerosolized medications are able to reach the alveoli with greater ease because of the reduced density of heliox compared with conventional air-oxygen mixtures. Only one small (13 randomized and 5 nonrandomized subjects) study has been published.[229] Subjects in this study were patients admitted to the pediatric intensive care unit with respiratory failure secondary to RSV bronchiolitis. Patients given heliox experienced a decrease in their clinical asthma scores. The therapy seemed to produce the most improvement in those who were sickest at the time treatment was begun. No complications were seen. Much more study is needed, but heliox therapy may hold some promise in the treatment of severely ill children with bronchiolitis.

Mechanical Ventilation and CPAP

Continuous positive airway pressure with mechanical ventilation is being used more frequently, as more infants with underlying respiratory or muscular handicaps are surviving after neonatal intensive care.[222,230]

Ribavirin

Ribavirin is a guanine analogue with broad-spectrum in vitro antiviral activity. Early studies of ribavirin in the treatment of severe RSV disease showed some efficacy. One of the most influential early studies was performed on subjects already intubated and ventilated for respiratory failure; improvement was seen in the ribavirin group compared with placebo.[231] The difficulty in studying ribavirin is that the method of its administration (nebulized by mask or through a ventilator setup 18 hours a day) precludes a simple placebo. If a study is to be properly blinded, control patients must be receiving some sort of nebulization. The study mentioned earlier has been criticized due to the choice of nebulized sterile water as the "placebo." Nebulized water is not entirely benign and provokes bronchospasm in some infants. The question, however, cannot be easily solved just by choosing 0.9% saline, either. The exact mechanics and physics of the condensation of nebulized fluids in the oropharynx and airway are complicated and speculative.

Most subsequent ribavirin studies have utilized nebulized normal saline as a control, and although probably not perfect, normal saline is a better control than is sterile water. Almost uniformly, studies using saline as a control have either failed to demonstrate a clinical benefit or have documented worsening of disease in recipients of ribavirin.[232] The recommendation from the American Academy of Pediatrics Section on Infectious Diseases has, therefore, vacillated somewhat. With each ensuing edition of the Red Book, the recommendation for ribavirin treatment is less firmly given.[233] Many experts currently believe that ribavirin need never be used in the treatment of RSV bronchiolitis, no matter how severe. It has utility in the treatment of children with severe immune suppression due to either cancer chemotherapy, bone marrow transplant, advanced AIDS, or severe combined immune deficiency (SCID). Aside from this group of patients, ribavirin can be considered on a case-by-case basis and at the discretion of local intensive care unit policies. It should probably not be utilized except in infants at high risk for severe or complicated RSV infection.

RSV should be proven by rapid diagnostic test or tissue culture isolation before embarking on ribavirin therapy. The toxicity of ribavirin appears to be negligible, but precautions should be taken to keep it from precipitating and thereby obstructing ventilating equipment. It has also caused birth defects in laboratory animals. Because of this, pregnant medical care personnel should be excused from caring for patients receiving aerosolized ribavirin, even though studies have not found evidence of ribavirin in either plasma or urine samples of health care professionals caring for patients on the drug.

Isolation techniques to avoid nosocomial spread of the virus should be observed.

Immunotherapy

Intravenous immunoglobulin (IVIG) selected for high-titer activity against RSV has been marketed as Respigam. Although RSV-IG has demonstrable efficacy in the prevention of RSV disease in high-risk babies, its use in treatment proved fruitless.[234] A humanized murine monoclonal antibody against RSV, called palivizumab (trade name Synagis), has also been shown to be useful in prophylaxis. To date, no studies on treatment of established RSV infection with this product have been published.

Leukotriene Receptor Antagonist

A single trial has reported the use of montclukast for therapy of wheezing illness after an episode of RSV bronchiolitis.[234a] Infants given montclukast were free of asthma symptoms 22% of the time compared with 4% of the time in infants on placebo. Further research with this class of medications is needed.

Digoxin

Congestive heart failure is sometimes suspected because the liver and spleen, pushed down by the diaphragm, often are palpable. However, cardiac catheterization of three infants with bronchiolitis indicated that congestive failure was not present in such cases.[235] Digoxin is not indicated unless some other evidence of congestive heart failure is observed, such as neck vein distension, dependent edema, or cardiomegaly. An ECG may be indicated to exclude left ventricular hypertrophy, which would be observed in left-sided congestive heart failure, and to recognize myocarditis.

Complications

Apnea

In young infants with bronchiolitis or pneumonia caused by RSV, apneic spells are not unusual,[202] as discussed in the beginning of this chapter.

Respiratory Failure

Some degree of hypoxemia is present in most infants, and hypercapnia occurs in the more severe cases. Mechanical ventilation may be needed in severe cases.

Cardiac Dysrhythmia

Although rare, several cases of supraventicular tachycardia in association with RSV bronchiolitis have been reported.[236] In addition, a single case of ventricular arrhthymia in an infant with RSV bronchiolitis has been published, which could represent a coincidental finding.[237]

Lung Damage

Bronchiectasis and unilateral hyperlucent lung (Swyer-James syndrome) have been reported as complicating bronchiolitis, apparently caused by adenovirus, in native Canadians and native Alaskans.[189,206] Exercise-induced bronchospasm or other abnormal pulmonary function tests are not unusual 10 years later.[238]

Pneumonia or Atelectasis

Complications of bronchiolitis in infants are often detected by chest roentgenogram. The pneumonia or atelectasis is often patchy and minimal and does not have a significant impact on the illness, because obstruction, rather than collapsed or fluid-filled alveoli, is the principal problem. The pneumonia or atelectasis is occasionally segmental or more extensive.

Immunocompromised Children

Life-threatening bronchiolitis caused by RSV can occur in older children who are immunocompromised by leukemia or a defect in cell-mediated immunity.[239]

Relation to Asthma

An association between acute bronchiolitis in infancy and recurrent wheezing later in life has been recognized for decades. It has always been a "chicken or egg" question as to whether early RSV infection actually predisposes a patient toward the development of asthma or whether severe disease with RSV infection comes about because of a preexisting predilection toward wheezing that exists in patients who subsequently develop asthma. The answer is likely to be a combination of the two.[239a] Certainly, infants at high familial and environmental risk for the development of asthma tend to wheeze more when they develop RSV bronchiolitis. This was documented in a prospective study of 24 infants with bronchiolitis, which demonstrated that nasal eosinophilia, family history of allergy, and personal history of allergy were all useful in predicting which patients would later develop typical asthma.[240]

On the other hand, animal models of RSV infection suggest that early infections with certain pathogens can "set" a person's immune system so that it responds somewhat differently to later infections than it would otherwise. This phenomenon was the cause of the greatly exaggerated RSV disease that occurred in patients who received formalin-inactivated RSV vaccine in the 1960s and then contracted wild-type RSV infection.[197] Larsen et al. have also documented long-term alterations in the neuronal control of airway smooth muscle following experimental RSV infection in an animal model.[241]

What is clear is that bronchiolitis in infancy, even mild bronchiolitis, is associated with wheezing later in childhood, even when variables of family and personal history of allergy and exposure to passive smoking are considered.

Prevention

Vaccines

Several theoretical problems need to be addressed in RSV vaccine development: (1) The worst disease occurs in very young infants. This is a problem because the immune system of a young infant is not as well equipped to respond to vaccination. (2) All adults have been infected with RSV, and therefore antibodies are passed to the fetus transplacentally. The presence of maternally derived passive antibody in neonatal serum could blunt the response to a vaccine. (3) Multiple doses of vaccine will probably be required, and parents are becoming both weary and leery of the number of vaccinations. Adding to the problem is that RSV doesn't make most parents' short list of feared childhood diseases because it doesn't get much press. (4) Most viruses against which we have developed effective vaccines are systemic illnesses or include viremia as a part of their pathogenesis. RSV is, for the most part, a mucosally restricted pathogen. This means that vaccination will probably need to produce mucosal

immunity in order to be maximally effective. (5) The first vaccination effort against RSV did not just fail; it was an unmitigated disaster. Therefore, vaccine research will have to be approached gingerly, and with an eye toward making sure that no harm is induced by the vaccine. (6) Immune correlates of protection are not well understood. (7) Finally, wild-type disease is not protective against reinfection, so the best that could be expected from a vaccine is attenuated disease.

At present, live-attenuated RSV vaccines seem to hold the most promise. Hundreds of potential candidates have been screened. Most strains have been either underattenuated (causing disease in recipients) or overattenuated (resulting in a poor antibody response).[242] However, there is a fairly good candidate on the horizon.[243] Subunit vaccines have shown some promise in a rodent model.[244] However, mice are semipermissive hosts and, as such, are easier to protect from disease than are human babies.

Passive Antibody

As mentioned earlier, two antibody preparations have been tested and shown to be useful in the prevention of RSV infection in infants at high risk of severe RSV disease. These antibody products are the only availiable mechanism for preventing severe RSV disease in infants at high risk. The first is a high-titer RSV-IG preparation that reduced the rate of RSV-associated hospitalization from 13.5% in the placebo group to 8.0% in the intervention group (a relative reduction of 41%).[245] The second is a humanized murine monoclonal antibody preparation called palivizumab that reduced the rate of RSV-associated hospitalization from 10.6% in the placebo group to 4.8% in the intervention group (a relative reduction of 55%).[246] Both of the preceding studies were restricted to children with bronchopulmonary dysplasia (BPD) or prematurity. In a subsequent study of 1,287 children with congenital heart disease, palivizumab was found to be both safe and efficacious in this population.[246a] The rate of RSV-associated hospitalization was 9.7% in the placebo group and 5.3% in the palivizumab group (a relative reduction of 45%).

Palivizumab is more convenient than RSV-IG because of the much smaller volume of antibody product that needs to be administered. It is given intramuscularly, rather than intravenously. This cuts down on both infusion-related costs and the rate of adverse events. RSV-IG, on the other hand, also reduced hospitalization due to other respiratory virus infections and reduced the rate of acute otitis media in recipients. Palivizumab contains only antibodies directed at the fusion protein of RSV and thus protects very specifically against RSV disease.

Guidelines for the use of these products, published by the American Academy of Pediatrics,[233,247] are summarized following.

Palivizumab prophylaxis should be considered for the following.

1. Children less than 2 years of age with chronic lung disease who have required medical therapy within 6 months of the start of the RSV season.
2. Infants born at 28 weeks gestational age or earlier who are or will be less than 12 months of age at the onset of the RSV season; infants born at 29 to 32 weeks gestational who are or will be less than 6 months of age at the onset of the RSV season.
3. Infants born between 32 and 35 weeks gestational age may be considered candidates for prophylaxis in the first 6 months of life if they have at least two additional risk factors for severe disease, such as neurologic impairment, immunodeficiency, day-care center attendance, multiple siblings, secondhand tobacco smoke exposure, and congenital abnormalities of the airways. Decisions should be made on a case-by-case basis.
4. Consideration may be given to the use of palivizumab in children 24 months of age or younger with hemodynamically significant congenital heart disease (whether cyanotic or acyanotic). Those most likely to benefit are children younger than 12 months of age who are currently receiving medication to control congestive heart failure, have moderate to severe pulmonary hypertension, or have cyanotic heart disease.[233]

Because of the enormous cost, most hospitals have modified the guidelines somewhat. The cost-benefit ratio and the "number needed to treat" improve when the products are given only to patients at highest risk. Except for children with BPD, RSV prophylaxis is unlikely to be cost effective after the first 12 months of life.[192] Other monoclonal antibody preparations have been developed and are undergoing clinical trials. It is important to remember that currently only about 15% of all RSV hospitalizations occur in children for whom prophylaxis with RSV antibodies is licensed.[192] In addition, palivizumab is only about 55% effective. Thus, for major inroads to be made in the prevention of RSV disease, vaccine development is crucial.

■ INFECTIOUS COMPLICATIONS OF ASTHMA

This section gives only basic concepts and guidelines; asthma is thoroughly discussed in textbooks of allergy.

Definitions

The term *asthma* is used in a number of different ways. In its broadest definition, asthma is used to mean wheezing for any reason, although it is generally not applied in this way. A more practical definition was given in the section on wheezing illnesses.

Factors Triggering Asthma

Infections

Frequent episodes of bronchitis may precede the recognition of acute bronchial asthma. Night cough, cough after exertion, frequent "colds" (rhinitis), or frequent episodes of bronchitis during the preschool years suggest the diagnosis of bronchial asthma precipitated by viral infections. Asthma in which infections are usually the precipitating factor in an attack is sometimes called intrinsic asthma.[248] A viral respiratory infection rather than a bacterial infection is the usual precipitating factor in infectious asthma. Rhinoviruses and RSV are the most common precipitating infections.[249] If both extrinsic allergens and infections appear to be involved as precipitating factors, this is sometimes called the mixed type of asthma.

Sinusitis

It is clear that sinusitis is a common co-morbidity in children with asthma. Radiographic evidence of sinusitis is present in a higher percentage of children with ashthma (20–30%) than in healthy children (approximately 5%).[250,251] However, the common perception that concomitant sinusitis causes exacerbation of lower airway disease in patients with asthma has not been proved.[252] Diagnostic criteria for sinusitis are the same as for children without asthma (see Chapter 5). When the diagnosis of sinusitis is made in a child experiencing an asthma exacerbation, both conditions should be treated.

Right Middle-Lobe Syndrome

Chronic or recurrent episodes of atelectasis or pneumonia of the right middle lobe are called right middle-lobe syndrome. This syndrome is discussed in the section of chronic or recurrent pneumonias in Chapter 8.

Aspergillosis

Allergic pulmonary aspergillosis is usually associated with eosinophilia and pneumonia and is discussed in the section of Chapter 8 on pulmonary infiltrates and eosinophilia.

Bronchiectasis and Emphysema

These conditions are uncommon and occur in severe cases after years of difficulty.

Corticosteroid-related Infections

Recent corticosteroid use may be a risk factor for increased severity of varicella in children.[253] A few case reports of disseminated fungal or tuberculous disease have been noted in asthmatic adults receiving corticosteroids. Both *Legionella* and *Pneumocystis* pneumonia have been reported in asthmatic children receiving long-term therapy with systemic corticosteroids.[254] In another study of children with asthma, use of short courses of prednisone did not appear to increase the risk of infection.[255]

■ REFERENCES

1. Fuhrman BP, Zimmerman JJ, eds. Pediatric critical care, 2nd ed. St Louis: Mosby-Year Book, 1998.
2. Levin DL, Morriss FC, eds. Essentials of pediatric intensive care, 2nd ed. New York: Churchill Livingstone, 1997
3. Rogers MC, ed. Textbook of Pediatric intensive care, 3rd ed. Baltimore: Williams and Wilkins, 1996.
4. Brayden RM, Paisley JW, Lauer BA. Apnea in infants with *Chlamydia trachomatis* pneumonia. Pediatr Infect Dis J 1987;6:423–5.
5. Church NR, Anas NG, Hall CB, et al. Respiratory syncytial virus-related apnea in infants. Am J Dis Child 1984;138:247–50.
6. Gray C, Davies F, Molyneux E. Apparent life-threatening events presenting to a pediatric emergency department. Pediatr Emerg Care 1999;15:195–9.
7. Spitzer AB, Boyle JT, Tuchman DN, Fox WW. Awake apnea associated with gastrointestinal reflux: a specific clinical response. J Pediatr 1984;104:200–5.
8. Riedel F, Kroener T, Stein K, et al. Rotavirus infection and bradycardia-apnea episodes in the neonate. Eur J Pediatr 1996;155:36–40.
9. Simon MW. Apnea associated with Epstein-Barr virus infection. Pediatr Infect Dis J 1994;13:82.
10. Breese BB, Disney FA, Talpey W. The nature of a small group practice. Pediatrics 1966;38:264–77.
11. Moffet HL. Common infections in ambulatory patients. Ann Intern Med 1978;89:743–5.
12. Burrows B, Huang N, Hughes R, et al. Pulmonary terms and symbols: a report of the ACCPATS joint committee on pulmonary nomenclature. Chest 1975;67:583–93.
13. Newth CJL. Recognition and management of respiratory failure. Pediatr Clin North Am 1979;26:617–43.
14. Downes JJ, Fulgencio T, Raphaely RC. Acute respiratory failure in infants and children. Pediatr Clin North Am 1972;19:423–45.
15. Mellis CM. Evaluation and treatment of chronic cough in children. Pediatr Clin North Am 1979;26:553–64.
16. Shuper A, Mukamel M, Mimouni M, et al. Psychogenic cough. Arch Dis Child 1983;58:745–7.
17. Hannaway PJ, Hopper GDK. Cough variant asthma in children. JAMA 1982;247:206–8.
18. Cloutier MM, Loughlin GM. Chronic cough in children: a manifestation of airway hyperreactivity. Pediatrics 1981;67:6–12.
19. Okada C, Horiba M, Matsumoto H, et al. A study of clinical features of cough variant asthma. Int Arch Allergy Immunol 2001;125(suppl):51–4.
20. Wald ER. Chronic sinusitis in children. J Pediatr 1995;127:339–47.
21. Orenstein SR, Shalaby TM, Putnam PE. Thickened feedings as a cause of increased coughing when used as treatment for gastroesophageal reflux in infants. J Pediatr 1992;121:913–5.
22. Blazer S, Naveh Y, Friedman A. Foreign body in the airway: a review of 200 cases. Am J Dis Child 1980;134:68–71.
23. Coffey JD Jr. Bilateral bronchial foreign bodies: a misadventure. Two aspirated peanut halves blocking each major bronchus. Clin Pediatr (Phila) 1977;16:749–50.
24. Newman DE. The radiolucent esophageal foreign body: an often-forgotten cause of respiratory symptoms. J Pediatr 1978;92:60–3.
25. Kosloske AM. Bronchoscopic extraction of aspirated foreign bodies in children. Am J Dis Child 1982;136:924–7.
26. Callahan CW. Etiology of chronic cough in a population of children referred to a pediatric pulmonologist. J Am Board Fam Pract 1996;9:324–7.
27. Holinger LD. Chronic cough in infants and children. Laryngoscope 1986;96:316–22.
28. Marx A, Torok TJ, Holman RC, et al. Pediatric hospitalizations for croup (laryngotracheobronchitis): biennial increases associated with human parainfluenza virus 1 epidemics. J Infect Dis 1997;176:1423–7.
29. Fulginiti VA. Acute supraglottitis (epiglottitis): to look or not [editorial]? Am J Dis Child 1988;142:597.
30. Newth CJL, Levison H, Bryan AC. The respiratory status of children with croup. J Pediatr 1972;81:1068–73.
31. Hodge KM, Ganzel TM. Diagnostic and therapeutic efficiency in croup and epiglottitis. Laryngoscope 1987;97:621–5.
32. Davis HW, Gartner JC, Galvis G, et al. Acute upper airway obstruction: croup and epiglottitis. Pediatr Clin North Am 1981;28:859–80.
33. Sofer S, Duncan P, Chernick V. Bacterial tracheitis: an old disease rediscovered. Clin Pediatr (Phila) 1983;22:407–11.

34. Henry RL, Mellis CM, Benjamin B. Pseudomembranous croup. Arch Dis Child 1983;58:180–3.

35. Denney JC, Handier SD. Membranous laryngotracheobronchitis. Pediatrics 1982;70:705–7.

36. Edwards KM, Dundon C, Altemeier WA. Bacterial tracheitis as a complication of viral croup. Pediatr Infect Dis 1983;2:390–1.

37. Liston SL, Gehrz RC, Siegel LG, et al. Bacterial tracheitis. Am J Dis Child 1983;137:764–7.

38. Koren G, Frand M, Barzilay Z, MacLeod SM. Corticosteroid treatment of laryngotracheitis versus spasmodic croup in children. Am J Dis Child 1983;137:941–4.

39. Denny FW, Murphy TF, Clyde WA Jr, et al. Croup: an 11-year study in a pediatric practice. Pediatrics 1983;71:871–6.

40. Henrickson KJ, Kuhn SM, Savatski LL. Epidemiology and cost of infection with human parainfluenza virus types 1 and 2 in young children. Clin Infect Dis 1994;18:770–9.

41. Peltola V, Heikkinen T, Ruuskanen O. Clinical courses of croup caused by influenza and parainfluenza viruses. Pediatr Infect Dis J 2002;21:76–8.

42. Ross LA, Mason WH, Lanson J, et al. Laryngotracheobronchitis as a complication of measles during an urban epidemic. J Pediatr 1992;121:511–5.

43. Krause I, Schonfeld T, Ben-Ari J, et al. Prolonged croup due to herpes simplex virus infection. Eur J Pediatr 1998;157:567–9.

44. DiGirolamo S, Anselmi M, Piccini A, et al. Aspecific membranous laryngitis after infectious mononucleosis. Int J Pediatr Otorhinolaryngol 1996;34:171–4.

45. Grattan-Smith T, Forer M, Kilham H, et al. Viral supraglottitis. J Pediatr 1987;110:434–5.

46. Molteni RA. Epiglottitis: incidence of extraepiglottic infection: report of 72 cases and review of the literature. Pediatrics 1976;58:526–31.

47. Johnson GK, Sullivan JL, Bishop LA. Acute epiglottitis: review of 55 cases and suggested protocol. Arch Otolaryngol 1974;100:333–7.

48. Lacroix J, Ahronheim G, Arcand P, et al. Group A streptococcal supraglottitis. J Pediatr 1986;109:20–4.

49. Lipson D, Kronick JB, Tewfik L, et al. Group B streptococcal supraglottitis in a 3-month-old infant. Am J Dis Child 1986;140:411–2.

50. Schwartz RH, Knerr RJ, Hermansen K, et al. Acute epiglottitis caused by beta-hemolytic group C streptococci. Am J Dis Child 1982;136:558–9.

51. Jacobs RF, Yasuda K, Smith A, et al. Laryngeal candidiasis presenting as laryngeal stridor. Pediatrics 1982;69:234–6.

52. Walsh TJ, Gray WC. Candida epiglottitis in immunocompromised patients. Chest 1987;91:482–5.

52a. Khabie N, Boyce TG, Roberts GD, Thompson DM. Laryngeal sporotrichosis causing stridor in a young child. Int J Pediatr Otorhinolaryngol 2003;67:819–23.

53. Esclamado RM, Richardson MA. Laryngotracheal foreign bodies in children: a comparison with bronchial foreign bodies. Am J Dis Child 1987;141:259–62.

54. Nussbaum E, Fleming PG, Wood RE, et al. Stridor due to radiotransparent esophageal foreign body. Am J Dis Child 1984;138:1081–3.

55. Waki EY, Madgy DN, Belenky WM, Gower VC. The incidence of gastroesophageal reflux in recurrent croup. Int J Pediatr Otorhinolaryngol 1995;32:223–32.

56. Contencin P, Maurage C, Ployet MJ, Seid AB, Sinaasappel M. Gastroesophageal reflux and ENT disorders in childhood. Int J Pediatr Otorhinolaryngol 1995;32(suppl):S135–44.

57. Winograd IM. Acute croup in an older child: an unusual toxic origin. Clin Pediatr 1977;16:884–7.

58. Amir J, Ashkenazi S, Schonfield T, et al. Laryngospasm as a single manifestion of epilepsy. Arch Dis Child 1983;58:151–3.

58a. Bork K, Hardt J, Schicketanz KH, Ressel N. Clinical studies of sudden upper airway obstruction in patients with hereditary angioedema due to C1 esterase inhibitor deficiency. Arch Int Med 2003;163:1229–35.

59. Newman KB, Mason UG III, Schmaling KB. Clincical features of vocal cord dysfunction. Am J Respir Crit Care Med 1995;152:1382–6.

60. Shackelford GD, Siegel MJ, McAlister WH. Subglottic edema in acute epiglottitis in children AJR 1978;131:603–5.

61. Mills JL, Spackman TJ, Borns P, et al. The usefulness of lateral neck roentgenograms in laryngotracheobronchitis. Am J Dis Child 1979;133:1140–2.

62. Walner DL, Ouanounou S, Donnelly LF, Cotton RT. Utility of radiographs in the evaluation of pediatric upper airway obstruction. Ann Otol Rhinol Laryngol 1999;108:378–83.

63. Stankiewicz JA, Bowes AK. Croup and epiglottitis: a radiologic study. Laryngoscope 1985;95:1159–60.

64. Eckel HE, Widemann B, Damm M, Roth B. Airway endoscopy in the diagnosis and treatment of bacterial tracheitis in children. Int J Pediatr Otorhinolaryngol 1993;27:147–57.

65. Greenes DS, Harper MB. Low risk of bacteremia in febrile children with recognizable viral syndromes. Pediatr Infect Dis J 1999;18:258–61.

66. Schloss MD, Gold JA, Rosales JK, et al. Acute epiglottitis: current management. Laryngoscope 1983;93:489–93.

67. Selbst SM. Epiglottitis: a review of 13 cases and a suggested protocol for management. J Fam Pract 1984;19:333–7.

68. Margolis CZ. Routine tracheotomy in H. influenzae type b epiglottitis. J Pediatr 1972;81:1150–3.

69. Smith DS. Editorial comment. J Pediatr 1972;81:1153.

70. Hatch DJ. Prolonged nasotracheal intubation in infants and children. Lancet 1968;1:1272–5.

71. Perches JM, Grosskrentz D, Chuang TH. Endotracheal intubation versus tracheostomy. South Med J 1966;59:1399–403.

72. Halldorsson TS, Bushnell LS, Connelley JP. Nasotracheal intubation as a substitute for tracheostomy. Clin Pediatr (Phila) 1967;6:1157–61.

73. Szold PD, Glicklich M. Children with epiglottitis can be bagged. Clin Pediatr (Phila) 1976;15:792–3.

74. Editorial correspondence: management of croup. J Pediatr 1973;83:166–9.

75. Waisman Y, Klein BL, Boenning DA, et al. Prospective randomized double-blind study comparing L-epinephrine and racemic epinephrine aerosols in the treatment of laryngotracheitis (croup). Pediatrics 1992;89:302–6.

76. Singer OP, Wilson WJ. Laryngotracheobronchitis: 2 years' experience with racemic epinephrine. Can Med Assoc J 1976;115:132–4.

77. Fogel JM, Berg IJ, Gerber MA, et al. Racemic epinephrine in the treatment of croup: nebulization alone versus neb-

ulization with intermittent positive pressure breathing. J Pediatr 1982;101:1028–31.

78. Rizos JD, DiGravio BE, Sehl AMJ, Tallon M. The disposition of children with croup treated with racemic epinephrine and dexamethasone in the emergency department. J Emerg Med 1998;16:535–9.

79. Butte MJ, Nguyen BX, Hutchison TJ, et al. Pediatric myocardial infarction after racemic epinephrine administration. Pediatrics 1999;104:e9.

80. Johnson DW, Jacobsen S, Edney PC, et al. A comparison of nebulized budesonide, intramuscular dexamethasone, and placebo for moderately severe croup. N Engl J Med 1998;339:498–503.

81. Geelhoed GC, Turner J, Macdonald WB. Efficacy of a small single dose of oral dexamethasone for outpatient croup: a double blind placebo controlled clinical trial. BMJ 1996;313:140–2.

82. Ausajo M, Saenz A, Pham B, et al. The effectiveness of glucocorticoids in treating croup: meta-analysis. Br Med J 1999;319:595–600.

83. Butt W, Koren G, England S, et al. Hypoxia associated with helium-oxygen therapy in neonates. J Pediatr 1985; 106:474–7.

84. Travis KW, Todres ID, Shannon DC. Pulmonary edema associated with croup and epiglottitis. Pediatrics 1977; 59:695–8.

85. Kanter RK, Watchko JF. Pulmonary edema associated with upper airway obstruction. Am J Dis Child 1984; 138:356–8.

86. Vinson DC, Lutz LJ. The effect of parental expectations on treatment of children with a cough: a report from ASPN. J Fam Pract 1993;37:430–1.

87. Chapman RS, Henderson FW, Clyde WA Jr, et al. The epidemiology of tracheobronchitis in pediatric practice. Am J Epidemiol 1981;114:786–97.

88. DeBaets F, Kint J, Pauwels R, Leroy J. IgG subclass deficiency in children with recurrent bronchitis. Eur J Pediatr 1992;151:274–8.

89. Silk H, Geha RS. Asthma, recurrent infections and IgG2 deficiency. Ann Allergy 1988;60:134–6.

90. Gaillard D, Jouet JB, Egreteau L, et al. Airway epithelial damage and inflammation in children with recurrent bronchitis. Am J Resp Crit Care Med 1994;150:810–7.

91. Nelson KE, Gavitt F, Batt MD, et al. The role of adenoviruses in the pertussis syndrome. J Pediatr 1975;86: 335–41.

92. Keller MA, Aftandelians R, Connor JD. Etiology of pertussis syndrome. Pediatrics 1980;66:50–5.

93. Beem MO, Saxon EM. Respiratory tract colonization and a distinctive pneumonia syndrome in infants infected with *Chlamydia trachomatis*. N Engl J Med 1977;296: 306–10.

94. Grayston JT, Campbell LA, Kuo C-C, et al. A new respiratory tract pathogen: *Chlamydia pneumoniae* strain TWAR. J Infect Dis 1990;161:618–25.

95. Hahn DL, Dodge RW, Golubjatnikov R. Association of *Chlamydia pneumoniae* (strain TWAR) infection with wheezing, asthmatic bronchitis, and adult-onset asthma. JAMA 1991;266:225–30.

96. Pruckl PM, Aspock C, Makristathis A, et al. Polymerase chain reaction for detection of *Chlamydia pneumoniae* in gargled-water specimens of children. Eur J Clin Microbiol Infect Dis 1995;14:141–2.

97. Colley JRT, Holland W, Corkhill RT. Influence of passive smoking and parental phlegm on pneumonia and bronchitis in early childhood. Lancet 1974;2:1031–4.

98. McCracken GH Jr, Ginsburg CM, Grossman M, Taussig L. Panel discussion: bronchitis and bronchiolitis. Pediatr Infect Dis 1986;5:766–9.

99. Taussig LM, Smith SM, Blemenfeld R. Chronic bronchitis in childhood: what is it? Pediatrics 1981;67:1–5.

100. Smith TF, Ireland TA, Zaatari GS, et al. Characteristics of children with endoscopically proved chronic bronchitis. Am J Dis Child 1985;139:1039–44.

101. Bowen AD, Oudjhane K, Odagari K, et al. Plastic bronchitis: large, branching, mucoid bronchial casts in children. AJR 1985;144:371–5.

102. Perez-Soler A. Cast bronchitis in infants and children. Am J Dis Child 1989;143:1024–9.

103. Yaari E, Yafe-Zimerman Y, Schwartz SB, et al. Clinical manifestations of *Bordetella pertussis* infection in immunized children and young adults. Chest 1999;115: 1254–8.

104. Brooksaler F, Nelson JD. Pertussis: a reappraisal and report of 190 confirmed cases. Am J Dis Child 1967;114: 389–96.

105. Olson LC. Pertussis. Medicine 1975;54:427–69.

106. Trollfors B. Clinical course of whooping cough in children younger than six months. Acta Paediatr Scand 1979; 68:323–8.

107. Congeni BL, Orenstein DM, Nankervis GA. Three infants with neonatal pertussis. Clin Pediatr (Phila) 1978;17: 113–8.

108. Sotomayor J, Weiner LB, McMillan JA. Inaccurate diagnosis with pertussis. Am J Dis Child 1985;139:724–7.

109. Keitel WA, Edwards KM. Acellular pertussis vaccines in adults. Infect Dis Clin North Am 1999;13:83–94.

110. Wright SW, Edwards KM, Decker MD, Zeldin MH. Pertussis infection in adults with persistent cough. JAMA 1995;273:1044–6.

111. Von Konig CHW, Rott H, Bogaerts H, Schmidt HJ. A serologic study of organisms possibly associated with pertusis-like coughing. Pediatr Infect Dis J 1998;17:645–9.

112. Hagiwara K, Ouchi K, Tashiro N, et al. An epidemic of pertussis-like illness caused by *Chlamydia pneumoniae*. Pediatr Infect Dis J 1999;18:271–5.

113. Onorato IM, Wassilak SG, Meade B. Laboratory diagnosis of pertussis: the state of the art. Pediatr Infect Dis J 1987; 6:145–51.

114. Mertsola J, Ruuskanen O, Eerola E, et al. Intrafamilial spread of pertussis. J Pediatr 1983;103:359–63.

115. Loeffelholz MJ, Thompson CJ, Long KS, Gilchrist MJ. Comparison of PCR, culture, and direct fluorescent antibody testing for detection of *Bordatella pertussis*. J Clin Microbiol 1999;37:2872–6.

115a. Sloan LM, Hopkins MK, Mitchell PS, et al. Multiplex LightCycler PCR assay for detection and differentiation of *Bordetella pertussis* and *Bordetella parapertussis* in nasopharyngeal specimens. J Clin Microbiol 2002;40: 96–100.

116. Wirsing von Konig CH, Gounis D, Laukamp S, et al. Evaluation of a single sample serological technique for diagnosing pertussis in unvaccinated children. Eur J Microbiol Infect Dis 1999;18:341–5.

117. Hoppe JE. Comparison of erythromycin estolate and erythromycin ethylsuccinate for treatment of pertussis. Pediatr Infect Dis J 1992;11:189–93.

118. Patamasucon P, Kaojarern S, Kusmiesz H, Nelson JD. Pharmacokinetics of erythromycin ethylsuccinate and estolate in infants under 4 months of age. Antimicrob Agents Chemother 1981;19:736–9.

119. Inman WH, Rawson NS. Erythromycin estolate and jaundice. Br Med J Clin Res Ed 1983;286:1954–5.

120. Bace A, Zrnic T, Bergovac J, et al. Short-term treatment of pertussis with azithromycin in infants and young children. Eur J Clin Microbiol Infect Dis 1999;18:296–8.

121. Lebel MH, Mehra S. Efficacy and safety of clarithromycin versus erythromycin for the treatment of pertussis: a prospective, randomized, single-blind trial. Pediatr Infect Dis J 2001;20:1149–54.

122. Bergquist SO, Bernander S, Dahnsjö H, et al. Erythromycin in the treatment of pertussis: a study of bacteriologic and clinical effects. Pediatr Infect Dis J 1987;6:458–61.

123. Honein MA, Paulozzi LJ, Himelright IM, et al. Infantile hypertrophic pyloric stenosis after pertussis prophylaxis with erythromycin: a case review and cohort study. Lancet 1999;354:2101–5.

124. Granstrom M, Olinder-Nielsen AM, Holmblad P, et al. Specific immunoglobulin for treatment of whooping cough. Lancet 1991;338:1230–3.

125. Kurt TL, Yeager AS, Guenette S, et al. Spread of pertussis by hospital staff. JAMA 1972;221:264–7.

126. Davis LE, Burstyn DG, Manclark CR. Pertussis encephalopathy with a normal brain biopsy and elevated lymphocytosis-promoting factor antibodies. Pediatr Infect Dis 1984;3:448–51.

127. Pittman M. Pertussis toxin: the cause of the harmful effects and prolonged immunity of whooping cough: a hypothesis. Rev Infect Dis 1979;1:401–12.

128. Kohn JL, Schwartz L, Greenbaum J, et al. Roentgenograms of the chest taken during pertussis. Am J Dis Child 1944;67:463–8.

129. Bass JW, Fajardo JE, Brien JH, et al. Sudden death due to epiglottitis. Pediatr Infect Dis 1985;4:447–9.

130. Lees AW. Atelectasis and bronchiectasis in pertussis. Br Med J 1950;2:1138–41.

131. Fawcitt J, Parry HE. Lung changes in pertussis and measles in childhood: a review of 1894 cases with a followup study of the pulmonary complications. Br J Radiol 1957;39:76–82.

132. Grant CC, McKay EJ, Simpson A, Buckley D. Pertussis encephalopathy with high cerebrospinal fluid antibody titers to pertussis toxin and filamentous hemagglutinin. Pediatrics 1998;102:986–90.

133. Centers for Disease Control. Pertussis surveillance, 1979–1981. MMWR 1982;31:333–6.

134. Setta F, Baecke M, Jacquy J, et al. Cerebella ataxia following whooping cough. Clin Neurol Neurosurg 1999;101:56–61.

135. Johnston ID, Stachan DP, Anderson HR. Effect of pneumonia and whooping cough in childhood on adult lung function. N Engl J Med 1998;338:581–7.

136. Jaworski MA, Moffatt MEK, Ahronheim GA. Disseminated herpes simplex associated with *H. influenzae* infection in a previously healthy child. J Pediatr 1980;96:426–9.

137. Bass JW. Pertussis: current status of prevention and treatment. Pediatr Infect Dis 1985;4:614–9.

138. Halperin SA, Bortolussi R, Langley JM, et al. A randomized, placebo-controlled trial of erythromycin estolate chemoprophylaxis for household contacts of children with culture-positive *Bordetella pertussis* infection. Pediatrics 1999;104:e42.

139. Granström G, Sterner G, Nord CE et al. Use of erythromycin to prevent pertussis in newborns of mothers with pertussis. J Infect Dis 1987;155:1210–4.

140. American Academy of Pediatrics. Pertussis. In: Pickering LK, ed. Red Book: 2003 Report of the Committee on Infectious Diseases. 26th ed. Elk Grove Village, IL: American Academy of Pediatrics, 2003:472–86.

141. Stewart GT. Whooping cough in relation to other childhood infections in 1977–9 in the United Kingdom. J Epidemiol Community Health 1981;35:139–45.

142. Rennels MB, Deloria MA, Pichichero ME, et al. Extensive swelling after booster doses of acellular pertussis-tetanus-diphtheria vaccines. Pediatrics 2000;105:e12.

143. Fine PEM, Clarkson JA. The recurrence of whooping cough: possible implications for assessment of vaccine efficacy. Lancet 1982;1:666–9.

144. Orenstein WA. Pertussis in adults: epidemiology, signs, symptoms, and implications for vaccination. Clin Infect Dis 1999;28(suppl):S147–50.

144a. Vitek CR, Pascual FB, Baughman AL, Murphy TV. Increase in deaths from pertussis among young infants in the United States in the 1990s. Pediatr Infect Dis J 2003;22:628–34.

145. Van Damme P, Burgess M. Immunogenicity of a combined diphtheria-tetanus-acellular pertussis vaccine in adults. Vaccine 2004;22:305–8.

146. Hethcote HW. Simulations of pertussis epidemiology in the United States: effects of adult booster vaccinations. Math Biosci 1999;158:47–73.

147. Gardner P. Indications for acellular pertussis vaccines in adults: the case for selective, rather than universal, recommendations. Clin Infect Dis 1999;28(suppl):S131–5.

148. Jordan WS, Denny FW, Badger GF, et al. A study of illness in a group of Cleveland families. XVII. The occurrence of Asian influenza. Am J Hyg 1958;68:190–221.

149. Neuzil KM, Mellen BG, Wright PF, et al. The effect of influenza on hospitalizations, outpatient visits, and courses of antibiotics in children. N Engl J Med 2000;342:225–31.

150. Paisley JW, Bruker FW, Lamer BA, et al. Type A2 influenza viral infections in children. Am J Dis Child 1978;132:34–6.

151. Wright PF, Ross KB, Thompson J, Karzon DT. Influenza A infections in young children. N Engl J Med 1977;296:829–34.

152. Moffet HL, Cramblett HG, Middleton GK, et al. Outbreak of influenza B in a children's home. JAMA 1962;182:834–8.

153. Price DA, Postlethwaite RJ, Longson M. Influenza A_2 infections presenting with febrile convulsions and gastrointestinal symptoms in young children. Clin Pediatr (Phila) 1976;15:361–7.

154. Paisley JW, Bruhn FW, Lauer BA, et al. Type A_2 influenza viral infections in children. Am J Dis Child 1978;132:34–6.

155. Dietzman DE, Schaller JG, Ray CG, et al. Acute myositis associated with influenza B infection. Pediatrics 1976;57: 255–8.

156. Middleton PJ, Alexander RM, Szymonski MT. Severe myositis during recovery from influenza. Lancet 1970;2: 533–5.

157. Liou YS, Barbour SD, Bell IM, et al. Children hospitalized with influenza B infection. Pediatr Infect Dis J 1987;6: 541–3.

158. Buescher EL. Respiratory disease and the adenoviruses. Med Clin North Am 1967;51:769–79.

159. Couch RB, Cote TR, Fleet WF, et al. Aerosol-induced adenovirus resembling the naturally occurring illness in military recruits. Am Rev Res Dis 1966;93:529–35.

160. Bisno AL, Barratt NP, Swanston WH, et al. An outbreak of acute respiratory disease in Trinidad associated with parainfluenza viruses. Am J Epidemiol 1970;91:68–77.

161. Evans AS. Infections with hemadsorption virus in University of Wisconsin students. N Engl J Med 1960;263: 233–7.

162. Johnson KM, Bloom HH, Mufson MA, et al. Acute respiratory disease associated with Coxsackie A21 virus infection. JAMA 1962;179:112–25.

163. Cordero L, Cuadrado R, Hall CB, Horstmann DM. Primary atypical pneumonia: an epidemic caused by *Mycoplasma pneumoniae*. J Pediatr 1967;71:1–12.

164. Rothbarth PH, Groen J, Bohnen AM, et al. Influenza virus serology—a comparative study. J Virol Methods 1999; 78:163–9.

165. Hall CB, Douglas RG Jr, Gelman JM, et al. Viral shedding patterns of children with influenza B infection. J Infect Dis 1979;140:610–3.

166. Ito Y, Ichiyama T, Kimura H, et al. Detection of influenza virus RNA by reverse transcription-PCR and proinflammatory cytokines in influenza-virus-associated encephalop-athy. J Med Virol 1999;58:420–5.

167. Grondahl B, Puppe W, Hoppe A, et al. Rapid identification of nine microorganisms causing acute respiratory tract infections by single-tube multiplex reverse transcription-PCR: feasibility study. J Clin Microbiol 1999; 37:1–7.

168. Centers for Disease Control and Prevention. Prevention and control of influenza: recommendations of the advisory committee on immunization practices. MMWR 2004;53:1–40.

169. National Institutes of Health Consensus Development Conference. Amantadine: does it have a role in the prevention and treatment of influenza? Clin Pediatr (Phila) 1980;19:416–8.

170. Cooper NJ, Sutton AJ, Abrams KR, et al. Effectiveness of neuraminidase inhibitors in treatment and prevention of influenza A and B: systematic review and meta-analysis of randomized controlled trials. Br Med J 2003;326:1235.

171. Williamson JC, Pegram PS. Respiratory distress associated with zanamavir [letter]. New Engl J Med 2000;342: 661–2.

172. Hayden FG, Atmar RL, Schilling M, et al. Use of the selective oral neuraminidase inhibitor oseltamivir to prevent influenza. N Engl J Med 1999;341:1336–43.

173. MacDonald KL, Osterholm MT, Hedberg CW, et al. Toxic shock syndrome: a newly recognized complication of in-fluenza and influenzalike illness. JAMA 1987;257: 1053–8.

174. Sperber SJ, Francis JB. Toxic shock syndrome during an influenza outbreak. JAMA 1987;257:1086–7.

175. Morishima T, Togashi T, Yokota S, et al. Encephalitis and encephalopathy associated with an influenza epidemic in Japan. Clin Infect Dis 2002;35:512–7.

176. Kolski H, Ford-Jones EL, Richardson S, et al. Etiology of acute childhood encephalitis at The Hospital for Sick Children, Toronto, 1994–1995. Clin Infect Dis 1998;26: 398–409.

177. Cunningham E, Kohli F, Venuto RC. Influenza-associated myoglobinuric renal failure. JAMA 1979;242:2428–9.

178. Rice J, Resar LM. Hematologic abnormalities associated with influenza A infection: a report of 3 cases. Am J Med Sci 1998;316:401–3.

179. LarayaCuasay LR, DeForest A, Huff D, et al. Chronic pulmonary complications of early influenza virus infection in children. Am Rev Resp Dis 1977;116:617–25.

180. Hobbins TE, Hughes TP, Rennels MB, et al. Bronchial reactivity in experimental infections with influenza virus. J Infect Dis 1982;146:468–71.

181. Hayden FG, Treanor JJ, Fritz RS, et al. Use of the oral neuraminidase inhibitor oseltamivir in experimental human influenza: randomized controlled trials for prevention and treatment. JAMA 1999;282:1240–6.

182. Poland GA, Hall CB. Influenza immunization of school-children: can we interrupt community epidemics? Pediatrics 1999;103:1280–2.

183. Park CL, Frank A. Does influenza vaccination exacerbate asthma? Drug Safety 1998;19:83–8.

184. James JM, Zeiger RS, Lester MR, et al. Safe administration of influenza vaccine to patients with egg allergy. J Pediatr 1998;133:624–8.

185. Belshe RB, Mendelman PM, Treanor J, et al. The efficacy of live attenuated, cold-adapted, trivalent, intranasal in-fluenzavirus vaccine in children. N Engl J Med 1998;338: 1405–12.

186. Boyce TG, Gruber WC, Coleman-Dockery SD, et al. Mucosal immune response to trivalent live attenuated intranasal influenza vaccine in children. Vaccine 1999;18: 82–8.

187. el-Madhun AS, Cox RJ, Soreide A, et al. Systemic and mucosal immune responses in young children and adults after parenteral influenza vaccination. J Infect Dis 1998; 178:933–9.

187a. Bergen R, Black S, Shinefeld H, et al. Safety of cold-adapted live attenuated influenza vaccine in a large cohort of children and adolescents. Pediatr Infect Dis J 2004; 23:138–44.

188. Leer JA, Green JL, Heimlich EM, et al. Corticosteroid treatment in bronchiolitis: a controlled, collaborative study in 297 infants and children. Am J Dis Child 1969; 117:495–503.

189. Wohl MEB, Chernick V. Bronchiolitis. Am Rev Resp Dis 1978;118:759–81.

190. Kern S, Uhl M, Berner R, et al. Respiratory syncytial virus infection of the lower respiratory tract: radiological findings in 108 children. Eur Radiol 2001;11:2581–4.

190a. Boyce TG, Weaver AL, St Savier JL, et al. Incidence of bronchiolitis-associated hospitalization among children in Olmsted County, Minnesota. Mayo Clin Proc 2004; 79:832–3

191. Shay DK, Holman RC, Newman RD, et al. Bronchiolitis-associated hospitalizations among US children, 1980–1996. JAMA 1999;282:1440–6.

192. Boyce TG, Mellen BG, Mitchel EF Jr, et al. Rates of hospitalization for respiratory syncytial virus infection among children in medicaid. J Pediatr 2000;137:865–70.

193. Simon G, Jordan WS. Infections and allergic aspects of bronchiolitis. J Pediatr 1967;70:533–8.

194. Hogg JC, Williams J, Richardson JB, et al. Age as a factor in the distribution of lower-airway conductance and in the pathologic anatomy of obstructive lung disease. N Engl J Med 1970;282:1283–7.

195. Griscom NT, Wohl MEB, Kirkpatrick JA Jr. Lower respiratory infections: how infants differ from adults. Radiol Clin North Am 1978;16:367–87.

196. Aherne W, Bird T, Court SDM, et al. Pathological changes in virus infections of the lower respiratory tract in children. J Clin Pathol 1970;23:7–18.

197. Kim HW, Canchola JG, Brandt CD, et al. Respiratory syncytial virus disease in infants despite prior administration of antigenic inactivated vaccine. Am J Epidemiol 1969;89:422–34.

198. Kapikian AZ, Mitchell RH, Chanock RM, et al. An epidemiologic study of altered clinical reactivity to respiratory syncytial (RS) vaccine in children previously vaccinated with an inactivated RS virus vaccine. Am J Epidemiol 1969;89:405–21.

199. Glezen WP, Paredes A, Allison JE, et al. Risk of respiratory syncytial virus infection for infants from low-income families in relationship to age, sex, ethnic group, and maternal antibody level. J Pediatr 1981;98:708–15.

200. Graham BS. Pathogenesis of respiratory syncytial virus vaccine-augmented pathology. Am J Respir Crit Care Med 1995;152(suppl):S63–6.

201. Welliver RC, Wong DT, Sun M, et al. The development of respiratory syncytial virus-specific IgE and the release of histamine in nasopharyngeal secretions after infection. N Engl J Med 1981;305:841–6.

202. Hall CB, Hall WJ, Speers DM. Clinical and physiological manifestations of bronchiolitis and pneumonia: cutcome of respiratory syncytial virus. Am J Dis Child 1979;133: 798–802.

203. Reynolds EOR. The effect of breathing 40 percent oxygen on the arterial blood gas tensions of babies with bronchiolitis. J Pediatr 1963;63:1135–9.

204. Henderson FW, Clyde WA Jr, Collier AM, et al. The etiologic and epidemiologic spectrum of bronchiolitis in pediatric practice. J Pediatr 1979;95:183–90.

205. Holdaway D, Romer AC, Gardner PS. The diagnosis and management of bronchiolitis. Pediatrics 1967;39:924–8.

206. Gold R, Wilt JC, Adhikari PK, et al. Adenoviral pneumonia and its complications in infancy and childhood. J Can Assoc Radiol 1969;20:218–24.

207. Welliver RC, Wong DT, Sun M, et al. Parainfluenza virus bronchiolitis. Am J Dis Child 1986;140:34–40.

207a. van den Hoogen BG, de Jong JC, Groen J, et al. A newly discovered human pneumovirus isolated from young children with respiratory tract disease. Nat Med 2001; 7:719–24.

207b. Williams JV, Harris PA, Tollefson SJ, et al. Human meta-pneumovirus and lower respiratory tract disease in otherwise healthy infants and children. N Engl J Med 2004; 350:443–50.

207c. Mullins J, Erdman D, Weinberg G, et al. Human metapneumovirus infection in children hospitalized for respiratory disease [abstract]. Infectious Diseases Society of America 40th Annual Meeting, Chicago, IL, 2002, abstract 774.

208. Tanner DD, Buckley PJ, Hong R, et al. Fatal cytomegalovirus bronchiolitis in a patient with Nezelof's syndrome. Pediatrics 1980;65:98–102.

209. Polmar SH, Robinson LD Jr, Minnefor AB. Immunoglobulin E in bronchiolitis. Pediatrics 1972;50:279–84.

210. Oymar K, Bjerknes R. Is serum eosinophil cationic protein in bronchiolitis a predictor of asthma? Pediatr Allergy Immunol 1998;9:204–7.

211. Shay DK, Holman RC, Roosevelt GE, et al. Bronchiolitis-associated mortality and estimates of respiratory syncytial virus-associated deaths among US children, 1979–1997. J Infect Dis 2001;183:16–22.

212. Eugene-Ruellan G, Freymuth F, Bahloul C, et al. Detection of respiratory syncytial virus A and B and parainfluenzavirus 3 sequences in respiratory tracts of infants by a single PCR with primers targeted to the L-polymerase gene and differential hybridization. J Clin Microbiol 1998;36:796–801.

213. Kelsche RC, Barr M Jr, Demuth GR. Mist therapy in lower respiratory infection: a controlled study. Am J Dis Child 1965;109:495–9.

214. Barker R, Levison H. Effects of ultrasonically nebulized distilled water on airway dynamics in children with cystic fibrosis and asthma. J Pediatr 1972;80:396–400.

215. Grady JJ, Bamman J. "Hypothermia" in a cool mist tent [letter]. J Pediatr 1976;88:691.

215a. Wainwright C, Altamirano L, Cheney M, et al. A multicenter, randomized, double-blind, controlled trial of nebulized epinephrine in infants with acute bronchiolitis. N Engl J Med 2003;349:27–35.

216. Kellner JD, Ohlsson A, Gadomski AM, Wang EE. Bronchodilators for bronchiolitis. Cochrane System Rev 2000; CD001266.

217. Reid L. Influence of the pattern of structural growth of lung on susceptibility to specific infectious diseases in infants and children. Pediatr Res 1977;11:210–5.

218. Roan Y, Galant SP. Decreased neutrophil beta adrenergic receptors in the neonate. Pediatr Res 1982;16:591–3.

219. Luga RA, Salyer JW, Dean JM. Albuterol in acute bronchiolitis—continued therapy despite poor response? Pharmacotherapy 1998;18:198–202.

220. O'Callaghan C, Milner AD, Swarbrick A. Paradoxical deterioration in lung function after nebulised salbutamol in wheezy infants. Lancet 1986;2:1424–5.

221. Brooks IJ, Cropp GJA. Theophylline therapy in bronchiolitis. Am J Dis Child 1981;135:934–6.

222. Outwater KM, Crone RK. Management of respiratory failure in infants with acute viral bronchiolitis. Am J Dis Child 1984;138:1071–5.

223. Hall CB, Powell KR, Schnabel KC, et al. Risk of secondary bacterial infection in infants hospitalized with respiratory syncytial virus infection. J Pediatr 1988;1113:266–71.

224. Liebelt EL, Qi K, Harvey K. Diagnostic testing for serious

bacterial infection in infants aged 90 days or younger with bronchiolitis. Arch Pediatr Adol Med 1999;153:525–30.

225. Andrade MA, Hoberman A, Glustein J, et al. Acute otitis media in children with bronchiolitis. Pediatrics 1998; 101:617–9.

226. Berger I, Argaman Z, Schwartz SB, et al. Efficacy of corticosteroids in acute bronchiolitis: short-term and long-term follow-up. Pediatr Pulmonol 1998;26:162–3.

227. Richter H, Seddon P. Early nebulized budesonide in the treatment of bronchiolitis and the prevention of postbronchiolitis wheezing. J Pediatr 1998;132:849–53.

228. Patel NR, Hammer J, Michani S, et al. Effect of inhaled nitric oxide on respiratory mechanics in ventilated infants with RSV bronchiolitis. Intensive Care Med 1999;25: 81–7.

229. Hollman G, Shen G, Zeng L, et al. Helium-oxygen improves clincal asthma scores in children with acute bronchiolitis. Crit Care Med 1998;26:1731–6.

230. Beasley JM, Jones SEF. Continuous positive airway pressure in bronchiolitis. Br Med J 1981;2:1506–8.

231. Smith DW, Frankel LR, Mathers LH, et al. A controlled trial of aerosolized ribavirin in infants receiving mechanical ventilation for severe respiratory syncytial virus infection. N Engl J Med 1991;325:24–9.

232. Guerguerian AM, Gauthier M, Lebel MH, et al. Ribavirin in ventilated respiratory syncytial virus bronchiolitis. A randomized, placebo-controlled trial. Am J Resp Crit Care Med 1999;160:829–34.

233. American Academy of Pediatrics. Respiratory syncytial virus. In: Pickering LK, ed. Red Book: 2003 Report of the Committee on Infectious Diseases. 26th ed. Elk Grove Village, IL: American Academy of Pediatrics, 2003: 523–8.

234. Rodriguez WJ, Gruber WC, Groothuis JR, et al. Respiratory syncytial virus immune globulin treatment of RSV lower respiratory tract infection in previously healthy children. Pediatrics 1997;100:937–42.

234a. Bisgard H. Study Group on Montelukast and Respiratory Syncytial Virus. A randomized trial of montelukast in respiratory syncytial virus postbronchiolitis. Am J Respir Crit Care Med 2003;167:379–83.

235. Ziegra SR, Keily B, Morales F. Cardiac catheterization in infants with bronchiolitis [abstract]. Am J Dis Child 1960; 100:528.

236. Armstrong DS, Menaham S. Cardiac arrhythmias as a manifestation of acquired heart disease in association with pediatric respiratory syncytial virus infection. J Pediatr Child Health 1993;29:309–11.

237. Huang M, Bigos D, Levine M. Ventricular arrhythmia associated with respiratory syncytial viral infection. Pediatr Cardiol 1998;19:498–500.

238. Kattan M, Keens TG, Lapierre LG, et al. Pulmonary function abnormalities in symptom-free children after bronchiolitis. Pediatrics 1977;59:683–8.

239. Padman R, Bye MR, Schidlow DV, et al. Severe RSV bronchiolitis in an immunocompromised child. Clin Pediatr (Phila) 1985;24:719–21.

239a. Martinez FD. Respiratory syncytial virus bronchiolitis and the pathogenisis of childhood asthma. Pediatr Infect Dis J 2003;22(2 suppl):S76–82 [letters].

240. Zweiman B, Schoenwetter WF, Hildreth EH. The relationship between bronchiolitis and allergic asthma: a prospective study with allergy evaluation. J Allergy 1966;37: 48–53.

241. Colasurdo GN, Hemming VG, Prince GA, et al. Human respiratory syncytial virus produces prolonged alteration of neural control in airways of developing ferrets. Am J Respir Crit Care Med 1998;157:1506–11.

242. Wright PF, Karron RB, Thompson J, et al. Evaluation of a live, cold-passaged, temperature-sensitive, respiratory syncytial virus vaccine candidate in infancy. J Infect Dis 2000;182:1331–42.

243. Whitehead SS, Firestone CY, Karron RA, et al. Addition of a missense mutation present in the L gene of respiratory syncytial virus (RSV) cpts530/1030 to RSV vaccine candidate cpts248/404 increases its attenuation and temperature sensitivity. J Virol 1999;73:871–7.

244. Crowe JE Jr. Respiratory syncytial virus vaccine development. Vaccine 2001;20(suppl):S32–7.

245. Groothius JR, Simoes EA, Hemming VG. Respiratory syncytial virus (RSV) infection in preterm infants and the protective effects of RSV immune globulin (RSVIG). Pediatrics 1995;95:463–7.

246. The Impact-RSV Study Group. Palivizumab, a humanized respiratory syncytial virus monoclonal antibody, reduces hospitalization from respiratory syncytial virus infection in high-risk infants. Pediatrics 1998;102:531–7.

246a. Feltes TF, Cabalka AK, Meissner HC, et al. Palivizumab prophylaxis reduces hospitalization due to respiratory syncytial virus in young children with hemodynamically significant congenital heart disease. J Pediatr 2003;143: 523–40.

247. Committee on Infectious Diseases. Prevention of respiratory syncytial virus infections: indications for the use of palivizumab and update on the use of RSV-IVIG. Pediatrics 1998;102:1211–6.

248. Horn MEC, Brain EA, Gregg I, et al. Respiratory viral infection and wheezy bronchitis in childhood. Thorax 1979;34:23–8.

249. Carlsten KH, Ørstavik I, Leegard J, et al. Respiratory virus infections and aeroallergens in acute bronchial asthma. Arch Dis Child 1984;59:310–5.

250. Rachelefsky GS, Goldberg M, Katz RM, et al. Sinus disease in children with respiratory allergy. J Allergy Clin Immunol 1987;80:268–73.

251. Kovatch AL, Wald ER, Ledesma-Medina J, et al. Maxillary sinus radiographs in children with nonrespiratory complaints. Pediatrics 1984;73:306–8.

252. Campanella SG, Asher MI. Current controversies: sinus disease and the lower airways. Pediatr Pulmonol 2001; 31:165–72.

253. Dowell SF, Bresee JS. Severe varicella associated with steroid use. Pediatrics 1993;92:223–8.

254. Abernathy-Carver KJ, Fan LL, Boguniewicz M, et al. *Legionella* and *Pneumocystis* pneumonias in asthmatic children on high doses of systemic steroids. Pediatr Pulmonol 1994; 18:135–8.

255. Grant CC, Duggan AK, Santosham M, DeAngelis C. Oral prednisone as a risk factor for infections in children with asthma. Arch Pediatr Adolesc Med 1996;150:58–63.

CHAPTER 8

Pneumonia Syndromes

■ GENERAL CONCEPTS AND METHODS

Pneumonia should be suspected when there is a history of cough, fever, and difficult or rapid breathing. Physical findings such as inspiratory crackles, decreased breath sounds, dullness to percussion, or grunting or painful breathing usually are reliable enough to be taken as presumptive evidence of pneumonia—physical examination of the chest is discussed further in Chapter 7. In general, the signs and symptoms that have a high degree of sensitivity (e.g., fever and tachypnea) lack specificity, while those that have a high degree of specificity (e.g., rales and pleuritic pain) lack sensitivity.[1]

Thus, if pneumonia is suspected, a chest x-ray should usually be obtained; the radiologic findings are usually regarded as definitive for confirmation of the presence and location of pneumonia, and they provide some assistance in distinguishing the probable cause.

The term *pneumonitis* literally means inflammation of the lungs; sometimes it is used interchangeably with pneumonia, and sometimes it is used to mean minimal pneumonia. The phrase *pulmonary infiltrate* is more precise and problem-oriented than *pneumonia* and may be used when the clinician suspects a noninfectious process. A recent review defines pneumonia in children as the presence of fever, acute respiratory symptoms, or both, plus evidence of parenchymal infiltrates on chest radiography.[1]

The most frequent etiologies for acute pneumonias discussed in this chapter are listed in Table 8-1.

Classification

The historic classification of pneumonias in the 1920s used the terms "typical" for classic pneumococcal pneumonia and "atypical" for almost all other pneumonias. When chest radiology became easily available in the 1930s, "silent pneumonia" and "walking pneumonia" were recognized, particularly during screening of military recruits. "Walking pneumonia" is now largely a lay term.

Pneumonias are now best classified as specific syndromes, using several variables:

1. *Onset and course*: Pneumonia can be acute or chronic, progressive or improving, recurrent or a first episode.
2. *Severity*: Pneumonia can be classified on the basis of severity, as estimated by clinical observations or by quantitation of respiratory acidosis and hypoxemia.
3. *Anatomic pattern*: Pneumonia can be classified as lobar, multilobar, segmental, subsegmental, lobular, interstitial, perihilar, nodular, or miliary. Combinations of these forms are also possible.
4. *Additional anatomic features*: Pleural thickening or effusion, cavitation, pneumatoceles, or pneumothorax may be present.
5. *Extrapulmonary features*: Eosinophilia in the peripheral blood smear and underlying chronic disease may be present. Pneumonia complicating cystic fibrosis or malignancy is discussed in Chapter 22.
6. *Etiology*: Most pneumonias in children are caused by infectious agents: viruses, bacteria (including mycobacteria), mycoplasmas, fungi, and protozoans. Etiologic diagnoses are not as easy to determine or as accurate as is sometimes implied, and proof of the etiology is not obtained in most cases.

To make a therapeutic decision in children, radiologic findings of the chest alone are not sufficient or accurate enough to distinguish a viral from a bacterial etiology.[2] However, the age of the child is a very important factor in selecting antibiotic therapy. The additional pulmonary features are also helpful, as confirmed viral pneumonias are rarely lobar, although they may be sublobular, and almost never produce hilar adenopathy, effusion, pneumothorax, pneumatoceles, or cavitation.[3]

It is helpful to give an accurate description for

TABLE 8-1. MOST FREQUENT ETIOLOGIES OF ACUTE PNEUMONIA SYNDROMES

PNEUMONIA SYNDROMES	MOST FREQUENT ETIOLOGIES
Lobar, segmental, spherical pneumonia or pneumonia with effusion	*Streptococcus pneumoniae*, Group A streptococcus, *Staphylococcus aureus*, *Haemophilus influenzae*
Bilateral interstitial pneumonia or mild subacute pneumonia with minimal infiltrates	*Mycoplasma pneumoniae*, *Chlamydia pneumoniae*, adenovirus (school-age), respiratory syncytial virus (infants), other viruses
Cold-agglutinin-positive pneumonia	*M. pneumoniae* or adenovirus
Fulminating pneumonia	Influenza virus, *S. pneumoniae*, Group A streptococcus, *S. aureus*, *M. pneumoniae*, cytomegalovirus, varicella (immunosuppressed child)
Pulmonary infiltrates with eosinophilia (PIE)	Unknown, *C. pneumoniae*, aspergillus
Miliary pneumonia	Tuberculosis, unidentified
Nodular pneumonia	Disseminated bacteremias (usually *S. aureus*), disseminated fungemias
Pneumonia complicating cystic fibrosis	*S. aureus*, *H. influenzae*, *Pseudomonas aeruginosa*, *Burkholderia cepacia*
Immunosuppressed state or malignancy	*S. aureus*, *P. aeruginosa*, *Pneumocystis jiroveci*, *Aspergillus*, other mycoses, *Mycobacterium tuberculosis*, other mycobacteria, cytomegalovirus, other viruses

the primary diagnosis or statement of the problem. The etiologic diagnosis should usually be expressed as a probability, along with a statement of other reasonable possibilities. Examples of such preliminary clinical diagnoses include:

- Acute lobar pneumonia; probably pneumococcal, possibly *Haemophilus influenzae.*
- Severe bilateral interstitial pneumonia; probably caused by influenza virus.
- Recurrent right middle-lobe pneumonia; probably pneumococcal; consider partial bronchial obstruction.
- Persistent right peripheral pneumonia with hilar adenopathy; probably tuberculous.
- Bilateral interstitial pneumonia complicating acute leukemia; consider cytomegalovirus.

The remainder of this section discusses the general principles involved in obtaining microbiologic specimens in pneumonias and the frequency of various etiologic agents. Subsequent sections discuss the various syndromes, such as lobar pneumonia, and the etiologic agents most commonly associated

with each. The physiologic principles involved in pneumonia, including respiratory insufficiency, are discussed in Chapter 7.

Etiologic Sources

Attempts to obtain a definitive etiologic diagnosis in pneumonia involve the use of culture, histology (smear or biopsy), skin tests, or serology. The significance of culture results in pneumonia depends on the source of the culture and the probability of finding the infectious agent from that source in normal individuals. One way to classify organisms is whether they may sometimes colonize the respiratory tract in the absence of disease. For organisms that do not colonize the respiratory tract, their isolation can be considered diagnostic of infection, regardless of the clinical setting (Box 8-1).

While considering such procedures as lung puncture or flexible bronchoscopy, the physician must weigh the balance between the likely value of the procedure and the risk to the patient.[4] In most clinical situations, a conclusive etiologic diagnosis

---

BOX 8-1 ■ Classification of Pathogens Based on Whether Isolation of the Organism from the Respiratory Tract is generally Diagnostic of Infection

Diagnostic	Nondiagnostic
Bacteria	
Mycobacterium tuberculosis	Nontuberculous
Legionella pneumophila	mycobacteria
Francisella tularensis	All other bacteria
Bordetella pertussis	
Nocardia spp.	
Mycoplasma spp.	
Viruses	
Influenza	All other viruses
Parainfluenza	
Respiratory syncytial virus	
Hantavirus	
Measles	
Enterovirus	
Adenovirus	
Fungi	
Histoplasma capsulatum	Candida species
Blastomyces dermatiditis	Aspergillus species
Coccidioides immitis	
Cryptococcus neoformans	
Pneumocystis jiroreci (carinii)	
Parasites	
Toxoplasma gondii	All others
Strongyloides stercoralis	

---

by a definitive procedure is not essential for optimal treatment and thus may entail an unnecessary risk to the patient. However, in immunocompromised children, invasive techniques such as lung biopsy may be indicated. Prospective randomized studies of risks and benefits have not been done even in adults.[4]

Conclusive Culture Sources

Cultures of blood, pleural fluid, material obtained by lung puncture, or lung biopsy specimens are usually considered conclusive.

Occasionally, one encounters statements about pneumonia that are not substantiated by any accurate data and in fact are examples of reverse logic. For example, the statement that 20% of patients with pneumococcal pneumonia have pneumococcal bacteremia requires some conclusive evidence that the other 80% without bacteremia had pneu-

mococcal pneumonia. Such statistics are usually not supported by any conclusive tests such as lung puncture. However, it can be accurate to say that 20% of a group of patients with lobar pneumonia had pneumococcal bacteremia.

Occasionally Significant Culture Sources

Material obtained from flexible fiberoptic bronchoscopy,[5,6] tracheostomy secretions,[7] rigid bronchoscopy aspiration, and transtracheal aspirations may occasionally be useful in identifying the etiologic agent. Transtracheal aspiration, although used in adults, has rarely been used in children because of their small, growing tracheas. In one study of children, the correlation between the types of bacteria recovered from transtracheal aspiration and those recovered from lung puncture was only fair.[8] Reported complications include transient hemoptysis, mediastinal or subcutaneous emphysema, and cardiac arrest, perhaps secondary to anoxia, vagal reflex, or vomiting with aspiration.[9]

Cultures of Dubious Significance

Direct orotracheal aspirates sometimes are useful in newborns with pneumonia.[10] Sputum culture is usually not useful, as children seldom produce sputum before about 6 years of age. After this age, specimen collection can sometimes be facilitated by techniques to induce sputum production, such as nebulized hypertonic saline. Occasionally, younger children do cough up and spit out tracheal secretions, especially if they have chronic pulmonary disease. However, sputum is an unreliable source for culture in children with acute pneumonia, because more than one potential pathogen can often be found even in normal individuals. In chronic pneumonias, even a 2-year-old may cough up purulent sputum, which may reveal budding yeasts (Fig. 8-1) or bacterial pathogens (as in cystic fibrosis).

Cultures of endotracheal tube secretions in patients on mechanical ventilators are similarly fraught with interpretational difficulties. One study suggests that endotracheal tube aspirates with negative Gram stains or with greater than 10 squamous epithelial cells per low-power field should be rejected.[11] Obtaining surveillance cultures from endotracheal tubes of all patients on mechanical ventilation does not predict the etiology of subsequent invasive disease.[12] Other than for epidemiologic purposes, this practice should be abandoned.

Nose or nasopharyngeal cultures usually yield a

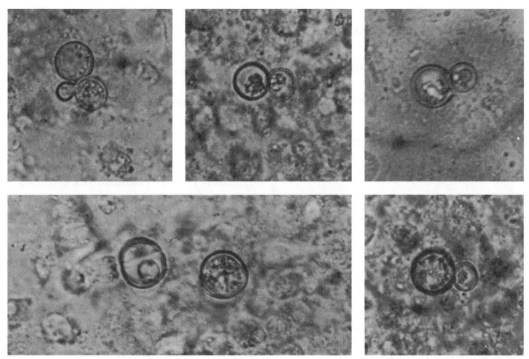

■ FIGURE 8-1 Blastomycosis. Yeast forms, including budding yeasts in unstained sputum, from a two-year-old child. *Cryptococcus* yeast forms have a very similar appearance in urine.

high frequency of potential pathogens and are not useful in diagnosing bacterial pneumonia. They may occasionally be useful if a viral pathogen, such as respiratory syncytial virus (RSV) or influenza, is suspected. Throat cultures are not useful in the etiologic diagnosis of pneumonia.

Gram Stain

A Gram stain of clinical material is often helpful. When the stain is done on material from a moderately significant culture source, it may help guide empiric therapy. The results of Gram staining may also aid interpretation of cultures obtained from sites that are often contaminated, such as the endotracheal tube, which may be cultured when ventilator-associated pneumonia is suspected. Endotracheal tubes are nearly always colonized with flora common to the intensive care unit, and therefore cultures are usually positive. If the Gram stain shows many neutrophils and a single bacterial morphology, the cultured organism is more likely to be a pathogen than if the Gram stain shows few white cells and mixed flora.

Detection of Antigens

Assaying sputum, pleural fluid, or serum for antigens is neither useful nor approved for the diagnosis of pneumonia. In 1999, the Food and Drug Administration (FDA) approved a rapid assay for the detection of pneumococcal antigen in the urine. However, this assay lacks specificity in children and is not recommended for use in that population.[13]

Bronchoalveolar Lavage

Bronchoalveolar lavage (BAL) often is a useful procedure in immunocompromised hosts with pulmonary infiltrates. In non-neutropenic patients with diffuse pulmonary infiltrates, the sensitivity of BAL is 80–90% and is highest in detecting *Pneumocystis jiroveci* (formerly *carinii*) pneumonia (PCP) in patients with human immunodeficiency virus (HIV) infection.[14] It is somewhat less sensitive in neutropenic cancer patients, and thus a negative result cannot rule out the possibility of an infectious cause of the infiltrates. For any patient population, the diagnostic yield in the case of focal infiltrates is relatively low.

Normal BAL cell counts in children have been published and are summarized in Box 8-2.[15]

Biopsy of the Lung or Pleura

Lung biopsy may be done thoracoscopically, by thoracotomy (open biopsy), or by needle. Open

---

BOX 8-2 ■ Normal Range of Bronchoalveolar Lavage Differential Cell Counts in Children*

WBC	7×10^4/mL to 50×10^4/mL
Macrophages	84–93%
Lymphocytes	7–13%
Neutrophils	1–4%
Eosinophils	0–0.2%

* Values are the approximate range of median values from five studies.

---

lung biopsy is most useful for the diagnosis of tuberculosis (TB) or of opportunistic microorganisms such as *Pneumocystis* in an immunocompromised host[16] or in chronic pneumonias (described later). It can be done using a limited thoracotomy (i.e., no rib resection).[17] A small pilot study in 13 immunocompromised patients with pneumonia showed that open lung biopsy yielded superior diagnostic information compared with BAL 5 of the patients had diagnoses established by open lung biopsy only.[18] However, we have occasionally seen patients in which the reverse was true (i.e., diagnosis was made by BAL with a negative lung biopsy).

Transbronchial lung biopsy using a flexible fiberoptic bronchoscope has been useful in distinguishing tumor from opportunistic infection in adults.[19] The use of this technique in children is limited because of an increased risk of bleeding and pneumothorax compared with adults.[14] In addition, transbronchial biopsy is contraindicated in patients receiving mechanical ventilation because of the risk of tension pneumothorax.[20]

Percutaneous needle biopsy under fluoroscopic guidance for histologic diagnosis is sometimes done in adults,[21] especially when malignancy is a consideration, but it is rarely done in children. Pleural biopsy is discussed in the section on pneumonia with effusion.

Thoracoscopy

Thorascopy has been used in children to rule out PCP, usually using sedation and local anesthesia.[22] It is also useful in evaluating intrathoracic tumors but is sometimes complicated by pneumothorax or bleeding. Its primary role is in decortication of loculated empyema and is discussed in the section on pneumonia with effusion.

Computed Tomography and Ultrasound

The use of computed tomography (CT) and ultrasound procedures is discussed in the sections on the syndromes where they are helpful. For example, ultrasound is most useful in detecting pleural effusion and in guiding thoracentesis. CT scanning is certainly more sensitive than plain chest films in picking up pleural effusions;[23] typically, however, any effusion small enough to be detected only by CT scanning is probably too small to be clinically significant. CT scanning also improves visualization of abscesses, and affords the clinician a better view of the mediastinum and its structures.[24]

Serum Antibodies

Serologic diagnosis is usually retrospective, except for cold agglutinins, which usually appear after one week of illness, often at about the time the patient seeks medical attention. Testing of paired sera is most useful for the diagnosis of *Chlamydia pneumoniae*, *Mycoplasma pneumoniae*, Q fever, and psittacosis. Serologic methods can be used for the detection of respiratory syncytial virus (RSV), influenza virus, parainfluenza virus, and adenovirus infection, but rapid antigen testing or viral culture methods are preferable.

Skin Tests

The intermediate-strength tuberculin test is very useful for the diagnosis of tuberculous pneumonia. However, serologic tests are better than skin tests for the diagnosis of current pneumonia caused by *Histoplasma* or *Coccidioides* species. Furthermore, skin tests for fungi may boost the antibody titer, resulting in a misleading rise.

■ ACUTE FOCAL PNEUMONIA

Acute lobar or segmental pneumonia is usually pneumococcal in all groups beyond the newborn period. It was once called typical pneumonia, in contrast to atypical pneumonia.

The following characteristics can be considered typical: *significant fever* above 102°F (38.8°C) is usually present; *chills* often are noted in older children and adults; and often, there is a *toxic appearance,* defined as appearing acutely ill, anxious, and distressed. Also, *definite chest signs* are usually present and lateralized including *consolidation,* which is defined by dullness to percussion, decreased breath sounds, increased fremitus (vibration felt on palpation of the chest wall, produced by the spoken voice), and, sometimes, bronchophony (increased intensity and clarity of voice sounds heard over a bronchus surrounded by consolidated lung tissue). *Fine end-inspiratory rales* are often present. *Rhonchi* are often described, which may be loud enough to make the end-inspiratory rales difficult to discern. *Pleuritic pain* or *splinting* may be noted.

The pain in lower-lobe pneumonia is sometimes mistaken for abdominal pain or is referred to the abdomen. The patient may be unwilling to breathe deeply to aid auscultation. Shallow breathing (splinting) and a rapid breathing rate are sometimes the only definite signs suggesting that the illness involves the chest. Grunting may be noted in infants or young children. Older children may fail to breathe deeply when asked to do so or complain of pain and cough when they do. On occasion, children with a round (spherical) pneumonia due to *S. pneumoniae* will present with fever only.

Pleurisy is often used as a lay term or older medical term for pleuritis or pleural pain. *Pleurodynia* refers to chest pain that is usually pleuritic but without pneumonia or pleural effusion and is characteristically caused by coxsackie B virus infection.[25]

In typical pneumonia, the chest roentgenogram shows a *dense infiltrate.* It may appear segmental or lobar or even spherical[26] (Fig. 8-2) but typically does not have multiple fluffy areas or bilateral thin linear infiltrates. Response to antibiotic therapy is often (but not always) dramatic, with the temperature falling from 104°F (40°C) to 98°F (36.7°C) after the first dose and remaining normal.

Possible Causes

The best evidence for the frequency of various causes of lobar pneumonia is that based on lung puncture or blood culture studies.

Streptococcus pneumoniae

The pneumococcus is almost always the cause of classic typical pneumonia as described earlier. However, the pneumococcus can also produce other forms of pneumonia, such as pneumonia that fails to respond promptly to antibiotics, pneumonia with effusion, and even interstitial pneumonia.[27] A retrospective review of 85 children between the ages of 5 months and 16 years with bacteremic pneumococcal pneumonia found that 70% of children had the "typical" illness described before, with high fever, leukocytosis (white blood cell [WBC] greater than 15,000/mcL), and lobar or segmental consolidation on chest x-ray.[28] Interestingly, however, one-fourth of the patients presented without any respiratory symptoms. Thirty-eight percent of patients had gastrointestinal tract symptomatology, but only 5 (6%) of the 85 children had gastrointestinal symptoms in the absence of respiratory symptoms.

Routine use of the conjugated heptavalent pneu-

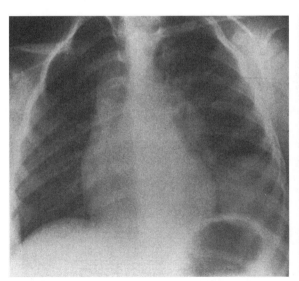
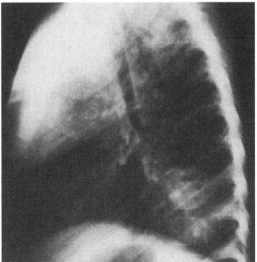

■ **FIGURE 8-2** Spherical pneumonia in the left lower lobe of a 4-year-old child. No special evaluation is necessary in this variation of a focal pneumonia, which responds to antibiotic therapy (Roentgenogram courtesy of Dr. Richard Logan).

mococcal vaccine will decrease the incidence of pneumococcal pneumonia, but it will not eliminate it. In a large, randomized controlled trial, the incidence of radiographically-confirmed pneumonia among vaccinees was decreased by 35%.[29]

H. influenzae Type B

The prevalence of *H. influenzae* type b (Hib) as a cause of pneumonia in children has greatly decreased because of widespread use of conjugated Hib vaccine. It is still a possible cause of lobar or segmental pneumonia in the unvaccinated child and is frequently accompanied by pleural effusion.[30,31] The onset is usually gradual but can be acute. Otitis media is frequent.[30] Purulent conjunctivitis is occasionally present. Hib can produce lobar or segmental pneumonia in older children and adults. The response to amoxicillin in recognized cases is typically poor. *H. influenzae* non-type b is also an occasional cause of pneumonia, especially in children younger than 10 years.

Uncommon Causes

Staphylococcus aureus is an uncommon cause of lobar pneumonia (see Box 8-3).[32] It should be considered in young or debilitated infants or when there is effusion or pneumatoceles, as discussed in a later section.

Group A streptococcal pneumonia often is associated with pleuritic pain and marked leukocytosis.[33] Often the organism cannot be recovered from the throat culture. A scarlatiniform rash may be present. Empyema and pneumatoceles occasionally occur, and *S. aureus* infection may be suspected. Group A streptococcal pneumonia tends to occur following a viral infection (especially varicella) and to have a fairly severe and protracted course.[34] In stark contrast to pneumonia caused by the pneumococcus, fever in Group A streptococcal pneumonia persists for days to weeks even in the face of appropriate antimicrobial therapy. Pneumonia caused by toxin-producing strains of *S. aureus* or Group A streptococcus may result in toxic shock syndrome (see Chapter 11).

Mycoplasma pneumoniae has to be considered as a possible cause of lobar pneumonia.[35] It is discussed further in the section on atypical pneumonia syndromes.

Primary pulmonary TB occasionally causes an acute lobar pneumonia, and in such a case, the tuberculin test is almost always positive at the time the pneumonia occurs.[36] All children with acute lobar pneumonia that is poorly responsive to empiric antibacterial therapy should have a tuberculin skin test placed. Tuberculosis also can be the basis for a segmental bacterial pneumonia, particularly in the right middle lobe, or for obstruction of a major bronchus by a lymph node. *Histoplasma* or other systemic fungi also can do this and should be considered in endemic areas.

The right middle-lobe syndrome and other recurrent or chronic lobar pneumonias are discussed later in this chapter.

Klebsiella pneumoniae is rarely documented as a cause of pneumonia in children by blood culture or lung puncture except in association with neonatal sepsis, nosocomial infection, or in immunocompromised hosts.

Meningococcal pneumonia without meningitis has been documented by blood cultures but is uncommon in children.[37] It may be more frequent in military populations 16–30 years of age and may follow influenza or adenovirus pneumonia. Serogroup Y is more likely to be associated with pneumonia than are the other serotypes. Septic shock may occur, but the typical purpuric rash may be absent.

Francisella tularensis is also a possible cause of acute focal pneumonia.[38] Most cases of tularemia follow the bite of a tick or a deerfly, and cause a systemic disease plus local inflammation at the site of the bite. The pneumonic form of tularemia usually occurs after inhalation of airborne organisms.

BOX 8-3 ■ Causes of Acute Focal Pneumonia

Usual
Streptococcus pneumoniae

Uncommon
H. influenzae type b (< 5 years old)
Nontypable H. influenzae
S. aureus
Group A streptococcus
Mycoplasma pneumoniae
Chlamydia pneumoniae

Rare
Francisella tularensis
Mycobacterium tuberculosis
Respiratory viruses (usually lobular): RSV,
    parainfluenza, adenovirus
Meningococcus
Enteric bacteria

Typically in these cases, there is an interesting exposure history; for example, beating a dead infected rabbit with sticks can be a cause of aerosolization. Pleuropulmonary involvement also occurs in typhoidal tularemia, which in children is sometimes acquired by ingestion of the agent.[39] Enteric bacteria such as *E. coli, Enterobacter,* and *Pseudomonas aeruginosa* are extremely rare causes of pneumonia unless there is an underlying disease or nosocomial acquisition in an intensive care unit.

Psittacosis with a lobar segmental pneumonia may present with an acute onset of chills and high fever. Patients with psittacosis usually do not have a leukocytosis.

Treatment

Antibiotic Therapy of Presumed Pneumococcal Pneumonia

Due to the ever-increasing numbers of penicillin-resistant pneumococci, therapy with ceftriaxone or cefotaxime should be instituted for an acute lobar pneumonia presumed to be due to the pneumococcus and requiring intravenous therapy (Table 8-2). If one is fortunate enough to isolate the organism from the blood, a pleural effusion, or another reliable sample (discussed earlier), sensitivity testing should be done, and therapy switched to penicillin for sensitive strains. For patients requiring intravenous therapy, administering penicillin by continuous infusion is an effective and cost-effective approach. The dose is generally 150,000–250,000 units/kg/day (with a maximum of 24 million units per day).[40] This provides constant serum levels that easily exceed the minimum inhibitory concentration (MIC) for all but highly penicillin resistant strains.[41] The outcome in patients with pneumococcal pneumonia is similar whether the organism is sensitive or resistant to penicillin.[42]

It is important to remember that resistance is relative and can often be overcome by higher doses of antibiotics. Success also depends on the ability of the antibiotic to achieve therapeutic levels at the site of infection (e.g., lung tissue or meninges). Confusion is compounded when some reports refer to both highly-resistant strains and intermediately-resistant strains as nonsusceptible, when in reality infections with intermediately-resistant strains are often easily treated by higher doses of penicillin or other beta-lactam antibiotics. The recent interpretive standards published by the National Committee for Clinical Laboratory Standards (NCCLS) address this issue by citing different MIC cutoffs depending on whether the isolate is from cerebro-

TABLE 8-2. INITIAL THERAPY OF PNEUMONIA

	TREATMENT		
AGE	OUTPATIENT	HOSPITALIZED	PRINCIPAL PATHOGENS
0–4 weeks	–	Ampicillin and gentamicin (+/– cefotaxime)	Group B streptococcus (++) Enteric gram negative bacilli (+)
1–5 months	Amoxicillin (or amoxicillin-clavulanate)	Cefotaxime*	Pneumococcus (++); viruses (++); S. aureus (+)
6 months–6 years	Amoxicillin (or amoxicillin-clavulanate)	Cefotaxime* +/– macrolide †	Pneumococcus (++); viruses (++); S. aureus (+); Group A streptococcus (+); Mycoplasma (+)
>6 years	Macrolide † (+/– amoxicillin)	Cefotaxime* and macrolide †	Mycoplasma (++); pneumococcus (+); S. aureus (+); Group A streptococcus (+); Chlamydia (+)
Immuno-compromised	–	Ceftazidime ‡ and vancomycin +/– macrolid +	Many

+ occasional cause; ++ common cause
* Or ceftriaxone or cefuroxime
† Erythromycin, azithromycin, or clarithromycin
‡ Or cefepime

TABLE 8-3. INTERPRETIVE STANDARDS FOR *S. PNEUMONIAE*

	SUSCEPTIBLE	INTERMEDIATE	RESISTANT
Penicillin	≤ 0.06	0.12–1	≥ 2
Amoxicillin or Amoxicillin-clavulanic acid	≤ 2	4	≥ 8
Cefotaxime or ceftriaxone (meningitis)	≤ 0.5	1	≥ 4
Cefotaxime or ceftriaxone (nonmeningitis)	≤ 1	2	≥ 4

spinal fluid (CSF) or some other source (see Table 8-3).[43] In general, it is rarely necessary to add vancomycin for therapy of pneumococcal pneumonia. Poor response to therapy is more likely due to inadequate drainage of an empyema. In contrast, as discussed in Chapter 9, the addition of vancomycin is advocated for meningitis caused by strains that are intermediate or resistant to cephalosporins.

One study of 26 children with culture proven pneumococcal pneumonia and complicated parapneumonic effusions found that children with penicillin-resistant isolates were younger than those with susceptible organisms. Bacteremia was also more common.[44]

Patients with presumed pneumococcal pneumonia who are well enough to be managed as outpatients can be given high-dose amoxicillin (80 mg/kg/day) or cefuroxime axetil, with close follow-up. Tetracycline should not be used for treatment of presumed pneumococcal pneumonia. Macrolides have relatively poor anti-pneumococcal activity as well. Fluoroquinolones are commonly used for community-acquired pneumonia in adults and adolescents. A report suggests that recent exposure to a fluoroquinolone antibiotic increases the risk of fluoroquinolone resistance and treatment failure of pneumococcal pneumonia.[45]

Patients who have a late diagnosis, who are seriously ill, or who have underlying disease should not be treated as outpatients.

Treatment of Young Children

Moderately ill children of preschool age should be admitted and treated with a parenteral antibiotic effective against both *S. pneumoniae* and beta-lactamase producing strains of *H. influenzae*. The third-generation cephalosporins are stable against these beta-lactamases and are therefore a good choice.

Supportive Therapy

Oxygen, bed rest, positioning, and other supportive therapies are discussed later. Chest physiotherapy is at best useless for the treatment of acute pneumonia in adults.[46,47]

Complications

Persistent Pneumonia

Persistent pneumonia is defined by persistence of consolidation on chest roentgenogram for more than 1 month. Pleural thickening, paralysis of the diaphragm, or atelectasis may explain some cases. Other causes of persistence of lobar or segmental densities are described in the section on chronic pneumonia.

Hemolytic-uremic Syndrome

Hemolytic-uremic syndrome (HUS) is an important, albeit uncommon, complication of pneumococcal pneumonia. Although occurring via a different mechanism, it presents similarly to other forms of HUS, with anemia, thrombocytopenia, and acute renal failure. Neuraminidase produced by *S. pneumoniae* removes N-acetylneuraminic acid from cell surface glycoproteins, exposing the T-antigen on red blood cells, platelets, and glomeruli. Immunoglobulin M (IgM) antibodies that are present in most human plasma react with the exposed T-antigen, resulting in hemolysis and damage to glomerular endothelial cells.[48]

Typically, cases occur in young children (1–2 years old) with severe or even fulminant pneumococcal pneumonia. Most patients have a positive direct Coomb's test.[49]

Because plasma products contain IgM antibodies that can activate the T-antigen, their use is contraindicated. In addition, if transfusions are necessary, the red blood cells should be washed to reduce the amount of IgM present.[50]

Poor Response to Antibiotic Therapy

This occasionally occurs in uncomplicated pneumococcal pneumonia. Patients with low white blood cell counts and multilobar involvement have the highest mortality rate. Poor clinical response may also occur in patients infected with highly penicillin-resistant strains of the pneumococcus. Occasionally, patients with pneumonia severe enough to require mechanical ventilation will have an initial response to therapy but then develop recrudescent fever. Such patients are often found to have secondary nosocomial pneumonia with a different organism (usually a gram negative).

Rare but serious complications include pericarditis, meningitis, endocarditis, arthritis, and peritonitis. Pleural effusion and empyema are described in the following section and should always be considered when there is failure of a lobar pneumonia to respond to adequate therapy (Fig. 8-3).

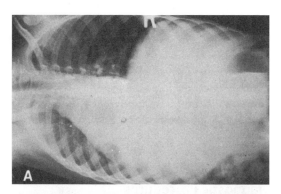

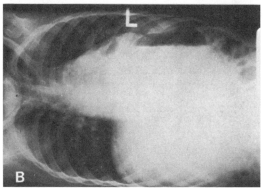

■ **FIGURE 8-3** Lateral decubitus position to show pleural effusion. **(A)** Right side up; **(B)** left side up. Left pleural effusion is best seen as a density in view A. Cavity can be seen behind heart on left side.

Effect on Lung Function in Adulthood

This question of the effect on lung function in adulthood was addressed by a prospective cohort study of 1392 British children followed from their births in 1958. Of these, 193 children had a history of pneumonia by the age of 7 years. At 35 years of age, pulmonary function testing was performed in all subjects. A history of pneumonia was associated with a small but significant decrease in forced expiratory volume in 1 second (FEV_1) and forced vital capacity (FVC), even after controlling for a history of wheezing and multiple other confounding factors. The effect was no greater for the subjects who had pneumonia at younger than 2 years than for those who had pneumonia between ages 2 and 7. It remains unclear whether pneumonia causes the deficit in lung function or whether pneumonia is more common among children who have poorer lung function before the disease.[51]

Follow-Up Chest Radiograph

In one study of 70 children, about 20% had residual pulmonary infiltrates 3–4 weeks after an acute pneumonia, and all who returned for follow-up had cleared the infiltrate within 3 months.[52] It was concluded that routine follow-up chest films are not necessary for children unless there is persistent respiratory difficulty or failure to thrive.

■ ACUTE PNEUMONIA WITH EFFUSION OR PNEUMATOCELE

Definitions

Pleural effusions in children typically accompany pneumonia, although they may be a result of noninfectious diseases. A pleural effusion in the setting of a known pneumonia is best referred to as a parapneumonic effusion.

Distinctions are traditionally made between effusions as exudates or transudates, which can be defined by the concentration of protein and lactic dehydrogenase (LDH). Exudates typically have a pleural fluid protein concentration greater than one-half that of the serum and usually also have an elevated LDH (greater than 200 units or greater than two-thirds of the upper limit of normal for serum LDH).[53] Other factors have also been used to classify an effusion as an exudate, such as glucose less than 40 mg/dl and pH less than 7.2.[54]

As a rule, children who have fluid in the chest

secondary to congestive heart failure, chronic renal failure, or low serum protein have these known predisposing causes, so that the finding of a transudate by analysis of the pleural fluid is not a surprise.

Empyema is traditional term for a thick purulent pleural effusion. An empyema may be simple, i.e., with free-flowing pus, or loculated. In addition, many exudates that are a result of an infectious disease in the chest at first appear straw-colored and serous and become thicker and cloudier over time. Whenever an entire hemi-thorax appears opaque, a large pleural effusion or hemothorax should be suspected.[55]

Radiographic Studies

Pleural effusion can be defined on a practical clinical basis as any fluid in the pleural space, as determined by thoracentesis. This definition should be distinguished from the radiologic criterion for a pleural effusion, because much more fluid (about 50 mL in children) is necessary to be visible on a chest film. Furthermore, demonstration of a pleural effusion by chest roentgenogram depends on proper positioning of the patient. A lateral decubitus or upright view is better than the supine view for demonstration of an effusion (Fig. 8-3).

A number of other imaging methods are useful to detect pleural fluid. Perhaps portable ultrasonic evaluation is the most convenient for detecting small amounts, which then can be tapped conveniently.[56] Ultrasound can also help differentiate effusion from consolidation.[57] Computed tomography is exceedingly useful in studying unusual pleural effusions detected by other methods, particularly in determining possible underlying disease.[58]

In adults, it usually takes approximately 200–500 mL of fluid to produce blunting of the costophrenic angle in an erect postero-anterior radiograph. This amount of fluid typically produces a noticeable increase in the density of the lower lung zone on the supine radiograph.[58] As the amount of effusion increases according to the upright film, the density in the supine radiograph also increases in stepwise fashion. The classic findings of increased density over the entire hemithorax with apical capping occurs only with a large pleural effusion (Fig. 8-4).[59] Another useful sign on the frontal film is the thorn sign, a thorn-like protrusion of fluid at the lateral end of the minor fissure.[60]

Fluid recovered by thoracentesis can be regarded as pleural fluid if it does not have the same hemato-

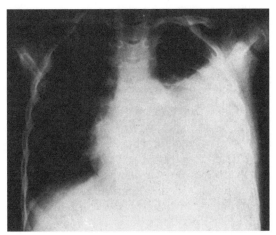

■ **FIGURE 8-4**   Empyema caused by *H. influenzae*. Note shift of trachea and right heart border to the right, suggesting fluid on the left. Pleural effusion should always be considered when there is opacification of the lower part of a hemithorax, especially if clinical response to therapy is poor.

crit as the patient's venous blood. The gross appearance of pleural fluid may be bloody (suggesting traumatic hemothorax or entry of the needle into a blood vessel), blood-tinged (often a result of slight bleeding from the procedure), cloudy and purulent (suggesting an exudate from an infectious process), or serous (suggesting a transudate). Patients who have had recent thoracic surgery may have a chylous effusion (milky-appearing) from disruption of the thoracic duct.

Even if the fluid obtained is not grossly purulent, it should be Gram-stained and cultured. A white cell count and differential study is useful. Measurement of protein content and LDH can be cancelled if the Gram stain shows bacteria.

Diagnostic Procedures

Several procedures may be of value in patients with suspected pleural effusions. Thoracentesis is the most common procedure if fluid is obviously present. Lung puncture is a closely related procedure, since attempts at lung puncture often yield unsuspected pleural fluid. Needle biopsy of the pleura is rarely done in children.

When pleural fluid is suspected, or even if the problem is distinguishing lung abscess or pneumonia from pleural effusion, thoracentesis should be done promptly (see Box 8-4).

Thoracentesis

Whenever there is radiologic evidence of pleural fluid in a patient with pneumonia, some of the fluid

---

BOX 8-4 ■ Management of Parapneumonic Effusions in Children

1. Suspect effusions when there is cough, dyspnea, and flatness to percussion in a lower lobe. Other findings include a decrease in tactile fremitus and the presence of egophony (upon auscultation the sound e is heard as an a).
2. Confirm with upright posteroanterior and lateral radiographs or ultrasound. "The sun should never set on a parapneumonic effusion." [63]
3. If density is in the pleural area but does not extend to the costovertebral angle, consider loculation.
4. Portable ultrasound scanning is useful to locate effusions and mark the place for the needle to be inserted.
5. Sedation is advisable.
6. Position patient sitting with spine straight (usually).
7. Anesthetize with 1–2% lidocaine and insert a 20-gauge needle on a 10-ml syringe or use Angiocath plastic tubing.
8. It is useful to *heparinize* the syringe and the sterile plastic container to avoid clotting of the fluid so tests can be done.
9. Use of a three-way stopcock is often helpful.
10. Avoid removing large volumes of fluid relative to the size of the child to avoid too-rapid reexpansion of the lung.
11. A postthoracentesis upright radiograph is advisable, as a small pneumothorax may be present.
12. Fluid should be sent for cell count, differential, Gram stain, and bacterial culture; if the illness has been over a week in duration, culture for fungi and tuberculosis also.
13. Unless the child has underlying disease that can cause transudates, such as heart disease or nephrotic syndrome, additional studies of the pleural fluid to distinguish a transudate are not needed.
14. When transudates such as that of congestive heart failure are considered a reasonable possibility, additional studies that might be helpful include pH, lactate dehydrogenase, and protein. Glucose and specific gravity usually do not add any new information, but confirm that the effusion is secondary to an infection as suspected.
15. In selected cases, rapidly centrifuging a specimen for cytology study for malignant cells might be appropriate.
16. Pleural effusions in children without chronic illness are almost always infectious exudates and not secondary to any of the long list of causes of effusions in adults.
17. Even when the pleural effusion is thin and straw colored, it is usually advisable to insert a chest tube for complete drainage; in infectious effusions, the fluid often becomes thicker and loculated and more difficult to drain if the chest tube is inserted later.
18. If the fluid is loculated, often thoracoscopy with lysis of adhesions or even open thoracotomy with decortication of the pleural rind is necessary.
19. In general, we are often slow to recognize an effusion, then delay the tap, then delay chest tube placement, and then leave the chest tube in too long.

---

should be removed for Gram stain and culture.[61] Thoracentesis is rarely associated with complications.[62] However, overly-rapid removal of large volumes may cause a sudden shift of the mediastinum with reflex changes in heart rate and, occasionally, cardiac arrest. Pneumothorax is rare.

The purpose of the procedure is to obtain enough fluid for diagnostic purposes, but occasionally respiratory excursions are improved by the removal of moderate volumes. Thoracentesis and exact bacteriologic diagnosis are especially needed in a severely ill patient. Even a small amount is useful for diagnostic study.

Fluid Studies

Thoracentesis is especially useful for culture of pus to determine the identity of the infecting organism so antibiotic therapy can be tailored. If the Gram stain is quickly available and reveals definite bacteria, the cell count, differential, protein measurement, glucose, and other studies add little. Both aerobic and anaerobic cultures should be ordered.

Rapid Antigen Testing

Type-specific antigens of pneumococci or *H. influenzae* can sometimes be detected in pleural fluid using various techniques, although these tests are unavailable in many centers and their sensitivity and specificity are unknown.

Intrapleural Fibrinolytic Therapy

Empyemas treated with closed chest tube drainage frequently loculate and then require a surgical procedure to remove the congealed pus. Several small trials have studied the idea of instilling fibrinolytic agents (such as urokinase) through the chest tube to prevent or even treat loculation.[64–66]

In children, only case series are reported.[67] In adults, this practice seems to be safe and to have a modest effect in shortening hospital stay and decreasing the need for surgical intervention. A systematic review concluded that because of the small size of these randomized trials there was insufficient evidence to support the routine use of intrapleural fibrinolytic therapy in the management of empyema.[68] A large, multicenter trial is currently underway.

Needle Biopsy of the Pleura

Percutaneous needle biopsy of the pleura is especially useful in the diagnosis of tuberculous pleurisy in adults. The procedure has also been used in children.[69]

Infectious Etiologies of Pleural Effusion

Sterile infectious effusions are relatively frequent. In a recent review of 76 cases of complicated parapneumonic effusions in children, 32 (42%) were sterile.[70] The most commonly identified agents were S. pneumoniae (31 patients), S. aureus (7 patients), and Group A streptococcus (5 patients). The proportion of cases caused by S. aureus increased from 6% in 1996–2000 to 30% in 2001. The more recent cases of S. aureus pneumonia were also more likely to be caused by methicillin-resistant strains.[70]

Thin Effusions

If the pleural fluid exudate is relatively clear, several etiologies are more likely (Box 8-5). Tuberculosis is a possibility if the fluid appears serous but the protein concentration is high. In tuberculous effusion, which reflects hypersensitivity, the tuberculin test is almost always positive.[71] Partially treated bacterial pneumonia with effusion is also a frequent cause of exudate that is not grossly purulent.

BOX 8-5 ■ Causes of Pneumonia with Effusion

Common
S. aureus
S. pneumoniae
Mycoplasma pneumoniae (small effusion)
Group B streptococci (newborn)
Sterile effusions (usually because of prior antibiotics)

Uncommon
Group A streptococci
Other streptococci
H. influenzae type b
Nontypable H. influenzae
Systemic fungi
Anaerobic enteric bacteria
Tuberculosis (adolescent)

Rare
F. tularensis
Pasteurella multocida
Atypical measles
Adenovirus (newborn)
Paragonimiasis (immigrant from Far East)
Aerobic enteric gram-negative rods
Hepatitis B
Hepatitis A
Yersinia, Listeria, Chlamydia
Cat scratch disease
Amebiasis
Dengue fever
Leptospirosis

Noninfectious
Congestive heart failure
Nephrotic syndrome
Cirrhosis (late complication of cystic fibrosis)
Vitamin A intoxication
Malignancy
Low serum protein diseases
Snake envenomation
Lymphatic abnormalities

Mycoplasma pneumoniae can cause small effusions in children.[72] In a study of young adults with mycoplasmal and viral pneumonia, small pleural effusions were found in about 20% of the 59 patients with serologic evidence of nonbacterial pneumonia.[73] Pleural effusions were seen in 6 (21%) of 29 patients with *Mycoplasma*, 1 (14%) of 7 with adenovirus, 1 (25%) of 4 with influenza virus pneumonia, and in 4 (21%) of 19 patients with elevated titers to cold agglutinins.[73] Another study of 56 patients with moderately severe disease from *M. pneumoniae* revealed that pleural effusions were detectable in 8 (14)%.[74] However, other studies have indicated that the frequency of pleural effusions in *Mycoplasma pneumoniae* in young adults is closer to 5%.[75]

Adenovirus, particularly type 7, can cause massive pleural effusions and disseminated disease, which may be fatal.[76] Epstein-Barr virus (EBV) is sometimes associated with a pleural effusion.[77] In infants and young children, the illness may not resemble infectious mononucleosis except for the presence of atypical lymphocytosis.[78] When a pleural effusion accompanies typical infectious mononucleosis in teenagers, a concurrent mycoplasmal pneumonia may be present.

A small pleural effusion can occur with viral hepatitis and may precede jaundice.[79] In an effusion secondary to hepatitis B, which is an immune-complex reaction, both blood and pleural fluid are positive for hepatitis B surface antigen, and serum transaminases are elevated even if jaundice has not yet appeared. Pleural effusion during the course of hepatitis A virus infection has been reported.[80] Cat scratch disease can produce a pleural effusion and anicteric hepatitis.[81] Leptospirosis can be associated with a pleural effusion; other features of the disease may lead to the correct diagnosis.[82] Yellow nail syndrome is an exceedingly rare lymphatic abnormality that may cause pleural, as well as pericardial, effusions.[83]

Purulent Effusions

Frankly purulent pleural fluid (empyema) is almost always caused by bacterial pneumonia. Before antibiotics were available, the pneumococcus or beta-hemolytic streptococci were the most common causes of empyema.[84 86] For a time thereafter, *Staphylococcus aureus* became the most common cause of empyema, but in recent years *S. pneumoniae* has again become prominent. The percentage of patients with pneumococcal pneumonia who have parapneumonic effusions is not as high as that seen with *S. aureus* (approximately 80% of children with *S. aureus* pneumonia have effusions);[32] but cases of pneumococcal pneumonia outnumber those of staphylococcal pneumonia by a large margin. In one series, 88% of culture-positive cases of parapneumonic effusion were due to *S. pneumoniae*.[87] A more recent study suggest that *S. aureus* may once again be surpassing the pneumococcus as a cause

of empyema.[88] As mentioned earlier, Group A streptococcus is an occasional cause. Rare causes include *F. tularensis*,[89] *H. influenzae* type b, and gram-negative enteric bacteria such as *Pseudomonas* or *Salmonella*.[90,91]

The viridans group of streptococci and diphtheroids (which are normal mouth flora) are rare causes of empyema associated with aspiration pneumonia, particularly in adults. *Pasteurella multocida* has caused empyema in a child with underlying pulmonary disease and exposure to animals.[92] *Nocardia* is a rare cause of pleural effusion, typically in compromised hosts. Other uncommon infectious causes of pleural effusions include *Yersinia*, *Chlamydia trachomatis*, and *Listeria*.[93–95]

Bacteroides or *Clostridium* species, anaerobic actinomyces, and anaerobic streptococci are occasional causes of empyema (particularly in adults), so that any fluid removed should be cultured anaerobically.[96,97] Blastomycosis, histoplasmosis, and coccidioidomycosis can be associated with thin to moderately purulent pleural effusions.[98–100] These fungi and cryptococci are special risks for immunosuppressed patients.[101–104] However, massive lung disease can sometimes occur in immunologically normal hosts who are exposed to a large inoculum of the fungus. Parasitic causes include paragonimiasis (in Far Eastern immigrants) and amebiasis.[105,106]

Noninfectious Causes

Noninfectious diseases also must be considered as possible causes of pleural exudates. Malignancy involving the pleura, especially lymphoma and neuroblastoma, sometimes produces effusions resembling those of tuberculosis. Rheumatoid disease, pancreatitis, and pulmonary infarction, which may occur in adults, are rare causes of thin exudates in children. Nitrofurantoin has been reported as a cause of allergic pneumonitis with effusion in adults. Trauma has been reported as a cause of effusion that may contain eosinophils.[107] Snake envenomation has been cited as a cause of pleural effusion.[108] Vitamin A intoxication is a rare cause in children.[109]

Intra-abdominal Abscess

Empyema is rarely the result of a perforated appendix.[110] Sometimes it is difficult to determine whether fluid is above or below the diaphragm if CT scanning is not readily available. Usually, it is better to do a thoracentesis and look for pleural fluid first, as removal of pleural fluid often results in the disappearance of radiologically apparent subdiaphragmatic fluid.

Pulmonary Embolism

Pulmonary embolism (PE) is uncommon in children, and when it occurs the diagnosis is usually delayed. The symptoms of tachypnea, chest pain, dyspnea, and fever are easily confused with pneumonia, which is usually the initial diagnosis. Most children with PE have one of several well-described risk factors, such as recent surgery, immobilization, malignancy, pregnancy, obesity, heart disease, the presence of a central venous catheter, oral contraceptive use, nephrotic syndrome, and sickle cell anemia.[111-114]

In children who develop PE without apparent risk factors, nearly all are found to have an antiphospholipid antibody or coagulation regulation protein abnormality (such as protein C or S deficiency).[115]

Tuberculous Pleural Effusions

Tuberculosis is much less common now in the United States than it used to be, and the relevant studies are now old. However, it remains common in the developing world, and physicians should consider the diagnosis in patients from endemic areas or with a suggestive exposure history. In one study of 202 children with tuberculous pleural effusion, published in 1958, the average duration of cough was 21 days. Difficulty breathing was noticed in only 25 (12%) of the children. The age range for pleural effusions indicated a rather even distribution between 1 and 13 years of age.[71] A newer report from Spain looked at 175 children with pulmonary tuberculosis; 22% of them had an effusion. On average, patients who had an effusion accompanying their pulmonary tuberculosis were older than those without effusion (13.5 vs. 7 years). In 41%, the effusion was the sole radiographic manifestation of pulmonary TB. Almost all of them had a tuberculin skin test (TST) greater than 5 mm.[116] Pleural effusions in TB are often accompanied by erythema nodosum. Sometimes, pleural effusions develop during chemotherapy for pulmonary tuberculosis.[117]

The most accurate way to confirm the diagnosis of a tuberculous effusion when it cannot be detected by examining the fluid for acid-fast bacilli is by pleural biopsy.[69] In the Spanish study, pleural fluid cultures were positive in 44%, biopsy cultures were positive in 67%, and the pleural biopsy yielded granulomatous changes in 78% of patients.[116] Pleural biopsy may not be necessary in a child with a suspected tuberculous effusion if the typical findings of pulmonary tuberculosis are present, especially if the organism can be cultured from another source, such as gastric aspirates.

Mycobacteria other than *Mycobacterium tuberculosis* can cause effusion, although this is most commonly associated with acquired immune deficiency syndrome (AIDS) in adults. Most often, the organism is of the *Mycobacterium avium* complex.[118]

Infectious Causes in the Newborn

In the newborn period, there are several causes of pneumonia associated with a pleural effusion. These include:

1. Group B streptococci[119]
2. Adenovirus with congenital pleural effusion[120]
3. *E. coli*[121]
4. Long-term ventilator therapy, especially with multiple courses of antibiotics; this can result in empyema caused by almost any of the nosocomial pathogens found in neonatal intensive care units.

Neonatal pneumonia and other pulmonary diseases in the newborn are discussed further in Chapter 19.

Pneumatoceles

Pneumatoceles occurring with empyema usually indicate staphylococcal pneumonia (Box 8-6).

BOX 8-6 ■ Causes of Pneumatoceles

Common
S. aureus

Rare
Group A streptococci
E. coli (newborn)
P. aeruginosa
B. cepacia (cystic fibrosis)
Pneumocystis jiroreci (carinii)
   (immunosuppressed)
Aspirated anaerobes
K. pneumoniae
H. influenzae

However, necrotizing pneumonia caused by other bacteria, including *H. influenzae, Pseudomonas,* and *Klebsiella,* can result in pneumatoceles.[122,123] Group A streptococci can produce pneumatoceles, and the throat culture may be negative for beta-hemolytic streptococci.[85] *E. coli* is an occasional cause of empyema, especially in the newborn period, and can produce pneumatoceles identical to those caused by staphylococci.[124] Rarely, septic emboli secondary to *Fusobacterium* infection produce pneumatoceles and may originate as exudative pharyngitis. Pneumatoceles can also occur with pneumococcal pneumonia, after hydrocarbon aspiration, and in *Pneumocystis* pneumonia.[84,125–127]

Chest Tubes

After thoracentesis has confirmed an empyema, a chest tube should be placed early so that the fluid can be removed thoroughly before it becomes too thick. The chest tube can be put into loculated fluid with guidance from ultrasound.

If it is a free-flowing effusion, as can be determined by lateral decubitus films (Fig. 8-3), the catheter can be put in a comfortable dependent location so that the patient can lie in comfort. Thoracoscopy can also be used for insertion of the chest tube.[128]

A large chest tube with continuous suction or straight drainage (no suction) should be inserted in all patients with anything more than small amounts of fluid. Small pigtail catheters drain transudates adequately, but should never be used in an attempt to drain parapneumonic effusions.[129] Decortication is rarely necessary if adequate chest tube drainage is used early.[130] The chest tube need not be inserted immediately if the fluid is serous, until the thoracentesis fluid has been analyzed. However, even if the fluid is thin, if it has the characteristics of an exudate, a chest tube should be put in, as the fluid may become more purulent except when tuberculosis is the cause.

The approach to loculated or thick and poorly draining pleural fluid is the subject of some debate. Studies show that early decortication reduces the duration of hospitalization and the length of illness.[88,131,132] However, others have reported that instillation of urokinase through an existing chest tube resulted in increased drainage and avoidance of surgery in 6 of 7[133] and in 8 of 9 [67] children with loculated pleural effusions. These authors recommend a trial of intrapleural urokinase instillation prior to surgical decortication. Clearly, much work remains to be done in defining the optimal approach to complicated pleural effusions in childhood.

Antibiotic Treatment

Antibiotic treatment should be directed at penicillin-resistant staphylococci and *S. pneumoniae* unless smear or culture indicates another organism. As a single agent, cefuroxime has reasonable activity against both *S. aureus* and the pneumococcus, although it is not the agent of choice for either organism. Thus, the combination of oxacillin (for superior *S. aureus* coverage) and cefotaxime (for superior *S. pneumoniae* coverage) is often used. In areas with a high incidence of community-acquired methicillin-resistant *S. aureus*, the use of vancomycin or clindamycin should be considered.[134] If the fluid has a fetid odor, the possibility of an anaerobic infection should be considered and clindamycin or metronidazole should be added.[54]

Complications

Pneumothorax may occur because of a bronchopleural fistula resulting from a break in a bronchial wall. Tension pneumothorax is suggested by a sudden increase in dyspnea and cyanosis. It may occur when the bronchial tear produces a valve-like effect, with entry of air into the pleural space on inspiration, and trapping of air by closure of the passage on expiration. This may produce collapse of the lung and a shift of the heart and mediastinum, especially in infants, who have a more movable mediastinum than do older children. Emergency release of the pressure should be done by insertion of a large needle and withdrawal of the free air until a chest tube can be inserted.

As with other severe infections, anemia is common in severe empyema of any cause; transfusion is only necessary if the child is symptomatic, which is uncommon.[135]

■ ATYPICAL PNEUMONIA SYNDROMES

Definitions

Criteria for the preliminary diagnosis of atypical pneumonia are the opposite of those for typical lobar pneumonia. The following features are usually regarded as atypical:

1. *Subacute onset.* The onset is gradual, with cough for several days before the patient seeks medical

attention. Toxicity is absent, and fever, if present, is low-grade.

2. *Prominent extrapulmonary features.* Headache, sore throat, and pharyngeal exudates may be present and are often more prominent than nonproductive cough or dyspnea.

3. *Minimal or disparate chest signs.* Rales may be bilateral or localized, but there is often a disparity between the auscultatory and radiologic findings. That is, the chest film often shows more extensive involvement than the clinician hears. On the other hand, sometimes the radiologic findings are minimal when the patient is cyanotic with a severe diffusion block.

4. *Chest infiltrate not focal.* The infiltrate is patchy or mottled, with various degrees of density, usually without a single dense area of consolidation.[136] There may be a wedge-shaped or linear infiltrate or a bilateral interstitial infiltrate.

5. *No clinical response to penicillins or cephalosporins.*

6. *No significant leukocytosis.*

7. *Slow course.* There is gradual improvement, sometimes with a long convalescence.

There are a number of other clinical patterns of pneumonias that are not typical of lobar pneumonia that can be excluded from the group of atypical pneumonia because of distinctive features. These pneumonias are discussed in other sections of this chapter: chronic or recurrent pneumonia, progressive or fulminating pneumonia, pneumonia with eosinophilia (Loeffler's syndrome), and miliary or multiple nodular pneumonia. Bronchiolitis with pneumonia and pertussis are discussed in Chapter 7.

Classification

It is useful to preserve the term atypical pneumonia as a broad preliminary clinical and radiologic diagnosis that can be subdivided into more specific problem-oriented diagnoses on the basis of certain features. Most patients with atypical pneumonia can be classified into one of the following subgroups or a combination of two of them. As noted earlier, most atypical pneumonias have a subacute onset.

Subacute Minimal Patchy Pneumonia

This subgroup is distinguished by a gradual onset over several days, usually with prominent extrapulmonary symptoms. The chest roentgenogram shows one or more patches of minimal foci of pneumonia. The most common causes are *Mycoplasma pneumoniae, Chlamydia pneumoniae,* and adenoviruses. Other causes are discussed in the following section on possible etiologies.

Subacute Dense Focal Pneumonia

This subgroup is distinguished by a subacute onset and an unexpectedly dense focal infiltrate that is segmental or smaller. Most of the other features of acute focal pneumonias (typical pneumonia), such as fever, toxicity, marked leukocytosis, and focal chest signs, are absent. Tuberculosis is an important consideration to exclude.

Acute Interstitial Pneumonia

This subgroup is distinguished by the absence of a solid focal or even minimal focal infiltrate. The infiltrate is sometimes described as reticular or patchy. There are many possible causes, most of which are viral and self-limited, but some of which are not viral or are progressive (Box 8-7).

Preliminary Diagnoses to Avoid

Mycoplasmal pneumonia should not be used as a preliminary diagnosis without proof of etiology, because many atypical pneumonias are not caused by *M. pneumoniae.* Furthermore, it is not possible to distinguish mycoplasmal pneumonia from other atypical types on clinical grounds.[138]

Nonbacterial pneumonia is a conclusion usually based on such observations as failure to respond to antimicrobial therapy, absence of leukocytosis, and sparse infiltrate. However, the term nonbacterial pneumonia should not be used, because it implies that bacterial causes have been excluded, when in fact this can rarely be done with certainty.

Possible Etiologies

The following etiologies are listed in approximate decreasing frequency of occurrence of the infectious agents within each microbiologic category.

Mycoplasmas

M. pneumoniae is probably the most frequent cause of atypical pneumonia, especially in school-age children and young adults.[139,140] Usually, the radiologic pattern is subacute with minimal densities, but occasionally it is an acute bilateral interstitial

BOX 8-7 ■ Possible Causes of Atypical
Pneumonia Patterns

Common
C. trachomatis (< 4 months)
RSV (< 5 years)
Mycoplasma pneumoniae (> 5 years)
Chlamydia pneumoniae (> 5 years)
Adenoviruses
Parainfluenza viruses
Influenza virus (in epidemics)
CMV; varicella-zoster virus (in
  immunosuppressed)
B. pertussis (usually not associated with
  pneumonia)

Uncommon
Hypersensitivity pneumonitis
Drug hypersensitivity
Herpes simplex virus
Pneumocystis jiroreci (carinii)
Chlamydia psittaci
H. influenzae
S. pneumoniae
Systemic fungi
Tuberculosis

Rare or Unproved
Ureaplasma urealyticum (< 3 months)
Mycoplasma hominis (< 3 months)
Q fever
Rhinoviruses; enteroviruses
Late-onset rubella syndrome
Human metapneumovirus[137]
SARS-coronavirus

It is often taught that mycoplasmal pneumonia has a classic radiographic appearance, which consists of bilateral reticular or interstitial infiltrates, with or without patchy infiltrates. However, almost any x-ray pattern is possible. Brolin and Wernstedt reported the radiographic findings of 56 patients with M. pneumoniae lower respiratory tract infection: 8 (14%) of patients had lobar findings and 21 (38%) had lobar or predominantly alveolar findings. Some had a combination of lobar/alveolar and interstitial infiltrates; if those are added, 36 (64%) of 56 patients had some component of lobar or alveolar infiltration. Twenty (36%) of the patients showed a purely interstitial pattern, and 33 (59%) had some component of interstitial infiltration. Interestingly, 22% had hilar adenopathy and 14% had a pleural effusion.[74]

M. pneumoniae pneumonia occurs most frequently in individuals 5–12 years old.[144] Subclinical infection is probably common before 5 years of age, but the organism is a relatively unusual cause of pneumonia in this group.[145] Most young adults have serum antibodies, which suggests a past infection and indicates that past infection is apparently not protective against future reinfection.

Chlamydiae

There are three medically important species in this genus. C. trachomatis is a frequent cause of acute bilateral afebrile pneumonia in infants less than 4 months of age and a less-frequent cause of pneumonia in older children and adults. Because it is sometimes associated with peripheral eosinophilia, it is discussed in the section on pulmonary infiltrates with eosinophilia (PIE syndrome).

C. psittaci infection (psittacosis) is uncommon in the United States, with only about 50 cases reported annually. Nevertheless, it is important to recognize because it responds to tetracycline. There is typically an exposure to parakeets or other birds.[146] Large outbreaks have been reported from turkey processing plants.[147] Psittacine birds (those with a bent beak) are more likely to be infected, and most birds with psittacosis are ill. C. psittaci infection in humans usually produces fever, chills, and severe headache; arthralgia is sometimes present. Typically, there has been the gradual onset of cough, and there is a patchy infiltrate on chest x-ray. Usually there is no leukocytosis, but eosinophilia is sometimes present. Elevated serum transaminase and alkaline phosphatase can occur.

pneumonia.[141] Rarely, it is lobar, as cited in the preceding section on focal pneumonias. The physician is often aware of an outbreak of atypical pneumonia syndrome ("walking pneumonia") in the community. Typically, there is a long incubation period (2–3 weeks) between illnesses in the same family, a feature that helps with the diagnosis.[139] However, cases seen in association with outbreaks may have incubation periods as short as one week. Occasionally, a point-source outbreak occurs,[142,143] but usually the illnesses involve separate members of a family over a long period of time.[139]

Otitis media with severe, painful, extremely red tympanic membranes is rarely caused by M. pneumoniae (as discussed previously). Urticarial or non-specific maculopapular rashes are also associated in some cases.[139] Eosinophilia exceeding 5% is not unusual.[140] More severe complications are discussed at the end of this section.

C. pneumoniae, originally classified as a strain of *C. psittaci* called the TWAR agent (named after the first two respiratory isolates, TW-183 and AR-39) is now recognized as a fairly common cause of respiratory disease in school-aged children, adolescents, and adults. Studies documenting its prevalence have been hampered by the lack of a diagnostic gold standard. The organism will not grow on cell-free media but is cultivatable in tissue culture. A nasopharyngeal swab is an appropriate specimen. The sample must be transported in culture transport media and processed within 24 hours of collection. The epidemiology of *C. pneumoniae* is similar to that of *M. pneumoniae* in that infection with this organism is rare in infancy, and becomes more common through childhood and peaks at adolescence. Most infections are probably asymptomatic.[148]

At all age points it appears to be somewhat less common than *M. pneumoniae*.[149] Respiratory disease caused by *C. pneumoniae* is very similar to that caused by *M. pneumoniae*. A prospective study of 667 college students with acute respiratory disease found 20 patients (3%) with *C. pneumoniae* and 29 patients (4%) with *M. pneumoniae* infection; patients with *C. pneumoniae* were less likely to have a temperature greater than 100° F (37.8° C) and were more likely to present with sore throat as a prominent complaint (80% vs. 52%). Hoarseness was seen in 30% of patients with *C. pneumoniae* infection but only in 3% of patients with *M. pneumoniae*.[150] Finally, the time from onset of symptoms to presentation for medical care was longer in patients with *C. pneumoniae* infection.

A variety of serologic tests are available that make a retrospective diagnosis. It may take 3–4 weeks to mount a measurable response; when convalescent titers are ordered too soon the diagnosis may be missed. Polymerase chain reaction (PCR) has been done experimentally, but the results are not always concordant with culture and serology. From 10–90% of patients positive for *C. pneumoniae* infection by PCR do not mount appropriate serologic responses.[151,152]

Some people harbor the organism for months after the acute infection. Such patients may be asymptomatic, or they may have problems with periodic wheezing and asthma. It has been suggested that some adults with severe, refractory wheezing may have chronic *C. pneumoniae* infection. In one study, resolution of infection correlated with improvement in asthma control.[153] Another study found that children with persistent *C. pneumoniae* PCR positivity suffered from more frequent asthma attacks.[154] *C. pneumoniae*-specific immunoglobulin E (IgE) was found in 12 (86%) of 14 culture-positive children with wheezing compared with only 1 (9%) of 11 culture-positive children without wheezing.[155] The precise relationship between *C. pneumoniae* infection and asthma is not understood.

Patients with cystic fibrosis can undergo pulmonary exacerbations in association with *C. pneumoniae* infection. In the one published study on this topic, *M. pneumoniae*, by contrast, was not found to be associated with exacerbations.[156]

Unusual Bacterial Causes

Some bacterial pneumonias are patchy or interstitial and do not respond to macrolides, the usual antibiotic therapy for *M. pneumoniae*. Tularemia is an example.[157]

Viruses

RSV is a frequent and important cause of atypical pneumonia, which is usually of the acute bilateral interstitial subgroup but can be patchy or even densely focal. The airway disease is more important than the alveolar involvement (Chapter 7).

A newly discovered virus, termed the human metapneumovirus (hMPV), was first isolated from nasopharyngeal aspirates of 28 children in the Netherlands who presented with respiratory tract symptoms and negative tests for known causes.[137] Like RSV, symptomatic infection appears to be most common in the first year of life. Symptoms ranged from mild respiratory problems to severe bronchiolitis or pneumonia, often accompanied by high fever and vomiting. Serologic testing suggests that infection within the first 5 years of life is nearly universal.

Adenoviruses, of which there are more than 40 serotypes, are a frequent cause of atypical pneumonia. Adenoviral pneumonia cannot be distinguished on clinical grounds from mycoplasmal pneumonia.[138] Occasionally, epidemics occur with severe disease, often with accompanying gastrointestinal signs.[158]

Influenza viruses almost always are associated with epidemics or large outbreaks. They can cause an atypical pneumonia usually associated with prominent extrapulmonary manifestations.

Parainfluenza virus type 3 can cause atypical pneumonia, especially in young children. It usually produces bronchiolitis (discussed in Chapter 7), possibly with minimal patchy pneumonitis, but occasionally produces bilateral interstitial pneumonia or perihilar pneumonia without bronchiolitis.

Rhinoviruses rarely cause atypical pneumonia.[159] Likewise, coxsackie A or B viruses are rarely associated. Coxsackievirus B has been recovered from the lungs of patients dying with pneumonia, and in the rare newborn or infantile case, the clinical syndrome is usually that of fulminant disease with concurrent myocarditis.

Measles virus is frequently associated with interstitial infiltrates when there is a classic measles illness.[160] It is not ordinarily considered a cause of atypical pneumonia, because the diagnosis is obvious in the classic case. However, pneumonitis is present before the eruption in about 20% of patients with classic measles.[160] Measles virus can cause fulminant pneumonia, as described in a later section.

Varicella-zoster virus can produce atypical pneumonia, especially in adults. The diagnosis should present no problem if the typical rash is present. The syndrome usually presents as chickenpox with pneumonia rather than as atypical pneumonia possibly caused by chickenpox virus. The virus can cause fulminating pneumonia in an immunosuppressed patient.

Cytomegalovirus (CMV) can produce an atypical pneumonia but more often produces an acute interstitial pneumonia in a patient with an immunologic problem (especially solid organ or stem cell transplant patients). In this population, CMV pneumonia is characterized by high fever, hypoxemia, and diffuse interstitial infiltrates. This is a serious disease with a high mortality rate. CMV also can cause interstitial pneumonia in very young infants, who appear to become colonized from their mother's genitourinary tract just before or during delivery.[161,162]

Herpes simplex can cause interstitial pneumonia, especially in immunosuppressed patients and newborns, that may become severe and extensive.[163,164]

Late-onset rubella syndrome is a rare cause of bilateral interstitial pneumonia.[165] It is typically associated with diarrhea, a skin rash, and hypoglobulinemia. It usually occurs between 3 and 12 months of age, with cough, tachypnea, and cyanosis and is associated with circulating immune complexes.

Infectious mononucleosis can produce hilar adenopathy as a part of the generalized lymphadenopathy, and a few patients have small pulmonary infiltrates.[166] Concurrent infection with *M. pneumoniae* might explain some cases of infectious mononucleosis with pneumonia, as both diseases are common in young adults.[167]

The recently discovered severe acute respiratory syndrome (SARS) coronavirus is discussed in the section on progressive or fulminating pneumonias.

Bacteria

Bordetella pertussis can be associated with an atypical pneumonia with subacute onset of cough, slight fever, and pulmonary infiltrates, especially linear lower-lobe interstitial infiltrates, perihilar infiltrates (shaggy heart border), or wedge-shaped upper-lobe infiltrates, perhaps with atelectasis. Lymphocytosis is usually present; when it is not, the clinical diagnosis is likely to be atypical pneumonia with perihilar infiltrate. Most children with pertussis have neither fever nor pulmonary infiltrates unless a secondary bacterial pneumonia (e.g., *S. aureus*) ensues. Pertussis-like illnesses are discussed in Chapter 7.

Other bacteria that can cause atypical pneumonia include the pneumococcus and *H. influenzae*. They are probably a more frequent cause of atypical pneumonia than are bacteria rarely causing human infection, such as *F. tularensis*. *P. aeruginosa*, acquired from water, can rarely cause atypical pneumonia.[168] *Legionella* is an important consideration, particularly in the immunocompromised host.

Mycobacteria

Mycobacterium tuberculosis is an uncommon but important cause of atypical pneumonia with a subacute onset, low-grade fever, and diffuse or linear infiltrates. Most often, the pneumonia is focal and dense, but the rest of the features are atypical, which would fit into the subgroup of a subacute dense focal pneumonia.

Occasionally other mycobacterium species are associated with an atypical pneumonia. Recently, nontuberculous mycobacteria (especially *M. avium* complex) have been associated with a diffuse pneumonia in patients exposed to hot tubs. Patients present subacutely with dyspnea, cough, hypoxia, and fever.[169] Some patients respond to corticosteroids alone, and thus the illness may be due to a hypersensitivity reaction to the organism.[170]

Rickettsiae

Coxiella burnetii, the cause of Query fever (Q fever), is a rare cause of atypical pneumonia.[171] The organism is excreted in large numbers at the time farm animals, particularly sheep, give birth. Long after the fact, viable organisms remain in the soil, and can be blown about by the wind. Thus, the patient need not have been in attendance at a birth but usually lives in a rural area and has some farm animal exposure history. The condition usually responds to doxycycline or erythromycin, which may be given because of suspected mycoplasmal pneumonia.

Inhalational Anthrax

In the past, this disease was very rare, and occurred primarily in those exposed to contaminated animal products (wool sorter's disease). Although still rare, recent bioterrorism-related cases were well publicized.[172] The illness presents in two stages. The first stage is that of an influenza-like illness with fever, cough, and chest pain. The second stage presents a few days later with abrupt onset of high fever, severe dyspnea, and shock. Chest x-ray classically demonstrates only a widened mediastinum, but progressive perihilar infiltrates can be present as well.[172] At least two drugs active against *B. anthracis* are recommended for treatment, (such as a fluoroquinolone plus rifampin). Despite appropriate therapy, the mortality rate is more than 50%.

Fungi

Histoplasma capsulatum and *Coccidioides immitis* are occasional causes of an atypical pneumonia. Patients may present with an acute interstitial pattern when there has been a single overwhelming exposure, but more often they present with a focal infiltrate of subacute onset.

Pneumocystis jiroveci can cause bilateral pulmonary infiltrates in immunocompetent infants 2–12 weeks of age.[173] Infants receiving high doses of systemic corticosteroids for prolonged periods of time are at increased risk,[173a] as are children with HIV infection (Chapter 20), transplant recipients (Chapter 22), and patients with primary cellular immunodeficiency (Chapter 23). Cough, tachypnea, and apneic episodes may occur, but fever is unusual, so that the clinical pattern resembles that of pertussis or chlamydial pneumonia. Serum IgM is usually elevated. Treatment is with trimethoprim-sulfamethoxazole, which is now used as routine prophylaxis for immunocompromised patients.

Miscellaneous Mycoplasma Species

Mycoplasma hominis and *Ureaplasma urealyticum* are uterine cervical flora that can colonize an infant just before or during delivery and lead to pneumonia.[161] One case of pneumonia with pleural effusion in a postpartum adolescent that was due to *M. hominis* has been reported.[174]

Noninfectious Causes

Congestive heart failure often resembles an atypical pneumonia. Pulmonary infarction or embolism is uncommon in children, as discussed in the section on pneumonia with effusion.

Allergies to *Actinomyces* species (which may contaminate air conditioners), to pigeons (pigeon breeder's disease), and to maple bark also may cause noninfectious atypical pneumonia with diffuse interstitial infiltrates. These pneumonias are discussed in the sections on chronic and recurrent pneumonia and PIE syndrome.

Toxic causes include silo filler's disease, caused by inhalation of nitrogen oxides, and other occupational inhalants. Medications such as phenytoin or nitrofurantoin are a rare cause of acute interstitial pneumonia.[175]

Collagen diseases occasionally associated with atypical pneumonia include rheumatic fever (Chapter 18) or rheumatoid arthritis (Chapter 10).

Laboratory Tests

Cold Agglutinins

Because the test is neither sensitive nor specific enough to establish a diagnosis, the use of cold agglutinins is in decline. In certain situations, however, the test may be helpful. If a specimen is desired, it may be obtained as soon as the pneumonia is recognized as "atypical," as agglutinins are often present at this point in the illness. This specimen can also be used as an acute serum for mycoplasmal and viral antibody studies.

Cold agglutinins are found in low titers (about 1:10) in about 10% of normal adults.[176] A titer of 1:32 or higher has been regarded as abnormal. *M. pneumoniae, C. pneumoniae,* and adenoviruses are the most likely causes of cold-agglutinin positive atypical pneumonia. However, RSV, parainfluenza viruses, and coxsackieviruses may also be to blame.[177] Cold agglutinin titers greater than 1:10 are unusual in influenza-virus infection but can occur in patients with pneumococcal pneumonia with bacteremia.[176]

A rapid bedside screening test for cold agglutinins can be performed by placing a few drops of blood into an anticoagulant tube and cooling it on ice. After inserting the specimen in ice, agglutination of red blood cells is visible as clumps when the tube is held up to a light source and rolled slowly. Quantification of a titer of cold agglutinins is not possible at the bedside, although blood with large quantities agglutinates more than does blood with low titers. In one study, 50% of children with acute respiratory disease and 75% of children with pneumonia and serologic evidence of *M. pneumoniae* infection had a positive screening test for cold agglutinins.[178] If a cold agglutinin test is positive in a preschool child, the pneumonia is probably viral. If it is positive in a school-aged child, the pneumonia is probably mycoplasmal. Quantification of cold agglutinin titers is of less utility in children less than 10 years of age.

Rapid Antigen Detection Methods

Some centers offer simultaneous fluorescent-antibody detection of the most common respiratory viruses, including RSV, influenza A and B, the parainfluenza viruses, and adenovirus. Enzyme-linked immunosorbent assay (ELISA) tests are also available for rapid detection of respiratory agents. Such rapid tests are especially useful if there is an established treatment, as for herpes simplex, varicella viruses, or *M. pneumoniae*, or a treatment that is possibly effective, as for influenza. Commercial ELISA tests for RSV and influenza A virus are readily available.

Serum Antibodies

The serum tested for cold agglutinins can also be used as an acute-phase serum for a battery of antibody studies in comparison with a later serum specimen. Antibodies that may be studied in paired sera include *M. pneumoniae, C. pneumoniae,* adenovirus, psittacosis, Q fever, influenza virus, and RSV. Occasionally, other agents known by recent laboratory studies to be prevalent in the community will be sought by the reference laboratory.

Often, complement-fixing antibodies to *M. pneumoniae* are present in low to moderate concentrations in the first serum obtained, which often is a week or so after the onset of the illness. Such low to moderate titers can be regarded as presumptive evidence of current infection with this organism, because these antibodies are usually not detectable in healthy children or adolescents. In one study, an IgM-capture assay drawn in the convalescent phase of illness was the single most reliable test in the diagnosis of *M. pneumoniae* infection.[179] However, in our experience, infections with other organisms can sometimes result in a nonspecific rise in mycoplasma IgM antibodies.

Mycoplasma Cultures

Culture of *M. pneumoniae* is technically difficult, less sensitive than serology, and not readily available.

Viral Cultures

Culture for viral agents is generally slow. RSV may grow within 3–4 days. Herpes simplex virus, likewise, may be fairly rapidly grown in cell culture. Other respiratory viruses may take a week or two. When virus cultures are available and inexpensive, they may be useful in selected cases, especially to identify viruses prevalent in the community. Some laboratories are able to do a "shell vial" assay for adenovirus, which uses centrifugation and detection of early gene products to speed up the process, in which case results may be available within 48 hours.[180]

Polymerase Chain Reaction

PCR testing for *M. pneumoniae* and *C. pneumoniae* on throat swabs or nasopharyngeal aspirates are available on an experimental basis. The sensitivity of such tests is a matter of debate. Evaluation of these tests is ongoing. PCR testing of cerebrospinal fluid, when positive, can establish the diagnosis of *M. pneumoniae* encephalitis.[181]

Treatment of Atypical Pneumonia

Treatment decisions should be based on diagnostic algorithms that begin with the age of the child, then consider clinical and epidemiologic factors, and finally take into account the results of laboratory studies and chest radiography.[1]

Indications for Antibiotics

Antibiotics are of no value in the treatment of viral pneumonia and have not been adequately studied to determine their value for the prevention of secondary bacterial pneumonia. In a study of military recruits with epidemic adenoviral pneumonia, the clinical distinction between viral and bacterial pneumonia was "extremely difficult if not impossible" using radiologic and laboratory techniques.[182] Similarly, there is usually great difficulty in being certain a child has an uncomplicated viral pneumonia.[183] Experienced physicians who have withheld antibiotics in such circumstances have sometimes observed that the course of the illness indicated a bacterial pneumonia, and early antibiotic therapy might have made the illness less severe. These are the basic reasons why antibiotics are usually given to children with atypical pneumonia of uncertain etiology, which is statistically likely to be viral.

Whether to use antibiotics for a child with an atypical pneumonia remains a complex decision, based on criteria of age, severity, reliability of the parents, ability to observe the child closely, and prevalent etiologic agents. Antibiotic treatment of the child with subacute mild pneumonia as if the condition were mycoplasmal is a reasonable general approach given the present state of knowledge and diagnostic techniques (see Table 8-2).

Chemotherapy

In many cases, the patient will already have been treated with amoxicillin or a cephalosporin without any clinical response. In mycoplasmal pneumonia treated early enough, tetracyclines or erythromycin seem to be effective in making some patients recover slightly faster than those in an untreated group.[184] However, in patients treated later than 1 week after onset, there is very little effect.[185] Tetracycline can be used for children older than 8 years of age, because there is no risk of staining the teeth. Both psittacosis and Q fever respond to tetracycline. Erythromycin is preferable for children less than 8 years of age who still have teeth developing. Erythromycin also is sometimes effective against staphylococci, *H. influenzae,* and pneumococci and is superior to tetracycline in such cases. If there is no response to one of these two antibiotics, changing to the other is usually of no value. A newer macrolide, clarithromycin,[186] and an azalide, azithromycin,[187] have both been tested in the treatment of community-acquired atypical pneumonias and have been found to be as effective as erythromycin. The incidence of gastric side effects seen with clarithromycin or azithromycin is considerably less than that seen with erythromycin. The macrolides

have only fair activity against *S. pneumoniae*; therefore, if the illness has some features of typical pneumonia, it is sometimes reasonable to prescribe both amoxicillin (to cover *S. pneumoniae*) and a macrolide (to cover *Mycoplasma*). For the older adolescent, fluoroquinolones are sometimes used and have the advantage of reasonably good activity against both of these organisms.

Management of Exposed Individuals

Administration of tetracycline to exposed family members appeared to result in subclinical infections rather than clinical illness.[188] This result suggests that when family contacts of individuals with cold-agglutinin-positive pneumonia show early manifestations of atypical pneumonia, prompt treatment with tetracycline or erythromycin may reduce the severity of clinical disease. The addition of azithromycin to environmental control assisted in the interruption of a *Mycoplasma* outbreak at an institution.[189]

Complications

Neurologic Complications

In mycoplasmal encephalitis, the patient typically has a history of progressive lower respiratory disease for 1–2 weeks before the onset of central nervous system manifestations, which range from headache and stiff neck to focal seizures and coma.[190] Typically, cold agglutinins are present, and serial *Mycoplasma pneumoniae* antibody titers are high or rising. The cell count of the cerebrospinal fluid is usually 30–300, with more than 90% neutrophils early and predominately lymphocytes later. *M. pneumoniae* has been recovered from the spinal fluid in some cases. PCR assays have been recently used. Paralytic disease (hemiplegia, ascending paralysis, cranial nerve paralysis, and myelitis) has been reported.[190,191] Myositis may also be present.

Arthritis

Arthralgia or arthritis is a rare complication of mycoplasmal pneumonia.[192] The association has been proven to be non-spurious by the finding of *M. pneumoniae*-specific IgM and IgG by ELISA and immunoblotting in children with arthropathy.[193]

Hematologic Abnormalities and Hypercoagulation

Mycoplasmal pneumonia is rarely fatal, but thrombosis, acute hemolytic anemia, or both may occur.[194,195] Two cases in which children with pre-existing hematologic abnormalities developed aplastic anemia in association with acute *M. pneumoniae* infection have been reported.[196] A child in Taiwan suffered a severe case of pulmonary *M. pneumoniae* infection complicated by lung abscess, pleural effusion, thrombocytopenia, and disseminated intravascular coagulation.[197]

Residual Pulmonary Disease

Severe mycoplasmal pneumonia may result in bronchiectasis, usually manifested as recurrent focal (or multifocal) pneumonia.[198] Severe adenovirus pneumonia also can result in residual pulmonary disease, including bronchiectasis.[158]

Dermatologic Problems

An erythematous macular or maculopapular rash in conjunction with acute *M. pneumoniae* infection is not uncommon, as discussed earlier. A more severe complication, Stevens-Johnson syndrome, has been reported at least 70 times.[199] In contrast, erythema multiforme is rare with mycoplasmal infection.

Other Complications

Pancreatitis is rarely seen in association with severe mycoplasmal infection.[200]

Double Infections

Sometimes, pneumonia is "atypical" because it is complicated by a second pathogen, resulting in confusing persistence of the illness or prominent findings in another organ system, such as diarrhea. A prospective study of 201 children with community-acquired pneumonia in Finland found that 9 patients (4%) had serologic evidence of concomitant *M. pneumoniae* and *C. pneumoniae* infection.[201] During the winter, persistence of fever in a child with typical or atypical pneumonia can be due to influenza. Conversely, influenza can predispose to these secondary pneumonias. RSV infection may occur concurrently with pertussis or shigellosis; salmonellosis or rotaviral diarrhea has been reported in conjunction with RSV infection.[202,203]

■ MILIARY AND NODULAR PNEUMONIAS

This section assumes that these pneumonias are acute or at least urgent when recognized, although the disease may really be chronic. Miliary or nodular pneumonia is an anatomic diagnosis based on a chest imaging study that shows multiple circular densities. *Miliary* refers to the size of a millet seed (millet is a grass cultured for hay). In general, miliary therefore refers to small densities (about 2 mm in diameter), whereas *nodular* refers to larger densities (usually about 6 mm in diameter).[204–206] For convenience, the general term nodular is used to include both finely and coarsely nodular disseminated patterns (Table 8-4).

Mechanisms

Any blood-borne infectious agent or particle can be disseminated evenly to the lungs. Relatively evenly distributed densities of the same size result from gradual release of small particles. In experimental

TABLE 8-4. CAUSES OF NODULAR AND MILIARY PNEUMONIA

TYPE OR SITUATION	POSSIBLE CAUSES
Miliary	
Acute interstitial pattern appears reticular or miliary	Usually viral
Hepatosplenomegaly present	Tuberculosis
Nodular	
Acute, severe	Septic emboli
In compromised host	Disseminated fungi, CMV, *Pneumocystis*
Ventilator or muscular weakness	Multiple aspirations

CMV, cytomegalovirus

miliary tuberculosis in rabbits caused by virulent or avirulent bovine tubercule bacilli, the miliary lesions become visible about 3 weeks after intravenous injection.[207] If dissemination of bacteria or emboli to the lung occurs irregularly, it usually produces a radiographic appearance of larger densities with more focal involvement of some parts of the lungs.

Classification

The syndromes associated with these radiologic findings are best classified according to the onset and course of the clinical illnesses.

Acute Nodular Pneumonia

The patient has high fever and appears moderately sick. The possible etiologies are discussed later.

Chronic Nodular Pneumonia

This type has a gradual onset, often with weight loss and low-grade fever, and the patient appears chronically ill.[208,209] Chronic nodular pneumonia is rare in children. Possible etiologies include miliary tuberculosis, disseminated fungal disease, pulmonary metastases, polyarteritis nodosa, Wegener's granulomatosis, and other collagen vascular diseases and even pneumoconioses. Pulmonary Langerhans cell histiocytosis is a rare cause of chronic nodules in children.[209,210] Alveolar proteinosis, pulmonary hemosiderosis, sarcoidosis, and diffuse interstitial fibrosis are discussed in the section on chronic pneumonia.

Asymptomatic Pulmonary Nodules

Such nodules are rare in children. The patient usually has had a chest roentgenogram taken for symptoms presumably unrelated to the finding. Multiple densities in these circumstances often are calcified. Histoplasmosis or coccidioidomycosis is the most likely cause of asymptomatic miliary calcifications. Miliary tuberculosis is a rare cause. Chickenpox can cause calcifications that are uneven, irregular, and numerous.[211] Alveolar microlithiasis is a rare cause of calcifications in children. The particles are fine and usually require overexposed films to be visible.[212]

Etiologies of Acute Miliary Pneumonias

Most patients with an acute miliary pattern on a chest film are treated as if they have miliary tuberculosis, at least until a more definite diagnosis can be made.[205,206] It is important to note the other features of miliary tuberculosis and other nodular pneumonias, which may help in differentiating them.

Acute Interstitial Pneumonia

Several viruses can cause an acute bilateral interstitial pneumonia that may be called reticular (like a fine net), as described in the section on atypical pneumonia. The reticular appearance may be slightly nodular, but follow-up films clarify the situation by showing either coalescence or clearing.

Acute Miliary Tuberculosis

Acute hematogenous tuberculosis is usually associated with a known exposure to active tuberculosis, but anywhere from 30–75% of patients do not have a positive tuberculin skin test on admission.[213, 214] Occasionally, children with pulmonary tuberculosis present with wheezing secondary to bronchial obstruction and are misdiagnosed with asthma. Empiric treatment with corticosteroids may allow the development of miliary disease.

Miliary tuberculosis is largely a disease of infancy; a review of 94 cases in childhood reported a mean age of 11 months.[215] Cough and fever were the most common symptoms, seen in 72% and 61%, respectively. Forty percent of patients had decreased appetite or weight loss. Vomiting and diarrhea were seen in a third of this cohort. Hepatomegaly and splenomegaly were seen in most cases, and lymphadenopathy was seen in almost half.[215] Dyspnea is seen only in the more severe cases. Additional focal pneumonia and hilar adenopathy are common. Tubercules may be seen in the retina. Skin lesions are not uncommon; many of these reveal granulomas on biopsy. A follow-up chest radiograph one week later will show that the miliary lesions are still present. The lesions are typically 0.5–2 mm in diameter, but lesions 4–8 mm can occur in disseminated tuberculosis. In adults, thrombocytopenia and inappropriate antidiuretic hormone secretion with hyponatremia have been reported.[216]

Frank meningitis is found in about 20% of children with disseminated tuberculous disease. More subtle involvement of the central nervous system (CNS) may be much more common; Gupta et al. performed magnetic resonance imaging (MRI) studies on 7 patients who had miliary pulmonary tuberculosis without any signs of CNS disease and found abnormalities in all.[217] Three patients had multiple lesions of greater than 3 mm in diameter, which were readily visualized. The others had lesions smaller than 3 mm in diameter; these were best visualized with contrast enhancement. The clinical significance of this finding is not known. The lesions regressed with therapy in all 7 patients.

Multiple Septic Emboli

Any bacteremia can result in multiple septic pulmonary emboli that may create a fine or coarse nodular pattern[218] or may produce a target sign, a density within a thin-walled cyst,[219] which represents cavitation as the necrotic process proceeds.[220] Brucellosis and tularemia, the examples often given, are now rare. In children, a focal *S. aureus* infection (e.g., endocarditis, osteomyelitis, or organ abscess) is probably the most common cause of septic emboli. The multiple septic foci in the lung are often larger than lesions of miliary tuberculosis, are often irregular in size or distribution, and may be connected or confluent. Typically, there is cough with purulent sputum, dyspnea, and an apparent source of bacteremia.

Disseminated Fungal Diseases

Histoplasmosis, coccidioidomycosis, aspergillosis, candidiasis, mucormycosis, paracoccidiodomycosis, and blastomycosis can look very similar to miliary tuberculosis by chest radiography (Fig. 8-5).[221–225] Any number of other, less common fungal pathogens have also been reported to

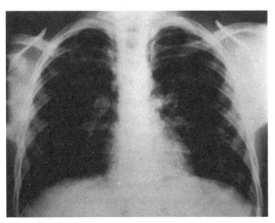

■ **FIGURE 8-5** Bilateral nodular pneumonia caused by histoplasmosis.

cause a similar roentgenographic pattern. *Pneumocystis jiroveci* pneumonia can produce bilateral nodular pneumonia and is discussed in the section on chronic pneumonia.

Viral Disease

CMV can produce diffuse nodular pulmonary infiltrates.[226] Severely immune suppressed patients may develop nodular pneumonias secondary to other herpes group viruses as well, including varicella zoster virus, herpes simplex virus,[227] and EBV. Any of the common respiratory viruses can produce a reticulonodular pattern on chest x-ray.

Multiple Aspirations

This is a common cause of nodular densities in children who are predisposed to aspirate. The densities are usually rather large and have a predilection for the lower lobes. The predisposing cause of the aspirations is usually evident.[228]

Lymphocytic Interstitial Pneumonitis

Lymphocytic interstitial pneumonitis (LIP), associated with EBV infection, produces a reticulonodular x-ray pattern in children with HIV infection (Chapter 20). Clubbing and diffuse lymphadenopathy are commonly associated. Children with LIP sometimes also have chronic or recurrent parotitis. Corticosteroids seem to provide benefit for the more severely affected patients.

Other Causes

Psittacosis and mycoplasmal infection occasionally produce acute nodular pneumonias.

In newborn babies, listeriosis can produce a miliary pattern, as can Group B streptococcal infection. Often these infections produce a finely reticulonodular pattern resembling the ground-glass appearance of respiratory distress syndrome.

Nocardiosis is an uncommon cause of nodular pneumonia. Aspergillosis is a cause of chronic nodular pneumonia, especially in patients with intracellular killing defects such as chronic granulomatous disease.[229] Infection with *Coxiella burnetii*, the agent of Q fever, can produce a reticulonodular x-ray pattern.

Leptospirosis is a zoonotic disease usually associated with a systemic infection characterized by a biphasic pattern, fever, hepatorenal involvement, and sometimes meningitis; however, 91 (59%) of

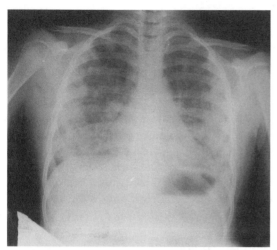

■ **FIGURE 8-6** Bilateral nodular pneumonia in a 10-year-old girl due to *Legionella pneumophila*. She had been receiving immunosuppressive therapy for idiopathic pulmonary hemosiderosis and developed fever and dyspnea 1 week after exposure to a hot tub.

154 cases recently reported had pulmonary involvement, and reticulonodular infiltration was seen in 40% of these patients.[230]

Legionella can cause acute pneumonia with a nodular pattern on chest x-ray, particularly in immunocompromised hosts (Fig. 8-6). [230a]

Noninfectious Causes

Pulmonary edema occasionally has a miliary appearance. Inhalation of toxic gases or acid fumes can produce an acute pneumonia with a miliary appearance (bronchiolitis fibrosis obliterans).[205] Wegener's granulomatosis can present as a chronic nodular pneumonia.[231] Langerhans cell histiocytosis can be a cause of bilateral reticular or reticulonodular pulmonary infiltrates.[232] This type of x-ray pattern is also common in hypersensitivity pneumonitis. Most cases of lipoid pneumonia produce bilateral air space consolidation, but a reticulonodular pattern is occasionally seen.[233] Unlike the disease in adults, which usually produces a confluent x-ray pattern, pulmonary alveolar proteinosis in childhood produces variable patterns on x-ray, including nodular, miliary, and scattered linear densities.[234]

Diagnostic Approach

A thorough history of risk factors for and possible exposures to tuberculosis should be taken. In children with tuberculosis, often the best way to obtain the organism is to isolate it from the sputum of the adult source case. An intermediate strength tuberculin test should be done, although patients with miliary tuberculosis are often anergic. Sputum should be obtained if possible for Gram stain, acid-fast stain, and culture for bacteria, mycobacteria, and fungi. In young children, a gastric aspirate is often performed instead. This is best done in the hospital with three consecutive early morning samples obtained by personnel trained in the procedure.[235,236]

Blood culture for bacteria should be done in acute nodular pneumonias. If miliary tuberculosis is suspected, spinal fluid should be examined for evidence of tuberculous meningitis.

Liver biopsy or bone marrow aspiration may be of value in chronic miliary pneumonias, because it may reveal evidence of tuberculosis or disseminated fungal disease. Serologic methods may make retrospective diagnoses in disseminated fungal diseases. Urine histoplasmosis antigen testing is usually positive in cases of disseminated histoplasmosis. BAL may be useful if other methods fail to reveal the diagnosis. In children with pulmonary tuberculosis, the yield with BAL is similar to that with gastric aspirates, but occasionally performing both tests increases the yield.[237,238] BAL has the advantage of being able to be performed as an outpatient procedure.

Lung puncture, transbronchial biopsy, and pleural biopsy are rarely indicated. These procedures are discussed at the beginning of this chapter.

Treatment
Chemotherapy

If there is reasonable suspicion of acute miliary tuberculosis, antimycobacterial therapy with 4 drugs (usually isoniazid, rifampin, pyrazinamide, and ethambutol) should be started. Usually, it is not necessary to add another antibiotic directed at bacteria such as staphylococci. However, this may be a reasonable step if the patient is seriously ill or diagnostic information is scant.

A change in the presumptive diagnosis of acute miliary tuberculosis can be made on the basis of results of these early tests and the course of the illness.

Corticosteroids

Patients with acute miliary tuberculosis have been treated with steroids in addition to appropriate antituberculous therapy, reportedly with good results.[239] However, no controlled studies have been done, and most experts reserve corticosteroid therapy for patients with confirmed CNS disease or severe hilar adenopathy causing bronchial obstruction.

■ PROGRESSIVE OR FULMINATING PNEUMONIAS

Progressive pneumonia can be defined as one that becomes radiologically and clinically worse in spite of antibiotic therapy that should be effective against the presumed etiologic agent. This situation often makes the physician consider methicillin-resistant *S. aureus* or gram-negative rods, including *Klebsiella* or *P. aeruginosa*, as the etiologic agent and change antibiotic therapy to treat these possibilities. However, the cause is often nonbacterial or even noninfectious (Box 8-8).

Fulminating pneumonia can be defined as a severe bilateral pneumonia with an unusually rapid progression, clinically or radiologically, over 24–48 hours. Usually, fine moist inspiratory rales are heard in all lung fields, as in acute pulmonary edema. Pneumonia in newborn infants and in compromised hosts is discussed in Chapters 19 and 22, respectively.

Possible Infectious Etiologies

Influenza Virus

Fulminating pneumonia is seen more frequently during influenza outbreaks, and some cases are clearly documented by recovery of the virus from the lung at autopsy. Usually, the pneumonia is bilateral and interstitial. In rapidly fatal cases, *S. aureus* is often also cultured from the lungs at autopsy, but *Pseudomonas aeruginosa* may be found in patients who have had mechanical ventilation. The white blood cell count is exceedingly variable but often is low in fatal cases.[240–242] Grossly bloody sputum, cyanosis, and irreversible progressive hypoxemia are characteristic of fatal cases. Myocarditis, intravascular coagulation, or invasive fungal pneumonia can occur.[243]

Bacterial pneumonia complicating influenza virus pneumonia can be particularly virulent, especially that caused by staphylococci or streptococci.[244,245] Influenza virus and some gram-positive bacteria may have a synergistic effect: the bacteria carry enzymes that catalyze the cleavage of viral

> **BOX 8-8 ■ Causes of Progressive or Fulminant Pneumonia**
>
> *Common*
> Influenza virus (during epidemics)
>
> *Uncommon*
> *B. pertussis*
> Measles virus
> Varicella zoster virus
> Adenovirus
> *Mycoplasma pneumoniae*
> *Chlamydia psittaci*
> Pulmonary vasculitis
> *Legionella pneumophila*
> *Listeria monocytogenes* (in newborns)
> *Coxiella burnetii* (Q fever)
> Neoplasia
> Group A streptococcus
> Group C streptococcus
> Hantavirus
> Nipah virus (exposure to pigs in Malaysia and Singapore)
> Hendra virus (exposure to horses in Australia)
> Rocky Mountain spotted fever
> Ehrlichiosis
> SARS-coronavirus
> Adult respiratory distress syndrome (ARDS)
>
> *In Immunosuppressed (Primarily)*
> Enteric gram-negative rods
> *Legionella*
> Tuberculosis
> Systemic fungi
> *Pneumocystis jiroreci (carinii)*
> Herpes simplex
> *Toxoplasma gondii*
> *Stenotrophomonas maltophilia*
> *Acinetobacter baumanii*
> *Mycobacteria chelonae*

proteins, which speeds infectivity of the virus; viral infectivity causes decreased ciliary motion, denudation, and leakage of fluids, creating an atmosphere that is conducive to bacterial growth. Staphylococcal toxic shock syndrome can be a fatal complication (Chapter 10).

SARS-coronavirus

In the spring of 2003, a worldwide outbreak of severe acute respiratory syndrome (SARS) occurred. Within a matter of weeks it was shown to be caused by a novel and highly transmissible coronavirus termed SARS-CoV.[245] The outbreak began in China and rapidly spread to 30 other countries. More than 8000 cases occurred, approximately 10% of them fatal.[245a]

The illness has a biphasic—or sometimes triphasic—course.[245b] After an incubation period of 2 to 10 days, patients initially present with nonspecific influenza-like symptoms of fever, myalgia, and headache. Lymphopenia is common. The respiratory phase starts within 2 to 4 days of onset of fever with a dry, nonproductive cough. The third phase, occurring in about 20% of patients, manifests as severe hypoxemia and the adult respiratory distress syndrome (ARDS). Chest radiographs of patients with SARS show patchy focal infiltrates or consolidation, often with a peripheral distribution, which may progress to diffuse infiltrates.[245b] Compared with adults and teenagers, SARS appears to have a less aggressive course in younger children.[245c]

The diagnosis can be made in reference laboratories by culture or reverse transcriptase-PCR (RT-PCR) of respiratory secretions or, in retrospect, by paired sera demonstrating an antibody response.[245] There is no proven antiviral therapy. Screening for suspect cases and strict infection control procedures are critical to preventing spread.[245b]

Other Viruses

Adenoviruses can produce a progressive fatal pneumonia.[246–248] The patient can be a normal host but often has an underlying disease. Conjunctivitis or pharyngitis is often found. In severe cases, rhabdomyolysis and hemoglobinuria can occur.[248]

Herpes simplex virus has been reported to cause a fulminating fatal pneumonia in a previously healthy 9-month-old child.[249]

Wild-type measles infection can produce a fulminating pneumonia, especially in immunosuppressed patients.[250] The disease also has been reported in apparently normal individuals.[251] In some hosts, there is no typical rash, especially if the patient has a severe underlying disease such as leukemia.[252]

EBV can also cause a progressive, but eventually reversible, pneumonia in infants and preschool children. Hepatosplenomegaly and atypical lymphocytes are typically present, but the heterophile test is almost always negative in this age group.[253]

Varicella zoster virus can produce a rapidly progressive, often fatal pneumonia in pregnant women.[254] Patients with compromised cellular immunity can also suffer a severe pneumonitis from this agent.

Hantavirus infection causes progressive and often fatal respiratory failure after an influenza-like prodrome. Most cases occur in adults. The disease, hantavirus pulmonary syndrome (HPS), was first described in 1994 after an outbreak of cases in the southwest US.[255] Isolated cases have since been described in other parts of the Americas. The primary risk factor for infection is exposure to rodents, the natural hosts of the virus. Features that help distinguish HPS from other causes of fulminant pneumonia include 3 clinical characteristics at admission (dizziness, nausea, and absence of cough) and 3 laboratory parameters (thrombocytopenia, acidosis, and elevated hematocrit).[256]

Gram-Negative Rods

P. aeruginosa, E. coli, Klebsiella, Enterobacter, and other gram-negative rods sometimes cause pneumonia. Predisposing factors include cystic fibrosis, burns, malignancy, chronic pulmonary disease, corticosteroid or immunosuppressive therapy, previous antimicrobial therapy, tracheostomy, mechanical ventilation, operative procedures on the kidney or bowel, and inhalation of contaminated aerosols from aerosol therapy or from contaminated heated whirlpool baths.[257,258]

In adults, *K. pneumoniae* can produce either progressive or fulminating pneumonia, particularly if the organism is resistant to the antibiotics being used. The condition is characterized by tenacious sputum, probably related to the extremely mucoid capsule of the organism. The white blood cell count is often low with a predominance of neutrophils. Sputum smear reveals neutrophils and gram-negative rods. In children, *K. pneumoniae* is a very rare cause of progressive pneumonia. Culture results must be interpreted with caution, because this organism is sometimes cultured from upper respiratory specimens of healthy infants. Prior treatment with amoxicillin (and probably other antibiotics) predisposes the upper respiratory tract to colonization with *Klebsiella.*

In adults, the radiologic appearance of a gram-negative pneumonia is usually focal or diffusely nodular.[258] *Pseudomonas* pneumonia often has diffuse nodular alveolar infiltrates that progress rapidly to cavitation. Infiltrative, localized, or cavitary pneumonia due to *Pseudomonas aeruginosa* is seen in adults and children with AIDS. *K. pneumoniae* usually causes dense lobar consolidation with a predilection for the upper lungs.[257] Often, there is bulging of the fissures and abscess formation with cavitation. Extensive pleural effusion with putrid empyema suggests *Bacteroides*. However, any gram-negative enteric rod can produce any of these radiographic patterns.

It may be difficult to distinguish coincidental colonization of the respiratory tract, which is frequent in chronically ill patients, from pulmonary infection. Gram-negative enteric bacilli may be found in sputum cultures without being the cause of pneumonia, and small amounts of coliforms may be present in the upper respiratory tract, particularly in patients receiving antibiotics. Contamination also may occur during collection of the specimen. If there is a significant delay before the specimen is cultured, the coliforms, which multiply at room temperature, overgrow the other flora. The bacteriologic diagnosis is certain only if the organism is recovered from lung puncture, pleural fluid, or blood or by finding the characteristic histologic pattern described above. Nevertheless, the physician often must begin treatment based on clues from the Gram stain, without a positive bacteriologic diagnosis, especially when the patient is extremely ill.

Mycoplasma

M. pneumoniae is an occasional cause of life-threatening pneumonia with severe cyanosis.[259] Oxygen therapy is important, and steroids may produce dramatic improvement.

Rare Causes

Psittacosis can manifest as a progressive pneumonia but usually responds to tetracycline.[260] Tuberculosis can cause either fulminating or progressive pneumonia.[261,262] Characteristically, rales are not heard.

Legionnaires' disease appears to be uncommon in children, but the childhood patterns of illness caused by *Legionella* species have not been fully defined. *L. pneumophila* is capable of causing fulminant necrotizing pneumonia in previously young, healthy adults. It has rarely been reported to cause disease complicating hematologic malignancies (see Chapter 22).

Histoplasmosis, blastomycosis, coccidioidomycosis, aspergillosis, and nocardiosis should also be considered.[263,264] *Pseudomonas pseudomallei* infection (melioidosis) can cause a progressive pneumonia and might be suspected in refugees or persons recently returned from Southeast Asia or India.[265] Leukocytosis may not be remarkable in spite of abscess formation in the liver and spleen as well as in the lungs. Initial treatment with ceftazidime is associated with decreased mortality as compared to older regimens.[266] Imipenem appears to be equally effective for initial treatment. Once the patient responds clinically, multi-drug oral therapy is provided for several months.[267]

Mucormycosis has been reported as a cause of rapidly progressive pneumonia in patients with diabetes mellitus.[268] Q fever, which usually causes an atypical pneumonia (discussed earlier), has been reported to cause rapidly progressive pneumonia.[269] Even with pneumonia, systemic symptoms such as headache, myalgia, and fever may predominate. Pneumonia may be present even in the absence of cough. In patients with AIDS, *Toxoplasma gondii* may cause a severe, progressive pneumonia.[270]

Tricuspid-valve endocarditis presents with pleuritic chest pain, fever, and pulmonary infiltrates and is easily confused with pneumonia. The patient is usually acutely ill with a systolic murmur that is loudest on inspiration. However, the peripheral stigmata of endocarditis are lacking.[271] Injection drug users and those with indwelling central venous catheters are at especially increased risk for this infection, but it occasionally occurs in those without known risk factors, in which case anemia and microscopic hematuria may be the only clues.[272]

Rocky Mountain spotted fever (RMSF) may present with progressive respiratory failure, mimicking a primary respiratory tract process. In one retrospective study, 15 (43%) of 35 patients with RMSF developed rales, abnormal chest roentgenograms, and impaired gas exchange, likely from noncardiogenic pulmonary edema.[273] In 8 patients (23%), the presence of respiratory symptoms led to an incorrect initial diagnosis and delay of appropriate therapy.

Cough (30%) and pulmonary infiltrates (10%) have also been reported in ehrlichiosis; rarely severe ARDS occurs.[274]

ARDS has also been reported in patients with Lyme disease[275] and babesiosis.[276]

Acute suppurative mediastinitis can be associated with marked leukocytosis or leukopenia, tachypnea, and a peculiar interrupted inspiration pattern.[277] In addition to antimicrobial therapy, operative drainage may be necessary.

Noninfectious Etiologies

Malignancies, particularly Hodgkin's or non-Hodgkin's lymphoma, are an occasional cause of progressive pulmonary infiltrates in children. Hemorrhage or infarction from an embolus is likewise an occasional cause.

Acute pulmonary edema secondary to congenital heart disease, acute myocarditis, or acute glomerulonephritis may be a cause of progressive pulmonary infiltrates in children. In addition, several types of pneumonia have been associated with subsequent development of acute glomerulonephritis.[278–281] *Mycoplasma* is perhaps the most commonly cited association.[282] Recurrent pneumonia and glomerulonephritis should bring to mind the possibility of C3 deficiency.[283]

Rarely, rheumatic pneumonia is fulminating. It is typically associated with some carditis.[284] Wegener's disease, Goodpasture's disease, systemic lupus erythematosis, and Henoch-Schönlein purpura can all present with both renal and pulmonary involvement.[285] Pathergic granulomatosis is a very rare disease that combines features of periarteritis nodosa, Wegener's granulomatosis, and allergic vasculitis.[286] High fever, conjunctivitis, focal pneumonia, and marked leukocytosis, with death in about 2 weeks has been reported. Thrombotic thrombocytopenia purpura can cause fulminating pneumonia in young adults.[287]

Churg-Strauss syndrome is a systemic disease that presents with hypereosinophilia, asthma, pulmonary infiltrates, and clinical evidence of vasculitis.[288] Some cases have been described in asthmatics receiving leukotriene receptor antagonists.[288a]

Laboratory Approach

Examination of sputum (if possible) or tracheal secretions for neutrophils and bacteria is important. Special stains for fungi or mycobacteria should be considered, as well as viral cultures. Urine antigen testing for *Histoplasma capsulatum* or *Legionella pneumophila* serotype 1 may be appropriate.

Blood cultures should be done. The white blood cell count is usually of no specific value. A low white count usually suggests that the basic pulmonary disease is not bacterial, but in some severe bacterial pneumonias the count is low, usually with a shift to the left.

Occasionally, chest CT will reveal diagnostic clues not appreciated on chest radiographs, such as a mass, cavity, adenopathy, parenchymal abscess, or bronchiectasis.

Urinalysis should be done to look for evidence of acute glomerulonephritis. An electrocardiogram or echocardiogram may be indicated to look for evidence of myocarditis or congenital heart disease. It is not uncommon for children with an undetected congenital heart defect or cardiomyopathy to present initially with a secondary pneumonia, which may result in severe respiratory distress due to low cardiac reserve.

In progressive pneumonia that is not responding to empiric antibiotics, the physician must strongly consider more invasive diagnostic techniques such as bronchoalveolar lavage or open lung biopsy, depending on the situation.

Treatment

Oxygen by mask is indicated immediately. Intubation and assisted ventilation may be urgently needed.

Other conditions such as pulmonary edema, huge pneumothorax, and extensive atelectasis should be excluded. If pulmonary edema is diagnosed, furosemide (and possibly an inotropic agent) is indicated.

Antibiotic therapy should be determined by the specific situation. Nafcillin (or cefuroxime) and gentamicin may be a good combination for suspected bacterial pneumonia in a patient without underlying immune deficiency who has a severe community-acquired pneumonia. Vancomycin should be added to the beta-lactam antibiotic if the patient acquired the infection in the hospital or if there is a high incidence of methicillin-resistant *S. aureus* in the community. Consideration should be given to the use of a macrolide to cover atypical causes. If there are epidemiologic or clinical clues to the possibility of psittacosis, RMSF, or ehrlichiosis, doxycycline should be added. Patients with cystic fibrosis or immune deficiency states have a higher likelihood of having a gram-negative pneumonia; ceftazidime plus gentamicin with or without vancomikin or another broad-spectrum anti-pseudomonal combination should be considered. Therapy should be guided by the results of history, physical examination, Gram stains, and cultures.

■ ASPIRATION PNEUMONIAS

Classification

Aspiration pneumonias can be classified according to what is aspirated, which can be relatively inert (water, saline, blood, buffered gastric contents), toxic (hydrocarbons, acid gastric contents), or oropharyngeal secretions.[289] *Aspiration pneumonitis* is a chemical injury caused by the inhalation of sterile gastric contents, whereas *aspiration pneumonia* is an infectious process caused by the inhalation of oropharyngeal secretions that are colonized by pathogenic bacteria.[289] Aspiration pneumonia secondary to oropharyngeal secretions can be classified as acute (as in a recently unconscious patient who is having the first episode of aspiration pneumonia) or chronic or recurrent (as in severely retarded children or long-term comatose or ventilator patients, who often are receiving antibiotics). The management of these different syndromes should be considered separately. For example, a single large aspiration in a child after cardiac surgery might best be treated very aggressively, as the underlying problem can be expected to improve over a week, so that antibiotic resistance would be less of a problem. On the other hand, a small aspiration pneumonia in a patient with permanent weakness might best be treated in a stepwise fashion, beginning with simple therapy directed at usual pharyngeal flora and proceeding to more potent and toxic therapy only after failure to improve on simple therapy.

Acute Aspiration Pneumonias

Hydrocarbon Pneumonia

Small children may swallow and aspirate hydrocarbon products such as kerosene. Because further aspiration might occur, vomiting should not be induced. This discussion is limited to the aspiration pneumonia that often results, but several toxic effects can occur. Prophylactic antibiotics do not appear to be of value clinically and are not recommended.[290] Oxygen and assisted ventilation may be needed.

If, after 24–48 hours, the patient develops fever and leukocytosis, therapeutic antibiotics for presumed bacterial superinfection may be indicated. Ceftriaxone or cefotaxime would be a reasonable single antibiotic to empirically treat infection with the usual pharyngeal flora, particularly *S. aureus*, *S. pneumoniae*, or *H. influenzae*.

Near Drowning

In general, the principles for antibiotics are the same as previously noted. That is, prophylactic antibiotics are not recommended, but antibiotics used empirically or based on appropriate cultures are reasonable when a secondary pulmonary infection occurs.[291] Neither steroid prophylaxis nor steroid therapy is supported by controlled studies.[291] Some experts think steroids may actually be harmful.[292]

Gastric Aspiration

In neurologically normal children, gastric aspiration usually occurs as a complication of anesthesia for surgical procedures. The overall incidence of clinically significant aspiration in children undergoing surgery is low: only 52 (0.1%) of 50,880 children who underwent general anesthesia in one report[293] and 24 (0.04%) of 63,180 in another.[294] Aspiration is more common in emergency surgeries than in scheduled procedures. In the studies cited above, the overall outcome was good; serious respiratory morbidity was unusual, and no deaths occurred. Stomach contents are generally sterile; therefore, prophylactic antibiotics are not advocated.[289] Corticosteroids do not affect the resolution of the injury.[295] Gastric emptying is slowest with breast milk, faster with low-fat milk, and faster still with a glucose solution.[296] Studies have shown that fasting longer than 2 hours after clear liquid ingestion changes neither the gastric volume nor the pH of the gastric contents.[297] Regardless of the duration of fasting, fewer than half of pediatric patients ever achieve a gastric volume less than 0.4 ml/kg of body weight, nor do they achieve a gastric pH greater than 2.5 (values that have been touted as "desirable" to minimize the risk of aspiration pneumonitis with sedation or anesthesia).

Gastric aspiration may occur on a chronic or recurrent basis in children with neurologic impairment, suck-swallow difficulties, and various rare defects such as bifid epiglottis.[298]

Particle Aspiration

Whenever solid particles have been aspirated, as in dirt aspiration, bronchoscopy is essential for their removal so that ventilation can be adequate.[299] Case reports of infants having respiratory failure from the inhalation of various powders used during diaper changes, including talcum and cornstarch, have been reported.[300]

Bacterial Aspiration Pneumonias

As mentioned earlier, aspiration pneumonia is to be differentiated from aspiration pneumonitis, in which gastric contents are aspirated. Unless the patient is on chronic antacids, H2 blockers, or proton pump inhibitors, gastric acidity renders stomach contents sterile. Aspiration pneumonitis, therefore, is a chemical process and generally does not require antibiotic therapy. In contrast, the basic defect leading to bacterial aspiration pneumonia is failure of the normal oropharyngeal defense mechanisms, particularly coughing. This causes the patient to aspirate colonized secretions from the oropharynx, leading to pneumonia in the dependent lung segments.[289] The patient typically has a depressed state of consciousness or has a neuromuscular defect that prevents adequate coughing.

Normal adults aspirate during sleep,[301] as can be demonstrated by dripping a radioactive tracer solution into the pharynx by a small nasopharyngeal tube. About half of normal adults demonstrate positive scans of peripheral pulmonary areas after normal deep sleep whereas about 70% of adults with depressed consciousness aspirate.[301]

Recurrent Pneumonia

In many patients with a long-term depressed state of consciousness or neuromuscular impairment, recurrent bacterial aspiration pneumonia may be inevitable. Extremely enlarged tonsils and adenoids can contribute to aspiration during sleep and to recurrent lower airway infection.[302]

Prevention by selection of foods, positioning, or suctioning may be the most important method of management. Some children with demonstrated esophageal reflux might benefit by gastric tube feedings. Inevitably, a subset of these patients will require surgical means to control chronic or recurrent aspiration. The traditional surgical procedure is the Nissen fundoplication, but bilateral submandibular gland excision and parotid duct ligation may be an effective surgical treatment for chronic or recurrent aspiration in children with neurologic impairment.[303]

Acute episodes of recurrent aspiration in the absence of recent antibiotic therapy can be treated using antibiotics directed at normal pharyngeal flora. Again, making a distinction between aspiration pneumonitis (due to aspiration of stomach contents), in which antibiotic therapy is usually unnecessary, and aspiration pneumonia (due to aspiration of oropharyngeal secretions), in which antibiotics are needed, is crucial. The decision to use or to withhold antibiotics is not always straightforward, and should be individualized. No good prospective studies are available to clarify the decision, so clinical judgment must be employed.

Percutaneous transtracheal aspiration has indicated that aspiration pneumonia in severely retarded institutionalized children is polymicrobial and often involves anaerobes.[304] These children are likely to harbor penicillin-resistant anaerobic organisms. A study comparing clindamycin, ticarcillin-clavulanate, and ceftriaxone for aspiration pneumonia in neurologically impaired children showed that antibiotics effective against penicillin-resistant anaerobes were superior to ceftriaxone, with satisfactory clinical and microbiological responses occurring in 89–91% of those treated with ticarcillin-clavulanate or clindamycin versus 50% of those treated with ceftriaxone.[305] When aerobic gram-negative enteric rods are present or suspected, gentamicin is effective.[306]

Acute Aspiration Pneumonia

Adequately controlled studies have not been done for acute aspiration pneumonia. In the child who has recently aspirated for the first time and whose underlying disease is acute and likely to improve, an aggressive course of antibiotics can be advocated. Waiting for worsening clinical findings before giving broad coverage for anaerobes and gram-negative rods may allow the pneumonia to become more severe. Reasonable options in this case include the combination of clindamycin and gentamicin or monotherapy with either piperacillin/tazobactam or meropenem.

■ PNEUMONIA WITH EOSINOPHILIA SYNDROME

Pulmonary infiltration with eosinophilia is a term coined to encompass all of the various clinical patterns with these findings.[307] Loeffler' syndrome was previously used to describe any type of pulmonary infiltrate associated with eosinophilia of the peripheral blood. Loeffler originally described transitory infiltrates with few symptoms and a benign course. Some of the causes of PIE syndrome are listed in Box 8-9. Because the presentation, clinical findings, prognosis, and treatment of PIE syndromes varies widely, a more complicated classification scheme has been proposed.[308] This new scheme contains the following classifications:

1. *Loeffler's syndrome* is now another term for simple pulmonary eosinophilia.
2. *Chronic eosinophilic pneumonia* (rare in children).
3. *Acute eosinophilic pneumonia.*
4. *Allergic granulomatosis* (Churg-Strauss syndrome).
5. *Allergic bronchopulmonary aspergillosis* (ABPA).
6. *Parasite-induced eosinophilia.*
7. *Drug reaction.*
8. *Idiopathic hypereosinophilic syndrome* (rare in children).
9. *Infant pulmonary eosinophilia.*

Eosinophilic pneumonia is more common in adults than it is in children. Because of its rarity, the typical clinical course is difficult to describe. Initial signs and symptoms are usually non-specific, and may include fever, cough, and dyspnea, with or without weight loss. In one report of 11 children with PIE, 8 had dyspnea, 6 had crackles on physical examination, and only 3 had wheezing.[309] Of these 11 cases, 3 were cases of acute eosinophilic pneumonia (one fatal), 2 were drug reactions, 2 were parasite induced, 2 were a new syndrome that was named infant pulmonary eosinophilia, 1 was Churg-Strauss syndrome, and 1 was atypical chronic PIE.

Eosinophilic pneumonia is defined by microscopic examination of the lung, which shows an eosinophilic infiltrate that may not be accompanied by eosinophilia in the peripheral blood. Eosinophils are usually present in broncheoalveolar lavage fluid, but rarely may be absent in that sample as well.[309] Idiopathic chronic eosinophilic pneumonia occurs in adults but is extremely rare in children.[310]

Possible Mechanisms

In some cases, the pulmonary infiltrates are caused by trapping of worm larvae in the smaller blood vessels of the lung. In other cases, both the pulmonary infiltrates and the blood eosinophilia appear to be hypersensitivity phenomena, such as during desensitization to poison ivy, or as a reaction to a medication. Patients with PIE usually have elevated levels of interleukin-5 (IL-5) in BAL fluid and in pleural fluid, if present.[311] Antidepressants, sulfa drugs such as sulfasalazine, and minocycline are some of the drugs more commonly associated with the development of PIE.

Chlamydial Pneumonia

C. trachomatis can produce afebrile bilateral pneumonia in young infants (usually 1–3 months of age) that is marked by the gradual onset and worsening of a chronic interstitial pneumonia, usually with mild to moderate peripheral eosinophilia.[312] Often, the infant has had a mild and persistent mucoid conjunctivitis since a few days after birth, a result of the *C. trachomatis* contracted from the mother's cervix. Conjunctival infection may occur despite appropriate perinatal eye prophylaxis. The disease can occur in very young infants that have been born by cesarean section.

The illness may resemble bronchiolitis because of the afebrile tachypnea and hyperinflated lungs with low diaphragms, but chlamydial pneumonia is more chronic. Scattered rales are sometimes heard, but wheezing is unusual. Radiographic findings include bilateral symmetrical interstitial infiltrates and reticulo-nodular infiltrates (probably atelectasis, as it clears rapidly).[313] Areas of moderate atelectasis may occur, but consolidation, pleural effusion, and cardiomegaly are not observed.[313] The chest x-ray findings are typically out of proportion to the clinical symptoms. The cough is staccato and persistent, and can be distinguished from the paroxysmal cough of pertussis by the pattern of breathing. Staccato cough is characterized by a breath between each cough, whereas the paroxysms of pertussis consist of a prolonged series of coughs, followed by a single deep breath, usually with a whoop. Mild leukocytosis with lymphocyte predominance may be seen; but unlike pertussis, absolute lymphocyte counts greater than 10,000 per mcL are rare. Occasionally, atypical lymphocytes are found in the smear.

Eosinophilia greater than 300 per mcL was found in 71% of cases in one series.[312] The serum IgM is typically very high for the baby's age, consistent with a chronic infection present since birth. IgA and IgG concentrations are usually elevated also.[312]

The clinical diagnosis is often obvious, but in the absence of conjunctival infection it is more difficult. Definitive etiologic diagnosis is established by recovering the organism in tissue culture. Because *C. trachomatis* is an obligate intracellular pathogen, culture samples must include cells, not just secretions. A direct fluorescent antibody (DFA) test is available and provides excellent sensitivity and specificity when used to diagnose conjunctival infection; its sensitivity drops off considerably when it is used on nasopharyngeal secretions in an attempt to diagnose *C. trachomatis* pneumonia. PCR testing is both more sensitive and more specific, and can be used where it is available. Serologic diagnosis is possible; the presence of specific IgM antibody to *C. trachomatis* is diagnostic. Paired sera may be used to demonstrate a four-fold rise in IgG antibody titer. In patients with concurrent chlamydial conjunctivitis, the etiologic diagnosis is probably established most quickly by sending a conjunctival scraping for DFA testing.

Erythromycin or sulfisoxazole stops the shedding of *Chlamydia* and appears to help the clinical illness.[314] The currently recommended therapy is oral erythromycin 40–50 mg/kg/day divided every 6 hours for 14 days. Because the administration of erythromycin to babies younger than 2 months of age has been associated with the development of idiopathic hypertrophic pyloric stenosis, parents should be informed of this potential risk. Both clarithromycin and azithromycin have excellent in vitro activity against *C. trachomatis*, and azithromycin is often used in the treatment of genital infection with this organism. Neither of these newer macrolides has been studied in the treatment of afebrile pneumonia of infancy. In vitro susceptibilities have not always correlated with in vivo efficacy in animal models of *C. trachomatis* pulmonary disease.[315] An intravenous formulation of azithromycin has been tested against genital chlamydial infection but not in the treatment of pneumonia.[316]

Bacterial superinfection is rare.[317] Myocarditis is likewise a rare complication.[318] Occasionally, an infant may present with apnea or develop it during the course of the disease. Chronic respiratory disease can develop with chronic cough and abnormal pulmonary function.[319] Infections in premature infants with *C. trachomatis* may result in chronic pulmonary disease resembling bronchopulmonary dysplasia.[320]

Other Infectious Causes

Corynebacterial Pneumonia

A case of PIE syndrome has been reported in which *C. pseudotuberculosis* was recovered in a transtracheal aspirate from a veterinary student who was exposed to horses.[321] *C. pseudotuberculosis* causes lymphadenitis in livestock but had not been reported previously in humans.

Parasites

Ascaris (human roundworm), *Toxocara canis* (dog roundworm), and *Toxocara cati* (cat roundworm) are the most frequent parasitic causes of PIE syndrome in the United States. Visceral larval migrans is the name for a syndrome caused by *T. canis* or *T. cati* that is associated with recurrent pneumonia or wheezing, hepatosplenomegaly, eosinophilia, hyperglobulinemia, and, rarely, eye infection.[322] Amebiasis, trichinosis, trichuriasis (whipworm), hookworm, and filariasis are also possible causes.

Strongyloides stercoralis can become disseminated in immunocompromised hosts and is important to recognize because it can be cured with ivermectin or thiabendazole when found in the stool before it disseminates.[323] Eosinophilia is found only in some cases.

Allergic Bronchopulmonary Aspergillosis (ABPA)

ABPA should always be considered if an asthmatic child develops the PIE syndrome.[324] Clinical findings include increased wheezing with low-grade fever, transient peripheral pulmonary infiltrates, and, occasionally, focal pneumonia or atelectasis. The child may spit up mucous plugs containing mycelia, and a sputum smear may reveal eosinophilia.[324] This disease can occur in young infants, having been reported as early as 6 months of age.[325] Chronic or recurrent aspergillosis may lead to bronchiectasis. Standard diagnostic criteria for establishing the presence of ABPA are listed in Chapter 22 in the section on cystic fibrosis.

Rare cases of a similar clinical syndrome associated with candidal infection rather than aspergillus have been reported.[326] Allergic bronchopulmonary mycosis is the general name for the same clinical pattern caused by fungi other than Aspergillus.[327]

Aspergillus Infection

The clinical picture of acute eosinophilic pneumonia is rarely caused by invasive pulmonary aspergillosis. In one case, a previously well child initially diagnosed with idiopathic eosinophilic pneumonia (later proven to be invasive aspergillosis with necrotizing granulomas) was found to have chronic granulomatous disease (CGD). She had two healthy siblings who also tested positive for CGD.[328] Another cautionary tale is that of a boy diagnosed with acute eosinophilic pneumonia who had an initial response to steroid therapy but then had rapid clinical deterioration and death from invasive aspergillosis.[329]

Noninfectious Causes

Hypersensitivity Pneumonia

The acute onset of bilateral interstitial pneumonia with associated eosinophilia can be caused by hypersensitivity to a number of antigens. These episodes occur several hours after exposure and usually last only a day or two. A number of inhalant allergens have been identified, most of which are molds: moldy hay (farmer's lung), moldy dust from air conditioners, thermophilic actinomyces in humidifiers, antigens in saunas, or dust from birds.[330–332]

Hypersensitivity pneumonias are of two types: (1) acute, diffuse alveolitis (extrinsic allergic alveolitis) with severe dyspnea, cough, fever, sweating, and basilar rales, as in pigeon-breeder's (bird-fancier's) lung; and (2) chronic and possibly localized infiltrates, with wheezing and low-grade fever, expectoration of mucous plugs, and peripheral eosinophilia, as in bronchopulmonary aspergillosis. Hypersensitivity pneumonias can cause chronic or recurrent pneumonias without eosinophilia as discussed in that section.

Asthma

Eosinophilia and pulmonary infiltrates can occur in patients with asthma, but the eosinophilia is usually minimal.

Other Causes

Polyarteritis nodosa, Hodgkin's disease or other lymphoma, Wegener's granulomatosis, Churg-Strauss syndrome, and other pulmonary vasculitides,[333] rheumatoid disease, nitrofurantoin or tetracycline hypersensitivity,[334] and tropical eosinophilia of unknown etiology are rare causes of the PIE syndrome and primarily afflict adults. Chest trauma may result in effusion and peripheral eosinophilia.

PIE has been reported in association with inhaled drugs of abuse, including Scotchguard™ [335] and crack cocaine.[336]

Idiopathic

Many children with the PIE syndrome recover completely with no specific cause being found. Probably some of these illnesses are caused by hypersensitivity to a self-limited infection or an inhaled allergen.

Diagnostic Approach

Examination of the stool for parasites is usually indicated. If ascariasis is suspected, examination of a gastric aspirate diluted in normal saline with sodium hydroxide may reveal *Ascaris* larvae.

If aspergillosis is suspected, a sputum smear and culture for *Aspergillus* is indicated. However, isolation of *Aspergillus* from respiratory secretions is not necessarily diagnostic of a causal association (see Box 8-1). Serologic tests for *Aspergillus* species may be available in some medical centers. Serum IgE levels are frequently extremely high in ABPA and may be useful for diagnosis and to follow the course of illness.[325] Eosinophilic cationic protein is elevated in the serum of patients with PIE, and levels decline with successful therapy.[337]

Tests for the diagnosis of chlamydial pneumonia in a young infant are discussed earlier. If hypersensitivity pneumonitis is suspected, the patient's serum can be tested at a reference laboratory for antibodies against a battery of suspected antigens.

Toxocara antibodies can now be detected by sensitive methods and should be looked for if visceral larval migrans is suspected.

Treatment

With the exception of acute eosinophilic pneumonia, which can be life-threatening, the syndrome usually has a benign etiology, and special therapy is unnecessary unless a specific cause is found. Allergic aspergillosis usually responds to corticosteroids. In fact, most cases of PIE are responsive to corticosteroid therapy. Chlamydial pneumonia is improved by treatment with erythromycin or sulfisoxazole. Parasitic causes can usually be treated with antiparasitic agents. Pulmonary failure, if it occurs, should be treated with mechanical ventilation. Some cases of PIE in the neonatal period have required extracorporeal membrane oxygenation (ECMO).

■ CHRONIC AND RECURRENT PNEUMONIA SYNDROMES

Chronic pneumonia can be defined as a pulmonary density that does not improve within one month. Recurrent pneumonia can be defined as more than one episode within a 1-year period or more than three episodes in a lifetime. Cough and fever are usually present at the onset but may not persist.

Many children with a chronic pulmonary lesion (especially a congenital anomaly) are thought to have recurrent pneumonias if chest roentgenograms are taken only during febrile respiratory infection.

Classification

Chronic pneumonias are best classified on the basis of the anatomic pattern, whether focal, interstitial, with hilar adenopathy, or with cysts, cavities, or spherical masses (Boxes 8-10 and 8-11).

Recurrent pneumonias are classified as focal or interstitial for purposes of discussion (Box 8-12).

Chronic Focal Pneumonias

Untreated or Undertreated Acute Pneumonia

Pneumonia due to a common pathogen that has been untreated or in which the treatment was never completed is a possible cause of chronic pneumonia. In treatment failures, resistant organisms may be responsible. Penicillin-resistant *S. pneumoniae* treated with antibiotics (such as TMP-SMX or a macrolide) that have moderate to poor activity

---

> **BOX 8-10 ■ Causes of Chronic Focal Pulmonary Disease**
>
> **Infectious**
> Mycobacterium tuberculosis
> Systemic fungi
> Nontuberculous mycobacteria
> Paragonimiasis
>
> **Noninfectious**
> Malignancy
> Atelectasis
> Foreign body
> Congenital anomalies of lung, thymus, or mediastinum
> Vascular rings
> Eventration of diaphragm (RLL)
> Plasma cell granuloma
> Inflammatory pseudotumor

---

against the pneumococcus may produce this clinical picture.

Tuberculosis

Pneumonia caused by *M. tuberculosis* is often detected when a chest x-ray is done because of a positive tuberculin test in an exposed but asymptomatic child, so the duration may be unknown. Alternatively, the infiltrate may be discovered when the child has an x-ray because of fever with mild respiratory signs and symptoms from another cause. Occasionally, tuberculosis presents as an acute febrile lobar pneumonia. Failure of the infiltrate to clear after antibiotic therapy may be noted before tuberculosis is suspected. Often, the infiltrate is wedge shaped and associated with regional hilar adenopathy. Tuberculosis is discussed further in a later section.

Nontuberculous Mycobacterial Pneumonia

M. avium-intracellulare complex and other mycobacteria can produce a tuberculosis-like disease, especially in children with defective cell-mediated immunity, but rarely in normal children.[338]

Fungal Pneumonia

Histoplasmosis, coccidioidomycosis, blastomycosis, cryptococcosis, and sporotrichosis can all produce a chronic focal pneumonia in children. The clinical presentation can be as varied as that in tu-

---

BOX 8-11 ■ Causes of Chronic Interstitial Pulmonary Disease; Pneumonia with Hilar Adenopathy; and Chronic Cavitary, Cystic, or Nodular Pneumonias

Causes of Chronic Interstitial Pulmonary Disease
Infectious
  Pneumocystis jiroveci
  CMV
  Lymphocytic interstitial pneumonitis (in patients with HIV infection)
  C. trachomatis
  Late-onset congenital rubella syndrome
Noninfectious
  Bronchopulmonary dysplasia
  Congestive heart failure
  Chronic interstitial fibrosis
  Lymphoid granulomatosis
  Pulmonary alveolar proteinosis
  Lipoid interstitial pneumonitis
  Bronchiolitis obliterans
  Desquamative interstitial pneumonia
  Pulmonary hemosiderosis
  Histiocytosis
  Sarcoidosis
  Juvenile rheumatoid arthritis
  Giant-cell pneumonitis
  Idiopathic fibrosing alveolitis (usual interstitial pneumonitis)

Causes of Pneumonia with Hilar Adenopathy
Common
  Mycobacterium tuberculosis
  Histoplasmosis
  Mycoplasma pneumoniae
  Chlamydia pneumoniae
Uncommon
  Nontuberculosis mycobacteria
  Fungi other than histoplasmosis

  Actinomycosis
  F. tularensis
  Lung abscess
  Anthrax
Noninfectious
  Lymphoma
  Other neoplasms

Causes of Chronic Cavitary, Cystic, or Nodular Pneumonias
Infectious
  Tuberculosis
  Systemic fungi
  Lung abscess
  Atypical measles
  Dog heartworm
  Paragonimiasis (Far East immigrant)
  Mycoplasma pneumoniae
  Necrotizing bacterial pneumonia, especially gram-negative rods such as Pseudomonads, Klebsiellae, and Pseudoallescheria boydii
  Actinomycosis
  Nocardiosis
Noninfectious
  Congenital anomalies
  Malignancy
  Traumatic cyst
  α-1 Anti-trypsin deficiency
  Anti-thyroid therapy
  Eosinophilic granuloma
  Pulmonary sarcoidosis

---

berculosis, from asymptomatic to a chronic cough with a low-grade fever to an acute lobar pneumonia. The radiographic appearance is often a chronic segmental consolidation but can be multiple nodules or a cavitary lesion. Hilar adenopathy is often noted, especially in histoplasmosis.

Unusual Pathogens

Coxiella burnetti (Q fever agent) and *Chlamydia psittaci* may cause chronic pneumonia. Systemic symptomas such as headaches and myalgias may dominate the clinical picture. The key to diagnosis is to ask the right questions regarding possible exposures (see Chapter 21).

Atelectasis

Chronic or recurrent focal pneumonias can be secondary to a focal anatomic abnormality, such as atelectasis. The underlying cause of the atelectasis might be a foreign body, a mucoid impaction of a small bronchus after an asthmatic attack or after pertussis, or a narrowed bronchus obstructed by secretions. Atelectasis can also be the result of compression of a bronchus due to cardiovascular anomalies, an enlarged lymph node, tumor, or postpneumonic inflammatory changes. Atelectasis can be round and give the impression that a tumor is present.[339]

Foreign Body

A radiolucent small foreign body, such as a peanut or a piece of Styrofoam, can cause a focal pneumonia. A history of choking is frequently reported[340] and wheezing is sometimes present. Inspiratory and expiratory roentgenograms sometimes show a shift of the mediastinum and an increased lucency on

BOX 8-12 ■ Causes of Recurrent Pneumonias

Recurrent Focal Densities
Asthma
Cystic fibrosis
Bronchiectasis
Right middle-lobe syndrome
Multiple aspiration pneumonia
Migratory foreign body
Congenital obstructing anomalies
Immunodeficiency diseases
Primary ciliary dyskinesia

Recurrent Interstitial Infiltrates
Asthma
Hypersensitivity pneumonias
Unilateral hyperlucent lung
Lymphocytic interstitial pneumonia (in patients with HIV infection)

the affected side. Computed tomography may be helpful in difficult cases.[341] Bronchoscopy is likely to be necessary to detect occult foreign bodies.[342]

Aspiration of the flowering head or spike (inflorescence) of a stalk of grass such as the Timothy grass can cause especially severe problems with persistent focal pneumonia, often with hemoptysis.[343] The aspiration is often forgotten, and bronchoscopic removal is often unsuccessful, leading to bronchiectasis and eventually to pulmonary resection. Acute symptoms of respiratory foreign-body aspiration are discussed in Chapter 7.

Congenital Anomalies

Many rare anomalies can give the impression of a chronic focal pneumonia and are often initially detected when a chest x-ray is taken during an episode of fever and respiratory symptoms. In addition, some conditions predispose to secondary bacterial pneumonia in the affected area of the lung due to trapping of secretions. These anomalies include hypoplasia of the lung, thymic tumors or cysts, posterior mediastinal accessory thymus, tracheal bronchus, cystic adenomatoid malformation, bronchogenic cysts, and congenital pulmonary sequestration of non-functioning lung tissue.[344,345]

Parasites

Paragonimiasis (lung fluke infection) can cause diffuse perihilar infiltrates, cysts, or hilar adenopathy in individuals from the Far East who eat contaminated freshwater crabs or crayfish.[346] Differentiation from smear-negative pulmonary tuberculosis may be difficult.[347] Diagnosis is by detection of the parasite in sputum or a gastric aspirate.

Neoplasms

Solid focal "pneumonias" occasionally are a result of a neoplasm, such as neuroblastoma.

Chronic Linear or Interstitial Infiltrates

Although these chronic pneumonias are rarely due to infections, infectious possibilities will be considered first.

Chlamydial Pneumonia

As described in the section on pulmonary infiltrates with eosinophilia, *C. trachomatis* typically produces subacute or chronic interstital pneumonia in children less than 6 months of age. This organism is also a rare cause of this syndrome in older children and adults, but eosinophilia is usually not present.[348]

Cytomegalovirus Pneumonia

Typically, CMV produces disease in immunosuppressed individuals, especially recipients of solid organ or stem cell transplants as described in Chapter 22. Infants may become colonized with CMV in the nursery or during delivery and develop a chronic interstitial pneumonia even without the usual iatrogenic immunosuppression associated with CMV disease.[349] Cough, wheezing, and tachypnea may occur without the usual chronic interstitial pneumonia, but most infants with symptoms appearing after 3 months of age have some underlying disease.[350]

Pneumocystis Pneumonia

Immunocompetent infants aged 2–12 weeks have been found to have chronic diffuse pneumonia with tachypnea caused by *Pneumocystis jiroveci*.[351] The median hospitalization was 3 weeks, with apparent clinical response to oxygen and trimethoprim-sulfamethoxazole.

Bronchopulmonary Dysplasia

Premature infants who have required mechanical ventilation can develop bronchopulmonary dysplasia (BPD) characterized by diffuse, often linear, infiltrates, focal hyperinflation, and chronic pulmonary insufficiency with exacerbations during intercurrent respiratory infections.[352,353] A new definition of BPD was recently proposed by a consensus panel and focuses on the need for supplemental oxygen for at least 28 days after birth.[354]

Congestive Heart Failure

This is a frequent cause of bilateral interstitial infiltrates in patients with congenital heart disease. Often, cardiomegaly and hepatomegaly are present.

Idiopathic Interstitial Pulmonary Diseases

This is a general term for a group of noninfectious pneumonias. Some chronic progressive forms are familial,[355] and circulating immune complexes may be involved in the pathogenesis of some of these.[356] Lung biopsy is necessary to make the diagnosis. Hydroxychloroquine, cyclosporine, or cyclophosphamide therapy produces improvement in some forms of this complex of diseases when corticosteroid therapy, the first choice, fails.[355]

Pulmonary alveolar proteinosis is characterized by progressive dyspnea with an oxygen diffusion block and cyanosis.[357] The chest x-ray may resemble that of pulmonary edema without cardiomegaly but often shows reticulonodular, miliary, or healing nodules.[358] The disease has been reported in children as young as 3 months of age. Recently, it has been discovered that mutations in the genes for granulocyte-macrophage colony-stimulating factor (GM-CSF) or its receptor can cause the syndrome, and the therapeutic use of aerosolized GM-CSF is promising.[359]

Several idiopathic diffuse interstitial lung diseases are seen exclusively in infancy. *Persistent tachypnea of infancy* presents with tachypnea and hypoxia and a normal chest x-ray.[360] The syndrome has an excellent prognosis and resolves over months to years. *Infantile cellular interstitial pneumonitis* usually is a reaction to another lung process; chest x-rays reveal a ground-glass pattern and lung biopsy shows infiltration of structural cells that have proliferated abnormally. The disease tends to go away when the underlying disease state resolves.[360] *Chronic pneumonitis of infancy* is a disease of unknown etiology that presents with tachypnea and hypoxemia. Biopsy shows cellular proliferation and an alveolar exudate consisting mainly of macrophages and eosinophilic debris. The prognosis of

chronic pneumonitis of infancy is guarded; many patients suffer progressive pulmonary deterioration.[361]

Desquamative interstitial pneumonia (DIP) is associated with the use of unfiltered cigarettes in adults; the incidence has been declining over the last decade. The incidence of DIP in childhood, however, has not changed. DIP is characterized by progressive dyspnea with an oxygen diffusion block and cyanosis, with the alveoli being filled with desquamated cells. This condition can occur in young infants with congenital rubella syndrome, apparently resulting from deposition of antigen-antibody complexes in the lungs.[362] It has also been associated with other infectious agents, including CMV.[363] Several cases have been observed in the first year of life, and it can be familial.[364] Steroid therapy often produces improvement, and sometimes chloroquine therapy is helpful.[365]

Usual interstitial pneumonia (idiopathic fibrosing alveolitis) is seen almost exclusively in adults. It typically has a fine reticular or finely nodular radiologic appearance but may appear linear. It can be familial and is sometimes reversed by corticosteroid therapy.[366]

Idiopathic pulmonary hemosiderosis is characterized by recurrent hemoptysis, bilateral diffuse mottled densities, and "honeycomb lung" and has been reported in infants as young as 9 months of age.[367] Goodpasture's syndrome appears to be a severe form of pulmonary hemosiderosis with renal involvement. The onset is associated with hemoptysis and iron-deficiency anemia, with uremia occurring later. In the 1990s a cluster of cases of acute pulmonary hemosiderosis and pulmonary hemorrhage in infants was initially attributed to exposure to the common mold *Stachybotrys atra*. However, the purported association remains unproven.[368,369]

Other Causes

Pulmonary Langerhans' cell histiocytosis is a rare cause of chronic diffuse interstitial pneumonia in children.[370] Lymphoid granulomatosis is a rare cause of progressive respiratory insufficiency with bilateral diffuse reticular pneumonia.[371] It has also been reported in association with hypogammaglobulinemia, HIV infection, and juvenile rheumatoid arthritis.[372,373] Lymphoid interstitial pneumonitis is a frequent occurrence in children with HIV/AIDS. It is associated with EBV infection and usually heralds a good prognosis in comparison with children who develop other opportunistic respiratory infections.[374] Diffuse chronic interstitial infiltrates can be an early presentation of sarcoidosis.[375]

Hilar Adenopathy

Hilar nodes typically appear as a rounded, lobulated mass and can be best seen at first by lateral chest roentgenograms[376] and further defined by computed tomography.[377]

Chronic pneumonia with hilar adenopathy in children is usually mycobacterial or fungal. Subacute pneumonia with hilar adenopathy can be caused by *Mycoplasma*.[378] The most common chronic pneumonia associated with hilar adenopathy in children is probably tuberculosis, discussed later. Histoplasmosis may be more common in areas of endemicity. Coccidioidomycosis and, less commonly, blastomycosis are possibilities to be considered. *Actinomyces* and nontuberculous mycobacteria are other rare causes.[379,380]

Sarcoidosis is a very rare cause of chronic pneumonia with hilar and paratracheal adenopathy in children.[375] Bilateral mottling and generalized adenopathy is usually present. Uveitis, hypercalcemia, bone lesions in the hands, and erythema nodosum are sometimes found. The disease can affect children as young as 2 years of age. Most large series have been reported from Virginia or the Carolinas.[375]

Lung abscess is another cause of hilar adenopathy, which disappears when the abscess is resolved.[381] Usually, the abscess can be identified as a circular mass, which eventually cavitates, as described in a later section.

Tularemia can cause hilar adenopathy and is discussed in the sections on acute focal pneumonia and pleural effusions.

Lymphomas or neoplasms of the mediastinum are a cause of hilar adenopathy and may be mistaken for chronic infections.[382]

Cysts, Cavities, or Spherical Masses

Spherical masses, with or without cavitation, are often of infectious origin in children.[383] A child with an acute febrile illness and a spherical density on a chest film may be suspected of having a tumor. However, such spherical masses are almost always infectious, as can be readily determined by their resolution during antibiotic therapy.[384]

Mycobacteria or Fungi

Tuberculosis is a possible cause of pulmonary cavitation in teenagers[384] and, rarely, in younger children.[385] Histoplasmosis, sporotrichosis, coccidioidomycosis, cryptococcosis, actinomycosis, nocardiosis, and blastomycosis should also be considered.[386,387] Sporotrichosis is a rare cause of chronic pulmonary disease with cavitation. Although the skin ulcerations usually respond dramatically to iodide therapy, the rare pulmonary form usually responds only to amphotericin B or itraconazole.

Cavities or Lung Abscess

The bacteria that produce necrotizing pneumonia include *S. aureus,* gram-negative enterics, and anaerobes.[388–393] Prior to the advent of good anaerobic culture techniques, *S. aureus* was the most frequently recovered organism. A review of the literature since then reveals that *Bacteroides fragilis* is the most common pathogen, followed by *S. aureus,* alpha-hemolytic streptococci, peptostreptococcus, and *Pseudomonas aeruginosa. E. coli* and *Klebsiella pneumoniae* are the most common gram-negative organisms found in lung abscesses. The pneumococcus is a rare cause of cavitary disease in childhood; a series of 3 pediatric cases in which typical lobar pneumonia was followed in several days by the appearance of pneumatoceles or frank abscess has been reported.[394] In adults, additional infection with anaerobes is usually present.[388] Group A streptococci have been recovered from lung abscesses.[395] *H. influenzae* and *M. pneumoniae* have been reported as rare causes of cavitary pneumonia or a lung abscess.[389,390] Fungi, especially *Aspergillus*, have to be considered in the immunocompromised host. In patients with HIV/AIDS, *Nocardia, Pneumocystis,* and *Rhodococcus equi* should be added to the differential diagnosis.[396]

Lung abscesses may appear to be cystic, cavitary, or solid, and in children are usually associated with underlying risks, most frequently neurologic or oncologic disorders. Abscess formation is also more common in patients with certain immune deficiencies. Bronchial obstruction, suppurative pneumonia, or dental infections also heighten the risk.[391,392] In infants and children, respiratory muscular weakness, a swallowing disturbance, or assisted ventilation may be reasons for aspiration which could lead to abscess formation.

The diagnosis of lung abscess is usually based

on radiologic demonstration of a circular density with an air-fluid interface. CT scan is excellent in defining abscesses and allowing the detection of smaller ones. Sputum or bronchoscopy-obtained secretions should be examined for *Aspergillus*, tubercle bacilli, and anaerobic bacteria. Percutaneous transtracheal aspiration studies indicate that anaerobes are common, and invasive techniques to obtain material for cultures can be used to aid therapy in severe or refractory cases.[393]

Treatment consists of antibiotic therapy based on stain and culture results and correction of the underlying conditions if possible. In general, empiric therapy should cover anaerobes and gram-negative bacilli. This can be accomplished by using clindamycin and ceftazidime, piperacillin-tazobactam, or nafcillin/gentamicin/metronidazole. Generally, intravenous therapy is continued until the patient is stable, usually less than a week. Total duration of therapy is usually 2–3 weeks, except in complicated cases, when therapy should continue for 2–3 weeks from stabilization. Amoxicillin-clavulanate or clindamycin (depending on the clinical situation) may be appropriate oral agents for completion of therapy. Lung abscesses can sometimes be drained by bronchoscopy or fluoroscopy-guided percutaneous aspiration, but such invasive procedures are usually not indicated, as many cases heal well without such drainage.[397] Radiographic resolution may take weeks to months. Follow-up chest x-rays to document the disappearance of the lesion should be obtained.

Parasites

Parasitic infection is a rare cause of cavitary disease. For example, paragonimiasis can be a cause of cavitary pneumonia in an adopted or immigrant child from the Far East.[346]

Nodular or coin-shaped densities may occur in human infection with the dog heartworm *Dirofilaria immitis*.[398] Dogs are the reservoir host, and the microfilariae are apparently transferred by mosquito bite from the dog's bloodstream to the human, where the mature adult later dies and becomes encapsulated in the lung. The mature adult cannot produce microfilariae in humans. About a hundred human infections have been confirmed, but none of these occurred in children. Cough, myalgia, and low-grade fever may occur. Eosinophils are noted in the lung lesions, but peripheral eosinophils rarely exceed 10%. Lung abscess due to amebiasis is not uncommon in the developing world. Patients with lung involvement almost always have concomitant liver abscesses.[399]

Pulmonary hydatid cysts due to infection with *Echinococcus granulosus* are not uncommon in endemic areas (parts of Africa, central Asia, and Australia). In children, the lung is the most common site of involvement, and there may be single or multiple cysts.[400] Surgery is the treatment of choice for most patients with pulmonary hydatid disease, and conservative surgical methods that preserve lung parenchyma are generally preferred.[401]

Noninfectious Causes

Neoplasms, especially lymphomas or metastatic malignancies, are an occasional cause of spherical pulmonary lesions in children. Langerhans' cell histiocytosis may be associated with multiple cysts in the lung, sometimes with pneumothorax (Fig.8-7).[402] Generalized or cervical adenopathy is likely to be present. Inflammatory pseudotumor is a rare cause of a circular pulmonary mass in children; it is usually asymptomatic.

Pulmonary cavitation can be the result of alpha$_1$-antitrypsin deficiency in children.

Trauma can cause lung cysts.[403] Other causes include bronchopulmonary dysplasia, Wegener's granulomatosis, autoimmune disease, and cystic bronchiectasis.[404] Antithyroid drugs can produce toxic side effects that can include cutaneous vasculitis and pulmonary cavitation.

Recurrent Focal Pneumonia

The child with only a few episodes of recurrent pneumonia often has no detectable defect and has

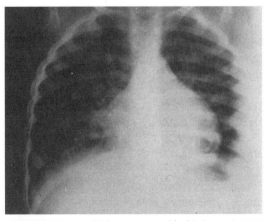

■ **FIGURE 8-7** Multiple cysts caused by histiocytosis. Note large cyst behind the heart. Pneumothorax may occur.

been categorized as a "normal but unlucky" child, if all findings are normal between episodes, growth and family history are normal, there is no history of other infections, and the child has a negative tuberculin skin test (see Box 8-12).[405] The next most frequent cause of recurrent focal or interstitial pneumonia is asthma.[405,406]

Right Middle-Lobe Syndrome

Recurrent or persistent pneumonia or atelectasis in the right middle lobe has been called the right middle-lobe syndrome, but the same pattern can occur in other lobes.[407] The underlying cause in children is often asthma, with obstruction by spasm and bronchial secretions. Hilar node or other extrinsic compression of a bronchus is another mechanism. Blastomycosis was found to be the cause in one patient, although fungal infection is usually not associated with the syndrome.[408] A seven-year follow-up study of 17 children who had the diagnosis in early childhood showed that 5 had ongoing respiratory problems: 4 had asthma and 1 had bronchiectasis. Pulmonary function tests were lower in those with continued respiratory disease.[409] Flexible bronchoscopy can be useful for removal of mucous plugs or secretions, even in young infants.[410] In one series of 21 cases, bronchoscopy was thought to be therapeutic in 14 (67%). Four patients eventually required lobectomy, and two had persistent but improving symptoms.[411]

Cystic Fibrosis

The underlying disease in chronic or recurrent pneumonias can be cystic fibrosis (see Chapter 22), which can be excluded by a sweat test. The type of pneumonia seen in cystic fibrosis is variable but is usually segmental or lobular.

Multiple Aspirations

An episode of aspiration can often be observed during hospitalization. An H-type tracheoesophageal fistula or aspiration caused by a swallowing abnormality can be excluded by a barium esophagram. Many cases of recurrent aspiration in children are related to a neuromuscular disturbance, particularly muscle weakness, as discussed in an earlier section.

Gastroesophageal Reflux

Some children with recurrent focal pneumonia have gastroesophageal reflux.[412]

Bronchiectasis

In patients with more than one episode of focal pneumonia, bronchiectasis should be suspected, particularly if the same area is involved and if each illness responds promptly to antibiotic therapy. In pediatrics, bronchiectasis is most commonly seen in association with cystic fibrosis. Occasionally, serial roentgenograms will demonstrate gradual resolution of an atelectasis, which is in reality a complete collapse with gradual hyperexpansion of an adjacent lobe as the diseased lobe atrophies. Prophylactic antibiotics are controversial. In a study of adults who had bronchiectasis but not cystic fibrosis, the condition was improved in a higher proportion of those who got amoxicillin prophylaxis than in controls. The frequency of exacerbations remained the same, but the severity was decreased.[413] The possible benefit of prophylactic antibiotics must be weighed against the risk of creating antimicrobial resistance.

Bronchiectasis is sometimes reversible. In one series, bronchograms were done in 60 consecutive acute pneumonias in soldiers.[414] Bronchiectasis was demonstrated in 8, of which 3 returned to normal within 4 months. Mild bronchial abnormalities were demonstrated in another 17 soldiers, and most returned to normal by 2 months.

Bronchiectasis and recurrent pneumonia can also result from a congenitally aberrant bronchus.[415] Other congenital or familial causes of bronchiectasis include cystic fibrosis, primary ciliary dyskinesia, alpha$_1$-antitrypsin deficiency, IgG or IgA deficiency, and complement or neutrophil defects.[416] Primary ciliary dyskinesia is discussed further in Chapters 5, 22, and 23.[417]

Specific infectious diseases, such as pertussis, *Mycoplasma*, or adenovirus infection, sometimes result in bronchiectasis or recurrent pneumonia, often with a unilateral hyperlucent lung.[418]

Migratory Foreign Body

Recurrent focal pneumonia can be caused by a migratory radiolucent foreign body.[419]

Congenital Anomalies

Recurrent pneumonias may be secondary to tracheomalacia, bronchomalacia, a vascular ring, or an H-type tracheoesophageal fistula.[420,421] Uncommon causes of chronic focal pneumonias include intralobar sequestration, an enteric-respiratory tract fistula, congenital cystic adenomatoid malformation, and paralysis or eventration of the diaphragm.

Immunologic Deficiency Diseases

Recurrent or progressive bacterial pneumonias occur in many such diseases, particularly in hypogammaglobinemia and in chronic granulomatous disease (see Chapter 23).[422]

Recurrent Linear or Interstitial Infiltrates

Asthma

The most common cause of recurrent interstitial pneumonia is acute bronchial asthma or asthmatic bronchitis, discussed in Chapter 7. These diagnoses are sometimes not easy to make on only the second or third episode, especially if there is little wheezing and the signs of the precipitating infection are prominent.

Hypersensitivity Pneumonitis

Also called extrinsic alveolitis, this disease is caused by allergic reactions to a variety of inhalants. The syndrome of hypersensitivity pneumonitis has been reported in children as young as 18 months of age. These pneumonias are sometimes associated with peripheral eosinophilia, in which case they would be categorized as PIE syndrome (see earlier section). So-called "farmer's lung," caused by hypersensitivity to antigens encountered on a farm, can be chronic and occur without eosinophilia. Like most hypersensitivity pneumonias, it responds well to corticosteroid therapy and avoidance of the inciting antigen.[423]

Pneumonias in Children with AIDS

Infants and young children with HIV infection frequently have recurrent or chronic pneumonia, as discussed in Chapter 20. Typically, hepatosplenomegaly, generalized lymphadenopathy, and failure to thrive are also present.

The three types of pneumonia are especially associated with AIDS in young children:[424–426]

1. *Pneumocystis jiroveci* pneumonia, which is usually a subacute, diffuse interstitial pneumonia.
2. Lymphoid interstitial pneumonitis, which typically has a chronic, diffuse, nodular pattern, and is often associated with early clubbing and very high EBV IgG.[425]

3. A subset of children with HIV infection is prone to recurrent *S. pneumoniae* infection. In some cases, this presents as recurrent pneumonia, although they may also develop bacteremia or grow the pneumococcus from unusual sites, including the parotid gland, the cervical lymph nodes, and even long bones.

Diagnostic Approach

The relative priority of these tests depends on the etiologies suspected. The beginning of this chapter discusses the use of laboratory tests and diagnostic procedures for pneumonia.

Skin Tests

An intermediate strength tuberculin skin test should be done routinely in a patient with chronic or recurrent pneumonia. Positive histoplasmin or coccidioidin skin tests only indicate past infection and so are not helpful. Testing of urine for *Histoplasma* antigen is probably worthwhile, although a negative result does not rule out histoplasmosis. The skin test for blastomycosis is unreliable. In a large outbreak involving normal children, it was positive in only 40% of patients with clinically suspected acute blastomycosis, but a serologic test detected 77% of cases.[427]

Smear and Culture

Tracheal or bronchial secretions obtained by endoscopic procedures described later are probably the best material for smear and culture. Sputum may be available from older children or even preschoolers if they have chronic lung disease. Flexible bronchoscopy may provide helpful specimens in young children.

Serologic Tests for Fungi

Serologic tests for histoplasmosis and coccidioidomycosis are usually helpful. Serologic tests for blastomycosis and sporotrichosis may be available in a reference laboratory. Serologic testing for blastomycosis is insensitive.

Radiographic Studies

An esophagram is useful in infants or young children when compression of the trachea or a major bronchus is suspected. Aspiration, defects in swallowing, or an H-type tracheoesophageal fistula may be observed during fluoroscopy as the radiopaque material is swallowed. Computed tomography is useful to identify cysts or cavities within apparently solid masses. An aortogram can demonstrate aberrant bronchial arteries to a sequestered lung segment. Radioisotopic lung scanning may be appropriate to find suspected ventilation or perfusion abnormalities.

Endoscopic Procedures

Direct laryngoscopy can be done in young infants for diagnostic purposes and for obtaining secretions for examination. Bronchoscopy is especially useful to confirm suspected tracheomalacia, foreign body, or external compression of the trachobronchial tree. It is also useful to obtain secretions for microscopic examination and culture and to aspirate obstructing mucous plugs or secretions. Bronchial brushing is especially useful for documenting pulmonary infection with opportunistic pathogens in immunocompromised hosts.

Biopsies

Lung puncture and pleural biopsy are discussed at the beginning of this chapter. Open or thoracoscopic lung biopsy may be advisable in difficult cases of chronic pneumonia.

HIV Serology

In a young child, chronic or interstitial pneumonia, hepatosplenomegaly, failure to thrive, or other recurrent infections should suggest the possibility of perinatally-acquired HIV infection (Chapter 20). Other immune deficiencies should also be considered (Chapter 23).

■ PULMONARY TUBERCULOSIS

Definitions

Tuberculosis (TB) is complex, but understanding a few definitions can simplify things greatly. *TB exposure* is defined as contact with an infectious case in the previous 3 months. The exposed child has a negative tubeculin skin test (TST), a normal physical examination, and a negative chest x-ray. The skin test is negative even in children who have become infected because it takes the child a few weeks to mount a delayed-type hypersensitivity response. Because children younger than 4 years old are at increased risk of rapid progression to disease, they

are treated with isoniazid for 3 months and repeat skin testing is done at that time. If the repeat test is negative, isoniazid can be discontinued. The same can be done for older children, especially household contacts; alternatively, isonizaid therapy can be omitted and a repeat skin test performed in 3 months.

Patients with *latent TB infection* (LTBI) have a positive skin test but no signs or symptoms, and they have a negative chest x-ray. Treatment is indicated, usually with isoniazid for 9 months. In the past, this had been referred to as "preventive therapy," which is an oxymoron; the term "treatment of LTBI" is more accurate and is preferred. The goal of therapy in this case is to prevent the child from progressing to *TB disease* (definition following). Although the child with LTBI is infected with *M. tuberculosis*, the organism load is much lower than in patients with tuberculosis disease, and thus a single agent is usually sufficient. Persons with LTBI are not contagious.

TB disease (sometimes referred to as *active TB*) is defined as disease in a person with infection in whom symptoms, signs, or radiographic manifestations caused by *M. tuberculosis* are apparent. *Primary disease* occurs as a complication of the initial infection, and this is the usual case in children. *Secondary* or *reactivation disease* occurs after a period of dormancy and is typical of disease in adults. Tuberculosis disease may or may not be contagious depending on the patient's age, site of organ involvement, symptoms, and duration of effective therapy. Adults with pulmonary tuberculosis are often contagious and are the usual source of transmission of infection to children. Distinguishing disease from infection is critical, because treatment of disease requires multi-drug therapy to avoid the creation of resistant organisms, which can be disastrous both from the perspective of the individual patient and from a public health standpoint.

Typical Childhood TB

Most childhood TB in the United States now presents as hilar adenopathy with or without peripheral pneumonia or is discovered by skin testing, usually because of a possible exposure. The source case often acquired the disease outside the United States or from a high-risk area within, such as a jail or a nursing home.

TB Outbreaks

In populations where the disease is rare, the frequency of various tuberculous presentations can be judged by outbreaks, which typically occur after a highly contagious index case joins a susceptible group.[428,429] In a British outbreak in 1984, there were 32 children found to have TB after contact with a woman who had extensive bilateral cavitary disease.[428] Of the 32 children, 75% had hilar adenopathy alone, 6% had tuberculous pneumonia, 6% had miliary tuberculosis, and 13% had a positive TST with a negative chest roentgenogram.

In an Oregon high school outbreak, the source case was a Korean teenager who had lived in the United States for one year.[429] When she was discovered to have cavitary tuberculosis, tuberculin testing of classroom contacts revealed 16 non-foreign-born classmates who were tuberculin positive. LTBI treatment was given, but four new cases of pulmonary tuberculosis developed, apparently in individuals who did not take the medication properly. More recently, 5 New York elementary school bus drivers were found to have TB. As a result, 3300 students in 49 schools were exposed. Amazingly, contact investigation revealed that only one of the bus drivers transmitted the infection to anyone; 10% of his contacts were skin test positive, and one case of active pulmonary disease in a child was discovered.[430]

Primary ("Ghon") Complex

The second most common form of childhood pulmonary tuberculosis (after isolated hilar adenopathy) is a peripheral pulmonary infiltrate with hilar adenopathy, often called the primary complex or the Ghon complex (Fig. 8-8). The hilar nodes may show calcium deposition, which usually indicates that the complex has been present at least 6 months but it may occur by as early as 2 months. Tuberculous nodes may compress a bronchus, resulting in atelectasis, or may erode through the bronchus, producing airway spread of the disease. Compression of the esophagus causing dysphagia may also occur. Bronchial obstruction may produce emphysema or, more commonly, a segmental fan-shaped x-ray lesion. Bronchial compression can cause wheezing and the child may be incorrectly diagnosed with asthma.

Laboratory Evaluation

Young children often do not cough and produce sputum. Although gastric washings can be done, searching for the contact source (usually a family member) and obtaining the isolate from that person's sputum is usually quicker and more reliable. This is best facilitated by prompt reporting of cases to the local health department. The yield from gastric washings, if properly done, may be as high as 40%; it is even higher in infants. Washings must be done first thing in the morning, just as the child is awakening, before the swallowed secretions from the previous night have left the stomach. Because *M. tuberculosis* is sensitive to sodium, a saline-free solution, such as sterile water, must be used. They should be done on three consecutive days. If a skilled bronchoscopist is available, that procedure may be done instead. A positive acid-fast stain from sputum, gastric washings, or bronchoscopy indicates the presumptive diagnosis of tuberculosis and means an isolate will likely be cultured that can be used for susceptibility testing.

DNA hybridization methods allow for immediate speciation and can be useful to separate *M. tuberculosis* from other mycobacteria. However, they are expensive, their sensitivity is not higher than culture, and they do not provide information regarding susceptibility. Nontuberculous mycobacteria are unlikely except in immunosuppressed patients and children with chronic cervical adenitis.

Tuberculin Skin Test

Indications

Persons in high-risk groups should have tuberculin tests yearly. The primary purpose of such routine testing is early recognition of tuberculous infection so that treatment can be given before progression or dissemination occurs. The other indications for testing are symptoms compatible with TB disease (e.g., chronic cough, fever, and lower respiratory tract disease) and suspected or known exposure to TB. A 48- to 72-hour follow-up examination for the illness is usually required, at which time the results of the test can be ascertained. It is wise to place a TST on patients with fever of unknown origin, even in the absence of respiratory symptoms. Children with presumed bacterial pneumonia who fail to respond to empiric antimicrobial therapy should have a TST placed. In the instance when primary pulmonary tuberculosis presents as pneumonia, the tuberculin test will be positive at its onset.

Routine screening of patients who are at low risk for tuberculosis (such as for school entry or at well-baby check-ups) is inappropriate; greater than 90% of all positive tests in such low-risk populations are falsely positive.[431] Because there is no follow-up

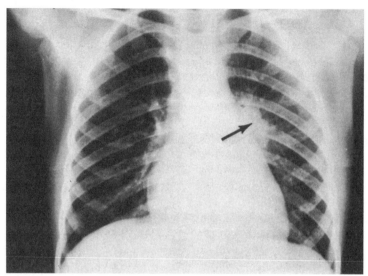

■ **FIGURE 8-8** Hilar adenopathy (*arrow*) with diffuse pneumonia in child with a primary complex caused by tuberculosis. (Photo courtesy of Dr. Justin Wolfson).

diagnostic test, all patients who test positive must receive 9 months of isoniazid (INH) therapy ("a decision to test is a decision to treat"). The Centers for Disease Control and Prevention (CDC) and the American Academy of Pediatrics (AAP) have long recommended abandonment of routine tuberculin testing in schools.[432,433]

The optimal way of controlling the disease is with thorough outbreak investigations and prompt and effective therapy for cases of TB disease. A child with LTBI is a harbinger that there is an untreated adult with contagious TB disease in the community. When a new case of active TB is recognized, the close contacts should have tuberculin tests and chest roentgenograms. The tuberculin-negative patients who are younger than 4 years old should then be given INH for 3 months with periodic evaluation before then, depending on their reliability and the risk.[434] If the TST and chest roentgenogram remain negative after 3 months, INH can be discontinued.

Methods

Unless otherwise specified, TST refers to the administration of 5 Tuberculin Units (intermediate strength) of purified proteins of the organism.[435] There are two methods of applying the antigen to the skin. The intradermal injection, called the Mantoux test, is the gold standard method and should always be used. Multiple-puncture methods should be abandoned because the amount of antigen on the tines is not standardized, which makes interpretation of the tests difficult.[436]

A convenient location for the test is midway between the wrist and elbow creases on the ulnar side of the right arm, using 0.1 mL of diluted purified protein derivative (PPD). The diluted PPD does not change in potency when stored at refrigerator temperature for up to 9 months except for a slight drop in potency the first day or so.[437] However, there is a risk of loss of potency through absorption of the antigen unless there has been stabilization with Tween.

Interpretation

The reaction should be measured at 48–72 hours and recorded in millimeters of induration (not erythema). Equivocal tests at 48 hours should be re-read at 72 hours, when nonspecific soft tissue swelling will have subsided. Interpretation of the TST is fraught with difficulty. Many experts believe that the ballpoint pen method is the most reliable way of measuring the diameter of the response. However, the area should be palpated first; there are no nerve endings at the tip of a ballpoint pen! Health care providers should read the TST. Studies have shown that parents frequently misread skin test results; in one high-risk population, only 22% of parents read skin test results accurately.[438]

Age, nutrition, concomitant viral infections, corticosteroid or other immunosuppressive therapy, and receipt of live virus vaccines can suppress the TST response. A 10-mm reaction was, at one time, considered positive regardless of circumstance. In an effort to increase both the sensitivity and the specificity of the test, however, newer guidelines suggest that the cut-off value should vary depending on epidemiologic and historical factors (Box 8-13).[439] Patients with known contact with contagious individuals, or those at high risk for dissemination should they become infected, are considered to have a positive TST if the reaction reaches 5 mm. For those who are at no particular risk and have no known exposure (i.e., those who, according to the CDC and AAP, should never have been tested in the first place), 15 mm is considered positive. For all others, the old standard of greater than or equal to 10 mm still applies.

It should be noted that there are certain parts of the country where exposure to non-tuberculous mycobacteria (NTM) in the soil is common. This type of exposure is likely to occasion a small reaction to a 5 TU PPD. Infection with one of the NTM (as, for example, in a cervical node) will produce a somewhat larger response (usually 6–9 mm). Sometimes, infection with NTM will produce a response greater than 15 mm, in which case interpretation may be difficult.[440] However, the majority of children infected with M. avium intracellulare (the most common of the NTMs in the United States) have responses less then 10 mm.[441]

Receipt of Bacille Calmette-Guerin (BCG) vaccine generally produces a response that is moderate and short-lived; most children who received BCG vaccine as newborns will have a negative TST by 3–5 years. Additionally, children who have a history of BCG receipt are usually from parts of the world where the prevalence of TB is very high; a positive test in such cases is more likely to result from exposure to TB than from a residual of BCG vaccination. Therefore, it is imperative that a positive TST not be ignored on the basis of past receipt of BCG vaccine. In fact, no modification of the guidelines is indicated: prior receipt of BCG vaccine should be disregarded.[442] A recent study in a pediatric population with high BCG vaccination coverage confirmed the utility of the TST in predicting true infection in this setting.[443]

Two other strengths of PPD are available but are seldom used. Measles vaccine, polio vaccine, measles, and chickenpox may temporarily suppress the tuberculin reaction,[435] but giving a vaccine and a tuberculin test on the same day does not invalidate the tuberculin test results.[432] Steroids or immunosuppressive agents also suppress the tuberculin reaction.

The accidental injection of the antigen subcutaneously, rather than the proper intradermal injection, is probably not an important source of error. In one study of children with primary pulmonary TB, the extent of induration was not significantly different in concurrently administered intradermal and subcutaneous intermediate-strength PPD tests.[444] Furthermore, 0.05 mL is as accurate as 0.1 mL when given intradermally.[445]

Anergy

A positive TST indicates past or present infection but is not useful as a guide to immunity. Individuals with a positive tuberculin test who have received 9 months of INH chemotherapy can be regarded as relatively immune but might have reactivation of disease under adverse host conditions. A negative TST is a relatively reliable indicator of susceptibility but can be the result of suppression by a disease such as chickenpox or rubella.

Tuberculin anergy (failure to react to the TST when infection is present) is not rare in adults. In

---

BOX 8-13 ■ Cut-Off Values for Positive Tuberculin Skin Test

5 mm
Children in close contact with known or suspected contagious tuberculosis
Children suspected to have tuberculosis disease, based on chest x-ray abnormalities or clinical evidence of tuberculosis

10 mm
Children at risk of dissemination, including those younger than age 4 years and those who have medical conditions such as HIV infection, diabetes, renal failure, or solid tumors
Children with increased exposure, including frequent exposure to HIV-infected persons, drug users, incarcerated persons, migrant farm workers, or nursing home residents
Children from areas endemic for tuberculosis and children who have contact with adults from these areas (Asia, Middle East, Africa, Latin America)

15 mm
Children 4 years of age and over without risk factors

one study, 25% of 200 adults with active pulmonary TB had less than 10 mm of induration in response to intermediate-strength PPD. The frequency of tuberculin anergy in children has not been adequately studied. Specific tuberculin anergy in adults in most cases appears to be a result of circulating inhibitors rather than loss of T cells or lack of T-cell sensitization.[446] Control antigens such as candida have been simultaneously applied in order to test general T-cell reactivity to antigens to which the child has previously been exposed. However, this practice is ineffective and is no longer recommended.[447] In some cases, anergy to *M. tuberculosis* is specific, which falsely leads the physician to believe that TB has been excluded from the differential diagnosis. A negative TST never excludes the diagnosis of tuberculosis. In fact, children with miliary or meningeal tuberculosis often have a negative TST. Children who are able to develop a delayed-type hypersensitivity response to tuberculosis (which the TST measures) are likely to be able to control the infection and usually present with either LTBI or granulomas in the lung or lymph nodes. In contrast, children who develop disseminated disease have been unable to mount a sufficient cell-mediated immune response to infection with *M. tuberculosis* and often will not respond to TST either.

Booster Effect

A booster effect may be observed when two tuberculin tests are given a week apart in individuals who have tuberculin hypersensitivity that has waned but is "boosted" by the first of the tests. The first test stimulates proliferation of memory T cells, so the second test is positive. The use of two tuberculin tests a week apart has been recommended to determine the true tuberculin status of those who are routinely and repeatedly tested (such as health care workers), but this is not necessary for testing in children. In the absence of actual *M. tuberculosis* infection, receipt of multiple TSTs does not provide enough antigenic stimulation to cause a false-positive TST. However, if routine testing is done more frequently than every 2 years, the booster effect may result in false positives from past non-tuberculous mycobacterial exposure or from previous BCG.

Whole-Blood Interferon-Gamma Assay

In 2001, the FDA approved the QuantiFERON®-TB test as an aid to the diagnosis of LTBI. The assay measures the amount of interferon-gamma released from sensitized lymphocytes after overnight incubation with PPD. A study of 1226 adults showed that the test performed well in comparison with TST and was better able to distinguish LTBI from a response to NTM and from previous BCG.[448] Other studies have reported less satisfactory results, particularly in patients with TB disease. The test has not yet been evaluated in children. CDC has published guidelines for use of the test as an adjunct to TST in detecting LTBI.[449] It should not be used in patients being evaluated for TB disease, as active TB is associated with suppression of the interferon-gamma response.

Management of LTBI in Children

Tuberculin "convertors" are defined as individuals who have had their TST change from negative to positive within the past 2 years. Tuberculin "reactors" are defined as individuals who have a positive TST.

By virtue of their young age, infants and children younger than 4 years old with LTBI have by definition been infected recently and are at high risk of progression to disease. Isoniazid therapy for LTBI appears to be more effective for children than adults, with several large clinical trials demonstrating risk-reduction of 70–90%.

INH at 10–15 mg/kg/day up to a maximum dose of 300 mg per day for 9 months is the currently favored regimen for patients with LTBI that is known or presumed to be due to an INH-sensitive strain. Therapy is instituted when a patient has met the guidelines for a positive TST, based on exposure history, age, and degree of risk (Box 8-13).

Every effort should be made to determine the strain's susceptibilities. This is usually accomplished by testing the strain isolated from the source case's sputum. If INH resistance in the source case's isolate is strongly suspected, rifampin should be added initially. For LTBI therapy in children when the source case is known to be infected with an INH-resistant organism, the AAP recommends a 6-month course of rifampin,[439] although this regimen has not been studied in children. Treatment of LTBI caused by multi-drug resistant strains should be performed in consultation with a TB expert.

Treatment of TB Disease

Empiric therapy of TB disease in children should be with at least 3 drugs (usually isoniazid, rifampin, and pyrazinamide). If suspicion for resistance in the source case is high, ethambutol should be added as well. All patients with TB disease in the United States should receive directly observed therapy (DOT), which means that a dispassionate third party (not a family member) observes the patient taking the medication. Guidelines for the treatment of TB disease are published and periodically updated by the CDC (www.cdc.gov).[434] Because of its complexity, TB disease should generally be managed with the assistance of a TB expert.

Use of Bacille Calmette-Guerin Vaccine

Efficacy

BCG is the most commonly administered vaccine in the world. It is currently given to newborns in over 100 countries.[450] BCG vaccine is effective at reducing disseminated infection and meningitis due to *M. tuberculosis*.[451] Studies regarding its efficacy in the prevention of pulmonary TB, however, have varied greatly. BCG does not prevent infection with *M. tuberculosis*. Variation in potency of different substrains of the vaccine also occurs. Controlled trials before 1955 using different BCG strains indicated protection of 0–80% of recipients. Because lasting protection is not assured, TB should always be considered as a possible cause of TB-like disease in BCG-vaccinated persons.

BCG vaccine is seldom used in the United States.[452] Its use can be recommended in the rare situation of constant exposure to a person with contagious pulmonary TB who is either being poorly treated or who is infected with a multiply drug-resistant strain, and when removal from exposure is not feasible. In these situations, physical separation is preferable. A TST should be done to ascertain tuberculin negativity before administration of BCG except in infants younger than 2 months of age.

Complications and Side Effects

BCG vaccination is generally well tolerated. Regional lymphadenitis, which sometimes progresses to a cold abscess, sometimes occurs. It is more common in children with HIV infection.[453] Osteomyelitis is rare.[454] Disseminated disease due to BCG (sometimes called BCGosis) can occur in patients with immune deficiency, especially severe combined immune deficiency (SCID)[455] or interferon-gamma receptor deficiency.[456] Disease caused by BCG is often not responsive to INH, and therapy with rifampin and ethambutol or ethionamide should be considered before INH in a patient with significant disease.

Contraindications

Any individual with a known defect of cell-mediated immunity should not be given BCG. Skin infections, superficial abrasions, burns, and corticosteroid therapy are also contraindications. Concurrent administration of INH is a contraindication, since this usually prevents effective infection by the vaccine organism. BCG should not be given to tuberculin-positive persons.

Public Health Considerations

Childhood TB is a public health emergency, as it represents ongoing transmission and failure of control measures in the community. Thus, every case of suspected TB disease should be promptly reported to the local health agency. In addition, LTBI in children younger than 4 years old should also be reported, since by virtue of their young age, acquisition (and thus transmission) has been relatively recent.

■ REFERENCES

1. McIntosh K. Community-acquired pneumonia in children. N Engl J Med 2002;346:429–37.
2. McCarthy PL, Spiesel SZ, Stashwick CA, et al. Radiographic findings and etiologic diagnosis in ambulatory childhood pneumonias. Clin Pediatr 1981;20:686–91.
3. Osborne D. Radiologic appearance of viral disease of the lower respiratory tract in infants and children. AJR 1978; 130:29–33.
4. Pratter MR, Irwin RS. The optimal approach to identifying the cause of lower respiratory tract infection: a resolvable controversy [editorial]. Chest 1983;83:714–5.
5. Fitzpatrick SB, March B, Stokes D, et al. Indications for flexible fiberoptic bronchoscopy in pediatric patients. Am J Dis Child 1983;137:595–7.
6. Pollock HM, Hawkins EL, Bonner JR, et al. Diagnosis of bacterial pulmonary infections with quantitative protected catheter cultures obtained during bronchoscopy. J Clin Microbiol 1983;17:255–9.
7. Brook I. Bacterial colonization, tracheobronchitis, and pneumonia following tracheostomy and long–term intubation in pediatric patients. Chest 1979;76:420–4.
8. Mimica I, Donoso E, Howard JE, et al. Lung puncture in the etiological diagnosis of pneumonia. Am J Dis Child 1971;122:278–82.
9. Pratter MR, Irwin RS. Transtracheal aspirations: guidelines for safety. Chest 1979;76:518–20.
10. Sherman MP, Goetzman BW, Ahlfors CE, et al. Tracheal aspiration and its clinical correlates in the diagnosis of congenital pneumonia. Pediatrics 1980;65:258–63.

11. Morris AJ, Tanner DC, Reller LB. Rejection criteria for endotracheal aspirates from adults. J Clin Microbiol 1993;31:1027–9.

12. Slagle TA, Bifano EM, Wolf JW, Gross SJ. Routine endotracheal cultures for the prediction of sepsis in ventilated babies. Arch Dis Child 1989;64:34–8.

13. Dowell SF, Garman RL, Liu G, et al. Evaluation of Binax NOW, an assay for the detection of pneumococcal antigen in urine samples, performed among pediatric patients. Clin Infect Dis 2001;32:824–5.

14. Wilson GJ, Dermody TS. Respiratory infections in immunocompromised children. Semin Pediatr Infect Dis 1995;6:156–65.

15. de Blic J, Midulla F, Barbato A, et al. Bronchoalveolar lavage in children. ERS Task Force on bronchoalveolar lavage in children. Eur Respir J 2000;15:217–31.

16. Wolff LJ, Bartlett MS, Baehner RL, et al. The causes of interstitial pneumonia in immunocompromised children: an aggressive systematic approach to diagnosis. Pediatrics 1977;60:41–5.

17. Stillwell PC, Cooney DR, Telander RL, et al. Limited thoracotomy in the pediatric patient. Mayo Clin Proc 1981;56:673–7.

18. Ellis ME, Spence D, Bouchama A, et al. Open lung biopsy provides a higher and more specific diagnostic yield compared to broncho-alveolar lavage in immunocompromised patients. Scand J Infect Dis 1995;27:157–62.

19. Jenkins R, Meyerowitz RL, Kavic T, et al. Diagnostic yield of transbronchoscopic biopsies. Am J Clin Pathol 1979;72:926–30.

20. Dichter JR, Levine SJ, Shelhamer JH. Approach to the immunocompromised host with pulmonary symptoms. Hematol Oncol Clin North Am 1993;7:887–912.

21. King EG, Bachynski JE, Mielke B. Percutaneous trephine lung biopsy. Chest 1976;70:212–6.

22. Rodgers BM, Moazam F, Talbert JL. Thorascopy in children. Ann Surg 1979;189:176–80.

23. Nagaoki K. Usefulness of chest CT in diagnosing pneumonia [Japanese]. Nippon Igaku Hoshasen Gakka Zasshi-Nippon Acta Radiologica 1997;57:258–64.

24. Correa AG. Diagnostic approach to pneumonia in children. Semin Resp Infect 1996;11:131–8.

25. Bain HW, McClean DM, Walker SJ. Epidemic pleurodynia (Bornholm disease) due to Coxsackie B5 virus. Pediatrics 1961;27:889–903.

26. Rose RW, Ward BH. Spherical pneumonias in children stimulating pulmonary and mediastinal masses. Radiology 1973;106:119–82.

27. Kantor HG. The many radiologic faces of pneumococcal pneumonia. AJR 1981;137:1213–20.

28. Toikka P, Virkki R, Jussi M, et al. Bacteremic pneumococcal pneumonia in children. Clin Infect Dis 1999;29:568–72.

29. Shinefield HR, Black S. Efficacy of pneumococcal conjugate vaccines in large scale field trials. Pediatr Infect Dis J 2000;19:394–7.

30. Ginsburg CM, Howard JB, Nelson JD. Report of 65 cases of *Haemophilus influenzae* b pneumonia. Pediatrics 1979;74:283–6.

31. Asmar BI, Slovis TL, Reed JO, et al. *Haemophilus influenzae* type b pneumonia in 43 children. J Pediatr 1978;93:389–93.

32. Chartrand SA, McCracken GH Jr. Staphylococcal pneumonia in infants and children. Pediatr Infect Dis 1982;1:19–23.

33. Kevy SV, Lowe BA. Streptococcal pneumonia and empyema in childhood. N Engl J Med 1961;264:738–43.

34. Trujillo M, McCracken GH. Prolonged morbidity in children with group A beta-hemolytic streptococcal pneumonia. Pediatr Infect Dis J 1982;1:19–23.

35. Cockcroft DW, Stilwell GA. Lobar pneumonia caused by *Mycoplasma pneumoniae*. Can Med Assoc J 1981;124:1463–8.

36. Shingadia D, Novelli V. Diagnosis and treatment of tuberculosis in children. Lancet Infect Dis 2003;3:624–32.

37. Witt D, Olans RN. Bacteremic W135 meningococcal pneumonia. Am Rev Respir Dis 1982;125:255–7.

38. Martone WJ, Marshall LW, Kaufmann AF, et al. Tularemia pneumonia in Washington, DC. JAMA 1979;242:2315–7.

39. Patt HA, Feigin RD. Diagnosis and management of suspected cases of bioterrorism: a pediatric perspective. Pediatrics 2002;109:685–92.

40. Bryan CS. Treatment of pneumococcal pneumonia: the case for penicillin G. Am J Med 1999;107:63S–68S.

41. MacGowan AP, Bowker KE. Continuous infusion of beta-lactam antibiotics. Clin Pharmacokinet 1998;35:391–402.

42. Pallares R, Linares J, Vadillo M, et al. Resistance to penicillin and cephalosporin and mortality from severe pneumococcal pneumonia in Barcelona, Spain. N Engl J Med 1995;333:474–80.

43. Performance standards for antimicrobial susceptibility testing: twelfth informational supplement. Wayne, Pa. Document number M100-S12. NCCLS 2002;22:110–2.

44. Hardie WD, Roberts NE, Reising SF, Christie CD. Complicated parapneumonic effusions in children caused by penicillin-nonsusceptible *Streptococcus pneumoniae*. Pediatrics 1998;101:388–92.

45. Davidson R, Cavalcanti R, Brunton JL, et al. Resistance to levofloxacin and failure of treatment of pneumococcal pneumonia. N Engl J Med 2002;346:747–50.

46. Britton S, Bejstedt M, Vedin L. Chest physiotherapy in primary pneumonia. Br Med J 1985;290:1703–4.

47. Kirilloff LH, Owns GR, Rogers RM, et al. Does chest physical therapy work? Chest 1985;88:436–44.

48. Feld LG, Springate JE, Darragh R, Fildes RD. Pneumococcal pneumonia and hemolytic uremic syndrome. Pediatr Infect Dis J 1987;6:693–5.

49. Erickson LC, Smith WS, Biswas AK, et al. *Streptococcus pneumoniae*-induced hemolytic uremic syndrome: a case for early diagnosis. Pediatr Nephrol 1994;8:211–3.

50. Gilbert RD, Argent AC. *Streptococcus pneumoniae*-associated hemolytic uremic syndrome. Pediatr Infect Dis J 1998;17:530–2.

51. Johnston I, Strachan DA, Anderson HR. Effect of pneumonia and whooping cough in childhood on adult lung function. N Engl J Med 1998;338:581–7.

52. Grossman LK, Wald ER, Nair P, et al. Roentgenographic followup of acute pneumonia in children. Pediatrics 1979;63:30–1.

53. Peterman TA, Speicher CE. Evaluating pleural effusions: a two-stage laboratory approach. JAMA 1984;252:1051–3.

54. Hamm H, Light RW. Parapneumonic effusion and empyema. Eur Respir J 1997;10:1150–6.

55. Fleisher GR, Fichman KR, Honig PJ. Hemothorax in a child. Clin Pediatr 1978;17:300–2.

56. Marks WM, Filly RA, Callen PW. Realtime evaluation of pleural lesions: new observations regarding the probability of obtaining free fluid. Radiology 1982;142:163–4.

57. Dorne HL. Differentiation of pulmonary parenchymal consolidation from pleural disease using the sonographic fluid bronchogram. Radiology 1986;158:41–2.

58. Willford ME, Hidalgo H, Putman CE, et al. Computed tomography of pleural disease. AJR 1983;140:909–14.

59. Woodring JH. Recognition of pleural effusion on supine radiographs: how much fluid is required? AJR 1984;142:59–64.

60. Oestreich AE, Haley C. Pleural effusion: the thorn sign: not a rare finding. Chest 1981;79:365–6.

61. Health and Public Policy Committee. Diagnostic thoracentesis and pleural biopsy in pleural effusions. Ann Intern Med 1985;103:799–802.

62. Stewart JR, Sarr MG. Thoracentesis. Surg Gynecol Obstet 1985;161:381–2.

63. Sahn SA, Light RW. The sun should never set on a parapneumonic effusion. Chest 1989;95:945–7.

64. Bouros D, Schiza S, Tzanakis N, et al. Intrapleural urokinase versus normal saline in the treatment of complicated parapneumonic effusions and empyema: a randomized, double-blind study. Am J Respir Crit Care Med 1999;159:37–42.

65. Bouros D, Schiza S, Patsourakis G, et al. Intrapleural streptokinase versus urokinase in the treatment of complicated parapneumonic effusions: a prospective, double-blind study. Am J Respir Crit Care Med 1997;155:291–5.

66. Davies RJ, Traill ZC, Gleeson FV. Randomised controlled trial of intrapleural streptokinase in community acquired pleural infection. Thorax 1997;52:416–21.

67. Krishnan S, Amin N, Dozor AJ, Stringel G. Urokinase in the management of complicated parapneumonic effusions in children. Chest 1997;112:1579–83.

68. Cameron R. Intra-pleural fibrinolytic therapy vs. conservative management in the treatment of parapneumonic effusions and empyema. Cochrane Database Syst Rev 2000 3:CD002312.

69. Levine H, Metzger W, Lacera D, et al. Diagnosis of tuberculous pleurisy by culture of pleural biopsy specimen. Ann Intern Med 1970;126:269–71.

70. Buckingham SC, King MD, Miller ML. Incidence and etiologies of complicated parapneumonic effusions in children. Pediatr Infect Dis J 2003;22:499–504.

71. Lincoln EM, Davies PA, Bovornkitti S. Tuberculous pleurisy with effusion in children: a study of 202 children with particular reference to prognosis. Am Rev Tuberc 1958;77:271–89.

72. Grix A, Giammona S. Pneumonitis with pleural effusion in children due to *Mycoplasma pneumoniae*. Am Rev Respir Dis 1974;109:665–71.

73. Fine NL, Smith LIZ, Sheedy PF. Frequency of pleural effusions in mycoplasma and viral pneumonias. N Engl J Med 1970;283:790–3.

74. Brolin L, Wernstedt L. Radiographic appearance of *mycoplasmal pneumoniae*. Scand J Resp Dis 1978;59:179–89.

75. George RB, Ziskind MM, Rasch JR, et al. Mycoplasma and adenovirus pneumonias: comparison with other atypical pneumonias in a military population. Ann Intern Med 1966;65:931–42.

76. Cho CT, Hiatt WO, Behbehani AM, et al. Pneumonia and massive pleural effusion associated with adenovirus type 7. Am J Dis Child 1973;126:92–4.

77. Fermaglich DR. Pulmonary involvement in infectious mononucleosis. J Pediatr 1975;86:93–5.

78. Andiman WA, McCarthy P, Markowitz RI, et al. Clinical, virologic, and serologic evidence of Epstein-Barr virus infection in association with childhood pneumonia. J Pediatr 1981;99:880–6.

79. Cocchi P, Silenzi M. Pleural effusion in HBsAG positive hepatitis. J Pediatr 1976;89:329–30.

80. Alhan E, Yildizdas D, Yapicioglu H, Necmi A. Pleural effusion associated with acute hepatitis A infection. Pediatr Infect Dis J 1999;18:1111–2.

81. Kamer HP, Treen B, Pankey GA, et al. Pleural effusion and anicteric hepatitis associated with cat scratch disease: documentation by cat scratch bacillus. Chest 1986;89:302–3.

82. Bowsher B, Callahan CW, Person DA, Ruess L. Unilateral leptospiral pneumonia and cold agglutinin disease. Chest 1999;116:830–2.

83. Paradisis M, Van Asperen P. Yellow nail syndrome in infancy. J Paediatr Child Health 1997;33:454–7.

84. Murphy D, Lockhart CH, Todd JK. Pneumococcal empyema: outcome of medical management. Am J Dis Child 1980;134:659–62.

85. Molteni RA. Group A beta-hemolytic streptococcal pneumonia: clinical course and complications of management. Am J Dis Child 1977;131:1366–71.

86. Fajardo JE, Chang MJ. Pleural empyema in children. South Med J 1987;80:593–6.

87. Freij BJ, Kusmeisz H, Nelson JD, McCracken GH Jr. Parapneumonic effusions and empyema in hospitalized children: a retrospective review of 227 cases. Pediatr Infect Dis J 1984;3:578–90.

88. Schulz KD, Fan LL, Pinsky J, et al. The changing face of pleural empyemas in children:epidemilogy and management 2004;113:1735–40.

89. Feldman KA, Enscore RE, Lathrop SL, et al. An outbreak of primary pneumonic tularemia on Martha's Vineyard. N Engl J Med 2001;345:1601–6.

90. Wolfe WG, Spock A, Bradford WD. Pleural fluid in infants and children. Am Rev Respir Dis 1968;98:1027–32.

91. Burney DP, Fisher RD, Schaffner W. *Salmonella* empyema: a review. South Med J 1977;70:375–7.

92. Goldenberg RI, Gushurst C, Controni G, et al. *Pasteurella multocida* pleural empyema. J Pediatr 1978;93:994–5.

93. Krober MS, Bass JW, Barcia PJ. Scarlatiniform rash and pleural effusion in a patient with *Yersinia pseudotuberculosis* infection. J Pediatr 1983;102:879–81.

94. Stutman HR, Rettig PJ, Reyes S. *Chlamydia trachomatis* as a cause of pneumonitis and pleural effusion. J Pediatr 1984;104:588–91.

95. Zawadsky PM, Reissman SE. *Listeria* pleural effusion in a noncompromised host. J Fam Pract 1985;20:79–80.

96. Landay MJ, Christensen EE, Bynum LJ, et al. Anaerobic pleural and pulmonary infections. AJR 1980;134:233–40.

97. Raff NU, Johnson JD, Nagar D, et al. Spontaneous clos-

tridial empyema and pyopneumothorax. Rev Infect Dis 1984;6:715–9.

98. Chesney PJ, Gourley GR, Peters ME, et al. Pulmonary blastomycosis in children. Am J Dis Child 1979;133: 1134–9.

99. Pinckney L, Parker BR. Primary coccidioidomycosis in children presenting with massive pleural effusion. AJR 1978;130:247–9.

100. Weissbluth M. Pleural effusion in histoplasmosis [letter]. J Pediatr 1976;88:894–5 and 1977;90:326–7.

101. Kinasewitz GT, Penn RL, George RB. The spectrum and significance of pleural disease in blastomycosis. Chest 1984;86:580–4.

102. Straus SE, Jacobson ES. The spectrum of histoplasmosis in a general hospital: a review of 55 cases diagnosed at Barnes Hospital between 1966 and 1977. Am J Med Sci 1980;279:147–58.

103. Bayer AS. Fungal pneumonias: pulmonary coccidioidal syndromes (part I). Chest 1981;79:575–83.

104. Young EJ, Hirsh DD, Fainstein V, et al. Pleural effusion due to *Cryptococcus neoformans*: a review of the literature and report of two cases with cryptococcal antigen determinations. Am Rev Respir Dis 1980;121:743–7.

105. Kubitschek KR, Peters J, Nickeson D, et al. Amebiasis presenting as pleuropulmonary disease. West J Med 1985;142:203–7.

106. Romeo DP, Pollock JJ. Pulmonary paragonimiasis: diagnostic value of pleural fluid analysis. South Med J 1986; 79:241–3.

107. Beckman JF, Bosniak S, Canter HG. Eosinophilia and elevated IgE concentrations in a serous pleural effusion following trauma. Am Rev Respir Dis 1974;110:484–9.

108. Halkin A, Jaffe R, Mevorach D, Bursztyn M. Thoracic complications following snake envenomization. Am J Med 1997;102:585–7.

109. Rosenberg HK, Berezin S, Heyman S, et al. Pleural effusion and ascites: unusual presenting features in a pediatric patient with vitamin A intoxication. Clin Pediatr 1982; 21:435–40.

110. Law DK, Murr P, Bailey WC. Empyema: a rare presentation of perforated appendicitis. JAMA 1978;240:2566–7.

111. Huang J, Yang J, Ding J. Pulmonary embolism associated with nephrotic syndrome in children: a preliminary report of 8 cases. Chin Med J 2000;113:251–3.

112. Vichinsky EP, Neumayr LD, Earles AN, et al. Causes and outcomes of the acute chest syndrome in sickle cell disease. N Engl J Med 2000;342:1855–65.

113. van Ommen CH, Heyboer H, Groothoff JW, et al. Persistent tachypnea in children: keep pulmonary embolism in mind. J Pediatr Hematol Oncol 1998;20:570–3.

114. Kjellin IB, Boechat MI, Vinuela F, et al. Pulmonary emboli following therapeutic embolization of cerebral arteriovenous malformations in children. Pediatr Radiol 2000;30: 279–83.

115. Nuss R, Hays T, Chudgar U, Manco-Johnson M. Antiphospholipid antibodies and coagulation regulatory protein abnormalities in children with pulmonary emboli. J Pediatr Hematol Oncol 1997;19:202–7.

116. Merino JM, Carpintero I, Alvarez T, et al. Tuberculous pleural effusion in children. Chest 1999;115:26–30.

117. Matthay RA, Neff TA, Iseman MD. Tuberculous pleural effusions developing during chemotherapy for pulmonary tuberculosis. Am Rev Respir Dis 1974;109:469–72.

118. Gribetz AR, Damsker B, Marchevsky A, et al. Nontuberculous mycobacteria in pleural fluid: assessment of clinical significance. Chest 1985;87:495–8.

119. Sokal MM, Fisher BJ. Neonatal empyema caused by group B beta-hemolytic streptococcus. Chest 1982;81:390–1.

120. Meyer K, Girgis N, McGravey V. Adenovirus associated with congenital pleural effusion. J Pediatr 1985;107: 433–5.

121. Gustavson EE. *Escherichia coli* empyema in the newborn. Am J Dis Child 1986;140:408.

122. Amitai I, Mogle P, Godfrey S, et al. Pneumatocele in infants and children: report of 12 cases. Clin Pediatr 1983; 22:420–2.

123. Chitayat D, Diamant SH, Lazevnick R, et al. *Hemophilus influenzae* type b pneumonia with pneumatocele formation. Clin Pediatr 1980;19:151–2.

124. Kuhn JP, Lee SB. Pneumatoceles associated with *Escherichia coli* pneumonias in the newborn. Pediatrics 1973; 51:1008–11.

125. Asmar BI, Thirumoorthi MC, Dajani AS. Pneumococcal pneumonia with pneumatocele formation. Am J Dis Child 1978;132:1091–3.

126. Bergeson PS, Hales SW, Lustgarten MD, et al. Pneumatoceles following hydrocarbon ingestion: report of three cases and review of the literature. Am J Dis Child 1975; 129:49–54.

127. Luddy RE, Champion LAA, Schwartz AD. *Pneumocystis carinii* pneumonia with pneumatocele formation. Am J Dis Child 1977;131:470.

128. Westcott JL. Percutaneous catheter drainage of pleural effusion and empyema. AJR 1985;144:1189–93.

129. Roberts JS, Bratton SL, Brogan TV. Efficacy and complications of percutaneous pigtail catheters for thoracostomy in pediatric patients. Chest 1998;114:1116–21.

130. McLaughlin FJ, Goldmann DA, Rosenbaum DM, et al. Empyema in children: clinical course and longterm followup. Pediatrics 1984;73:587–93.

131. Rizalar R, Somuncu S, Bernay F, et al. Postpneumonic empyema in children treated by early decortication. Eur J Pediatr Surg 1997;7:135–7.

132. Doski JJ, Lou D, Hicks BA, et al. Management of parapneumonic collections in infants and children. J Pediatr Surg 2000;35:265–8.

133. Kornecki A, Sivan Y. Treatment of loculated pleural effusion with intrapleural urokinase in children. J Pediatr Surg 1997;32:1473–5.

134. Palavecino E. Community-acquired methicillin-resistant *Staphylococcus aureus* infections. Clin Lab Med 2004;24: 403–18.

135. Abshire TC. The anemia of inflammation. Pediatr Clin North Am 1996;43:623–37.

136. Osborne D. Radiologic appearance of viral disease of the lower respiratory tract in infants and children. AJR 1978; 130:29–33.

137. van den Hoogen BG, de Jong JC, Groen J, et al. A newly discovered human pneumovirus isolated from young children with respiratory tract disease. Nat Med 2001;7: 719–24.

138. Mufson MA, Manko MA, Kingston Jr, et al. Eaton agent pneumonia clinical features. JAMA 1961;178:369–74.

139. Broughton RA. Infections due to *Mycoplasma pneumoniae* in childhood. Pediatr Infect Dis 1986;5:71–85.

140. Andrews CE, Hopewell P, Burrell RE, et al. An epidemic of respiratory infection due to *Mycoplasma pneumoniae* in a civilian population. Am Rev Respir Dis 1967;95:972–9.

141. Nastro JA, Littner MR, Tashkin DP, et al. Diffuse, pulmonary interstitial infiltrate and mycoplasmal pneumonia. Am Rev Respir Dis 1974;110:659–62.

142. Broome CV, LaVenture M, Kaye HS, et al. An explosive outbreak of *Mycoplasma pneumoniae* infection in a summer camp. Pediatrics 1980;66:884–8.

143. Khatib R, Schnarr D. Pointsource outbreak of *Mycoplasma pneumoniae* infection in a family unit. J Infect Dis 1985; 151:186–7.

144. Brunner H, Prescott B, Greenberg H, et al. Unexpectedly high frequency of antibody to *Mycoplasma pneumoniae* in human sera as measured by sensitive techniques. J Infect Dis 1977;135:524–30.

145. Michelow IC, Olsen K, Lozano J. Epidemiology and clinical characteristics of community-acquired pneumonia in hospitalized children Pediatrics 2004;113:701–7.

146. Schaffner W, Drutz DJ, Duncan GW, et al. The clinical spectrum of endemic psittacosis. Arch Intern Med 1967; 119:433–43.

147. Centers for Disease Control. Psittacosis at a turkey processing plant–North Carolina, 1989. MMWR 1990;39: 460–9.

148. Aldous MB, Grayston JT, Wang SP, Foy HM. Seroepidemiology of *Chlamydia pneumoniae* TWAR infection in Seattle families, 1966-1979. J Infect Dis 1992;166:646–9.

149. Heiskanen-Kosma T, Korppi M, Laurila A, et al. *Chlamydia pneumoniae* is an important cause of community-acquired pneumonia in school-aged children: serological results of a prospective, population-based study. Scand J Infect Dis 1999;31:255–9.

150. Thom DH, Grayston JT, Wang SP, Kuo CC, Altman J. *Chlamydia pneumoniae* strain TWAR, *Mycoplasma pneumoniae*, and viral infections in acute respiratory disease in a university student health clinic population. Am J Epidemiol 1990;132:248–56.

151. Verkooyen RP, Willemse D, Hiep-van Casteren SC, et al. Evaluation of PCR, culture, and serololgy for the diagnosis of *Chlamydia pneumoniae* respiratory infections. J Clin Microbiol 1998;36:2301–7.

152. Menendez R, Cordoba J, de La Cuadra P, et al. Value of the polymerase chain reaction assay in noninvasive respiratory samples for diagnosis of community-acquired pneumonia. Am J Resp Crit Care Med 1999;159: 1868–73.

153. Hahn DL, Bukstein D, Luskin A, Zeitz H. Evidence for *Chlamydia pneumoniae* infection in steroid-dependent asthma. Ann Allergy Asthma Immunol 1998;80:45–9.

154. Cunningham AF, Johnston SL, Julious SA, et al. Chronic *Chlamydia pneumoniae* infection and asthma exacerbations in children. Eur Resp J 1998;11:345–9.

155. Emre U, Sokolovskaya N, Roblin PM, et al. Detection of anti-*Chlamydia pneumoniae* IgE in children with reactive airway disease. J Infect Dis 1995;172:265–7.

156. Emre U, Bernius M, Roblin PM, et al. *Chlamydia pneumoniae* infection in patients with cystic fibrosis. Clin Infect Dis 1996;22:819–23.

157. Halsted CC, Kulasinghe HP. Tularemia pneumonia in urban children. Pediatrics 1978;61:660–2.

158. James AG, Lang WR, Liang AY, et al. Adenovirus type 21 bronchopneumonia in infants and young children. J Pediatr 1979;95:530–3.

159. George RB, Mogabgab WJ. Atypical pneumonia in young men with rhinovirus infections. Ann Intern Med 1969; 71:1073–8.

160. Kohn JL, Koiransky H. Successive roentgenograms of the chest of children during measles. Am J Dis Child 1929; 28:258–70.

161. Dworsky ME, Stagno S. Newer agents causing pneumonitis in early infancy. Pediatr Infect Dis 1982;1:188–95.

162. Boyce TG, Wright PF. Cytomegalovirus pneumonia in two infants recently adopted from China. Clin Infect Dis 1999;28:1328–30.

163. Hull HF, Blumhagen JD, Benjamin D, et al. Herpes simplex viral pneumonitis in childhood. J Pediatr 1984;104: 211–5.

164. Dominguez R, Rivero H, Gaisie G, et al. Neonatal herpes simplex pneumonia: radiographic findings. Radiology 1984;153:395–9.

165. Tardieu M, Grospierre B, Durandy A, et al. Circulating immune complexes containing rubella antigens in late onset rubella syndrome. J Pediatr 1980;97:370–3.

166. Waterhouse BE, Lapidus PH. Infectious mononucleosis associated with a mass in the anterior mediastinum. N Engl J Med 1967;277:1137–8.

167. Dearth JC, Rhodes KH. Infectious mononucleosis complicated by severe *Mycoplasma pneumoniae* infection. Am J Dis Child 1980;134:744–6.

168. Rose HD, Franson TR, Sheth NK, et al. *Pseudomonas* pneumonia associated with use of a home whirlpool spa. JAMA 1983;250:2027–9.

169. Khoor A, Leslie KO, Tazelaar HD, Helmers RA, Colby TV. Diffuse pulmonary disease caused by nontuberculous mycobacteria in immunocompetent people (hot tub lung). Am J Clin Pathol 2001;115:755–62.

170. Embil J, Warren P, Yakrus M, et al. Pulmonary illness associated with exposure to *Mycobacterium-avium* complex in hot tub water. Hypersensitivity pneumonitis or infection? Chest 1997;111:813–6.

171. Maltezou HC, Raoult D. Q fever in children. Lancet Infect Dis 2002;2:686–91.

172. Borio L, Frank D, Mani V, et al. Death due to bioterrorism-related inhalational anthrax: report of 2 patients. JAMA 2001;286:2554–9.

173. Stagno S, Pifer LL, Hughes WT, et al. *Pneumocystis carinii* pneumonitis in young immunocompetent infants. Pediatrics 1980;66:56–62.

173a. Aviles R, Boyce TG, Thompson DM. *Pneumocystis carinii* pneumonia in a 3-month-old infant receiving high-dose corticosteroid therapy for airway hemangiomas. Mayo Clin Proc 2004;79:243–5.

174. Word BM, Baldridge A. *Mycoplasma hominis* pneumonia and pleural effusion in a postpartum adolescent. Pediatr Infect Dis J 1990;9:295–6.

175. Michael JR, Rudin ML. Acute pulmonary disease caused by phenytoin. Ann Intern Med 1981;95:452–4.

176. Young LE. The clinical significance of cold hemagglutinins. Am J Med Sci 1946;211:23–9.

177. Sussman SJ, Magoffin RL, Lennette EH, et al. Cold agglu-

tinins, Eaton agent, and respiratory infections of children. Pediatrics 1966;38:571–7.

178. Griffin JP. Rapid screening for cold agglutinins in pneumonia. Ann Intern Med 1969;70:701–5.

179. Waris ME, Toikka P, Saarinen T, et al. Diagnosis of *Mycoplasma pneumoniae* pneumonia in children. J Clin Microbiol 1998;36:3155–9.

180. Espy MJ, Hierholzer JC, Smith TF. The effect of centrifugation on the rapid detection of adenovirus in shell vials. Am J Clin Pathol 1987;88:358–60.

181. Ieven M, Demey H, Ursi D, et al. Fatal encephalitis caused by *Mycoplasma pneumoniae* diagnosed by the polymerase chain reaction. Clin Infect Dis 1998;27:1552–3.

182. Ellenbogen C, Graybill JR, Silva J Jr, et al. Bacterial pneumonia complicating adenoviral pneumonia: a comparison of respiratory tract bacterial culture sources and effectiveness of chemoprophylaxis against bacterial pneumonia. Am J Med 1974;56:169–78.

183. Turner RB, Lande AE, Chase P, et al. Pneumonia in pediatric outpatients: cause and clinical manifestations. J Pediatr 1987;111:194–200.

184. Shames JM, George RB, Holliday WB, et al. Comparison of antibiotics in the treatment of mycoplasmal pneumonia. Arch Intern Med 1970;125:680–4.

185. Stevens D, Swift PGF, Johnston PGB, et al. *Mycoplasma pneumoniae* infections in children. Arch Dis Child 1978;53:38–42.

186. Block S, Hedrick J, Hammerschlag MR, et al. *Mycoplasma pneumoniae* and *Chlamydia pneumoniae* in pediatric community-acquired pneumonia: comparative efficacy and safety of clarithroycin vs. erythromycin estolate. Pediatr Infect Dis J 1995;14:471–7.

187. Schonwald S, Gunjaca M, Kolacny-Babic L, et al. Comparison of azithromycin and erythromycin in the treatment of atypical pneumonias. J Antimicrob Chemother 1990;25 Suppl A:123–6.

188. Jensen KJ, Senterfit LB, Scully WE et al. *Mycoplasma pneumoniae* infections in children: an epidemiologic appraisal in families treated with oxytetracycline. Am J Epidemiol 1967;86:419–32.

189. Klausner JD, Passaro D, Rosenberg J, et al. Enhanced control of an outbreak of *Mycoplasma pneumoniae* pneumonia with azithromycin prophylaxis. J Infect Dis 1998;177:161–6.

190. Hodges GR, Fass RJ, Saslaw S. Central nervous system disease associated with *Mycoplasma pneumoniae* infection. Arch Intern Med 1972;130:277–82.

191. Rothstein TL, Kenny GE. Cranial neuropathy, myeloradiculopathy, and myositis: complications of *Mycoplasma pneumoniae* infection. Arch Neurol 1977;36:476–7.

192. Lambert HP. Syndrome with joint manifestations in association with *Mycoplasma pneumoniae* infection. Br Med J 1968;3:156–7.

193. Cimolai N, Malleson P, Thomas E, Middleton PJ. *Mycoplasma pneumoniae* associated arthropathy: confirmation of the association by determination of the antipolypeptide IgM response. J Rheumatol 1989;16:1150–2.

194. Maisel JD, Babbitt LH, John TJ. Fatal *Mycoplasma pneumoniae* infection with isolation of organisms from lung. JAMA 1967;202:287–90.

195. Turtzo DF, Ghatak PK. Acute hemolytic anemia with *Mycoplasma pneumoniae* pneumonia. JAMA 1976;236:1140–1.

196. Stephan JL, Galambrun C, Pozzetto B, Grattard F, Bordigoni P. Aplastic anemia after *Mycoplasma pneumoniae* infection: a report of two cases. J Pediatr Hematol Oncol 1999;21:299–302.

197. Chiou CC, Liu YC, Lin HH, Hsieh KS. *Mycoplasma pneumoniae* infection complicated by lung abscess, pleural effusion, thrombocytopenia, and disseminated intravascular coagulation. Pediatr Infect Dis J 1997;16:327–9.

198. Goudie BM, Kerr MR, Johnson RN. *Mycoplasma* pneumonia complicated by bronchiectasis. J Infect Dis 1983;7:151–2.

199. Tay YK, Huff JC, Weston WL. *Mycoplasma pneumoniae* infection is associated with Stevens-Johnson syndrome, not erythema multiforme (von Hebra). J Amer Acad Dermatol 1996;35:757–60.

200. Parenti DM, Steinberg W, Kang P. Infectious causes of acute pancreatitis. Pancreas 1996;13:356–71.

201. Heiskanen-Kosma T, Korppi M, Laurila A, et al. *Chlamydia pneumoniae* is an important cause of community-acquired pneumonia in school-aged children: serological results of a prospective, population-based study. Scand J Infect Dis 1999;31:255–9.

202. Dagan R, Hall CB, Menegus MA. Atypical bacterial infections explained by a concomitant virus infection. Pediatrics 1985;76:411–4.

203. Santosham M, Yolken RH, Quiroz E, et al. Detection of rotavirus in respiratory secretions of children with pneumonia. J Pediatr 1983;103:583–5.

204. Gould DM, Dalrymple GV. Radiologic analysis of disseminated lung disease. Am J Med Sci 1959;238:621–37.

205. Felson B. Acute miliary disease of the lung. Radiology 1952;59:32–48.

206. Buechner HA. The differential diagnosis of miliary diseases of the lungs. Med Clin North Am 1959;43:89–112.

207. Medlar EM, Pesquera GS, Ordway WH. A comparison of roentgenograms with the pathology of experimental pulmonary tuberculosis in the rabbit. Am Rev Tuberc 1944;50:1–23.

208. Scadding JG. Chronic lung disease with diffuse nodular or reticular radiographs shadows. Tubercle 1952;33:352–65.

209. Herman PG, Hillman B, Pinkus G, et al. Unusual noninfectious granulomas of the lung. Radiology 1976;121:287–92.

210. O'Neill TJ, Johnson MC, Edwards DA. Multicentric mixed pattern pneumonia in a young adult. JAMA 1979;242:1288–9.

211. Darke CS, Middleton RSW. Calcification of the lungs after chickenpox. Br J Dis Chest 1967;61:198–204.

212. Clark RB, Johnson FC. Idiopathic pulmonary alveolar microlithiasis. Pediatrics 1961;28:650–4.

213. Gurkan F, Bosnak M, Dikici B, et al. Miliary tuberculosis of children: a clinical review. Scand J Infect Dis 1998;30:359–62.

214. Schuit KE. Miliary tuberculosis in children: clinical and laboratory manifestations in 19 patients. Am J Dis Child 1979;133:583–5.

215. Hussey G, Chisholm T, Kibel M. Miliary tuberculosis in children: a review of 94 cases. Pediatr Infect Dis J 1991;10:832–6.

216. Cockcroft DW, Donevan RE, Copland GM, et al. Miliary tuberculosis presenting with hyponatremia and thrombocytopenia. Can Med Assoc J 1976;115:871–3.

217. Gupta RK, Kohli A, Gaur V, et al. MRI of the brain in patients with miliary pulmonary tuberculosis without signs of central nervous system involvement. Neuroradiology 1997;39:699–704.

218. Thomas AV, Sodeman TH, Bentz RR. Bifidobacterium (Actinomyces) eriksonii infection. Am Rev Respir Dis 1974; 110:663–8.

219. Zelefsky MN, Lutzker LG. The target sign: a new radiologic sign of septic pulmonary emboli. Am J Roentgenol 1977;129:453–5.

220. Musher DM, Franco M. Staphylococcal pneumonia: a new perspective. Chest 1981;79:172–5.

221. Libshitz HI, Pagani JJ. Aspergillosis and mucormycosis: two types of opportunistic fungal pneumonia. Radiology 1981;140:301–6.

222. Kohlschütter A, Pelet B. Pulmonary candidiasis treated with 5-fluorocytosine. Arch Dis Child 1974;49:154–6.

223. Sarosi GA, Davies SF. State of the art: blastomycosis. Am Rev Respir Dis 1979;120:911–38.

224. Goodwin RA Jr, Des Prez RM. State of the art: histoplasmosis. Am Rev Respir Dis 1978;117:929–56.

225. Drutz DJ, Catanzaro A. State of the art: coccidioidomycosis II. Am Rev Respir Dis 1978;117:727–71.

226. Kim YJ, Gururaj VJ, Mirkovic RR. Concomitant diffuse nodular pulmonary infiltration in an infant with cytomegalovirus infection. Pediatr Infect Dis 1982;1:173–6.

227. Feldman S, Stokes DC. Varicella zoster and herpes simplex virus pneumonias. Sem Resp Infect 1987;2:84–94.

228. Kaplan SL, Gnepp DR, Katzenskein ALA, et al. Multiple pulmonary nodules due to aspirated vegetable particles. J Pediatr 1978;92:448–50.

229. Chusid MJ, Sty JR, Wells RG. Pulmonary aspergillosis appearing as chronic nodular disease in chronic granulomatous disease. Pediatr Radiol 1988;18:232–4.

230. Courtin JP, De Francia M, Du Couedic I, et al. Respiratory manifestations of leptospirosis: a retrospective study of 91 cases (1978–1984). Revue de Pneumologie Clinique 1998;54:382–92.

230a. Watson AM, Boyce TG, Wylam ME. Legionella pneumonia: infection during immunosuppressive therapy for idiopathic pulmonary hemosiderosis. Pediatr Infect Dis J 2004;23:82–4.

231. Shin MS, Young KR, Ho KJ. Wegener's granulomatosis upper respiratory tract and pulmonary radiographic manifestations in 30 cases with pathogenetic consideration. Clin Imaging 1998;22:99–104.

232. Bianchi M, Cataldi M. Pneumothorax secondary to pulmonary histiocytosis X. [Italian] Minerva chirurgica 1999;54:531–6.

233. Lee KS, Muller NL, Hale V, et al. Lipoid pneumonia: CT findings. J Comp Assist Tomography 1995;19:48–51.

234. McCook TA, Kirks DR, Merten DF, et al. Pulmonary alveolar proteinosis in children. Am J Roentgenol 1981;137:1023–7.

235. Pomputius WF 3rd, Rost J, Dennehy PH, Carter EJ. Standardization of gastric aspirate technique improves yield in the diagnosis of tuberculosis in children. Pediatr Infect Dis J 1997;16:222–6.

236. Lobato MN, Loeffler AM, Furst K, et al. Detection of Mycobacterium tuberculosis in gastric aspirates collected from children: hospitalization is not necessary. Pediatrics 1998;102:E40.

237. Singh M, Moosa NV, Kumar L, Sharma M. Role of gastric lavage and broncho-alveolar lavage in the bacteriological diagnosis of childhood pulmonary tuberculosis. Indian Pediatr 2000;37:947–51.

238. Somu N, Swaminathan S, Paramasivan CN, et al. Value of bronchoalveolar lavage and gastric lavage in the diagnosis of pulmonary tuberculosis in children. Tuberc Lung Dis 1995;76:295–9.

239. Gerbeaux J, Baculard A, Couvrer J. Primary tuberculosis in childhood. Am J Dis Child 1965;110:507–18.

240. Connor E, Powell KR. Fulminant pneumonia caused by concomitant infection with influenza B virus and Staphylococcus aureus. J Pediatr 1985;106:447–50.

241. Glezen WP. Influenza B and staphylococcal pneumonia [letter]. J Pediatr 1985;107:651–2.

242. Winterbauer RH, Ludwig WR, Hammar SP. Clinical course, management, and long-term sequelae of respiratory failure due to influenza viral pneumonia. Johns Hopkins Med J 1977;141:148–55.

243. Fischer JJ, Walker DH. Invasive pulmonary aspergillosis associated with influenza. JAMA 1979;241:1493–4.

244. Gerber GJ, Farmer WC, Fulkerson LL. Beta-hemolytic streptococcal pneumonia following influenza. JAMA 1978;240:242–3.

245. Ksiazek TG, Erdman D, Goldsmith CS, et al. A novel coronavirus associated with severe acute respiratory syndrome. N Engl J Med 2003;348:1953–66.

245a. Centers for Disease Control and Prevention. Update: severe acute respiratory syndrome—worldwide and United States, 2003. MMWR 2003;52:664–5.

245b. Sampathkumar P, Temesgen Z, Smith TF, Thompson RL. SARS: epidemiology, clinical presentation, management, and infection control measures. Mayo Clin Proc 2003; 78:882–90.

245c. Hon KLE, Leung CW, Cheng WTF, et al. Clinical presentation and outcome of severe acute respiratory syndrome in children. Lancet [serial online]. April 2003. Available at: http//image. thelancet. com/extras/03let4127web. pdf.

246. Kim KS, Gohd RS. Fatal pneumonia caused by adenovirus type 35. Am J Dis Child 1981;135:473–5.

247. Dagan I, Schwartz RH, Insel RA, et al. Severe diffuse adenovirus 7a pneumonia in a child with combined immunodeficiency: possible therapeutic effect of human immune serum globulin containing specific neutralizing antibody. Pediatr Infect Dis 1984;3:246–51.

248. Wright J, Couchonnal G, Hodges GR. Adenovirus type 21 infection: occurrence with pneumonia, rhabdomyolysis, and myoglobinuria in an adult. JAMA 1979;241:2420–1.

249. Sofer S, Pagtakhan RD, Hoogstratten J. Fatal lower respiratory tract infection due to herpes simplex virus in a previously healthy child. Clin Pediatr 1984;23:406–9.

250. Stogner SW, King JW, Black-Payne C, Boccini J. Ribavirin and intravenous immune globulin therapy for measles pneumonia in HIV infection. South Med J 1993;86:1415–8.

251. Lipsey AI, Kahn MJ, Bolande RP. Pathologic variants of congenital hypogammaglobulinemia: an analysis of 3 patients dying of measles. Pediatrics 1967;39:659–74.

252. Koffler D. Giant cell pneumonia. Arch Pathol 1964;78: 267–73.

253. Andiman WA, McCarthy P, Markowitz RI, et al. Clinical, virologic, and serologic evidence of Epstein-Barr virus infection in association with childhood pneumonia. J Pediatr 1981;99:880–6.

254. Landsberger EJ, Hager WD, Grossman JH III. Successful management of varicella pneumonia complicating pregnancy: a report of three cases. J Reproduct Med 1986; 31:311–4.

255. Duchin JS, Koster FT, Peters CJ, et al. Hantavirus pulmonary syndrome: a clinical description of 17 patients with a newly recognized disease. N Engl J Med 1994;330: 949–55.

256. Moolenaar RL, Dalton C, Lipman HB, et al. Clinical features that differentiate hantavirus pulmonary syndrome from three other acute respiratory illnesses. Clin Infect Dis 1995;21:643–9.

257. Hoffman NR, Preston FS Jr. Friedlander's pneumonia: a report of 11 cases and appraisal of antibiotic therapy. Dis Chest 1968;53:481–6.

258. Unger JD, Rose HD, Unger GF. Gram-negative pneumonia. Radiology 1973;107:283–91.

259. Koletsky RJ, Weinstein AJ. Fulminant *Mycoplasma pneumoniae* infection: report of a fatal case and a review of the literature. Am Rev Respir Dis 1980;122:491–6.

260. Prouty RL, Jordan WS Jr. Family epidemic of psittacosis with occurrence of fatal case. Arch Intern Med 1956;98: 365–71.

261. Chapman CB, Whorton CM. Acute generalized miliary tuberculosis in adults: clinicopathological study based on 63 cases diagnosed at autopsy. N Engl J Med 1946;235: 239–48.

262. Hui C, Wu CL, Chan MC, et al. Features of severe pneumonia in patients with undiagnosed pulmonary tuberculosis in an intensive care unit. J Formos Med Assoc 2003; 102:563–9.

263. Griffith JE, Campbell GD. Acute miliary blastomycosis presenting as fulminating respiratory failure. Chest 1979; 75:630–2.

264. Gururaj VJ, Marsh WW, Aiyar SR. Fulminant pulmonary coccidioidomycosis in association with Coxsackie B$_4$ infection. Clin Pediatr 1985;24:406–8.

265. Pattamasukon P, Pichyangkura C, Fischer GW. Melioidosis in childhood. J Pediatr 1975;87:133–6.

266. White NJ, Dance DA, Chaowagul W, et al. Halving of mortality of severe melioidosis by ceftazidime. Lancet 1989;2:697–701.

267. Samuel M, Ti TY. Interventions for treating melioidosis. Cochrane Database Syst Rev 2001;2:CD001263.

268. Rubin SA, Chaljub G, Winer-Muram HT, Flicker S. Pulmonary zygomycosis: a radiographic and clinical spectrum. J Thorac Imag 1992;7:85–90.

269. Marrie TJ. *Coxiella burnetii* (Q fever) pneumonia. Clin Infect Dis 1995;21 Suppl 3:S253–64.

270. Rottenberg GT, Miszkiel K, Shaw P, Miller RF. Case report: fulminant *Toxoplasma gondii* pneumonia in a patient with AIDS. Clin Radiol 1997;52:472–4.

271. Frontera JA, Gradon JD. Right-side endocarditis in injection drug users: review of proposed mechanisms of pathogenesis. Clin Infect Dis 2000;30:374–9.

272. Nandakumar R, Raju G. Isolated tricuspid valve endocarditis in nonaddicted patients: a diagnostic challenge. Am J Med Sci 1997;314:207–12.

273. Donohue JF. Lower respiratory tract involvement in Rocky Mountain spotted fever. *Arch InternMed* 1980;140: 223–7.

274. Case records of the Massachusetts General Hospital. Weekly clinicopathological exercises. Case 37-2001. A 76-year-old man with fever, dyspnea, pulmonary infiltrates, pleural effusions, and confusion. N Engl J Med 2000;345:1627–34.

275. Kirsch M, Ruben FL, Steere AC, et al. Fatal adult respiratory distress syndrome in a patient with Lyme disease. JAMA 1988;259:2737–9.

276. Horowitz ML, Coletta F, Fein AM. Delayed onset adult respiratory distress syndrome in babesiosis. Chest 1994; 106:1299–301.

277. Feldman R, Gromisch DS. Acute suppurative mediastinitis. Am J Dis Child 1971;121:79–81.

278. Tanaka H, Onodera N, Ito R, et al. Acute glomerulonephritis associated with pneumonia: a possible *Chlamydia pneumoniae* etiology? Pediatr Int 1999;41:698–700.

279. Yoh K, Kobayashi M, Hirayama A, et al. A case of superantigen-related glomerulonephritis after methicillin-resistant *Staphylococcus aureus* (MRSA) infection. Clin Nephrol 1997;48:311–6.

280. Jose MD, Bannister KM, Clarkson AR, et al. Mesangiocapillary glomerulonephritis in a patient with *Nocardia* pneumonia. Nephrol Dial Transplan 1998;13:2628–9.

281. Campbell JH, Warwick G, Boulton-Jones M, et al. Rapidly progressive glomerulonephritis and nephrotic syndrome associated with *Mycoplasma pneumoniae* pneumonia. Nephrology Dial Transplantation 1991;6:518–20.

282. Said MH, Layani MP, Colon S, et al. *Mycoplasma pneumoniae*-associated nephritis in children. Pediatr Nephrol 1999;13:39–44.

283. Borzy MS, Gewurz A, Wolff L, Houghton D, Lovrien E. Inherited C3 deficiency with recurrent infections and glomerulonephritis. Am J Dis Child 1988;142:79–83.

284. Serlin SP, Rimsza ME, Gay JH. Rheumatic pneumonia: the need for a new approach. Pediatrics 1975;56:1075–8.

285. von Vigier RO, Trummler SA, Laux-End R, et al. Pulmonary renal syndrome in childhood: a report of twenty-one cases and a review of the literature. Pediatr Pulmonol 2000;29:382–8.

286. Collins JO, Rosenburg HA, Warren P. Disseminated pathergic granulomatosis in a 4-month-old infant: a case report. Pediatrics 1967;40:975–9.

287. Howard TP. Fulminant respiratory failure: a manifestation of thrombotic thrombocytopenic purpura. JAMA 1979;242:350–1.

288. Conron M, Beynon HL. Churg-Strauss syndrome. Thorax 2000;55:870–7.

288a. Choi IS, Koh YI, Joo JY, et al. Churg-Strauss syndrome may be induced by leukotriene modifiers in severe asthma. Ann Allergy Asthma Immunol 2003;91:98.

289. Marik PE. Aspiration pneumonitis and aspiration pneumonia. N Engl J Med 2001;344:665–71.

290. Eade NR, Taussig LM, Marks MI. Hydrocarbon pneumonitis. Pediatrics 1974;54:351–7.

291. Faudel I, Bancalari E. Neardrowning in children: clinical aspects. Pediatrics 1976;58:573–9.

292. Modell JH. Drowning. N Engl J Med 1993; 328:253–6.

293. Borland LM, Sereika SM, Woelfel SK, et al. Pulmonary aspiration in pediatric patients during general anesthesia: incidence and outcome. J Clin Anesth 1998;10:95–102.

294. Warner MA, Warner ME, Warner DO, et al. Perioperative pulmonary aspiration in infants and children. Anesthsiology 1999;90:66–71.

295. Gates S, Huang T, Cheney FW. Effects of methylprednisolone on resolution of aspiration pneumonitis. Arch Surg 1983;118:1262–5.

296. Sethi AK, Chatterji C, Bhargava SK, et al. Safe pre-operative fasting times after milk or clear fluid in children: a preliminary study using real-time ultrasound. Anaesthesia 1999;54:51–9.

297. Ingebo KR, Rayhorn NJ, Heckt RM, et al. Sedation in children: adequacy of two-hour fasting. J Pediatr 1997; 131:155–8.

298. Stroh B, Rimell FL, Mendelson N. Bifid epiglottis. Int J Pediatr Otorhinolaryngol 1999;47:81–6.

299. Bergeson, PS, Hinchcliffe WA, Crawford RF, et al. Asphyxia secondary to massive dirt aspiration. J Pediatr 1978;92:506–7.

300. Silver P, Sagy M, Rubin L. Respiratory failure from cornstarch aspiration: a hazard of diaper changing. Pediatr Emerg Care 1996;12:108–10.

301. Huxley EJ, Viroslav J, Gray WR, et al. Pharyngeal aspiration in normal adults and patients with depressed consciousness. Am J Med 1978;64:564–8.

302. Konno A, Hoshin T, Togawa K. Influence of upper airway obstruction by enlarged tonsils and adenoids on recurrent infection of the lower airway in childhood. Laryngoscope 1980;90:1709–16.

303. Gerber ME, Gaugler MD, Myer CM III, Cotton RT. Chronic aspiration in children: when are bilateral submandibular gland excision and parotid duct ligation indicated? Arch Otolaryngol Head Neck Surg 1996;122: 1368–71.

304. Brook I, Finegold SM. Bacteriology of aspiration pneumonia in children. Pediatrics 1980;65:1115–20.

305. Brook I. Treatment of aspiration or tracheostomy-associated pneumonia in neurologically impaired children: effect of antimicrobials effective against anaerobic bacteria. Int J Pediatr Otorhinolaryngol 1996;35:171–7.

306. Brook I. Bacteriology and treatment of gram-negative pneumonia in longterm hospitalized children. Chest 1981;79:432–7.

307. Reeder WH, Goodrich BE. Pulmonary infiltration with eosinophilia (PIE syndrome). Ann Intern Med 1952;36: 1217–40.

308. Allen JN, Davis WB. Eosinophilic lung diseases: state of the art. Am J Respir Crit Care Med 1994;150:1423–38.

309. Oermann CM, Panesar KS, Langston C, et al. Pulmonary infiltrates with eosinophilia syndromes in children. J Pediatr 2000;136:351–8.

310. Rao M, Steiner P, Rose JS, et al. Chronic eosinophilic pneumonia in a one-year-old child. Chest 1975;68: 118–20.

311. Godding V, Bodart E, Delos M, et al. Mechanisms of acute eosinophilic inflammation in a case of acute eosinophilic pneumonia in a 14-year-old girl. Clin Exp Allergy 1998; 28:504–9.

312. Tipple MA, Beem MO, Saxon EM. Clinical characteristics of the afebrile pneumonia associated with *Chlamydia tra-chomatis* infection in infants less than 6 months of age. Pediatrics 1979;63:192–7.

313. Radkowski MA, Kranzler JK, Beem MO, et al. *Chlamydia* pneumonia in infants: radiography in 125 cases. AJR 1981;137:703–6.

314. Beem MO, Saxon E, Tipple MA. Treatment of chlamydial pneumonia of infancy. Pediatrics 1979;63:198–203.

315. Beale AS, Faulds E, Hurn SE, Tyler J, Slocombe B. Comparative activities of amoxycillin, amoxycillin/clavulanic acid and tetracycline against *Chlamydia trachomatis* in cell culture and in an experimental mouse pneumonitis. J Antimicrob Chemother 1991;27:627–38.

316. Garey KW, Amsden GW. Intravenous azithromycin. Ann Pharmacother 1999;33:218–28.

317. Mundel G, Katz I, Eshel G, et al. Superinfection of *Chlamydia trachomatis* pneumonia by *Staphylococcus aureus.* Clin Pediatr 1982;21:499–501.

318. Ringel RE, Givner LB, Brenner JI, et al. Myocarditis as a complication of infantile *Chlamydia trachomatis* pneumonitis. Clin Pediatr 1983;22:631–3.

319. Harrison HR, Taussig LM, Fulginiti VA. *Chlamydia trachomatis* and chronic respiratory disease in childhood. Pediatr Infect Dis 1982;1:29–33.

320. Numazaki K, Chiba S, Kogawa K. et al. Chronic respiratory disease in premature infants caused by *Chlamydia trachomatis.* J Clin Pathol 1986;39:84–8.

321. Keslin MH, McCoy EL, McCusker JJ, et al. *Corynebacterium pseudotuberculosis:* a new cause of infectious and eosinophilic pneumonia. Am J Med 1979;67:228–31.

322. Zinkham WH. Visceral larval migrans. Am J Dis Child 1978;132;627–33.

323. Harris RA Jr, Musher DM, Fainstein V, et al. Disseminated strongyloidosis: diagnosis made by sputum examination. JAMA 1980;244:65–6.

324. Wang JLF, Patterson R, Mintzer R, et al. Allergic bronchopulmonary aspergillosis in pediatric practice. J Pediatr 1979;94:376–81.

325. Imbeau SA, Cohen M, Reed CE. Allergic bronchopulmonary aspergillosis in infants. Am J Dis Child 1977;131: 1127–30.

326. Miyagawa H, Yokota S, Kajimoto K, et al. A case report of pulmonary infiltration with eosinophilia syndrome induced by *Candida albicans.* [Japanese] Arerugi 1992;41: 49–55.

327. Hendrick DJ, Ellithorpe DB, Lyon F, et al. Allergic bronchopulmonary helminthosporiosis. Am Rev Resp Dis 1982;126:935–8.

328. Trawick D, Kotch A, Matthay R, Homer RJ. Eosinophilic pneumonia as a presentation of occult chronic granulomatous disease. Eur Respir J 1997;10:2166–70.

329. Ricker DH, Taylor SR, Gartner JC Jr, Kurland G. Fatal pulmonary aspergillosis presenting as acute eosinophilic pneumonia in a previously healthy child. Chest 1991; 100:875–7.

330. Katz RM, Kniker WT. Infantile hypersensitivity pneumonitis as a reaction to organic antigens. N Engl J Med 1973; 288:233–7.

331. Cunningham AS, Fink JN, Schlueter DP. Childhood hypersensitivity pneumonitis due to dove antigens. Pediatrics 1976;58:436–42.

332. Heersma JR, Emanuel DA, Wenzel FJ, et al. Farmer's lung in a 10-year-old girl. J Pediatr 1969;75:704–6.

333. Fulmer JD, Kaltreider HB. The pulmonary vasculitides. Chest 1982;82:615–24.

334. Ho D, Tashkin DP, Bein ME, et al. Pulmonary infiltrates with eosinophilia associated with tetracycline. Chest 1979;76:33–6.

335. Kelly KJ, Ruffing R. Acute eosinophilic pneumonia following intentional inhalation of Scotchguard. Ann Allergy 1993;71:338–9.

336. Nadeem S, Nasir N, Israel RH. Loffler's syndrome secondary to crack cocaine. Chest 1994;105:1599–600.

337. Hamada H, Sakatani M, Yamamoto S, et al. Evaluation of eosinophilic cationic protein levels in patients with eosinophili pneumonia. [Japanese] Nihon Kokyuki Gakkai Zasshi 1998;36:864–70.

338. Powell DA, Walker DH. Nontuberculous mycobacterial endobronchitis in children. J Pediatr 1980;96:268–70.

339. Schneider HJ, Felson B, Gonzalez LL. Rounded atelectasis. AJR 1980;134:225–32.

340. Wiseman NE. The diagnosis of foreign body aspiration in childhood. J Pediatr Surg 1984;19:531–5.

341. Berger PE, Kuhn JP, Kuhns LR. Computed tomography and the occult tracheobronchial foreign body. Radiology 1980;134:133–5.

342. Banks W, Potsic WP. Elusive unsuspected foreign bodies in the tracheobronchial tree. Clin Pediatr 1977;16:31–5.

343. Dudgeon DL, Parker FB, Fritteli G, et al. Bronchiectasis in pediatric patients resulting from aspirated grass inflorescences. Arch Surg 1980;115:979–83.

344. Chernick V, Boat TF, eds. Kendig's Disorders of the Respiratory Tract in Children, 6th ed. Philadelphia: WB Saunders, 1997.

345. Laberge JM, Bratu I, Flageole H. The management of asymptomatic congenital lung malformations. Paediatr Respir Rev 2004;5(Suppl A):S305–12.

346. Fischer GW, McGrew GL, Bass JL. Pulmonary paragonimiasis in childhood: a cause of persistent pneumonia and hemoptysis. JAMA 1980;243:1360–2.

347. Narain K, Devi KR, Mahanta J. Pulmonary paragonimiasis and smear-negative pulmonary tuberculosis: a diagnostic dilemma. Int J Tuberc Lung Dis 2004;8:621–2.

348. Komaroff AL, Aronson MD, Schachter J. *Chlamydia trachomatis* infection in adults with community acquired pneumonia. JAMA 1981;245:1319–22.

349. Whitley RJ, Brasfield D, Reynolds DW, et al. Protracted pneumonitis in young infants associated with perinatally acquired cytomegalovirus infection. J Pediatr 1976;89:16–22.

350. Smith SD, Sho CT, Brahmacupta N, et al. Pulmonary involvement with cytomegalovirus infections in children. Arch Dis Child 1977;52:441–6.

351. Thomas CF Jr, Limper AH. *Pneumocystis* pneumonia. N Engl J Med 2004;350:2487–98.

352. O'Brodovich HM, Mellins RB. Bronchopulmonary dysplasia: unresolved neonatal acute lung injury. Am Rev Respir Dis 1985;132:694–709.

353. Goetzman BW. Understanding bronchopulmonary dysplasia. Am J Dis Child 1986;140:332–4.

354. Jobe AH, Bancalari E. Bronchopulmonary dysplasia. Am J Respir Crit Care Med 2001;163:1723–9.

355. Farrell PM, Gilbert EF, Zimmerman JJ, et al. Familial lung disease associated with proliferation and desquamation of type II pneumonocytes. Am J Dis Child 1986;140:262–6.

356. Dreisin RB, Schwarz MI, Theofilopoulas AN, et al. Circulating immune complexes in the idiopathic interstitial pneumonias. N Engl J Med 1978;298:353–7.

357. Teja K, Cooper PH, Squires JE, et al. Pulmonary alveolar proteinosis in four siblings. N Engl J Med 1981;305:1390–2.

358. McCook TA, Kirks DR, Merten DF, et al. Pulmonary alveolar proteinosis in children. AJR 1981;137:1023–7.

359. deMello DE, Lin Z. Pulmonary alveolar proteinosis: a review. Pediatr Pathol Mol Med 2001;20:413–32.

360. Deterding RR, Fan LL, Morton R, et al. Persistent tachypnea of infancy (PTI)—a new entity. Pediatr Pulmonol 2001;23:72–3.

361. Katzenstein AL, Gordon LP, Oliphant M, et al. Chronic pneumonitis of infancy: a unique form of interstitial lung disease occurring in early childhood. Am J Surg Pathol 1995;19:439–47.

362. Boner A, Wilmott RW, Dinwiddie R, et al. Desquamative interstitial pneumonia and antigen-antibody complexes in two infants with congenital rubella. Pediatrics 1983;72:835–9.

363. Schroten H, Manz S, Kohler H, et al. Fatal desquamative interstitial pneumonia associated with proven CMV infection in an 8-month-old boy. Pediatr Pulmonol 1998;25:345–7.

364. Tal A, Maor E, BarZiv J, et al. Fatal desquamative interstitial pneumonia in three infant siblings. J Pediatr 1984;104:873–6.

365. Leahy F, Pasterkamp H, Tal A. Desquamative interstitial pneumonia responsive to chloroquine. Clin Pediatr 1985;24:230–2.

366. Midwinter RE, Apley J, Burnam D. Diffuse interstitial pulmonary fibrosis with recovery. Arch Dis Child 1966;41:295–8.

367. Repetto G, Lisbon C, Emparanza E, et al. Idiopathic pulmonary hemosiderosis: clinical, radiological, and respiratory function studies. Pediatrics 1967;40:24–32.

368. Centers for Disease Control and Prevention. Update: pulmonary hemorrhage/hemosiderosis among infants—Cleveland, Ohio, 1993-1996. MMWR 2000;49:180–4.

369. Terr AI. *Stachybotrys*: relevance to human disease. Ann Allergy Asthma Immunol 2001;87(Suppl 3):57–63.

370. Colby TV, Lombard C. Histiocytosis X in the lung. Hum Pathol 1983;114:847–56.

371. Pearson ADJ, Kirpalani H, Ashcroft T, et al. Lymphomatoid granulomatosis in a 10-year-old boy. Br Med J 1983;286:1313–4.

372. Church JA, Isaacs H, Saxon A, et al. Lymphoid interstitial pneumonitis and hypogammaglobulinemia in children. Am Rev Respir Dis 1981;124:491–6.

373. Lovell D, Lindsley C, Langston C. Lymphoid interstitial pneumonia in juvenile rheumatoid arthritis. J Pediatr 1984;105:947–50.

374. Spira R, Lepage P, Msellati P, et al. Natural history of human immunodeficiency virus type 1 infection in children: a five-year prospective study in Rwanda. Pediatrics 1999;104:e56.

375. Pattishall EN, Strope GL, Spinola SM, et al. Childhood sarcoidosis. J Pediatr 1986;108:169–77.

376. Chang CH, Zinn TW. Roentgen recognition of enlarged

hilar lymph nodes: an anatomical review. Radiology 1976;120:291–6.

377. Sone S, Higashihara T, Morimoto S, et al. CT anatomy of hilar lymphadenopathy. AJR 1983;140:887–92.

378. Demos TC, Studio JD, Puczynski M. *Mycoplasma* pneumonia: presentation as a mediastinal mass. AJR 1984; 143:981–2.

379. Spinola SM, Bell RA, Henderson FW. Actinomycosis: a cause of pulmonary and mediastinal mass lesions in children. Am J Dis Child 1981;135:336–9.

380. Kelsey DS, Chambers RT, Hudspeth AS. Nontuberculous mycobacterial infection presenting as a mediastinal mass. J Pediatr 1981;98:431–2.

381. Rohlfing BM, White EA, Webb WR, et al. Hilar and mediastinal adenopathy caused by bacterial abscess of the lung. Radiology 1978;128:289–93.

382. Gaebler JW, Kleiman MB, Cohen M, et al. Differentiation of lymphoma from histoplasmosis in children with mediastinal masses. J Pediatr 1984;104:706–9.

383. Wallace LS, Robinson AE. Unusual radiological manifestations of acquired pulmonary cysts in children. JAMA 1982;248:85–7.

384. Marais BJ, Gie RP, Schaaf HS, et al. The natural history of childhood intra-thoracic tuberculosis: a critical review of literature from the pre-chemotherapy era. Int J Tuberc Lunc Dis 2004;8:392–402.

385. Curtis AB, Ridzon R, Vogel R. Extensive transmission of *Mycobacterium tuberculosis* from a child. N Engl J Med 1999;341:1491–5.

386. Bennish M, Radkowski MA, Ripon JW. Cavitation in acute histoplasmosis. Chest 1983;84:496–7.

387. Cohen I. Isolated pulmonary cryptococcosis in a young adolescent. Pediatr Infect Dis 1985;4:416–8.

388. Leatherman JW, Iber C, Davies SF. Cavitation in bacteremic pneumococcal pneumonia: causal role of mixed infection with anaerobic bacteria. Am Rev Respir Dis 1984; 129:317–21.

389. Liechty E, Kleiman MB, Ballantine TVN, et al. Primary *Hemophilus influenzae* lung abscesses with bronchial obstruction. J Pediatr Surg 1982;17:281–4.

390. Siegler DIM. Lung abscess associated with *Mycoplasma pneumoniae* infection. Br J Dis Chest 1973;67:123–7.

391. Levine MM, Ashman R, Heald F. Anaerobic (putrid) lung abscess in adolescence. Am J Dis Child 1976;130:77–81.

392. Stern RC, Berkowitz RJ, Shurin SB, et al. Multiple microaerophilic streptococcal lung abscesses after orthodontic treatment. Pediatrics 1982;70:722–4.

393. Brook I, Finegold SM. Bacteriology and therapy of lung abscess in children. J Pediatr 1979;94:10–2.

394. McCarthy VP, Patamasucon P, Gaines T, Lucas MA. Necrotizing pneumococcal pneumonia in childhood. Pediatr Pulmonol 1999;28:217–21.

395. Frieden TR, Biebuyck J, Hierholzer WJ Jr. Lung abscess with group A beta-hemolytic streptococcus: case report and review. Arch Intern Med 1991;151:1655–7.

396. Eng RH, Bishburg E, Smith SM. Evidence for the destruction of lung tissues during *Pneumocystis carinii* infection. Arch Intern Med 1987;147:746–9.

397. Asher MI, Spier S, Beland M, et al. Primary lung abscess in childhood: the longterm outcome of conservative management. Am J Dis Child 1982;136:491–4.

398. Merrill JR, Otis J, Logan WD Jr, et al. The dog heartworm

399. Pluche KD, Jensen WA. Pleuropulmonary amebiasis. Semin Respir Infect 1997;12:106–12.

400. Czermak BV, Unsinn KM, Gotwald T, et al. *Echinococcus granulosus* revisited: radiologic patterns seen in pediatric and adult patients. AJR 2001;177:1051–6.

401. Cangir AK, Sahin E, Enon S, et al. Surgical treatment of pulmonary hydatid cysts in children. J Pediatr Surg 2001; 36:917–20.

402. Roland AS, Merdinger WF, Froeb HF. Recurrent spontaneous pneumothorax: a clue to the diagnosis of histiocytosis X. N Engl J Med 1964;270:73–7.

403. Ellis R. Traumatic lung cysts. JAMA 1976;236:1976–7.

404. Godwin JD, Webb WR, Savoca CJ, et al. Multiple, thin-walled cystic lesions of the lung. AJR 1980;135: 593–604.

405. Rubin BK. The evaluation of the child with recurrent chest infections. Pediatr Infect Dis 1985;4:88–98.

406. Eigen H, Laughlin JJ, Homrighausen J. Recurrent pneumonia in children and its relationship to bronchial hyperreactivity. Pediatrics 1982;70:698–704.

407. Rosenbloom SA, Ravin CE, Putman CE, et al. Peripheral middle lobe syndrome. Radiology 1983;149:17–21.

408. Kinzy JD, Powers WP, Baddour LM. Case report: *Blastomyces dermatitidis* as a cause of middle lobe syndrome. Am J Med Sci 1996;312:191–3.

409. De Boeck K, Willems T, Van Gysel D, et al. Outcome after right middle lobe syndrome. Chest 1995;108:150–2.

410. Nussbaum E. Pediatric flexible bronchoscopy and its application in infantile atelectasis. Clin Pediatr 1985;24: 379–82.

411. Livingston GL, Holinger LD, Luck SR. Right middle lobe syndrome in children. Int J Pediatr Otorhinolaryngol 1987;13:11–23.

412. Berquist WE, Rachelefsky GS, Kadden M, et al. Gastroesophageal reflux associated recurrent pneumonia and chronic asthma in children. Pediatrics 1981;68:29–35.

413. Currie DC, Garbett ND, Chan KL, et al. Double-blind randomized study of prolonged higher-dose oral amoxicillin in purulent bronchiectasis. Q J Med 1990;76: 799–816.

414. Bachman AL, Hewitt WR, Beckley HC. Bronchiectasis: a bronchographic study of sixty cases of pneumonia. Arch Intern Med 1953;91:78–96.

415. McLaughlin FJ, Strieder DJ, Harris GBC, et al. Tracheal bronchus: association with respiratory morbidity in childhood. J Pediatr 1985;106:751–5.

416. Davis PB, Hubbard VS, McCoy K, et al. Familial bronchiectasis. J Pediatr 1983;102:177–85.

417. Turner JAP, Corkey CWB, Lee JYC, et al. Clinical expression of immotile cilia syndrome. Pediatrics 1981;67: 805–10.

418. Daniel TL, Woodring JH, Vandiviere HM, et al. Swyer-James syndrome: unilateral hyperlucent lung syndrome. Clin Pediatr 1984;23:393–7.

419. Hargis JL, Hiller FC, Bone RC. Migratory pulmonary infiltrates secondary to aspirated foreign body. JAMA 1978; 240:24–69.

420. Coghill TH, Moore FA, Accurso FJ, et al. Primary tracheomalacia. Ann Thorac Surg 1983;35:538–41.

421. Lynch JI. Bronchomalacia in children: considerations

governing medical vs surgical treatment. Clin Pediatr 1970;9:279–82.

422. Carson NU, Chadwick DL, Brubacker CA, et al. Thirteen boys with progressive septic granulomatosis. Pediatrics 1965;36:405–12.

423. Bureau MA, Fecteau C, Patriquin H, et al. Farmer's lung in early childhood. Am Rev Respir Dis 1979;119:671–5.

424. Rubenstein A, Morecki R, Silverman B, et al. Pulmonary disease in children with acquired immune deficiency syndrome and AIDS-related complex. J Pediatr 1986;108:498–503.

425. Chayt KJ, Harper ME, Marselle LM, et al. Detection of HTLV-III RNA in lungs of patients with AIDS and pulmonary involvement. JAMA 1986;256:2356–9.

426. Rubenstein A. Pediatric AIDS. Current Probl Pediatr 1986;26:360–409.

427. Klein BS, Vergeront JM, Weeks RJ, et al. Isolation of *Blastomyces dermatitidis* in soil associated with a large outbreak of blastomycosis in Wisconsin. N Engl J Med 1986;314:529–34.

428. Bosley ARJ, George G, George M. Outbreak of pulmonary tuberculosis in children. Lancet 1986;1:1141–3.

429. Centers for Disease Control. INH-resistant tuberculosis in an urban high school Oregon. MMWR 1980;29:194–6.

430. Yusuf HR, Braden CR, Greenberg AJ, et al. Tuberculosis transmission among five school bus drivers and students in two New York counties. Pediatrics 1997;100:e9.

431. American Academy of Pediatrics Committee on Infectious Diseases. Screening for tuberculosis in infants and children. Pediatrics 1994;93:131–4.

432. American Thoracic Society/Centers for Disease Control and Prevention/Infectious Diseases Society of America. Targeted tuberculin testing and treatment of latent tuberculosis infection. Am J Respir Crit Care Med 2000;161:S221–47.

433. American Academy of Pediatrics Committee on Infectious Diseases. Update on tuberculosis skin testing of children. Pediatrics 1996;97:282–4.

434. American Thoracic Society/Centers for Disease Control and Prevention/Infectious Diseases Society of America. Treatment of tuberculosis. Am J Respir Crit Care Med 2003;167:603–62.

435. Enarson DA. Use of the tuberculin skin test in children. Paediatr Respir Rev 2004;5(Suppl A):S135–7.

436. Lee E, Holzman RS. Evolution and current use of the tuberculin test. Clin Infect Dis 2002;34:365–70.

437. Kendig EL Jr. Tuberculin testing in the pediatric office and clinic [commentary]. Pediatrics 1979;64:965–6.

438. Cheng TL, Ottolini M, Getson P, et al. Poor validity of parent reading of skin test induration in a high risk population. Pediatr Infect Dis J 1996;15:90–2.

439. American Academy of Pediatrics. Tuberculosis. In: Pickering LK, ed. Red Book: 2003 Report of the Committee on Infectious Diseases, 26th ed. Elk Grove Village, IL: American Academy of Pediatrics, 2003:642–60.

440. Cohen Y, Zeharia A, Mimouni M, et al. Skin indurations in response to tuberculin testing in patients with nontuberculous mycobacterial lymphadenitis. Clin Infect Dis 2001;33:1786–8.

441. Correa AG, Starke JR. Nontuberculous mycobacterial disease in children. Semin Respir Infect 1996;11:262–71.

442. Mandalakas AM, Starke JR. Tuberculosis screening in immigrant children. Pediatr Infect Dis J 2004;23:71–2.

443. Lockman S, Tappero JW, Kenyon TA, et al. Tuberculin reactivity in a pediatric population with high BCG vaccination coverage. Int J Tuberc Lung Dis 1999;3:23–30.

444. Rosenberg M, Gotlieb RP. Current approach to tuberculosis in childhood. Pediatr Clin North Am 1968;14:513–47.

445. Furcolow ML, Watson KA, Charron T, et al. A comparison of the Tine and MonoVacc tests with the intradermal tuberculin test. Am Rev Resp Dis 1967;96:1009–27.

446. Sbarao JA. The FDA's final decision concerning the tuberculin multiple puncture test [correspondence]. Am Rev Respir Dis 1979;120:1390–1.

447. Squier CL, Goetz AM, Wagener MM, Muder RR. The anergy panel: an ineffective tool to validate tuberculin skin testing. Am J Infect Control 2004;32:243–5.

448. Mazurek GH, LoBue PA, Daley CL, et al. Comparison of whole-blood interferon gamma assay with tuberculin skin testing for detecting latent *Mycobacterium tuberculosis* infection. JAMA 2001;286:1740–7.

449. Centers for Disease Control and Prevention. Guidelines for using the QuantiFERON®-TB test for diagnosing latent *Mycobacterium tuberculosis* infection. MMWR 2003;52(RR02):15–8.

450. World Health Organization. BCG vaccine: WHO position paper. Wkly Epidemiol Rec 2004;79:27–38.

451. Nelson LJ, Wells CD. Global epidemiology of childhood tuberculosis. Int J Tuberc Lung Dis 2004;8:636–47.

452. Centers for Disease Control and Prevention. The role of BCG vaccine in the prevention and control of tuberculosis in the United State. MMWR 1996;45(RR04):1–18.

453. Hesseling AC, Schaaf HS, Hanekom WA, et al. Danish bacille Calmette-Guerin vaccine-induced disease in human immunodeficiency virus-infected children. Clin Infect Dis 2003;37:1226–33.

454. Corrales IF, Cortes JA, Mesa ML, Zamora G. Sternal osteomyelitis and scrofuloderma due to BCG vaccination [Spanish]. Biomedica 2003;23:202–7.

455. Talbot EA, Perkins MD, Silva SF, Frothingham R. Disseminated bacille Calmette-Guerin disease after vaccination: case report and review. Clin Infect Dis 1997;24:1139–46.

456. Sasaki Y, Nomura A, Kusuhara K, et al. Genetic basis of patients with bacille Calmette-Guerin osteomyelitis in Japan: identification of dominant partial interferon-gamma receptor 1 deficiency as a predominant type. J Infect Dis 2002;185:706–9.

CHAPTER 9

Neurologic Syndromes

■ GENERAL

Acute infection of the central nervous system (CNS) is the most likely cause of a febrile illness with manifestations of CNS involvement (Table 9-1). Stiff neck or crying when handled suggests meningeal irritation. Bulging fontanel, headache, or vomiting suggests increased intracranial pressure. Papilledema is unusual in any of the acute neurologic infections but should be excluded before doing a lumbar puncture. If severe papilledema is present, a more chronic process may be involved.

A change in consciousness, such as confusion or disorientation, is an alarming sign that suggests a disturbance of cerebral cortical function that may have many causes, including cerebral anoxia, inflammation, or edema. Any of the findings in Table 9-1 should be regarded as suggesting a medical emergency until further evaluated.

■ CLASSIFICATION

Purulent Meningitis

Purulent meningitis is best defined by a cerebrospinal fluid (CSF) that is cloudy and contains more than 1000 neutrophils/mcL. Whether or not a bacterial etiology is proven by culture, purulent meningitis is almost always bacterial. When the term "meningitis" is not further modified, it usually means purulent meningitis (Table 9-2).

Nonpurulent Meningitis

A CSF leukocyte count of 10–500/mcL, usually predominantly lymphocytes, can be defined as nonpurulent meningitis and this usually indicates a nonbacterial process (aseptic meningitis syndrome), but not always. Patients with CSF cell counts in the intermediate range (500–1000/mcL) can usually be classified as having presumed bacterial meningitis or aseptic meningitis syndrome on the basis of the cell count and differential, glucose, protein, Gram stain, and state of consciousness.

Definitions of aseptic meningitis syndrome are discussed further in that section.

Acute Encephalitis

Acute encephalitis is defined in this book as a severe and nontransient disturbance of consciousness with a CSF cell count like that of nonpurulent meningitis. Fever is usually present. Ordinarily, the number of leukocytes is less than 300 but sometimes exceeds 1000 per mcL. A disturbance of consciousness should be considered nontransient if it persists for more than 8 hours and should be distinguished from febrile delirium, which occurs only at the time of a high fever.

Acute Encephalopathy

In this book, the acute onset of severe and nontransient disturbance of consciousness and a normal CSF white cell count (fewer than 10/mcL) is defined as acute encephalopathy. Other manifestations of brain disease, such as convulsions and abnormal focal neurologic signs, are variably present. Fever is often absent. Otherwise, encephalopathy has the same clinical pattern as encephalitis except for a normal CSF white cell count. This distinction between encephalitis and encephalopathy is a useful one, as the causes of encephalitis are usually infectious or postinfectious, whereas the causes of encephalopathy are usually toxic, metabolic, or vascular. Encephalitis and encephalopathy are discussed in detail later in this chapter.

This classification is not perfect, and there is definite overlapping, but it is a helpful preliminary classification that has remained useful with years of use.[1] It is also useful to search in both the encephalitis and encephalopathy sections for answers.

Rarely, we have used two preliminary problem-oriented diagnoses such as purulent meningitis or encephalitis (in a case of La Crosse encephalitis) or acute encephalitis or encephalopathy (in a case when the cause was never found). The term

TABLE 9-1. MANIFESTATIONS OF CENTRAL NERVOUS SYSTEM INFECTIONS

SIGNS OR SYMPTOMS	SUGGESTS
Severe headache	Increased intracranial pressure
Persistent vomiting	
Bulging fontanel	
Stiff neck	Meningeal irritation
Crying when handled	
Disturbed consciousness (lethargy, irritability)	Brain involvement
High fever	Infection

"meningoencephalitis" is used too often when the patient can be classified as having nonpurulent meningitis or acute encephalitis, using the state of consciousness to distinguish them.

OTHER CNS SYNDROMES

Other syndromes associated with paralysis, ataxia, tetanus-like rigidity, or ventriculitis are discussed in later sections. The relative frequency of these syndromes in hospital admissions depends on the age of the child, on the season, and on whether a lumbar puncture is done before admission. In community hospitals, aseptic meningitis is more frequent than purulent meningitis, especially in the summer and fall months. Referral hospitals have more admissions for purulent meningitis than for aseptic meningitis, probably because such clinically severe illness often requires referral. All of these various syndromes occur most frequently in young infants.

■ DIFFERENTIAL DIAGNOSIS

Meningismus

"Meningismus" is a term best used to describe a stiff neck secondary to local or reflex irritation, which may occur from streptococcal pharyngitis or pneumonia. Rheumatoid arthritis and tetanus also may be associated with nuchal rigidity and normal spinal fluid. This diagnosis should not be made unless the spinal fluid is normal.[2,3] The term "meningismus" is sometimes used as a synonym for "nuchal rigidity" or "stiff neck," a usage that should be avoided, as it spoils its meaning of "stiff neck with normal spinal fluid," which is a cumbersome substitute for "meningismus."

Retropharyngeal Abscess

Deep cervical adenitis and retropharyngeal abscess may produce meningismus and are discussed in Chapter 6.

TABLE 9-2. CLASSIFICATION OF MAJOR INFECTIOUS NEUROLOGIC SYNDROMES

SYNDROME	LEUKOCYTES (PER mcL)	SPINAL FLUID FINDINGS PROTEIN (MG/DL)	GLUCOSE (MG/DL)	CONSCIOUSNESS
Purulent Meningitis	>1000 (mostly "polys")	>100 (high)	<40 (low)	Lethargic to comatose
Nonpurulent Meningitis				
Normal glucose subgroup	10–500 (Usually lymphocytes)	Normal	>40	Irritable; variable
Low glucose subgroup		Usually high	<40	Lethargic to comatose
Acute Encephalitis	10–1000	Sometimes high	Varies	Severely disturbed
Acute Encephalopathy	<10	Normal	Normal	Severely disturbed

Pseudotumor Cerebri

An increased pressure, manifested by a bulging fontanel or papilledema, with infection, tumor, sinus thrombosis, and obstruction of the ventricular system specifically excluded, is defined as benign intracranial hypertension or pseudotumor cerebri. Tetracycline is a possible cause. A bulging fontanel may also be produced by early congestive heart failure.

■ LUMBAR PUNCTURE

Indications and Risks

When meningitis is suspected, lumbar puncture is an emergency procedure. Lumbar puncture (LP) is relatively simple in children and should be done when bacterial meningitis is suspected, because the risk of undiagnosed or inadequately treated meningitis is significant. If the results are normal, but the child's clinical condition is worsening and still suggests meningitis, then the tap should be repeated.[4] Clinical suspicion should not be ignored; we have seen bacterial meningitis (confirmed by culture) in patients with a classical presentation but normal initial CSF profile.

Before lumbar puncture is done, the optic fundi should be examined to exclude papilledema. Papilledema takes time to develop, and its absence does not rule out elevated intracranial pressure (ICP). Clinical features that suggest elevated ICP include focal neurologic signs, postural or respiratory abnormalities, absent oculocephlic (doll's eyes) reflexes, dilated or unequal pupils, ophthalmoplegia, protracted seizures, or severe obtundation or coma (Glasgow Coma Scale less than 8).[5,6] Patients with these signs or symptoms should receive an emergency computed tomography (CT) scan prior to lumbar puncture in order to minimize the risk of cerebral herniation. Unfortunately, even a normal CT scan is not entirely protective; several cases of children who experienced herniation following lumbar puncture despite a normal CT scan have been reported.[6,7] Spinal subdural hematomas[8] and even intracranial hematomas have been reported,[9] but these complications are extremely rare. Overall the procedure is safe. Although the decision regarding performance of a lumbar puncture should be made thoughtfully, in the vast majority of patients the benefits of early lumbar puncture far outweigh the small risks. The practice of routinely ordering head CT scans prior to lumbar puncture has no support in the literature and may cause unnecessary delay in institution of treatment.

Several diseases may require special caution or delay in doing a lumbar puncture. Reye syndrome is a disease in which lumbar puncture should sometimes not be done because of increased pressure.[4] Papilledema is usually not present, but cerebral edema may be extreme. An elevated serum transaminase concentration and elevated blood ammonia is helpful in making the diagnosis if the clinical findings are compatible, as described in the section on acute encephalopathy. Fortunately, Reye syndrome is now quite rare. Children with posterior fossa tumors may present with fever and nuchal rigidity, but a careful history will usually indicate that the illness began several days or even weeks earlier. Suspicion of a brain abscess may be a reason for the physician to postpone a lumbar puncture if a brain CT scan can be obtained on an emergency basis. A cautious lumbar puncture 30 minutes after a mannitol infusion, as described later, with withdrawal of less than 1 mL of fluid, is probably the best way to deal with this dilemma when increased pressure is suspected but cannot be evaluated.

Patients with hemophilia A (or B) may safely undergo the procedure if they are given infusions of factor VIII (or factor IX) prior to beginning; no complication occurred in a series of 58 patients managed in this way.[10]

Technique

Use of a scalp vein needle without a stylet appears to be simpler for newborns. However, the possibility of the needle cutting a core of skin and injecting the dermal cells into the lumbar space has been suggested as a cause of epidermoid CNS tumors. Therefore, this method is not recommended. An alternative method, in which the stylet is removed after the needle has been advanced through the skin and subcutaneous tissues, has been suggested as a way to minimize the number of traumatic lumbar punctures without increasing the risk of spinal epidermoid tumors, but this hypothesis has not been proved. Lumbar puncture in newborn infants requires special caution. Studies have indicated the newborn should not be positioned with the neck flexed lying in the lateral position, and the sitting position is probably preferable to avoid respiratory deterioration.[11,12]

The measurement of pressure is not indicated when acute infection is suspected, and attempts to measure pressure with a manometer may result in a bloody tap. Pressure can be estimated by counting the number of drops over a specified period of time. At patient temperatures lower than 40°C, using a 22-gauge 1.5 inch needle, the number of drops of CSF delivered in 21 seconds is an estimate of CSF pressure in cm of H_2O. For a 22-gauge, 3.5 inch needle, the counting time is 39 seconds, while for a 20 gauge, 3.5 inch needle, the counting time is 12 seconds. If the patient's temperature is higher than 40°C, the counting periods are shorter: 20, 37, and 11 seconds, respectively. These estimates are accurate if the patient is calm and in the lateral recumbent position.[13]

In larger children, measurement of the opening pressure can be more easily obtained without compromising the integrity of the LP, and should be done.

If the fluid appears cloudy or purulent, an immediate rapid intravenous infusion or injection of a third-generation cephalosporin, followed by vancomycin infusion, is indicated without delay, as described later in the section on emergency treatment of meningitis.

Cell Count

A Wright stain of a smear should be examined under oil for an accurate differential count. When the tap has been traumatic, the presence of red blood cells suggests that some of the white blood cells have come from the peripheral blood. Various formulas based on experimental studies have been used to try to calculate the effect of contamination of CSF by peripheral blood, but the calculations are complicated by the decreased survival time of white blood cells (WBC), especially neutrophils.[14,15]

Contamination with more than 100,000 red cells/mcL occasionally can obscure the recognition of purulent bacterial meningitis, and the use of peripheral white to red blood cell ratios to interpret the CSF often underestimates the CSF white count.[16,17] Many authors who have studied this problem suggest "corrected white blood cell counts of blood-contaminated fluids (should) be viewed with skepticism and not be given undue weight in clinical decisions."[17] However, a review of 92 children who had a traumatic LP, 30 of whom had bacterial meningitis, showed that all patients with bacterial meningitis had an observed to predicted ratio of WBC greater than 1. In fact, 28 (93%) of the 30 had a ratio greater than 10, and 24 (80%) had ratios greater than 100.[18] Additionally, a predominance of neutrophils in the CSF (97% vs. 11%), hy-poglycorrhachia, (73% vs. 3%) and positive Gram stains (80% vs. zero) were found more commonly in the patients with meningitis.

It is sometimes important to differentiate a traumatic tap from subarachnoid hemorrhage. Blood contamination of the CSF tends to decrease from the first tube to the last, and often produces a difference that can be seen by the naked eye. Additionally, centrifugation of the fluid usually produces a clear supernatant in traumatic tap, whereas xanthochromia persists in cases of subarachnoid hemorrhage. The best test for differentiating a traumatic tap from subarachnoid hemorrhage is the D-dimer assay; D-dimer assay is negative in traumatic tap.[19] The CSF protein is also frequently elevated beyond that expected by calculations in the cleared tube of a "bloody tap."

A study of the spinal fluid of 108 term neonates in whom infection was very carefully excluded showed a mean of 7.3 WBC/mcL, with a median of 4 and a range of 0 – 130.[20] The patient with 130 WBC was clearly an outlier, however. Older studies defined normal as a maximum of 7/mcL with as many as 4 of these being polymorphonuclear cells.[21] After 6 weeks of age, the maximum count in normal CSF can be taken as 5, of which 2 can be "polys."[21] In an earlier study, in the first week of life, normal term infants had a maximum of 32 leukocytes with a mean of 8/mcL.[22] Preterm infants had a maximum of 29 leukocytes, with a mean of 9/mcL.

Glucose and Protein

In general, glucose and protein values should be determined whenever spinal fluid is obtained. The importance of these values and the mechanisms involved in creating abnormal ones are discussed in the sections on purulent meningitis and nonpurulent meningitis. The CSF glucose can be considered abnormal when it is less than 40 mg/dL or less than 40% of the blood glucose.[23]

Smears

Centrifugation of the spinal fluid before microscopic examination may be helpful, but it is usually not practical when small amounts of fluid have been obtained. One drop of sediment from the centrifuged CSF should be allowed to dry on each of two slides and fixed by brief gentle flaming. One specimen is Gram stained and examined for bacteria. The other is stained with Wright stain for a differential count if necessary.

A Gram stain should be done on all spinal fluid specimens with an increased number of white blood cells. Bacteria are most likely to be observed in purulent fluid and are rarely seen in CSF with low leukocyte counts. The exceptions include some cases of neonatal meningitis, where there may be a poor leukocyte response, with only a few hundred leukocytes per mcL, yet many bacteria. Early infection with meningococci or pneumococci occasionally produces a positive Gram stain of the CSF, confirmed by culture, before any remarkable CSF pleocytosis occurs.[24] The ability to detect bacteria on the Gram stain depends on their CSF concentration, which is correlated with the concentration of bacteria in the blood.[25]

Contamination of tubes or other equipment is rare. In such cases, a variety of stained bacteria are typically seen.

CSF Culture

Although the main purpose is culture of the spinal fluid for bacteria, an extra tube can be held in the laboratory until the cell count, the glucose, and the protein are determined, in case this information suggests the need for further studies such as culture for viruses or tuberculosis (TB).

The microbiology laboratory may delay reporting the species obtained from the spinal fluid until all the metabolic studies are complete. However, the physician can make clinical judgments sooner and can presume, for example, that a pure culture of a gram-negative diplococcus is going to be meningococcus, even though definitive identification may require several days.

The frequency of various bacterial contaminants of CSF cultures has been studied.[26] *Staphylococcus epidermidis* and diphtheroids are the most common contaminants, but in special circumstances (especially CSF shunts) they can be pathogens.

Positive CSF Culture with Minimal CSF Abnormalities (Seeded Meningitis)

Sometimes, the physician finds a positive CSF culture with minimal other abnormalities. This problem was the subject of a short clinical report, but most large series of patients with meningitis include a few examples.[24] Bacteremia is usually found if a blood culture has been taken and involves the organism recovered on culture of the CSF, although the cell count, Gram stain glucose, and protein are normal. Usually, patients with these findings are very sick and are suspected of having a bacteremia of unknown source. Typically, the patient is hospitalized and treated for sepsis and often gets a second lumbar puncture 12–36 hours later that reveals purulent meningitis.[27] Occasionally, this pattern is observed early in endocarditis (Chapter 18) or in bacteremia in an outpatient (Chapter 10).

The working diagnosis for severely ill patients should be "probable sepsis" until objective evidence of CSF abnormalities or a positive CSF culture is found. The diagnosis of meningitis should generally not be made with normal CSF findings, but a word is needed to describe a positive CSF culture in this situation. Bacteria in the CSF can be called "bacterrhachia," analogous to "bacteremia" and "hypoglycorrhachia." Bacterrhachia without CSF pleocytosis is further discussed later.

The pattern of "seeding" of the CSF during bacteremia without any other CSF abnormalities is typically not associated with the complications of purulent bacterial meningitis. The prognosis depends rather on the disease causing the bacteremia.

Antigen Detection

Various methods have been developed to detect bacterial antigens in the CSF.[28] It was hoped that these tests would be positive when prior antibiotics prevented a positive culture. In reality, these tests for bacterial antigens (latex agglutination, enzyme-linked immunosorbent assay [ELISA], or other) rarely help and should not be ordered routinely. Antigen detection studies can be ordered when the patient has received previous antibiotics but can be delayed until the Gram stained smear is found negative by a qualified technologist.

Other CSF Tests

Tests for bacterial endotoxin (Limulus lysate test), bacterial enzymes (transaminase, lactic acid dehydrogenase), bacterial products (lactic acid), and acute-phase reactants (C-reactive protein), among other things, have been studied in an attempt to aid in the differentiation of viral meningitis from partially-treated bacterial meningitis. Many of these substances are elevated in the CSF, but either the sensitivity and specificity are not sufficient to aid in diagnosis or the test is reflected in other, simpler tests. For example, lactate levels increase linearly with lactate-producing cells; therefore, they correlate with leukocytosis,[29] which is a lab value the clinician already has at hand. In adults, neither CSF lactate nor CSF C-reactive protein, nor a combination of the two yields anything better than 60% positive predictive value for bacterial meningitis.[30] The enthusiasm for such tests has been based on their good correlation with clear-cut cases of bacterial meningitis or normals. However, the results are typically equivocal in patients with negative cultures and an equivocal conventional CSF glucose, protein, and cell count.

As yet, no test has been shown to correlate better with cultures than the combination of protein, glucose, and white cell count with a differential study.[31,32] If available, enteroviral polymerase chain reaction (PCR) on CSF can be helpful in distinguishing viral meningitis from bacterial meningitis obscured by previous oral antibiotic therapy.[33] This test is particularly cost-effective during enteroviral season (summer and fall).[34]

Serum Tests

Serum tests have actually fared much better than CSF tests in navigating the muddy waters. In one large study of 325 children with bacterial meningitis and 182 with proven or suspected viral meningitis, the serum C-reactive protein level (CRP) averaged 11.5 mg/dL in those with bacterial disease versus less than 20 mg/dL in those with viral CNS infections. Serum CRP was the only test that reliably discriminated gram-stain negative bacterial meningitis from meningitis of viral etiology; a serum CRP of less than 2.0 mg/dL had a negative predictive value of 99% for bacterial meningitis.[35] In another study, 18 children with bacterial meningitis had a mean serum procalcitonin value of 54.5 mg/L, whereas 41 children with viral meningitis had a mean value of 0.32 mg/L. The highest value found in a child with viral meningitis was 1.7 mg/L, and the lowest found in a child with a positive CSF culture was 4.8 mg/L; thus, there was no overlap between the two groups.[36] Although the preliminary data look fairly promising, these laboratory tests have not yet become commonplace in clinical practice.

■ FEVER AND CONVULSIONS

Definitions

Several diagnostic phrases are used to describe a variety of clinical situations with fever and convulsions.[37] "Fever and convulsions" is the most neutral expression and therefore the best syndrome diagnosis when no etiologic diagnosis is yet possible. "Seizures precipitated by fever" is an etiologic diagnosis indicating that the patient is known to have a convulsive disorder and now has had a convulsion precipitated by fever. "Simple febrile convulsion" is best regarded as an etiologic diagnosis that should be based on exclusion of many other possibilities. In a child with a first convulsion with fever, the following criteria should be present for the etiologic diagnosis of simple febrile convulsion:

1. Fever at the time of the convulsion.
2. Brief generalized (nonfocal) seizure, usually lasting less than 5 minutes and not longer than 15 or 20 minutes, in a child 6 months to 5 years of age. No recurrence of seizure within the first 24 hours.
3. Prompt recovery to normal state of consciousness without definite neurologic abnormalities, such as paralysis or weakness. If the state of consciousness does not return to normal within about 30 minutes after the convulsion, the patient should be considered to have an acute encephalopathy or a CNS infection until proven otherwise.
4. Family history of febrile convulsions or past convulsion with fever supports the diagnosis of simple febrile seizure but is not in itself sufficient to establish the diagnosis.
5. Exclusion of increased intracranial pressure by examination of the optic fundi.
6. Exclusion of CNS infections such as meningitis or encephalitis, when lumbar puncture is indicated.
7. Exclusion of metabolic causes of convulsions, such as hypoglycemia, hypocalcemia, or hyponatremia, when indicated.
8. Normal developmental history.

The principal advantage of the use of the diagnosis of simple febrile seizure is that it avoids the term "epilepsy," which is often associated with much misunderstanding and fear among laypersons. The major disadvantage is that the improper use of this diagnosis may lull the physician into symptomatic therapy without searching for treatable, and sometimes urgent, specific causes.

Emergency Management

A quick history should be obtained to look for recent head injury (in which case sedation may be contraindicated) and current or recent medications such as anticonvulsants or toxin or poison ingestion. *A quick physical examination* should be done to check for evidence of head injury and to clear the airway and position the child with the head turned to avoid aspiration. *Fever reduction* by pharmacologic means should be begun immediately if the temperature is above 40°C (104°F). *Oxygen* may be indicated if the patient is cyanotic, and the airway should be checked to be sure it is clear.

Anticonvulsant drugs should be given to stop the convulsion if it has not already stopped. A short-acting anticonvulsant such as lorazepam is given in a dose of 0.05–0.10 mg/kg. This dose can be repeated if the seizure persists. On a rare occasion, phenytoin (or fosphenytoin) at a dose of 15–20 mg/kg will be required. This drug should be administered slowly to avoid hypotension and cardiac rhythm problems.

Phenobarbital can also be used, at an intravenous dose of 10–20 mg/kg (loading dose) to stop prolonged seizures.[38] If the patient has intermittent seizures but has stopped convulsing before any medications are given, 5 mg/kg can be given instead of 10 mg/kg to prevent further seizures.[39]

For stopping a prolonged seizure (defined here as longer than 15 or 20 minutes), intravenous lorazepam, phenobarbital, or phenytoin is usually recommended.[38–43] These drugs all have potential dangers. All primary care physicians and emergency rooms should have a written plan or protocol readily available for the control of prolonged seizures.

Possible Etiologies

CNS Infection

Between 15–25% of all patients with meningitis will have seizure with fever either at the time of presentation or sometime during the course of the disease. Patients with meningitis almost always have symptoms other than seizure that suggest the diagnosis. Meningitis or encephalitis should always be excluded by examination of the spinal fluid if there is any question of the state of consciousness or meningeal irrigation.

Non-CNS Infection

Infection not involving the CNS with seizure precipitated by fever or toxins, such as shigellosis, pneumococcal bacteremia, or infection with human herpesvirus type 6 (HHV-6) is another category of causes. There was a lot of enthusiasm for HHV-6 as a cause of febrile seizures after it was discovered that one third of patients up to the age of two years presenting to the emergency department with the clinical syndrome of simple febrile seizure had HHV-6 infection.[44]

However, a subsequent case-control study found evidence of acute HHV-6 infection in 15 (43%) of 35 patients with febrile seizures and in 15 (45%) of 33 controls.[45] The conclusion of these authors was that HHV-6 infection is not a major factor in the pathogenesis of febrile seizures. A more plausible interpretation might be that HHV-6 infection is a frequent cause of high fever in the age group at risk for febrile seizures, and that some children are predisposed to the development of seizures with fever.

Toxic and Metabolic Causes

Convulsion secondary to a specific cause such as lead encephalopathy or hypoglycemia can accompany fever caused by an infection and need to be excluded if suggestive clinical findings are present.

Seizure Disorder

Idiopathic convulsive disorder ("epilepsy") with seizure precipitated by fever is the proper diagnosis if there is an abnormal electroencephalogram (EEG) obtained at least a week after the seizure or if convulsions also occur without fever.

Simple Febrile Convulsion

This is by far the most common cause of seizure with fever, occurring in approximately 4% of children between the ages of 6 months and 5 years. Simple febrile seizures are a benign condition whose main complication is recurrence, which happens in about one-third of patients. Recurrence risk is difficult to predict, but seems to be higher in children who present at a younger age.[46] The diagnosis of simple febrile seizure is fairly straightforward in older toddlers who have a classic history and physical examination, but it is more difficult in younger patients.

Diagnostic Approach

Lumbar Puncture

There has been much discussion about the need for lumbar puncture in the evaluation of seizure and fever; clearly, the yield is low in cases where the diagnosis of simple febrile seizure is clinically suggested. However, meningitis can present with seizure and fever, and in young children, other signs of meningitis may be subtle. Because of this, the American Academy of Pediatrics (AAP) practice parameter recommends that excluding CNS infection by lumbar puncture be strongly considered in children younger than 12 months, and considered for children between 12 and 18 months of age.[47]

A recent review of 503 cases of meningitis (97% of which were proven or suspected to be bacterial) showed that 115 presented with seizures (23%). Of these patients, 105 (91%) were obtunded or comatose, and thus obvious candidates for lumbar puncture. Of the other 10, 6 had nuchal rigidity, 1 had prolonged focal seizures, and 1 had multiple seizures and a petechial rash, all independent reasons to obtain spinal fluid by lumbar puncture. Two were suspected, on clinical grounds, of having viral meningitis.[48]

In an older review of 152 children with purulent meningitis, 27 (18%) had fever and seizures.[49] Of these 27 children, 11 (41%) had no recorded meningeal irritation, no change of consciousness, and no bulging fontanelle; all of these children were less than 18 months of age. It is often stated that clinicians with experience can exclude meningitis on clinical grounds; however, science supporting this statement is absent. In fact, one of the authors of this last study argued that after years of experience it is still difficult to exclude meningitis in young children on clinical grounds alone, and he would do a lumbar puncture on all children under 16 months of age who present with fever and a convulsion.[50]

In a retrospective review of 709 outpatients undergoing lumbar puncture, 225 (32%) had fever and a convulsion as the reason for the puncture.[51] Only five had abnormal CSF, and most of these also had signs of meningeal irritation. A prospective emergency department study that allowed physicians to decide which patients required lumbar puncture (and thus biased the results toward finding a higher percentage of children with meningitis) found a total of 7 cases of meningitis (3 bacterial) in 102 patients who underwent lumbar puncture. There were 98 patients who were thought not to need the test. Most of the children with meningitis had lethargy, irritability, or vomiting; all had features of complex febrile seizure.[52] The "catch-22" is this: those who clearly have simple febrile seizure

need not undergo lumbar puncture; however, absence of meningitis is one of the criteria for establishing the diagnosis of simple febrile seizure. The author of *Clinical Pediatric Neurology* says that "a brief, generalized seizure from which the child recovers rapidly and completely is not caused by meningitis, especially if the fever subsides spontaneously..."[53] Certainly, lumbar puncture in a child with fever and a convulsion can be selectively obtained, and other findings must be considered.

Criteria suggested for electing lumbar puncture are:

1. Any clinical suspicion of meningitis
2. Under 18 months of age
3. Unusually slow recovery of normal function after a febrile seizure[54]
4. Complex febrile seizure, especially focal seizure.

Electroencephalogram

An EEG is usually not indicated immediately after the convulsion.[54] It will often be abnormal even after a simple febrile convulsion, although an expert can often distinguish between a simple postictal abnormality and abnormalities suggesting epilepsy. If the EEG reveals epileptogenic activity several weeks after the seizure, the correct diagnosis is more likely to be "convulsive disorder precipitated by fever." The pattern of activity seen on acute EEG is not predictive of recurrence risk.[55]

Other Tests

Skull roentgenogram and blood glucose, calcium, sodium, or blood urea nitrogen (BUN) measurements are unlikely to reveal an abnormality and are not recommended unless there is some clinical basis for suspecting an abnormality.[54,56–58]

Hospitalization is not recommended except for severe or multiple seizures or when the parents are too frightened or otherwise unable to observe the child.[54]

Prevention

Antipyretic Medication

Various antipyretic medications, given at the onset of fever and at a fixed interval throughout the course of a febrile illness, have been tested in prophylaxis against febrile seizures. Prospective randomized trials of acetaminophen[59] and ibuprofen[60] have failed to show a reduction in the number of recurrences. Although antipyresis may have other beneficial effects, there appears to be no scientific basis for the use of antipyretics in the prevention of febrile seizures.

Anticonvulsant Medication

About one-third of patients will develop recurrence of febrile seizure, and half of those patients go on to a third episode. These recurrences can be decreased by continuous anticonvulsant therapy with either phenobarbital or valproic acid, but these medications are not without risk. Prophylaxis against recurrent febrile seizure with phenobarbital has been shown to lower achievement scores even 5 years out.[61] Valproic acid is more effective at prevention of seizures,[62] but carries the risk of idiopathic and irreversible severe hepatotoxicity.[63]

In one study, diazepam, taken at the onset of fever, was also shown to decrease the incidence of febrile seizures; 39% of recipients, however, developed side effects of the medication.[64] Other studies failed to duplicate the beneficial effect.[62] Some authorities believe that prophylaxis is even less likely to be needed if the convulsion is associated with roseola, shigellosis, or viral meningitis, because these illnesses have a tendency to be associated with convulsions. A lower recurrence rate among children whose first febrile seizure was associated with HHV-6 (the causative agent of roseola) has been confirmed by a prospective clinical trial.[65] A major factor to consider is that in the grand majority of cases, febrile seizure, even if it recurs, is a benign disorder with an excellent prognosis. The risk of most prophylactic regimens outweighs the potential benefits.

Exceptions could include children with neurologic disease, those with focal seizures, a family history of epilepsy, or a febrile seizure lasting more than 15 minutes or followed by a neurologic abnormality.[66]

Postictal Pleocytosis

Occasionally the question arises as to whether seizure activity alone may be responsible for the finding of leukocytes in the CSF. In approximately 5% of cases, WBCs may be found in the CSF within 72 hours of a seizure, and most commonly within 12 hours of a seizure.[67–69] The maximum number of WBCs in the spinal fluid is usually less than 15 per mcL, but may rarely be as high as 80 per mcL.[70] Mildly increased protein may also be observed after

seizures in about 10% of cases.[67] Postictal pleocytosis can occur after simple, complex partial, or generalized tonic-clonic seizures.[68] Clearly, this is a diagnosis of exclusion, and infectious causes should be pursued vigorously.

■ PURULENT MENINGITIS

Definitions

Purulent meningitis is a medical emergency. It is usually manifested by clinical signs of acute neurologic infection and cloudy spinal fluid. Typically, the CSF has more than 1000 leukocytes/mcL with a predominance of neutrophils, low glucose (often 0–10 mg/dL), and elevated protein (usually more than 100 mg/dL). Some patients with early bacterial meningitis have cell counts, glucose, and protein in the same range found in nonpurulent meningitis; that is, aseptic meningitis syndrome, which is discussed in the following section. Prior oral antibiotic treatment decreases yield of CSF culture, but does not significantly alter the CSF parameters; total number of white blood cells, glucose levels, and protein levels are not affected. In order to avoid jumping to etiologic conclusions, it is useful to use the terms "purulent" and "nonpurulent" meningitis until a bacterial etiology is confirmed or excluded by culture. In the patient with apparent purulent meningitis but a negative Gram stain, the possibility of a parameningeal infection (such as a brain abscess or subdural empyema) should be considered.

Ventriculitis may occur without meningitis, particularly if the CSF flow is obstructed. This is most likely as a complication of neurosurgical shunting operations for hydrocephalus and is discussed later in this chapter.

Age

In the past, purulent meningitis occurred predominately in children. The advent of the protein conjugate *H. influenzae* type b vaccine has had a dramatic effect on the epidemiology of bacterial meningitis. In 1986, 62% of bacterial meningitis in the United States occurred in children younger than 2 years of age and 79% occurred in children younger than 18. By 1995, children younger than 2 years old accounted for 25% of all cases of bacterial meningitis and those younger than 18 accounted for 48%.[71]

It is reasonable to assume that widespread use of the protein conjugate pneumococcal vaccine will decrease the incidence of bacterial meningitis in young children even further.

Risk Factors

Males are slightly more likely to acquire meningitis than are females. There is a suggestion that meningitis is more common in poor populations. The incidence of pneumococcal meningitis is 8- to 24-fold higher in blacks, irrespective of socioeconomic status or crowding.[72] Patients with asplenia/polysplenia, sickle cell disease, or other hemoglobinopathies that lead to splenic dysfunction are at higher risk than the general population. Patients with malignancies or immunodeficiencies have a higher rate of meningitis and are more likely to be infected with uncommon bacteria. Malnourishment causes immune dysregulation that is the probable cause of increased risk in these children.[73] Patients with occult or known dermal sinuses or dural defects are at increased risk. Children with cochlear implants have a 30-fold increased risk for pneumococcal meningitis.[74] Finally, systemic diseases, especially diabetes mellitus or chronic renal disease, may confer a higher risk of meningitis.

Clinical Presentation

Patients suffering from purulent meningitis are generally ill-appearing. They usually have some combination of fever, headache, nausea, vomiting, photophobia, and neck stiffness. They may be irritable or lethargic. Obtundation and coma are late signs. On physical examination, nuchal rigidity may be found; this finding is less common in infants. Classically, Kernig and Brudzinski signs are sought. Kernig sign is elicited as follows: with the patient in the supine position with the hip flexed 90 degrees (knee pointing straight up), the knee joint is extended by slowly raising the foot upwards. Kernig sign is positive if this motion causes extreme discomfort. With the patient remaining supine, Brudzinski sign is positive if the hips are involuntarily flexed when the examiner bends the head down toward the chest. As with simple testing for nuchal rigidity, Kernig and Brudzinski signs are meant to help the physician detect inflammation of the meninges. Although these signs are often discussed, rigorous examination of their clinical utility is largely lacking. One prospective study of 295 adults with suspected meningitis found that neither the Kernig sign nor the Brudzinski sign was of clinical utility in differentiating patients with meningitis from those without meningitis.[75]

Possible Infectious Causes

Most purulent meningitis is caused by *Neisseria meningitidis, Streptococcus pneumoniae,* or *Haemophilus influenzae* type b (Hib). The epidemiology of meningitis has changed drastically since the introduction of the Hib vaccine. Prior to the vaccine, *H. influenzae* was by far the most common cause, especially in children between the ages of 1 month and 5 years. The incidence of Hib meningitis dropped from 19.4 cases per 100,000 in 1980 to 3.7 cases per 100,000 in 1991.[76] The vaccine was introduced in October of 1990. There has been a continued decline in the number of cases of Hib meningitis to even lower levels. The vaccine induces protection against nasopharyngeal carriage, which allows even the unvaccinated some measure of protection. From 1–23 months of age, pneumococcal meningitis is slightly more common than meningococcal meningitis. In children between the ages of 2 and 18 years, *N. meningitidis* accounts for 59% of cases; in adults *S. pneumoniae* predominates.[71]

In the first 30 days of life, the most common causes are Group B streptococci and enteric bacteria (particularly *E. coli*). Other bacteria that rarely cause meningitis except in the newborn period include other enteric gram-negative rods, *Listeria monocytogenes,* and *Staphylococcus aureus.* These agents also are an occasional cause of meningitis in the first few months of life, especially in prematurely born or debilitated infants.

Unusual infectious causes are discussed in the section on therapy of unusual infections.

Early Diagnosis

In young infants, it is important to do a lumbar puncture and examine the spinal fluid whenever the neck is questionably stiff or the anterior fontanel is questionably bulging and the patient appears ill. Disturbed consciousness (lethargy, irritability) and crying when handled are especially important symptoms suggesting early meningitis, as nuchal rigidity may be absent or appear late in young infants.

Treatment Before Lumbar Puncture

In rare cases, the illness may be so severe that supportive therapy should be started before the diagnostic studies. Any of the three major pathogens of meningitis can cause septic shock or cerebral edema. For example, in patients in whom meningococcemia is suspected because of hypotension and

---

BOX 9-1 ■ Emergency Treatment of Meningitis

1. *Do rapid history and examination*, including vital signs, testing for meningeal irritation, pupillary size and reflexes, "choked" optic disks, and capillary refill of nail beds.
2. *Take blood pressure.* If hypotensive, reinflate cuff and obtain an antecubital intravenous route for fluid therapy of shock before doing the lumbar puncture. Give 25 mL/kg of saline or Ringer's lactate solution over a 5- to 30-minute period. Administer a third-generation cephalosporin as a bolus and start vancomycin to infuse over one hour. Blood for culture and other studies can be obtained at the time the intravenous infusion is begun. If hypotension or a petechial rash is noted, all attendants should put on masks if they have not already done so.
3. If the patient has signs of rapidly deteriorating level of consciousness, *the trachea should be intubated and hyperventilation begun.* Examine pupils. If pupils are unequal or dilated and react sluggishly to light, give 0.5 g/kg of 20% mannitol over 30 minutes before doing a lumbar puncture. Deep coma, convulsions, apnea, cardiopulmonary arrest, or Cheyne-Stokes breathing are also usually indications for a mannitol infusion. In these cases, a CT scan should probably be obtained prior to the lumbar puncture. Obviously, intravenous antibiotic therapy should not be delayed until after an imaging study.
4. *Examine optic fundi.* If choked optic disks are not present, proceed with the lumbar puncture. Do not measure pressure. Minimal or questionable blurring of the disks is not unusual in meningitis, and the lumbar puncture is less risky than delay in the diagnosis. Coincidental high fever in a child with chronic, severely increased intracranial pressure (as from brain tumor, lead poisoning, or abscess) is very uncommon and typically produces obvious severe papilledema.
5. *Cloudy fluid is obtained.* Send cerebrospinal fluid (CSF) for study. As soon as puncture is finished, draw a blood culture from a large vein and give one-half to two-thirds the daily dose of a third-generation cephalosporin (such as ceftriaxone or cefotaxime). As before, start vancomycin as well until the identity and sensitivity of the organism causing the meningitis is known. Keep the IV route if it is practical, until a secure line can be started in another vein. The bolus of antibiotic allows the physician to move the patient and to feel less urgency about securing an IV, provided hypotension is not present.
6. *Begin flow sheet.* Every 15–30 minutes, record the pulse, blood pressure, respiratory rate and regularity, state of consciousness, pupil size and reaction to light, and spontaneous movements.

---

purpura, good intravenous access should be established and treatment of shock begun before doing a lumbar puncture. Meningococcemia can occur without meningitis, and the early treatment of septic shock is more important than determining if meningitis is present. An intravenous bolus of ceftriaxone can be given as soon as access is established. Some patients with evidence of life-threatening cerebral edema may be treated with mannitol before a lumbar puncture is done. Priorities in the emergency management of purulent meningitis are listed in Box 9-1.

In patients who are going to be transported to a hospital, if lumbar puncture cannot be done locally, presumptive antibiotic therapy should be begun without obtaining CSF if meningitis is suspected and transport will delay treatment.[77]

Children with purulent meningitis should generally be admitted to the critical care unit for close neurological monitoring, at least for the first 24 hours of illness, when complications such as shock, herniation, cerebral infarction, and seizures are most common.

Spinal Fluid Examination

Indications and technique of lumbar puncture and examination of the spinal fluid are described in an earlier section. Complete examination of the CSF should be done in order to detect any abnormality that may be helpful in the diagnosis. A Gram-stained smear should be examined even when few or no white blood cells are found. A few organisms can sometimes be found that originate on the slide or in the stain, but in rare instances, many organisms are found in spinal fluids that have no pleocytosis, especially in pneumococcal meningitis. The meningococcus is the organism most frequently missed on smear but found on culture, and *H. influenzae* is often misinterpreted as another organism.

Glucose and protein should be determined and are discussed in the following section.

Antibiotic therapy should not be delayed until the spinal fluid studies are available, especially if the fluid is grossly cloudy. As soon as the CSF is obtained, a third-generation cephalosporin such as ceftriaxone, 80 mg/kg as a loading dose,[78] should be given as an intravenous bolus. If there is likely to be a delay in starting the infusion into a small vein, the antibiotic should be given into a large vein, such as an antecubital or external jugular vein, or even intramuscularly if an intravenous route is not readily obtainable. As soon as an intravenous line is available, vancomycin should also be administered.

Prior Antibiotic Therapy

Often, patients are receiving oral antibiotic therapy (as for otitis media) when the clinical and CSF findings of purulent (or nonpurulent) meningitis occur. This should not be called "partially treated meningitis." "Meningitis during antibiotic therapy" is more accurate and does not imply a missed bacterial meningitis.

Meningitis during antibiotic therapy represents one of the most frequent and difficult situations in pediatrics. Prior antibiotic therapy is associated with a longer duration of symptoms,[78–80] especially in children with *H. influenzae* type b infection, which led to the theory that *H. influenzae* meningitis has two forms, one rapid and one slower in onset.[80] It has been suggested that the slower-onset form has a lower mortality rate,[80] but bacteriologically confirmed *H. influenzae* meningitis with prior oral antibiotics has a higher incidence of neurologic sequelae.[81]

The definitive study of the effects of prior oral or intramuscular antibiotic therapy on modifying the CSF findings in bacterial meningitis has not been done, nor is it likely to be done. The design needed was described by Wheeler in a 1970 editorial.[82] In 1975, in a chart review, the authors concluded "little more can be learned by a chart review of cases with positive cultures" and indicated that a prospective study with better diagnostic methods was needed.[80]

The prospective (and unlikely) study that would approach the issues directly would involve following, without antibiotic therapy, children who had developed clinical signs of meningitis while receiving oral antibiotics, who have CSF findings of 10–1000 white blood cells/mcL (with or without

a predominance of "polys"), normal or abnormal glucose, and normal or abnormal protein.

In the absence of such a study to evaluate variables of age, dose and duration of antibiotics, and the predictive value of low glucose, high protein, or CSF leukocyte count, clinicians decide whether to treat "as if" the patient had a bacterial meningitis by making an individualized clinical judgment based on these variables.

An infant less than 1 year of age is more likely to be treated for bacterial meningitis because the risk of brain damage is greater in the developing brain. Similarly, either a low glucose or an elevated protein in the CSF is much more likely to reflect a bacterial than a viral meningitis. As described later in the section on atypical presentations, however, the actual number and type of cells is sometimes the opposite of the expectation, even when no prior antibiotics have been given. Finally, patients with typical purulent meningitis (low glucose, high protein, high number and percent of neutrophils) have negative cultures in about 5–10% of cases with no preceding antibiotics and have just as bad a prognosis as those with positive cultures.[79]

In the absence of the definitive prospective study, several types of imperfect alternate studies are sometimes cited, although they do not provide conclusive guidance:

1. *Proved bacterial meningitis.* The CSF findings in proved *H. influenzae* meningitis do not differ significantly between patients with and without prior antibiotics when the culture is positive.[80] One study concluded an oral antibiotic preceding admission would not alter the CSF findings in most patients to an extent that would preclude establishing a diagnosis of *H. influenzae* meningitis.[81] In a study in Denmark that included 569 patients with pneumococcal, meningococcal, or *Haemophilus* meningitis, prior antibiotic therapy did not statistically change the frequency of CSF WBC counts below 1000/mcL, nor was there any increase in mortality rate or late sequelae.[83]

2. *Examining CSF after IV therapy.* Studies regarding the effect of antibiotics on CSF parameters have reached conflicting results. In one study, full appropriate IV antibiotic therapy of established bacterial meningitis for 44–68 hours did not alter the findings characteristic of bacterial meningitis (i.e., low CSF glucose, predominance of polymorphonuclear leukocytes) on the sec-

ond lumbar puncture.[84] In that study, three children with meningococcal meningitis had a normal CSF glucose and negative culture after 48 hours of therapy, but the remaining 65 children showed no statistically significant alterations in CSF cytology or biochemistry after about 48 hours' treatment. However, in another study of 42 patients, which was done to compare ampicillin and chloramphenicol against *H. influenzae* meningitis, many test values in both groups fell into a range of normal for glucose, protein, and total WBC count after 1–4 days of therapy.[85]

3. *Comparing bacterial with nonbacterial meningitis.* In some studies, the two groups compared were defined by positive or negative CSF cultures, and the CSF findings are statistically significantly different in terms of mean values, although overlap of values for each measure is present. In one study that included 38 children given antibiotic therapy in the 48-hour period before lumbar puncture, two patients with a positive CSF culture had cell and differential counts characteristic of "aseptic meningitis," with a slightly decreased glucose and definitely elevated protein.[86] No patient with a positive bacterial culture had all CSF findings compatible with aseptic disease, but the range of cell count, percentage of polymorphonuclear cells, glucose, and protein clearly overlapped those of the prior-antibiotic group whether or not the culture was positive. These authors interpreted their data to support Wheeler's 1970 editorial that "there is a small but important group" in whom prior antibiotic therapy may significantly alter the CSF laboratory values. However, others have speculated that it would be rare for prior antibiotics to alter all measurements simultaneously.[87] There is no evidence that bacterial antigen tests are more sensitive than Gram stain for the detection of meningitis in patients pretreated with antibiotics.[88]

Investigators continue to search for a biologic marker that would clearly differentiate viral meningitis from bacterial meningitis with antibiotic treatment. One study showed that CSF ferritin levels were greater than 18 ng/mL in 46 (98%) of 47 cases of bacterial meningitis, and that these levels did not correlate with CSF neutrophil count, CSF protein concentration, serum ferritin levels, or the age of the patient.[89] Furthermore, in 16 (84%) of 19 patients who had additional lumbar punctures performed, the ferritin levels remained elevated for an average of 15 days, despite appropriate intravenous antibiotic therapy. However, 15 (3%) of the 441 control patients also had ferritin levels greater than 18 ng/mL; 12 had bacteremia or pneumonia, 2 had relapsed CNS leukemia, and 1 had hemorrhagic herpes encephalitis.

Another group of investigators measured the N-acetyl neuraminic acid (NANA) levels in the CSF of 68 patients with bacterial meningitis, 37 of whom had pyogenic organisms and 31 of whom had tuberculous meningitis. They found that free NANA levels were elevated only in patients with pyogenic meningitis, and that the increase was not related to cell count or CSF glucose levels.[90] Unfortunately, however, this paper did not address the fate of the NANA levels after antibiotic treatment, so it does not directly address the question.

In spite of the various interpretations of the available studies, reasonable guidelines for continuing antibiotic therapy in a child developing meningitis while receiving antibiotics can be proposed, recognizing that experienced clinicians disagree. We suggest continuing IV antibiotic therapy if any of the following is present:

1. Significant neurologic signs such as lethargy, vomiting, paresis, convulsions
2. Age less than 1 year (some would include older infants)
3. CSF glucose or protein clearly abnormal
4. CSF WBC count exceeding 300/mcL or exceeding 60% polymorphonuclear cells
5. Any early complication of bacterial meningitis.

If the patient is neurologically normal at 72 hours when the CSF culture is negative and maximum temperature is less than 101°F (38.4°C), antibiotics can be discontinued. If bacteria are seen on initial Gram stain and found on review, or if neurologic abnormalities are present, therapy should be continued for the usual duration.

A second lumbar puncture may be indicated if significant fever or neurologic signs persist, with consideration of appropriate studies for the numerous causes of nonpurulent meningitis. A CT scan may be indicated for persistent fever or neurologic abnormalities.

Fortunately, most patients with viral meningitis will be clinically very much improved after 72 hours. A patient with bacterial meningitis sufficiently modified by prior antibiotics who has none of the above criteria for continuing antibiotics is likely to be fully cured by 72 hours of further IV antibiotics.

In a school-age child with a good state of consciousness and no significant neurologic signs, with fewer than 300 cells/mcL (predominately mononuclear), with normal CSF glucose and protein, the clinician can elect to stop antibiotics and observe carefully. If the patient is not definitely improved in 8–12 hours, the CSF can be reexamined, with the various causes of nonpurulent meningitis kept in mind for further study.

Atypical Presentations

Bacterial meningitis may not develop in the usual clinical pattern (Table 9-3). Probably the most common atypical presentation is mistaken for pneumonia; fever and rapid breathing, presumably caused by central hyperventilation, dominate the clinical picture. Weakness or ataxia also is presumably of CNS origin.

Even after the newborn period, signs of meningeal irritation were absent in 16 (1.5%) of 1064 of patients in one series.[91] Acute hearing loss has been reported as the presenting sign in a 6-year-old with meningitis after a posttraumatic basilar skull fracture.[92]

It is important to note that fever is not uniformly present in children with bacterial meningitis. Neonates with meningitis are at least as likely to have a normal or low temperature as they are to have an elevated temperature at the time of presentation. In children outside the neonatal period, more than 85% will have fever at the time of presentation.[93]

TABLE 9-3. ATYPICAL PRESENTATIONS OF MENINGITIS

CLINICAL
Fever and tachypnea
Weakness or ataxia
Absent meningeal signs
Hemiparesis
LABORATORY FINDINGS
Many bacteria; few leukocytes
Few (<100) CSF leukocytes
Predominance of CSF lymphocytes
CSF within normal limits

In one review of children older than 6 years old with bacterial meningitis, 11 (44%) of 25 were afebrile on presentation, suggesting that fever may be less common in older children.[94] Overall, the classic triad of fever, stiff neck, and mental status changes occurs in only one-half to two-thirds of patients with bacterial meningitis.[93]

Bacterrhachia Without Pleocytosis

Atypical CSF findings include spinal fluid with cell count, glucose, and protein within normal limits, a situation where bacteremia "seeds" the meninges and the bacteria are culturable before the inflammatory reaction has occurred. A review found that 7 (3%) of 261 children with bacterial meningitis had CSF findings within normal limits when first seen.[95] All appeared sick enough to be hospitalized, and all but one child were immediately treated for sepsis, indicating that children with bacteremia producing positive CSF cultures and normal CSF findings usually appear sick enough to be hospitalized and treated for suspected septicemia. Another report described the atypical finding of cloudy spinal fluid with innumerable pneumococci and few leukocytes.[96]

Low CSF cell counts (nonpurulent meningitis) may also occur with bacteremia. The prognosis in this situation depends on the prognosis for the bacteremic disease more than on the prognosis for meningitis if appropriate antibiotic therapy is given. Early meningococcemia or infective endocarditis may produce a "seeding" of the CSF with fewer than 100 leukocytes/mcL and normal CSF glucose and protein.

Other Atypical Patterns

Prior antibiotic therapy is probably the most frequent factor causing delay in diagnosis of bacterial meningitis.[97] Previous immunization with the polysaccharide *H. influenzae* type b vaccine occasionally resulted in a more gradual onset in *H. influenzae* meningitis, presumably related to partial protection by antibodies stimulated by the vaccine. This clinical pattern has not been seen following receipt of the protein-conjugate Hib vaccine.

A predominance of mononuclear cells with low glucose and high protein can occur with *Listeria* or tularemia.[98] On the other hand, several virus infections (such as enteroviruses or La Crosse virus) may present with a leukocyte count above 1000/mcL, although the CSF glucose and protein are typically normal or near normal (see section on purulent meningitis with negative culture).

Eosinophilic meningitis is discussed in the section on non-purulent meningitis.

Initial Antibiotic Therapy

Purulent meningitis is an extremely serious disease, and the outcome can range from complete recovery to brain damage or death. For this reason, no area in pediatric infectious diseases has had so many changing recommendations for antibiotic therapy. The epidemiology of the disease has also changed, due mostly to the efficacy of the conjugated Hib vaccine, but also to the overuse of antibiotics and subsequent spread of penicillin-resistant *S. pneumoniae* isolates. The two most likely pathogens in children outside the neonatal period are the pneumococcus and *N. meningitidis*; empiric therapy should be directed against these two pathogens. Third-generation cephalosporins such as ceftriaxone or cefotaxime penetrate CSF well and have good activity against all isolates of *N. meningitidis*; they are also active against all penicillin-susceptible and most penicillin-resistant isolates of *S. pneumoniae*. Unfortunately, a recent rise in the percentage of pneumococcal isolates that are only intermediately sensitive to these cephalosporins has mandated the inclusion of vancomycin in the empiric treatment of suspected bacterial meningitis in children outside the neonatal period. Vancomycin is a large molecule that crosses the blood-brain barrier poorly; therefore, children should be given large doses (20 mg/kg/dose) to enhance penetration into CSF. Once an organism has been identified and susceptibilities are available, therapy should be tailored appropriately.

Empiric therapy for neonates should be directed against Group B streptococci and the enteric gram-negative rods. The combination of ampicillin and gentamicin, or ampicillin and cefotaxime, are reasonable choices. Some experts would use all 3 drugs initially if purulent spinal fluid is obtained. Ceftriaxone should probably be avoided in the first 6 weeks of life because of its propensity to displace bilirubin from albumin binding sites and to cause "sludging" of bile in the gall bladder; both of these effects raise serum bilirubin levels.

Specific Antibiotic Treatment

Pneumococcal Meningitis

As soon as *S. pneumoniae* is identified as the cause of meningitis and penicillin- and cephalosporin-resistance have been excluded by an oxacillin disk diffusion, minimal inhibitory concentration (MIC) test, and/or the e-test, penicillin alone is sufficient therapy and is less expensive than ampicillin. The dose is 250,000 units/kg per day divided into four to six doses. Penicillin-allergic patients can be treated with ceftriaxone, unless there is a history of anaphylaxis, in which case beta-lactam agents should probably be avoided. Vancomycin plus rifampin may be used in this unusual circumstance.

Patients infected with penicillin-resistant strains should be treated with a third-generation cephalosporin. In the event the isolate is intermediately or completely resistant to third-generation cephalosporins as well, vancomycin should be continued for the entire course of therapy. The cephalosporin should not be discontinued, as levels achieved in the spinal fluid may exceed the minimum inhibitory concentration of even "resistant" strains. For cases of meningitis caused by highly resistant strains, some experts advocate a repeat lumbar puncture 48–72 hours into therapy to document sterilization of the CSF.

Meningococcal Meningitis

Penicillin, ampicillin, or third-generation cephalosporins are effective. Penicillin is the drug of choice for susceptible strains. Usually, patients allergic to penicillin can be treated with a third-generation cephalosporin. Prophylaxis of household and other intimate contacts (such as daycare contacts) should be carried out as detailed in Table 21-9. There are several drugs that have been shown to eradicate carriage of meningococci; these drugs are effective prophylactic agents. Rifampin 600 mg twice a day for four total doses is effective in adults; children can be given 10 mg/kg/dose for four doses. Children less than one year should get 5 mg/kg/dose instead. A single dose of 500 mg of ciprofloxacin has been shown to be effective in adults and is considerably less cumbersome. One intramuscular dose of ceftriaxone is also effective,[99] and may be considered in cases where compliance to the other regimens is likely to be poor, or in situations where the other agents are contraindicated, as, for example, for prophylaxis of a pregnant woman.

A deficiency of the terminal components of complement is sufficiently common in systemic meningococcal infection that the patient should be screened for this disorder with a CH_{50}.[100] It is more common in patients of African-American descent.

A second case of invasive meningococcal infection is especially suspicious. The family should be screened if the patient has a complement deficiency.

H. influenzae Meningitis

As alternatives to ceftriaxone listed in Table 9-4, cefotaxime can be used for initial empiric therapy, depending on cost and availability.[77]

Unusual Bacterial Causes

Other bacterial causes are usually related to trauma, the newborn period, or to some host defect. Recommended initial chemotherapy is shown in Table 9-5.

Nafcillin appears to be the best of the penicillinase-resistant penicillins for penetration of the CSF.[101] Clindamycin penetrates CSF poorly. *Bacteroides* meningitis also has been successfully treated with oral metronidadole.[102]

Duration of Therapy

For the patient with uncomplicated bacterial meningitis, antibiotic therapy should be given for at least 10 days except for meningococcal meningitis, where 5–7 days is sufficient.[78] Patients should generally be afebrile for 48–72 hours before therapy is

TABLE 9-4. INITIAL EMPIRIC THERAPY OF BACTERIAL MENINGITIS

AGE / CONDITION	COMMON BACTERIAL PATHOGENS	RECOMMENDED EMPIRIC THERAPY
0–4 wk*	Group B streptococcus, E. coli, *K. pneumoniae,* Salmonella, other gram-negative bacilli, Listeria, Enterococcus	Ampicillin 300 mg/kg/day div Q6h PLUS cefotaxime 200 mg/kg/day div Q6h (†)
4–12 wk	Group B streptococcus, *S. pneumoniae, N. meningitidis, E. coli, H. influenzae,* Listeria	Ampicillin 300 mg/kg/day div Q6h PLUS cefotaxime 300 mg/kg/day div Q6h (†, ‡)
3 mo to 18 yr	*S. pneumoniae, N. meningitidis, H. influenzae*	Cefotaxime¶ 300 mg/kg/day div Q6h (max daily dose 12 g) PLUS vancomycin 60 mg/kg/day div Q6h or Q8h
Immunocompromised host	*S. pneumoniae, N. meningitidis,* Listeria monocytogenes, gram-negative bacilli including Pseudomonas	Ampicillin 300 mg/kg/day div Q6h (max daily dose 12 g) PLUS cefepime 150 mg/kg/day div Q8h (max daily dose 6 g) PLUS vancomycin 60 mg/kg/day div Q6h or Q8h
Basilar skull fracture	*S. pneumoniae, H. influenzae,* Group A streptococcus	Cefotaxime¶ 300 mg/kg/day div Q6h (max daily dose 12 g) PLUS vancomycin 60 mg/kg/day div Q6h or Q8h
Head trauma; post-neurosurgery	*S. aureus, S. epidermidis,* gram-negative bacilli (including Pseudomonas)	Cefepime 150 mg/kg/day div Q8h (max daily dose 6 g) PLUS vancomycin 60 mg/kg/day div Q6h or Q8h
Cerebrospinal fluid shunt infection	*S. epidermidis, S. aureus, P. acnes,* gram-negative bacilli (including Pseudomonas)	Cefepime 150 mg/kg/day div Q8h (max daily dose 6 g) PLUS vancomycin 60 mg/kg/day div Q6h or Q8h

*Dosing may be different for premature or low-birth weight infants.
† If suspect Group B streptococcus, enterococcus, or Listeria, add gentamicin 7.5 mg/kg/day div Q8 hr.
‡ If suspect S. pneumoniae, add vancomycin 60 mg/kg/day div Q6 hr.
¶Or ceftriaxone 100 mg/kg/day div Q12 hr (max daily dose 4 g)
Note: All doses assume normal renal function.

TABLE 9-5. ANTIBIOTICS FOR UNUSUAL BACTERIA CAUSING MENINGITIS

BACTERIA	ANTIBIOTIC	ALTERNATE
Listeria	Ampicillin + gentamicin	TMP-SMX
MSSA	Nafcillin	Vancomycin
MRSA	Vancomycin	Linezolid
S. epidermidis	Vancomycin	Linezolid
Viridans streptococci	Cefotaxime	Vancomycin
Enterococci	Ampicillin + gentamicin	Vancomycin + gentamicin
E. coli; Klebsiella	Cefotaxime	Meropenem
Pseudomonas	Cefepime	Meropenem
Stenotrophomonas	TMP-SMX	Levofloxacin
Bacteroides	Metronidazole	Meropenem

TMP-SMX, trimethoprim-sulfamethoxazole

MSSA, methicillin-susceptible *Staphylococcus aureus*

MRSA, methicillin-resistant *Staphlycoccus aureus*

stopped. If therapy is begun late, or if the prognosis is otherwise poor, 14 days of IV therapy should be given. Duration of therapy for gram-negative meningitis should probably be longer; 21 days is considered standard.

In our opinion, treatment of bacterial meningitis should be completed in the hospital by the intravenous route. When there is unusually severe illness, when the patient is a young infant, or when there is a delay in diagnosis and treatment, the clinician should choose the longer duration and the higher doses of antibiotics, using the surest route. CSF protein and WBC do not usually return to normal until well after therapy has been completed; normalization of CSF parameters should not be used as a criterion for duration of therapy.

Relative Importance of Antibiotic Therapy

The management of meningitis requires more than the choice of the best antibiotic, the best dose, and the best route. Indeed, antibiotic therapy of meningitis is relatively standardized; the anticipation, early recognition, and effective treatment of complications, particularly cerebral edema, must be emphasized.

Neonatal Meningitis

Meningitis occurring in the first month of life differs from meningitis in older individuals in a number of important respects:

1. *Poor prognosis.* The diagnosis is often late because of minimal symptoms. Also, brain complications are more likely and more severe, because the central nervous system is still developing.

2. *Misleading clinical response.* Newborn infants often have a prompt return of the temperature to normal, suck well, and appear to be fairly normal yet may ultimately develop hydrocephalus or signs of brain damage. Repeat lumbar punctures should be done to follow the response to therapy early in the course.

3. *Infecting organisms.* Group B streptococci and *E. coli* are the usual pathogens, but *Listeria*, other streptococci, staphylococci, *Hemophilus,* and many gram-negative bacillary species are also possible.[103] *E. coli* is almost never a cause of meningitis after the first 6 weeks of life, although rare exceptions might occur in a very premature infant or an infant with an underlying disease, such as severe congenital heart disease.

4. *Chemotherapy.* A collaborative study showed no evidence of difference between ampicillin plus amikacin (representing aminoglycosides) and ampicillin plus moxalactam (representing a third-generation cephalosporin).[104] Each regimen has its benefits and its drawbacks: the combination of ampicillin and an aminoglycoside (gentamicin, tobramycin) is synergistic for Group B streptococcal infection and effective against gram-negative meningitis as well, but in

some hospitals monitoring of serum levels is cumbersome, and aminoglycosides have well-known renal and ototoxicity. Ampicillin plus a third-generation cephalosporin (usually cefotaxime) is more convenient and less toxic, but is probably less reliable against Group B streptococci, especially those that are ampicillin tolerant (discussed later). Many experts would use all three days initially (ampicillin plus gentamicin plus cefotaxime).

A 72- to 96-hour follow-up lumbar puncture should be done in neonatal meningitis to ensure sterility as a guide to efficacy and prognosis.

In the newborn or very young infant with meningitis caused by Group B streptococci, ampicillin and gentamicin appear to be synergistic and should be used for 14 days or longer.[78] Although penicillin-resistant Group B streptococci have not been identified, some isolates are penicillin tolerant (the minimum bactericidal concentration is more than 4 times greater than the minimum inhibitory concentration). Therefore, high doses of penicillin (450,000 U/kg/day) or ampicillin (300 mg/kg/day) should be used. The incidence of side effects with high-dose penicillin or ampicillin is no higher than that seen with lower doses. For gram-negative enteric bacilli, adding gentamicin to cefotaxime may produce a synergistic effect. Some gram-negative bacilli (especially *Enterobacter* and *Citrobacter*) possess a chromosomal, inducible beta-lactamase and can develop resistance to beta-lactams during therapy, even if initial susceptibility testing is favorable.[105] For these pathogens, a carbapenem (meropenem) or fourth-generation cephalosporin (cefepime) plus an aminoglycoside (gentamicin or tobramycin) is appropriate therapy. Other gram-negatives (especially *Klebsiella* and *Serratia*) may also harbor extended-spectrum beta-lactamases that can render semi-synthetic penicillins and cephalosporins useless. When caring for newborns with gram-negative meningitis of any kind, consultation with an infectious diseases specialist is advised. Patients with gram-negative meningitis should be treated for 21 days or longer.

5. *Other therapy.* The poor outcomes seen with gram-negative meningitis have led some to consider trials of intraventricular or intrathecal antibiotic therapy. A multicenter, randomized, controlled trial of intravenous ampicillin and gentamicin with or without intrathecal gentami-

cin was conducted in 117 infants with gram-negative enteric meningitis. There were no significant differences in the mortality, morbidity, or time to CSF sterilization between the two groups.[106]

Seizures in neonates with gram-negative meningitis have multiple potential causes, including poor cerebral perfusion, infarcts, edema, and hypoglycemia. The development of cerebral abscesses is common and should be screened for with computed tomography. Drainage by a neurosurgeon may be necessary.

Early Complications

The complications of meningitis can be divided into early complications (those that occur during the first 24 hours and may be the immediate cause of death) and late complications (those usually recognized after several days or later) (Table 9-6). The early complications are cerebral edema, septic shock, disseminated intravascular coagulation, myocarditis, hyponatremia with water intoxication (which aggravates cerebral edema), and convulsions.[107] Sensorineural deafness is also an early complication but may not be detected until later. Cerebral edema and endotoxic shock are the principal causes of death after patients have reached the hospital and are receiving antibiotics. In order to detect early signs of these severe complications, the physician should be sure the indicators of shock and cerebral edema (described below) are charted on a flow sheet every 15 minutes in the early hours of treatment, just as one would chart such vital data in a hospitalized diabetic in severe acidosis.

Diagnosis of Cerebral Edema

The recognition of cerebral edema is based on progressive changes in several physical findings[108] (Table 9-7). A flow sheet is useful to follow the course (Fig. 9-1). In cerebral edema, the state of consciousness changes from alert but irritable, to lethargic but arousable, to stuporous, and finally to deep coma. Pupillary reflexes change from midposition, equal, and reactive to light to dilated and sluggish and, finally, to dilated and fixed. The optic discs are usually not a useful guide, because rapid changes in pressure are often not reflected by anything more than minimal blurring of the discs. Such a minimal blurring in acute purulent meningitis is not a contraindication to a careful lumbar puncture.

TABLE 9-6. ACUTE COMPLICATIONS OF BACTERIAL MENINGITIS

COMPLICATION	THERAPY
Brain swelling	Mannitol, urea, or corticosteroids
Septic shock*	Plasma volume replacement
Disseminated intravascular coagulation*	
Myocarditis	Digitalization
Pericarditis	Pericardiocentesis
Hyponatremia	Reduce water intake
Convulsions	Depends on mechanism
Hemiparesis; focal signs	Observation if no increased pressure
Endophthalmitis; endocarditis	
Carotid artery thrombosis	
Cortical blindness; opsoclonus	
Brain abscess	

* Septic shock and disseminated intravascular coagulation are discussed in Chapter 10.

TABLE 9-7. PROGRESSION OF SIGNS OF BRAIN SWELLING

LEVEL OF CONSCIOUSNESS	PUPILS	RESPONSE TO STIMULATION	BREATHING
Alert but irritable	Mid position, equal, briskly reactive	Crying, withdrawal	Regular
Lethargic but arousable			Irregular, periodic
Stuporous	Dilated, sluggish	Stiffening, rigidity	Cheyne-Stokes
Deep coma	Dilated, fixed	Flaccid	

Marked papilledema or choked discs implies a more dangerous situation, and a chronic illness such as lead encephalopathy should be considered, as discussed earlier under Indications and Risks. Eye movements change from fixation on distant objects when the neck is rotated, to rotation in concert with the head, as if staring (doll's eye movement) late in the course of the disease. Response to pain changes from purposeful withdrawal of the extremity to which the painful stimulus is applied, to non-purposeful withdrawal and stiffening with decerebrate rigidity, to complete flaccidity.

The pattern of breathing is an important guide to increased intracranial pressure. In cerebral edema, the breathing pattern changes from regular to irregular to the Cheyne-Stokes pattern. Cheyne-Stokes respirations are characterized by periods of deep and rapid respirations alternating with periods of slow, shallow respirations or apnea. The late changes in breathing and eye movements are related to compression of the brainstem and are often not seen if the child receives early chemotherapy.

The fontanel may change from flat to bulging. Convulsions may occur. Patients with meningitis who have had convulsions should not be kept deeply sedated, because this obscures changes of consciousness that are a guide to the severity of cerebral edema. Lateral rectus palsy may be seen in severe or chronic cerebral edema and is not of localizing value.

There is one report of 5 children who developed cutaneous flushing, an obvious but transient red-

Time (15-minute, then 30-minute intervals)	Level of Consciousness	Pupils	Response to Stimulation	Respiration	Pulse	B.P.	Temp.	Other
7:00								
7:15								
7:30								
7:45								
8:00								
8:30								
9:00								
9:30								
10:00								

■ **FIGURE 9-1** Flow sheet for observation for brain swelling. Use Table 9-7 for signs to be recorded.

dening of the skin, at the same time they experienced neurologic deterioration secondary to increased intracranial pressure. The epidermal flushing involved the upper chest, face, or arms, and lasted from 5–15 minutes. The exact origin of this response is unknown, but it is postulated that it may be a centrally mediated response to sudden elevations in ICP.[109]

These changes associated with cerebral edema resemble the progression of stages during induction of general anesthesia and have also been described in patients with brain tumors when herniation is imminent. This progression can sometimes be reversed by drugs such as mannitol that create an osmotic gradient between the brain and the plasma. Osmolar agents rapidly remove water from all of the extravascular space, but it is the removal of water from the swollen brain cells that may be lifesaving. Increased cerebral blood flow also occurs during mannitol infusion and may be a factor in its cerebral effects.[110]

Corticosteroids such as dexamethasone also reduce cerebral edema, according to studies of patients with brain tumors.

Other agents have been shown to decrease intracerebral pressure in experimental meningitis in animal models, including the calcium-channel blocking agent nimodipine.[111]

The use of mannitol or dexamethasone in patients with meningitis and progressive worsening of brain signs has not yet been proved effective in any prospective controlled comparative study. The evidence for its effectiveness is derived primarily from repeated observation of reversal of the signs of brain deterioration in individual patients when this therapy is given.

Cerebral Herniation

The fatal consequence of cerebral edema is cerebral herniation and typically occurs within 8 hours of admission.[112] This is the usual cause of death in the first 24 hours of *H. influenzae* meningitis.[113] However, it is not always fatal when treated (e.g., with mannitol), as described later in this section. Prevention by limiting intravenous fluids, as described later, is better than having to treat the cerebral edema, but fluid restriction has no immediate effect in an urgent cerebral edema situation. In addition, cerebral perfusion pressure is dependent on adequate systemic blood pressure; fluid restriction is thus inappropriate in the patient with hypotension and shock.

Relation of Cerebral Edema to CSF Manometric Pressure

The presence of cerebral edema should be recognized by clinical observations. The actual measurement of opening pressure at the time of lumbar puncture is much more easily accomplished in older patients who are lucent enough to be cooperative with the examination (i.e., those who likely have normal pressures). In smaller children and in babies, attempting to measure the CNS pressure by manometry increases the risk of needle manipulation and may produce intrathecal bleeding. This blood in the spinal fluid may make the CSF cell count and protein results, which are of critical importance in a patient with suspected meningitis, difficult to interpret. Free back-flow is often not obtained if the patient is straining. Localized cerebral edema may be present in the absence of increased spinal fluid pressure as measured in the lumbar area.[114] Finally, the finding of a normal opening pressure does not rule out the presence of increased pressure a few hours later, after intravenous fluids have begun to correct dehydration.

Treatment of Cerebral Edema

Mannitol, urea, and dexamethasone appear to be effective in reducing cerebral edema from causes other than meningitis. The use of these agents has not been adequately studied in meningitis.

Mannitol has some theoretical advantages: there is no commitment to continuous therapy, and there is no risk of adrenal suppression or gastric ulceration or of masking fever, as is the case with dexamethasone. Moreover, there is no preparation time because of addition of diluents required, and no confusion about possible renal insufficiency, as in the case of urea. Urea is seldom used.

Mannitol is usually given intravenously as a 25% solution, 0.25–0.5 g/kg/dose, over a 20- to 30-minute period, for trauma.[115] A review of supportive therapy recommended mannitol at 0.5–2.0 g/kg/

dose over a 30-minute period, repeated as necessary.[107]

A decrease in CSF pressure has been noted in brain tumors within 1/2 hour of starting the infusion, with the lowest pressure reached after 2–4 hours (Fig. 9-2). Pressure returned to previous levels by 6–10 hours. Mannitol can be repeated as soon as 4–6 hours after the last infusion if signs of cerebral edema are again noted. However, after about 48 hours, or six to eight doses, the patient's long-term prognosis is likely to be unchangeable. The decrease in cerebral edema produced by mannitol or urea is only temporary, and the result depends on improvement of the disease process itself.

Prevention of Cerebral Edema

There has been some controversy over the role of fluid restriction in the prevention of cerebral edema in patients with meningitis. Prospective studies have shown that as many as 88% of patients with meningitis develop the syndrome of inappropriate antidiuretic hormone secretion (SIADH).[116] Furthermore, studies done in patients who were never fluid restricted showed that the development of SIADH correlated with poor neurologic outcomes.[117] However, the diagnosis of SIADH should never be made in a patient who is dehydrated (because the release of ADH in the setting of dehydration is not inappropriate). Restriction of fluids in

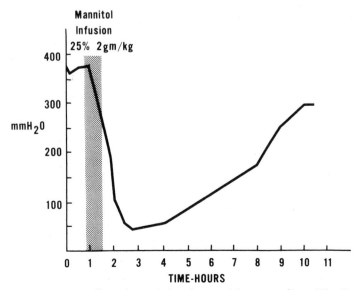

■ **FIGURE 9-2** Effect of mannitol on intracranial pressure. (From Wise BL, Chafer N. J Neurosurg 1962;19:1038–43.)

the setting of even mild dehydration may decrease cerebral perfusion. A prospective study of 50 children with meningitis suggested a worse outcome in patients who were fluid restricted.[118]

After restoring circulatory perfusion, restricting fluid therapy to approximately two-thirds maintenance in patients with hyponatremia would be a rational approach. Fluid restriction should be continued only until it can be demonstrated that the patient does not have SIADH, after which fluids are liberalized. This can usually be accomplished within 24–36 hours by careful monitoring of the patient's input, output, serum sodium concentrations, and urine specific gravities and osmolalities. Serum sodium concentration should be monitored at least twice every 24 hours, especially in patients with documented sodium levels less than 130 mg/dL. Use of less than one-half the calculated maintenance dose as a preliminary guide may contribute to low blood volume, hypotension, or cerebral vascular sludging and venous thrombosis and is therefore to be avoided.

Initial Treatment of Poor Perfusion (Compensated Shock)

Often, children with meningitis have poor circulatory perfusion when first seen, as judged by poor capillary refilling in nail beds and cool extremities. This is not the same as septic shock, which is a later, more severe, situation. Treatment consists of a rapid intravenous infusion of Ringer's lactate, 10–20 mL/kg/dose, repeated as necessary, to restore circulatory blood volume and improve brain perfusion.

Septic Shock

Shock is usually recognized by low systemic blood pressure and a fast, weak pulse. The extremities may be warm, so that septic shock is sometimes called "warm shock." Slow filling of the capillary nail beds may be a useful guide to septic shock.

Treatment of Shock

The therapy of septic shock is controversial and is discussed in more detail in Chapter 10. The optimal therapy is plasma volume expansion, which can be done using plasma or 5% albumin, with an estimated initial dose of 25 mL/kg/dose. Patients with meningitis and shock need to receive enough fluid to keep systolic blood pressures adequate, and to

keep urine output above 0.5 mL/kg/hour. Central venous pressure should be monitored. Pressor agents such as dopamine can be used to support blood pressure when needed but are not a substitute for adequate filling volume.

The total amount of plasma or 5% albumin given should be based on the blood pressure and on the central venous pressure. When the blood pressure is low or unobtainable, blood volume replacement should be given until blood pressure is adequate or central venous pressure is high.

Disseminated Intravascular Coagulation

The patient with meningococcemia is much more likely to develop disseminated intravascular coagulation (DIC) with purpura than is a patient with bacterial meningitis of another cause. This problem is discussed further in Chapter 10.

Myocarditis

Congestive heart failure, manifested by rapid pulse, enlarging tender liver, or pulmonary edema, is not always caused by over-treatment of endotoxin shock by excessive intravenous fluids. Myocarditis, presumably secondary to endotoxin, has been demonstrated in some cases by autopsy findings of petechiae, cell infiltrates, and muscle fiber necrosis. Digoxin may be of value.

Purulent pericarditis may also occur, especially as a complication of *H. influenzae* meningitis. Small, self-limited effusions were detected in 20% of 100 consecutive cases.[119] They were usually not significant clinically.

Hyponatremia

Decreased serum sodium concentration may be noted as early as the time of admission to the hospital, although it usually appears after the patient has had some intravenous therapy. This hyponatremia is probably secondary to brain disease and is mediated by an "inappropriate" excessive secretion of ADH. Use of 0.5 normal saline as the maintenance intravenous fluid is reasonable, with continued fluid restriction. Mannitol should be avoided when the patient is severely hyponatremic, because it increases sodium losses. It is an error to focus on correction of serum sodium and the mechanism of inappropriate ADH secretion to the neglect of the basic complication of cerebral edema and its treatment.

Convulsions

In a patient with meningitis, convulsions may occur because of cerebral edema, hyponatremia, subdural effusion, fever, and, by unexplained mechanisms, the disease itself. It is important to consider all possible underlying causes that might be improved by treatment other than anticonvulsants. Barbiturates in low to moderate doses may actually improve the state of consciousness in a patient with constant seizures. However, high doses of barbiturates or other anticonvulsants can obscure the persistence of a physiologic disturbance that should be corrected, such as cerebral edema or subdural effusions.

Hemiparesis or Focal Signs

Focal or lateralized signs observed during the first few days of purulent meningitis have several possible etiologies.[120] Usually, mild focal signs such as slight asymmetry of strength or reflexes improve with observation and specific antibiotics and presumably have a vascular or inflammatory basis. However, hemiparesis or total paralysis may be caused by bleeding from DIC, indicating potential residual damage. Focal signs can also be caused by subdural effusions or asymmetric cerebral edema. CT scanning is indicated in the patient with focal neurologic signs.

Subdural Effusion

In young children with bacterial meningitis subdural effusions are very common, occurring in 44 (39%) of 113 children aged 1–18 months old in one study. Only one child had a documented subdural empyema.[121]

Long-term follow-up (median 5.5 years) demonstrated no increased incidence of seizures, hearing loss, neurologic deficits, or developmental delay. The authors concluded that specific invasive therapy is not indicated in infants with meningitis and subdural effusion who are otherwise improving. The rare child with a subdural empyema will usually not improve clinically on antibiotics alone or will have an initial improvement followed by relapse. In the older child, whose cranial sutures are closed, subdural effusions are potentially more serious, especially if large or if associated with midline brain shift. Neurosurgical consultation for possible drainage should be obtained immediately.

Brain Abscess

Except for gram-negative meningitis in the neonatal period, brain abscess is extremely rare in the first week of purulent meningitis. Operative drainage is not usually necessary unless intracranial pressure is increasing.

Anemia

As with other severe infections, meningitis is frequently accompanied by the anemia of inflammation.[122]

Diagnostic Approach

EEG

One retrospective study of neonates with meningitis concluded that a markedly abnormal EEG during the acute phase of meningitis correlated with long-term poor neurologic outcome.[123] The study looked at 75 EEGs in 29 neonates; babies with normal or near-normal EEGs had good outcomes. This study also suggested that in a population of neonates, EEG may be useful for detecting subtle or subclinical seizure activity.[123]

Brain Scans

The availability of CT and magnetic resonance imaging (MRI) scanning has revolutionized CNS diagnosis. Scanning is useful for detecting brain abscess or subdural effusion (neither of which usually needs to be drained), large lateral ventricles (implying ventricular obstruction and ventriculitis), small lateral ventricles (cerebral edema), and diminished attenuation or focal hemorrhage (neither particularly treatable nor closely correlated with prognosis).[124] Imaging may be useful for the patient who is not responding as expected after several days of adequate therapy; to look for cerebral edema when there is no clinical emergency and a chronic process is suspected; and to evaluate possible hydrocephalus. It is also useful for the patient with focal neurologic signs. However, routine brain scanning in all patients with meningitis is not indicated: one prospective study of serial CT scans in meningitis concluded that clinical management was not influenced by scan results, which failed to reveal any significant abnormalities not suspected on neurologic examination.[125] Another study of 58 children with meningitis showed that positive findings with obvious clinical significance were found in only 6 (10%) of 58 CT scans, all of which were occasioned by complex or prolonged seizures or prolonged fever.[126] The procedure demonstrates what clinicians and pathologists have always known: purulent meningitis exerts a profound effect on the brain parenchyma as well as on the meninges. If imaging is deemed necessary, contrast-enhanced MRI is probably the best imaging modality.[127]

Hearing Loss

Sensorineural hearing loss is the most common adverse neurologic outcome in children who recover from bacterial meningitis. This complication occurs in about 10% of patients, with about half of these cases being bilateral.[128] It is most common with meningitis due to *S. pneumoniae* (31%), as compared with *N. meningitidis* (11%) or *H. influenzae* (6%).[128] It appears to be unrelated to the number of days of illness before admission or the type of antibiotic therapy but is correlated with ataxia, severe neurologic deficits, or initial CSF glucose of less than 20 mg/dL.[128] It is thought that hearing loss is secondary to inflammation that results not only from the infection itself, but also from the bacterial products released by lysis during antibiotic therapy.

Pretreatment with dexamethasone decreases the concentrations of some inflammatory mediators and leads to decreased hearing loss in animal models of experimental meningitis, especially meningitis caused *by H. influenzae*. Some clinical studies also documented better hearing outcomes in patients pretreated with dexamethasone versus placebo.[129] Most of the patients in these trials were suffering from *H. influenzae* infection, as the trials were carried out when Hib was the most common pathogen. Even though some aspects of the pathogenesis of disease are similar, extrapolation of data obtained from children with *H. influenzae* meningitis to those with *S. pneumoniae* or *N. meningitidis* infection may not be straightforward. A small, prospective trial of dexamethasone vs. placebo in children with pneumococcal meningitis showed a trend toward better audiologic outcomes in the dexamethasone recipients.[130] Limitations of the study include that the numbers were small and that ampicillin/sulbactam was the antimicrobial therapy employed. It has already been demonstrated that hearing outcomes vary with differing antimicrobial regimens.

A large, prospective, multicenter trial demonstrated that hearing loss, when it occurred, was present within the first several hours of illness.[131] There is also the theoretical concern about the ability of dexamethasone to tighten the blood-brain barrier that is opened due to the inflammation of meningitis. This would normally be considered good, as it decreases the transport of plasma proteins, etc.; however, in this era of increasingly resistant *S. pneumoniae* isolates, the concern is that the transport of large molecules such as vancomycin would also be decreased. In a rabbit model of meningitis, CSF concentrations of vancomycin have been shown to be lower in rabbits that received concomitant dexamethasone.[132]

Most experts advise pretreatment with dexamethasone in cases where the suspicion of *H. influenzae* infection is high (e.g., contact with a known case, gram-negative rods on Gram stain, patient from a group that gets no vaccinations for religious reasons). A recent randomized, placebo-controlled trial in adults with bacterial meningitis demonstrated decreased morality in the dexamethasone-treated group.[133] However, the use of steroids in the treatment of bacterial meningitis remains controversial. The preponderance of the clinical evidence suggests that benefit for patients with pathogens other than *H. influenzae*, if indeed a benefit exists, is small enough to be clinically difficult to demonstrate. The risk of having meningitis secondary to a multiply-resistant pneumococcus that requires vancomycin therapy, on the other hand, is tangible.

Hearing loss, if it is going to occur, is present within 48 hours of presentation. Children with bacterial meningitis should thus have their hearing tested prior to discharge from the hospital or shortly thereafter. If it is normal, no further testing is necessary. If abnormal, repeat testing should be performed, because about one-third of children will regain hearing over the ensuing 6 months. For infants under about 1 year of age, routine electrical auditory testing is advisable. Behavioral hearing testing by a pediatric audiologist in a soundproof room is the best method for a cooperative child.

Prognosis

Purulent meningitis is still one of the most important medical emergencies. It should be suspected and diagnosed early by prompt lumbar puncture and treated vigorously. Management includes anticipation and treatment of cerebral edema and shock as early complications. Late complications and permanent brain damage remain significantly frequent.

The clinician should usually avoid predictions to the family about prognosis and about intellectual recovery and should instead advise parents to wait and see how the child does, using follow-up examinations and, later, specialized testing if necessary as a guide.

Later Complications

These complications occur from a few days to a few weeks after onset and include subdural effusion, hydrocephalus, and brain damage with mental retardation.

Subdural Effusion

The subdural space normally contains no fluid. Subdural effusions occur in about a third of children with meningitis, according to subdural taps done routinely.[121] The best explanation of the pathogenesis of subdural effusion is that protein enters the subdural space from dural blood vessels, which are abnormally permeable in meningitis. The protein then brings in fluid from the vessels by osmotic action. In early papers, it was suggested that subdural effusions are more likely to occur when relatively large amounts of spinal fluid are removed at lumbar puncture. Although this has not been clearly documented, the theoretical risk has resulted in the consensus that the volume of fluid removed at lumbar puncture should be kept to the minimum necessary for study (a total of 2–3 mL).

Subdural effusions are least frequent after meningococcal meningitis[135] and, after correction for age, are about equally frequent in *H. influenzae* and *S. pneumoniae* meningitis.

A subdural effusion is not likely to occur until several days after the onset of purulent meningitis but rarely is found on the first day that meningitis is recognized, particularly if there has been preceding antibiotic therapy.

Because small asymptomatic effusions are common, and because asymptomatic moderate effusions typically resolve without drainage, they need not be looked for and drained routinely, as was done in the past. Effusions are often blamed for persistent fever, vomiting, or other complications of meningitis; subdural effusions are common enough that you might expect to find them in patients with these clinical features. Causation is more difficult

to establish. Prospective studies suggest that the neurologic outcome is no worse for those with effusions than for those without.[121] Effusions presumably also occur in older children with closed fontanels and usually resolve without drainage. Subdural punctures are rarely done when small effusions are detected on older infants, because the procedure is much more invasive if the anterior fontanel is closed. CT scans demonstrate that even large effusions may resolve completely.[137]

Clinical indications to obtain CT scans consist primarily of persistent or recurrent neurologic abnormalities after 48 hours of therapy. These include focal neurologic signs, continuing lethargy, seizures, bulging fontanel, or increase in head circumference.[138] Usually, the fever is higher than expected for the day of the illness. CT scans can only detect effusions of about 30 mL or larger, but smaller effusions are unlikely to be clinically significant.[138] Transillumination is a simple, less expensive way to detect the thin layer of fluid and can be used to supplement the CT scan (Fig. 9-3).

If an effusion is found concurrently with any of the above neurologic findings, subdural needle aspiration through an open fontanel should be considered to see if improvement occurs. A second aspiration is usually not indicated unless the first aspirate is positive on culture or unless neurologic findings are relieved and then recur later to an equally severe degree. Large volumes of fluid (25

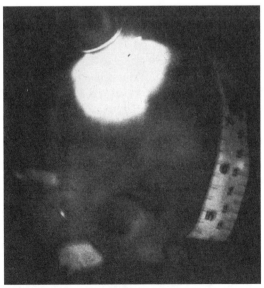

■ FIGURE 9-3 Transillumination is useful to detect subdural effusions. (Photo courtesy of Dr. Raymond Chun.)

mL or more) should not be removed rapidly, because this may result in rapid expansion of the compressed brain, which may be manifested by pallor, tachycardia, or even apnea. Persistent subdural effusions have been treated by neurosurgical shunting of the fluid from the subdural space into the peritoneal cavity. However, the more conservative approach of waiting for absorption of the fluid may be just as effective in most cases.

Subdural Empyema

This term is used when the effusion is purulent, containing more than 5000 leukocytes/mcL. It is more likely to be associated with a positive culture and severe neurologic damage.[138] Subdural empyema can also occur as a complication of severe sinusitis or mastoiditis without presenting as a purulent meningitis.[139] In contrast to patients with simple effusions, patients with subdural empyema usually present with focal signs, especially hemiparesis. Imaging may reveal shift of the midline structures, requiring an immediate neurosurgical referral for drainage.

Slow Improvement During Days 3 to 7

During the first 2 days of treatment for purulent meningitis, the patient often improves significantly in terms of state of consciousness and fever. From the third to the seventh day, improvement is steady but less rapid, as the temperature may remain somewhat elevated, the neck somewhat stiff, and the child irritable (Fig. 9-4). The physicians need patience during this time. They should not do unnecessary procedures (such as a CT scan or a repeat lumbar puncture, which often leads to a third). Solid clinical reasons should make the clinician "do something" diagnostic, but this is typically a time of "worry, but watch carefully."

Follow-up Lumbar Puncture

A follow-up LP should be performed 3–4 days into therapy in neonates with gram-negative meningitis and in patients infected with drug-resistant pneumococci, and should be considered in anyone who has a poor response to therapy. Neonates with bacterial meningitis of any etiology should have a repeat LP at the end of therapy. However, routine follow-up examination of the spinal fluid is unnecessary as a test of cure.[77,140] Sometimes, equivocal results on the follow-up examination as the result

of laboratory variation or a traumatic (bloody) tap prolong hospitalization and lead to another lumbar puncture, both of which are clinically unnecessary.

Patients with neurosyphilis generally get a follow-up LP at 6 months and those with cryptococcal meningitis are "re-tapped" two weeks into therapy. Meningitis caused by multidrug resistant *Mycobacterium tuberculosis* is a vexing problem; follow-up LP may be required on more than one occasion.

Persistent Pleocytosis or Low Glucose

Persistent pleocytosis alone should not be used as a reason for prolonging therapy beyond 14 days. Repeat lumbar puncture to be sure the CSF glucose has risen to normal is not essential, if the response has otherwise been adequate. The frequency distributions of glucose, protein, and leukocyte counts show wide variation after successful treatment of meningitis.[140]

Persistent Fever

The most frequent causes of fever beyond the expected range are drug fever, unrelated infections, phlebitis, arthritis, and unknown etiology.[141] Sometimes prolonged fever is diagnosed and evaluated based on an unrealistic expectation of the rapidity of defervescence. Prolonged and even secondary fevers (fever occurring after a period of defervescence) are not uncommon in children with bacterial meningitis, even in the absence of complications. A brain CT scan is not automatically indicated. Several studies have documented that approximately 10–13% of patients with meningitis have fever beyond 8 days, and about 15–20% develop secondary fevers.[142] The presence of prolonged or secondary fever does not correlate with adverse neurologic outcome, nor does it correlate with relapse or recrudescence.[143] If the child is neurologically well, and progressive improvement in clinical condition (other than fever) is noted, watchful waiting is the best approach. Plotting a graph of the child's fever curve may also reveal a decrease in the temperature index, which is encouraging. Small undetected collections of serous fluid containing antigen-antibody complexes may be present in a joint, pleural space, pericardial space, or intracranially. This theoretical explanation is based on the detection of larger fluid collections in some patients with persistent fever.

Antibiotic therapy need not be continued be-

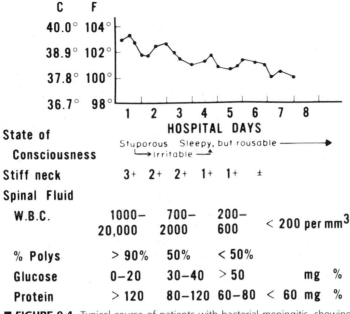

C	F											

(Chart showing temperature over Hospital Days 1–8, ranging from 40.0°C/104°F down through 36.7°C/98°F)

State of Consciousness			

Stuporous → Irritable → Sleepy, but rousable →

Stiff neck	3+	2+	2+	1+	1+	±

Spinal Fluid

W.B.C.	1000–20,000	700–2000	200–600	< 200 per mm^3
% Polys	> 90%	50%	< 50%	
Glucose	0–20	30–40	> 50	mg %
Protein	> 120	80–120	60–80	< 60 mg %

■ **FIGURE 9-4** Typical course of patients with bacterial meningitis, showing usual range of clinical and cerebrospinal fluid findings.

yond the previously recommended times if the clinical condition is satisfactory.

Hydrocephalus

Hydrocephalus may be communicating or obstructive. Obstructive hydrocephalus can occur within a few days of the onset of the illness if there is thick pus in the ventricles that blocks CSF flow out of the ventricular system, especially in newborns or very small infants. Obstructive hydrocephalus occurring early in the illness is usually manifested by acutely increased intracranial pressure, with slow pulse, rising blood pressure, and apnea. Emergency treatment consists of insertion of a needle into the ventricles to remove CSF and relieve pressure.

Communicating hydrocephalus usually is not noted until 2 weeks or more after the onset of the illness. It occurs more frequently in patients with a delay in beginning therapy. It may also occur in young infants with meningococcal meningitis, where the onset of the disease may be slow even without modification by preceding antibiotic therapy. Hydrocephalus is sometimes first suspected by noting a "setting sun" appearance of the eyes (Fig. 9-5), and an enlarging head can be confirmed by daily measurement of the head circumference. A CT scan or sonogram is useful to determine whether the ventricles are dilated throughout (communicat-

ing) or if there is obstruction of the aqueduct with a small fourth ventricle. Hydrocephalus is a more common complication of tuberculous or cryptococcal meningitis.

Brain Damage with Mental Retardation

Severe intellectual damage is probably the most dreaded complication of meningitis. Other neurologic deficits that may result include seizures, paralysis, and deafness. Many mechanisms can con-

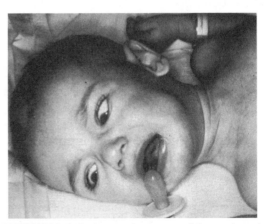

■ **FIGURE 9-5** Setting sun appearance of the eyes in early hydrocephalus. The pupils and iris are the "sun," with increased visibility of the white sclera as the "sky."

tribute to this damage. Cerebral anoxia with subsequent infarction may occur because of shock or apnea or increased intracranial pressure. Direct infectious or toxic destruction of brain tissue may also occur.

Statistical data are usually not helpful in discussing the prognosis of an individual patient with the parents. Bad prognostic factors include coma, hypothermia, shock, age less than 12 months, anemia, and seizures that are intractable or last (or have their onset) greater than 72 hours into antibiotic therapy. In most patients with sequelae, functional improvement tends to occur to at least some extent over time.

Hemorrhage, Thrombosis, or Infarct

With CT scanning, these findings are recognized more often, but no specific therapy is available. Infarctions are more common with meningitis caused by *S. pneumoniae*. Hemiparesis may be present but sometimes resolves with time. Occlusion of the internal carotid artery has been reported.[120]

Immune or Reactive Arthritis

Sterile arthritis representing a presumed antigen-antibody reaction has been recognized as a complication of infections such as hepatitis B, yersiniosis, salmonellosis, meningococcemia, and gonorrhea. During the course of *H. influenzae* meningitis, a sterile high-protein arthritis with fever is occasionally observed, which typically responds promptly after removal of the fluid. Arthritis during the first few days, on the other hand, is usually septic.[144,145]

Other Complications

Transient or permanent cortical blindness, quadriplegia, acute endocarditis, and endophthalmitis are basically not preventable. Brain abscess can occur, especially in neonatal enteric bacterial meningitis.[146] Movement disorders, such as athetosis, as well as convulsive disorders, can occur.[147]

Purulent Meningitis With Negative Culture

Bacterial Meningitis

This is presumed to be the usual cause of purulent meningitis with a negative spinal fluid culture. In many cases, the culture is negative because of preceding antibiotic therapy,[148] and in a few cases,

cultures may be negative because of improper collection or delay in delivery to the laboratory. This is discussed further in the following section on aseptic meningitis syndrome. *Listeria monocytogenes* may not be positive on culture until 72 hours of incubation.

Congenital Dermal Sinus

The CSF culture may be negative, or a skin or other "contaminant" bacterium may be found, so the culture is regarded as negative when the source is a congenital dermal sinus. Any child suffering from meningitis who is noted to have a midline dimple over any part of the vertebral column should have an MRI performed to look for the presence of an associated dermal sinus. If present, the sinus tract should be resected after recovery from the meningitis to prevent a second episode.

Anaerobic Meningitis

Anaerobes are a very rare cause of bacterial meningitis and would result in a negative conventional culture.[149] Anaerobic meningitis is usually associated with prior CNS or otolaryngologic surgical procedures or penetrating trauma. The diagnosis is sometimes suspected by the finding of pneumocephaly on imaging studies.[150] The principal predisposing cause in a child would be chronic sinusitis or chronic otitis media. An illustrative case of an 18-year-old with infectious mononucleosis who developed Lemierre's syndrome and associated meningitis has been reported. The blood culture grew *Fusobacterium necrophorum*, but the CSF culture grew *Prevotella bivia*. CT scan showed pan-sinusitis.[151] Another report tells of a previously healthy child who developed *Fusobacterium necrophorum* meningitis secondary to purulent otitis media with the same organism.[152] A 3-year-old who injured her eye with a toothbrush developed meningitis secondary to *Veillonella parvula*, a gram-negative anaerobic coccus found in the mouth flora.[153]

Reactive Meningitis (Parameningeal Infection)

Acute sinusitis or other bacterial infection near the meninges may produce more than 1000 WBC/mcL, predominately neutrophils, whereas the glucose and protein are usually normal or nearly normal, and the Gram stain typically reveals no organisms. In the absence of prior antibiotics, parameningeal infection should be suspected, and head imaging should be obtained.

Amebic Meningitis

Amebic meningitis is exceedingly rare. However, the physician should be aware that purulent meningitis with a negative culture can be due to amebae such as *Naegleria* species.[154] The patient sometimes has a history of swimming in lake water, which may be the source of the ameba. It has been suggested that the route of inoculation is through the nose to the olfactory bulbs. The CSF cell count is usually in the purulent meningitis range, with a predominance of neutrophils. Erythrocytes are often present and may provide a useful clue. The spinal fluid glucose may be normal or slightly depressed. The CSF protein is usually elevated.

This diagnosis can be made by isolating the ameba from the brain or by observing the motile organism in the spinal fluid (Fig. 9-6). Specific chemotherapy with amphotericin B, miconazole, and rifampin has cured several cases,[154,155] but the prognosis is extremely poor. In animal models, passive antibody prior to infection is protective,[156] and antibody given intracisternally as therapy prolongs survival but does not prevent death.[157]

Contaminated CSF Collection

In this situation, there are no CSF findings of purulent meningitis except a smear showing bacteria, which may be traced to commercial lumbar puncture kits.[158] False positive gram staining due to contamination of the ethanol the slides were stored in has been reported. If contaminated gentian violet is placed on a hot slide, false positive Gram stains may result; this problem is solved by placing gentian violet on slides that have cooled.[159]

Cerebravascular Accidents

Hemorrhage or thrombosis of the brain occasionally results in a CSF leukocytosis beyond what can be explained on the basis of the red blood cells present. It should be remembered that erythrocytes become hemolyzed in the CSF, resulting in the supernatant CSF becoming xanthochromic.

Herpes Simplex Encephalitis

As discussed later in this chapter, herpes simplex encephalitis can resemble bacterial meningitis with negative bacterial cultures.

Mycoplasma Meningitis

Mycoplasma pneumoniae produces CNS involvement in approximately 1 in 1000 patients. The primary manifestation is usually encephalitis, but meningitis and meningoencephalitis may also be seen. In meningitis secondary to *Mycoplasma pneumoniae* the cells may be predominantly neutrophils and the protein may be elevated, but the glucose is normal.[160] Typically, there is a preceding definite middle or lower respiratory infection, as discussed in Chapter 8.

Mycoplasma hominis is carried in the genital tract of 12–50% of pregnant women. Prevalence of infection and frequency of antibody titers increase with increasing parity.[161] *M. hominis* cannot be seen on Gram stain and is difficult to isolate on routine microbiology laboratory media. Waites et al. found evidence of CNS infection with *M. hominis* in 5 of 100 predominantly preterm babies being evaluated for meningitis. In 4 babies, the organism was repeatedly isolated over several weeks.[162] In another study of infants with good prenatal care, *M. hominis* was isolated from 9 (3%) of 318 infants who under-

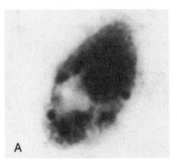
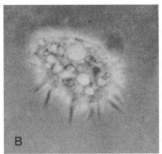
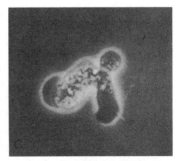

■ **FIGURE 9-6** (**A**) Naegleria as seen in cerebrospinal fluid. (Photo courtesy of Drs. James Seidel and Zane Price. From N Engl J Med 1982 306;346–8.) (**B**) Hartmanella (Acanthamoeba) culbertsoni. (**C**) Naegleria aeroba. (B and C courtesy of Dr. Clyde G. Culbertson.)

went lumbar puncture. Most cleared the infection without specific therapy. In all these studies, the lack of a control group of healthy infants makes interpretation of the findings difficult.

Mollaret's Meningitis

This is an uncommon syndrome of recurrent aseptic meningitis, usually seen in adults and rarely teenagers, characterized by cloudy spinal fluid, usually with a neutrophilic pleocytosis and normal glucose and protein. The presence of "Mollaret cells," once thought to be endothelial but now known to be of the monocyte/macrophage family, is pathognomonic. This syndrome is now thought to be secondary to HSV-2. This conclusion is based on the PCR finding of HSV-2 DNA in the CSF of three patients with the disorder and on the known propensity of herpes group viruses to cause recurrent disease.[163]

Intravenous Immunoglobulin

Several cases of aseptic meningitis after receipt of high-dose immune globulin have been reported. Bacterial meningitis is often suspected initially because of the neutrophilic predominance.[164,165] In a review of 11 cases,[165] the mean CSF leukocyte count was 1123 per mcL (median, 451) with a mean of 74% neutrophils (median 87%).

Neonatal Intraventricular Hemorrhage

After the red blood cells have been lysed, the white blood cells and protein may remain for several days after an intraventricular hemorrhage. The CSF glucose also is usually depressed early or several weeks later, and this may persist. The finding of xanthochromic fluid is the principal clue to this cause of suspected meningitis with negative cultures.

Chronic Meningitis

Persistently low CSF glucose concentrations may occur, particularly in enteric bacterial meningitis of newborns. This finding may indicate brain dysfunction rather than persistence of infection.[166]

Most chronic meningitis is of fungal or mycobacterial origin.[167] Malignant infiltrations usually occur in patients with known malignant disease. In adults, other noninfectious causes include vasculitis, sarcoidosis, systemic lupus erythematosus, Sjögren's syndrome, and drug reactions. Other causes are discussed under recurrent meningitis.

Relapsing or Recurrent Meningitis

Recurrent episodes of purulent meningitis with negative cultures can be categorized under the diagnosis of Mollaret's meningitis. An extremely rare cause of chronic CSF pleocytosis in teenagers with recurrent oral, genital, or ocular lesions is Behçet's syndrome.[168] An intracranial epidermoid cyst or other tumor can cause recurrent sterile meningitis.[169,170]

An immunoglobulin deficiency is rarely a cause of repeated episodes of meningitis. Deficiency of a terminal component of complement or of properdin is a cause of recurrent meningococcal meningitis.[171,172]

A neurenteric fistula associated with presacral mass and an abnormal sacrum is seen in Currarino syndrome, which can be a cause of recurrent or polymicrobial meningitis. Most patients have a history of constipation because of associated anal stenosis. A congenital encephalocele may extend into the sinuses and result in recurrent meningitis. The diagnosis is made with a fine-cut MRI of the sinuses.

Posttraumatic or Post-Operative Meningitis

An abnormal communication with the CSF, such as a skull or spinal wound, skull fracture, or a congenital dermal sinus in the sacral or occipital areas, should be sought early in all cases of persistent, relapsing, or recurrent meningitis.[173,174] Recurrent pneumococcal meningitis suggests an occult CSF leak through a dural tear held open by a skull fracture.[173] Imaging of the sacral spine may reveal abnormalities in patients with recurrent meningitis caused by enteric gram-negative rods, or in babies with polymicrobial gram-negative meningitis.

CSF rhinorrhea after trauma may be localized by radiographic techniques and repaired if spontaneous closure does not occur.[175–177]

■ NONPURULENT MENINGITIS

Definitions

Nonpurulent meningitis (aseptic meningitis syndrome) can be separated from the general category of presumptive CNS infections by the absence of severe cerebral manifestations, such as a severe disturbance of consciousness, and by a spinal fluid cell count of 10–500 leukocytes/mcL (see Table 9-2).

Usually, encephalitis can be distinguished clinically from nonpurulent meningitis. In one study of both these syndromes, mild impairment of consciousness, febrile convulsions, or mental dysfunction associated with high fever alone were not accepted as definite evidence of encephalitis.[178]

Obviously, patients with 500–1000 WBC/mcL need to be fit in to one of the categories on the basis of other criteria. This classification is intended as a preliminary one, and exceptional cases occur. In mumps virus meningitis, the CSF WBC count sometimes exceeds 1000/mcL but is typically mostly lymphocytes. In enterovirus outbreaks, especially of Coxsackie-virus meningitis, the protein may be slightly elevated or the glucose slightly depressed or the cell count may be above 500/mcL with a slight predominance of neutrophils, even on an early repeat tap. In a study of 150 children in an epidemic of echovirus meningitis, only 3% had an initial CSF glucose below 40 mg/dL and none were less than 20 mg/dl.[179] However, 23% of the children had an initial CSF white blood cell count exceeding 1000/mcL, 21% had a predominance of neutrophils, and 12% had a CSF protein exceeding 80 mg/dL. (These abnormalities did not necessarily occur concurrently.)[179] Thus, the preliminary categories are not absolutely perfect in predicting the possible etiologies, and patients who have findings atypical of purulent or nonpurulent categories should be judged individually by clinical findings and according to whether there is enterovirus disease in the community. Many such patients, especially infants, get treated for bacterial meningitis until their diagnosis is clarified.

"Aseptic meningitis syndrome" is the term now used most frequently. "Viral meningitis" and "meningoencephalitis" are terms with significant disadvantages. All of these terms can be further defined.

Aseptic meningitis syndrome was originally defined by Wallgren as an acute illness with meningeal signs and symptoms, a small or large number of cells in the cerebrospinal fluid, and absence of bacteria on direct smear or culture of CSF with no general or local parameningeal infection, and a relatively short benign course (Table 9-8).[180] Aseptic meningitis syndrome is now usually defined on the basis of CSF findings that allow the prediction that bacterial pathogens will not be found; namely, a moderate number of leukocytes that are predominately lymphocytes and a smear negative for bacteria (Fig. 9-7). The CSF glucose and protein may or may not be abnormal by this definition. The Centers for Disease Control and Prevention (CDC) include recovery without antibiotics in its recording of definitive cases of aseptic meningitis.

The diagnosis of viral meningitis should not be regarded as equivalent to aseptic meningitis syndrome, which is a syndrome that has many other possible etiologies that are extremely important to consider (Table 9-9). "Nonpurulent meningitis" is a better problem-oriented diagnosis because it makes the clinician more likely to consider such important etiologic possibilities as tuberculosis or partially treated bacterial meningitis.

The term "meningoencephalitis" has the disadvantage of failing to distinguish patients who should be said to have "encephalitis," which has severe cerebral signs and a higher probability of brain damage. A severe and persistent (at least 8 hours) disturbance of consciousness is an early and relatively reliable indication of a poor prognosis. Nonpurulent meningitis and acute encephalitis also differ in probable etiologies.

A single virus can produce a spectrum of severity of illness, from asymptomatic to mild to severe to fatal. Coxsackieviruses, for example, can cause a spectrum of severity from headache and fever, to nonpurulent meningitis, to paralytic poliomyelitis-like syndrome, to acute and fatal encephalitis. However, from the starting point of a single patient's illness, it is useful to make a presumptive diagnosis of either nonpurulent meningitis or acute encephalitis and then analyze the etiologic possibilities.

Importance of CSF Glucose

A decreased CSF glucose concentration (hypoglycorrhachia) is usually present in purulent meningitis. It has little more than supportive diagnostic value because the purulent spinal fluid and Gram stain already indicate the presumptive diagnosis of bacterial meningitis. The decreased CSF glucose appears to be related to decreased glucose transport across the blood-CSF barrier and conversion of the brain metabolism from oxidative to the less efficient glycogenolysis. Thus, a lowered glucose suggests more severe brain involvement.

In nonpurulent meningitis, a low CSF glucose is correlated with more chronic or more serious etiologic agents, such as *Mycobacterium tuberculosis*. Therefore, in patients with nonpurulent meningitis, a decreased CSF glucose has special diagnostic value. It is thus useful to divide nonpurulent meningitis into two subgroups: those with and those without decreased CSF glucose (Table 9-2). It is

TABLE 9-8. DEFINITIONS OF SOME ACUTE CENTRAL NERVOUS SYSTEM SYNDROMES

SYNDROME	SIGNS
Aseptic meningitis syndrome (Wallgren's original definition)	Acute meningeal signs and symptoms
	Cerebrospinal fluid (CSF) pleocytosis, small or large number of cells
	No bacteria by smear or culture
	No general or local parameningeal infection
	Relatively short benign course
Aseptic meningitis syndrome (current usage)	Acute meningeal signs and symptoms usually, but no significant disturbance of consciousness
	CSF pleocytosis, nonpurulent, mostly lymphocytes
	No bacteria by smear
	Recovery without antibiotic therapy
Acute encephalitis	Acute, severe, nontransient disturbance of consciousness
	CSF pleocytosis, nonpurulent, mostly lymphocytes
	No bacteria, normal CSF glucose
Acute encephalopathy	Acute, severe, nontransient disturbance of consciousness
	No CSF pleocytosis
	No bacteria, normal CSF glucose

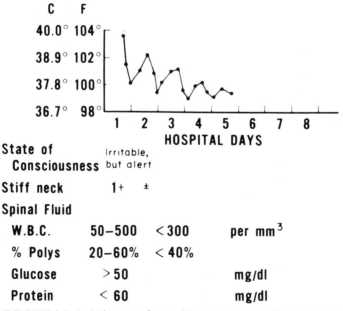

■ **FIGURE 9-7** Typical course of coxsackievirus meningitis, showing normal glucose and protein and predominance of lymphocytes in cerebrospinal fluid after a few days of illness.

TABLE 9-9. NONPURULENT MENINGITIS: CLASSIFICATION OF ETIOLOGIES

TYPE OF ETIOLOGY	CAUSES
Infectious	Viral meningitis (e.g. echo virus, coxsackie virus, mumps)
	Early bacterial meningitis (especially meningococcal or neonatal, and embolization to the meninges in bacterial endocarditis)
	Partially treated bacterial meningitis
	Brain abscess and other adjacent infections, including sinusitis and mastoiditis
	Uncommon infections (leptospirosis, syphilis, toxoplasmosis, trichinosis)
	Low CSF glucose group (tuberculosis, cryptococcosis and other fungi, occasionally mumps, listeriosis, lymphocytic choriomeningitis, meningeal neoplasm)
	H. influenzae vaccine-modified meningitis
	Lyme disease
Noninfectious	Poisons (lead, arsenic)
	Medications (immune giobulin, nonsteroidal anti-inflammatory drugs)
	Trauma (subdural hematoma; intrathecal injections)
	Hypersensitivity (serum sickness)
	Kawasaki disease

useful to define CSF glucose as definitely lowered if it is less than 40% of the blood glucose, or as less than 40 mg/dL if the blood glucose is not known.

An elevation of CSF protein concentration is often also present when there is a decreased CSF glucose. However, a slightly elevated protein may be a result of laboratory variability, of slight bleeding during the lumbar puncture, or of previous traumatic lumbar punctures or operative procedures.

Low-Glucose Subgroup

Bacterial Meningitis

When a patient develops nonpurulent meningitis while receiving an antibiotic, the most reliable clue to bacterial meningitis may be a significantly decreased CSF glucose. In this situation, the protein may also be elevated. Because prior antibiotic therapy may prevent recovery of the infecting organism on culture, the frequency of this etiology is unknown, but it is probably the most frequent cause of hypoglycorrhachia in children.[181] This situation is discussed in detail in the section on purulent meningitis.

Early bacterial meningitis may also produce this CSF pattern. *Listeria monocytogenes* produces nonpurulent meningitis with predominately lymphocytes in a small proportion of cases. The CSF glucose is almost always low and the protein almost always high in such cases.[182]

Bacterial meningitis can also present as nonpurulent meningitis with a normal CSF glucose, as discussed later.

Tuberculous Meningitis

Tuberculous meningitis presents subacutely in 3 clinical stages. Stage 1 consists of nospecific signs such as fever and headache. In stage 2 the patient develops mental confusion and early focal signs, such as cranial nerve palsies. In stage 3 the patient progresses to obtundation and coma. The prognosis is directly related to the clinical stage at the time therapy is begun. Thus, it is critical to make the diagnosis as early as possible.

Tuberculous meningitis usually results in hypoglycorrhachia. In a series of 405 children with tuberculous meningitis from 1987–1998, 80% had depressed CSF glucose levels. CSF protein was greater than 100 mg/dL in 65%. Half of patients had less than 60 WBC per mcL, 45% had 60–500 WBC/mcL, and 5% had more than 500 WBC/mcL. Just over half had evidence of pulmonary involvement, and only 16% had a positive tuberculin skin test (TST). Nearly 70% had a positive family history of tuberculosis.[183]

Another study reported a higher percentage of pulmonary involvement: 87% of 214 children with tuberculosus (TB) meningitis in that series had an abnormal chest x-ray.[184] Family or exposure history was found in 66%, and the TST was greater than 10 mm in only 30%.

A study comparing 110 children with tuberculous meningitis to 94 patients with non-TB aseptic meningitis syndrome identified 5 clinical features that suggested TB:

1. prodromal stage of one week or longer
2. optic atrophy
3. focal neurologic deficit
4. abnormal movements, and
5. less than 50% of CSF white blood cells of the polymorphonuclear phenotype

When tuberculous meningitis is suspected, three factors should be evaluated: TST, chest roentgenogram, and exposure history (including past travel to or residence in a high-risk area). If the TST is negative (less than 5 mm), the chest roentgentogram is normal, and there is no history of exposure to tuberculosis (or residence in high-risk areas), then tuberculous meningitis is much less likely. In contrast to past teaching, pulmonary tuberculosis that has been present long enough to calcify (more than about 6 months) may still be associated with dissemination.[185] Thus, even if the three factors listed above are negative, tuberculous meningitis should be considered if the CSF glucose is low and there is a CSF lymphocytosis.

A second lumbar puncture and CSF examination should be done if the CSF glucose is borderline low on the first test, because during the course of untreated tuberculous meningitis, there is almost always a progressive fall in the glucose, a rise in the protein, and a continuation of the CSF lymphocytosis.

Studies of early detection or surrogate markers of tuberculous meningitis have been published. A good method is needed primarily because AFB stain is positive in only about 15% and culture in only about 30% of cases.[184] In one study, 80–85% of children with TB meningitis were shown by ELISA to have immunoglobulin G (IgG) or immunoglobulin M (IgM) to antigen A60 in serum, and 60–75% had antibodies in the CSF; unfortunately, no controls were reported.[186] Another report looked at detection of H37Rv antigen in CSF; this test was 90% sensitive and 96% specific for the diagnosis.[187] Finally, a PCR for the detection of *Mycobacterium tuberculosis* DNA in CSF has been developed and tested; the sensitivity ranges from 60–85%, and the specificity ranges from 94–100%, depending on the report.[188,189] Only the PCR test is commercially available.

Fungal Meningitis

Cryptococcal meningitis, generally only seen in patients with advanced immunodeficiency, may have an indolent onset and may present with subtle signs and symptoms, such as intermittent headache with or without low-grade fever. This condition is associated with a low glucose and a high protein.[190,191] The sensitivity of the India ink test to detect budding yeast forms in the CSF is about 50%; however, either serum or CSF cryptococcal antigen testing will be positive in nearly every patient with cryptococcal meningitis.[192]

The organism often grows out in a few days on most of the solid media usually used for the culture of *Mycobacterium tuberculosis*.

Candida albicans can cause a nonpurulent meningitis with low CSF glucose, high protein, and, usually, a predominance of CSF neutrophils.[193] Premature infants with many prior courses of antibiotics are most frequently affected.

Coccidioidomycosis uncommonly presents as a meningitis in patients with illness severe enough to require hospitalization.[194] Blastomycosis and histoplasmosis rarely produce meningitis, and when they do, disseminated disease is usually also present with hepatosplenomegaly in histoplasmosis and chronic pulmonary disease in blastomycosis. Urine histoplasma antigen is positive (greater than 1 unit) in approximately 80% of patients with disseminated disease.[195]

In immunosuppressed patients, aspergillosis, mucormycosis, or superficial fungi occasionally produce meningitis.

Serologic and antigen studies for fungi, as well as CSF smears for fungi, should be done if the features of presumed tuberculous meningitis are atypical. The CSF can be tested for cryptococcal antigen or coccidioidal antibody for rapid diagnosis. It is important to detect fungal causes of nonpurulent meningitis, because therapy with appropriate anti-fungal agents can be lifesaving.

Viral Meningitis

Viruses can lower the CSF glucose,[196,197] although this is uncommon. Mumps meningitis is occasionally associated with slightly decreased CSF glucose concentration,[198] although most studies indicate glucose below 40 mg/dL in only about 3%.[197,199] Mumps virus can be cultured from CSF or saliva. Paired sera can be used to demonstrate an antibody titer rise.

Echoviruses and coxsackieviruses have produced low CSF glucose and elevated protein along with their typical lymphocytic pleocytosis, thus resembling tuberculous meningitis, especially in infants.[200,201] One study of 17 babies 2 months of age or younger with coxsackievirus type B1 meningitis reported that 64% had hypoglycorrhachia.[202] The patients' clinical and CSF results improve steadily in such cases (Fig. 9-7).

Lymphocytic choriomeningitis virus can lower the CSF glucose. The CSF protein may be elevated.[203] The virus can sometimes be cultured from CSF, but usually the diagnosis is made on the basis of an antibody titer rise.

Amebic Meningitis

Free-living amebae such as *Naegleria* species can produce lower CSF glucose and high protein. The cells are usually predominately neutrophils, as discussed in the section on purulent meningitis with negative culture. Chemotherapy may be helpful, so this is an important diagnosis to consider despite its rarity.

Unusual Infectious Causes

Toxoplasmosis can present with nonpurulent meningitis with a lymphocytic predominance and depressed CSF glucose.[204] Listeriosis can produce nonpurulent meningitis with cranial nerve palsies and low CSF glucose, resembling the basilar meningitis (rhombencephalitis) of tuberculous meningitis.[205]

Chronic enteroviral (usually echovirus) meningitis in children with agammaglobulinemia typically has fewer than 1000 white blood cells/mcL, elevated CSF protein, and depressed CSF glucose (between 15 and 45 mg/dL).[206] These patients often improve after intravenous immunoglobulin ther-

apy. Pleconaril, previuosly available on a compassionate use basis for chronic or severe enteroviral infections,[207] is no longer available from the manufacturer.

Noninfectious Causes

Chemical meningitis can result from injections into the subarachnoid space and may produce lowered glucose as well as pleocytosis. Spinal anesthetics or even corticosteroids may be implicated.[208]

Cerebral neoplasms, particularly meningeal neoplasms, can produce a low CSF glucose. There also may be an increase in leukocytes in the CSF. Intracranial bleeding or hematoma also can be a cause of low CSF glucose with pleocytosis.

Normal-Glucose Subgroup

Viral Meningitis

Viruses are the most common, but not the only, cause nonpurulent meningitis with a normal CSF glucose. In three large series with viral cultures of patients with nonpurulent meningitis in the 1950s, the most common causes were coxsackieviruses (20–50%), echoviruses (10–15%), and mumps virus (5–15%). Mumps virus is now a rare cause. The typical course of coxsackievirus meningitis is shown in Figure 9-7.

In the United States, coxsackieviruses and echoviruses characteristically are found in the summer and fall, although echoviruses may be found all year. Wintertime outbreaks of echovirus meningitis have been reported.[209] Young infants may be more likely to have echoviruses as a cause of nonpurulent meningitis, especially in outbreaks.[210,211] The prognosis for full intellectual functioning after recovery in infants less than 3 months old with enteroviral meningitis is as good as for matched controls.[212] Outcomes may be worse in babies infected within the first week of life, however.

Newly recognized enteroviruses are no longer classified as echoviruses or coxsackieviruses, so that enterovirus types (such as enterovirus type 71) are now being reported as causes of nonpurulent meningitis.[213] A report comparing the clinical symptomatology of patients with enterovirus 71 infection versus those with coxsackievirus A16 infection during a large outbreak showed that, in general, enterovirus 71 infection was more severe. A total of 7% of the group with enterovirus 71 infection had aseptic meningitis, 10% had encephalitis, 5% were classified as encephalomyelitis, and the mortality rate was 7%; all deaths were attributed to pulmonary edema. In contrast, 94% of the Coxsackie A16 infections were uncomplicated, only 6% had aseptic meningitis syndrome, and there were no deaths.[214]

Outbreaks of enterovirus disease associated with day-care centers and neonatal nurseries have been reported.[215,216]

Vaccination history should be obtained. Immunization has made mumps virus infection much less common now than it was in the past, but a history of mumps exposure should be sought, especially in the unvaccinated child, and the patient should be examined carefully for parotid enlargement. An elevated serum amylase in the presence of suspected parotid enlargement is supportive evidence for the diagnosis of mumps. Mumps virus or enteroviruses can often be recovered on culture in a virus diagnostic laboratory, so viral cultures of the throat, rectum, and CSF should be done if facilities are available.[196] Enteroviral PCR on CSF is performed in some laboratories and can be very helpful in this setting.[217]

Antibody studies using two sera, one obtained as soon as possible after the onset and the second obtained 3–6 weeks later, are useful for diagnosis of a number of viruses: mumps, lymphocytic choriomeningitis, California group (La Crosse) encephalitis, Eastern equine encephalitis, Western equine encephalitis, St. Louis encephalitis, and West Nile virus encephalitis. However, with the exception of La Crosse virus and West Nile virus, infection with these viruses is relatively uncommon in the United States, except in occasional localized outbreaks.

Pet hamsters or mice can be a source of lymphocytic choriomeningitis virus infection. Adenovirus is a rare cause of aseptic meningitis.[218] Measles encephalitis is rarely associated with a predominance and persistence of a CSF neutrophilic pleocytosis.[219] Rotavirus gastroenteritis has been associated with nonpurulent meningitis in a patient with minimal CSF pleocytosis and detection of rotavirus antigen in the CSF. Typical rotavirus particles were seen in the CSF by immunoelectron microscopy.[220]

Infectious mononucleosis is sometimes complicated by a CSF pleocytosis and a variety of neurologic complications, as discussed in the section on encephalitis.

Unknown Etiology

In the three large studies mentioned previously, about 30–50% of patients with nonpurulent men-

ingitis had negative cultures and negative serologic studies for viruses. Probably some of these patients had a viral etiology for their illness, but viruses are often difficult to isolate from the CSF.

Mycoplasma

Mycoplasma pneumoniae can cause nonpurulent meningitis, often with preceding respiratory symptoms.[221] Usually, the CSF glucose and protein levels are normal and the CSF leukocyte count is in the nonpurulent range, with a predominance of lymphocytes. The organism can also be a rare cause of encephalitis, polyneuritis, paralysis, and psychosis, as discussed in these sections. PCR can be used to detect *M. pneumoniae* in spinal fluid specimens, although not all cases with meningeal or encephalitic involvement are PCR positive.[222] CSF PCR is more likely to be positive in encephalitis. In all cases, the duration of illness prior to the development of CNS symptoms is an important predictor of the sensitivity of PCR; the shorter the duration, the more likely the PCR will be positive.[223]

The genital mycoplasmas *Mycoplasma hominis* and *Ureaplasma urealyticum* are rare causes of nonpurulent meningitis in the newborn period.[224] In many cases, sepsis is suspected since there may be no CSF pleocytosis. Intraventricular hemorrhage and hydrocephalus also have been reported to be associated with recovery of these microorganisms from the CSF, especially in preterm infants.[224]

Lyme Disease

Borrelia burgdorferi can cause nonpurulent meningitis, sometimes with a cranial neuritis. Neurologic symptoms are typically preceded by a rash at the site of the tick bite. In one study of 201 children with Lyme disease, 2% were diagnosed with aseptic meningitis.[224] CSF PCR is relatively insensitive, but serology is usually positive.[225,226]

Rickettsial Diseases

Rocky Mountain spotted fever and ehrlichiosis (see Chapter 11) are both typically associated with a mononuclear pleocytosis of 10–100 WBC/mL.[224a,224b] In patients with a history of travel to sub-equatorial Africa, African tick bite fever is a possible cause of fever, headache, and stiff neck. The disease is caused by the recently identified *Rickettsia africae* and responds rapidly to treatment with doxycycline.

Infectious Mononucleosis

As discussed in Chapter 3, Epstein-Barr virus (EBV) can produce nonpurulent meningitis as the predominant clinical manifestation.

Cat-Scratch Disease

Occasionally, central nervous system complications occur in cat-scratch disease. Encephalitis is more common than aseptic meningitis. Usually, there is regional adenopathy, as described in Chapter 6.

Parameningeal Infection

Sometimes, infection near the central nervous system, particularly ethmoid or sphenoid sinusitis, produces a sterile, nonpurulent meningitis.[227] Typically, the CSF glucose and protein are normal, and neutrophils are usually the predominant cell in the pleocytosis.

Chlamydia species

The increased frequency and study of sexually transmitted *Chlamydia trachomatis* has led to the recognition of its rare association with nonpurulent meningitis.[228]

C. pneumoniae has also rarely been associated with aseptic meningitis syndrome.[229]

Early Bacterial Meningitis ("Seeded Meningitis")

In bacteremic patients, the CSF may contain bacteria from the blood, with minimal cellular pleocytosis and normal CSF glucose and protein, as discussed previously.

Leptospirosis

Leptospira were the apparent cause of about 4% of 430 cases of nonpurulent meningitis in one study. The illness can be associated with conjunctival injection, muscle pain and tenderness, and a rash. Jaundice, tender liver, microscopic hematuria, pyuria, and proteinuria may also be present, as discussed in Chapter 13. Involvement of the CNS in the process of systemic leptospirosis is common, usually mild, and mostly unrecognized. Isolated CNS involvement, without other signs and symptoms, is extraordinarily rare.[230] Spinal fluid xanthochromia is common, but decreased CSF glucose is rare.[231] Culture is possible but usually not practical, so serologic studies should be done if there is

a history of exposure to animal urine (see Chapter 21). A leptospiral PCR has now been tested experimentally but is not readily available.[232]

Brain Abscess

With brain abscess, the CSF protein may be elevated, but the CSF glucose is normal, as discussed in a later section of this chapter.

Tuberculosis

A tuberculin skin test, chest roentgenogram, and a thorough history of exposure to tuberculosis should be done for most patients with the aseptic meningitis syndrome even if the initial CSF glucose and protein are normal. A second lumbar puncture should be done in all patients who have not improved after several days' observation in order to be certain the CSF glucose is not falling and the protein rising, as normally occurs in the course of tuberculous meningitis. Transient CSF lymphocytosis with normal glucose and protein and spontaneous recovery has been reported rarely with recovery of the tubercle bacillus from the spinal fluid.[233]

Bacterial Meningitis Modified by Prior Antibiotics

Nonpurulent meningitis with a normal glucose is sometimes the result of bacterial meningitis occurring during antibiotic therapy.[82] The frequency of this situation is unknown, as discussed in detail in the section on purulent meningitis. Some published studies have stated that prior antibiotic therapy does not "significantly" modify the CSF findings in bacterial meningitis. However, these studies compared the *mean* values for patients with proved bacterial meningitis with and without preceding antibiotic therapy, although the *range* of CSF glucose, protein, cell count, and differential overlapped. Further confirmation of this overlap can be found in studies of antibiotic therapy with proved bacterial meningitis.[85,234] In these studies, the mean CSF glucose was often normal after a few days of appropriate antibiotic therapy for bacterial meningitis. The mean CSF protein is usually still elevated at this time, but the range of the protein was as low as 25 mg/dL.

In addition, prior antibiotic therapy reduces the concentration of bacteria in the CSF of some patients.[235] Conclusive evidence that preceding antibiotic therapy sometimes modifies the CSF findings and results in a nonpurulent meningitis with normal CSF glucose and protein can be seen in individual case histories. Occasional patients with this clinical pattern have been observed and have not had antibiotics continued. Relapse has followed within a day or two, with more typical findings of bacterial meningitis and a positive culture. The frequency of antibiotic-modified bacterial meningitis is unknown. Use of nonculture techniques, such as detection of bacterial antigens, has not been helpful in clarifying this issue.

Noninfectious Causes

Nonpurulent meningitis with a normal glucose can have a number of possible noninfectious inflammatory causes. These include chemicals injected into the subdural space for diagnosis or therapy (such as myelography) and oral medications (such as tolmetin).[236,237] Nonsteroidal anti-inflammatory drugs and antibiotics such as trimethoprim-sulfamethoxazole can produce this pattern of disease.[238]

Kawasaki Disease

This multi-system disease is discussed in Chapter 11. Usually, fever and an erythematous rash are the predominant findings, but a sterile CSF pleocytosis can be present. Of patients with Kawasaki disease who undergo lumbar puncture, more than one-third have a pleocytosis.[239]

Eosinophilic Meningitis

Nonpurulent meningitis may rarely be associated with eosinophils in the CSF, peripheral blood eosinophilia, or both. Parasitic causes include cysticercosis, toxocariasis, toxoplasmosis, trichinosis, disseminated strongyloidiasis, and numerous parasites in other countries.[240,241]

An emerging cause of eosinophilic meningitis in the United States is neural larva migrans caused by inadvertent ingestion of the raccoon roundworm, *Baylisascaris procyonis*.[242] Patients described in the literature are young children (usually boys) with a history of geophagia (soil ingestion) or with extensive exposure to raccoons. Presentation may be indolent or fulminant. Symptoms are usually those of encephalitis, and include progressive lethargy, somnolence, and confusion. Seizures and developmental delay may occur. Fever is variable. Neuroretinitis secondary to larval invasion of the eye is frequently seen. There is usually a mild CSF pleocytosis with the presence of eosinophils. Peripheral eosinophilia may be present as well. Diagnosis is made by demonstrating the presence of antibodies to *B. procyonis* in the serum or CSF. Treatment is with a larvicidal agent with good CNS penetration, such as albendazole. However, based on cases reported to date, the prognosis is grave, with or without treatment.[242]

Other possible causes include chronic lymphocytic choriomeningitis virus meningitis,[243] foreign bodies (such as ventriculoperitoneal shunts), hypereosinophilic syndrome, lymphoma, and demyelinating diseases.[244] We have seen inexperienced laboratory technicians report neutrophils as eosinophils.

Diagnostic Approach

Bacterial culture of the spinal fluid should be done. The use of viral cultures and paired sera for viral antibodies is discussed in the section on acute encephalitis.

A rapid slide test for heteroph antibodies is simple and appropriate if there is any suspicion of infectious mononucleosis. If suspicion of EBV infection is high and the rapid test is negative, EBV serologies should be performed.

Cold agglutinins are non-specific but immediately available, and mycoplasma serology to detect IgM antibody may be ordered when mycoplasmal meningitis is suspected.

Treatment

Antibiotics

The following general rules are useful for the treatment of nonpurulent meningitis. If an antibiotic has not been given before the lumbar puncture, antibiotic therapy need not be used. Exceptions to this rule include the patient who appears seriously ill or is a young infant or a newborn. Even young infants can have viral meningitis, but the clinical and CSF response in bacterial meningitis of newborns or young infants can be atypical.[245] If the patient has received antibiotic therapy before the lumbar puncture, the patient should be treated with an antibiotic as if it were a partially treated bacterial meningitis, as described further in the section on purulent meningitis. Exceptions to this rule include the older child who does not appear sick and who can be observed carefully in the hospital, particularly when coxsackievirus or echovirus infections are known to be frequent in the community. A second lumbar puncture 24 hours later in a hospitalized patient not given antibiotics will sometimes clarify the diagnosis.[246] However, a recent retrospective study of children presenting with aseptic meningitis syndrome during the summer showed that 57% of children with aseptic meningitis (defined as WBC in the CSF with a negative culture and no prior antibiotic therapy) had a polymorphonuclear predominance at the time of first lumbar puncture, and that the duration of illness prior to lumbar puncture did not significantly alter that result. In other words, the polymorphonuclear predominance may last longer than 24 hours in children with nonpurulent meningitis and negative CSF cultures.[247]

An alternative policy followed by some clinicians for patients with nonpurulent meningitis and no preceding antibiotics is to treat the patient with intravenous antibiotics until the CSF culture is known to be negative, usually about 2–3 days.[82] This policy has the disadvantage that many patients with nonpurulent meningitis are still febrile and relatively sick after 3 days. The clinician might then consider continuing antibiotic therapy, although doubting the diagnosis of bacterial meningitis, and have difficulty interpreting the results of another CSF examination. In addition, about 10–15% of patients with purulent meningitis will have no growth on CSF cultures even in the absence of prior antibiotic therapy.[79] Therefore, it may occasionally be appropriate to continue antibiotics in spite of a negative culture in nonpurulent meningitis. A positive enteroviral PCR on spinal fluid, as mentioned previously, can help with the decision to stop antibiotics.[217]

Supportive Treatment

Inappropriate ADH secretion has been reported in about 10% of children hospitalized with nonpurulent meningitis.[248] The intravenous administration of hypotonic fluids in hospitalized children should generally be avoided to prevent iatrogenic hyponatremia.[249]

Antituberculous Therapy

Children nearly always acquire tuberculous meningitis from adults with pulmonary tuberculosis. There is no time to await culture results and susceptibility studies in tuberculous meningitis. Unless the source of the child's illness is known with certainty and that contact's organism is known to be suscepti-

ble, initial therapy should cover the possibility of a resistant organism.

For tuberculous meningitis, isoniazid, rifampin, pyrazinamide, and streptomycin are usually given for 2 months, followed by 10 months of isoniazid and rifampin for susceptible strains. Consultation with an expert in the management of tuberculosis is recommended.

Corticosteroids

Dexamethasone has been useful in reducing the increased intracranial pressure in tuberculous meningitis, with clinical improvement in the first 72 hours of therapy.[250,251] The spinal fluid cell count, glucose, and protein returned to normal sooner in steroid-treated patients than in controls, but no improvement in morbidity or mortality rates was shown to be related to these changes. Gastrointestinal bleeding was more common in the steroid-treated group. Increased survival appears to be related to decreased intracranial pressure early in the illness. The equivalent of 1–2 mg/kg/day of prednisolone is usually given for 4–8 weeks.[252]

Antifungal Chemotherapy

Amphotericin B is the most effective therapy for meningitis caused by cryptococcus or other fungi. Nephrotoxicity is a potential problem. The newer lipid preparations of amphotericin are less nephrotoxic but are also much more costly. Standard therapy of cryptococcal meningitis consists of intravenous amphotericin B, 0.7–1 mg/kg/day, plus oral flucytosine, 100 mg/kg/day, for 6–10 weeks. An alternative to this regimen consists of these two agents for 2 weeks, followed by at least 10 weeks of fluconazole. Flucytosine can never be given as a single agent, because resistance is predictable and rapid.

In patients with HIV infection or other immune compromise, fluconazole is continued for life.[253]

Careful attention to the management of intracranial pressure is critical; patients with cryptococcal meningitis may require frequent spinal taps to reduce the pressure.

■ ACUTE ENCEPHALITIS

Definitions

Acute encephalitis typically produces signs suggesting acute central nervous system infection: fever, disturbed consciousness, and increased intracranial pressure. However, signs of meningeal irritation are often absent. As defined in this book, a severe and non-transient disturbance of consciousness is the essential characteristic of both encephalitis and encephalopathy. This disturbance is not always present at the time of admission to a hospital but is usually noted within 24 hours. Acute psychoses related to infections are discussed later in this chapter.

Spinal fluid pleocytosis is the characteristic used to make the clinical distinction between encephalitis and encephalopathy. If spinal fluid pleocytosis of more than 10 leukocytes/mcL is present, then the presumptive diagnosis should be encephalitis. This clinical definition is especially useful because the acute encephalitides are often related to infections, whereas the acute encephalopathies are usually not infectious but rather have toxic, metabolic, or vascular etiologies. High fever is characteristic of acute encephalitis, but fever is often absent in acute encephalopathy. The differentiating features of encephalitis and encephalopathy are summarized in Table 9-10.

Purulent meningitis is often associated with depressed consciousness but usually is easily distinguished from acute encephalitis, which does not produce purulent spinal fluid. Aseptic meningitis syndrome can be distinguished from acute encephalitis by the absence of a severe or lasting disturbance of consciousness.

Febrile delirium, defined by its transient occurrence during high fever, is often found in bacter-emias, infective endocarditis, shigellosis, and typhoid fever.[256]

Frequency

Because most cases go unreported, it is difficult to get accurate data about the frequency of encephalitis or encephalopathy or the frequency of the various etiologies of either. In addition, most sporadic cases never have an etiology proved. Approximately 1500 cases of encephalitis are reported per year in the US, with about 200 deaths.[257] It is estimated that the number of cases of encephalitis is about 10 times higher than the number reported.[258] The incidence in children is about 2–4 times that in adults, and is thought to be around 16 cases per 100,000 person-years.[1,259] With the emergence of West Nile virus the current incidence is somewhat higher.[260,261]

Infectious Etiologies

Epidemic acute encephalitis is usually caused by an arbovirus such as West Nile virus or La Crosse virus (a member of the California encephalitis group of viruses). The term arbovirus is short for *arthropod-borne* and includes viruses of multiple genera; their geographic distributions are discussed in Chapter 21. Sporadic acute encephalitis has many possible causes, but herpes simplex virus is the most important, as chemotherapy is available and greatly affects outcome. Many causes of acute encephalitis are pos-

TABLE 9-10. DIFFERENTIATION OF ACUTE ENCEPHALITIS AND ACUTE ENCEPHALOPATHY

CHARACTERISTIC	ACUTE ENCEPHALITIS	ACUTE ENCEPHALOPATHY
Acute onset	Present	Present
Disturbed consciousness	Present	Present
CSF lymphocytosis	Present	Absent
Increased CSF pressure	Variable	Usual
High fever	Usual	Often absent
Meningeal irritation	Variable	Usually absent
Increased CSF protein	Variable	Variable
Usual etiologies	Infection or unknown	Toxic, metabolic, vascular, or unknown
Usual prognosis	Variable, depending on etiology	Variable, depending on etiology

sible, and there is some overlap with the causes of acute encephalopathy (Boxes 9-2,3).[261-277]

Herpes Simplex Virus

Outside of the newborn period, the classic clinical findings are temporal lobe symptoms, focal paralysis, lateralized seizures, and CSF pleocytosis with some erythrocytes. Mucosal or cutaneous lesions are present in less than 10% of documented cases, but this can be coincidental.[278]

Temporal lobe symptoms include curious bizarre behavior and hallucinations of taste and smell. Focal paralysis, particularly cranial nerve paralysis, or aphasia may occur. Facial nerve paralysis is common. Such focal paralyses also can occur in tuberculosis, which usually produces a low CSF glucose, and brain abscess, which often has a distant focus of infection as its source. Lateralized seizures or motor changes may be explained by the tendency for HSV to spread contiguously from cell to cell. Lateralized seizures also may occur in brain abscess, La Crosse virus infection, and many other diseases. Fever is almost always present (90%).[279]

In the spinal fluid, WBCs, usually predominately lymphocytes, are present in numbers from 10–300/mcL. Red blood cells are also frequently found in small numbers. A severe fulminating HSV encephalitis, called acute necrotizing hemorrhagic encephalopathy, is manifested by severe focal signs with many red blood cells as well as WBCs in the spinal fluid. Uncommonly (5%), no leukocytes are present in the CSF, so this etiology must be considered in patients preliminarily classified as having acute encephalopathy.[279]

Abnormalities on EEG (characteristic spike and slow wave complexes at 2–3 second intervals) occur earlier in the course of the disease than do imaging abnormalities. MRI is more sensitive than CT scan for finding focal abnormalities. Focal CT or MRI scans can occur in nonherpetic viral encephalitis, tumors, and even congenital metabolic disturbances, such as urea cycle disorders.[280]

Serum and CSF serology and antibody ratios are not reliable.[281] Of 113 biopsy-proved cases, 32 (28%) did not develop a serum antibody titer rise; therefore serology is not useful even as a retrospective tool.

Brain Biopsy and PCR

Once the most reliable method of establishing the diagnosis of herpesvirus encephalitis, brain biopsy

---

BOX 9-2 ■ Possible Causes of Acute Encephalitis

Frequent
No etiology found

Less Common
Herpes simplex virus 1 and 2
Arboviruses (epidemic)
Enteroviruses
Varicella zoster virus (chickenpox, zoster)
Mumps, measles, rubella
Epstein-Barr virus
Cytomegalovirus
Mycoplasma pneumoniae
Tuberculous meningitis
Rickettsia rickettsiae (Rocky Mountain spotted fever)
Borrelia burgdorferi (Lyme disease)
HHV-6
Bartonella henselae (cat scratch disease)
Pertussis
Influenza virus

Rare
Listeria
Adenovirus
Lymphocytic choriomeningitis virus
Toxoplasmosis
Trichinosis
Psittacosis
Ehrlichiosis
Chlamydia pneumoniae
Brucellosis
Cryptococcosis, histoplasmosis, coccidiodomycosis, blastomycosis
Hendra virus
Nipah virus
Progressive multifocal leukoencephalopathy (JC virus)
Naegleria fowleri
Plasmodium falciparum (cerebral malaria)
Rabies (unrecognized contact)
Neural larva migrans (*Baylisascaris procyonis*)
Acute onset of a usually chronic neurologic disorder

Noninfectious
Postinfectious or postvaccinal reactions (acute disseminated encephalomyelitis, acute hemorrhagic leukoencephalitis)
Drug-induced, intrathecal injections
Serum sickness, rupture of dermoid or epidermoid cyst
Granulomatous angiitis, lymphoid granulomatosis
Systemic lupus erythematosis, metastatic malignancy

is now seldom employed. PCR of CSF for herpesvirus has replaced the brain biopsy in clinical practice. PCR is favored because it is non-invasive and highly sensitive. Sensitivity and specificity of PCR are both about 92%,[282] but they depend greatly on the experience of the laboratory performing the test. Occasionally, the HSV PCR can be negative early in the patient's course.[282] Thus, patients with suspected HSV encephalitis and a negative PCR should continue to receive antiviral therapy and undergo a repeat lumbar puncture in 4–7 days.

One advantage of brain biopsy is the ability to establish other diagnoses. There are other clinical syndromes, such as tumor, toxoplasmosis, and infection with other viruses (which usually require culture confirmation) that can be found at the time of brain biopsy. On the other hand, false-negative brain biopsies can occur, although they are believed to be rare (fewer than 5%).[281]

Treatment for HSV

Acyclovir is now the standard treatment for all age groups and is superior to vidarabine.[278,283] It is safe, but renal toxicity can occur with too-rapid administration.[278] For central nervous system infection, the dose is 45–60 mg/kg/dose intravenously divided every 8 hours for 21 days. Although well-tolerated by neonates, the higher dose often precipitates reversible renal failure in older children and adults.

A repeat lumbar puncture should be performed at the end of therapy. If the PCR is still positive, an additional 7 days of therapy should be given. If a clinical recurrence is noted, the course should be repeated. In severe encephalitis, the clinician may want to use empiric acyclovir until the clinical picture becomes clearer, but it has been recommended that acyclovir should not be used empirically when there are no focal neurologic findings.[284]

Arbovirus Encephalitides

La Crosse virus (a member of the California encephalitis virus group) is the most common cause of arthropod-borne virus encephalitis in childhood. La Crosse virus is responsible for almost all infections by California encephalitis group viruses in the United States. In some places, the terms "California virus encephalitis" and "California encephalitis" are used; these should be abandoned in favor of La Crosse virus encephalitis, in part because these infections are most common in the Midwestern and mid-Atlantic states, so the term is misleading. Most

cases are relatively mild and resolve in about a week. Focal signs are present in 15–25% of cases, which may make the disease resemble herpesvirus encephalitis. The mortality rate is less than 1%; however, residual neurologic deficits are found in up to 12% of patients.[285] The tree-hole mosquito is both the reservoir of the virus in nature and the vector for transmission of infection to humans. The virus is able to persist in nature due to 1) transovarial transmission and overwintering in infected eggs and 2) horizontal transmission to small mammals (especially chipmunks and squirrels), which serve as amplifying hosts of the virus. The disease is most frequent in late summer. Outbreaks have been traced to sources of standing water such as found in holes in trees or in old tires.[286]

Other arboviruses are transmitted by the bites of different mosquitoes. St. Louis encephalitis virus affects adult more frequently than children. As with La Crosse encephalitis, the ratio of asymptomatic to symptomatic disease approximates 100:1.[287] Eastern equine encephalitis (EEE) is a fulminant disease with a high mortality rate. CSF white blood cell counts tend to be higher in EEE than in the other encephalitides (as high as 2000 cells/mL), and a predominance of polymorphonuclear leukocytes is not uncommon.[287] Western equine encephalitis is also associated with significant morbidity.

West Nile virus encephalitis was first reported in the United States in August 1999, when it caused an outbreak in New York City. Initially confined to the Northeast, in subsequent summers it has spread further west.[261] In 2002, most of the 3,700 reported cases occurred in Illinois, Michigan, Ohio, and Louisiana. In 2003, Colorado, South Dakota, and Nebraska reported the most cases.[287a] Overall, there were more than 9,800 reported cases and 264 deaths. In 2004, most cases were reported from Arizona and California.[287a] After an incubation period of 5–15 days, patients present with fever, headache, stiff neck, altered mental status, rash, photophobia, and myalgia. Muscle weakness is common and helps distinguish West Nile virus infection from other causes of encephalitis.[287b] Illness is most severe in the elderly.[288] Diagnosis is by serology or by PCR of spinal fluid. Treatment is supportive. Prevention rests with avoiding mosquito bites, which can be accomplished with the use of insect repellent containing 20–30% DEET.

Many of the clinical findings of an acute arbovirus encephalitis closely resemble those of herpes simplex encephalitis.[289] Diagnosis is usually established by acute and convalescent serology. Convalescent serology should be done in 4–6 weeks. The first sample should be saved so the assays can be run in tandem. An elevated serum IgM to La Crosse virus is nearly always present at the time of presentation.[290]

Infectious Mononucleosis

Neurologic manifestations have been reported in about 2–5% of patients with infectious mononucleosis, but true acute encephalitis is uncommon.[291–293] EBV has been recovered from the spinal fluid of a child with encephalitis complicating heterophile-positive infectious mononucleosis.[294] In most cases, the central nervous system involvement is not the only symptom.[295] CSF usually has a lymphocytic pleocytosis, an elevated protein, and a normal glucose concentration. Diagnosis can be established by finding EBV DNA in the spinal fluid using PCR technology.[287]

Mycoplasmal Encephalitis

Like EBV, *Mycoplasma pneumoniae* can produce many different neurologic complications, including acute encephalitis.[296,297] In a series of 50 hospitalized children with acute encephalitis who underwent microbiological investigation, *M. pneumoniae* was the most common etiologic agent identified. It was found in 9 (18%) of 50 cases (45% of the 20 cases in which an etiologic agent was identified).[298]

About 20% of patients have no preceding respiratory symptoms.[296] Typically, the spinal fluid has about 50–300 WBC/mcL, with a predominance of neutrophils early in the illness. One study found that 5% of patients sick enough to be hospitalized with *M. pneumoniae* infection had CNS involvement.[299]

Rickettsia rickettsii

Rocky Mountain spotted fever (RMSF) is an acute systemic disease caused by infection with *Rickettsia rickettsii*, which is transmitted by the bite of a tick. The tick must be attached for at least 6 hours for infection to occur. The disease is heralded by fever, headache, nausea and vomiting, and myalgia. The characteristic rash usually appears first on the ankles, but it can rapidly spread centripetally and involves the palms and soles. Signs of encephalitis occur in about one-fourth of patients with RMSF.[300] RMSF should be considered in any patient with encephalitis and a rash. Other common manifestations include adult respiratory distress syndrome (ARDS), renal failure, coagulopathy, hyponatremia, thrombocytopenia, and elevated liver enzymes. CSF specimens usually reveal a low WBC count (less than 100/mcL), a lymphocyte predominance, and an elevated protein. Doxycycline is the treatment of choice. RMSF is discussed further in Chapter 11.

Human Herpesvirus type 6 (HHV-6)

HHV-6 is a ubiquitous virus whose spectrum of disease continues to enlarge. It is the most common cause of roseola infantum (discussed in Chapter 11). It can occasionally be associated with encephalitis; focal seizures and a focal neurologic examination are not uncommon, thus resembling HSV infection. The diagnosis can only be established by the concomitant isolation of the virus from CSF and the finding of a four-fold or greater rise in serum antibody titer between acute and convalescent samples. CSF PCR may be positive in asymptomatic reactivation, and thus by itself cannot be used to make the diagnosis of active disease. The virus is relatively resistant to acyclovir, and it is not known whether treatment is of any benefit.

Enteroviruses

Usually a cause of nonpurulent meningitis, as discussed earlier, the enteroviruses can also cause encephalitis. The syndrome is usually associated with a macular or maculopapular rash and seizures. Macular lesions may occur on the palms and soles as well. Petechiae are occasionally found on the trunk and lower extremities, but purpura is not seen. PCR can be used to identify the viral genome in CSF.

Post-infectious Encephalitis

This group includes encephalitis following measles, mumps, influenza, chickenpox or zoster, rubella, and vaccination against smallpox. Other infectious agents, such as EBV, may be associated as well.

Also referred to as acute disseminated encephalomyelitis (ADEM), post-infectious encephalitis is estimated to account for 10–15% of cases of acute encephalitis in the United States.[300a] Presentation is similar to infectious encephalitis, but the onset is typically 1–3 weeks after recovery from a respiratory or other illness. Examination of CSF usually demonstrates a mild mononuclear cell pleocytosis and slightly elevated protein, but CSF is completely normal in one-third of patients.[300a] The most useful test is T2-weighted MRI, which usually shows bilateral, asymmetrical, patchy areas of demyelination in the white matter, basal ganglia, or spinal cord.[300b] Although no clinical trials have been performed, corticosteroids are often used and anecdotally appear to be of benefit.[300b] Occasionally relapses occur, which make distinction between ADEM and multiple sclerosis difficult.

Other Rare Infections

Measles is associated with an acute encephalitis during the rash (and measles may not always be an obvious clinical diagnosis).[301] In addition, encephalitis may occur 1–6 months after mild measles or measles immunization in the immunocompromised host.[302,303] Finally, it is associated with a slowly progressive subacute sclerosing panencephalitis 1–10 years after the measles virus infection.

Kawasaki disease, which resembles an infectious disease, can be associated with acute encephalitis and with acute cerebral vasculitis.[304] Encephalitis can be caused by toxoplasmosis,[305] lymphocytic choriomeningitis virus,[306] rabies,[307] adenovirus,[291] hepatitis A virus,[308] and Legionnaires' disease.[309]

Influenza Virus

Encephalitis that occurs at the height of culture-proven influenza virus infection has been reported; virus has not been recovered from either CSF or brain tissue.[310]

A recent influenza epidemic in Japan was associated with a large number of cases of encephalitis/encephalopathy.[310a] Of 148 cases reported, 121 (82%) were in children younger than 5 years old. Most patients developed CNS disease either on the day that influenza signs appeared or on the next day. Three categories of patients were described: 6 patients (4%) had a Reye syndrome-like illness with hypoglycemia and hyperammonemia; 14 (10%) had encephalitis (defined as more than 8 WBC/mcL in the CSF); and 128 (86%) had encephalopathy without CSF pleocytosis. An attempt to detect influenza in the CSF by reverse transcriptase-PCR (RT-PCR) was made in 18 patients; only 3 (17%) of specimens yielded positive results. The case-fatality rate was 32%. Predictors of poor outcome included platelet count less than 50,000/mcL and AST more than 1000 IU/L. None of the patients had received the influenza vaccine. Encephalitis/encephalopathy has been described in association with both influenza A and influenza B virus infections.[310b]

Tuberculosis

Although it usually presents subacutely, tuberculous meningitis should always be considered a possible cause of acute encephalitis, because both a disturbed consciousness and CSF lymphocytes may be present.[311] Either decreased glucose or elevated protein in the CSF should alert the physician to this important possibility.

Reye Syndrome

Occasionally, a mild CSF pleocytosis occurs in Reye syndrome, which is best diagnosed by evidence of severe liver involvement, particularly elevated levels of serum aminotransferas and ammonia. Usually, however, there is no pleocytosis, so Reye syndrome is discussed in the section on acute encephalopathies.

Diagnostic Approach

Brain scans and EEG may be helpful to localize a lesion or to detect unrecognized seizures but do not help much for specific diagnosis, except in the case of ADEM where demyelinating lesions on MRI can be diagnostic. IgM-specific antibodies can provide an early diagnosis and are often available for EBV, toxoplasmosis, and La Crosse virus encephalitis. IgM-specific serology or fluorescent antibody tests may be available in some areas for the rapid diagnosis of *Mycoplasma pneumoniae*, *Legionella*, hepatitis A, and other infectious agents. Influenza can be diagnosed by sending a nasopharyngeal swab for rapid antigen testing or culture. All but the most mildly affected patients with encephalitis should have spinal fluid sent for HSV PCR, as discussed earlier.

Therapy

Acyclovir

As discussed earlier, IV acyclovir is often used with or without a specific diagnosis while awaiting the results of PCR testing for HSV. Many times this is a rational choice, as specific therapy for most other causes is not available, and the prognosis of HSV encephalitis without treatment is abysmal.

Corticosteroids

No adequate studies have been done. In encephalitis secondary to a cerebral vasculitis or in post-infectious encephalitis, a clinical trial of corticosteroids may be indicated. Some experience suggests that corticosteroids, given in concert with effective antibiotics, may be helpful in patients suffering from encephalitis due to *Mycoplasma pneumoniae*.[312]

■ ACUTE ENCEPHALOPATHY

Definitions

Acute encephalopathy is defined as the recent onset of severe, continuing (more than 12 hours) change of consciousness with no definite CSF pleocytosis (fewer than 10 WBC/mcL). The CSF protein may be elevated. The condition is distinguished from acute encephalitis by this absence of CSF pleocytosis (see preceding sections). In general, encephalopathies are not usually related to infections, whereas encephalitides often are.

Acute encephalopathy is usually not used as a syndrome diagnosis when the cause of the change of consciousness is known; for example, a known head injury or poisoning. Convulsions may occur in this syndrome and may be focal or generalized, brief or persistent. Fever and signs of meningeal irritation are usually absent, but if present, physicians should not exclude this as a working diagnosis. Acute psychoses related to infections are discussed later in this chapter.

Other diagnostic phrases sometimes used to describe this syndrome are "acute cerebral edema" or "acute toxic encephalopathy." However, "acute encephalopathy" is used in this section as a more general and less restrictive preliminary diagnosis of a syndrome that has many possible causes. When known possible causes (trauma, hypertension, diabetic coma, poisoning) have been excluded, the preliminary diagnosis can be acute encephalopathy of obscure origin.

Possible etiologies of acute encephalopathy, with appropriate references, are shown in Box 9-3.

Reye Syndrome

Encephalopathy and fatty degeneration of the viscera as a disease entity in childhood was described by Reye and others in 1963.

In Reye's report, there were usually minor respiratory symptoms and vomiting for several days followed by convulsions.[313] Wild delirium and seizures were common. Firm hepatomegaly, hyperpnea, dilated pupils, tachycardia, and a characteristic posture with clenched hands, flexed elbows, and extended legs were observed. Other findings were occasional brief apparent abdominal pain and a poorly described rash that may be mistaken for chickenpox. Vomiting is often the most persistent and prominent finding. Laboratory findings included elevated serum amino transferas and ammonia, hypoglycemia, and low CSF glucose with no leukocyte. Autopsy findings include swollen brain and fatty infiltration of the liver and kidney.[313]

Because Reye syndrome is now rare, any child with that presumptive diagnosis should undergo testing for the many inborn metabolic errors that can mimic Reye syndrome.

The etiology of Reye syndrome is unknown. Its association with treatment of influenza or chickenpox with salicylates is well known.[314] Although part of the dramatic decline in Reye syndrome incidence could be attributable to differences in the currently circulating strains of influenza, most of the decline can be attributed to decreased aspirin use.[315]

Treatment

Treatment should be specific for the cause of the encephalopathy, whenever this is possible to determine. Consultation with an expert in metabolic disorders is critical.

Mannitol treatment of cerebral edema, as outlined in the section on meningitis, may be of temporary value for many encephalopathies. Intravenous glucose may be indicated for hypoglycemia. When carefully analyzed and controlled for the stage of severity of Reye syndrome, no therapy has been proved to be of value.[316]

■ ACUTE PARALYSIS AND WEAKNESS SYNDROMES

Infectious agents are a frequent cause of paralysis or weakness in children. Most children with paralysis or weakness can be given a preliminary problem-oriented diagnosis as shown in Table 9-11.

Acute Flaccid Paralysis (Paralytic Poliomyelitis)

This syndrome can be defined as nonpurulent meningitis with asymmetric flaccid (lower motor neu-

---

BOX 9-3 ■ Possible Etiologies of Acute Encephalopathy

Metabolic
Inborn errors of metabolism
Urea cycle defects, organic acidemias, Leigh disease,[274] aminoacidopathies (MSUD), Wernicke encephalopathy, mitochondrial disease (MELOS)
Adrenoleukodystrophy
Uremia
Intrahepatic shunts
Postdialysis
Diabetic acidosis
Hyperosmolar nonketotic coma
Water intoxication
Respiratory acidosis
Hypoglycemia, hyponatremia, hypernatremia, hypocalcemia
Hypoxia
CO_2 narcosis
Acidosis
Late relapse after hypoxia[268]

Toxic
Carbon monoxide, lead,[262] heavy metals, mushrooms, Jimson weed, ethanol,[263] antiemetics,[264] drug abuse or narcotic overdose,[265] salicylates,[266] insect repellents,[267] diphenhydramine overdose, sedative hypnotic overdose, organophosphates

Infections
Viral agents listed under acute encephalitis; respiratory viruses such as influenza[269] or adenovirus[270]
Brain abscess
Cat scratch disease[271]
Cerebral malaria
Infectious hepatitis
Listeriosis[272]

Intracranial Disease
Epidural hematoma
Subdural hematoma
Subarachnoid hemorrhage
Tumor
Intracranial hemorrhage (ruptured berry aneurysm)
Head injury
Cerebral edema

Vascular
Stroke
Hypertension
Migraine

Demyelinating Disease
Acute demyelinating encephalomyelitis (ADEM)
Acute multiple sclerosis[273]
Central pontine myelinolysis

Idiopathic
Henoch-Schönlein purpura
Hemolytic-uremic syndrome
Reye syndrome
Hemorrhagic shock and encephalopathy[275–277]
Acute distention of a hollow viscus (intussusception, acute bladder hydrops)

---

ron) paralysis. Although the term poliomyelitis technically refers to inflammation of the gray matter of the spinal cord (polio = gray; myelitis = inflammation of the spinal cord), the term has been widely associated with poliovirus infection. This clinical syndrome can be caused by other agents, and, in fact, is less and less likely to be due to poliovirus infection; for this reason, the term acute flaccid paralysis is preferred. Histologically there is destruction of the anterior horn cells of the spinal cord. This clinical syndrome also has been called "infantile paralysis," because at one time, it was most frequent in young children.

Poliovirus Infection

Before polio vaccine was available, wild poliovirus was the cause of most cases of aseptic meningitis in the summer. Outbreaks of "polio" occurred, but for every patient with paralysis, there were many with asymptomatic infection or with aseptic meningitis syndrome without paralysis, called "nonparalytic poliomyelitis." Rarely, paralysis of muscles of breathing or involvement of the medullary centers resulted in death.[317] The diagnosis of poliomyelitis traditionally has relied on recovery of the wild-type poliovirus in stool or rectal swab culture. These cul-

TABLE 9-11. PROBLEM-ORIENTED DIAGNOSIS OF INFECTIOUS PARALYTIC DISEASES

SYNDROME	PARALYSIS TYPE	CEREBROSPINAL FLUID	OTHER
Polio-like illness	Focal, flaccid	Lymphocytosis	Fever, stiff neck
Ascending paralysis	Usually symmetric	Normal or elevated protein	Sensory and nerve conduction changes
Descending paralysis	Typically includes cranial nerves	Usually normal	
Isolated cranial-nerve paralysis	Focal	Usually normal	
Acute hemiplegia	Usually spastic	Variable	
Acute paraplegia	Fixed level at cord	Variable	

tures are most likely to be positive in the first two weeks after onset of disease. Thereafter, serology looking for IgM directed against poliovirus is much more sensitive.[318]

Polio Vaccine Virus

Until recently, live attenuated polio vaccine virus (Sabin vaccine virus) has accounted for about 10 or so cases of paralytic disease each year in the United States. Each year, about four cases occurred in recipients of the vaccine, about five cases occurred in contacts of recipients, and about 1 case occurred in an immunodeficient person.[319] Paralytic poliomyelitis was most likely to occur at the time of the infant's first oral vaccine, presumably because pre-existing immunity from prior vaccine(s) prevented the development of disease after later doses. This syndrome, called vaccine-associated paralytic poliomyelitis (VAPP), has disappeared in the United States since use of the live-attenuated vaccine has been abandoned in favor of the inactivated poliovirus vaccine (Salk vaccine). However, cases of VAPP continue to occur in other countries. Investigations suggest that a form of "provocation poliomyelitis" (the occurrence of clinically significant poliovirus disease related to injections given after contact with poliovirus) may be responsible for the high rate of VAPP in some countries, specifically Romania.[320] The association of intramuscular injections and VAPP was strongest for patients who received 10 or more injections in the 30 days following vaccination (odds ratio = 57).

Enteroviruses

Since polio vaccine has been widely used, and since specific laboratory diagnosis of many viral infections has become available, it has been recognized that several other enteroviruses are rare causes of acute flaccid paralysis. These viruses include coxsackieviruses and certain enterovirus serotypes. Coxsackievirus A7, enterovirus type 70, and enterovirus type 71 have been documented as causes of outbreaks of paralytic disease involving more than three individuals.[321–324] Enterovirus 71 may be particularly virulent; outbreaks associated with central nervous system disease have been reported. In Taiwan, 4 (10%) of 41 children with culture-proven enterovirus 71 infection had acute flaccid paralysis.[325] In Brazil, of 426 children with acute neurologic syndromes of any type, enterovirus 71 was recovered from 24 (6%) of them.[326] In a 1987 outbreak in the United States due to enterovirus 71, 27 (60%) of 45 children with culture-proven cases had neurologic involvement: 6 (13%) children had paralysis and 1 (2%) had Guillain-Barre syndrome.[327]

Coxsackieviruses are probably the most frequent non-poliovirus cause of what is usually a mild paralytic disease.[328] A series of 44 patients with coxsackievirus B infection and limb paralyses has been reported from Africa. Single limb paralysis was self-resolving and mild, but those who presented with paralysis of more than one limb had a poorer prognosis, with only 1 (7%) of 15 demonstrating complete recovery 5 months after the illness.[329]

Japanese Encephalitis Virus

Japanese encephalitis virus is another possible cause of acute flaccid paralysis, especially in areas where infection with the virus in endemic. In a series of 22 children in Vietnam with acute flaccid paralysis, 1 (5%) had wild-type poliovirus infection, 3 (14%) had infections with a nonpolio enterovirus, and 12 (55%) proved to have Japanese encephalitis virus infection. Only one (1%) of a control group of 88 age-matched children had evidence of Japanese encephalitis virus infection.[330]

Other Viruses

Mumps virus, HSV, and St. Louis encephalitis virus have been reported to cause acute flaccid paralysis.[331,332] In one case, a 7-year-old boy who developed subtotal and permanent upper extremity paralysis after a respiratory tract infection was found to have HSV-1 DNA in PCR of spinal fluid.[333]

Poliomyelitis-Like Syndrome and Asthma (Hopkins syndrome)

A syndrome that has a poor prognosis for recovery of the paralyzed limb is a poliomyelitis-like syndrome complicating asthma. The etiology is unknown.[334] Perhaps some cases had unrecognized *Mycoplasma*-induced asthma. One case of Hopkins syndrome associated with serologic evidence of *Mycoplasma pneumoniae* infection has been reported.[335]

Mycoplasma

Mycoplasma pneumoniae can cause stiff neck, CSF pleocytosis, and flaccid paralysis, especially after the respiratory symptoms.[336] It can also cause transverse myelitis.[337]

Malaria

Infection with *Plasmodium falciparum* sometimes includes a syndrome known as cerebral malaria. A variety of nervous system symptoms can develop, including, rarely, transient muscle paralysis that resembles periodic paralysis.[338]

Nutritional Deficiency

A 4-year-old child, unimmunized against poliovirus, who presented with sudden inability to stand or walk, fever, respiratory infection, muscle tenderness, and weakness in the lower limbs, was given a preliminary diagnosis of paralytic poliomyelitis until a plain film of the left thigh revealed features of scurvy. Parenteral vitamin C therapy resulted in normal ambulation within 2 weeks.[339]

Ascending Paralysis

Acute ascending paralysis can be defined as the sudden onset of paralysis of both legs with evidence of progression of the paralysis to involve the arms, the muscles of breathing, or the cranial nerves. There are many possible etiologies of ascending paralysis.

Guillain-Barré Syndrome

The diagnosis of Guillain-Barré syndrome is usually made by exclusion of specific causes of ascending paralysis. This syndrome is characterized by decreased conduction velocity of peripheral nerves as measured by an oscilloscope and by cyto-albuminologic dissociation (high CSF protein, with normal or only slightly elevated leukocytes in the CSF). These findings may not be noted on the first lumbar puncture but are present within a week of onset. There usually is complete recovery and return to normal activities, provided the patient receives adequate supportive care. Mechanical ventilation may be necessary if the respiratory muscles are involved. This syndrome may even occur in young infants.[340]

Until quite recently, the cause of Guillain-Barré syndrome was completely unknown, although it was often regarded as an infectious disease caused by an unknown agent. Although there are undoubtedly a number of antecedents to this condition, infection with *Campylobacter jejuni* has emerged as the most common; it is estimated that 30–40% of cases are preceded by this infection.[341] The hypothesis is that the lipopolysaccharides of *Campylobacter* species contain ganglioside-like epitopes, and that antibodies formed in response to the infection attack the molecularly similar sites on peripheral nerves after the infection has resolved. This is known as "molecular mimicry."[342]

Other pathogens associated with Guillain-Barre syndrome with some frequency include HSV, EBV, varicella-zoster virus (VZV), cytomegalovirus (CMV), and *M. pneumoniae*. The 1976 "swine flu" influenza vaccine was credibly linked with Guillain-Barre syndrome.[343] Other vaccines (particularly rabies, tetanus, and influenza vaccine) have been anecdotally reported to be associated with Guillain-Barre syndrome, but careful epidemiologic studies have shown that if a true association exists, it is extremely rare.[343a,343b] Guillain-Barré syndrome is often the erroneous diagnosis in a child with degenerative polyneuropathy.[344]

Tick Paralysis

Tick paralysis is caused by a neurotoxin injected by an attached tick and is cured by removing the tick.[345,346] The ascending paralysis then rapidly reverses. As in the Guillain-Barré syndrome, nerve conduction velocity may be slowed. Characteristically, the disease occurs in the warm seasons when ticks are found and occurs more frequently in girls, because the tick is more likely to be overlooked in long hair.

Herpes Simplex Virus

Human herpesvirus infection appears to be an occasional cause of ascending paralysis as demonstrated by recovery of the virus from the spinal fluid.[347] In one adult with this disease, the initial spinal fluid obtained at the time of flaccid paralysis of the legs revealed 13,000 WBC/mcL with a predominance of neutrophils, and a spinal fluid glucose of 2 mg/dL but no growth of bacteria (and no preceding antibiotics).[347]

Cercopithicine herpesvirus 1

Cercopithicine herpesvirus 1 (B virus, Herpes virus B) infection of humans, usually acquired by the bite of a macaque monkey, can produce an ascending paralysis that is usually, but not always, fatal.[348] Acyclovir may be lifesaving.[349]

Other Causes

Buckthorn berry ingestion can produce an ascending flaccid paralysis. A careful history should be obtained of any berry ingestion. Most cases have been reported from Texas, New Mexico, and northern Mexico in children who have eaten the coyotillo berry.[350]

Paralytic shellfish poisoning (red tide) can also cause ascending paralysis, as can Addison's disease.[351] One case of a patient with severe tonsillopharyngitis without abscess who developed Guillain-Barre syndrome and facial palsy has been reported.[352] A neonate who presented in the second week of life with microcephaly, microphthalmia, and progressive ascending motor and sensory deficit that led to complete paralysis and death at age

27 days was found to have *Toxoplasma gondii* trophozoites within CSF macrophages.[353]

Acute Paraparesis and Paraplegia

Acute paraparasis is sudden bilateral weakness, and paraplegia is paralysis of both legs. If the paralysis increases to involve the trunk and upper extremities, the diagnosis should be changed to ascending paralysis and the etiologies listed in that section should be considered.

Transverse Myelopathy

Transverse myelopathy (often called transverse myelitis) is the cause of paraplegia presumed to be due to an infectious agent when a vascular accident cannot be demonstrated. The term "myelopathy" is preferred because evidence of inflammation is not always found. Synchronous viral or mycoplasmal infections are sometimes found, but proof of causation is lacking.[354] Possible viral associations include all common childhood viral infections (such as chickenpox) plus hepatitis A virus, CMV, EBV,[355] *Borrelia burgdorferi* (Lyme disease),[356] and *Mycoplasma pneumoniae*.[357,358] This condition is rarely reported as a complication of bacterial meningitis.[359] The meningovascular form of syphilis may mimic transverse myelopathy and requires immediate treatment. One case of transverse myelopathy secondary to the inadvertent administration of benzathine penicillin into an artery has been reported.[360] In a patient with freshwater exposure from an area endemic for schistosomiasis, the possibility of spinal cord schistosomiasis should be considered. Praziquantel is the treatment of choice.[361]

The role of corticosteroids in the treatment of infectious or post-infectious transverse myelitis is unclear, but they are often given. Careful monitoring and supportive care are critical.

Spinal Epidural Abscess

Spinal epidural abscess is rare, but it is important to identify because it may respond to operative drainage of the abscess and antibiotics.[362] The disease may start insidiously with what has been termed "spinal ache." A thorough spinal examination in which all the spinous processes are tapped by the examiner may disclose the location of a subtle ache. This is followed by root pain, and finally by weakness or paralysis. The neck is often stiff, and fever is usually present. Frank meningitis may occur later. The CSF protein is almost always elevated, sometimes greater than 1000 mg/dL, with few WBCs found early in the course. However, lumbar puncture should not be performed when an epidural abscess is suspected. In a series of 12 hemodialysis patients with spinal epidural abscess, plain films, CT scans without contrast, and bone scans were of low diagnostic yield. MRI had a sensitivity of 80%, and myelography or CT-myelography revealed the diagnosis in all twelve.[363] MRI is most commonly used to make this diagnosis and should be obtained emergently if the diagnosis is suspected.

Staphylococcus aureus is the most common cause, followed by aerobic and anaerobic streptococci. Treatment is urgent. Despite a recent anecdote of a good outcome in a child with very early spinal epidural abscess who was treated by medical management alone, if this diagnosis is suspected, a neurosurgeon should be consulted. The combination of surgical intervention and aggressive antimicrobial therapy seems to offer the best hope of recovery. After surgical drainage, intravenous antibiotics are given for a minimum of 3–4 weeks, often followed by a course of oral antibiotics. A recent review suggested that relapse is less likely if a total of 8 weeks of therapy is given.[364] The prognosis of spinal epidural abscess is poor; the case fatality rate is about one-third, and another third have permanent neurologic sequelae. This disease should always be considered in a patient with paralysis of both legs, particularly if furuncles, diabetes, or any skin infection is present.

Rabies

Rabies sometimes develops from a mild illness with paresthesias into paralysis, especially in the bitten extremity. It may progress to a flaccid quadriplegia. A CSF pleocytosis is typically present.[307]

Anterior Spinal Artery Thrombosis

Anterior spinal artery thrombosis may cause acute paraplegia.[365] Pain is often the initial symptom, followed by weakness or paralysis of the legs. The paralysis may be flaccid at first because of spinal shock but soon becomes flaccid at the level of the lesion and spastic below that level. Vibratory and position sense are spared, but pain and temperature sense are lost. Urinary retention, hyperactive reflexes, and positive Babinski signs are usually present. There is usually no ascending progression of the disease. Later, there is generally gradual improvement as the vascular supply to the cord increases. If the ischemia is severe or permanent, however, flaccid paralysis may persist because of degeneration of the anterior horn cells.

Neuromyelitis Optica

Transverse myelitis may occur with optic neuritis (neuromyelitis optica or Devic syndrome).[366] Spinal fluid shows mild monocytosis and increased protein. It is rare in children, but may follow common childhood infections, and typically responds to corticosteroid therapy. The largest report of childhood neuromyelitis optica was a series of 9 patients. This series revealed an average age of onset of 7 years, a mild respiratory illness prodrome in all patients, and complete and sustained recovery in all nine.[367] This pattern of illness differs from that seen in adults, which has a much worse prognosis.

This disease has some similarities to multiple sclerosis, which is a very rare cause of sensory or motor disturbances or of optic neuritis in children.[368] Neuromyelitis has been reported to accompany zoster in immunosuppressed patients[369] and coincidentally with pulmonary tuberculosis without CNS involvement.[370] Finally, Devic syndrome has been seen with secondary syphilis.[371]

Conversion Hysteria

Probably the most frequent cause of sudden weakness or "paralysis" of the legs in older children is conversion hysteria. The muscle strength and tone and the deep tendon reflexes are normal. Often, evidence of normal function of the legs can be elicited while distracting the patient.

Descending and Cranial Nerve Paralysis

Food-Borne and Wound Botulism

Food-borne botulism is usually associated with the ingestion of home-canned or home-processed foods; asparagus, green beans, and peppers are the most common items. Fewer than 5% of reported outbreaks are associated with restaurants, but they are responsible for about 40% of the cases. Items implicated in restaurant outbreaks include improperly canned jalapeno peppers (79 cases),[372] baked potatoes wrapped in foil (30 cases),[373] sautéed onions (28 cases),[374] and improperly stored commercial cheese sauce (8 cases).[375] In each case, these foods were prepared by ordinary cooking procedures (which do not kill *C. botulinum* spores) and then stored for hours to days under relatively anaerobic conditions at temperatures warm enough to encourage the outgrowth of spores and production of toxin but not hot enough to kill the heat-labile toxin. The foods were then eaten without having been thoroughly reheated. The incubation period is usually between 18 and 36 hours.

Wounds can also become infected with *C. botulinum* and serve as a nidus for toxin-production. This is now most commonly associated with injection of contaminated black tar heroin, although half of cases in the United States are seen in teenagers, many of whom suffered from compound fractures of limb bones.[376]

The clinical manifestations of foodborne and wound botulism are the same, with the following exceptions: in wound botulism, fever is more common and gastrointestinal symptoms are lacking. The paralysis almost always begins with the cranial nerves, with impaired swallowing, speaking, and/or seeing (Fig. 9-8). Findings may be subtle, but it is not possible to have botulism without the presence of multiple cranial nerve palsies. Ptosis and diplopia are common. Dry mouth and sore throat may occur. Weakness and paralysis of the extremities may develop later, but usually deep tendon reflexes are normal. Mental status is maintained. Sudden and unexpected death may result from cardiac arrhythmias caused by the toxin. Approximately 15% of patients require ventilatory support. Equine trivalent botulinum antitoxin is effective if given early in the illness and is available from the Centers for Diseases Control and Prevention through state health departments. About 9% of patients develop hypersensitivity reactions, so it should not be given when the diagnosis is doubtful.[377]

Single-fiber electromyography may be the most sensitive of the neurophysiologic tests.[378] The characteristic finding is an incremental response to rapid repetitive stimulation at 50 Hz. Because binding of the toxin to the neuromuscular junction is irreversible, recovery requires the regrowth of nerve endings, which may take several months.

Herpes Simplex Virus

This virus has been recognized as an important cause of cranial nerve paralysis in children, teenagers, and young adults. Facial nerve palsy is espe-

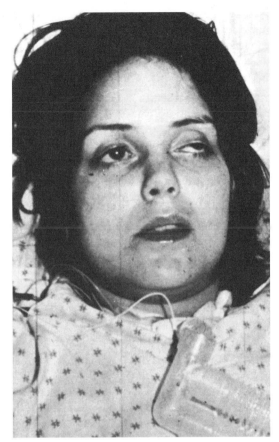

■ **FIGURE 9-8** Cranial nerve paralysis in patient with botulism. Note deviation of the left eye, droopy eyelid (ptosis), and facial asymmetry. Tubing from a tracheotomy to a ventilator can also be seen. (Photo courtesy of Drs. William Terranova and Joel Breman. From Moffet HL. Clinical Microbiology. Philadelphia: JB Lippincott, 1980.)

cially common, but the oculomotor and trigeminal nerves have also been involved.[379] Benign intracranial hypertension may be associated with facial nerve paralysis (Bell palsy) and recovery of herpes simplex virus.

Other Infectious Causes

Mycoplasma pneumoniae can cause isolated cranial nerve paralysis. Lyme disease, discussed in Chapter 11, can cause cranial neuropathies, including unilateral or bilateral facial paralysis.[380]

Varicella-zoster virus, CMV, influenza virus, mumps, and EBV infection have all been observed concurrently with peripheral facial nerve (Bell) palsy.[381,382] In Japan, 396 patients with Bell palsy had serologic testing for VZV, HSV, and adenoviruses; positive titers were found in 8%, 4%, and 4%, respectively.[383] No controls were studied. Evidence of viral infection was more likely to be found in younger patients.

In one case, facial palsy was the presenting feature of cat-scratch disease.[384] Patients with Bell palsy may have a CSF pleocytosis, or benign intracranial hypertension may be present.[385,386] In adults, 7th cranial nerve paralysis is the most common manifestation of neurosarcoidosis.[387] Orbital myositis is a possible cause detectable by enlarged orbital muscles on CT scan.[388]

Ramsay Hunt syndrome (herpes zoster oticus) is caused by reactivation of VZV from the geniculate ganglion.[383a] It results in unilateral facial nerve palsy, sensorineural hearing loss, and vestibulocochlear dysfunction. Vesicles may be visible in the ear canal. Prompt treatment with acyclovir may improve the outcome.[383a]

Bell palsy can also be caused by otitis media.

Benign recurrent isolated cranial sixth-nerve palsy is a diagnosis made by exclusion of other, serious causes.[389,390] Melkersson-Rosenthal syndrome is an uncommon condition in which recurrent facial nerve palsy is associated with recurrent orofacial edema and lingua plicata (a fissured tongue).[391] Sometimes, one or more of the descriptive triad may be missing. Granulomatous cheilitis is the pathologic hallmark of this condition.

Acute Hemiplegia

Unilateral paralysis of the arm and leg is usually a spastic paralysis caused by an intracranial lesion. Hemiplegic migraine can occur in a teenager or young adult.[392] Despite the fact that cerebral vascular accidents are rare in children, cerebral vascular disease accounted for two-thirds of all acute hemiplegia in a series of 57 infants and children in Taiwan.[393] In Japan, about half of cerebrovascular accidents in pediatric patients are caused by moyamoya disease,[394] which is a progressive arterial disease of unknown pathogenesis that can be familial. Protein C deficiency may increase the risk of cerebrovascular occlusive accidents.[395] Hemiplegia has also been reported in patients with sickle cell disease.[396] Rupture of a berry aneurysm is more likely in a child or a young adult than is thrombosis and can occur in the first year of life.[397] Carotid artery thrombosis is unusual.[398] Thrombosis of a cerebral vessel also can complicate cyanotic congenital heart disease with polycythemia.

It is important to take a history for trauma that

may have been forgotten. There are several reports of children developing vertebral artery dissection and stroke after using trampolines.[398a] As these children did not sustain a fall, the mechanism is presumably from rapid shearing forces during jumping. Similarly, there are multiple reports of chiropractic manipulation leading to vertebral artery dissection and stroke.[398b]

Although multiple sclerosis is rare in childhood, acute hemiparesis was the most common presenting feature in a recent review.[399] Two cases of human herpesvirus 7 (HHV-7) infection manifested as exanthem subitum and acute hemiplegia have been reported.[400] One 4-year-old boy presented with acute hemiplegia, ataxia, and dysarthria and 24 hours later exhibited a typical varicella exanthem. MRI findings were consistent with multiple cerebral ischemic infarcts. It was suggested that he may have seeded his central nervous system vessels during the secondary viremia stage of varicella zoster virus infection.[401] Four children developed acute hemiplegia weeks to months after chickenpox. Although a definitive link could not be established, 2 of these had middle cerebral artery lesions reminiscent of those seen with herpes zoster opthalmicus.[402] Acute hemiplegia secondary to a large infarct in a 16-month-old with HIV encephalopathy has been reported.[403]

Infantile acquired hemiplegia is characterized by fever, convulsions, and hemiplegia and may complicate a variety of acute infections.[404-406] Residual hemiplegia is usually mild. Occasionally, the infant dies, and autopsy reveals vascular lesions.

Brain abscess can produce hemiplegia, as discussed in a later section.

One of us recently cared for a teenager who presented with a 3-day history of headache, left-sided neck pain, and decreased movement of his left upper extremity. MRI demonstrated a cervical epidural abscess, and intraoperative cultures and blood cultures grew Group A streptococcus. Spinal epidural abscess is discussed in the previous section on Acute Paraparesis and Paraplegia.

Cerebral vasculitis may be secondary to sinusitis and typically is associated with hemiparesis, fever, convulsions, and, occasionally, a stiff neck with CSF pleocytosis.[407] MRI scanning may be helpful in eliciting a cause for acute hemiplegia,[408] and gadolinium-enhanced MRI is better suited to reveal small lesions such as capsular infarctions.[394] Magnetic resonance angiography may be used.

Variants of Guillain Barré syndrome can occur

that involve only cranial nerves or begin with involvement of the arms.[409]

Injury to an extremity may result in apparent paralyses (painful paralysis).

Weakness, Myalgia, and Myositis

Infant Botulism

In a weak young infant, botulism is a possible infectious etiology.[410–413] Botulinum toxin has been found in honey, and cases of infant botulism have been traced directly to its ingestion. For this reason, honey should never be fed to a baby younger than 12 months old. Although there has been some concern about corn syrups (sometimes employed by mothers in the therapy of "constipation"), the latest information suggests that these syrups are not likely to be a source of botulism. In most cases the exact exposure is never ascertained. Cases in which exposure to dust precipitated the disease have been reported. The other diagnostic possibilities in a baby with a botulism-like syndrome include hereditary muscular disorders, sepsis, and neonatal myasthenia gravis.[413] The peak age of botulism is 2–4 months, by which time congenital myasthenia gravis will have already made itself known.

Babies with botulism are almost always afebrile, which helps to differentiate this condition from sepsis. Weakness dominates the clinical picture. As with the other forms of botulism, bulbar symptoms are always present but are sometimes subtle. Repeatedly shining a light into the patient's eye and watching the pupillary reflex will reveal a diminished response with repeated testing; muscular fatigability with repetitive contraction is a hallmark of infant botulism. The spectrum of botulism may range from sudden infant death to a mild outpatient illness with "failure to thrive" and hypotonia. Constipation is a prominent early feature but is historically often overlooked. Mothers will often report poor feeding. In hospitalized infants, ptosis, expressionless facies, and loss of suck and gag reflexes may be seen.

The diagnosis can be confirmed by recovery of botulinum toxin or *Clostridium botulinum* from the stool. In the past, scientific support for horse-serum derived antitoxin was scant; however, administration of a human-derived botulinum antitoxin has been shown by a 5-year prospective placebo-controlled study to reduce length of hospital stay in hospitalized infants with botulism. The average length of stay was reduced from 5.5 days to 2.5 days at a savings of $70,000 in costs per case. It should be administered as soon as the diagnosis is strongly suspected, rather than awaiting laboratory confirmation. The antitoxin is available from the California Department of Health Services (1-510-540-2646). Mechanical ventilation may be necessary. Babies who survive the acute phase of the illness usually recover full neurologic function, but recovery may be prolonged.

Up to 1 in 20 cases of SIDS were attributable to infant botulism in one California study.[414] Infant botulism is less common in other parts of the country, however.

Influenza and Other Viruses

Influenza virus[415–417] clearly causes myalgia, myositis, and myoglobinuria, as described in Chapter 7. Myalgia occurs to a lesser degree in other viral infections.[418]

Septic Myositis

In staphylococcal bacteremia, myalgia and myositis may be prominent.[419]

Other Causes

In toxic shock syndrome due to either *S. aureus* or *S. pyogenes* (Chapter 10), myalgia and myositis are often prominent. Myalgia is also prominent in Rocky Mountain spotted fever and in dengue fever. Withdrawal of corticosteroid therapy can cause myalgia.

Rhabdomyolysis

Severe muscle involvement can result in muscle necrosis and myoglobinuria (resembling hemoglobinuria [rhabdomyolysis]). This is the severe end of the spectrum of myositis and can be caused by influenza virus, enteroviruses, superimposed beta-hemolytic streptococcal infection, and tularemia.[420–422]

Management of Acute Paralysis

The extent and severity of the paralysis should be defined and recorded, so that progression can be recognized. Etiologies with a specific treatment should be looked for, especially poisonings such as botulism and acute infections such as epidural abscess. Those with botulism should be treated as soon as possible with botulinum antitoxin. Antibiotic therapy should not be used in patients with botulism unless an obvious secondary infection occurs, because antibiotics can actually worsen the disease by releasing toxin from lysed bacteria.

Acute respiratory failure is the principal cause of death in most of these syndromes. Weakness of the diaphragms and intercostal muscles leads to inadequate lung expansion. Weak cough and swallowing lead to obstruction of the respiratory tract by secretions, producing atelectasis. Tracheal intubation with suctioning and mechanical ventilation followed by tracheotomy are the chief emergency measures the physician should be prepared to use. Respiratory muscle paralysis may not occur until several days after the onset of paralysis in another area but unfortunately may be the first indication that the paralysis is ascending. Aspiration pneumonia and atelectasis may to some extent be prevented by suctioning and positioning.

■ ACUTE INFECTIOUS PYSCHOSES

Acute infectious psychoses are characterized by the acute onset of disorientation or hallucinations concurrently with manifestations of a mild fever in the absence of high fever, stiff neck, ataxia, coma, semicoma, or other manifestations of the CNS syndromes previously described in this chapter. Usually, there is no headache. Hallucinations or bizarre behavior are the predominant manifestations.

Differential Diagnosis

Infectious mononucleosis is a common infectious cause of apparent psychosis.[423] Visual aberration and a detached feeling have been described (the "Alice-in-Wonderland syndrome").[424] One adolescent female became frankly psychotic and attempted suicide during infection with EBV; her mental status returned to normal with resolution of the infection.[425] *Mycoplasma pneumoniae* has also been etiologically linked to acute psychotic episodes.[426,427] Several cases in which neurocysticercosis has been associated with acute psychosis have been reported.[428] Patients with HSV encephalitis can present with temporal lobe syndrome-like symptoms, in which extreme disinhibition and bizarre behavior might be misinterpreted as acute psychosis. A 13-year-old boy with typhoid fever and infection-associated hemophagocytic syndrome presented with psychosis, fever, and pancytopenia.[429]

Intracranial abscesses have been associated with behavioral changes described as "feeling goofy," confusion, and incoherent speech; but these patients have had other clues to intracranial suppuration.[430]

Antibiotic therapies of various types have been associated with acute psychosis. Treatment of an infection with procaine penicillin can be associated with brief, immediate hallucinations due to inadvertent intravenous injection, apparently related to the procaine component, and often associated with a seizure (Hoigne's syndrome).[431] Psychosis in association with both oral[432] and intravenous[433] trimethoprim-sulfamethoxazole has been reported. Fluoroquinolones have also been temporally associated with acute psychotic episodes.[434,435] A series of 6 patients who developed a self-limiting psychosis after receiving mefloquine for malaria has been reported. All were neurologically normal prior to receiving the drug, developed symptoms within 8–24 hours of taking it, and recovered completely.[436] Decongestants containing pseudoephedrine can produce hallucinations.[437]

Acute Noninfectious Causes

Temporal-lobe epilepsy should be considered as an acute noninfectious cause. Sleepwalking and night terrors have been associated with febrile illnesses.[438] Childhood migraine can produce time and body distortion and hallucinations.[439]

Poisoning or drug abuse, as with Jimson weed, narcotics, methamphetamine and others can produce hallucinations.[440]

■ VENTRICULITIS AND INFECTED SHUNTS

Ventriculitis can be conveniently and arbitrarily defined as more than 25 leukocytes/mcL or as a positive culture from cerebrospinal fluid obtained from a ventricle of the brain. The level of spinal fluid protein is usually elevated but that of glucose is often normal rather than decreased. Increased leukocytes and protein are often secondary to infection but can be due to a recent neurosurgical procedure, increased pressure from obstruction, or drugs put into the ventricles. CSF eosinophilia is relatively common in children with CNS shunts and is a marker both for subsequent shunt failure and infection.[441]

Predisposing Causes

Infection of the ventricles of the brain occurs in patients with meningitis or with an artificial ventricular shunt. In most cases, the infection is a complication of hydrocephalus treated by the insertion of plastic tubing, which shunts the spinal fluid from a lateral ventricle to the vena cava or peritoneal cavity (Fig. 9-9). Because most shunt infections occur within the first 8–24 weeks after surgical placement,[442] it is thought that most infections result from the tube's acting as a foreign-body focus for infection by skin bacteria introduced at the time of surgery. Obstruction of the tubing, as by a malfunctioning valve, predisposes the shunt to infection. Usually, the bacteria in the valve or tubing pass through the tubing to the peritoneum or blood. A prospective study showed that 6 (3%) of 173 shunts were culture positive at the time of implantation surgery; all 6 of them developed malfunction during the first few weeks.[443] In a series of 727 shunt insertions or revisions, patient age of less than 2 years at the time of implantation of the shunt was the single most important risk factor for infection.[444] In a recent study of 820 consecutive ventriculoperitoneal shunt placements in children, 92 shunts (11%) became infected a median of 19 days after insertion. Premature birth, previous shunt infection, and intraoperative use of the neuroendoscope were independent risk factors for shunt infection.[445]

Prophylactic intravenous antibiotics at the time of shunt placement appeared to decrease the risk of shunt infections in the first few months in one study, but intraventricular vancomycin or intravenous nafcillin did not help in other studies.[447,448] In one study, a large dose of ceftriaxone was given perioperatively to 100 consecutive shunt placement patients; over the ensuing 4 years no shunt infections were diagnosed in the cohort.[449] This study was uncontrolled, and subsequent controlled studies have been unable to replicate the findings. A prospective, randomized, placebo-controlled trial of a prophylactic second-generation cephalosporin showed an infection rate of 8% in the treatment group versus 13% in the control group;[450] however,

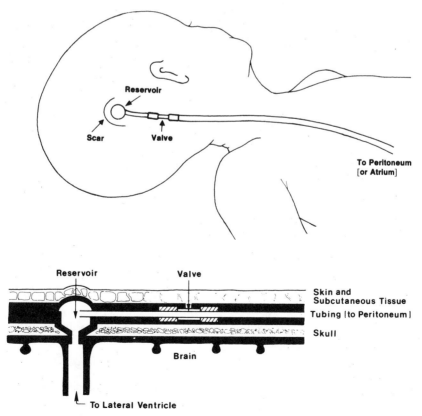

■ **FIGURE 9-9** Typical location (*top*) and tubing and reservoir parts (*bottom*) of a ventriculoperitoneal shunt.

the control rate of 13% was higher than the expected background infection rate in shunting procedures, which is usually from 4–8%. A meta-analysis looking at this question found that of 12 randomized, properly-performed prospective trials, only one showed a statistically significant benefit from perioperative antimicrobial prophylaxis. However, in aggregate, they found an approximately 50% reduction in shunt infections between patients in the treatment arms.[451] The scientific basis for the value of prophylactic antibiotics is debatable, but most neurosurgeons use them. Because of the consequences of infection, use of a perioperative antibiotic (such as intravenous cefazolin) is reasonable. By extrapolation with prophylaxis for other surgical procedures, a single preoperative dose given 30 minutes prior to skin incision provides adequate tissue levels throughout the surgery, and postoperative doses are usually unnecessary.[452]

One group of investigators hypothesized that the reason shunt infections were more common in premature neonates was that their humoral immune system is not fully functioning. To test this hypothesis, they administered IVIG at a dose of 1 gm/kg to 30 neonates the night prior to shunt implantation, and gave a placebo infusion to 30 others. No patient who received IVIG developed a shunt infection over the following 6 months, whereas the infection rate per procedure in the control group was approximately 5%.[453] These numbers did not reach statistical significance, and further study on this type of prophylaxis has not been published.

Ventriculitis is probably frequent with bacterial meningitis but has no immediate clinical importance unless pus or edema obstructs the ventricles, as can occur in newborn and young infants with very thick exudates and small aqueducts.

Ordinary bacterial meningitis can occur in a patient with a shunt. *H. influenzae* meningitis, for example, may respond to usual therapy without removal of the shunt.[454] Our experience has been that such patients appear less seriously ill than the usual child with meningitis, probably because the cerebral edema effects are relieved to a large extent by a functioning shunt. Shunt infections secondary to *H. influenzae* (either type b or untypable) occur much later than do infections with staphylococci, presumably because they are secondary to hematogenous spread rather than to contamination of the shunt during surgery.[455] Infections due to Hib, of course, are rare in the conjugate vaccine era, but nontypable strains are still occasionally seen.

Shunt Infections

Obstruction of the shunt can be diagnosed by clinical findings and confirmed by CT scan, which usually shows an increase in the size of the lateral ventricles.[456] However, diagnosis of shunt infections may be difficult for many reasons.

Minimal Systemic Signs

Much of the delay is due to the lack of signs of toxicity usually expected with meningitis. Fever to 103°F or higher is common, but the patient often looks well enough that spinal fluid examination is postponed. Signs of ventricular obstruction and increased intracranial pressure, such as vomiting, may occur later. Nuchal rigidity is usually absent. Headache and malaise are common but nonspecific. In the child with recurrent shunt infection, the astute parent can often correctly diagnose a presumptive infection based on similar manifestations to previous episodes.

Variable Location of Infection

It is important to understand the anatomy and the type of shunt equipment used in an individual patient's shunt (see Fig. 9-9).[457] It is also extremely important that the spinal fluid specimens be precisely labeled as to source when sent to the laboratory. A negative examination and culture of spinal fluid obtained from one area is not sufficient to exclude a shunt infection in another area. The infection can be a wound infection, a ventriculitis, a peritonitis, or embolization of the blood or peritoneum from the valve or the tubing. For example, the finding of normal spinal fluid in a ventricle does not exclude infection in the valve. Similarly, normal spinal fluid in the ventricle does not exclude meningeal infection. Lumbar puncture may be indicated if ventricular cultures are negative, because acute hematogenous meningitis can be milder in patients with shunts, since intracranial pressure is relieved by the shunt. Cultures of CSF obtained by lumbar puncture, on the other hand, may be negative in the face of a positive shunt culture.

Minimal CSF Findings

An elevated protein concentration may be the result of obstruction of the ventricles as well as of infection. The cellular response in ventriculitis is typically much less than that found in purulent meningitis: cell counts may be only 10–600 WBC/mcL. This may be attributable to the low virulence of the organism, but more likely it is due to the difference between the ventricles and meninges in terms of inflammatory response capabilities. A low spinal fluid glucose sometimes helps distinguish an infectious ventriculitis from a postoperative inflammation, but it is not a regular finding early in the course. Normal spinal fluid glucose concentration is the rule, rather than the exception.

Culture of Possible Contaminants

The culture may reveal an organism of low virulence, such as *S. epidermidis*, which is a frequent skin contaminant in cultures. The organism may be regarded by the physician as a contaminant, particularly since the patient usually does not appear "septic," although fever is usually present. Recovery of *S. epidermidis* from spinal or ventricular fluid of a patient with a shunt should be regarded as potentially significant, as this is the most frequent cause of ventriculitis in such patients.[458] *Propionibacterium acnes* ("anaerobic diphtheroid"), which is normal flora of the skin, is also capable of causing shunt infections, and its recovery should not be regarded as evidence of contamination.[459] Of course, both *S. epidermidis* and *Propionibacterium* spp can contaminate CSF cultures of patients with shunts. Recovery of such organisms from more than one culture (taken either from different sites during the same surgery or from the same site during different surgeries) increases the likelihood of true infection.

One of the things that causes confusion is that most microbiology laboratories utilize thioglycolate broth cultures in addition to the standard agar cultures in the evaluation of possible shunt infection. Broth cultures increase the sensitivity of culture a great deal; if only one organism is present in a sample the broth culture will turn positive. The cost of this increased sensitivity is that contaminants will also be identified more frequently. A review of 1188 shunt-derived spinal fluid samples shed some light on the interpretation of these "broth-only" isolates. There was no instance in which *S. epidermidis* grown in the broth only was considered to be causing true infection. The clinical significance of *Propionibacterium* spp was a little less clear; in several cases, the broth was the only positive culture in patients with real infection.[460] These data suggest that if a coagulase-negative staphylococcus is grown in a single culture from the thioglycolate broth but does not grow on solid agar, it can be reasonably assumed to be a contaminant.

In addition to coagulase-negative staphylococci and *Propionibacterium* spp., common pathogens include *S. aureus*, viridans streptococci, enterococci, and *Corynebacteria*. Gram negative organisms, such as *E. coli*, are less frequent causes. *Candida albicans*, as well as other species of *Candida*, can infect shunts.[461] Fungal infection of shunts seems to be more common in premature neonates who receive a shunt because of complications of intraventricular hemorrhage.[462]

Minimal Local Signs

In peritonitis, the peritoneal signs may at first be minimal because the bacteria, such as *S. epidermidis*, are of low virulence.[463] Tenderness may be localized around the site of the peritoneal insertion of the tube, which is often tender even in the absence of infection because of the flow of spinal fluid into a loculation within the peritoneal cavity. However, fever and obvious peritoneal irritation eventually develop.[464] Cyst formation, colon perforation, development of an inguinal hernia, appendicitis, or volvulus around the tubing can also occur,[465] as can simple kinking of the tube.

In wound infections, the infection around the tubing, which is subcutaneous during most of its route, may erode through the surface of the skin. It is necessary to determine whether the erythema and tenderness over the tube is caused by a foreign-body reaction or an infection with a low-virulence organism.

Ascites and pseudocyst formation may occur without infection.[466,467]

Diagnostic Strategies

Cultures can be obtained through the reservoir (if there is one) or by needle aspiration of the valve. Pumping the valve and culturing the blood can be done in the case of the less commonly used ventriculo-atrial shunt. Peritoneal tap is rarely helpful. Lumbar puncture is needed only if systemic meningitis is suspected.

If the Gram stain of ventricular fluid shows bacteria, antibiotics based on the stain can be begun. Otherwise, antibiotics should be withheld until two sets of cultures are obtained, as it is essential to obtain the infecting organism.

Treatment Strategies

In addition to the use of antibiotics, there are essentially three options for management of shunt infections:

1. remove the shunt and utilize an external ventricular drainage device for decompression (usually for 7–10 days), followed by reinsertion of another shunt;
2. remove the infected shunt and replace it immediately with a new indwelling device; and
3. leave the shunt in place (antibiotic therapy only).

Bisno and Sternau compiled the results from 20 different studies comparing these three strategies. Of 227 infections treated with shunt removal and insertion of an external drainage device, 213 (94%) were cured, compared with 114 (71%) of 161 infections treated with immediate shunt replacement, and 95 (37%) of 254 infections in which shunts were left in place.[468]

Given these data, the first strategy is recommended for most patients with CNS shunt infections. Treatment with antibiotics alone may sometimes be tried for very low-grade infections, or if the shunt is apparently in the last possible location. Sometimes the reservoir is a vital route to treat leukemia or carcinomatous meningitis, in which case the second strategy may be used. For ascending infections in which the source is the periotoneal cavity, an alternative is to externalize the distal end of the peritoneal shunt, although many such patients will require a complete shunt revision.

Treatment

It is difficult to interpret the results of reviews of treatment because of the many changes in approach from early cases to more recent cases.[469,470] Each short series every 4 years is helpful only in indicating what has been successful in some cases.

Good communication is essential between the neurosurgeon, who knows the anatomy and the mechanics of the shunt, and the medical consultant.

The tubing acts as a foreign body in perpetuating the infection and usually must be removed. However, this step may allow pressure to increase within the ventricles and tends to perpetuate the infection unless the obstruction is relieved by repeated ventricle or reservoir puncture or by temporary externalization of the peritoneal catheter.[471] As dis-cussed previously, the best approach is to remove all tubing and utilize an external ventricular device for several days. Fluid can be obtained daily or every other day for cell count, Gram stain, and culture. Once sterility of the fluid is documented, a new shunt can be inserted, usually after 7–10 days. Penetration of some antibiotics into the ventricles is poor. Local instillation of antibiotics is sometimes helpful in eradicating the organism,[471] but is not used routinely.

There are more similarities to subacute bacterial endocarditis than to meningitis. Unlike acute bacterial meningitis, there is usually time (12–24 hours) to get adequate cultures. Study of the organism's minimum inhibitory and bactericidal concentrations is useful. Testing the patient's ventricular fluid for antibacterial activity against the isolate also is useful. A penicillin and an aminoglycoside are often synergistic. Vancomycin and rifampin have been useful in *S. epidermidis* infections,[472–475] but rifampin may not be necessary.[474]

Removal of Shunt

The entire shunt usually has to be removed to control the infection.[476] However, antibiotic therapy is occasionally attempted first. In general, *S. epidermidis* and other skin bacteria are more likely to be eradicated without removal of the shunt than are enteric gram-negative bacteria and *Pseudomonas aeruginosa*, which almost always require removal of the shunt.[476] In our experience, it is best to remove the shunt even with the less virulent organisms.

Systemic Antimicrobials

As noted, the situation is analogous to subacute bacterial endocarditis in several respects. First, antibiotic therapy must wait until sufficient cultures are obtained, so that therapy can be based on sensitivity studies. Second, antibiotics must be bactericidal, because the usual host resistance factors are of little help. Third, dosages must be as high as possible without toxicity because of poor penetration into the infected areas. Finally, therapy must be long enough to prevent relapse.

For most Gram positive infections, 10–14 days of antibiotics is sufficient, provided that the infected shunt has been removed. For *S. aureus*, a minimum of 14 days of therapy should be given. The usual practice is to treat with antibiotics for 7–10 days while the external drain is in place, and then for an additional 24–48 hours after the new shunt has been placed. Gram negative infections and those due to fungi require longer courses of therapy (usually 21 days). Bactericidal activity of ventricular fluid against the patient's own organism, minimal bactericidal concentration, and antibiotic concentration and duration in the ventricular fluid may be useful to determine, as described in the section on infective endocarditis (Chapter 18).

Intraventricular Antibiotics

Whether intraventricular antibiotics are helpful in eradicating infection has not been studied systematically. They may occasionally be necessary to treat a difficult infection, but are not usually necessary if the approach described above (removal, use of an external drainage device, and delayed reinsertion) is used. In addition, they are not without complications. If they are used, an antibiotic that is not irritating to the brain tissue should be injected. A reservoir is useful to avoid needling brain tissue (see Fig. 9-9). If a functioning shunt is present, the intraventricular antibiotic may run off very rapidly if there is increased pressure. Penicillin may produce convulsions if present in concentrations above 1000 units/mL. However, penicillin derivatives and cephalosporins have been injected into the ventricles in infants with hydrocephalus and ventriculitis without adverse effects, with some cures.[477] Kanamycin, gentamicin, or polymyxin B have been used for infections caused by gram-negative rods. The dose depends on the estimated volume of the ventriculitis.

Dosages for children and adults for penicillins or cephalosporins for intraventricular use are described in the larger series.[459,477] The doses are calculated by estimating the ventricular volume and inserting enough drug to produce a CSF concentration at least as high as the maximum desired serum concentrations. For example, 1 mg of gentamicin in 100 mL of CSF results in 10 ug/mL.

Oral trimethoprim-sulfamethoxazole and rifampin with intrathecal vancomycin (10–20 mg per dose) has been successful in some patients without removing the shunt.[478]

In patients without any obstruction, intraventricular drugs are diluted by newly formed spinal fluid and absorbed through the arachnoid villi or run out through the shunt. In patients with obstructive hydrocephalus, drugs may remain in the ventricles for many days, with additive increases in concentration if more drug is injected. If intraventricular antibiotics are used, measurement of antibiotic concentrations in ventricular fluid is important. Determination of bactericidal titer of the ventricular fluid against the patient's own organism may be useful, if available.

Reduce Intraventricular Pressure

Ventricular pressure should be relieved when necessary by insertion of a needle through the burr hole originally made to insert the tubing or through the diaphragm of a reservoir. If the external ventricular device becomes dislodged in a patient who was previously shunt-dependent, it should be replaced without delay. This is particularly true for those at increased risk for tonsillar herniation, such as a patient with an Arnold-Chiari malformation.

Reduction of intraventricular pressure by needling the system after high pressures have been built up may result in tearing small vessels and bleeding. Continuous external ventricular drainage may be necessary when spinal fluid production is high and obstruction is complete.[471] In some patients, improvement may occur only after the CSF production is decreased as a result of damage from the infection.

Complications

Nephritis with hematuria, proteinuria, and azotemia may occur in ventriculo-atrial (VA) shunts but not in ventriculo-peritoneal (VP) shunts. The finding of decreased serum complement and the results of electron microscopy and immunofluorescence studies suggest an immunologic mechanism.[479] Candida albicans shunt infections can follow immediately after therapy for bacterial shunt infections.

Brain damage may occur due to destructive effects of long-term infection, which may only be suppressed by antibiotics. This is especially true in infections caused by more virulent organisms, such as Enterobacter spp. Sometimes, a chronic, slowly progressive intellectual deterioration occurs in spite of the absence of any documentation of infection or pressure. This phenomenon might be the result of antigen-antibody reaction or to atrophy after ischemia.

■ TETANUS-LIKE ILLNESSES

Tetanus is a clinical syndrome manifested by generalized muscle rigidity, characteristically with episodes of muscle spasms. Due to the advent of modern intensive care, the mortality rate is lower than it used to be; in most series, it is between 10 and 50%. Intensive care in a large medical center should be given if possible. The patient often has a tightly clenched jaw secondary to masseter spasm (trismus), which gave rise to the name "lockjaw." *Clostridium tetani*, the etiologic agent of tetanus, is a strictly anaerobic organism that is difficult to recover in most clinical laboratories. Therefore, patients might be given the descriptive diagnosis of "tetanus-like illness" until the diagnosis can be either confirmed by culture or the clinical course or excluded by demonstrating drug toxicity by use of an antidote.

Tetanus is extremely rare in children in the United States. Between 1995 and 1997, there were 124 cases of tetanus reported, and only 5% of those occurred in patients younger than 20 years. The overall annual incidence in the U.S. is approximately 0.15 cases per million population.[480]

Classification

Episodic Generalized Rigidity

Generalized rigidity is the usual clinical pattern of tetanus and is the severe form of the disease implied when the term "tetanus" is used unmodified.

Neonatal Episodic Rigidity

Neonatal tetanus occurs in the first month of life, usually with the tetanus bacilli infecting the umbilical stump after a home delivery. Use of nonsterile instruments to cut the cord, dressing the cord with dirty rags, and the direct application of mud or animal feces onto the umbilical stump are major risk factors in third-world countries. Poor sucking is an early symptom.[481] Neonatal tetanus is usually considered separately in tetanus statistics because of the extremely high mortality rate. Due to widespread vaccination, neonatal tetanus is rare in the United States, but it is responsible for nearly 300,000 deaths worldwide each year. Neonates born to women who did not receive a complete primary tetanus vaccine series are at increased risk. Such groups include foreign-born persons and those who object to vaccination for philosophical reasons.[482,483]

Obstetricians should specifically inquire about tetanus vaccination status in pregnant women; unvaccinated patients should receive tetanus and diphtheria toxoid vaccine (dT) during pregnancy.[484,485]

Prognosis is poorest for the babies who present at the youngest age. Poor prognosis is also heralded by presentation with risus sardonicus (a grimacing facial expression, literally "sardonic smile") and/or opisthotonus (hyperextension of the neck and spine).[486]

Localized Rigidity

Localized tetanus can occur in the region of the wound, usually in an extremity.

Mild Rigidity

"Modified tetanus" is a term sometimes applied to mild or atypical tetanus, especially that in a patient who has had some previous immunization.[487] The mild form of the disease is more likely to occur in children than it is in adults.[488] The diagnosis cannot be certain unless both previous immunization and infection with *C. tetani* are documented.[489] Serum for measurement of antitoxin should be obtained before antitoxin therapy is given to a patient with apparent tetanus after immunizations.[487,489] Rarely, generalized tetanus can occur with antitoxin levels previously assumed to be protective.[490]

Physiologic Principles

Tetanus is produced by an exotoxin that acts directly on the anterior horn cells of the spinal cord to block the inhibitory transmitter at synapses, producing repeated muscle contractions or spasms lasting a few seconds to minutes. Once the toxin is fixed to neural tissue, it cannot be released, so antitoxin cannot reverse the effects of already attached toxin. Antitoxin treatment of tetanus acts primarily to neutralize any new toxin produced by the organism. Toxigenic strains of *C. tetani* contain a plasmid that codes for neurotoxin production, whereas nontoxigenic strains lack that plasmid.

Muscle spasm is best detected in unopposed muscles such as the jaw and the abdominal muscles. The mechanism of death is almost always respiratory failure. The patient is unable to breathe because of muscle spasms. Management consists of drugs to relax the muscles to allow the patient to breathe and, in some cases, mechanical ventilation. If breathing can be maintained for the period of time required for the toxin effects to wear off (usually 3 weeks or longer) without severe pneumonia, the patient will probably recover.

The toxin is a poor antigen and does not stimulate adequate antibody production by the patient. An attack of the disease does not produce immunity, and some narcotic addicts have had the disease several times. Therefore, active immunization with tetanus toxoid should be given to prevent further attacks.[491]

Many people in China, India, and the Galapagos Islands have antibodies to tetanus toxin without ever having been immunized by tetanus toxoid, apparently from being immunized by ingested tetanus bacteria and subclinical illness.[492]

Early Clinical Diagnosis

Muscle Spasms

Tetanus should be suspected in any patient who has generalized muscle spasms. There may be difficulty walking or pain in the abdomen or back due to muscle spasm. Occasionally, the neck stiffness is prominent enough to lead the physician to do a lumbar puncture.

Trismus

Spasm of the masseter muscle is the usual early manifestation that allows the physician to make a presumptive diagnosis of tetanus. When the physician attempts to examine the pharynx, it is found that the patient cannot open the mouth well. The presence of trismus, episodic muscle spasms that may be painful, and exclusion of drug ingestion (particularly phenothiazines) is sufficient to allow the physician to make a presumptive diagnosis of tetanus.

Convulsions

Generalized seizures can be the presenting finding in tetanus. The trismus and increased muscle tone after the convulsion should suggest the diagnosis.

Wound Infection

Many patients with tetanus have an infected laceration or other wound. Although is it popularly believed that deep puncture wounds are more likely to be associated with tetanus, many patients have a history of only minor trauma. Others have sources of the toxin that are more difficult to recognize, such as necrotic umbilical stump of a newborn infant, otitis media (especially in neglected otitis in individuals with no medical care), phlebitis or skin or muscle abscesses complicating repeated non-sterile injections by drug addicts, recent gastrointestinal surgery, crushing injuries, burns, septic abortions, infected decubitus ulcers, animal bites, or dental infections.[491] A few patients have no identifiable source of the toxin, and undoubtedly some of the reported sources of infection are coincidental.

Immunization History

Most patients with tetanus have never been immunized against it. Some have had their first injection of toxoid at the time the injury was treated, which is inadequate to prevent tetanus.[491] Such patients should start a schedule to receive the entire primary series. They may also require tetanus immune globulin, as outlined in Table 17-2.

Culture

Bacteriologic confirmation is difficult, because the organism is such a strict anaerobe, and unnecessary, since the clinical findings are usually sufficient to be certain of the diagnosis. The organism can occasionally be isolated from draining wounds or ears. Therapy should not be delayed in order to await cultural confirmation, but phenothiazine toxicity should be excluded.

Other Causes of Rigidity

Generalized Rigidity

An adverse reaction to a phenothiazine should be suspected when a patient with this syndrome has received Chlorpromazine, prochlorperazine, or trimethylbenzamide.[493,494] Immediate reversal of the effect occurs after the intravenous administration of 25–100 mg of diphenhydramine (Benadryl)[495] or physostigmine.[496] The mechanism of action is not known.

Spinal cord tumors occasionally present as persistent spinal rigidity. However, this occurs gradually and usually does not present any confusion with tetanus. Krabbe disease is rare. It usually begins at about 5 months of age with rigidity and tonic spasms. It is primarily familial and has the histologic findings of diffuse cerebral sclerosis.

Stiff-person syndrome is a rare neurologic disorder with autoimmune features. It is most common in adult females and responds to IVIG therapy.[496a] Maple syrup urine disease begins at about 3–5 days of age with rigidity and, later, opisthotonus and may be confused with neonatal tetanus. Convulsions may occur. Maple syrup urine disease may be suspected by the maple syrup odor of the urine. The disease is fatal at about the age of 3 months if not recognized and treated with a special diet.

Other causes of episodic generalized rigidity include strychnine poisoning, black widow spider bite, hypocalcemic tetany, and any convulsive disorder causing tonic convulsions.

A physician in Italy has described a genetic disorder that presents with trismus, muscular hypertonia, and occasionally opisthotonus that resembles that of tetanus. However, the syndrome is also characterized by dysmorphic facial features, camptodactyly, and dysregulation of body temperature.[497]

Isolated Trismus

Infections near the masseter muscle, as of the teeth, throat, or parotid gland, can produce trismus.[498] Rabies often causes spasms related to swallowing, but this is not true trismus.

Treatment

Diphenhydramine Trial

If there is a suspicion of phenothiazide ingestion, diphenhydramine should be given intravenously.[495] This should not be done if the patient is having spasms that may interfere with breathing.

Sedation

Sedation should be begun as soon as a patient is suspected of having tetanus and before diagnostic studies are done. If a painful procedure is done before the patient is completely relaxed, it may precipitate spasms, which may interfere with breathing. Lumbar punctures, injections, venipunctures, and unessential parts of the physical examination are all contraindicated if severe spasms are occurring in a patient with a clinical presumption of tetanus. Fortunately, the onset of tetanus is usually gradual, so that the early signs of muscle rigidity are present for a day or so before the spasms become so frequent and lasting that they interfere with breathing, and usually, patients are ambulatory when first seen by a physician. The spasms get worse over the first few days and require higher and higher doses of sedation.

At the time a patient is first seen, it is not possible to know whether the illness will be a severe one, which will require 3 or more weeks of sedation,

muscle-paralyzing agents such as vecuronium, and mechanical ventilation, or whether the patient can be managed by a less complicated program of sedation alone. Therefore, the physician should sedate the patient sufficiently, and admit the patient to the intensive care unit.

Benzodiazepines are now the drug of choice for spasms associated with tetanus; they are effective anti-seizure agents as well. Diazepam (Valium) or lorazepam (Ativan) are usually used. Doses are described in the section on febrile convulsion.

Airway and Assisted Ventilation

It is both difficult and a dangerous waste of time to attempt to force an airway or to ventilate a patient while a spasm is occurring. It is of no value to do a tracheotomy or intubate to provide an airway unless the patient is adequately relaxed. It is an error to attempt intubation or do a tracheotomy during a tetanic spasm, because the physiologic problem is muscle spasm, not obstructed airway. In the case of cyanosis from a long spasm of the chest muscles, immediate intravenous medication should be given to paralyze the muscles: succinylcholine or a short-acting barbiturate such as thiopental. Then the patient should be ventilated by bag and mask. Intubation may not be needed.

Antitoxin

This should not be given until the patient's muscle spasms are controlled by sedation. It is a common error to give antitoxin higher priority than sedation to prevent chest muscle spasms. Sedation is of primary importance and should be given without delay. Antitoxin (tetanus immune globulin) is probably only of value to neutralize any toxin still being released. Human antitoxin should be given, in a dose of 500 units intramuscularly. Although its value is not clearly established, in a retrospective review of 545 cases, patients treated with antitoxin had a significantly lower case-fatality rate.[499] If it is not available, IVIG can be used.

Antibiotics

Penicillin eradicates the organism, but may act as an agonist to tetanospasmin by inhibiting gamma-aminobutyric acid. Therefore, metronidazole is currently the drug of choice. The dose is 15 mg/kg for loading, followed by 30 mg/kg/day divided q 6 hours. Attempting to eradicate *C. tetani* is, like antitoxin therapy, less urgent than muscle relaxation. In an open-label study, response to treatment, duration of hospital stay, and mortality were all improved by metronidazole therapy.[500]

Other Measures

Debridement of the infected wound is indicated following the same surgical principles as any other situation. It should be limited to removal of dead tissue until viable tissue is reached, which should not be sacrificed. Hyperbaric oxygen is of no value.

Complications

Aspiration pneumonia is usually the first complication of tetanus. It may occur within the first couple of days or a week later. In prior years, when patients were treated with penicillin for tetanus, the pneumonia was usually caused by a penicillin-resistant organism, usually *S. aureus*. Other complications include urinary retention with urinary infection.

Prevention

Approximately 50 cases of tetanus are reported annually in the United States, and despite improvements in intensive care treatments, the disease has a high fatality rate of from 10–50%. The mortality rate is highest in newborns, intravenous drug abusers, and in the elderly. In the most recent report, 87% of all patients with tetanus were not fully vaccinated. All of the deaths from tetanus in the United States are preventable by immunization.

Active immunization with tetanus toxoid is indicated in childhood, with boosters throughout life. Immunization of women of childbearing age is effective in preventing tetanus of the newborn.[501] Passive immunization with tetanus immune globulin is effective when medical care is sought for a wound. This should be administered, in concert with a dT booster, to anyone with a tetanus-prone wound and an unknown or incomplete vaccination history. Tetanus immune globulin need not be administered to anyone who has solid proof of a complete vaccination history. dT boosters, however, should be given to patients with tetanus-prone wounds who have not had a booster shot in the previous 5 years and to all patients for whom it has been more than 10 years. since their last booster. A summary of the approach to tetanus prophylaxis after wounds is presented in Table 17-2.

Antibiotic therapy for wounds is not an adequate substitute for active immunization before injury.

■ ACUTE ATAXIA AND VERTIGO

Acute ataxia is defined as the sudden loss of balance in sitting or walking by a previously well individual. "Acute cerebellar ataxia" is a diagnosis often used to describe a pattern of acute ataxia in young children;[502–504] however, it is more useful to regard acute ataxia in children as a syndrome with many possible etiologies until the physician has excluded these causes. Only after the patient improves with no etiology found should the diagnosis be "acute cerebellar ataxia" or "acute post-infectious cerebellitis."

Infectious Causes

Bacterial Meningitis

Although this is a rare cause of acute ataxia, it should always be considered because of its potential severity. Spinal fluid findings of purulent meningitis with a positive CSF culture have been documented in children with acute ataxia but no meningeal signs.[505] A few of the reported cases have had no fever or no meningeal signs. Possibly bacterial meningitis can occur simultaneously with acute cerebellar ataxia, but these case reports suggest that ataxia can be the major or only neurologic symptom.

Acute Postinfectious Cerebellitis

Acute postinfectious cerebellitis (acute cerebellar ataxia) is a common pattern of ataxia. At least half of patients have antecedent symptoms compatible with an infection. However, the condition is most common in children between the ages of 1 and 5 years, a time that coincides with a high incidence of viral infection, and thus proof of causation is difficult. The association of varicella and acute cerebella ataxia, however, has been well studied and is well established. In the largest series of consecutive cases of acute post-viral cerebellitis, varicella infection accounted for 19 (26%) of 73 cases.[506] Other infectious diseases and agent temporally associated with acute benign cerebellar ataxia of childhood include acute histoplasmosis,[507] HSV, coxsackieviruses, *Mycoplasma pneumoniae,* infectious mononucleosis,[508] mumps,[509] and legionellosis.[510] One child with ataxia secondary to neurobrucellosis has been reported.[511] There is a case report of echovirus type 9 recovered from the spinal fluid of a patient with the typical illness,[512] but CSF cultures for viruses otherwise have been negative. EBV infection has been found with acute ataxia, with normal CSF except for elevated lactic dehydrogenase.[513] In a large outbreak of enterovirus 71 infection in Taiwan, 20 (49%) of 41 children with neurologic manifestations presented with rhombencephalitis which was characterized by jerks, tremors, or ataxia.[325]

In the typical pattern, the child is 1–5 years of age. Often, there is a prodrome of mild respiratory or gastrointestinal symptoms occurring for a day or two before the ataxia is noted. The onset of ataxia is sudden, and reaches maximal severity within the first 24 hours. Ataxia that waxes and wanes or progresses more slowly is likely to represent a different clinical syndrome. Fever is uncommon. Most patients maintain a normal level of consciousness, no matter how severe the ataxia becomes. Hypotonia may or may not be present. Absent reflexes suggest Miller-Fisher syndrome, discussed below. Nystagmus is rare. A few patients have focal cerebral signs or increased pressure sufficient to justify studies to exclude an intracranial tumor.[502] The transient nature of the disease suggests that edema or a vascular mechanism may be the basis of the cerebellar signs. Long-term outcome is almost uniformLy excellent.[506]

Brainstem Encephalitis

This condition is defined by more severe cerebral disease with primary involvement of the cerebellum. Many cases that might be called brainstem encephalitis have been reported in series of acute cerebellar ataxia. This pattern also may follow a specific infection such as that caused by measles, adenovirus, or enteroviruses. The cranial nerves are often involved. Complete recovery is less likely than in acute postinfectious cerebellitis. Brainstem encephalitis is usually characterized by some mononuclear pleocytosis in the spinal fluid, whereas acute cerebellar ataxia usually has few or no cells.

Noninfectious Causes

Poisoning

Phenytoin, phenothiazides (e.g., Compazine), benzodiazepines, chlordiazepoxide, and ethyl alcohol are the most common causes of drug-induced ataxia in children.[514] Some mouthwashes contain enough alcohol and taste good enough that a toddler may ingest enough to become ataxic and even hypoglycemic.[263] Anti-seizure medications such as carbamazepime (Tegretol) taken in large amounts precipitate nystagmus and ataxia.[515] Excessive use of antihistamines in toddlers with common colds can produce ataxia. In a series of 40 children with ataxia, drug screening proved to be the most useful diagnostic test, helping to establish the diagnosis in over 60% of cases.[516]

Brain Tumor

Brain tumor is a common solid tumor in children. Typically, the ataxia is chronic, with a gradual onset and a progressive course, but it occasionally resembles the acute ataxias. Brain tumor is usually associated with increased CSF pressure if it produces ataxia, because in cerebellar or pons tumors, obstruction to CSF flow usually occurs very early. When the tumor is not in the midline, there are usually some lateralizing signs. A subdural hematoma can produce the same kind of mass effect as a neoplasm.

Occult Neuroblastoma

Ataxia is a rare presentation of neuroblastoma and is usually associated with intention tremor and opsoclonus (multidirectional, chaotic movements of the eyes).[517] The combination of opsoclonus and myoclonus (so-called Kinsbourne syndrome) should always make the clinician think of neuroblastoma. A case where this combination of symptoms was associated with T-cell lymphoma of the brain has also been reported.[518]

Other Causes

Congenital cerebellar hypoplasia may have the early onset of delayed development of balance, with delayed sitting and walking because of ataxia. Usually, some gradual improvement occurs as the patient learns to compensate for the cerebellar dysfunction. Vermal aplasia, seen in Joubert syndrome and Dandy-Walker malformation, is another congenital ataxia disorder.

There are many genetic disorders that cause ataxia. Most of these produce either ongoing or progressive disease. Many have other features that may be more prominent than the ataxic component. Progressive degenerative ataxia usually has an insidious onset of ataxia with progression of the disease slowly over a period of years. In one series,

Friedreich ataxia presented before the age of 10 years in 36 (38%) of 95 cases.[519] Ataxia-telangiectasia is discussed in Chapter 23. Metabolic disorders such as maple syrup urine disease, Hartnup disease, and others may produce either recurrent or progressive ataxia. Paroxysmal tonic upgaze of childhood with ataxia is the somewhat cumbersome name attached to a rare childhood disorder that is thought to be autosomal dominantly inherited.[520] There are two forms of inherited ataxia, called episodic ataxia types I and II; type II is more frequently responsive to acetazolamide.[521]

Basilar migraine produces gait ataxia in about half of sufferers. Visual loss, vertigo, alternating hemiparesis, and paresthesias can also occur. The syndrome peaks in the teenage years and is more common in girls.[522] The neurologic symptoms are often followed by a severe, pulsatile headache. Because the tendency toward basilar migraine is inherited in an autosomal dominant fashion, there is often a family history.

Tick paralysis (see the section on ascending paralysis) can present as ataxia.

Miller-Fisher syndrome, a syndrome of ataxia, areflexia, and ophthalmoplegia, is a variant of Guillain-Barre syndrome. Antibodies to the lipopolysaccharide of a particular serotype of *C. jejuni* (Penner serotype 2) cross react with ganglioside epitopes of the cranial nerves and deep cerebellar nuclei, causing ophthalmoplegia and cerebellar ataxia.[523]

Multiple sclerosis may begin with ataxia as early as 2 years of age.[524] In early childhood multiple sclerosis, the female to male preponderance seen in adults may be reversed, especially in those who develop the disease before 24 months of age. Prognosis is unfavorable in this group. The most common presenting symptom in children less than 6 years of age is ataxia.[525]

Wernicke encephalopathy, caused by thiamine deficiency and usually associated with alcoholism, is an uncommon cause of ataxia in childhood; however, at least 31 cases have been reported. Most patients had underlying disorders such as malignancy.[526] Only 6 (19%) of the 31 patients demonstrated the classic triad of mental status changes, ocular signs, and ataxia. Patients on long-term total parenteral nutrition who are not receiving intravenous vitamins, even if they are on oral vitamin supplements, are at risk.[527]

■ VERTIGO SYNDROMES

Defined as a true twirling or spinning sensation, vertigo can produce ataxia, often with nystagmus.

It often is caused by an abnormality of the vestibular system.[528,529] Most vertigo syndromes occur in adults, but occasionally the question is raised whether the young child really has vertigo (the sensation of spinning) but cannot verbalize it. In general, Meniere's syndrome and vestibular neuronitis are exceedingly rare in children younger than 15 years of age.[529,530] However, outbreaks of vestibular neuronitis, which is usually associated with an upper respiratory infection, have been reported; some of these outbreaks apparently included preschool children. The syndrome of epidemic vertigo has been associated with atypical lymphocytes in the peripheral blood smear, 5–15 lymphocytes/mcL in the CSF, and weakness.[531] A definitive etiology has never been proven. In a case-control study of a large outbreak of vertigo that occurred in Wyoming in 1992, 74% of cases versus 54% of controls had serologic evidence of recent enterovirus infection.[532] It is presumed to be central, rather than labyrinthine, in origin.

Benign recurrent vertigo is a syndrome marked by abrupt onset of severe vertigo that lasts from a few minutes to several hours. Some attacks are associated with, or followed by, headache. This disorder is thought to be a migraine variant, and sufferers often benefit from migraine prophylaxis. Benign paroxysmal vertigo is characterized by brief, multiple sporadic episodes of ataxia, often with anxiety, nystagmus, and vomiting.[533] Headache is not an initial symptom. Patients may have pallor and appear panicked. It usually occurs between 1 and 3 years of age and attacks last less than 5 minutes. Over time, attacks of vertigo may be replaced by attacks of severe headache, readily distinguishable as migrainous.

Bacterial labyrinthitis is commonly an extension from middle ear or meningeal infection and usually is associated with hearing loss. Viral infection of the labyrinth probably also occurs, with similar symptoms. Vestibular symptoms are sometimes seen in patients with infectious mononucleosis. A case of vertigo occurring during the course of mumps virus infection has been reported.[534]

Antibiotics can produce vestibular toxicity that may result in vertigo. Streptomycin has been particularly indicted, but all the aminoglycosides may have this effect. Minocycline can produce dizziness and ataxia even when given in recommended dosages.

Sometimes simple partial seizures may be manifested as vertigo. Vertigo in association with tinnitus and decreased hearing suggests Meniere disease. It is uncommon in childhood.

Patients with postural tachycardia syndrome, sometimes referred to as orthostatic intolerance or autonomic dysfunction syndrome, usually present with fatigue, exercise intolerance, dizziness, nausea, pallor, and recurrent syncope.[535,536] Some patients will complain of vertigo or ataxia upon standing as well.

Vertigo can be the presenting symptom of multiple sclerosis in teenagers.[537]

Ramsay Hunt syndrome (herpes zoster oticus) can result in vertigo and is discussed in the preceeding section on Descending and Cranial Nerve Paralysis.[383a]

Diagnostic Plan and Treatment

Lateralizing signs and increased intracranial pressure should be looked for carefully. Lumbar puncture should be considered to exclude bacterial meningitis if there is no evidence of increased intracranial pressure. Examination of the spinal fluid may also indicate intracranial bleeding. Skull films may be indicated to exclude separation of the sutures. An EEG is rarely helpful. Consultation with an otolaryngologist for special tests of eighth-nerve function is indicated for any persistent vertigo. Careful examination of the ear canal for vesicles should be done, and serologic testing for varicella IgM should be considered.

Treatment depends on the identification of a specific cause.

■ BRAIN ABSCESS

Predisposing Causes

Most brain abscesses in children occur with cyanotic congenital heart disease or are secondary to spread from sinusitis, chronic otitis, or mastoiditis.[538–542] In one report, 12% of cerebral and 63% of extra-axial brain abscesses were complications of sinusitis.[543] Other predisposing causes include dental infections, head trauma, and cranial operations. Meningitis is rarely associated with brain abscess, except in neonates with gram-negative meningitis, in which case it is relatively common. Sometimes brain abscess develops after seemingly minor trauma, especially to the eye.[544] A prospective study showed that 72% of children undergoing esophageal dilatation for stenosis became bacteremic, mostly with alpha-hemolytic streptococci;[545]

brain abscess is a rare complication.[546] Patients with cystic fibrosis and immunosuppressed hosts also are at greater risk for brain abscess.

Clinical Patterns

Brain abscesses can be classified on the basis of the anatomic location or the etiologic agent. From the clinician's point of view, the clinical pattern of illness is the most important starting point. A brain abscess usually presents with pressure (like a brain tumor) or with lateralizing signs (like a focal lesion).

Brain Tumor-like Presentation

A brain abscess can produce manifestations of a mass or tumor and should always be considered in the differential diagnosis of brain tumors because of its better prognosis. The source of infection can be found in 60–80% of patients with proved abscesses.[540] The source may be an adjacent infection near the brain, particularly otitis media, mastoiditis, and sinusitis. Identification of a site of infection is usually useful in identifying the location of a contiguous abscess. The source may also be a metastatic infection, as from pulmonary infection, endocarditis, or an abscess elsewhere.

Nonpurulent Meningitis

Brain abscess should be considered as a rare cause of nonpurulent meningitis and only if there are lateralizing signs or increased intracranial pressure. If the brain abscess has not ruptured to produce purulent meningitis, the spinal fluid white cell count is usually in the non-purulent range (20–500/mcL) with elevated protein and a normal glucose. Brain abscesses are usually, but not always, associated with a CSF pleocytosis.

Fever and Hemiparesis with Cyanotic Congenital Heart Disease

The CSF may be normal, but the combination of fever, hemiparesis, and cyanotic heart disease should be considered to indicate a brain abscess until proved otherwise.[541] The absence of fever, however, does not rule out the possibility of a brain abscess; only about half of patients with brain abscess have fever. In addition, the presence of a right-to-left cardiac shunt may be previously undiagnosed, such as with a patent foramen ovale.[541a]

Occasionally, a cerebral thrombosis mimics a

brain abscess in a patient with cyanotic heart disease, particularly if polycythemia is present. Papilledema and dilated, tortuous retinal veins may occur in children with cyanotic congenital heart disease because of the polycythemia and decreased oxygen saturation, without a brain abscess.[542]

Hemiparesis and Purulent Meningitis

A ruptured brain abscess may produce the combination of lateralized paralysis and purulent meningitis. This is usually fatal within a few hours. However, if the CSF glucose is normal and many erythrocytes are found in addition to the neutrophils, acute necrotizing hemorrhagic encephalopathy secondary to HSV should be considered (see the section on encephalitis), although this disease is rare.

Possible Etiologies

Anaerobic Bacteria

Cultures of brain abscesses indicate that anaerobic streptococci are the most common agents.[547] *Bacteroides* species are probably more frequent than published reports indicate, because these anaerobes are very difficult to grow. *Actinomyces* species also can produce brain abscess. Therefore, anaerobic cultures should always be done of pus obtained in a brain abscess.

Aerobic Bacteria

Many different aerobic organisms have been found in brain abscesses. Gram-positive cocci are especially common, particularly *Streptococcus milleri* group (which may be alpha-, beta-, or non-hemolytic). Other streptococci, enterococci, *S. aureus*, and *S. epidermidis* are also frequently seen. *Nocardia* is found in about 2% of brain abscesses.[548] The pneumococcus is a rare cause. A report of the systemic complications of *Pseudomonas aeruginosa* conjunctivitis in a neonatal intensive care unit included a case of brain abscess.[549] Gram-negative enteric bacteria also are sometimes recovered, particularly in neonates.

Multiple or Unusual Pathogens

Mixed flora were recovered in about one-third of those cultured in one series. Anaerobes are often found in mixed culture with aerobes. Fungi or atypical mycobacteria are uncommon causes of brain abscesses. Multiple brain abscesses were found in one 2-month-old with typhoid fever.[550] Toxoplasmosis of the CNS can resemble a brain abscess and should be considered in immunocompromised patients.[551] Immunosuppressed patients also acquire fungal brain abscesses; a review of 12 brain abscesses in children with cancer revealed that the most common organisms in this set of patients were *Aspergillus fumigatus*, *Listeria monocytogenes*, *Fusarium* spp, and *Candida lusitaneae*.[552]

Diagnostic Approach

Imaging Studies

MRI is the imaging modality of choice, although CT scans with intravenous contrast also offer excellent resolution. Brain scanning has revolutionized the diagnosis of brain abscess and has undoubtedly led to a significant lowering of the mortality rate.[553] Many small abscesses have been successfully treated with antibiotic therapy without surgical intervention.[553,554]

Brain abscess has been studied experimentally in dogs using CT to monitor the effects of direct intracerebral inoculation of bacteria.[555,556] Stages have been defined as early cerebritis (1–3 days after inoculation); late cerebritis, days 4–9; early capsule formation, days 10–13; and late capsule formation, from day 14 on.[555,556] Cerebritis is patchy but later develops into a characteristic (but not specific) lesion surrounded by a uniform ring, which is enhanced if steroids are withdrawn.[553] The abscess can also be a dense nodule. CT scanning has allowed a clearer definition of cerebritis, which was previously a clinical definition. Cerebritis may be defined as a focal brain infection that has not progressed to an abscess. There are clinical or radiologic findings of a focus, with sterile CSF, usually with normal glucose, elevated protein, and about 10–500WBC/mcL.[557]

Radionuclide Scan

This procedure may be available in some hospitals that do not have CT scanning facilities. This scan may indicate a focus of cerebritis that may not be exerting a mass effect. Apparent abscesses or cerebritis complicating bacterial meningitis may resolve with proper antibiotic therapy without any neurosurgical intervention (Fig. 9-10).

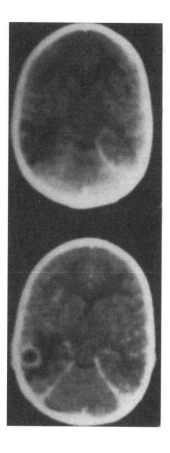

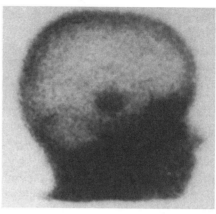

■ **FIGURE 9-10** Brain abscess in child with congenital cyanotic heart disease. Radionucleotide scan (*right*) shows increased activity in right temporal region. Computed tomography (CT) without contrast (*upper left*) shows low-density lesion, and CT scan with contrast (*lower left*) shows typical ring enhancement and surrounding low-density edema. (Photo courtesy of Dr. Richard Shore.)

Other Approaches

Use of arteriograms or ventriculograms may occasionally be appropriate, but have largely been replaced by MRI and CT scanning. EEG adds little to the diagnostic evaluation. Lumbar puncture should be mentioned only to emphasize its danger. It does not localize the lesion and often results in serious complications, particularly herniation. If papilledema is present, or if a brain abscess is suspected clinically, a CT should be obtained before a lumbar puncture is performed.

Treatment

Surgical Drainage

Like abscesses in other locations, surgical drainage remains the treatment of choice for brain abscesses, especially those that are large and well developed. Excision is associated with high risks and is usually not attempted. Stereotactic CT-guided aspiration is usually successful; in a series of 21 patients with 58 abscesses, this approach, combined with 8 weeks of antimicrobial therapy, resulted in good outcomes for all 21 patients.[558] Repeat aspirations may be necessary in some cases. A Japanese study of 11 patients with brain abscess attempted to answer the question: "How small must a brain abscess be before it can be decided that further aspiration is not necessary?" The authors conclusion was that once an abscess becomes less than 2 cm in diameter and the size is not increasing on serial CT scans, it will probably be successfully treated with antimicrobial therapy alone.[559] These results and clinical experience suggest that with the help of good imaging, sometimes surgical procedures to aspirate brain abscesses can be postponed or even omitted. Usually, antibiotic therapy is done first, followed by aspiration when the abscess is better localized and the patient stabilized. Gas in an abscess appears to be an indication for surgical excision.[560]

Systemic Antibiotics

Antibiotic therapy should be given to try to localize the infection. The choice depends on age and possibly upon the source of infection. Nafcillin or vancomycin (dosed at anti-meningitic doses) plus cefotaxime and metronidazole appears to be a reasonable initial choice. Anti-pseudomonal antibiotics may be considered if the abscess is secondary to chronic otitis media (for example, ceftazidime can be substituted for cefotaxime). Depending upon whether staphylococci, anaerobic streptococci, or gram-negative bacteria are recovered, the therapy can be adjusted. Many clinicians opt to continue coverage for anaerobic infection even if anaerobes are not isolated. The duration of therapy should be guided by the patient's clinical course, follow-up imaging studies, and whether or not the abscess was drained. In general, 6–12 weeks of therapy is appropriate.

Local Antibiotics

In unusually difficult cases, injection of antibiotics into the cavity can be done to try to sterilize the area before operation, following the same principles as discussed in the section on ventriculitis.[561] However, this is rarely necessary.

■ PSEUDOTUMOR CEREBRI

Pseudotumor cerebri can be defined as an elevated intracranial pressure, normal ventricular system, and normal spinal fluid.[562] It has also been called "benign intracranial hypertension," with a clinical picture including sudden onset of headache, papilledema, frequent sixth-nerve paralysis, and absence of convulsions or focal neurologic abnormalities.[563]

Possible Causes

Corticosteroid withdrawal, vitamin A intoxication, venous sinus thrombosis,[564] oral contraceptives, systemic lupus erythematosus, and tetracycline[565] are but a few of the noninfectious causes. Respiratory infections have been concurrently present but are probably coincidental.

Treatment

A therapeutic lumbar puncture in which the closing pressure is taken to half of the opening pressure is curative in many cases. Occasionally another lumbar puncture will be required. When medications are used, most experts recommend acetazolamide at 10 mg/kg/day. If these measures fail, a two-week course of dexamethasone is occasionally tried. In severe cases, insertion of a lumbar drain may be required. However, for many cases, observation has been an acceptable approach.

■ REFERENCES

1. Nicolosi A, Hauser WA, Beghi E, Kurland LT. Epidemiology of central nervous system infections in Olmsted County, Minnesota, 1950–1981. J Infect Dis 1986;154: 399–407.
2. Reik L Jr. Disorders that mimic CNS infections. Neurol Clin 1986;4:223–48.
3. Stein MT, Trauner D. The child with a stiff neck. Clin Pediatr 1982;21:559–63.
4. Byers RK. To tap or not to tap: further comments. Pediatrics 1973;51:561.
5. Heldrich FJ, Walker SH, Crosby RMN. Risk of diagnostic lumbar puncture in acute bacterial meningitis. Pediatr Emerg Care 1986;2:180–2.
6. Shetty AK, Desselle BC, Craver RD, Steele RW. Fatal cerebral herniation after lumbar puncture in a patient with a normal computed tomography scan. Pediatrics 1999; 103:1284–7.
7. Rennick G, Shann F, deCampo J. Cerebral herniation during bacterial meningitis in children. Br Med J 1993; 306:953–5.
8. Egede LE, Moses H, Wang H. Spinal subdural hematoma: a rare complication of lumbar puncture: case report and review of the literature. Md Med J 1999;48:15–7.
9. Mohanty A, Basudev MK, Chandra PS. Extradural hematoma complicating lumbar puncture following a craniotomy: a case report. J Neurosurg Sci 1998;42:233–7.
10. Silverman R, Kwiatkowski T, Bernstein S, et al. Safety of lumbar puncture in patients with hemophilia. Ann Emerg Med 1993;22:1739–42.
11. Weisman LE, Merenstein GB, Steenbarger JR. The effect of lumbar puncture position in sick neonates. Am J Dis Child 1983;137:1077–9.
12. Gleason CA, Martin RJ, Anderson JV, et al. Optimal position for a spinal tap in preterm infants. Pediatrics 1983; 71:31–5.
13. Ellis RW 3rd, Strauss LC, Wiley JM, et al. A simple method of estimating cerebrospinal fluid pressure during lumbar puncture. Pediatrics 1992;89:895–7.
14. Rubenstein JS, Yogev R. What represents pleocytosis in blood contaminated ("traumatic tap") cerebrospinal fluid in children? J Pediatr 1985;107:249–51.
15. Steele RW, Marmer DJ, O'Brien MD, et al. Leukocyte survival in cerebrospinal fluid. J Clin Microbiol 1986;23: 965–6.
16. Mehl AL. Interpretation of traumatic lumbar puncture: predictive value in the presence of meningitis. Clin Pediatr 1986;25:575–7.
17. Novak RW. Lack of validity of standard corrections for white blood cell counts of blood contaminated cerebrospinal fluid in infants. Am J Clin Pathol 1984;82:95–7.
18. Bonadio WA, Smith DS, Goddard S, Burroughs J, Khaja G. Distinguishing cerebrospinal fluid abnormalities in children with bacterial meningitis and traumatic lumbar puncture. J Infect Dis 1990;162:251–4.
19. Lang DT, Berberian LB, Lee S, Ault M. Rapid differentiation of subarachnoid hemorrhage from traumatic lumbar puncture using the D-dimer assay. Am J Clin Pathol 1990; 93:403–5.
20. Ahmed A, Hickey SM, Ehrett S, et al. Cerebrospinal fluid

values in the term neonate. Pediatr Infect Dis J 1996;15: 298–303.

21. Portnoy JM, Olson LC. Normal cerebrospinal fluid values in children: another look. Pediatrics 1985;75:484–7.

22. Sarff LD, Platt LH, McCracken GH Jr. Cerebrospinal fluid evaluation in neonates: comparison of high risk infants with and without meningitis. J Pediatr 1976;88:473–7.

23. Donald PR, Malan C, van der Walt A. Simultaneous determination of cerebrospinal fluid glucose and blood glucose concentrations in the diagnosis of bacterial meningitis. J Pediatr 1983;103:413–5.

24. Onorato IM, Wormser GP, Nicholas P. "Normal" CSF in bacterial meningitis. JAMA 1980;244:1469–71.

25. La Scolea LJ Jr, Dryja D. Quantitation of bacteria in cerebrospinal fluid and blood of children with meningitis and its diagnostic significance. J Clin Microbiol 1984;19: 187–190.

26. Olson DA, Hoeprich PD. Analysis of bacterial isolates from cerebrospinal fluid. J Clin Microbiol 1984;19: 144–6.

27. Fischer GW, Brenz RW, Alden ER, et al. Lumbar punctures and meningitis. Am J Dis Child 1975;129:590–2.

28. Ballard TL, Roe MH, Wheeler RC, et al. Comparison of three latex agglutination kits and counterimmunoelectrophoresis for detection of bacterial antigens in a pediatric population. Pediatr Infect Dis J 1987;6:630–4.

29. Kolmel HW, von Maravic M. Correlation of lactic acid level, cell count and cytology in cerebrospinal fluid of patients with bacterial and non-bacterial meningitis. Acta Neurol Scand 1988;78:6–9.

30. Komorowski RA, Farmer SG, Knox KK. Comparison of cerebrospinal fluid C-reactive protein and lactate for the diagnosis of meningitis. J Clin Microbiol 1986;24:982–5.

31. Rutledge J, Benjamin D, Hood L, et al. Is the CSF lactate measurement useful in the management of children with suspected bacterial meningitis? J Pediatr 1981;98:20–4.

32. Lannigan R, MacDonald MA, Marrie TJ, et al. Evaluation of cerebrospinal fluid lactic acid levels as an aid in differential diagnosis of bacterial and viral meningitis in adults. J Clin Microbiol 1980;11:324–7.

33. Ahmed A, Brito F, Goto C, et al. Clinical utility of the polymerase chain reaction for diagnosis of enteroviral meningitis in infancy. J Pediatr 1997;131:393–7.

34. Nigrovic LE. Chiang VW. Cost analysis of enteroviral polymerase chain reaction in infants with fever and cerebrospinal fluid pleocytosis. Arch Pediatr Adol Med 2000; 154:817–21.

35. Sormunen P, Kallio MJ, Kilpi T, Peltola H. C-reactive protein is useful in distinguishing Gram stain negative bacterial meningitis from viral meningitis in children. J Pediatr 1999;134:725–9.

36. Gendrel D, Raymond J, Assicot M, et al. Measurement of procalcitonin levels in children with bacterial or viral meningitis. Clin Infect Dis 1997;24:1240–2.

37. Ouellette EM. The child who convulses with fever. Pediatr Clin North Am 1974;21:467–81.

38. Committee on Drugs, American Academy of Pediatrics: emergency drug doses for infants and children. Pediatrics 1988;81:462–5.

39. Mitchell WG. Status epilepticus and acute serial seizures in children. J Child Neurol 2002;17 Suppl 1:S36–43.

40. Lacey DJ, Singer WD, Horwitz SJ, et al. Lorazepam ther-

apy in status epilepticus in children and adolescents. J Pediatr 1986;108:771–4.

41. Delgado-Escueta AV, Waterlain C, Treiman DM, et al. Current concepts in neurology: Management of status epilepticus. N Engl J Med 1982;306:1337–40.

42. Earnest MP, Marx JA, Drury LR. Complications of intravenous phenytoin for acute treatment of seizures. JAMA 1983;249:762–5.

43. Reuter D, Brownstein D. Common emergent pediatric neurologic problems. Emerg Med Clin North Am 2002; 20:155–76.

44. Hall CB, Long CE, Schnabel KC, et al. Human herpesvirus-6 infection in children. A prospective study of complications and reactivation. N Engl J Med 1994;33: 432–8.

45. Hukin J, Farrell K, MacWilliam LM, et al. Case-control study of primary human herpesvirus 6 infection in children with febrile seizures. Pediatrics 1998;101:E3.

46. Van Stuijvenberg M, Steyerberg EW, Derksen-Lubsen G, Moll HA. Temperature, age, and recurrence of febrile seizure. Arch Pediatr Adolesc Med 1998;152:1170–5.

47. The Subcommittee on Febrile Seizures. Practice Parameter: the neurodiagnostic evaluation of a child with a first simple febrile seizure. Pediatrics 1996;97:769–72.

48. Green SM, Rothrock SG, Clem KJ, Zurcher RF, Mellick L. Can seizures be the sole manifestation of meningitis in febrile children? Pediatrics 1993;92:527–34.

49. Samson JH, Apthorp J, Finley A. Febrile seizures and purulent meningitis. JAMA 1969;210:1918–9.

50. Finley AH. Lumbar puncture in children who have had fever and a convulsion [letter]. Lancet 1980;2:83.

51. Gururaj NU, Russo RM, Allen JE, et al. To tap or not to tap... What are the best indicators for performing a lumbar puncture in an outpatient child? Clin Pediatr 1973; 12:488–93.

52. Al Eissa YA. Lumbar puncture in the clinical evaluation of children with seizures associated with fever. Pediatr Emerg Care 1995;11:347–50.

53. Fenichel GM. In: Clinical Pediatric Neurology. A signs and symptoms approach. Philadelphia: WB Saunders Co, 1997.

54. Wolf SM. Laboratory evaluation of the child with a febrile convulsion. Pediatrics 1978;62:1074–6.

55. Kuturec M, Emoto SE, Sofijanov N, et al. Febrile seizures: is the EEG a useful predictor of recurrence? Clin Pediatr Phila 1997;36:31–6.

56. Wears RL, Luten RC, Lyons RG. Which laboratory tests should be performed on children with apparent febrile convulsions? An analysis and review of the literature. Pediatr Emerg Care 1986;2:191–6.

57. Joffe A, McCormick M, DeAngelis C. Which children with febrile seizures need lumbar punctures? Am J Dis Child 1983;137:1153–6.

58. Gerber MA, Berliner BC. The child with a "simple" febrile seizure: appropriate diagnostic evaluation. Am J Dis Child 1981;135:431–3.

59. Uhari M, Rantala H, Vainionpaa L, Kurttila R. Effect of acetaminophen and of low intermittent doses of diazepam on prevention of recurrences of febrile seizures. J Pediatr 1995;126:991–5.

60. Van Stuijvenberg M, Derksen-Lubsen G, Steyerberg EW, et al. Randomized, controlled trial of ibuprofen syrup

administered during febrile illnesses to prevent febrile seizure recurrences. Pediatrics 1998;102:E51.

61. Sulzbacher S, Farwell JR, Temkin N, et al. Late cognitive effects of early treatment with phenobarbital. Clin Pediatr Phila 1999;38:387–94.

62. Rantala H, Tarkka R, Uhari M. A meta-analytic review of the preventive treatment of recurrences of febrile seizures. J Pediatr 1997;131:922–5.

63. Dreifuss FE, Santilli N, Langer DH, et al. Valproic acid hepatic fatalities: a retrospective review. Neurology 1987; 37:379–85.

64. Rosman NP, Colton T, Labazzo J, et al. A controlled trial of diazepam administered during febrile illnesses to prevent recurrence of febrile seizures. N Engl J Med 1993; 329:79–84.

65. Jee SH, Long CE, Schnabel KC, et al. Risk of recurrent seizures after a primary human herpesvirus 6-induced febrile seizure. Pediatr Infect Dis J 1998;17:43–8.

66. Elliott J. Consensus on "rational approach" to childhood febrile seizures. JAMA 1980;244:111–2.

67. Wong M, Schlaggar BL, Landt M. Postictal cerebrospinal fluid abnormalities in children. J Pediatr 2001;138: 373–7.

68. Devinsky O, Nadi S, Theodore WH, Porter RJ. Cerebrospinal fluid pleocytosis following simple, complex partial, and generalized tonic-clonic seizures. Ann Neurol 1988; 23:402–3.

69. Edwards R, Schmidley JW, Simon RP. How often does a CSF pleocytosis follow generalized convulsions? Ann Neurol 1983;13:460–2.

70. Schmidley JW, Simon RP. Postictal pleocytosis. Ann Neurol 1981;9:81–4.

71. Schuchat A, Robinson K, Wenger JD, et al. Bacterial meningitis in the United States in 1995. N Engl J Med 1997; 337:970–6.

72. Fraser DW, Darby CP, Koehler RE, et al. Risk factors in bacterial meningitis: Charleston County, South Carolina. J Infect Dis 1973;127:271–7.

73. Feigin RD, Shearer WT. Opportunistic infection in children. Part I. In the compromised host. J Pediatr 1975; 87:507–14.

74. Reefhuis J, Honein MA, Whitney CG, et al. Risk of bacterial meningitis in children with cochlear implants. N Engl J Med 2003;349:435–45.

75. Thomas KE, Hasbun R, Jekel J, Quagliarello VJ. The diagnostic accuracy of Kernig's sign, Brudzinski's sign, and nuchal rigidity in adults with suspected meningitis. Clin Infect Dis 2002;35:46–52.

76. Adams WG, Deaver KA, Cochi SL, et al. Decline of childhood Haemophilus influenzae type b (Hib) disease in the Hib vaccine era. JAMA 1993;269:221–6.

77. Klein JO, Feigin RD, McCracken GH Jr. Report of the task force on diagnosis and management of meningitis. Pediatrics 1986;78(Suppl):959–82.

78. McCracken GH Jr, Nelson JD, Kaplan SL, et al. Consensus report: Antimicrobial therapy for bacterial meningitis in infants and children. Pediatr Infect Dis J 1987;6:501–5.

79. Mathies AW Jr, Leedom JM, Thrupp LD, et al. Experience with ampicillin in bacterial meningitis. Antimicrob Agents Chemother 1966;1965:610–7.

80. Davis SD, Hill HR, Feigl P, et al. Partial antibiotic therapy in Haemophilus influenzae meningitis: Its effect on cerebrospinal fluid abnormalities. Am J Dis Child 1975;129: 802–7.

81. Kaplan SL, Smith EO, Wills C, et al. Association between preadmission oral antibiotic therapy and cerebrospinal fluid findings and sequelae caused by Haemophilus influenzae type b meningitis. Pediatr Infect Dis 1986;5: 626–32.

82. Wheeler WE. The lumbar tapper's dilemma [editorial]. J Pediatr 1970;77:747.

83. Bohr V, Rasmussen N, Hansen B, et al. 875 cases of bacterial meningitis: diagnostic procedures and the impact of preadmission antibiotic therapy III. J Infect 1983;7: 193–202.

84. Blazer S, Berant M, Alon U. Bacterial meningitis: effect of antibiotic treatment on cerebrospinal fluid. Am J Clin Pathol 1983;80:386–7.

85. Schulkind ML, Altemeier WA III, Ayoub EM. A comparison of ampicillin and chloramphenicol therapy in Hemophilus influenzae meningitis. Pediatrics 1971;48:411–6.

86. Converse GM, Gwaltney JM Jr, Strassburg DA, et al. Alteration of cerebrospinal fluid findings by partial treatment of bacterial meningitis. J Pediatr 1973;83:220–5.

87. Lewin EB. Partially treated meningitis. Am J Dis Child 1974;128:145–7.

88. Finlay FO, Witherow H, Rudd PT. Latex agglutination testing in bacterial meningitis. Arch Dis Child 1995;73: 160–1.

89. Katnik R. A persistent biochemical marker for partially treated meningitis/ventriculitis. J Child Neurol 1995;10: 93–9.

90. Darbari A, Bhandari NR, Agrawal BK, Bhambal SA. Cerebrospinal fluid N-acetyl neuraminic acid estimation for early diagnosis and differentiation of bacterial meningitis. Indian Pediatr 1991;28:513–9.

91. Geiseler PJ, Nelson KE. Bacterial meningitis without clinical signs of meningeal irritation. South Med J 1982;75: 448–50.

92. Stephens J, San Joaquin VH. Deafness as the presenting sign of posttraumatic pneumococcal meningitis. Pediatr Infect Dis 1984;3:239–41.

93. Kaplan SL. Clinical presentations, diagnosis, and prognostic factors of bacterial meningitis. Infect Dis Clin North Am 1999;13:579–94.

94. Bonadio WA, Mannenbach M, Krippendorf R. Bacterial meningitis in older children. Am J Dis Child 1990;144: 463–5.

95. Polk DB, Steele RW. Bacterial meningitis presenting with normal cerebrospinal fluid. Pediatr Infect Dis J 1987;6: 1040–2.

96. Onorato IM, Wormser GP, Nicholas P. "Normal" CSF in bacterial meningitis. JAMA 1980;244:1469–71.

97. Dunn DW. Factors contributing to delay in diagnosis of bacterial meningitis. South Med J 1984;77:1115–7.

98. Harper JL, Florman AL. Tularemic meningitis in a child with mononuclear pleocytosis. Pediatr Infect Dis 1986; 5:595–7.

99. Schwartz B, al-Tobaiqi A, Al-Rewais A, et al. Comparative efficacy of ceftriaxone and rifampin in eradicating pharyngeal carriage of group A Neisseria meningitidis. Lancet 1988;1:1239–42.

100. Leggidaro RJ, Winkelstein JA. Prevalence of complement

deficiencies in children with systemic meningococcal infections. Pediatr Infect Dis 1987;6:75–6.

101. Fossieck BE Jr, Kane JG, Diaz CR, et al. Nafcillin entry into human cerebrospinal fluid. Antimicrob Agents Chemother 1977;11:965–7.

102. Law BJ, Marks MI. Excellent outcome of *Bacteroides* meningitis in a newborn treated with metronidazole. Pediatrics 1980;66:463–5.

103. McCracken GH Jr, Mize SG, Threlkeld N. Intraventricular gentamycin therapy in gram-negative bacillary meningitis of infancy. Lancet 1980;1:787–91.

104. McCracken GH Jr, Threlkeld N, Mize SG, et al. Moxalactam therapy for neonatal meningitis due to gram-negative enteric bacilli: a prospective controlled evaluation. JAMA 1984;252:1427–32.

105. Pfaller MA, Jones RN, Marshall SA, et al. Inducible amp C beta-lactamase producing gram-negative bacilli from blood stream infections: frequency, antimicrobial susceptibility, and molecular epidemiology in a national surveillance program (SCOPE). Diagn Microbiol Infect Dis 1997;28:211–9.

106. McCracken GH Jr, Mize SG. A controlled study of intrathecal antibiotic therapy in gram-negative enteric meningitis of infancy. Report of the neonatal meningitis cooperative study group. J Pediatr 1976;89:66–72.

107. Kaplan SL, Fishman MA. Supportive therapy for bacterial meningitis. Pediatr Infect Dis J 1987;6:670–7.

108. Williams CRS, Swanson AG, Chapman JT. Cerebral edema with acute purulent meningitis: report of treatment with hypertonic intravenous urea. Pediatrics 1964;34:220–7.

109. Hornig GW. Flushing in relation to a possible rise in intracranial pressure: documentation of an unusual clinical sign. Report of five cases. J Neurosurg 2000;92:1040–4.

110. Shenkin HA, Bouzarth WF. Clinical methods of reducing intracranial pressure: role of the cerebral circulation. N Engl J Med 1970;282:1465–71.

111. Paul R. Reduction in intracranial pressure by nimodipine in experimental pneumococcal meningitis. Crit Care Med 2000;28:2552–6.

112. Horwitz SJ, Boxerbaum B, O'Bell J. Cerebral herniation in bacterial meningitis in childhood. Ann Neurol 1980;7:524–8.

113. MacDonald NE, Keene DL, Humphreys MP, et al. Fulminating *Haemophilus influenzae* b meningitis. Can J Neurol Sci 1984;11:78–81.

114. Rockoff MA. Does lumbar CSF pressure accurately reflect intracranial pressure? Pediatrics 1981;67:746–7.

115. Marshall LF, Smith RW, Rauscher LA, et al. Mannitol dose requirements in brain-injured patients. J Neurosurg 1978;48:169–72.

116. Feigin RD, Dodge PR. Bacterial meningitis: newer concepts of pathophysiology and neurologic sequelae. Pediatr Clin North Am 1976;23:541–56.

117. Feigin RD, Stechenberg BW, Chang MJ, et al. Prospective evaluation of treatment of *Hemophilus influenzae* meningitis. J Pediatr 1975;87:677–94.

118. Singhi SC, Pratibha D, Singhi MD, et al. Fluid restriction does not improve the outcome of acute meningitis. Pediatr Infect Dis J 1995;14:495–503.

119. Laird WP, Nelson JD, Huffines FD. The frequency of

120. McMenamin JB. Internal carotid artery occlusion in *Haemophilus influenzae* meningitis. J Pediatr 1982;101:723–5.

121. Snedeker JD, Kaplan SL, Dodge PR, et al. Subdural effusion and its relationship with neurologic sequelae of bacterial meningitis in infancy: a prospective study. Pediatrics 1990;86:163–70.

122. Abshire TC. The anemia of inflammation. A common cause of childhood anemia. Pediatr Clin North Am 1996;43:623–37.

123. Chequer RS, Tharp BR, Dreimane D, et al. Prognostic value of EEG in neonatal meningitis: retrospective study of 29 infants. Pediatr Neurol 1992;8:417–22.

124. Bodino J, Lylyk P, Del Valle M, et al. Computed tomography in purulent meningitis. Am J Dis Child 1982;136:495–501.

125. Cabral DA, Flodmark O, Farrell K, et al. Prospective study of computed tomography in acute bacterial meningitis. J Pediatr 1987;111:201–5.

126. Daoud AS, Omari H, al-Sheyyab M, Abuedteish F. Indications and benefits of computed tomography in childhood bacterial meningitis. J Trop Pediatr 1998;44:167–9.

127. Kanamalla US, Ibarra RA, Jinkins JR. Imaging of cranial meningitis ventriculitis. Neuroimaging Clin North Am 2000;10:309–31.

128. Dodge PR, Davis H, Feigin RD, et al. Prospective evaluation of hearing impairment as a sequela of acute bacterial meningitis. N Engl J Med 1984;311:869–74.

129. Lebel MH, Freij BJ, Syrogiannopoulos GA, et al. Dexamethasone therapy for bacterial meningitis: results of two double-blind, placebo-controlled trials. N Engl J Med 1988;319:964–71.

130. Kanra GY, Ozen H, Secmeer G, et al. Beneficial effects of dexamethasone in children with pneumococcal meningitis. Pediatr Infect Dis J 1995;14:490–4.

131. Vienny H, Despland PA, Lutschg J, et al. Early diagnosis and evolution of deafness in childhood bacterial meningitis: a study using brainstem auditory evoked potentials. Pediatrics 1984;73:579–86.

132. Cabellos C, Martinez-Lacasa J, Martos A, et al. Influence of dexamethasone on efficacy of ceftriaxone and vancomycin therapy in experimental pneumococcal meningitis. Antimicrob Agents Chemother 1995;39:2158–60.

133. de Gans J, van de Beck D, et al. Dexamethasone in adults with bacterial meningitis, N Engl J Med 2002;347:1549–56.

134. Feigin RD. Use of corticosteroids in bacterial meningitis. Pediatr Infect Dis J 2004;23:355–7.

135. Rabe EF. Subdural effusion in infants. Pediatr Clin North Am 1967;14:831–50.

136. Tuncer O, Caksen H, Arslan S, et al. Cranial computed tomography in purulent meningitis of childhood. Int J Neurosci 2004;114:167–74.

137. Mofenson HC, Greensher J, Khan WA. Spontaneous resolution of a massive subdural effusion following meningitis. Clin Pediatr 1979;18:304–6.

138. Syrogiannopoulos GA, Nelson JD, McCracken GH Jr. Subdural collections of fluid in acute bacterial meningitis: a review of 136 cases. Pediatr Infect Dis 1986;5:343–52.

139. Weisberg L. Subdural empyema. Clinical and computed

tomographic correlations. Arch Neurol 1986;43: 497–500.

140. Durack DT, Spanos A. End of treatment spinal tap in bacterial meningitis. JAMA 1982;248:75–8.

141. TzouYien L, Nelson JD, McCracken GH Jr. Fever during treatment for bacterial meningitis. Pediatr Infect Dis 1984;3:319–22.

142. Daoud AS, Zaki M, al-Saleh QA. Prolonged and secondary fever in childhood bacterial meningitis. Eur J Pediatr 1989;149:114–6.

143. Schaad UB, Nelson JD, McCracken GH Jr. Recrudescence and relapse in bacterial meningitis of childhood. Pediatrics 1981;67:188–95.

144. Rush PJ, Shore A, Inman R, et al. Arthritis associated with *Haemophilus influenzae* meningitis: septic or reactive? J Pediatr 1986;109:412–5.

145. Likitnukul S, McCracken GH Jr, Nelson JD. Arthritis in children with bacterial meningitis. Am J Dis Child 1986; 140:424–7.

146. Sutton DL, Ouvrier RA. Cerebral abscess in the under 6 month age group. Arch Dis Child 1983;58:901–5.

147. Burstein L, Breningstall GN. Movement disorders in bacterial meningitis. J Pediatr 1986;109:260–4.

148. Geiseler PJ, Nelson KE, Levin S. Community acquired purulent meningitis of unknown etiology: a continuing problem. Arch Neurol 1981;38:749–53.

149. Heerema MS, Ein ME, Musher DM, et al. Anaerobic bacterial meningitis. Am J Med 1979;67:219–27.

150. Penrose-Stevens A, Ibrahim A, Redfern RM. Localized pneumocephalus caused by *Clostridium perfringens* meningitis. Br J Neurosurg 1999;13:85–6.

151. Busch N, Mertens PR, Schonfelder T, et al. Lemierre's post-tonsillitis sepsis with meningitis and intravascular consumption coagulopathy as a complication of infectious mononucleosis with pansinusitis. Dtsch Med Wochenschr 1996;121:94–8.

152. Pace-Balzan A, Keith AO, Curley JW, et al. Otogenic *Fusobacterium necrophorum* meningitis. J Laryngol Otol 1991; 105:119–20.

153. Nukina S, Hibi A, Nishida K. Bacterial meningitis caused by *Veillonella parvula*. Acta Pediatr Jpn 1989;31:609–14.

154. Simon MW, Wilson HD. The amebic meningoencephalitides. Pediatr Infect Dis 1986;5:562–9.

155. Seidel JS, Harmatz P, Visevara GS, et al. Successful treatment of primary amebic meningoencephalitis. Engl J Med 1982;306:346–8.

156. Ferrente A, Rowan-Kelly B. The role of antibody in immunity against experimental Naegleria meningoencephalitis ('amoebic meningitis'). Immunology 1988;64:241–4.

157. Lallinger GJ, Reiner SL, Cooke DW, et al. Efficacy of immune therapy in early experimental *Naegleria fowleri* meningitis. Infect Immun 1987;55:1289–93.

158. Peterson E, Thrupp L, Uchiyama N, et al. Factitious bacterial meningitis revisited. J Clin Microbiol 1982;16: 758–60.

159. Ericcson CD, Carmichael M, Pickering LK, et al. Erroneous diagnosis of meningitis due to false positive Gram stains. South Med J 1978;71:1524–5.

160. Hodges GR, Fass RJ, Saslaw S. Central nervous system disease associated with *Mycoplasma pneumoniae* infection. Arch Intern Med 1972;130:227–82.

161. Embree J. *Mycoplasma hominis* in maternal and fetal infections. Ann NY Acad Sci 1988;549:56–64.

162. Waites KB, Rudd PT, Crouse DT, et al. Chronic *Ureaplama urealyticum* and *Mycoplasma hominis* infections of central nervous system in preterm infants. Lancet 1988; 1:17–21.

163. Picard FJ, Dekaban GA, Silva J, Rice GP. Mollaret's meningitis associated with herpes simplex type 2 infection. Neurology 1993;43:1722–7.

164. Boyce TG, Spearman P. Acute aseptic meningitis secondary to intravenous immunoglobulin in a patient with Kawasaki syndrome. Pediatr Infect Dis J 1998;17:1054–6.

165. De Vlieghere FC, Peetermans WE, Vermylen J. Aseptic granulocytic meningitis following treatment with intravenous immunoglobulin. Clin Infect Dis 1994;18: 1008–10.

166. Groover RV, Sutherland JM, Landin BH. Purulent meningitis of newborn infants: eleven-year experience in the antibiotic era. N Engl J Med 1961;264:1115–21.

167. Willhelm C, Ellner JJ. Chronic meningitis. Neurol Clin 1986;4:115–41.

168. O'Duffy JD, Goldstein NP. Neurologic involvement in seven patients with Behçet's disease. Am J Med 1976;61: 170–8.

169. Givner LB, Baker CJ. Anaerobic meningitis associated with a dermal sinus tract. Pediatr Infect Dis 1983;2: 385–7.

170. Roach ES, Laster DW. Prolonged course of meningitis due to an arachnoid cyst. Arch Neurol 1981;38:720–1

171. Vogler LB, Newman SL, Stroud RM, et al. Recurrent meningococcal meningitis with absence of the sixth component of complement: an evaluation of underlying immunologic mechanisms. Pediatrics 1979;64:465–7.

172. Merino J, Rodriguez-Valverde V, Lamelas JA, et al. Prevalence of deficits of complement components in patients with recurrent meningococcal infections. J Infect Dis 1983;148:331.

173. Surpure JS, Strickland S. Spontaneous cerebrospinal fluid rhinorrhea with recurrent meningitis. Clin Pediatr 1979; 18:700,703–4.

174. Fyfe DA, Rothner DA, Orlowski J, et al. Recurrent meningitis with brain abscess in infancy. Am J Dis Child 1983; 137:912–3.

175. Park JI, Strelzow W, Friedman WH, et al. Current management of cerebrospinal fluid rhinorrhea. Laryngoscope 1983;93:1294–1300.

176. Curries JT, Vincent LM, Kowalsky RJ, et al. CSF rhinorrhea: detection and localization using overpressure cisternography with Tc99mDTPA. Radiology 1985;154: 795–9.

177. Steele RW, McConnell JR, Jacobs RF, et al. Recurrent bacterial meningitis: coronal thin-section cranial computed tomography to delineate anatomic defects. Pediatrics 1985;76:950–3.

178. Beghi E, Nicolosi A, Kurland LT, et al. Encephalitis and aseptic meningitis, Olmsted County, Minnesota, 1950–1981 I: Epidemiology. Ann Neurol 1984;16: 283–94.

179. Singer JI, Maur PR, Riley JP, et al. Management of central nervous system infections during an epidemic of enteroviral aseptic meningitis. J Pediatr 1980;96:559–63.

180. Adair CV, Gauld RL, Smadel JE. Aseptic meningitis, a

disease of diverse etiology: clinical and etiologic studies on 854 cases. Ann Intern Med 1953;39:675–704.

181. Silver TS, Todd JK. Hypoglycorrhachia in pediatric patients. Pediatrics 1976;58:67–71.

182. Visintine AM, Oleske JM, Nahmias AJ. *Listeria monocytogenes* infection in infants and children. Am J Dis Child 1977;131:393–7.

182a. Newton RW. Tuberculous meningitis. Arch Dis Child 1994;70:364–6.

183. Lee LV. Neurotuberculosis among Filipino children: an 11 year experience at the Philippine Children's Medical Center. Brain Dev 2000;22:469–74.

184. Yaramis A, Gurkan F, Elevli M, et al. Central nervous system tuberculosis in children: a review of 214 cases. Pediatrics 1998;102:E49.

185. Zarabi M, Sane S, Girdany BR. The chest roentgenogram in the early diagnosis of tuberculous meningitis in children. Am J Dis Child 1971;121:389–92.

186. Singh P, Baveja CP, Talukdar B, et al. Diagnostic utility of ELISA test using antigen A60 in suspected cases of tuberculous meningitis in paediatric age group. Indian J Pathol Microbiol 1999;42:11–4.

187. Srivastava KL, Bansal M, Gupta S, et al. Diagnosis of tuberculous meningitis by detection of antigen and antibody in CSF and sera. Indian Pediatr 1998;35:841–50.

188. Bonington A, Strang JI, Klapper PE, et al. Use of Roche AMPLICOR *Mycobacterium tuberculosis* PCR in early diagnosis of tuberculous meningitis. J Clin Microbiol 1998; 36:1251–4.

189. Seth P, Ahuja GK, Bhanu NV, et al. Evaluation of polymerase chain reaction for rapid diagnosis of clinically suspected tuberculous meningitis. Tuber Lung Dis 1996; 77:353–7.

190. Diamond RD, Bennett JE. Prognostic factors in cryptococcal meningitis: a study in 111 cases. Ann Intern Med 1974;80:176–81.

191. Stockstill MT, Kauffman CA. Comparison of cryptococcal and tuberculous meningitis. Arch Neurol 1983;40:81–5.

192. van der Horst CM, Saag MS, Cloud GA, et al. Treatment of cryptococcal meningitis associated with the acquired immunodeficiency syndrome. National Institute of Allergy and Infectious Diseases Mycoses Study Group and AIDS Clinical Trials Group. N Engl J Med 1997;337: 15–21.

193. Lilien LD, Ramamurchy RS, Pildes RS. *Candida albicans* meningitis in a premature neonate successfully treated with 5 fluorocytosine and amphotericin B: a case report and review of the literature. Pediatrics 1978;61:57–61.

194. Lyons RW, Andriole VT. Fungal infections of the CNS. Neurol Clin 1986;4:159–70.

195. Wheat LJ, Garringer T, Brizendine E, Connolly P. Diagnosis of histoplasmosis by antigen detection based upon experience at the histoplasmosis reference laboratory. Diagn Microbiol Infect Dis 2002;43:29–37.

196. Wildin S, Chonmaitree T. The importance of the virology laboratory in the diagnosis and management of viral meningitis. Am J Dis Child 1987;141:454–7.

197. Karandanis D, Shulman JA. Recent survey of infectious meningitis in adults: review of laboratory findings in bacterial, tuberculous, and aseptic meningitis. South Med J 1976;69:449–57.

198. Wilfert CM. Mumps meningoencephalitis with low cerebrospinal fluid glucose, prolonged pleocytosis and elevation of protein. N Engl J Med 1969;280:855–9.

199. Oetgen WJ. Mumps and hypoglycorrhachia. Pediatrics 1978;61:158.

200. Malcom BS, Eiden JJ, Hendley JO. ECHO virus type 9 simulating tuberculous meningitis. Pediatrics 1980;65: 725–6.

201. Chesney PJ, Quennec P, Clark C. Hypoglycorrhachia and Coxsackie B3 meningoencephalitis. Am J Clin Pathol 1978;70:947–8.

202. Chiou CC, Liu WT, Chen SJ, et al. Coxsackievirus B1 infection in infants less than 2 months of age. Am J Perinatol 1998;15:155–9.

203. Green WR, Sweet LK, Prichard RW. Acute lymphocytic choriomeningitis: a study of twenty-one cases. J Pediatr 1949;35:688–701.

204. Grines C, Plouffe JF, Baird IM, et al. Toxoplasma meningoencephalitis with hypoglycorrhachia. Arch Intern Med 1981;141:935.

205. Bach MC, Davis KM. Listeria rhombencephalitis mimicking tuberculous meningitis. Rev Infect Dis 1987;9:130–3.

206. McKinney RE Jr, Katz SL, Wilfert CM. Chronic enteroviral meningoencephalitis in agammaglobulinemic patients. Rev Infect Dis 1987;9:334–56.

207. Rotbart HA, Webster AD. Treatment of potentially life-threatening enterovirus infections with pleconaril. Clin Infect Dis 2001;32:228–35.

208. Plumb VJ, Dismukes WE. Chemical meningitis related to intrathecal corticosteroid therapy. South Med J 1977; 70:1241–3.

209. Mori I, Matsumoto K, Hatano M, et al. An unseasonabale winter outbreak of echovirus type 30 meningitis. J Infect 1995;31:219–23.

210. Sumaya CV, Corman LI. Enteroviral meningitis in early infancy: significance in community outbreaks. Pediatr Infect Dis 1982;1:151–4.

211. Jarvis WR, Tucker G. Echovirus type 7 meningitis in young children. Am J Dis Child 1981;135:1009–12.

212. Wilfert CM, Thompson RJ Jr, Sunder TR, et al. Longitudinal assessment of children with enteroviral meningitis during the first three months of life. Pediatrics 1981;67: 811–5.

213. Goldberg F, Weiner LB. Cerebrospinal fluid white blood cell counts and lactic acid dehydrogenase in enterovirus type 71 meningitis. Clin Pediatr 1981;20:327–30.

214. Chang LY, Lin TY, Huang YC, et al. Comparison of enterovirus 71 and coxsackie-virus A16 clinical illnesses during the Taiwan enterovirus epidemic, 1998. Pediatr Infect Dis J 1999;18:1092–6.

215. Vieth UC, Kunzelmann M, Diedrich S, et al. An echovirus 30 outbreak with a high meningitis attack rate among children and household members at four day-care centers. Eur J Epidemiol 1999;15:655–8.

216. Chambon M, Bailly JL, Beguet A, et al. An outbreak of echovirus type 30 in a neonatal unit in France in 1997: usefulness of PCR diagnosis. J Hosp Infect 1999;43:63–8.

217. Ahmed A, Brito F, Goto C, et al. Clinical utility of the polymerase chain reaction for diagnosis of enteroviral meningitis in infancy. J Pediatr 1997;131:393–7.

218. Kelsey DS. Adenovirus meningoencephalitis. Pediatrics 1978;61:291–3.

219. Jarvis WR. Measles meningoencephalitis: an unusual presentation. Am J Dis Child 1979;133:751.

220. Wong CJ, Price Z, Bruckner DA. Aseptic meningitis in an infant with rotavirus gastroenteritis. Pediatr Infect Dis 1984;3:244–6.

221. Hodges GR, Fass RJ, Saslaw S. Central nervous system disease associated with Mycoplasma pneumoniae infection. Arch Intern Med 1972;130:277–82.

222. Narita M, Matsuzono Y, Togashi T, Kajii N. DNA diagnosis of central nervous system infection by Mycoplasma pneumoniae. Pediatrics 1992;90:250–3.

223. Narita M, Itakura O, Matsuzono Y, Togashi T. Analysis of mycoplasmal central nervous system involvement by polymerase chain reaction. Pediatr Infect Dis J 1995;14:236–7.

224. Gerber MA, Shapiro ED, Burke GS, et al. Lyme disease in children in southeastern Connecticut. N Engl J Med 1996;335:1270–4.

224a. Walker DH. Rocky Mountain spotted fever: a seasonal alert. Clin Infect Dis 1995;20:1111–7.

224b. Jacobs RF, Schutze GE. Ehrlichiosis in children. J Pediatr 1997;131:184–92.

224c. Jensenius M, Fournier PE, Vene S, et al. African tick bite fever in travelers to rural sub-equatorial Africa. Clin Infect Dis 2003;36:1411–7.

225. Meissner HC, Gellis SE, Milliken JF Jr. Lyme disease first observed to be aseptic meningitis. Am J Dis Child 1982;136:465–7.

226. Jorbeck HJA, Gustafsson PM, Lind HCF, et al. Tickborne Borrelia meningitis in children. Acta Paediatr Scand 1987;76:228–33.

227. Reik L Jr. Disorders that mimic CNS infections. Neurol Clin 1986;4:223–48.

228. Goldman JM, McIntosh CS, Calver GP, et al. Meningoencephalitis associated with Chlamydia trachomatis infection. Br Med J 1983;286:517–8.

229. Sundelof B, Gnarpe H, Gnarpe J. An unusual manifestation of Chlamydia pneumoniae infection: meningitis, hepatitis, iritis, and atypical erythema nodosum. Scand J Infect Dis 1993;25:259–61.

230. Torre D, Giola M, Martegani R, et al. Aseptic meningitis caused by Leptospira australis. Eur J Clin Microbiol Infect Dis 1994;13:496–7.

231. Pierce JF, Jabbari B, Shraberg D. Leptospirosis: a neglected cause of nonbacterial meningoencephalitis. South Med J 1977;70:150–2.

232. Romero EC, Billerbeck AE, Lando VS, et al. Detection of leptospira DNA in patients with aseptic meningitis by PCR. J Clin Microbiol 1998;36:1453–5.

233. Edmond RTD, McKendrick GDW. Tuberculosis as a cause of transient aseptic meningitis. Lancet 1973;2:234–6.

234. Taber LH, Yow MD, Nieberg FG. The penetration of broadspectrum antibiotics into the cerebrospinal fluid. Ann NY Acad Sci 1967;145:473–81.

235. Feldman WE. Effect of prior antibiotic therapy on concentrations of bacteria in CSF. Am J Dis Child 1978;132:672–4.

236. DiMario FJ Jr. Aseptic meningitis secondary to metrizamide lumbar myelography in a 4-month-old infant. Pediatrics 1985;76:259–62.

237. Ruppert GB, Barth WF. Tolmetin induced aseptic meningitis. JAMA 1981;245:67–8.

238. Boyce TG, Smidt RG, Edmonson MB. Fever as an adverse reaction to oral trimethoprim-sulfamethoxazole therapy. Pediatr Infect Dis J 1992;11:772–3.

239. Dengler LD, Capparelli EV, Bastian JF, et al. Cerebrospinal fluid profile in patients with acute Kawasaki disease. Pediatr Infect Dis J 1998;17:478–81.

240. Bia FJ, Barry M. Parasitic infections of the central nervous system. Neurol Clin 1986;4:171–206.

241. Gould IM, Newell S, Green SH, et al. Toxocariasis and eosinophilic meningitis. Br Med J 1985;291:1239–40.

242. Gavin PJ, Kazacos KR, Tan TQ, et al. Neural larva migrans caused by the raccoon roundworm Baylisascaris procyonis. Pediatr Infect Dis J 2002;21:971–5.

243. Chesney PJ, Katcher ML, Nelson DB, et al. CSF eosinophilia and chronic lymphocytic choriomeningitis virus meningitis. J Pediatr 1979;94:750–2.

244. Snead OC III, Kalavsky SM. Cerebrospinal fluid eosinophilia. J Pediatr 1976;89:83–4.

245. Marier R, Rodriguez W, Chloupek AJ, et al. Coxsackie B5 infection and aseptic meningitis in neonates and children. Am J Dis Child 1975;129:321–5.

246. Feigin RD, Shackelford PG. Value of repeat lumbar puncture in the differential diagnosis of meningitis. N Engl J Med 1973;289:571–4.

247. Negrini B, Kelleher KJ, Wald ER. Cerebrospinal fluid findings in aseptic versus bacterial meningitis. Pediatrics 2000;105:316–9.

248. Chemtob S, Reece ER, Mills EL. Syndrome of inappropriate secretion of antidiuretic hormone in enteroviral meningitis. Am J Dis Child 1985;139:292–4.

249. Moritz ML, Ayus JC, McJunkin JE, et al. La Crosse encephalitis in children. N Engl J Med 2001;345:148–9.

250. Sheller JR, Des Prez RM. CNS tuberculosis. Neurol Clin 1986;4:143–58.

251. O'Toole RD, Thorton GF, Mukherjee MM, et al. Dexamethasone in tuberculous meningitis: relationship of cerebrospinal fluid effects to therapeutic efficacy. Ann Intern Med 1969;70:39–48.

252. Prasad K, Volmink J, Menon GR. Steroids for treating tuberculous meningitis. Cochrane Database Syst Rev 2000;3:CD002244.

253. Saag MS, Graybill RJ, Larsen RA, et al. Practice guidelines for the management of cryptococcal disease. Infectious Diseases Society of America. Clin Infect Dis 2000;30:710–8.

254. Kolski H, Ford-Jones EL, Richardson S, et al. Etiology of acute childhood encephalitis at The Hospital for Sick Children, Toronto, 1994–1995. Clin Infect Dis 1998;26:398–409.

255. Correspondence. Viral encephalitis. N Engl J Med 1963;273:1110.

256. Henry WD, Mann AM. Diagnosis and treatment of delirium. Can Med Assoc J 1965;93:1156–66.

257. Centers for Disease Control. Annual Summary 1984: reported morbidity and mortality in the United States. MMWR 1986;32:124.

258. Whitley RJ. Viral encephalitis. N Engl J Med 1990;323:242–50.

259. Koskimiemi M, Tautonen J, Lehtokoski-Lehtiniemi E,

Vaheri A. Epidemiology of encephalitis in children: a 20-year survey. Ann Neurol 1991;29:492–7.

260. Romero JR, Newland JG. Viral meningitis and encephalitis: traditional and emerging viral agents. Semin Pediatr Infect Dis 2003;14:72–82.

261. Roos KL. West Nile encephalitis and myelitis. Curr Opin Neurol 2004;17:343–6.

262. Subcommittee on Accidental Poisoning. Prevention, diagnosis, and treatment of lead poisoning in childhood. Pediatrics 1969;44:291–8.

263. Weller-Fahy ER, Berger LR, Troutman WG. Mouthwash: a source of acute ethanol intoxication. Pediatrics 1980; 66:302–5.

264. Schwartz JF, Patterson JH. Toxic encephalopathy related to antihistamine-barbiturate antiemetic medication. Am J Dis Child 1978;132:37–9.

265. Moore RA, Rumack BH, Conner CS, et al. Naloxone: underdosage after narcotic poisoning. Am J Dis Child 1980; 134:156–8.

266. Dove DJ, Jones T. Delayed coma associated with salicylate intoxication. J Pediatr 1982;100:493–6.

267. Roland EH, Jan JE, Rigg JM. Toxic encephalopathy in a child after brief exposure to insect repellents. Can Med Assoc J 1985;132:155–6.

268. Antony JH. Relapsing encephalopathy after hypoxia. J Pediatr 1978;92:433–4.

269. Delorme, L, Middleton PJ. Influenza A virus associated with acute encephalopathy. Am J Dis Child 1979;133: 822–4.

270. Kim KS, Gohd RS. Acute encephalopathy in twins due to adenovirus type 7 infection. Arch Neurol 1983;40: 58–9.

271. Lewis DW, Tucker SH. Central nervous system involvement in cat scratch disease. Pediatrics 1986;77:714–9.

272. Brun-Buisson CJ, de Gialluly E, Gheradi R, et al. Fatal nonmeningitic *Listeria* rhombencephalitis: report of two cases. Arch Intern Med 1985;145:1982–5.

273. Gall JC, Hayles AB, Siekert RG, et al. Multiple sclerosis in children: clinical study of 40 cases with onset in childhood. Pediatrics 1958;21:703–9.

274. Eisengart MA, Powers JM, Rose AL. Subacute necrotizing encephalomyelopathy: rapidly fatal course of Leigh disease in a 5-year-old child. Am J Dis Child 1974;127: 730–2.

275. Levin M, Hjelm M, Kay JDS, et al. Haemorrhagic shock and encephalopathy: a new syndrome with a high mortality in young children. Lancet 1983;2:64–7.

276. Anonymous. Hemorrhagic shock and encephalopathy [editorial]. Lancet 1985;2:534–6.

277. Soler S, Phillip M, Hershkowitz J, et al. Hemorrhagic shock and encephalopathy syndrome: its association with hyperthermia. Am J Dis Child 1986;140:1252–4.

278. Arvin AM, Johnson RT, Whitley RT, et al. Consensus: management of the patient with herpes simplex encephalitis. Pediatr Infect Dis 1987;6:2–5.

279. Whitley RJ, Soong SJ, Linneman C Jr, et al. Herpes simplex encephalitis: clinical assessment. JAMA 1982;247: 317–20.

280. Charney EB, Orecchio EJ, Zimmerman RA, et al. Computerized tomography in infantile encephalitis. Am J Dis Child 1979;133:803–5.

281. Nahmias AJ, Whitley RJ, Visintine AN, et al. Herpes simplex virus encephalitis: laboratory evaluations and their diagnostic significance. J Infect Dis 1982;145:829–36.

282. Weil AA, Glaser CA, Amad Z, Forghani B. Patients with suspected herpes simplex encephalitis: rethinking an initial negative polymerase chain reaction result. Clin Infect Dis 2002;34:1154–7.

283. Whitley RJ, Alford CA, Hirsch MS, et al. Vidarabine versus acyclovir therapy in herpes simplex encephalitis. N Engl J Med 1986;314:144–9.

284. Whitley RJ. Indications for empiric acyclovir in patients with encephalitis [response to question in a letter]. Pediatr Infect Dis J 1987;6:699–700.

285. McJunkin JE, de los Reyes EC, Irazuzta JE, et al. La Crosse encephalitis in children. N Engl J Med 2001;344:801–7.

286. Boyce TG, Craig AS, Schaffner W, Dermody TS. Fever and encephalopathy in two school age boys. Pediatr Infect Dis J 1998;17:935:935–40.

287. Roos KL. Encephalitis. Neurologic Clinics 1999;17: 813–33.

287a. Centers for Disease Control and Prevention. West Nile virus activity—United States, August 4–10, 2004. MMWR 2004;53:719–20.

287b. Horga MA, Fine A. West Nile virus. Pediatr Infect Dis J 2001;20:801–2.

288. Marfin AA, Gubler DJ. West Nile encephalitis: an emerging disease in the United States. Clin Infect Dis 2001;33: 1713–9.

289. Balfour HH Jr, Siem RA, Bauer H, et al. California arbovirus (La Crosse) infections I: clinical and laboratory findings in 66 children with meningoencephalitis. Pediatrics 1973;52:680–91.

290. Calisher CH, Pretzman CI, Muth DJ, et al. Serodiagnosis of La Crosse virus infections in humans by detection of immunoglobulin M class antibodies. J Clin Microbiol 1986;23:667–71.

291. West TE, Papasian CJ, Park BH, et al. Adenovirus type 2 encephalitis and concurrent Epstein-Barr virus infection in an adult man. Arch Neurol 1985;42:815–7.

292. Russell J, Fisher M, Zivin JA, et al. Status epilepticus and Epstein-Barr virus encephalopathy: diagnosis by modern serologic techniques. Arch Neurol 1985;42:789–92.

293. Silverstein A, Steinberg G, Nathanson M. Nervous system involvement in infectious mononucleosis: the heralding and/or major manifestation. Arch Neurol 1972;26: 353–8.

294. Halstead CC, Chang RS. Infectious mononucleosis and encephalitis: recovery of EB virus from the spinal fluid. Pediatrics 1979;64:257–8.

295. Connelly KP, DeWitt LD. Neurologic complications of infectious mononucleosis. Pediatr Neurol 1994;10: 181–4.

296. Lerer RJ, Kalavsky SM. Central nervous system disease associated with *Mycoplasma pneumoniae* infection: report of five cases and review of the literature. Pediatrics 1973; 52:658–68.

297. Novelli VM, Matthew DJ, Dinwiddie RD. Acute fulminant toxic encephalopathy associated with *Mycoplasma pneumoniae* infection. Pediatr Infect Dis 1985;4:413–5.

298. Kolski H, Ford-Jones EL, Richardson S, et al. Etiology of acute childhood encephalitis at The Hospital for Sick Children, Toronto, 1994–1995. Clin Infect Dis 1998;26: 398–409.

299. Ponka A. Central nervous system manifestations associated with serologically verified *Mycoplasma pneumoniae* infection. Scand J Infect Dis 1980;12:175–84.

300. Horney LF, Walker DH. Meningoencephalitis as major manifestations of Rocky Mountain spotted fever [abstract]. South Med J 1988;81:915.

300a. Johnson RT. Acute encephalitis. Clin Infect Dis 1996;23: 219–26.

300b. Hynson JL, Kornberg AJ, Coleman LT, et al. Clinical and neuroradiologic features of acute disseminated encephalomyelitis in children. Neurology 2001;56:1308–12.

301. Michener RC, Henley WL. Focal convulsions associated with subclinical measles infection. Clin Pediatr 1983;22: 643–5.

302. Valmari P, Lanning M, Tuokko H, et al. Measles virus in the cerebrospinal fluid in postvaccination immunosuppressive measles encephalopathy. Pediatr Infect Dis J 1987;6:59–63.

303. Lyon G, Ponsot G, Lebon P. Acute measles encephalitis of the delayed type. Ann Neurol 1977;2:322–7.

304. Case Records of the Massachusetts General Hospital. Case 43-1986. N Engl J Med 1986;315:1143–54.

305. Bach MC, Armstrong RM. Acute toxoplasmic encephalitis in a normal adult. Arch Neurol 1983;40:596–7.

306. Green WR, Sweet LK, Prickard RW. Acute lymphocytic choriomeningitis: a study of twenty-one cases. J Pediatr 1949;35:688–701.

307. Morrison AJ Jr, Wenzel RP. Rabies: a review and current approach for the clinician. South Med J 1985;78:1211–8.

308. Hammond GW, MacDougall BK, Plummer F, et al. Encephalitis during the prodromal stage of acute hepatitis A. Can Med Assoc J 1982;126:269–70.

309. Harris LF. Legionnaires' disease associated with acute encephalomyelitis. Arch Neurol 1981;38:462–3.

310. Rantala H, Uhari M. Occurrence of childhood encephalitis: a population-based study. Pediatr Infect Dis J 1989; 8:426–30.

310a. Morishima T, Togashi T, Yokota S, et al. Encephalitis and encephalopathy associated with an influenza epidemic in Japan. Clin Infect Dis 2002;35:512–7.

310b. Newland JG, Romero JR, Varman M, et al. Encephalitis associated with influenza B virus infection in 2 children and a review of the literature. Clin Infect Dis 2003;36: e87–95.

311. Miller JD, Ross CAC. Encephalitis: a four-year survey. Lancet 1968;1:1121–6.

312. Koskiniemi M. CNS manifestations associated with *Mycoplasma pneumoniae* infections: summary of cases at the University of Helsinki and review. Clin Infect Dis 1993; 17:S52–7.

313. Reye RDC, Morgan G, Baral J. Encephalopathy and fatty degeneration of the viscera: a disease entity in childhood. Lancet 1963;2:749–52.

314. Hurwitz ES, Barrett MJ, Bregman D, et al. Public Health Service study of Reye's syndrome and medications: report of the main study. JAMA 1987;257:1905–11.

315. Belay ED, Bresee JS, Holman RC, et al. Reye's syndrome in the United States from 1981 through 1997. N Engl J Med 1999;340:1377–82.

316. Corey L, Rubin RJ, Hattwick MAW. Reye's syndrome: clinical progression and evaluation of therapy. Pediatrics 1977;60:708–14.

317. Ferris BG Jr, Auld PAM, Cronkhite L, et al. Life-threatening poliomyelitis: Boston, 1955. N Engl J Med 1960;262: 371–80.

318. Herremans T, Koopmans MP, vanderVoort HG, vanLoon AM. Lessons from diagnostic investigations of patients with poliomyelitis and their direct contacts for the present surveillance of acute flaccid paralysis. Clin Infect Dis 1999;29:849–54.

319. Nkowane BM, Wassilak SGF, Orenstein WA. Vaccine-associated paralytic poliomyelitis United States: 1973 through 1984. JAMA 1987;257:1335–40.

320. Strebel PM, Ion-Nedelcu N, Baughman AL, et al. Intramuscular injections within 30 days of immunization with oral poliovirus vaccine—a risk factor for vaccine-associated paralytic poliomyelitis. N Engl J Med 1995;332: 500–6.

321. Centers for Disease Control. Paralytic disease-Puerto Rico. MMWR 1973;22:143–4.

322. Samuda GM, Chang WK, Yeung CY, et al. Monoplegia caused by enterovirus 71: an outbreak in Hong Kong. Pediatr Infect Dis J 1987;6:206–8.

323. Wadia NH, Katrak SM, Misra VP, et al. Polio-like motor paralysis associated with acute hemorrhagic conjunctivitis in an outbreak in 1981 in Bombay, India: clinical and serologic studies. J Infect Dis 1983;147:660–8.

324. Chonmaitree T, Menegus MA, Schervish-Swierkosz EM, et al. Enterovirus 71 infection: report of an outbreak with two cases of paralysis and a review of the literature. Pediatrics 1981;67:489–93.

325. Huang CC, Liu CC, Chang YC, et al. Neurologic complications in children with enterovirus 71 infection. N Engl J Med 1999;341:936–42.

326. Takimoto S, Waldman EA, Moreira RC, et al. Enterovirus 71 infection and acute neurological disease among children in Brazil (1988–1990). Trans R Soc Trop Med Hyg 1998;92:25–8.

327. Alexander JP Jr, Baden L, Pallansch MA, et al. Enterovirus 71 infections and neurologic disease—United States, 1977–1991. J Infect Dis 1994;169:905–8.

328. Magoffin RL, Lennette EH, Schmidt NJ. Association of Coxsackie viruses with illness resembling mild paralytic poliomyelitis. Pediatrics 1961;28:602–13.

329. Yui LA, Gledhill RF. Limb paralysis as a manifestation of coxsackie B virus infection. Dev Med Child Neurol 1991; 33:427–38.

330. Solomon T, Kneen R, Dung NM, et al. Poliomyelitis-like illness due to Japanese encephalitis virus. Lancet 1998; 351:1094–7.

331. Magoffin RL, Lennette EH, Hollister AC Jr, et al. An etiologic study of clinical paralytic poliomyelitis. JAMA 1961; 175:269–78.

332. Sabin AB. Paralytic poliomyelitis: old dogmas and new perspectives. Rev Infect Dis 1981;3:543–64.

333. Kyllerman MG, Herner S, Bergstrom TB, Ekholm SE. PCR diagnosis of primary herpesvirus type I in poliomyelitis-like paralysis and respiratory tract disease. Pediatr Neurol 1993;9:227–9.

334. Wheeler SD, Ochoa J. Poliomyelitis-like syndrome associated with asthma: a case report and review of the literature. Arch Neurol 1980;37:52–3.

335. Acharya AB, Lakhani PK. Hopkins syndrome associated

with *Mycoplasma* infection. Pediatr Neurol 1997;16: 54–5.

336. Warren P, Fischbein C, Mascoli N, et al. Poliomyelitis-like syndrome caused by *Mycoplasma pneumoniae*. J Pediatr 1978;93:451–2.

337. MacFarlane PI, Miller V. Transverse myelitis associated with *Mycoplasma pneumoniae* infection. Arch Dis Child 1984;59:80–2.

338. Roman GC, Senanayake N. Neurological manifestations of malaria. Arq Neuropsiquiatr 1992;50:3–9.

339. Ramar S, Sivaramakrishnan V, Manoharan K. Scurvy—a forgotten disease. Arch Phys Med Rehabil 1993;74:92–5.

340. Carroll JE, Jedziniak M, Guggenheim MA. Guillain-Barré syndrome: another cause of the "floppy infant." Am J Dis Child 1977;131:699–700.

341. Allos BM. *Campylobacter jejuni* infection as a cause of the Guillain-Barre syndrome. Infect Dis Clin North Am 1998; 12:173–84.

342. Sheikh KA, Ho TW, Nachamkin I, et al. Molecular mimicry in Guillain-Barre syndrome. Ann NY Acad Sci 1998; 845:307–21.

343. Hughes RA, Rees JH. Clinical and epidemiologic features of Guillain-Barre syndrome. J Infect Dis 1997;176 Suppl 2:S92–8.

343a. Tuttle J, Chen RT, Rantala H, et al. The risk of Guillain-Barre syndrome after tetanus-toxoid-containing vaccines in adults and children in the United States. Am J Pub Health 1997;87:2045–8.

343b. Lasky T, Terracciano GJ, Magder L, et al. The Guillain-Barre syndrome and the 1992–1993 and 1993–1994 influenza vaccines. N Engl J Med 1998;339:1797–802.

344. Evans OB. Polyneuropathy in childhood. Pediatrics 1979; 64:96–105.

345. Gorman RJ, Snead OC. Tick paralysis in three children. Clin Pediatr 1978;17:249–51.

346. Andersen RD. Colorado tick fever and tick paralysis in a young child. Pediatr Infect Dis 1983;2:43–4.

347. Klastersky J, Cappel R, Sroeck JM, et al. Ascending myelitis in association with Herpes simplex virus. N Engl J Med 1972;287:182–4.

348. Breen GE, Lamb SG, Otaki AT. Monkeybite encephalomyelitis: report of a case with recovery. Br Med J 1958; 2:22–3.

349. Ostrowski SR, Leslie MJ, Parrott T, et al. B-virus from pet macaque monkeys: an emerging threat in the United States? Emerg Infect Dis 1998;4:117–21.

350. Calderon-Gonzales R, Rissi-Hernandez H. Buckthorn polyneuropathy. N Engl J Med 1967;277:69–71.

351. Pollen RH, Williams RH. Hyperkalemic neuromyopathy in Addison's disease. N Engl J Med 1960;263:273–8.

352. Morgan N, Brookes GB. Central nervous system complications of acute tonsillitis. J Laryngol Otol 1997;111: 274–6.

353. Al-Shahwan S, Rossi ML, al-Thagafi MA. Ascending paralysis due to myelitis in a newborn with congenital toxoplasmosis. J Neurol Sci 1996;139:156–9.

354. Novak RW, Jones G, Ch'ien LT. Acute transverse myelopathy in childhood: a study of four cases. Clin Pediatr 1978;17:894–896–899.

355. Tsutsumi H, Kamazaki H, Nakata S, et al. Sequential development of acute meningoencephalitis and transverse myelitis caused by Epstein-Barr virus during infectious mononucleosis. Pediatr Infect Dis J 1994;13:665–7.

356. Rousseau JJ, Lust C, Bangerle PF, et al. Acute transverse myelitis as presenting neurological feature of Lyme disease. Lancet 1986;2:1222–3.

357. Tyler KL, Gross RA, Cascino GD. Unusual viral causes of transverse myelitis: hepatitis A virus and cytomegalovirus. Neurology 1986;36:855–8.

358. Klimek JJ, Russman BS, Quintiliani R. *Mycoplasma pneumoniae* meningoencephalitis and transverse myelitis in association with low cerebrospinal fluid glucose. Pediatrics 1976;58:133–5.

359. Seay AR. Spinal cord dysfunction complicating bacterial meningitis. Arch Neurol 1984;41:545–6.

360. Weir MR, Fearnow RG. Transverse myelitis and penicillin. Pediatrics 1984;71:988.

361. Boyce TG. Acute transverse myelitis in a 6-year-old girl with schistosomiasis. Pediatr Infect Dis J 1990;9:279–84.

362. Enberg RN, Kaplan RJ. Spinal epidural abscess in children: early diagnosis and immediate surgical drainage is essential to forestall paralysis. Clin Pediatr 1974;13: 247–53.

363. Obrador GT, Levenson DJ. Spinal epidural abscess in hemodialysis patients: report of three cases and review of the literature. Am J Kidney Dis 1996;27:75–83.

364. MacKenzie AR, Laing RB, Smith CC, et al. Spinal epidural abscess: the importance of early diagnosis and treatment. J Neurol Neurosurg Psychiatr 1998;65:209–12.

365. Steegmann AT. Syndrome of the anterior spinal artery. Neurology 1952;2:15–35.

366. Arnold TW, Meyers GJ. Neuromyelitis optica (Devic syndrome) in a 12-year-old male with complete recovery following steroids. Pediatr Neurol 1987;3:313–5.

367. Jeffery AR, Buncic JR. Pediatric Devic's neuromyelitis optica. J Pediatr Ophthalmol Strabismus 1996;33:223–9.

368. Duquette P, Murray TJ, Pleines J, et al. Multiple sclerosis in childhood: clinical profile in 125 patients. J Pediatr 1987;111:359–63.

369. Merle H, Smadja D, Cordoba A. Optic neuromyelitis and bilateral acute retinal necrosis due to varicella zoster in a patient with AIDS. J Fr Ophthalmol 1998;21:381–6.

370. Silber MH, Willcox PA, Bowen RM, Unger A. Neuromyelitis optica (Devic's syndrome) and pulmonary tuberculosis. Neurology 1990;40:934–8.

371. Vidal-Marsal F, Garcia-Saavedra V, Gonzalea J, Richart-Jurado C. Devic's syndrome during secondary syphilis [letter]. An Med Interna 1989;6:497–8.

372. Terranova W, Breman JG, Locey RP, Speck S. Botulism type B: epidemiologic aspects of an extensive outbreak. Am J Epidemiol 1978;108:150–6.

373. Angulo FJ, Getz J, Taylor JP, et al. A large outbreak of botulism: the hazardous baked potato. J Infect Dis 1998; 178:172–7.

374. MacDonald KL, Spengler RF, Hatheway CL, et al. Type A botulism from sauteed onions: clinical and epidemiologic observations. JAMA 1985;253:1275–8.

375. Townes JM, Cieslak PR, Hatheway CL, et al. An outbreak of type A botulism associated with a commercial cheese sauce. Ann Intern Med 1996;125:558–63.

376. Rapoport S, Watkins PB. Descending paralysis resulting from occult wound botulism. Ann Neurol 1984;16: 359–61.

377. Black RE, Gunn RA. Hypersensitivity reactions associated with botulinal antitoxin. Am J Med 1980;69:567–70.

378. Padua L, Aprile I, Monaco ML, et al. Neurophysiological assessment in the diagnosis of botulism: usefulness of single-fiber EMG. Muscle Nerve 1999;22:1388–92.

379. Adour KK, Bell DN, Hilsinger RL Jr. Herpes simplex virus in idiopathic facial paralysis (Bell's palsy). JAMA 1975; 233:527–30.

380. Glasscock ME III, Pensak ML, Gulya AJ, et al. Lyme disease: a cause of bilateral facial paralysis. Arch Otolaryngol 1985;111:47–9.

381. Djupesland G, Berdal P, Johannesson TA, et al. Viral infection as a cause of acute peripheral facial palsy. Arch Otolaryngol 1976;102:403–6.

382. Grose C, Hele W, Henle G, et al. Primary Epstein-Barr-virus infections in acute neurologic diseases. N Engl J Med 1975;292:392–5.

383. Kukimoto N, Ideda M, Yamada K, et al. Viral infections in acute peripheral facial paralysis. Nationwide analysis centering on CF. Acta Otolaryngol Suppl 1988;446: 17–22.

383a. Grose C, Bonthius D, Afifi AK. Chickenpox and the geniculate ganglion: facial nerve palsy, Ramsay Hunt syndrome and acyclovir treatment. Pediatr Infect Dis J 2002;21: 615–7.

384. Walter RS, Eppes SC. Cat scratch disease presenting with peripheral facial nerve paralysis. Pediatrics 1998;101: e13.

385. Chutorian AM, Gold AP, Braun CW. Benign intracranial hypertension and Bell's palsy. N Engl J Med 1977;296: 1214–5.

386. Sandstedt P, Hyden D, Odkvist LM, et al. Peripheral facial palsy in children: a cerebrospinal fluid study. Acta Paediatr Scand 1985;74:281–5.

387. Lower EE, Broderick JP, Brott TG, Baughman RP. Diagnosis and management of neurological sarcoidosis. Arch Intern Med 1997;157:1864–8.

388. Purcell JJ Jr, Taulbee WA. Orbital myositis after upper respiratory tract infection. Arch Ophthalmol 1981;99: 437–8.

389. Sullivan SC. Benign recurrent isolated VI nerve palsy of childhood. Clin Pediatr 1985;24:160–1.

390. Werner DB, Savino PJ, Schatz NJ. Benign recurrent sixth nerve palsies in childhood: secondary to immunization or viral illness. Arch Ophthalmol 1983;101:607–8.

391. Greene RM, Rogers RS 3rd. Meldersson-Rosenthal syndrome: a review of 36 patients. J Am Acad Dermatol 1989;21:1263–70.

392. Schraeder PL, Burns RA. Hemiplegic migraine association with an aseptic meningeal reaction. Arch Neurol 1980; 37:377–9.

393. Chou YH, Wang PJ, Lin MY, et al. Acute hemiplegia in infancy and childhood. Chung Hua Min Kuo Hsiao Erh Ko I Hsueh Hui Tsa Chih 1994;35:45–56.

394. Okuno T. Acute hemiplegia syndrome in childhood. Brain Dev 1994;16:16–22.

395. VanKuijck MA, Rotteveel JJ, vanOostrom CB, Novakova K. Neurological complications in children with protein C deficiency. Neuropediatrics 1994;25:16–9.

396. Nantulya FN. Neurological complications asssociated with sickle cell anemia: an experience at the AgaKhan Hospital, Nairobi. East Afr Med J 1989;66:669–77.

397. Keren G, Barzilay Z, Cohen BE. Ruptured intracranial arterial aneurysm in the first year of life: a case report. Arch Neurol 1980;37:392–3.

398. Fisher RG, Friedmann KR. Carotid artery thrombosis in persons fifteen years of age or younger. JAMA 1959;170: 1918–9.

398a. Wechsler B, Kim H, Hunter J. Trampolines, children, and stroke. Am J Phys Med Rehabil 2001;80:608–13.

398b. Nadgir RN, Loevner LA, Ahmed T, et al. Simultaneous bilateral internal carotid and vertebral artery dissection following chiropractic manipulation: case report and review of the literature. Neuroradiology 2003;45:311–4.

399. Sanchez-Calderon M, deSantos T, Martin S, et al. Multiple sclerosis in childhood: our experience and a review of the literature. Rev Neurol 1998;27:237–41.

400. Torigoe S, Koide W, Yamada M, et al. Human herpesvirus 7 infection associated with central nervous system manifestations. J Pediatr 1996;129:301–5.

401. Tsolia M, Skardoutsou A, Tsolas G, et al. Pre-eruptive neurologic manifestations associated with multiple cerebral infarcts in varicella. Pediatr Neurol 1995;12:165–8.

402. Ichiyama T, Houdou S, Kisa T, et al. Varicella with delayed hemiplegia. Pediatr Neurol 1990;6:279–81.

403. Kugler SL, Barzilai A, Hodes DS, et al. Acute hemiplegia associated with HIV infection. Pediatr Neurol 1991;7: 207–10.

404. Zilkha A, Mendelsohn F, Borofsky LG. Acute hemiplegia in children complicating upper respiratory infections: report of three cases with angiographic findings. Clin Pediatr 1976;15:1137–42.

405. Baker FJ, Kotchmar GS Jr, Foshee WS, et al. Acute hemiplegia of childhood associated with Epstein-Barr-virus infection. Pediatr Infect Dis 1983;2:136–8.

406. Young RSK, Coulter DL, Allen RJ. Capsular stroke as a cause of hemiplegia in infancy. Neurology 1983;33: 1044–6.

407. Wise GR, Farmer TV. Bacterial cerebral vasculitis. Neurology 1971;21:195–200.

408. Connoly B, King MD, Stack J. MRI in acute hemiplegia in childhood. J Comput Assist Tomogr 1995;19:492–4.

409. Eiben RM, Gersony WM. Recognition, prognosis and treatment of the Guillian-Barré syndrome (acute idiopathic polyneuritis). Med Clin North Am 1963;47: 1371–80.

410. Arnon SS. Infant botulism: anticipating the second decade. J Infect Dis 1986;154:201–6.

411. Long SS. Botulism in infancy. Pediatr Infect Dis 1984;3: 266–71.

412. Hatheway CL. Laboratory procedures for cases of suspected infant botulism. Rev Infect Dis 1979;1:647–51.

413. Brown LW. Differential diagnosis of infant botulism. Rev Infect Dis 1979;1:625–8.

414. Arnon SS, Damus K, Chin J. Infant botulism: epidemiology and relation to sudden infant death syndrome. Epidemiol Rev 1981;3:45–66.

415. Stevens D, Burman D, Clarke SKR, et al. Temporary paralysis in childhood after influenza B. Lancet 1974;2:1354.

416. Ruff RL, Secrist D. Viral studies in benign acute childhood myositis. Arch Neurol 1982;39:261–3.

417. Kessler HA, Trenholme GM, Harris AA, et al. Acute myopathy associated with influenza A/Texas/1/77 infection:

isolation of virus from a muscle biopsy specimen. JAMA 1980;243:461–2.

418. Horton L, Gorman RL. Benign acute childhood myositis: an unusual cause of refusal to walk. Pediatr Emerg Care 1986;2:170–2.

419. Adamski GB, Garin EH, Ballinger WE, et al. Generalized nonsuppurative myositis with staphylococcal septicemia. J Pediatr 1980;96:694–7.

420. Porter CB, Hinthorn DR, Couchonnal G, et al. Simultaneous Streptococcus and picornavirus infection: muscle involvement in acute rhabdomyolysis. JAMA 1981;245: 1545–7.

421. Josselson J, Pula T, Sadler JH. Acute rhabdomyolysis associated with an echovirus 9 infection. Arch Intern Med 1980;140:1671–2.

422. Kaiser AB, Rieves D, Price AH, et al. Tularemia and rhabdomyolysis. JAMA 1985;253:241–3.

423. Rubin RL. Adolescent infectious mononucleosis with psychosis. J Clin Psychiatry 1978;39:773–5.

424. Copperman SM. "Alice in Wonderland" syndrome as a presenting symptom of infectious mononucleosis in children: a description of those affected young people. Clin Pediatr 1977;16:143–6.

425. Jarvis MR, Wasserman AL, Todd RD. Acute psychosis in a patient with Epstein-Barr virus infection. J Am Acad Child Adolesc Psychiatr 1990;29:468–9.

426. Moskal MJ, Kaylarian VH, Doro JM. Psychosis complicating *Mycoplasma pneumoniae* infection. Pediatr Infect Dis 1984;3:63–6.

427. Arnold SE. Psychosis and *Mycoplasma pneumoniae*. Hillside J Clin Psychiatry 1987;9:231–5.

428. Signore RJ, Lahmeyer HW. Acute psychosis in a patient with cerebral cysticercosis. Psychosomatics 1988;29: 106–8.

429. Chien YH, Lee PI, Huang LM, et al. Typhoid fever presenting as infection-associated hemophagocytic syndrome: report of one case. Chung Hua Min Kuo Hsiae Erh Ko I Hsueh Hui Tsa Chih 1999;40:339–40.

430. Liston SL, Waeckerle JF, Robinson W. Intracranial abscesses with behavioral changes. Arch Otolaryngol 1979; 105:343–6.

431. Silber TJ, D'Angelo L. Psychosis and seizures following the injection of penicillin G procaine: Hoigne's syndrome. Am J Dis Child 1985;139:335–7.

432. Gregor JC, Zilli CA, Gotlib IH. Acute psychosis associated with oral trimethoprim-sulfamethoxazole therapy. Can J Psychiatry 1993;38:56–8.

433. Mermel LA, Doro JM, Kabadi UM. Acute psychosis in a patient receiving trimethoprim-sulfamethoxazole intravenously. J Clin Psychiatry 1986;47:269–70.

434. James EA, Demian AZ. Acute psychosis in a trauma patient due to ciprofloxacin. Postgrad Med J 1998;74: 189–90.

435. Mulhall JP, Bergmann LS. Ciprofloxacin-induced acute psychosis. Urology 1995;46:102–3.

436. Sowunmi A, Adio RA, Oduola AM, et al. Acute psychosis after mefloquine. Report of six cases. Trop Geogr Med 1995;47:179–80.

437. Sankey RJ, Nunn AJ, Sills JA. Visual hallucinations in children receiving decongestants. Br Med J 1984;288: 1369.

438. Kales JD, Kales A, Soldatas CR. Sleepwalking and night terrors related to febrile illness. Am J Psychiatry 1979; 136:1214–5.

439. Golden GS. The Alice in Wonderland syndrome in juvenile migraine. Pediatrics 1979;63:517–9.

440. Greydanus DE, Patel DR. Substance abuse in adolescents: a complex conundrum for the clinican. Pediatr Clin North Am 2003;50:1179–223.

441. Tung H, Raffel C, McComb JG. Ventricular cerebrospinal fluid eosinophilia in children with ventriculoperitoneal shunts. J Neurosurg 1991;75:541–4.

442. Mancao M, Miller C, Cochrane B, et al. Cerebrospinal fluid shunt infections in infants and children in Mobile, Alabama. Acta Paediatr 1998;87:667–70.

443. Vanaclocha V, Saiz-Sapena N, Leiva J. Shunt malfunction in relation to shunt infection. Acta Neurochir Wien 1996; 138:829–34.

444. Piatt JH Jr, Carlson CV. A search for determinants of cerebrospinal fluid shunt survival: retrospective analysis of a 14-year institutional experience. Pediatr Neurosurg 1993;19:233–41.

445. McGirt MJ, Zaas A, Fuchs HE, George TM, Kaye K, Sexton DJ. Risk factors for pediatric ventriculoperitoneal shunt infection and predictors of infectious pathogens. Clin Infect Dis 2003;36:858–62.

446. Horgan MA, Piatt JH Jr. Shaving of the scalp may increase the rate of infection in CSF shunt surgery. Pediatr Neurosurg 1997;26:180–4.

447. Younger JJ, Simmons JCH, Barrett FF. Failure of single-dose intraventricular vancomycin for cerebrospinal fluid shunt surgery prophylaxis. Pediatr Infect Dis J 1987;6: 212–3.

448. Schmidt K, Gjerris F, Osgaard O, et al. Antibiotic prophylaxis in cerebrospinal fluid shunting: a prospective randomized trial in 152 hydrocephalic patients. Neurosurgery 1985;17:1–5.

449. Arnaboldi L. Antimicrobial prophylaxis with ceftriaxone in neurosurgical procedures: a prospective study of 100 patients undergoing shunt operations. Chemotherapy 1996;42:384–90.

450. Zentner J, Gilsbach J, Felder T. Antibiotic prophylaxis in cerebrospinal fluid shunting: a prospective randomized trial in 129 patients. Neurosurg Rev 1995;18:169–72.

451. Langley JM, LeBlanc JC, Drake J, Milner R. Efficacy of antimicrobial prophylaxis in placement of cerebrospinal fluid shunts: meta-analysis. Clin Infect Dis 1993;17: 98–103.

452. Antimicrobial prophylaxis in surgery. Med Lett Drugs Ther 2001;43:92–7.

453. Ersahin Y, Mutluer S, Kocaman S. Immunoglobulin prophylaxis in shunt infections: a prospective randomized study. Childs Nerv Syst 1997;13:546–9.

454. Petrak RM, Pottage JC Jr, Harris AA, et al. *Haemophilus influenzae* meningitis in the presence of a cerebrospinal fluid shunt. Neurosurgery 1986;18:79–81.

455. Ronan A, Hogg GG, Klug GL. Cerebrospinal fluid shunt infections in children. Pediatr Infect Dis J 1995;14: 782–6.

456. Murtagh FR, Quencer RM, Poole CA. Cerebrospinal fluid shunt function and hydrocephalus in the pediatric age group. Radiology 1979;132:385–8.

457. Post EM. Currently available shunt systems: a review. Neurosurgery 1985;16:257–60.

458. Shurtleff DB, Foltz EL, Weeks RD, et al. Therapy of *Staphylococcus epidermidis*: infections associated with cerebrospinal fluid shunts. Pediatrics 1974;53:55–62.

459. Browne MJ, Dinndorf PA, Perek D, et al. Infectious complications of intraventricular reservoirs in cancer patients. Pediatr Infect Dis 1987;6:182–9.

460. Meredith FT, Phillips HK, Reller LB. Clinical utility of broth cultures of cerebrospinal fluid from patients at risk for shunt infections. J Clin Microbiol 1997;35:3109–11.

461. Gower DJ, Crone K, Alexander E Jr, et al. *Candida albicans* shunt infection: report of two cases. Neurosurgery 1986; 19:111–3.

462. Chiou CC, Wong TT, Lin HH, et al. Fungal infection of ventriculoperitoneal shunts in children. Clin Infect Dis 1994;19:1049–53.

463. Younger JJ, Simmons JCH, Barrett FF. Occult distal ventriculoperitoneal shunt infections. Pediatr Infect Dis 1985;4:557–8.

464. Hubschmann OR, Countee RW. Gram-positive peritonitis with infected ventriculoperitoneal shunts. Surg Gynecol Obstet 1979;149:69–71.

465. Grosfeld JL, Cooney DR, Smith J, et al. Intraabdominal complications following ventriculoperitoneal shunt procedures. Pediatrics 1974;54:791–6.

466. Young RA, Glazier MC, Mealey J Jr, et al. Cerebrospinal fluid ascites complicating ventriculoperitoneal shunting. J Neurosurg 1984;61:180–3.

467. Briggs JR, Hendry GMA, Minns RA. Abdominal ultrasound in the diagnosis of cerebrospinal fluid pseudocysts complicating ventriculoperitoneal shunts. Arch Dis Child 1984;59:661–4.

468. Bisno AL, Sternau L. Infections of central nervous system shunts. In: Bisno AL, Waldvogel FA, eds. Infections Associated with Indwelling Medical Devices. Washington, DC: American Society for Microbiology, 1994:91–109.

469. Yogev R. Cerebrospinal fluid shunt infections: a personal view. Pediatr Infect Dis 1985;4:113–8.

470. Odio C, McCracken GH Jr, Nelson JD. CSF shunt infections in pediatrics: a seven-year experience. Am J Dis Child 1984;138:1103–8.

471. McLaurin RL, Frame PT. Treatment of infections of cerebrospinal fluid shunts. Rev Infect Dis 1987;9:595–603.

472. Pau AK, Smego RA Jr, Fisher MA. Intraventricular vancomycin: observations of tolerance and pharmacokinetics in two infants with ventricular shunt infections. Pediatr Infect Dis 1986;5:93–6.

473. Osborn JS, Sharp S, Hanson EJ, et al. *Staphylococcus epidermidis* ventriculitis treated with vancomycin and rifampin. Neurosurgery 1986;19:824–7.

474. Odio C, Umana M, Salas J, et al. Treatment of CSF shunt infections [abstract]. Abstracts of the 1986 Interscience Conference on Antimicrobial Agents and Chemotherapy, New Orleans, 1986.

475. Vichyanond P, Olson LC. Staphylococcal CNS infections treated with vancomycin and rifampin. Arch Neurol 1984;41:637–9.

476. Sells CJ, Shurtleff DB, Loeser JD. Gram-negative cerebrospinal fluid shunt-associated infections. Pediatrics 1977; 59:614–8.

477. Wold SL, McLaurin RL. Cerebrospinal fluid antibiotic levels during treatment of shunt infections. J Neurosurg 1980;52:41–6.

478. Frame PT, McLaurin RL. Treatment of CSF shunt infections with intrashunt plus oral antibiotic therapy. J Neurosurg 1984;60:354–60.

479. Rames L, Wise B, Goodman JR, et al. Renal disease with *Staphylococcus albus* bacteremia: a complication in ventriculoatrial shunts. JAMA 1970;212:1671–7.

480. Bardenheier B, Prevots DR, Khetsuriani N, Wharton M. Tetanus surveillance—United States, 1995–1997. MMWR CDC Surveill Summ 1998;47:1–13.

481. Adams JM, Kenney JD, Rudolph AJ. Modern management of tetanus neonatorum. Pediatrics 1979;64:472–7.

482. Craig AS, Reed GW, Mohon RT, et al. Neonatal tetanus in the United States: a sentinel event in the foreign-born. Pediatr Infect Dis J 1997;16:955–9.

483. Neonatal tetanus—Montana, 1998. MMWR 1998;47: 928–30.

484. American College of Obstetricians and Gynecologists. Immunization during pregnancy. ACOG Technical Bulletin 160. Washington, DC: American College of Obstetricians and Gynecologists, 1991.

485. Centers for Disease Control and Prevention. General recommendations on immunization: recommendations of the Advisory Committee on Immunizations Practices (ACIP). MMWR 1996;45(RR-5):1–24.

486. Gurkan F, Bosnak M, Dikici B, et al. Neonatal tetanus: a continuing challenge in the southeast of Turkey: risk factors, clinical features, and prognostic factors. Eur J Epidemiol 1999;15:171–4.

487. Editorial. Can modified tetanus occur? N Engl J Med 1962;266:1117–8.

488. Khajehdehi P, Rezaian GR. Tetanus in the elderly: is it different from that in younger age groups? Gerontology 1998;44:172–5.

489. Edsall G. Suspected tetanus in a previously immunized person [letter]. N Engl J Med 1965;273:1051.

490. Passen EL, Andersen BR. Clinical tetanus despite a "protective" level of toxin-neutralizing antibody. JAMA 1986; 255:1171–3.

491. Stoll BJ. Tetanus. Pediatr Clin North Am 1979;26: 415–31.

492. Veronesi R, Bizzini B, Focaccia R, et al. Naturally acquired antibodies to tetanus toxin in humans and animals from the Galapagos Islands. J Infect Dis 1983;147:308–11.

493. Holmes C, Flaherty RJ. Trimethobenzamide HCl (Tigan) induced extrapyramydal dysfunction in a neonate. J Pediatr 1976;89:669–70.

494. Scime IA, Tallant EJ. Tetanus-like reactions to prochlorperazine (Compazine): report of eight cases exhibiting extrapyramidal disturbances after small doses. JAMA 1959;171:1813–17.

495. Smith NU, Miller MM. Severe extrapyramidal reaction to perphenazine treated with diphenhydramine. N Engl J Med 1961;264:396–7.

496. Wang SF, Marlowe CL. Treatment of phenothiazine overdosage with physostigmine. Pediatrics 1977;59:301–3.

496a. Murison BB. Stiff-person syndrome. Neurologist 2004; 10:131–7.

497. Crisponi G. Autosomal recessive disorder with muscle contractions resembling neonatal tetanus, characteristic face, camptodactyly, hyperthermia, and sudden death: a new syndrome? Am J Med Genet 1996;24:365–71.

498. Gremse DA, Waterspiel JN. Acute poststreptococcal poly-myalgia with trismus. Pediatrics 1987;80:953–4.

499. Blake PA, Feldman RA, Buchanan TM, et al. Serologic therapy of tetanus in the United States, 1965–1971. JAMA 1976;235:42–4.

500. Ahmadsyah I, Salim A. Treatment of tetanus: an open study to compare the efficacy of procaine penicillin with metronidazole in the treatment of moderate tetanus. Br Med J 1985;29:640–50.

501. Schoefield FD, Tucker VM, Westbrook GR. Neonatal tetanus in New Guinea: effect of active immunization in pregnancy. Br Med J 1961;2:785–9.

502. King G, Schwartz GA, Slade HW. Acute cerebellar ataxia of childhood: report of 9 cases. Pediatrics 1958;21:731–44.

503. Lasater GM, Jabbour JT. Acute ataxia of childhood: a summary of fifteen cases. Am J Dis Child 1959;97:61–5.

504. Aigner BR, Siekert RG. Differential diagnosis of acute ataxia in children. Proc Staff Meet Mayo Clin 1959;34:573–81.

505. Yabek SM. Meningococcal meningitis presenting as acute cerebellar ataxia. Pediatrics 1973;52:718–20.

506. Connolly AM, Dodson WE, Prensky AL, Rust RS. Course and outcome of acute cerebellar ataxia. Ann Neurol 1994;35:673–9.

507. Shearer WT, Kobayashi G, Prensky AL. Presumptive histoplasmosis presenting as a cerebral ataxia with spontaneous recovery. Pediatrics 1975;57:150–2.

508. Erzurum S, Kalavsky SM, Watanakunakorn C. Acute cerebellar ataxia and hearing loss as initial symptoms of infectious mononucleosis. Arch Neurol 1983;40:760–2.

509. Nussinovitch M, Volovitz B, Varsano I. Complications of mumps requiring hospitalization in children. Eur J Pediatr 1995;154:732–4.

510. Nigro G, Pastoris MC, Fantasia MM, et al. Acute cerebellar ataxia in pediatric legionellosis. Pediatrics 1983;72:847–9.

511. al Eissa YA. Clinical and therapeutic features of childhood neurobrucellosis. Scand J Infect Dis 1995;27:339–43.

512. McAllister RM, Hummeler K, Coriell LL. Acute cerebellar ataxia: report of a case with isolation of Type 9 ECHO virus from the cerebrospinal fluid. N Engl J Med 1959;261:1159–62.

513. Cleary TG, Henle W, Pickering LK. Acute cerebellar ataxia associated with Epstein-Barr virus infection. JAMA 1980;243:148–9.

514. Munoz-Garcia D, Del Ser T, Bermejo F, Portera A. Truncal ataxia in chronic anticonvulsant treatment: association with drug-induced folate deficiency. J Neurol Sci 1982;55:305–11.

515. Lifshitz M, Gavrilov V, Sofer S. Signs and symptoms of carbamazepime overdose in young children. Pediatr Emerg Care 2000;16:26–7.

516. Gieron-Korthals MA, Westberry KR, Emmanuel PJ. Acute childhood ataxia: 10-year experience. J Child Neurol 1994;9:381–4.

517. Roberts KB, Freeman JM. Cerebral ataxia and "occult neuroblastoma" without opsoclonus. Pediatrics 1975;56:464–5.

518. al Ghamdi H, Sabbah R, Martin J, Patay Z. Primary T-cell lymphoma of the brain in children: a case report and literature review. Pediatr Hematol Oncol 2000;17:341–3.

519. DeMichele G, DiMaio L, Filla A, et al. Childhood onset of Friedreich ataxia: a clinical and genetic study of 36 cases. Neuropediatrics 1996;27:3–7.

520. Guerrini R, Belmonte A, Carrozzo R. Paroxysmal tonic upgaze of childhood with ataxia: a benign transient dystonia with autosomal dominant inheritance. Brain Dev 1998;20:116–8.

521. Kim HJ, Jeon BS. Acetazolamide-responsive hereditary paroxysmal ataxia: report of a family. J Korean Med Sci 1998;13:196–200.

522. Golden GS, French JH. Basilar artery migraine in young children. Pediatrics 1975;56:722–6.

523. Yuki N. Molecular mimicry between gangliosides and lipopolysaccharides of *Campylobacter jejuni* isolated from patients with Guillain-Barre syndrome and Miller Fisher syndrome. J Infect Dis 1997;176 Suppl 2:S150–3.

524. Bejar JM, Ziegler DK. Onset of multiple sclerosis in a 24-month-old child. Arch Neurol 1984;41:881–2.

525. Ruggieri M, Polizzi A, Pavone L, Grimaldi LM. Multiple sclerosis in children under 6 years of age. Neurology 1999;53:478–84.

526. Vasconcelos MM, Silva KP, Vidal G, et al. Early diagnosis of pediatric Wernicke's encephalopathy. Pediatr Neurol 1999;20:289–94.

527. Hahn JS, Berquist W, Alcorn DM, et al. Wernicke encephalopathy and beriberi during total parenteral nutrition attributable to multivitamin infusion shortage. Pediatrics 1998;101:e10.

528. Eviatar L, Eviatar B. Vertigo in children: differential diagnosis and treatment. Pediatrics 1977;59:833–8.

529. Beddoe GM. Vertigo in childhood. Otolaryngol Clin North Am 1977;10:139–44.

530. Meyerhoff WL, Paparella MM, Shea D. Meniere's disease in children. Laryngoscope 1978;88:1504–11.

531. Pedersen E. Epidemic vertigo: clinical picture, epidemiology and relation to encephalitis. Brain 1959;82:566–80.

532. Simonsen L, Khan AS, Gary HE Jr. Outbreak of vertigo in Wyoming: possible role of an enterovirus infection. Epidemiol Infect 1996;117:149–57.

533. Dunn DW, Snyder CH. Benign paroxysmal vertigo of childhood. Am J Dis Child 1976;130:1099–100.

534. Acomacchio F, D'Eredita R, Marchiori C. MRI evidence of labyrinthine and eighth-nerve bundle involvement in mumps virus sudden deafness and vertigo. ORL J Otorhinolaryngol Relat Spec 1996;58:295–7.

535. Stewart JM. Orthostatic hypotension in pediatrics. Heart Dis 2002;4:33–9.

536. Jacob G, Costa F, Shannon JR, et al. The neuropathic postural tachycardia syndrome. N Engl J Med 2000;343:1008–14.

537. Molteni RA. Vertigo as a presenting symptom of multiple sclerosis in childhood. Am J Dis Child 1977;131:553–4.

538. Jadavji T, Humphreys RP, Prober CG. Brain abscesses in infants and children. Pediatr Infect Dis 1985;4:394–8.

539. Fischer EG, McLennan JE, Suzuki Y. Cerebral abscess in children. Am J Dis Child 1981;135:746–9.

540. Idries ZH, Gutman LT, Kronfol NM. Brain abscesses in infants and children. Clin Pediatr 1978;17:738–46.

541. Kagawa M, Takeshita M, Yato S, et al. Brain abscess in

congenital cyanotic heart disease. J Neurosurg 1983;58: 913–7.

541a. Friedlander RM, Gonzalez RG, Afridi NA, Pfannl R. Case records of the Massachusetts General Hospital. Weekly clinicopathological exercises. Case 16-2003. A 58-year-old woman with left-sided weakness and a right frontal brain mass. N Engl J Med 2003;348:2125–32.

542. Peterson RA, Rosenthal A. Retinopathy and papilledema in cyanotic congenital heart disease. Pediatrics 1972;49: 243–9.

543. Giannoni C, Sulek M, Friedman EM. Intracranial complications of sinusitis: a pediatric series. Am J Rhinol 1998; 12:173–8.

544. Ecklund JM, Mauer PK, Ellenbogen RG. Cerebral abscess after presumed superficial periorbital wound. Mil Med 1999;164:444–5.

545. Bautistia-Casasnovas A, Varella-Cives R, Estevez-Martinez E, et al. What is the infection risk of esophageal dilatation? Eur J Pediatr 1998;157:901–3.

546. Leahy WR, Toyka KV, Fishbeck KH Jr, et al. Cerebral abscess in children secondary to esophageal dilatation. Pediatrics 1977;59:300–1.

547. Brook I. Bacteriology of intracranial abscess in children. J Neurosurg 1981;54:484–8.

548. Fleetwood IG, Embil JM, Ross IB. *Nocardia asteroides* cerebral abscess in immunocompetent hosts: report of three cases and review of surgical recommendations. Surg Neurol 2000;53:605–10.

549. Shah SS, Gallagher PG. Complications of conjunctivitis caused by *Pseudomonas aeruginosa* in a newborn intensive care unit. Pediatr Infect Dis J 1998;17:97–102.

550. Hanel RA, Araujo JC, Antoniuk A, et al. Multiple brain abscesses caused by *Salmonella typhi*: case report. Surg Neurol 2000;53:86–90.

551. Connor E, Menegus M, Cecalupo A, et al. Central nervous system toxoplasmosis mimicking a brain abscess in a compromised pediatric patient. Pediatr Infect Dis 1984; 3:552–5.

552. Antunes NL, Harihan S, DeAngelis LM. Brain abscesses in children with cancer. Med Pediatr Oncol 1998;31: 19–21.

553. Whelan MA, Hilal SK. Computed tomography as a guide in the diagnosis and follow-up of brain abscesses. Radiology 1980;135:663–71.

554. Rennels MB, Woodward CL, Robinson WL, et al. Medical cure of apparent brain abscesses. Pediatrics 1983;72: 220–4.

555. Britt RH, Enzmann DR. Clinical stages of human brain abscesses on serial CT scans after contrast infusion. J Neurosurg 1983;59:972–89.

556. Britt RH, Enzmann DR, Placone RC Jr, et al. Experimental anaerobic brain abscess. J Neurosurg 1984;60:1148–59.

557. Liston TE, Tomasovic JJ, Stevens EA. Early diagnosis and management of cerebritis in a child. Pediatrics 1979;65: 484–6.

558. Barlas O, Sencer A, Erkan K, et al. Stereotactic surgery in the management of brain abscess. Surg Neurol 1999; 52:404–10.

559. Yamamoto M, Fukushima T, Hirakawa K, et al. Treatment of bacterial brain abscess by repeated aspiration—follow-up by serial computed tomography. Neurol Med Chir Tokyo 2000;40:98–104.

560. Young RF, Frazee J. Gas within intracranial abscess cavities: an indication for surgical excision. Ann Neurol 1984; 16:35–9.

561. Wright RL, Ballantine HT. Management of brain abscess in children and adolescents. Am J Dis Child 1967;114: 113–22.

562. Weisberg LA, Chutorian AM. Pseudotumor cerebri of childhood. Am J Dis Child 1977;131:1243–8.

563. Rose A, Matson DD. Benign intracranial hypertension in children. Pediatrics 1967;39:227–37.

564. Imai WK, Everhart FR Jr, Sanders JM Jr. Cerebral venous sinus thrombosis: report of a case and review of the literature. Pediatrics 1982;70:965–70.

565. Walters BNJ, Gubbay SS. Tetracycline and benign intracranial hypertension: report of five cases. Br Med J 1981; 282:19–20.

CHAPTER 10

Fever and Shock Syndromes

■ GENERAL CONCEPTS

Definitions

Despite its frequency, there is no generally accepted definition of fever. A practical definition is a temperature above 38°C (100.4°F) by mouth or above 38.4°C (101°F) by rectum. Lower temperatures have been proposed as a definition of fever but are not practical and contribute to excessive concern, especially because it is not abnormal for a child to have a rectal temperature between 100°F and 101°F in the afternoon or after exercise.[1]

Fever is not equivalent to hyperthermia. Fever is an adaptive response that is well regulated by the body and is not dangerous in and of itself (although the *cause* of the fever may be quite serious). Temperatures due to fever almost never exceed 41°C (105.8°F). In contrast, hyperthermia is an elevated body temperature caused by a dysregulation of the normal mechanisms and can be very dangerous, with temperatures exceeding the body's set point. Examples include heat stroke (in which body temperature is elevated by external means) and malignant hyperthermia (caused by markedly increased heat production via uncoupling of oxidative phosphorylation).

Normal body temperature shows a diurnal variation, being lowest before awakening and highest in the late afternoon or evening. Fever curves usually follow this diurnal pattern also.

Conversion between Centigrade and Fahrenheit degrees can be made using the following formulas:

$$(C \times 9/5) + 32 = F$$
$$(F - 32) \times 5/9 = C$$

■ MECHANISMS

Body temperature is a dynamic balance between heat production and heat loss. In the case of infections, fever is probably produced both by vasoconstriction and by increased heat production. These functions are controlled by the thermoregulatory center in the hypothalamus, which responds to stimulation by pyrogens. Experimental studies have increased the understanding of the exogenous pyrogens of bacteria and the endogenous pyrogens produced by leukocytes. Currently recognized endogenous pyrogens include interleukin-1, TNF-α, interleukin-6, and interferon.[2]

Elevated core body temperature is the cardinal symptom of fever, but multiple other processes are involved. Fever is a well-regulated and complex physiologic response, involving generation of a host of cytokines and acute phase reactants and activation of numerous physiological, endocrinologic, and immunologic mechanisms.[2]

The increase in body temperature is modulated by the up-regulation of the thermostatic set point in the hypothalamus. The primary thermoregulatory mechanism used to maintain an elevated temperature is the redirection of blood flow from cutaneous to deep vascular beds, which minimizes heat loss through the skin.[3]

■ DANGERS AND BENEFITS

Convulsions can occur in children who have fever during relatively minor illnesses, as discussed in the section on febrile convulsions in Chapter 9. Body temperatures in excess of 42°C have multiple harmful effects. However, body temperature caused by the fever mechanism almost never reaches this level, unless there is failure of the thermoregulatory mechanims.[4]

Body temperatures above 42°C are nearly always the result of hyperthermia, not fever. Temperatures this high have numerous damaging cellular effects—most deaths from hyperthermia are due to cardiac arrhythmias.[3]

Fever has been postulated to have several effects that might be expected to be useful in the control of infectious diseases: white cell mobility is increased, some viruses and bacteria are killed, natural killer cell activity is increased, killing of bacteria by antibiotics is enhanced, and the effects of interferon are augmented. Despite these theoretical benefits, there is no clear evidence that fever has a measurable favorable influence on the course of any infectious disease in humans.

Temperature Measurement

Axillary temperature measurement is slow, has poor sensitivity in detecting fever, and is not recommended for use in infants and children in outpatient settings.[5] In rapidly breathing patients, even when there is no obvious mouth breathing, oral temperatures may be erroneously low.[6] The so-called tempadots (papers that are placed on the child's forehead) and temperature-taking pacifiers are inaccurate and should not be used. Tympanic membrane thermometers ("ear thermometers") have the advantage of being rapid, noninvasive, and painless; however, their accuracy has been questioned in several studies. Mothers' estimation of high fever in young children (< 2 years old) and their estimation that a child has no significant fever are very accurate most of the time, without the use of a thermometer.[7] However, the determination of so-called tactile fever should not be relied on in infants in the first 2 months of life.[8]

Medical lore holds that children with severe central nervous system (CNS) abnormalities have decreased temperature regulation and exaggerated fever responses, and this is supported by some studies.[9,10]

Corticosteroids, like antipyretics, can obscure the presence of fever. Sometimes, high fever occurs in children receiving high doses of corticosteroids, and other times, fever is obscured by steroids, especially in tuberculosis.[11]

Symptomatic Treatment

In each child with a fever, the physician should first ask whether any symptomatic treatment is really necessary. The phrase *fever phobia* has been used to describe undue worry by parents about fever.[12,13] A recent study showed that fever phobia persists despite efforts at education. About 25% of parents became worried enough about their child's fever that they measured his/her temperature five or more times a day, and an equal percentage of parents slept in the same room as the child with fever.[14] Fear of fever has also been documented to exist among medical professionals.[15]

Guidelines in counseling parents have been recommended for use for children over 6 months of age.[1,13] These include retaking the temperature after the child rests for one-half hour, defining 105°F as a high fever, teaching parents that normal body temperature regulation will keep the fever from going "out of control," and using antipyretic therapy only when fever makes the child uncomfortable.[13] Sponging has been recommended only if the temperatures are over 40°C (104°F) and then only if the temperature has not improved within 1 hour of giving an antipyretic. The child is not to be awakened for temperature taking or antipyretic administration because sleep is more important. The parents are taught that temperature taking or "breaking the fever" is not a substitute for more important observations, such as watching for dyspnea, change in consciousness, or pain.[1,13]

In general, excessive clothing or blankets should be removed to a point of comfort. Hydration with oral fluids is usually advised but should not be forced.

Sponging with tepid (but not cold) water is a comfortable and effective method that is traditional for high fever. One study showed that over the first 30 minutes sponging was more effective than either acetaminophen or ibuprofen, but by 60 minutes it was inferior to both of these agents.[16]

Sometimes hospitalized patients with high fevers are placed on cooling blankets to decrease their body temperature. A study of febrile adults in an intensive care unit found that the use of cooling blankets plus acetaminophen was no more effective in reducing fever than the use of acetaminophen alone. In addition, the use of cooling blankets was associated with wide fluctuation in temperatures and with rebound hypothermia.[17]

Unlike antipyretics, external cooling acts not by reducing the elevated set point but by overwhelming metabolically expensive effector mechanisms that have been evoked by the elevated set-point.[18]

For patients with hyperthermia, external cooling may be lifesaving. However, for patients with fever, the use of cooling blankets is nonsensical, as it causes forced peripheral vasoconstriction at a time when the body is attempting to dissipate heat by vasodilatation.

Antipyretics

Acetaminophen is similar to aspirin as an antipyretic and is less toxic to animals. Acetaminophen alone is comparable in efficacy to tepid water sponging and when used together, there is some additive effect.[19] The pediatric community has amassed a considerable amount of clinical experience using acetaminophen since aspirin (the old standard of care) was dropped as a pediatric antipyretic because of its association with Reye's syndrome.

Over the past decade, ibuprofen has been used with increasing frequency. Early reports about ibuprofen appeared to show that it reduced fever more rapidly and kept the fever down for a longer period of time than acetaminophen.[20, 21] However, a careful reading of those studies shows that the dosages of acetaminophen used were below the standard dose, which may have biased them toward finding ibuprofen to be superior. Furthermore, more recent studies have failed to find a difference, even when using a suboptimal dose of acetaminophen: no difference in time to lowest temperature, extent of temperature decrease, rate of temperature decrease, or duration of fever was found in groups taking 10 mg/kg of either preparation.[22]

Finally, although many pediatricians advise parents to alternate acetaminophen and ibuprofen, presumably to give a more frequent dose of antipyretics, there are no data supporting either the safety or the utility of this approach.[23] Until such a study has been performed, there is no rationale for the alternating antipyretic approach. Advising such a course of action is unwise; furthermore, it implies that absolute fever control is medically necessary, which it is not.

Complications of Fever Treatment

Sometimes, the treatment of fever produces more problems than the fever. Complications of treatment include antipyretic overdosage, particularly aspirin poisoning (salicylism), which was more common in the past. Acetaminophen can produce delayed liver toxicity or the rare complications of dermatitis, hypoglycemia, agranulocytosis, thrombocytopenia, and methemoglobinemia. Overdosage may produce prolongation of the prothrombin time, vomiting, hepatic failure, and death after 2–7 days. The toxicity of aspirin and acetaminophen have been reviewed in detail.[24]

Children administered ibuprofen have a higher rate of gastrointestinal bleeding than those treated with acetaminophen. Renal side effects have been reported, too, especially in children with preexisting renal problems or intravascular volume contraction.[25] There has been some concern that the use of ibuprofen for antipyresis in children with varicella may increase the risk of necrotizing fasciitis caused by Group A streptococcal superinfection. The evidence in favor of this association is one case-control study and one retrospective cohort study. The case-control study showed an odds ratio of 11.5 for ibuprofen use in children with necrotizing fasciitis versus the control group;[26] in many of these cases, ibuprofen use was initiated *after* the child had developed symptoms of secondary infection. This fact is used by many to say that perhaps ibuprofen use was simply a marker for more severe infection. However, studies in a rabbit model suggest that ibuprofen is capable of preventing neutrophil adhesion, suppressing azurophil granule secretion, and decreasing the production of superoxide,[27] all of which are mechanisms by which ibuprofen potentially could increase the risk of progression of an existing superinfection. The cohort study showed that if ibuprofen was dispensed to a child within the 30 days prior to the onset of varicella, the rate of bacterial skin superinfection was 3.1 times higher; if only superinfections severe enough to warrant hospitalization were included, that ratio rose to 5.1.[28] Problems with this study include that there is no evidence the children actually *took* the medication and that the confidence intervals of both odds ratios are wide, and the *P* values nonsignificant. Nevertheless, the suggestion of a possible association, coupled with the severity of the disease in question and the ready availability of an alternative antipyretic agent would seem to argue against the use of ibuprofen in children with varicella.

Poisoning can occur from inhalation of alcohol used to sponge the skin and may produce hypoglycemia and coma.[29,30]

In hospitalized patients who are being treated with an antibiotic, the use of antipyretics for moderate fever can interfere with the interpretation of the effectiveness of the antibiotic. However, if the infecting organism is known and the therapy known to be appropriate, then use of antipyretics for discomfort is appropriate.

■ CLASSIFICATION OF FEVER PATTERNS

Interpretation of fever patterns is difficult for many reasons: children are given antipyretics, which may alter the pattern; or consecutive temperatures may be taken by differing routes. Nevertheless, if a pattern of fever can be discerned, this information may provide additional diagnostic clues to the clinician. The classical fever pattern descriptions, along with the syndromes with which they have been associated, are shown in Table 10-1.[2]

Classification of Fever Syndromes

It is helpful to have a classification of fever syndromes for use in the problem-oriented approach. The classification in Table 10-2 was developed by Dechovitz and Moffet in 1968 by analyzing the records of 155 children hospitalized for fever and is the basis for subsequent individual sections in this chapter.[31]

Prolonged unexplained fever is defined as a documented fever higher than 38.4°C (101°F) occurring daily for more than 10 days. This pattern is often called "fever of unknown origin (FUO)."

Fever without localizing signs is defined as a fever of less than or equal to 10 days' duration, with no signs of the source of the infection on physical examination and normal urine. Newborn infants younger than 2 months old are excluded from this category, and children from 2 months to 2 years of age are considered a special subgroup because of an increased risk for occult bacteremia. At the time this classification was devised, many physicians were using the diagnosis of FUO wrongly to describe children with fever of brief duration without localizing signs. Of course, not every child with fever has a urinalysis and/or urine culture done in practice, but it is useful to retain this requirement in the definition to remind the clinician that the possibility of a urinary infection has not been excluded.

Fever with Nonspecific signs is defined as a fever of less than or equal to 10 days' duration and some abnormal physical findings that direct investigation to a specific area.

Fever complicating a chronic disease is defined as fever in a patient with a disease known to have a predilection for a particular febrile complication. Many chronic diseases have a particular expected febrile complication, such as subacute bacterial endocarditis or brain abscess, which must be considered in fever with congenital heart disease.

Fever in an immunocompromised host should be considered a separate category because the diagnostic considerations must be broadened to include opportunistic infections and because the urgency of providing specific therapy is usually greater (see Chapters 20, 22, and 23).

TABLE 10-1. SOME FEVER PATTERNS AND ASSOCIATED CAUSES

PATTERN	USUAL ASSOCIATED DISEASES
Continuous fever*	Pneumonia, typhoid, CNS disorders, tularemia, rickettsioses, falciparum malaria
Intermittent fever (quotidian)†	Abscesses, IE, brucellosis, JRA
Double quotidian‡	Salmonellosis, miliary TB, Neisserial IE
Saddle-back (biphasic) fever¶	Dengue, yellow fever, Colorado tick fever, relapsing fever, influenza, LCMV infection, leptospirosis
Intermittent hectic fever§	Cholangitis, JRA
Pel-Ebstein fever**	Hodgkin's, relapsing fever, brucellosis
Typhus inversus††	Military TB, hepatic abscess, IE, salmonellosis

* Sustained fever with only slight remissions not exceeding 2°F
† Exaggeration of the normal diurnal pattern, with low temperatures in the morning and high temperatures in the late afternoon
‡ Two spikes per day
¶ Several days of fever, afebrile for about 24 hours, then several additional days of fever
§ Sporadic episodes of fever mixed with periods of normal temperatures
** Fever for a week or longer, afebrile for similar period, then febrile again
†† Reversal of normal diurnal pattern (highest temperature elevation in the early morning)
CNS, central nervous system; IE, infective endocarditis; JRA, juvenile rheumatoid arthritis; TB, tuberculosis; LCMV, lymphocytic choriomeningitis virus
Modified from Mackowiak PA, Bartlett JG, Borden EC, et al. Concepts of fever: recent advances and lingering dogma. Clin Infect Dis 1997;25:119–38.

TABLE 10-2. CLASSIFICATION OF FEVER SYNDROMES

PATIENT GROUP	CHARACTERISTICS
Fever without localizing signs	Does not appear seriously ill
	No abnormalities on physical examination
	Normal urinalysis
	Duration ≤ 10 days
	Increased risk of occult bacteremia in those < 2 years old
Fever with nonspecific signs	Signs such as hepatosplenomegaly or abdominal mass are present but not diagnostic
Fever of unknown origin (prolonged unexplained fever)	Signs may be present but are not diagnostic. Initial studies (e.g., chest x-ray, throat culture, blood culture, and urine culture) are negative. Duration > 10 days
Fever complicating chronic disease	Patient has chronic disease with expected complication to be excluded
Fever in an immunocompromised host	Differential diagnosis includes opportunistic pathogens
	Patient's increased susceptibility necessitates a more rapid and/or invasive diagnostic approach
Fever secondary to a specific infection	Diagnosis of a specific, often localized, infection can be made by initial physical examination
Suspected septicemia	Child appears seriously ill or hypotensive
Neonatal fever	Suspect septicemia in infants < 2 months old. Hypothermia is equally important
Recurrent fever	Multiple separate episodes of documented high fever
Periodic fever	Recurrent fevers that occur at regular or predictable intervals (often 21 to 28 days)
Pseudofever	Temperatures < 38°C oral or < 38.4°C rectal in a well-appearing child

Recurrent fever is defined as separate episodes of definite high fever.

Periodic fever is defined as recurrent episodes of definite fever that occur at regular or predictable intervals.

Influenza-like illness is defined as fever with prominent respiratory symptoms of cough and sore throat without remarkable respiratory signs such as dyspnea or rales and usually including myalgia. This syndrome is discussed in Chapter 7. "Viral syndrome" is an inadequate working diagnosis, as it lacks the specificity of the previous diagnostic phrases.

Pseudofever is the term used when parents bring a child to medical attention for temperatures that are above their concept of "normal" but do not meet the definition of fever given earlier; that is, temperature greater than 37°C (98.6° F) but less than 38°C (100.4° F) oral or 38.4°C (101°F) rectal. Because this is not true fever at all or is just diurnal or exercise temperature variation, the clinician should try to avoid reiterating the parent's use of the word *fever*. It is helpful to explain to the parents that this is a normal variation of temperature, especially when the child's appearance and examination are normal, as discussed later.

■ FEVER WITHOUT LOCALIZING SIGNS

Definition

Fever without localizing signs is a tentative or working diagnosis and is best defined as:

1. Documented fever (rectal temperature of 38.4°C [101°F] or higher)
2. Brief duration (less than or equal to 10 days and usually only a few days)

3. No localizing signs sufficient to account for the fever
4. Normal urinalysis including microscopic examination and negative urine culture.

A urine dipstick examination that includes testing for leukocyte esterase and bacterial products such as nitrites might be substituted for a microscopic study. However, if a clean-catch urine has been obtained, the additional time involved in the more thorough study is usually minimal. It is not rare to discover important urinary tract disease when a proper urinalysis is done after a number of febrile illnesses attributed to respiratory infections (see Chapter 14).

The preliminary diagnosis of fever without localizing signs should be reserved for patients who do not appear seriously ill. Suspected septicemia should be the preliminary diagnosis if the patient is seriously ill or hypotensive.

Fever without localizing signs (FWLS) also should be defined to exclude the newborn and young infant in the first 2 months of life (Table 10-2). Neonatal fever is a better preliminary descriptive diagnosis and raises the question of sepsis, discussed in Chapter 19.

Fever without localizing signs as a preliminary diagnosis helps to avoid using more exact, but less certain, diagnoses. Other descriptive diagnoses with a similar meaning include "fever only," "undifferentiated febrile illness," "undiagnosed fever," and "fever, not seriously ill-appearing." All of these preliminary diagnoses are acceptable, but the term *fever without localizing signs* is being used more widely and is readily understood.

Inadequate Definitions

Although "flu syndrome" has been used to describe this pattern, it is not accurate, because influenza-like illnesses characteristically have prominent respiratory symptoms, especially cough and sore throat, as described in Chapter 7. "Viremia" has also been used to describe this syndrome, but this term is neither useful nor accurate, because documentation of a virus in the blood is rarely possible using currently available methods.

"Upper respiratory infection" (URI) is also an inappropriate diagnosis, because these patients do not have sufficient upper respiratory signs or symptoms to account for the magnitude of the fever. URI is too vague a diagnosis even when respiratory symptoms are present.

Clinical Course

The preliminary diagnosis of fever without localizing signs may be changed to another diagnosis as the course of the illness evolves. There are several courses the illness may take:

1. Development of new signs. When these signs occur, the physician may make a diagnosis of a specific localized infection, a viral exanthem such as roseola, or a working diagnosis of fever with nonspecific signs, indicating an area for investigation. Fever with nonspecific signs such as splenomegaly is discussed in a subsequent section of this chapter.
2. Persistence of fever. When fever persists for more than 10 days, the working diagnosis of prolonged unexplained fever or fever of unknown origin (FUO) is applicable, as described in a later section.
3. Complete, uneventful recovery. When the patient recovers uneventfully from the illness, the retrospective diagnosis can be undifferentiated febrile illness or self-limited febrile illness, as discussed later. In one study of 102 children with fever without localizing signs, about 70% had an uneventful recovery, whereas about 30% developed signs of a specific infectious disease.[31]

"Self-limited febrile illness" is a retrospective descriptive diagnosis used for a fever persisting for several days from which the patient recovers without antibiotic therapy and without any localized infection, rash, or other signs.[32] A urinary tract infection must be reliably excluded to make this diagnosis. If antibiotic therapy is used, the term *self-limited* is not appropriate. This syndrome is usually presumed to be a viral illness and has also been called "3-day fever," "acute undifferentiated febrile illness," "systemic infection," and "febrile illness of short duration."

Causes

Common Viruses

Coxsackieviruses and echoviruses are probably the most common causes of self-limited febrile illnesses in the United States.[33] Parainfluenza viruses also appear to be a common cause of this syndrome.[34] Adenovirus and influenza virus sometimes cause this syndrome (especially in young infants) but more frequently result in sufficient respiratory symptoms to be classified as an influenza-like illness.[35]

Bacteria

Many bacterial infections can be self-limited without antibiotic therapy (ear infections, streptococcal pharyngitis). Even bacteremias such as pneumococcemia, discussed later in this section, can be self-limited.

Uncommon

In endemic areas of the United States, arboviruses are an occasional cause of self-limited febrile illnesses during the season of the year that humans can be exposed to the arthropod vector. Such viruses include La Crosse encephalitis virus (California encephalitis virus) and equine encephalitis viruses.

Other uncommon causes of self-limited febrile illnesses in the United States include lymphocytic choriomeningitis virus infection,[36] Colorado tick fever (a virus),[37] and tick-borne relapsing fever, a spirochetal disease in the western United States.[38]

Ehrlichiosis

There are two forms of ehrlichiosis: human monocytic ehrlichiosis (HME) and human granulocytic ehrlichiosis (HGE). HME is much more common. It is caused by a rickettsial organism known as *Ehrlichia chaffeensis* that can cause fever in humans after a tick bite.[39,40] Formerly recognized only in dogs, the human disease was originally described as resembling Rocky Mountain spotted fever (RMSF) without a rash, and therefore was sometimes referred to as Rocky Mountain spotless fever. This name, for several reasons, should not be used. First, the same name is being applied to patients who become infected with *Rickettsia rickettsiae* and develop symptoms of RMSF but without a rash. Second, some patients do develop a rash during the course of ehrlichiosis. In fact, rash seems to be more common in children than it is in adults and was found in two-thirds of childhood cases of HME in the largest series published to date.[41]

Fever and myalgia are seen in most patients, and about a fourth have headache, vomiting, and diarrhea.[41] Laboratory findings that suggest the diagnosis include thrombocytopenia, lymphopenia or leukopenia, anemia, and hyponatremia. Liver enzymes are commonly mildly elevated. This diagnosis needs to be seriously considered in patients who present during "tick season" with fever, myalgia, and headache, with or without rash, who have suppression of one or more cell lines on complete blood count. Doxycycline is the drug of choice in all age groups.[42] The illness can be quite severe and even life-threatening.[43] Some patients with long-term cognitive or subtle neurologic abnormalities have been identified,[41] but most make a complete recovery with appropriate therapy. The diagnosis is established by demonstrating a fourfold rise in antibody titers to *E. chaffeensis*, or by an acute titer over 1:64 in a patient with a clinically compatible illness. Polymerase chain reaction (PCR) is very sensitive but is not widely available.[43a] Morulae (cytoplasmic vacuoles containing the organisms) are usually not demonstrable. Therapy must be started before the diagnosis is confirmed. HGE, caused by *Anaplasma* (formerly, *Ehrlichia*) *phagocytophila*,[43b] clinically resembles HME but granulocytopenia, rather than lymphopenia, is observed. Because this pathogen is carried by the *Ixodes* species of tick, its distribution resembles that of Lyme disease.[43c]

Unknown

Unknown or unidentified viruses may be a cause of this syndrome, but most children do not have any virus recovered when studied using available techniques. Other infectious agents such as Epstein-Barr virus (EBV) or cytomegalovirus (CMV) are often not detected, because no specific diagnostic studies are done when the child does not seem very sick and is afebrile within a few days.

Development of Focal Infections

Pharyngitis

Frequently in young children, infections are manifested only by fever, with considerable delay in localization of the infection. Frontal headaches and abdominal pain may develop and provide a clue to the diagnosis. It is wise to perform a throat culture for Group A streptococci in most young children with fever without localizing signs in the first day or two of the fever (see Table 2-4). However, even school-age children sometimes do not develop signs of exudative pharyngitis until a day after the onset of fever (see Fig. 2-4).[32] Because of such delays in localization of infection, the physician should not omit follow-up physical examination in a patient with continued fever on the assumption that the patient has a benign, self-limiting viral illness.

Pneumonia

Unrecognized pneumonia is one of the most frequent focal causes of fever without localizing signs. Abdominal pain (probably really pleuritic or referred from the diaphragm) and vomiting may mislead the clinician toward the abdomen.

Other

Although the majority of infections observed will not be serious, a few patients will be found to have such serious illnesses as osteomyelitis, septic arthritis, or meningitis. One value of the preliminary diagnosis of fever without localizing signs is the emphasis on the need to repeat the physical examination looking for localizing signs of infection.

In a 1968 study of hospitalized children, the earliest indication of a localized infection was usually the development of abnormalities on physical examination.[31] In fact, about 20% of the 105 patients hospitalized because of undiagnosed fever had evidence of a specific localized infection on the first physical examination after admission. Presumably, they had developed these signs of a specific infection *after* the physical examination that led to the hospitalization. After throat culture and urinalysis were negative, further laboratory studies rarely provided the first clue to the final diagnosis. A notable exception was the chest x-ray, which revealed six unsuspected cases of pneumonia, usually lobar or segmental, which presumably were pneumococcal.

In children, the most frequent infections that are likely to be recognized by new localized signs are exanthems (especially roseola syndrome, presumed enteroviral rashes, or occasionally rickettsial disease); exudative tonsillitis, otitis media, or stomatitis; meningitis (purulent or aseptic); pneumonia, parotitis or cervical adenitis; and arthritis or osteomyelitis. These localized infections are discussed further in other chapters.

Laboratory Approach

Exposures

In a child older than 2 years, the history and physical examination usually allow the clinician to decide if a laboratory workup is needed. If other family members or school contacts have been having self-limited febrile illnesses, this is an important clue to the probability of a viral etiology, and it is likely that no further laboratory studies are required.

No laboratory test should be done *routinely* in a child with fever without localizing signs. Sometimes, minor symptoms might suggest some value to a particular test, especially if the general appearance or magnitude of the fever (above 39.5°C [103°F]) is suspicious.

Throat Culture

This may reveal Group A streptococci if sore throat is present early in the illness and the fever is above 38.8°C (102°F), as discussed earlier.

Urinalysis and Culture

This has already been mentioned in the definition of fever without localizing signs. Usually, fever secondary to a urinary infection is accompanied by urinary symptoms, but these may not be recognized in a younger child. The yield for finding a positive urine culture is low (2%) in febrile children,[44] but urinary tract infections are important to diagnose and treat.

White Blood Cell Count and Differential

This study may be useful in a teenager with fever and fatigue to detect atypical lymphocytosis in the typhoidal presentation of infectious mononucleosis. It also may be useful for the sicker-appearing child with a higher fever, although leukocytosis is nonspecific and may only stimulate a more careful reexamination or possibly other simple specific studies.

Chest Roentgenogram

In the younger, sicker-appearing child, especially one with leukocytosis and some cough, an unrecognized bacterial pneumonia may be present without many clinical signs. Reexamination after the diagnosis may reveal some slight splinting or tachypnea (beyond that attributable to the fever), but often it does not. A chest roentgenogram was the most useful study that detected a focal infection unsuspected by physical examination in one large study of febrile children.[31] This is a lesson frequently relearned even by experienced clinicians. It is reasonable to include a chest x-ray in the evaluation of the child with FWLS, even in the absence of respiratory signs or symptoms if the fever has been present for three or more days.

Lumbar Puncture

If there is any clinical suspicion of a CNS infection in febrile infants or young children, a lumbar puncture is indicated. In children beyond infancy, more definite signs are usually present with CNS infections. With increased experience, the physician becomes more skillful at recognizing these findings. However, in situations in which parents are unreliable about observing the young child or seeking care promptly, lumbar puncture should be done for less-obvious medical indications.

Management

In the child over 2 years of age with fever without localizing signs, clinical decisions concerning hospitalization and therapy can be based on the clinical findings, ability of parents to judge changes, and convenience and reliability of follow-up contacts. Usually, the child can be followed by telephone if done carefully, with return visits as necessary for reexamination and without antibiotic therapy if there is no specific likely explanation for the fever. New symptoms or signs may be noted on follow-up, the illness may resolve without a diagnosis, or hospitalization may be needed for further study.

Instructions to Parents

The parents can be told that a bacterial infection is unlikely but that the child should be reexamined if significant new symptoms develop, such as difficulty in arousing the child, difficult breathing, changes in sleep patterns, or pain or tenderness in any area. Parents can make the other clinical observations (such as playfulness) described later. They should be told to note the general appearance and alertness of the child and to call the physician if the child appears worse by the preceding criteria or if a rash is noted. The availability of the physician for follow-up should be emphasized. A return visit in 24 hours should be required for some patients, such as those who have very high fever (>39.5°C). For other children, the parents should be instructed to bring the child back for another examination if the fever is still present in 3 to 4 days. Fluids should be encouraged; solids are unnecessary but permissible. Symptomatic treatment of fever may be indicated, as described earlier in this chapter.

■ HIGH FEVER IN NEONATES, INFANTS, AND TODDLERS

Historical Factors

Beginning in the early 1970s, there was an increasing appreciation of the occurrence of unrecognized ("occult" or "outpatient") bacteremia in young children (younger than 2 years and younger than 3 months became established as the major age breakpoints). Within recent years, the cutoff age for hospital admission for suspected sepsis in babies with fever has been changed to 2 months in some centers, and to 4–6 weeks in others. Prospective studies have looked at many clinical, laboratory, and epidemiologic variables, so that more accurate information is now available about one of the most difficult clinical diagnostic problems: high fever in young children.

It is not surprising that age breakpoints have become so helpful in assessing the probabilities for various infections, as pediatrics is a field that makes progressively finer age distinctions at younger ages.

Age Differences

Infants younger than 2 months are susceptible to more diseases and are often treated similarly to newborns, but they also may have many of the same diseases as older infants. Early in this period, there is less social eye contact and less social smiling, and as a consequence, the general appearance is harder to evaluate.[45] Additionally, babies are unable to communicate, which makes interpretation and diagnosis of their illnesses somewhat trickier. Finally, young infants often develop similar, nonspecific signs and symptoms in response to a wide variety of illnesses; this makes distinguishing the cause of the fever difficult.

Most physicians have routinely hospitalized infants less than 2 months of age because of fever, regardless of the results of preliminary laboratory studies. This policy is discussed later. In one series of 169 children aged 3 months or younger, serious infections were found in 8 (36%) of 22 infants with a temperature of 40°C (104°F) or higher and in 15 (10%) of 147 infants with fever of 37.5°C to 39.9°C (100°F to 103.9°F) who were brought to an emergency room.[46]

In another series of infants less than 6 months of age, the frequency of serious illness was higher in those with very high temperatures.[47] This general correlation of magnitude of fever with seriousness of illness has been found in many studies, but additional clinical and laboratory findings can be used to develop more predictive accuracy than the fever alone. An exception to this rule is a temperature 41.1°C (106°F) or more, which is frequently associated with serious illness regardless of other findings.[48] In general, hospitalization can be individualized rather than routine for those older than 1 month old, depending on the findings and the ability and accessibility of the parents (Table 10-3).

Causes

Viral Infections

In a study of 182 young infants with fever, enteroviruses (coxsackieviruses and echovirus) were the most frequent cause,[49] as is the case in older infants and preschool children.[50] During influenza virus outbreaks, high fever and lethargy secondary to influenza virus infections can mimic septicemia in young infants.[51]

In a study of 258 febrile children in Finland, 66% of whom were less than 2 years of age, fever from respiratory virus infection was just as likely to be as high and to last as long as in serious bacterial infections, with 37% of the children having fever lasting 5 days or longer.[52] In another study of very young infants with fever, nonpurulent meningitis (presumably viral) was the most frequent cause found, but nearly 70% of infants had no cause found and presumably had self-limited viral infections.[53]

Focal Bacterial Infections

In one study, urinary tract infections were a frequent cause of fever in young infants, particularly

---

TABLE 10-3. MODIFIED ROCHESTER CRITERIA AND MODIFIED PHILADELPHIA CRITERIA FOR IDENTIFICATION OF FEBRILE INFANTS 28–90 DAYS WHO ARE AT LOW RISK FOR SERIOUS BACTERIAL INFECTION

	ROCHESTER	PHILADELPHIA
Clinical appearance	"Well-appearing"	Yale observational score < 10
History	≥ 37 weeks gestation	Absence of recognizable immunodeficiency
	• Discharged from birth hospitalization with mother (or before)	
	• No hyperbilirubinemia	
	• No antibiotics (either perinatally or more recently)	
	No underlying illness	
Physical examination	No evidence of focal infection (soft tissue, bone, joint, or ear)	No evidence of focal infection (soft tissue, bone, joint, or ear)
Laboratory evaluation		
CBC	• WBC 5000 to 15,000/μL	WBC < 15,000/μL
	• Band count ≤ 1500/μL	Band to neutrophil ratio < 0.2
Urinalysis	≤ 10 WBC/hpf	< 10 WBC/hpf; negative Gram stain
Cerebrospinal fluid	None	< 8 WBC/μL; negative Gram stain
Chest x-ray	None	No infiltrate*
Stool studies	≤ 5 WBC/hpf*	"Normal"*

Abbreviations: CBC = complete blood count; WBC = white blood count; hpf = high-powered field.
* These studies were obtained selectively.

in uncircumcised boys.[49] Salmonellosis, with or without diarrhea, was also observed in this study. Other studies have indicated other focal infections such as bone and joint infections.

Occult Bacteremia

Occult bacteremia is a condition in which a young child is febrile, physical examination reveals no obvious source for the fever, and the child is judged well enough to be managed as an outpatient, but blood culture obtained at the time of evaluation yields a pathogenic bacterium. This condition is most commonly caused by the pneumococcus, but cases of unsuspected bacteremia with meningococcus, *Haemophilus influenzae* type b, nontyphi *Salmonella* species, and other bacteria also occur. The incidence of occult bacteremia secondary to Hib has decreased because of the widespread use of conjugated Hib vaccine. The prognosis of occult bacteremia has, therefore, changed; this is discussed in more detail later. Occult bacteremia is an important cause of fever in infants up to about 2 years of age.[54–56] The child typically has high fever without localizing signs, although a few patients have upper respiratory findings and a few have had a seizure. Historically, the incidence of occult bacteremia in children between the ages of 6 and 24 months who present with FWLS has been estimated to be approximately 5%; a more recent, large study found a lower incidence of 1.9%.[57] To a certain extent, the prevalence of occult bacteremia in a study of children with FWLS depends on the stringency of the inclusion criteria used in the study. Bass et al. found that about 16% of children in their study had occult bacteremia; their study enrolled only children with fever greater than 39.5°C *and* a white blood cell (WBC) count greater than 15,000/μL, or children with fever greater than 40.0°C.[58] However, the overall incidence of occult bacteremia continues to decline based on the widespread use of conjugated vaccines against both Hib and *Streptococcus pneumoniae*.

Marked leukocytosis (greater than 25,000/μL) is often found with pneumococcal bacteremia. In one series of 111 infants and children with pneumococcal bacteremia, 41 (37%) had a WBC count higher than 25,000/μL.[54] There were fifteen patients with no clearly defined source of the bacteremia, and seven of these had an initial WBC count higher than 24,000/μL. In another series of twelve patients with unexpected pneumococcal bacter-

emia, all had a white cell count higher than 20,000/μL.[55] In another report of twenty-two patients with occult pneumococcal bacteremia, nine had WBC counts higher than 20,000/μL.[56] Although very high WBC counts are frequently seen with pneumococcal bacteremia, this finding is not universal; thus one is not able to rule out bacteremia based on a lower WBC count.

Febrile convulsions occasionally occur in pneumococcal bacteremia.[54–56] Hyponatremia, petechiae, and vomiting were also observed in some of these patients.[54–56]

The prognosis of occult bacteremia is changing; in general it is better than might be expected given the presence of bacteria in the blood stream. Older, retrospective studies warned the physician of a 5–10% risk of bacterial meningitis, a 10% risk of localized bacterial infection, and another 30% risk of continued bacteremia and fever.[59] One study that helped to prompt the widespread use of intramuscular ceftriaxone in the outpatient setting estimated that the risk of meningitis in occult bacteremia was 9.8% in patients given no antibiotic therapy, 8.2% in patients treated with oral antibiotics, and 0.3% in those given parenteral antibiotic treatment.[60] This study was a Bayesian meta-analysis of published studies available at the time. Of importance is that all cases of bacterial meningitis that resulted from untreated or insufficiently treated occult bacteremia were caused by Hib. Because Hib is no longer the second most common cause of occult bacteremia, the outcome of pneumococcal bacteremia has become the statistic of most interest. The course of unrecognized pneumococcal bacteremia is varied, but it is better than that of occult bacteremia due to Hib or to the meningococcus. Hib is about 12 times more likely than *S. pneumoniae* to cause meningitis in patients who present with occult bacteremia.[61]

Two recent large studies paint a clearer picture of risks in the current environment. The first was a prospective evaluation of children between 3 and 36 months of age with fever of 39°C or higher who had no obvious focus of infection and were discharged home from the emergency department. This study focused primarily on determining the prevalence of occult bacteremia in this population. Blood cultures were obtained from 9,465 children who fit this description; (1.6%) children had blood cultures that were positive for pathogenic organisms.[62] The second was a retrospective study of FWLS in children from 2–24 months of age in a pediatric emergency department. This study found bacteremia in 111 (1.8%) of 5,901 children; 83% were caused by the pneumococcus, and 96% of those underwent resolution of their bacteremia without therapy.[57] *Salmonella* was the second most common isolate, accounting for 5.4% of occult bacteremia, followed by Group A streptococci. No cases of either Hib or meningococcal occult bacteremia were seen.

Bacteremia caused by the meningococcus, *Salmonella, Staphylococcus aureus,* and even gram-negative enteric bacteria are uncommon causes of fever in infants.[63–65] Hib bacteremia has become very rare. The child typically becomes sicker within hours or develops localizing signs. The clinical manifestations of septicemia with these bacteria are discussed later in the section on septicemia and bacteremia.

Clinical Evaluation

The separation of febrile infants with early serious infections from those with benign self-limited illnesses is one of the most difficult decisions in the care of children. Every experienced pediatrician has known the feeling of not recognizing an early serious infection.

Prospective studies have been done, especially by McCarthy and colleagues, to help give guidelines for both clinical and laboratory evaluation.[66–70] Unfortunately, rapid and unexpected change is typical of illness in young children. No laboratory tests or clinical observations detect all of the children who progress to a serious illness, so that follow-up clinical observations by the physician and parents are essential.

What observations help the parent or physician detect a worsening course? In studies directed at this question, the child's playfulness and eye contact were helpful guides.[69,70] Other useful criteria were the degree of alertness and of consolability, essential observations needed to determine potential severity. Other definable components include the infant's use of its eyes to observe people, spontaneous arm and leg movement, appropriate smiling or crying, playing, sucking, reaching, and vocalizing. Generally, patients as a group can be divided into those who are at high risk and those who are at low risk of bacteremia or invasive disease. However, this ability does not extend to the individual patient level; in other words, some children initially designated as being at low risk for serious infection prove to develop serious infection, and some children initially thought to be at high risk prove to have trivial self-limiting illnesses.

Duration of Fever

In young children at risk for occult bacteremia, the duration of fever correlates inversely with the presence of bacteremia. A prospective study of 6,619 children with FWLS showed that a greater proportion of those with fever for less than one day had positive blood cultures than those with fever for greater than one day.[71] The incidence in those with fever for less than 2 days, in turn, was higher than for those with fever for longer than 2 days. Presumably, patients with occult bacteremia become ill quite suddenly and seek medical attention more quickly than do patients without bacteremia.

Afebrile Bacteremia

In a review of 182 children with bacteremia during an 18-month period, 24 (13%) were afebrile at the time of evaluation in the emergency room.[72] However, half had received recent antipyretics because of a history of fever. Of the five afebrile children who also had no recent history of fever, localizing signs of meningitis, pneumonia, or orbital cellulitis were present in four, and the other appeared clinically "toxic." This study serves to remind clinicians what they already know: Absence of fever can accompany clinical findings of significant infection.

Response to Acetaminophen

Improvement in clinical appearance and reduction of fever after an appropriate dose of acetaminophen does not exclude the possibility of severe illness.[73] A prospective trial of 154 children with FWLS, 19 of whom had positive blood cultures, showed that the response to acetaminophen did not differ between the groups; furthermore, the appearance of the child when afebrile (often cited as a differentiating factor by practicing physicians) was shown to be identical.[74] Only those with meningitis remained ill appearing when fever was reduced. Perhaps the clinician should be more wary when a child remains ill appearing after fever reduction, but response to acetaminophen or ibuprofen can be misleading and thus should not be used as a diagnostic test.

Laboratory Approach
White Blood Cell Count and Differential

Most prospective studies have confirmed the value of the WBC count that was observed in retrospective reviews of "outpatient bacteremia" and occult pneumococcemia in the 1970s.[53,75–80] It appears to be the simplest and most reliable of the laboratory tests, is applicable to office practice, and can be used together with clinical and social factors either to help decrease the concern for serious disease or to stimulate further laboratory studies.

A marked leukocytosis (greater than 25,000/μL) with a predominance of neutrophils is often taken as presumptive evidence for a bacterial infection, although this criterion has not been adequately studied in a prospective fashion, because the final etiologic diagnosis is often unknown. The most widely used screening values (in conjunction with high fever) are a count of 15,000/μL or more and total segmented neutrophils of 10,000/μL or more.

Bass et al.'s careful, multicenter, prospective study of children with high fever clearly showed an increased risk of occult bacteremia with increasing peripheral WBC count. Bacteremia was documented in none of 99 children with a WBC count less than 10,000/μL; in 21 (8%) of 265 children with a WBC count from 10,000/μL to less than 20,000/μL; in 30 (24%) of 127 children with a WBC count from 20,000/μL to less than 30,000/μL; and in 9 (43%) of 21 children with a WBC count more than 30,000/μL.[58]

Vacuolization and Toxic Granulation

The value of these morphologic changes in segmented neutrophils is unclear. They were found to be sensitive and specific predictors of bacteremia in one study[80] but of no predictive value in another.[81]

C-Reactive Protein

Although C-reactive protein is usually elevated in children with occult bacteremia, sensitivity and specificity are insufficient to make the test of any clinical utility.[82,83]

Chest Roentgenogram

The principles discussed earlier for the child over 2 years of age with fever without localizing signs also apply to the infant with fever. In the older infant, unsuspected pneumonia may be discovered by a chest x-ray to be the cause of high fever and marked leukocytosis. Outpatient management may be practical for some older infants.

Lumbar Puncture

Meningitis is likely to be subtler in terms of clinical findings as the age of the infant decreases. A lumbar puncture may also reveal nonpurulent meningitis, giving an explanation for the fever that can be managed as described in Chapter 9. Lumbar puncture should not be withheld for fear of producing meningitis in a bacteremic child.[86]

Urinalysis and Urine Culture

A collaborative study to determine the frequency of urinary infection in febrile infants indicated a rate of 4%, all in girls.[87] Another study found uncircumcised boys to be at higher risk than circumcised boys.[49] As discussed in Chapter 14, bagged urine specimens often reflect the periurethral flora. When there is no indication of the source of the fever, especially if the temperature is 103°F or higher, a catheterized urine for microscopic study and culture is reasonable. Although the yield is low,[87] it is the young infant who is at highest risk for renal damage from unrecognized infection, especially if there is an underlying congenital urinary tract anomaly (Chapter 14).

Outpatient Blood Cultures

Studies of outpatients in the early 1970s showed that blood cultures were positive in a small percentage of children with fever, particularly those under 2 years of age with higher fever (104°F, 40°C) or leukocytosis (greater than 20,000/L).[63] S. pneumoniae and H. influenzae were the most frequent species detected, but Group A streptococci, S. aureus, Salmonella, and meningococci were also detected, along with a number of skin contaminants. One emergency room study reported that 25% of the positive blood cultures were attributable to contaminants.[64] In the newer study mentioned previously, however, only 2.1% of positive blood cultures were thought to be secondary to contamination.[57] Using continuously monitored blood culture systems such as BACTEC may be helpful in differentiating true pathogens from contaminants: The mean time to positivity in patients with true pathogens was 15 hours; it was 31 hours in those with contaminants.[57]

In other studies, some of the children did not seem seriously ill or had seemingly trivial illnesses, but a high fever (140°F, 40°C) or a high leukocyte count (20,000/μL) was clearly a risk factor.

These studies led to the definition and recognition of occult bacteremia. Many pediatricians in private practice have been skeptical that outpatient blood culture is superior to careful follow-up, especially because many bacteremic children do not develop serious illness rapidly or without clinical findings on follow-up examination. In one study of 4,151 visits to private practices, with 145 children aged 3–24 months deemed "at risk" for occult bacteremia, blood cultures, sedimentation rates, and WBC counts were seldom used, but hospitalizations were rare, and no deaths or notable sequelae were encountered.[88]

Bacteremia with *H. influenzae* is certainly a potentially serious disease. One study of 69 children with culture-proven Hib bacteremia found that on follow-up, 36 (52%) of the children were still clinically ill; 17 developed meningitis, 5 got pneumonia, 3 had epiglottitis, 5 had cellulitis, 3 had septic arthritis, and 3 were persistently febrile. Even the patients who felt well at follow-up were apparently not safe; 3 (9%) of 33 were still bacteremic despite being afebrile, and 5 (15%) developed a secondary focus of infection.[89] This is in sharp contrast to the 96% spontaneous cure rate observed with pneumococcal bacteremia in the retrospective emergency department study cited earlier.[57]

The criteria have not been entirely clarified for the use of blood cultures in the office of the private pediatrician or the walk-in clinic, which may deal with a different patient population. One of the best analyses of this dilemma deserves quotation: "When good observation or a well-functioning relationship with the medical system does not exist, the blood culture may serve an 'administrative' function by bringing to attention those infants in need of prompt recall and re-evaluation."[90]

For some physicians, "obtaining a blood culture binds anxiety" (by giving the feeling that one is 'doing something'), but it is not by itself therapeutic for the infant."[90] At the present time, most investigators emphasize that blood cultures obtained selectively, using some clinical and laboratory criteria, do result in the detection of infants at higher risk of developing serious disease. However, it has also been noted that the same criteria for obtaining blood cultures can be applied for using outpatient antibiotic therapy until culture results are known.[91] The efficacy of such treatment is unknown, and the patient must still be followed carefully. The rate of false-positive blood cultures (2% to 40%) and the cost of cultures also make them only another test, the value of which depends on the clinician's judg-

ment and experience with its use. Sloppy, injudicious, and unwise use and interpretation of blood cultures in the setting of fever can lead to enormous costs, both financial and psychological. In one extreme example, 41% of positive blood cultures contained only contaminants; despite this, phone calls, return visits, extra diagnostic procedures, and hospital admissions resulted, amassing a cost of $78,904, or $642 for every true pathogen isolated.[92] It should be noted that, in most centers, the rate of false positive blood cultures is less than 5%.

Antibiotics in Febrile Outpatients

Antibiotics are usually not indicated in children over 2 years of age with fever without localizing signs, because most of these illnesses are viral. If an antibiotic is used and fever persists, there may be continued confusion and changing of antibiotics. In addition, antibiotics may disguise localizing signs of infection and sometimes allow unrecognized progression of tissue damage. Antibiotics do not reduce bacterial complications of acute viral diseases. In addition, antibiotics can be a cause of persistent fever and rarely may have serious, even life-threatening, toxicities.

Criteria for Antibiotic Use

In children younger than 2 years of age, it has been suggested that a nontoxic infant who meets the criteria for an outpatient blood culture merits antibiotic therapy.[91,93] Some studies of antibiotics in febrile infants have been done. In the oldest studies, an injection of procaine-benzathine penicillin followed by oral penicillin V was better than a placebo for nonhospitalized infants at high risk of bacteremia.[94] Oral amoxicillin was no different from a placebo in another study of febrile infants.[95] A meta-analysis of all published trials that compared oral antibiotics (usually amoxicillin) with no treatment in children whose cultures eventually grew *S. pneumoniae* showed a modest benefit of oral antibiotics. A total of 656 cases of pneumococcal occult bacteremia were identified. The incidence of serious bacterial infections was 3.3% in the group given oral antibiotics versus 9.9% in those left untreated. Meningitis developed in 7 (2.7%) of 257 children in the untreated control group, but only in 3 (0.8%) of the 399 children given oral antimicrobials.[96] The numbers concerning the incidence of meningitis were too small to reach statistical significance, but a trend was demonstrated. It must be remembered that this study included only those with proven bacteremia, not a population of children with FWLS, the majority of whom do not have occult bacteremia.

It has become increasingly popular to give children who present with high fever and/or a WBC count over 15,000/μL an injection of intramuscular ceftriaxone. Although emergency department physicians could not agree about which patients need WBC counts, which patients need blood cultures, or which patients require other diagnostic evaluations, 75% of them agreed on IM ceftriaxone as their first choice for patients at high risk for occult bacteremia.[97] The popularity of IM ceftriaxone in the setting of FWLS stems from a couple of studies: (1) The study that cited a 9.8% risk of progression to meningitis in children without therapy of occult bacteremia also found that none of 139 patients who received IM ceftriaxone developed meningitis.[97a] (2) A multicenter prospective trial of IM ceftriaxone versus oral amoxicillin for patients with occult bacteremia reported that there were three patients with persistently positive blood cultures and two children with positive spinal fluid cultures among those who were randomized to the oral amoxicillin arm, but none in the ceftriaxone group. The paper went on to state that probable or definite serious bacterial infections occurred in six children in the oral amoxicillin group, but in only three children in the ceftriaxone group. Finally, fever persisted longer in those who received oral amoxicillin.[98]

How do we account for these differences, if ceftriaxone is not, indeed, superior? In the first study, all the patients who developed meningitis had Hib infection. Occult bacteremia due to Hib, as mentioned earlier, is a disappearing disease. In the second study, the children in the parenteral group received 50 mg/kg of ceftriaxone, whereas the children in the oral treatment group received 20 mg/kg/dose of amoxicillin for 6 doses (60 mg/kg/d for 2 days). These dosages are probably not equivalent. In the era of increasing penicillin resistance among isolates of the pneumococcus, a larger dose of amoxicillin would be prudent to ensure levels that exceed the minimum inhibitory concentration of most isolates. A careful reading of the second study also reveals some problems with outcome assignment. One of the patients in the amoxicillin group grew *S. pneumoniae* from spinal fluid that was obtained *before* amoxicillin was administered.

Additionally, two children in the ceftriaxone group had cerebrospinal fluid (CSF) pleocytosis at the time of follow-up; in the setting of proven bacteremia, these findings are indicative of bacterial meningitis, despite negative CSF cultures. Reassigning these patients gives a total of five serious bacterial infections (four meningitis) in the ceftriaxone group and five serious bacterial infections (two meningitis) in the amoxicillin group, results that surely cannot be construed to support the supposed superiority of ceftriaxone.[98a]

Moreover, the incidence of bad outcomes from occult bacteremia is decidedly lower in the post-Hib era. Thus, differences in efficacy between IM ceftriaxone and oral amoxicillin, even if they exist, are not likely to be *clinically* significant. One large meta-analysis comparing the two regimens concluded that the differences are so small that a study that included more than 7,500 bacteremic children (approximately 300,000 with FWLS) would be required to demonstrate superiority of one regimen over the other.[98b] Drawbacks to the widespread use of IM ceftriaxone, on the other hand, are obvious and include pain, expense, potentially serious drug reactions, and widespread increases in antibiotic resistance patterns of common bacteria. Giving IM ceftriaxone in this setting effectively asks the parents to judge whether they think their child is developing partially treated bacterial meningitis, a daunting task even for the trained professional.[98a] There is no support for the unfortunately widespread practice of administering IM ceftriaxone without obtaining blood cultures.

The problem becomes stickier still if one extends it to its true setting; that is, in clinical practice, the physician doesn't know which children with fever are bacteremic and which are not. In this setting, the use of either IM ceftriaxone or oral amoxicillin is not convincingly effective. Both forms of treatment trend toward being beneficial, but statistical significance is not reached. A meta-analysis of empiric antibiotic therapy for children with fever reached the conclusion that approximately 414 children would need to be treated unnecessarily in order to prevent 1 serious bacterial infection.[99] It is clear that widespread use of empiric antibiotics for children with FWLS is likely to treat many children who cannot possibly benefit from the therapy.

Recommendations

An expert panel met and published practice guidelines in 1993.[100] Their recommendations were based on a review of available literature and discussion of the issues. They recommended the following: (1) hospitalization and intravenous antibiotics for all children less than 28 days and for all toxic-appearing infants and children, (2) febrile infants between 28 and 90 days of age may be defined to be at low risk by specific clinical and laboratory criteria (Table 10-3) and, if so judged, can be managed as outpatients if close follow-up is ensured, (3) children 3–24 months old with fever less than 39°C without a source need neither antibiotics nor laboratory tests, (4) children 3–24 months of age with fever greater than 39°C and a WBC count of 15,000/μL or greater should be considered for blood culture and antibiotic treatment pending culture results, and (5) urine cultures should be obtained in all boys 6 months of age or less and all girls 2 years of age or less who are treated with antibiotics.

The choice of empiric antibiotic for those who are judged to be at highest risk for true occult bacteremia should be either high-dose amoxicillin (80–150 mg/kg/day divided TID) or ceftriaxone 50 mg/kg as a single intramuscular dose, to be given after blood culture and possibly CSF culture is obtained. Follow-up examination is of utmost importance and should be scheduled for the next morning.

Hospitalization

Hospitalization is more likely to be indicated if the child is very young or appears "toxic" or if the parents are too anxious or too unreliable to be alert for changes in the general appearance as described earlier. Symptoms of dyspnea, somnolence, or areas of pain or tenderness also call for hospitalization.

Hospitalization need not be done routinely for the infant less than 2 months of age, as iatrogenic risks and financial costs argue against *routine* admission.[45,101] Infants who are deemed to be at higher risk for severe infection because of prematurity, poor growth, or other parameters are routinely hospitalized. Clinical and laboratory criteria (Table 10-3) for identifying babies over 1 month of age who are at low risk for serious bacterial infection have been identified, studied, and even established as the standard of care in some hospital emergency departments.[102,103] The Rochester criteria have a greater focus on the babies' health history, whereas the Philadelphia criteria place more weight on clinical appearance and laboratory findings (Table 10-3).

Most pediatricians routinely hospitalize babies who develop fever during the first 28 days of life, probably because of a perception that the risk of severe infection is higher in these babies. Strictly speaking, this perception is true. There is no magic shift in immune function that occurs at the age of 29 days, however, and children between the ages of 28 days and 2 months with high fever remain candidates, on a case-by-case basis, for hospitalization. Some authors are attempting to apply the approach of screening with selective treatment even to babies less than 28 days of age. In one study, only one (0.8%) of 131 febrile neonates younger than 28 days who appeared well, had no focal physical examination findings, had a peripheral WBC count of between 5,000 and 15,000/μL, a neutrophil band form count of less than 5,000/μL, a spun urine specimen that had less than 10 WBCs per high-power field, and a C-reactive protein of less than 20 mg/dL had a bacterial infection.[104] Further study along these lines will be required before the standard of care is altered. Most experts agree that babies less than 28 days old with fever should undergo a complete work-up for sepsis, be hospitalized, and be given intravenous antibiotics expectantly. Treatment is generally ampicillin plus either gentamicin or cefotaxime. If the reason for hospitalization is related more to parents' ability to observe or return, then observation without antibiotics is satisfactory.

■ FEVER OF UNKNOWN ORIGIN (FUO)

Prolonged unexplained fever is a more precise diagnosis than FUO, particularly when the original definition of FUO is not observed. FUO is a convenient working diagnosis if properly defined. The review and classification of fever by Dechovitz and Moffet in 1968 was stimulated by the prevalent misuse of the diagnosis of FUO in children now classified as having fever without localizing signs.[31]

Fever of unknown origin was classically defined by three criteria:[105]

1. Documented fever of at least 38.4°C (101°F) rectally and usually higher.
2. Prolonged fever of at least 2 weeks' duration in some definitions[106] and at least 3 weeks' in others.
3. Unexplained fever with no diagnosis after simple laboratory tests after 1 week of study in a hospital.

These criteria were developed for use in adults

and at a time when sophisticated radiographic screening techniques were not readily available. These criteria are neither practical nor particularly useful in the modern practice of pediatrics. In general, diagnoses are established much sooner now than they were in the past.

Old lists of causes of FUO are more a guide to the utility of early studies than a true list of late-diagnosed diseases. Indeed, the subgroup here called fever with nonspecific signs, discussed later, has clues about anatomic areas to investigate and includes many diagnoses on the old list of causes of FUO.

The list of causes of FUO changes depending on the definition used for "prolonged." If the duration of fever is set at 7 days, for example, one is likely to include many more cases of respiratory illnesses and other self-limited viral illnesses that lack classic features. If the duration is set to 3 weeks, as in the past, all self-limited infections will be excluded, and the percentage of patients with serious illnesses will increase. It seems to us that a reasonable clinical definition of FUO in childhood would be the presence of fever greater than 38.3°C (101°F) for more than 10 consecutive days in a patient without an obvious focus of infection by physical examination and screening laboratory evaluation.

It is useful to preserve the concept of a syndrome of fever that is documented, prolonged, and unexplained. Many other working diagnoses that describe this syndrome have been used, including fever (or pyrexia) of unexplained origin, fever of obscure origin, fever of undetermined origin, obscure fever, persistent perplexing pyrexia, and prolonged undiagnosed fever. Many of these terms lack an important component of this clinical picture, which is that the fever is prolonged. This is a problem with the currently used appellation, fever of unknown origin, as well, although the term is widely understood. In contrast, fever of recent onset should be regarded as a different syndrome, because it is usually benign and self-limited.

"Pseudo-FUO" has been used for patients with a history of fever that cannot be documented, often in families with stress, misinformation, or behavioral problems.[107]

Causes

The frequencies of the various possible causes of prolonged undiagnosed fever are considerably different in children than in adults, and children are not included in most reviews of fever in adults. There are only a few reviews to consult for the possible causes of prolonged fever in children.[106–109] The possible causes are described following and are listed in Box 10-1.[106–122]

The text follows the sequence of the table. For completeness, some very rare possibilities are listed, which often are based on a few case reports. It may seem difficult to see how some of these possibilities were not diagnosed earlier, but retrospective analysis always seems simpler.

Juvenile Rheumatoid Arthritis (JRA)

One of the most common causes of prolonged fever in children is acute rheumatoid disease.[109] Rheumatoid arthritis is defined by rheumatologists using rather strict criteria on the basis of definite arthritis involving multiple joints and lasting over a period of at least several months. In adults or older children, rheumatoid arthritis usually presents as a problem of arthritis. This form of rheumatoid arthritis occasionally resembles acute rheumatic fever or infectious arthritis. In young children, however, rheumatoid arthritis may present as a diagnostic problem of prolonged fever without definite arthritis. This form of the disease is commonly referred to as "systemic-onset juvenile rheumatoid arthritis" or Still's disease. No specific laboratory test is available, and the diagnosis is a clinical one, often delaying therapy.

Any form of rheumatoid arthritis occurring in children younger than 16 years of age is called JRA.

JRA is especially difficult to identify when it has its onset during or at the end of another illness, as it often does, thus appearing to be a complication or continuation of the first illness.

Because acute JRA with a systemic form of onset is one of the most frequent causes of prolonged fever in children, and because the diagnosis usually must be based on clinical findings, it is discussed in detail later in a separate section.

Other Collagen Vascular Diseases

Systemic lupus erythematosus or acute rheumatic fever are a rare causes of prolonged unexplained fever. Usually, however, polyarthritis or polyarthralgia is prominent, as described in Chapter 16. In polyarteritis nodosa in children, abdominal pain and hypertension are usually present.[110]

I. Noninfectious inflammatory diseases

1. Juvenile rheumatoid arthritis (systemic onset type)
2. Less-common collagen vascular diseases (systemic lupus erythematosus, acute rheumatic fever, polyarteritis nodosa)
3. Inflammatory bowel disease (Crohn's disease, ulcerative colitis)

II. Infectious Diseases

1. Abscess (especially abdominal)
2. Other focal infections (low-grade or antibiotic-modified, such as osteomyelitis, nonbacterial meningitis, extrapulmonary tuberculosis such as mesenteric lymphadenitis, sinusitis)
3. Nonfocal bacterial infections (endocarditis, cat-scratch disease, *Salmonella* enteric fever, chronic meningococcemia, chronic *H. influenzae* bacteremia, miliary tuberculosis, brucellosis, tularemia)
4. Viral infections (EBV, CMV, lymphocytic choriomeningitis virus, chronic echovirus, adenovirus, hepatitis viruses)
5. Other microorganisms
   Rickettsiae (Rocky Mountain spotted fever, ehrlichiosis, Q fever)
   Spirochetes (Lyme disease, leptospirosis, *Borrelia* relapsing fever)
   Mycoplasmas (*M. pneumoniae*)
   Parasites (toxoplasmosis, visceral larval migrans, malaria, babesiosis)
   Fungi (disseminated systemic mycoses)
   Unclassified (sarcoidosis)

III. Malignancies

1. Occult solid tumors (neuroblastoma, Wilms' tumor, retinoblastoma)
2. Hematologic tumors (lymphoma and Hodgkin's disease)

IV. Miscellaneous

1. Factitious
2. Metabolic (drug fever, milk allergy, dehydrated diabetes insipidis)
3. Genetic (familial Mediterranean fever, infantile cortical hyperostosis [Caffey's disease], hypothalamic dysfunction, ectodermal dysplasia, familial dysautonomia, hemoglobinopathy crisis)
4. Never diagnosed

Inflammatory Bowel Disease

Crohn's disease can begin with chronic fever before bowel symptoms appear. There is usually a normocytic anemia and at least a mildly elevated erythrocyte sedimentation rate (ESR).[106]

Occult Abscesses

Abdominal abscesses can be a cause of prolonged fever in children (see Chapter 12). Liver abscess can be pyogenic or amebic and is best diagnosed by a scanning method as described in chapter 12. In pyogenic abscess, the children usually have an underlying disease or are infants who have had umbilical catheterization or septicemia. Typically, the liver is enlarged and tender.

Intraabdominal abscesses can occur in the spleen, kidney, psoas muscle, and above or below the liver, as well as in the liver. Computed tomography (CT) is usually the diagnostic study of choice.

Typically, there are clinical clues that the source of the fever is in the abdomen. In a series that used abdominal CT scans to look for the cause of FUO, 22 (79%) of 28 patients ultimately shown to have intraabdominal abscesses had previous findings suggesting disease in the abdomen, and only two of the remaining six had a source of fever found on CT scan in the absence of abdominal findings.[111]

Other Focal Infections

Meningitis, osteomyelitis, and other focal infections are much more frequent causes of prolonged fever in children than adults.[108,109] Careful physical examination will sometimes detect subtle findings, giving a clue to the location of the infection. The diagnostic approach to suspected focal infection is discussed following. Other focal infections include extrapulmonary tuberculosis, such as mesenteric adenitis.[112]

Bacteremias

Prolonged fever can be caused by *Salmonella* species, especially *S. typhi* and *S. paratyphi*. Indeed, the form of many diseases that is manifested by fever alone is often called the typhoidal form of that disease. Blood cultures for bacteria ought to detect bacteremia, but sometimes they are not done or are interfered with by antibiotics.

Infective endocarditis is occasionally associated with negative blood cultures (see Chapter 18). Compared with adults, children with endocarditis are more frequently known to have structurally abnormal hearts. Chronic or unrecognized bacteremia can occur in chronic meningococcemia (usually with arthralgias), brucellosis, tularemia, and even *H. influenzae* infection.[113] Many other species can produce FUO without resulting in focal infection.

The spirillum bacteria of rat bite fever cannot be cultured on ordinary media and require mouse inoculation. However, in the United States, rat bite fever is almost always caused by *Streptobacillus moniliformis*. Similarly, mycobacteria cannot be grown from ordinary blood culture bottles, although nontuberculous mycobacteria can be grown in special bottles if requested. Miliary tuberculosis is technically a bacterial disease, but the diagnosis in children is likely to be made by liver or bone marrow acid-fast stains; it should be suspected when there is an exposure to tuberculosis, usually in the presence of hepatosplenomegaly.

Brucellosis

Brucellosis is a very rare cause of continued fever.[114] Chills, headache, weight loss, mild arthralgia, and muscle aches are often present. Leukopenia with atypical lymphocytosis may occur. The patient almost always has had a special exposure to cattle or swine, or has a family member who is a farmer or veterinarian.[115] However, children with brucellosis are more likely than adults to have no recognized exposure. Dogs, especially beagles, are another possible source of *Brucella* in humans. Raw milk is rarely a source in the United States in recent years because of the control of brucellosis in cattle by testing and slaughtering infected animals. However, imported goat cheese has been a source, so that a history should be obtained of imported food exposure in patients with unexplained fever.

The diagnosis is confirmed by culture of the organism from the blood or from bone marrow. The latter has a higher yield.[116] The brucella agglutinin test measures antibodies to *B. melitensis, B. suis*, and *B. abortus,* reflecting infection acquired from cattle, swine, and goats, respectively. A separate antibody test is required to diagnose *B. canis* infection.[117] A single high titer of agglutinating antibodies (≥ 1: 160) to the organism is suggestive but not diagnostic.

Viruses

EBV can produce a typhoidal form of infectious mononucleosis as well as many atypical presentations (Chapter 3) and is one of the most common diagnoses made in children referred to an infectious diseases physician for prolonged unexplained fever. CMV has been a cause of FUO in most of the series reported in children. Lymphocytic choriomeningitis virus is a rare cause of prolonged fever in children. Other common viruses rarely cause FUO, although adenoviruses, echoviruses, and coxsackieviruses can sometimes cause fever for as long as 10–14 days.

Cat-Scratch Disease (Bartonella henselae Infection)

Although the principal manifestation of *Bartonella henselae* infection is regional adenitis, it is increasingly being implicated in FUO. Patients with prolonged fever in association with cat-scratch disease often have hepatic and/or splenic microabscesses that can easily be visualized by abdominal ultrasound. In one series of pediatric cases of FUO, three of seven children ultimately diagnosed as having cat-scratch disease had prolonged fever as the only manifestation.[118] Most children with hepatosplenic involvement in cat-scratch disease, have abdominal pain, although it may be vague and unimpressive.[119] A recent report that described the course of fever in 13 children with hepatosplenic cat-scratch disease found that fever lasted from 3–16 weeks. All hepatic and splenic lesions resolved without sequelae except for residual splenic calcification in one child.[120]

Parasitic Causes

An appropriate travel history is critical to considering the possibility of malaria. In nonendemic settings, more than 60% of malaria cases are initially misdiagnosed.[121] Malaria usually occurs after travel to a tropical area without the use of chemoprophylaxis, although breakthrough cases are not uncommon. Examination of at least three thick and thin blood smears by an experienced laboratorian is necessary to exclude the diagnosis. Very rarely, malaria is acquired in the United States via blood transfusion or when it is passed (via mosquito bite) from someone who returned from travel to an endemic area.[122] Hepatosplenomegaly is sometimes present in malaria. Malaria is so common that any patient with fever who has been in a malarious area during the previous two months (usual incubation period, 2 weeks) should be considered to have malaria until proven otherwise.[123]

Tick exposure is usually known in babesiosis. A

history of residence in or travel to an endemic area is helpful. This includes certain areas of Massachusetts, Rhode Island, New York, and Connecticut.[124] It can also be transmitted by blood transfusion. Other parasitic causes of FUO include toxoplasmosis, detectable by serology, and visceral larval migrans, associated with eosinophilia.

Other Microorganisms

Rickettsiae, particularly those responsible for RMSF, ehrlichiosis, and Q fever, can cause FUO. Spirochetes, such as leptospirosis, borrelial relapsing fever (in the western United States), and Lyme disease are discussed in Chapter 21. *Mycoplasma pneumoniae* without remarkable respiratory disease has been reported as a cause of FUO in an adult.[125]

Malignancies

Neuroblastoma is one of the commonest malignancies in young children and may be the most frequent malignant cause of FUO. Testing the urine for increased excretion of catecholamines or vanillyl mandelic acid may be useful if neuroblastoma is considered. However, the diagnostic approach to FUO is best done in a systematic fashion, as described later. Lymphoma also can have persistent fever as a prominent presenting complaint, but usually lymph node, spleen, or liver enlargement is present. Leukemia occasionally presents with fever, but usually some peripheral hematologic abnormality is present.[109] Ewing's sarcoma may have prominent fever as an early manifestation, but bone mass or tenderness usually makes the illness resemble osteomyelitis rather than FUO. Retinoblastoma is apparently a rare cause of continued fever.[126]

Other proliferative disorders, such as benign giant lymph-node hyperplasia of a mesenteric node, associated with refractory anemia and hyperglobulinemia and detected by a small bowel roentgenogram, have been reported as a cause of continued fever.[127]

Kawasaki Disease

When children are first hospitalized for evaluation of high fever, they may not have developed enough of the findings of Kawasaki disease for that diagnosis to be suspected. As discussed in Chapter 11, swelling of the dorsum of the hands and feet is a helpful sign in Kawasaki disease. Early findings typically include a scarlet-fever-like rash, conjunctival injection, and cervical lymphadenopathy, which may lead to ineffective antibiotic use for the mistaken diagnosis of cervical adenitis.

Miscellaneous Causes

Factitious fever is occasionally the result of heating of the thermometer by an older child or parent.[128] Testing the urine temperature immediately after voiding and retaking the temperature immediately under supervision can help confirm the diagnosis.

Drug fever can be caused by many common medications, including beta-lactam antibiotics, isoniazid, anticonvulsants, sulfonamides, and a long list of others.[129] Eosinophilia is often present. No characteristic fever pattern is found, and little risk is associated with rechallenge with the suspected drug if no cardiovascular disease is present.[129]

The case of a 14-year-old girl with fever for 2 months and vague left arm pain, who was eventually diagnosed as having Takayasu's arteritis, has been reported.[130] A series of three children between the ages of 3 and 11 years with sarcoidosis that presented with prolonged fever has been described.[131] Kikuchi's disease (histiocytic necrotizing lymphadenitis) was found to be the cause of prolonged fever with generalized lymphadenopathy in an 8-year-old boy, and in a 13-year-old boy, fever and leukopenia had been present for a month.[132,133]

Inflammatory pseudotumor of the abdomen or pelvis can cause prolonged fever along with weight loss, anemia, and elevated sedimentation rate.[134]

Genetic and metabolic causes listed in Box 10-1 often have other signs of the generalized disease and are referenced in the reviews cited and under recurrent fever later in this chapter.

Unknown and undiagnosed causes are found in as many as 25% of children with FUO.[106]

Diagnostic Approach

The following actions should be considered and are listed in order of usefulness:

1. Stop medications. Drug fever is especially likely in the unexpected persistence of fever following antibiotic therapy of a febrile illness. In drug fever, the temperature typically returns to normal when the drug is eliminated from the system, which usually occurs within a duration equivalent to five half-lives (within 48 hours for most commonly used agents).

2. Observation of the fever in the hospital for 24–48 hours without antipyretics is advisable to document it and observe the pattern before undertaking elaborate diagnostic procedures. Repeated physical examinations should be done, especially for transient arthritis, limitation of the range of joint motion, or transient rash, all of which suggest systemic-onset JRA, discussed in the next section. Careful funduscopic exam should be done to look for choroid tubercles.

3. Blood cultures are useful to exclude subacute bacterial endocarditis and may detect an unexpected bacteremia, as in chronic meningococcemia, a rare cause of persistent fever and rash in children.

4. Complete blood count, tuberculin skin test, sedimentation rate, and urine culture should be done. A test for occult blood in the stool is a simple way to screen for inflammatory bowel disease (but may be negative early in the disease process).

5. Radiologic examination of the chest and a renal ultrasound examination should be done. Radiologic examination of joints is of no value in the diagnosis of systemic onset JRA. Bony changes of arthritis are almost never seen unless clinical evidence of arthritis has been present for weeks or months. Occasionally, radiologic examination may be useful to detect changes of decreased bone density, particularly if the history of past joint symptoms is vague or unreliable. Bony changes due to leukemia may be discovered.

6. Serologic tests. Of all the serologic tests that may be sent in the evaluation of prolonged unexplained fever, measurement of serum antibodies to Epstein-Barr virus is most likely to be diagnostic. A heterophile antibody test is helpful if it is positive, but a negative test does not exclude the diagnosis. By the time a child reaches the point of being evaluated for prolonged unexplained fever, EBV antibody titers, rather than a heterophile antibody test should be obtained. Antibody titers to CMV should also be sent. *B. henselae* antibody titers should be sent if there is a history of cat ownership or cat contact and can be considered on a case-by-case basis for others. Repeated testing for *B. henselae* antibodies may need to be obtained, as early testing may produce false-negative results. False-positive results also occur and may

distract the clinician from considering other possibilities. Serology for histoplasmosis and coccidioidomycosis may be indicated. In areas of histoplasmosis endemicity, disseminated disease can be diagnosed by sending a urine sample for histoplasmosis antigen testing. Where a clinical suspicion exists, antibody titers for RMSF, ehrlichiosis, leptospirosis, tularemia, and others may be helpful; however, a reasoned, directed approach is superior to a "shotgun" approach. For some conditions such as RMSF, it may take weeks to develop an antibody response. Thus, if there is a reasonable clinical suspicion of RMSF, the patient should be treated empirically with doxycycline.

It is very difficult to confirm the diagnosis of acute rheumatoid disease by serologic tests, because autoantibodies to IgG are rarely detected in this stage of the illness in children. Latex fixation and other tests for rheumatoid factors that are commonly found in patients with manifest rheumatoid joint disease are almost universally negative in acute juvenile rheumatoid disease of the systemic-onset type. Antinuclear antibodies also are rarely found in such patients.

7. Bone marrow aspiration should be considered with examination of the smear for acid-fast bacilli, yeast forms, and bacteria, as well as for malignancy. Culture of the marrow for fungi, mycobacteria, and other bacteria should be done.

8. Lumbar puncture will sometimes reveal either viral meningitis or bacterial meningitis that has been suppressed by antibiotics. The test may already have been done because of cervical arthralgia and high fever of systemic-onset JRA.

9. Radiography. In adults, scanning using CT has been useful in some patients with suspected intraabdominal malignancy or abscess, especially of the liver. Scanning of the abdomen also may be useful in children if there is some evidence of liver tenderness or abnormal liver function or other intraabdominal findings. Abdominal and pelvic ultrasound may also reveal abscesses, masses, or the focal granulomas of systemic cat-scratch disease. Immunoscintigraphy may be helpful if available; in one retrospective study of young children with FUO, a site of infection was found in 11 (37%) of 30 patients by this test. Five of the children in whom immunoscintigraphy was not helpful eventually proved to have systemic-onset JRA;

patients with a clinical diagnosis of suspected endocarditis also had negative scans.[135]

Radioactive gallium (^{67}Ga) can be useful for the detection of abscesses, especially in the abdomen, by scanning for increased uptake of the isotope in a focus of inflammation. A prospective study of 30 children with fever for more than 2 weeks without a known cause who underwent gallium scanning showed that it was much more likely to be helpful in patients who had some sign or symptom of focal disease; scans were unrevealing in 24 (96%) of 25 patients who had an illness that was entirely systemic in nature.[136]

10. Biopsy of the liver or a lymph node should be considered in selected cases if there is abnormal enlargement.

11. Empiric trial. A trial of antimicrobial therapy is rarely useful and makes interpretation of subsequent culture results difficult. It should not be done except in life-threatening situations such as suspected disseminated tuberculosis. In children, a nonsteroidal antiinflammatory trial may be justified when there is a strong suspicion of systemic JRA.

■ SYSTEMIC JUVENILE RHEUMATOID ARTHRITIS

Juvenile rheumatoid arthritis with systemic onset is a common cause of prolonged unexplained fever in children. No specific laboratory tests are conclusive, so the diagnosis must usually be based on a constellation of clinical and laboratory findings, as described following.

Clinical Findings

High Fever

Typically, the temperature ranges from as low as about 35°C (94°F or 95°F) to as high as about 41°C (104°F to 105°F). The fever spikes may occur once a day (quotidian) or twice a day (double quotidian).[137] Classically, a fever spike occurs in the late afternoon or early evening. There is no response of the fever to antibiotics. Usually, there is no response to ordinary doses of aspirin (Fig. 10-1). The temperature usually spikes up abruptly and goes back to normal rapidly as well, a pattern that is correctly described as "hectic fever."

Transient Rash

The rash usually is faint, evanescent, and maculopapular or macular. It is usually red or salmon-colored, typically occurring at the height of fever, often on the trunk or over joints.[137–140] Often, large, flat, red macules with pale centers are seen. The rash may be linear from scratching (Fig. 10-2). The major characteristic of the rash is its evanescent character; often, it is present only for a few minutes

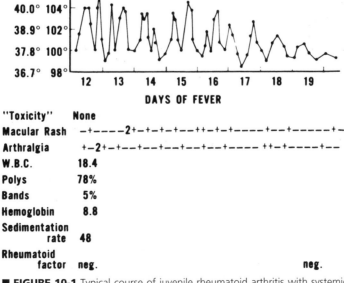

■ **FIGURE 10-1** Typical course of juvenile rheumatoid arthritis with systemic onset, showing fever spike twice a day (double quotidian fever).

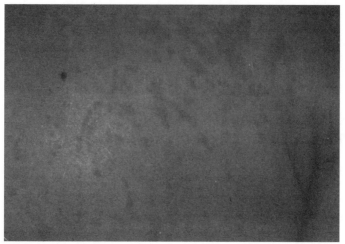

■ **FIGURE 10-2** Typical rash in rheumatoid arthritis of systemic onset. (Photo from Dr. Richard Hong)

or hours. The rash appears to be related in some cases to pressure. Occasionally, it is pruritic.

Arthralgias and Myalgias

Arthralgia is often present but may not be easy to detect.[139,141,142] It is often noted on flexing the spine. A lumbar puncture is occasionally done in these patients, because the stiff neck or back and the higher fever make the physician want to exclude meningitis. Arthralgia is also often noted in shoulders and knees when the range of motion of these joints is tested. Often, the young child will refuse to walk and will want to be held on the lap without being moved, which appears to cause discomfort. At the beginning of the illness, objective evidence of arthritis is often transient or absent in the systemic-onset type of rheumatoid disease. Usually, arthritis appears within weeks or months, but the course is highly variable.

Isomorphic Response (Koebner Phenomenon)

This is a wheal that appears on the skin a few minutes after the physician makes a superficial scratch mark.[140] The phenomenon provides some support for a diagnosis of rheumatoid disease but is not specific.

Other Clinical Findings

Abdominal pain occasionally is severe enough to resemble an acute abdomen. The pain may result from enlarged mesenteric nodes, as demonstrated at laparotomy in some studies. In such cases, generalized lymphadenopathy is usually present. Liver and spleen enlargement occasionally is prominent.[143]

Laboratory and Other Findings

The erythrocyte sedimentation rate is markedly elevated. A leukocytosis of greater than 20,000/uL (as high as 100,000/uL) with a predominance of neutrophils may be found after the fever has been present for several days or weeks. Anemia may not be present at first, but usually the hemoglobin progressively falls from about 12 to 8 or 9 g/dL. Thrombocytosis of 500,000 to 1,000,000/uL may be found.

Rheumatoid factor is not found in JRA of systemic onset and is of supportive value in the diagnosis only in older children with polyarticular arthritis.

Although not specific for JRA, patients with the systemic onset form often will have extremely high serum ferritin levels when disease is active.[144]

A chest roentgenogram may reveal cardiac enlargement, or the electrocardiogram may reveal changes suggesting myocarditis or pericarditis (see Complications). Echocardiography may be useful to detect small pericardial effusions.[145]

Therapy

High doses of aspirin, beginning with 100 mg/kg per day and increasing to a salicylate level of about

25 mg/dL, are usually effective in returning the temperature to normal or to a low-grade fever in several days, with marked relief of joint and other inflammatory symptoms.[146] Many rheumatologists favor naproxen sodium (5–10 mg/kg/dose BID) or other non-salicylate-containing anti-inflammatory agents.

Complications

Confusing complications can occur, usually after a few weeks of high fever but occasionally earlier.[139,147] These include:

1. Pericarditis with effusion and sometimes tamponade[148]
2. Myocarditis (less common)
3. Pleural effusions, usually small
4. Interstitial pneumonitis (may precede joint signs)[149]

Course

In most cases, the diagnosis of systemic-onset JRA is confirmed by the eventual appearance of chronic or recurrent polyarthritis, since the arthritis usually occurs within 6 months.[139,141] Occasionally, the diagnosis proves erroneous or is never confirmed. A study was done of the course of 43 children with a diagnosis of rheumatoid arthritis that could not be confirmed during the first hospitalization.[141] This diagnosis was based predominantly on findings of arthralgia or synovitis and elevated erythrocyte sedimentation rate, often with fever, rash, and lymphadenopathy. Five children eventually developed typical rheumatoid polyarthritis and 15 eventually had another diagnosis including psoriasis, ulcerative colitis, rheumatic fever, ankylosing spondylitis, osteochondritis, probable septic arthritis, Raynaud's disease, systemic lupus erythematosus, dermatomyositis, and scleroderma.[141] Of the 43 children, 23 (53%) had a course that led to the continuing working diagnosis of probable rheumatoid arthritis. These 23 children could be classified into three patterns, according to their course: 10 had a benign systemic course with rash, fever, and lymphadenopathy with minimal symptoms or signs in the joints but never developed chronic polyarthritis; 9 had an oligoarthritic course, with chronic arthritis but with less than four joints involved; 4 had a transient polyarthritic course with few or no systemic findings. Their polyarthritis was of too short a duration (less than 3 months) to meet criteria for rheumatoid arthritis.

■ FEVER WITH NONSPECIFIC SIGNS

Fever with various nonspecific signs can be defined as a definite fever of at least 38.4°C rectal (101°F) of less than 10 days' duration with abnormal physical findings that indicate an area for diagnostic study. "Fever with nonspecific signs" is a general category, and the specific sign or signs should be stated such as "fever and splenomegaly," "fever with hepatosplenomegaly," or a similar phrase. Further discussion is found in the appropriate section as shown in Table 10-4. It seems apparent that many cases included in pediatric series of FUO really had fever with nonspecific signs. This may partially account for the fact that at least one large series found EBV infection to be the most common cause of pediatric FUO.[125]

Causes of Fever and Hepatosplenomegaly

Infections are the most important causes of fever and hepatosplenomegaly. Some cases may be cured by early diagnosis and proper chemotherapy. Miliary tuberculosis is discussed in chapter 8. Infectious mononucleosis-like syndromes are discussed in Chapter 3. If malignancy is the cause, peripheral hematologic abnormalities are usually suggestive, but sometimes lymph node or liver biopsy, or even splenectomy, is necessary for diagnosis.

Epstein-Barr Virus or Cytomegalovirus Infection

In many cases, fever and mild-to-moderate hepatosplenomegaly are the only signs of EBV or CMV infection. The diagnosis is readily established by testing for serologic response to these viruses.

Systemic Bartonellosis (Bartonella henselae Infection)

Often in cat-scratch disease with hepatosplenic involvement, no obvious hepatosplenomegaly is seen. However, subtle splenomegaly can sometimes be found on careful physical examination.

Acute Disseminated Histoplasmosis

Fever and hepatosplenomegaly are the major findings in acute disseminated histoplasmosis, which occurs most commonly in young infants or debilitated adults (Fig. 10-3). The chest film is typically

TABLE 10-4. CHAPTERS GIVING FURTHER DISCUSSION OF FEVER WITH NONSPECIFIC SIGNS

NONSPECIFIC SIGN	DIFFERENTIAL DIAGNOSIS	CHAPTER
Liver or spleen enlargement	Disseminated fungal or mycobacterial infection	10
	Malignancy	10
Jaundice	Hepatitis	13
	Neonatal hepatitis	19
Pleuritis; pericarditis	Rheumatoid disease	10
	Pneumonia	8
	Carditis	18
Rash	Viral or bacterial infection, noninfectious	11
Abdominal distention or pain	Appendicitis, cholecystitis, or pancreatitis	12
	Urinary tract infection	14
	Pneumonia	8
	Discitis or pelvic osteomyelitis	16
Generalized lymphadenopathy	Infectious mononucleosis-like illness	3
	HIV infection	20

normal but occasionally reveals miliary lesions. Histoplasmosis antibodies are usually present when the patient is first seen. Urine testing for histoplasmosis antigen is almost uniformly positive (> 1 arbitrary unit). Hematologic abnormalities are usually present and often are prominent enough to receive the major diagnostic consideration. In other cases, bowel involvement is severe and may lead to misdiagnoses such as infantile inflammatory bowel disease.

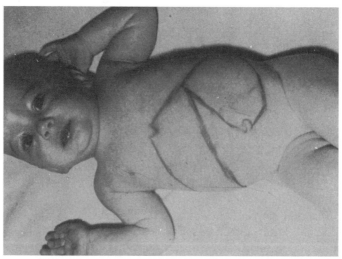

■ **FIGURE 10-3** A 4-month-old child with massive hepatosplenomegaly and thrombocytopenia caused by disseminated histoplasmosis.

Hemolytic anemia with reticulocytosis, leukopenia, and thrombocytopenia may be the major presenting pattern.[150] Because fever and hepatosplenomegaly are often present, acute leukemia may be considered. The bone marrow does not reveal an abnormal number of blast cells, but the yeast-phase oval *Histoplasma* organisms can usually be found. Disseminated intravascular coagulation is a possible complication of disseminated histoplasmosis.[150]

Culture from bone marrow requires about 10 days, and this may delay treatment too long in the disseminated form of the disease. Thus, a careful examination of a bone marrow smear should be done when disseminated histoplasmosis is suspected. The yeast forms of the organism can usually be identified by their typical morphology in stained smears. The clinician should tell the technician what is suspected, although a hematology technician may recognize the organism in such a stain even without a warning. Disseminated histoplasmosis in infancy thus resembles acute leukemia, with thrombocytopenia, hepatosplenomegaly, anemia, leukopenia, but without excessive blast forms. Histoplasma budding yeast forms should be looked for in all cases of suspected leukemia in which leukemia cannot be confirmed by bone marrow examination. Fluorescent antibody stains of the bone marrow smear may be extremely useful if disseminated histoplasmosis is suspected,[150] but they are unlikely to be available except in geographic areas where the disease is frequent.

Disseminated Infection with Other Fungi

Disseminated coccidioidomycosis may occur in children living in the southwestern United States. Blastomycosis can also have a disseminated form. The diagnostic approach is the same as that described previously for histoplasmosis.

Disseminated fungal diseases occurring in immunosuppressed patients are discussed in Chapters 22 and 23.

Hemophagocytic Syndrome

This syndrome (also called hemophagocytic lymphohistiocytosis or HLH) consists of fever, hepatosplenomegaly, lymphadenopathy, peripheral pancytopenia, and increased numbers of histiocytes that have engulfed platelets, myeloid elements, and erythrocytes.[151] EBV is one of the causes of this syndrome, which may resemble Langerhans cell histiocytosis.

Malignant Infiltrations

Leukemia, lymphoma, histiocytosis, neuroblastoma, and metastatic tumors are the most frequent malignant causes of fever with enlarged liver, spleen, or lymph nodes. If there is a family history of a similar illness in a sibling or a cousin who eventually died, the patient probably has familial reticuloendotheliosis.[152] Eosinophilia may be present in reticuloendotheliosis or lymphomatous malignancies.

Storage Diseases

In Niemann-Pick disease, Gaucher's disease, and other lipidoses, the fever is usually caused by an unrelated concurrent infection.

Malaria or Babesiosis

Both of these diseases may present with fever and hepatosplenomegaly. Travel history may raise the suspicion of malaria. A new form of babesiosis has been reported in adolescents and young adults living in parts of northern California.[153] This disease is probably underdiagnosed because of its relative obscurity.

Collagen Vascular Diseases

Systemic-onset JRA is sometimes associated with marked enlargement of the liver and was discussed earlier.

Diagnostic Approach

In patients with fever and nonspecific signs such as hepatosplenomegaly, prompt diagnosis and specific therapy may be lifesaving if the cause is infectious. Malaria, histoplasmosis, and tuberculosis deserve special emphasis, because specific chemotherapy exists, and these diseases are often not considered. If history and physical examination do not indicate a different priority, the following tests should be done in approximately this order:

1. **Peripheral blood smear.** A peripheral blood smear may reveal blast forms, atypical lymphocytes, malarial forms, or an extreme predominance of lymphocytes, suggesting leukemia. If malaria is a possibility, thick and thin smears should be performed and reviewed by a parasitologist.
2. **Complete blood count.** Any combination of

suppression of the three cell lines (red blood cells, WBCs, and platelets) may be found in patients with malignant bone-marrow infiltration or infection. Hypersplenism may produce a low platelet count.

3. **Infectious mononucleosis tests.** For evaluation of infectious mononucleosis, a rapid slide test should be done. If positive, this may allow cancellation of the bone marrow examination. If the slide test is negative, serologic tests for EBV, toxoplasmosis, and CMV should be done, even if atypical lymphocytes are not present on the blood smear.

4. **Chest roentgenogram.** Evidence of mediastinal adenopathy or unsuspected pulmonary disease may be shown by a chest x-ray.

5. **Tuberculin skin test.** The tuberculin skin test is discussed in chapter 8. As a reminder, a negative test does not rule out the possibility of tuberculosis.

6. **Ultrasonography.** Fever and hepatosplenomegaly may be secondary to renal malignancy or infected hydronephrosis pushing the liver or spleen down and forward. An ultrasound scan is usually indicated early in the evaluation.

7. **Serologic tests for fungi.** Histoplasmosis or coccidioidomycosis, in the appropriate geographic area, should be evaluated by serology. The use of skin testing for fungi is not useful because the test is rarely positive in acute disseminated forms of disease, and a positive test may simply reflect prior exposure. In areas where histoplasmosis is endemic, urine histoplasmosis antigen testing is usually readily available and may be as sensitive as bone marrow aspiration for the diagnosis of disseminated histoplasmosis.

8. **Bone marrow smear and culture.** By examination of the bone marrow smear, many diagnoses can be made, including leukemia, storage diseases, and infections such as histoplasmosis. Culture of the marrow should routinely be done. Even as little as 1/2 mL of marrow, inoculated using the same technique as for a blood culture, is likely to yield more positive results than a peripheral blood culture. It is especially useful for the recovery of histoplasma and intracellular bacteria such as *Salmonella* and in patients with special susceptibility to opportunistic infections, as in leukemia[154] or AIDS.

9. **Scanning.** Radionuclide or CT scanning may be especially useful.

10. **Biopsies.** Biopsy of the liver or a lymph node is reasonable as an early procedure, especially if there is clinical or laboratory evidence of liver disease or lymphadenopathy.

■ RECURRENT AND PERIODIC FEVER

In the evaluation of the child with recurrent fever, perhaps the most important step is the separation of fever that recurs at random intervals from fever that recurs at predictable intervals, as the conditions associated with each are entirely different.[154a] Recurrent fever can be defined as recurrent, nonpredictable episodes of definite fever of at least 38.4°C (101°F), confirmed by medical personnel, with intervening periods of entirely normal temperature. The term *periodic,* on the other hand, means occurring at fixed intervals. This term should not be used to mean happening *occasionally*, as the term is used in daily speech. The parents of children with true periodic fever can sometimes predict the onset of the next fever within hours or a day. Daily fever for more than 10 days was discussed in the section on fever of unknown origin. Episodes of fever with temperature less than 38.4°C (101°F) are discussed later.

Common Causes of Recurrent Fever

Recurrent Respiratory Infection

The most frequent cause of recurrent episodes of fever in young children is probably unrelated respiratory infections, as discussed in Chapters 2 and 23. The child with recurrent bronchitis may also have signs of allergy and later develop asthma, as discussed in Chapter 7. Typically, the patient has mild respiratory findings, such as cough or rhinitis, noted with each episode. Usually, the child improves gradually, whether or not antibiotic therapy is used. Often, antibiotic therapy is resorted to late in an infection when natural resolution is about to begin. Consequently, administration of an antibiotic is associated with resolution of symptoms in the minds of the parents.

Occasionally, successive viral infections may occur with fever as the only symptom. Enteroviruses, EBV, CMV, HHV-6, and other viruses can all result in fever only, as discussed earlier. However, it is unusual for a child to have three or more successive viral illnesses in which fever is the only symptom.

Recurrent Urinary Infection

It is important not to assume that recurrent fever is a result of respiratory infection simply because mild respiratory symptoms are present. Urinary infections are sometimes overlooked because the urine is not examined, especially in small children who often have mild respiratory symptoms and who are usually difficult about furnishing urine specimens.

Factitious Fever

Children about 8 years of age and older sometimes produce abnormal thermometer readings by heating or rubbing the thermometer. The parent may produce the false thermometer readings. Hospitalization may be necessary to detect this diagnosis.

Individual Idiosyncrasy

The only explanation in some cases of recurrent fever is an individual idiosyncrasy. As medical knowledge increases, fewer patients will have to be placed in this category.

Uncommon Causes

Rare Infections

Relapsing fever is a disease caused by the *Borreliae,* a group of spirochetes.[155,156] The disease is usually transmitted by ticks and is found primarily in the northwestern United States. Headache, arthralgia, myalgia, and severe fatigue are often present. There may be from 1–3 relapses of fever lasting from 2–7 days, alternating with afebrile periods of 2–4 days. Diagnosis is best made by examination of peripheral blood during a febrile episode.

Immune Deficiency Syndromes

Immune deficiency syndromes are not associated with recurrent fever unless definite clinical infection is present (Chapter 23).

Chronic Diseases with Recurrent Infections

Cystic fibrosis, which is associated with recurrent pneumonia, is discussed in Chapter 22. Cystic fibrosis is not particularly associated with recurrent episodes of fever unless pneumonia is also present.

Rheumatoid Disease

The ultimate diagnosis in some patients with recurrent episodes of fever is JRA, which was discussed earlier. It should be considered when there are recurrent episodes of fever, especially if arthralgia or a rash is also present.

Inflammatory Bowel Disease

Children with Crohn's disease may present with prolonged, unexplained fever or, less commonly, with recurrent episodes of fever. They usually have anemia and an elevated sedimentation rate.

Allergies

Many children with recurrent respiratory infections later are recognized to have asthma. The fever in these patients is caused by infection rather than allergy. However, allergy to drugs or food can be a rare cause of fever. Foods such as milk can be a cause of recurrent fever episodes, but the episode is typically accompanied by gastrointestinal manifestations.

Temperature Regulation Defects

Some patients with static encephalopathies or other neurologic diseases may have an exaggerated febrile response to ordinary respiratory infections.[157] Ectodermal dysplasia of the anhidrotic type is a cause of recurrent fever because of the absence of sweat glands.[158] Familial dysautonomia (Riley-Day syndrome) is a very rare disease producing drooling and difficult swallowing in infancy, as well as episodes of unexplained fever.[159] The diagnosis can be made by examination of the tongue, which lacks fungiform papillae.[160]

Causes of Periodic Fever

Periodic Fever, Adenitis, Pharyngitis, and Aphthous Stomatitis (PFAPA)

PFAPA is a relatively recently described syndrome of unknown etiology that causes episodes of fever lasting 3–5 days that recur at approximately 4-week intervals.[161] This condition is uncommon, but it is by no means rare. Patients with this condition develop high fevers (103°F–105°F) that begin abruptly, last for several days, and then disappear. During the febrile episode patients appear somewhat ill; activity level is decreased, appetite is decreased, and pallor may be noted. Physical examination often reveals tender cervical adenitis and nonexudative pharyngitis. Aphthous ulcers may or may not be present. Laboratory values are nonspecific, but may include a slightly elevated erythrocyte sedimentation rate. Throat cultures are repeatedly negative. Between episodes, patients appear completely well. Growth and development are normal. Any weight lost during febrile episodes is quickly regained.

These children do not seem to be more susceptible to infections; if anything, the opposite seems to be the case, as they are often reported (aside from the febrile episodes) to be sick less often than their siblings. Primary care pediatricians and family practitioners alike will often attribute this pattern to recurrent respiratory infection; it is only when the mother produces a calendar and demonstrates the extreme predictability of the febrile episodes that recurrent viral infection seems unlikely.

Episodes of fever are reproducibly aborted by a single oral dose of prednisone, 1–2 mg/kg, given at the onset of the fever. Occasionally, a second dose 12–24 hours later is necessary. This strategy saves the patient and the family an immense amount of inconvenience. However, treatment with prednisone sometimes produces the unwanted effect increasing the frequency of the febrile episodes. Anecdotally, tonsillectomy has been reported to be curative in several patients.[162] Cimetidine, originally reported to be possibly beneficial,[163] is no longer promising.[161] With or without treatment, the syndrome has a universally good prognosis; in most patients, the febrile episodes continue for several years and then the condition self-resolves. Resolution is often heralded by a gradual lengthening of the time between episodes.[161]

Familial Mediterranean Fever (FMF)

FMF is an autosomal recessive disease and an uncommon cause of periodic fever. In most cases, the episodes do not occur with precise periodicity. Episodes of fever are almost always accompanied by abdominal pain; arthralgia and chest pain are also relatively common. Symptoms typically last only a day or two. The disease usually occurs in persons of Armenian, Arabic, Turkish, or Jewish background. The gene responsible for FMF has been cloned, and genetic testing at a reference laboratory can detect at least one mutation in about three-quarters of cases.[164]

In adults and children, episodes can usually be prevented with daily colchicine, but relapse occurs if the drug is stopped.[165] Importantly, the use of prophylactic colchicine significantly decreases the risk of developing amyloidosis, the major long-term risk in patients with FMF.[166] The usual dose in adults is 1 mg daily.

Cyclic Neutropenia

Cyclic neutropenia is a disorder of blood cell maturation that causes recurrent episodes of neutropenia. These episodes are accompanied by fever even when an infection is not present. Patients may also experience malaise and headache. As with PFAPA, stomatitis can be a prominent part of the clinical picture, as can adenitis and pharyngitis. Periodontal disease is common. The periodicity is usually shorter than with PFAPA, with fevers occurring every 18–21 days. During periods of neutropenia, the patient is at increased risk of acquiring infections; therefore, it is important to establish or rule out this diagnosis in patients with periodic fever. Most cases are sporadic, but an autosomal dominant form has also been described.[167] Family members may know of a relative who died of unknown causes or of a sudden severe infection in early childhood.

Treatment is with G-CSF, which significantly increases neutrophil counts, decreases the frequency of infections, and improves periodontal disease. It does, however, tend to shorten the interval between episodes to about 14 days.[168]

Most patients do not develop life-threatening infections, but occasionally sepsis with unusual organisms, such as *Clostridium septicum*, occurs.[169]

Hyper-IgD Syndrome (HIDS)

HIDS is an extremely uncommon cause of recurrent fever associated with elevated levels of IgD. The clinical syndrome often includes headache, abdominal pain, skin rashes, and arthralgias or true arthritis. Patients may also have diarrhea. The attacks usually last 4–6 days and recur every 4–6 weeks, although the interval can be quite variable. The diagnosis can be established by obtaining IgD levels; affected patients usually have continuously high levels (greater than 100 IU/mL). No specific therapy has been shown to be effective.[170]

Tumor Necrosis Factor Receptor-Associated Periodic Syndrome (TRAPS)

This autosomal dominant condition, originally termed Familial Hibernian Fever and thought to involve only one family in Ireland, has been discovered to be due to a TNF-alpha receptor abnormality. Attacks of disease usually begin within the first 18 months of life and sometimes within the first 6 months. In addition to fever, patients have systemic symptoms, including rash in 84%, unilateral conjunctivitis or periorbital edema in 44%, abdominal discomfort in 88%, and myalgia in 80%. About two-thirds have headache, half have arthralgia, and about 40% have pleuritic chest pain.[171] Treatment is investigational, but use of an anti-TNF alpha agent (etanercept) appears promising.[170]

Laboratory Approach

Identification of the cause of a single episode of fever is useful in the patient with recurrent episodes of fever. This can be done by noting exposure to infectious disease, physical examination for signs of a specific infectious disease, WBC count and differential, urinalysis, and culture of the throat for streptococci. Erythrocyte sedimentation rate or C-reactive protein may be useful. In some conditions (e.g., Crohn's disease, tuberculosis, occult bacterial infection, and systemic-onset JRA) these markers remain elevated in between febrile episodes. In contrast, children with PFAPA, hyper-IgD, and FMF have elevated inflammatory markers only when febrile. The child with recurrent viral infections usually has a normal ESR, even during the illness. Viral cultures or specific serologic testing may be helpful in certain cases.

When there is a suspicion that the patient's fever pattern may be periodic, establishing that fact with fever charts is helpful. The patient should be examined during a febrile episode. Careful examination of the mouth and oropharynx should be performed. The diagnosis of cyclic neutropenia should be ruled out by obtaining a complete blood count during a febrile episode and repeating this laboratory test when the child is well and again at the time of the next fever. If the absolute neutrophil count is normal on all three occasions, cyclic neutropenia is effectively eliminated from the diagnostic possibilities.

Most children with periodic fever have PFAPA, and not all patients with PFAPA demonstrate all components of the syndrome. Our experience has been that a trial of prednisone as described earlier is usually effective at eliminating the clinical features of PFAPA, even in patients who lack one or more features. If the diagnosis of PFAPA is in doubt, cyclic neutropenia has been eliminated, and the patient has diarrhea, abdominal pain, skin rashes, and

other features suggestive of Hyper-IgD syndrome, an IgD level can be obtained. Young children with periodic fever, rash, conjunctivitis, and abdominal or chest pain can be investigated for the presence of the missense codon in the TNF-alpha receptor gene at a reference laboratory. Similarly, genetic testing is available for FMF, but not all mutations are detected. Thus, in patients with a classic presentation, a trial of colchicine is reasonable.

■ NONFEVER (PSEUDOFEVER)

Parents will sometimes bring children in for evaluation of "fever" that a child has had for weeks or even months. Typically, the child experienced a definite illness with real fever, but without a definitive diagnosis. Thereafter, the parent feels compelled to check the child's temperature frequently, often several times a day. The parent may bring a piece of paper with temperatures carefully recorded. Temperatures will be in the range of an oral temperature not higher than 38.0°C (100.4°F) or a rectal temperature usually not higher than 38.5°C (101.1°F). If graphed, the temperature curve may show wide swings (attributable to the normal diurnal variation and sometimes due to a mix of axillary and rectal measurements), and the "spikes" are interpreted as a fever, even though the absolute level is lower than 38.5°C rectally. The child does not appear sick. Physical examination is entirely normal. This nonfever category is similar to the syndrome called pseudo-FUO, mentioned in the section on FUO.[107]

Causes

Parental anxiety, often supported by the physician, is the usual reason for repeated temperature measurement. Strenuous exercise, a large meal, ovulation, or exposures to chemicals are other possible causes of nonfever. Important diseases to be excluded include urinary infection and tuberculosis.

Diagnostic Approach and Management

Elaborate diagnostic studies are not warranted for the patient with nonfever, if no abnormal physical findings are present. The physician should perform repeated physical examination at times of "fever," along with confirmation of the temperature elevation. Simple diagnostic studies, such as routine blood count, urinalysis and culture, erythrocyte sedimentation rate, tuberculin test, and chest roentgenogram, may be reasonable in selected patients.

The parents should be told about the normal diurnal temperature variation and the effect of exercise on the temperature. If simple screening studies are negative, the temperature should not be taken unless the child has other indications of illness. Sometimes it requires a great deal of persuasion to convince a parent to stop taking the child's temperature. Some parents become heavily "invested" in this activity and in believing that there is something wrong with the child. Multiple visits for reassurance purposes may be necessary.

■ FEVER COMPLICATING CHRONIC DISEASES

Fever complicating a chronic disease is a useful descriptive diagnosis when a fever is documented in a patient with a chronic disease known to have one or more febrile complications. The diagnosis should be phrased as "fever complicating ..." specifying the disease involved. The following section gives some of the more frequent examples and is not intended to include every possibility. These febrile complications should always be considered first when a patient with one of these diseases develops a fever.

The complicating infections are discussed in more detail in the appropriate chapters, as shown in Table 10-5.

Fever After Hospitalization

Nosocomial Respiratory or Gastrointestinal Infections

A new episode of fever after hospitalization is relatively common in children. In one study of 50 new episodes of fever in hospitalized children, intercurrent respiratory infection, such as Group A streptococcal infection or parainfluenza virus infection, was the most common cause.[34] In the appropriate season, nosocomial RSV infection is fairly common, especially if appropriate infection control measures are not undertaken. In a community hospital especially, fever after hospitalization usually represents intrahospital transmission of a common community infection.[172]

Postoperative, Posttraumatic, and Postinstrumentation Fever

Causes of fever from these sources are discussed in the chapters dealing with the anatomic system

---

TABLE 10-5. CHAPTERS GIVING FURTHER DISCUSSION OF FEVER COMPLICATING CHRONIC DISEASES

CHRONIC DISEASE	CAUSE TO BE EXCLUDED	CHAPTER(S)
Heart disease	Endocarditis, recurrent rheumatic fever, brain abscess	18
Malignancy	Sepsis, line infection	10, 22
Shunted hydrocephalus	Ventriculitis	9
Chronic renal disease	Urinary tract infection; peritonitis	14, 22
Cystic fibrosis	Pneumonia	8, 22
Solid organ or hematopoietic stem cell transplant	Sepsis, opportunistic infection of specific organ system	22
Hemoglobinopathies	Sepsis from encapsulated organisms	22
Injection drug use	Hepatitis B and C, infective endocarditis, HIV infection	13, 18, 20
HIV infection	Multiple common and opportunistic pathogens	20
Congenital immunodeficiency syndromes	Multiple common and opportunistic pathogens	23

involved. Thus, bladder catheter-related infections are discussed in Chapter 14, fever after cardiac surgery is discussed in Chapter 18, and postoperative or aspiration pneumonia is discussed in Chapter 8. Infections secondary to intravenous cannulas or contaminated intravenous fluids are discussed later in this chapter in the section on septicemia and bacteremia. Fever can occur secondary to trauma and was observed about 5 days after injury in 40% of children with closed fracture of the femoral shaft.[173]

Malignant Hyperthermia

This is a complication of general anesthesia that had about a 65% mortality rate before the use of dantrolene for treatment.[174] Hyperthermia, muscle rigidity, metabolic acidosis, and rapid pulse and breathing occur during or soon after general anesthesia. The role of the primary care physician is to help detect a family history of this disease, as it is usually familial with unclear genetic factors, so that the patient can be evaluated before anesthesia for potential risk.[174]

■ INTRAVASCULAR DEVICE INFECTIONS

Definitions

Types of Intravascular Devices

This section emphasizes central venous catheters (CVC) of the type developed by Broviac and Hickman.[176,177] These Silastic catheters may have more than one lumen and typically have a subcutaneous tunnel and skin exit site, with the distal tip ending in a large central vein (superior vena cava, subclavian) or right atrium. It is important to distinguish these long-term intravenous access devices from shorter term CVCs that are not tunneled subcutaneously. This section deals to a lesser extent with peripheral venous catheters or monitoring devices, to which the same principles apply. A CVC is usually inserted for administration of antibiotics, chemotherapy for oncology patients, or parenteral hyperalimentation.

Types of Catheter-Related Infections

Contaminated intravenous (IV) solutions or tubing, exit-site infection, tunnel infections, pocket infection, catheter colonization, catheter-related bacter-emia, and septic phlebitis are examples of line-related infections.

Culture Methods

Central Venous Line Cultures

Prior to withdrawing blood from a CVC, the tip should be cleaned with Betadine and allowed to dry. A sufficient volume of blood, depending on the child's weight, is withdrawn from a central line and cultured. In the bacteremic patient, the yield is directly related to the volume of blood obtained for culture; a common mistake is to obtain too little blood. If the CVC contains more than one port, it is important to culture each port separately, as results are sometimes disparate.[178]

Peripheral Venous Cultures

After preparing the skin with Betadine, blood is obtained from a peripheral vein and cultured. Often, obtaining a peripheral culture at the same time as the CVC culture will provide additional information that is helpful in defining the extent and possibly the source of the infection. Infections that originate in a site other than the catheter and produce bacteremia should cause both the peripheral venous culture and the CVC culture to be positive with the same organism. Furthermore, if the cultures are obtained at the same time and monitored in an automated system such as BACTEC, both cultures will become positive at about the same time. Time to positivity depends on the inoculum of bacteria in the blood sample,[179] which depends on the amount of blood placed into the culture bottle; therefore, the preceding rule of thumb assumes that similar amounts of blood were cultured from each site.

By contrast, infections that originate in the CVC and then cause bacteremia can be detected because the CVC culture becomes positive prior to the peripheral culture. If the CVC culture turns positive 120 minutes before the peripheral culture, the sensitivity is 94% and the specificity 91% in identifying catheter-related bacteremia.[179] This distinction can sometimes be made clinically, if another source of infection is obvious. Time to positivity as a guide to the source of the bacteremia is probably most useful in caring for children with oncologic problems who are neutropenic secondary to chemotherapy, in whom signs and symptoms of infection may be subtle.[180]

Peripheral venous cultures may also be helpful in differentiating catheter-related bloodstream infection from culture contamination or catheter colonization. In these cases, CVC cultures are positive for coagulase-negative staphylococci, diphtheroids, or more than one organism, whereas peripheral cultures are sterile. Unfortunately, a pure growth of coagulase-negative staphylococcus from a CVC could represent either contamination or a line-centered infection, and differentiating the two is next to impossible. Line infection with negative peripheral cultures still presents a health hazard to the patient, particularly one with a suppressed immune system. In fact, one study that evaluated clinical outcomes in 59 patients with CVC-related bacteremia and 91 patients with catheter infection without bacteremia revealed that there were no differences in APACHE II score, WBC count, length of hospital stay, time from admission to fever, time from fever to treatment, normalization of WBC, days of antibiotics, gender, presence of comorbidities, or (most importantly) mortality rate between the two groups.[181]

Removed Catheter Tips

Quantitative or semiquantitative cultures can be done from the cutoff distal 6 cm of the catheter by rolling the tip on a culture plate (Maki method) or by adding 1 mL of broth to the dry tip and culturing a 0.1 mL specimen on a plate.[182] The method with the highest sensitivity involves sonication of the catheter tip in broth prior to plating.[183]

If the catheter tip is available to culture, obviously a clinical decision has been made that removal was needed. More practical kinds of culture methods are needed to give information before the CVC is removed.

Quantitative Blood Cultures

Studies of quantitative cultures from the peripheral venous and from CVC-obtained blood suggest the utility of counting the microorganism using the lysis centrifugation method (Isolator; DuPont) or by inoculating 0.5 mL on the surface of an agar plate at the bedside.[184-186] Quantitative blood culture methods are costly and not readily available; the evidence suggests that time to positivity is a reasonable and inexpensive surrogate for quantitative blood culture techniques (see previous).

Management

Fever in a Child with a CVC

Several groups have reported their experience and recommendations for these children.[177,184-190] Some adults have brief self-limited bacteremia from CVCs,[191] but routine blood cultures of asymptomatic patients does not seem to be helpful clinically. On the basis of the references cited earlier, a broad plan for the management of the child with a CVC who develops fever is shown in Box 10-2. In general, empiric antimicrobial therapy for suspected bloodstream infection while awaiting culture results should be based on the severity of the patient's clinical disease, the nature and severity of the patient's underlying condition, and local knowledge of the relative frequency and susceptibility patterns of nosocomial pathogens.

Criteria for Removal of CVC

Recovery from infection with almost any type of bacterium is aided by removal of the infected device. In some cases, removal alone is curative. However, in most cases, the CVC is needed for the management of whatever condition prompted the placement of the line; thus, in certain situations clinicians will try to "salvage the line" (i.e., treat the infection without removing the line). The Infectious Diseases Society of America has published clinical guidelines for treatment of infected intravascular devices.[183]

In general, nontunneled catheters should usually be removed if thought to be infected. For infections of tunneled catheters (e.g., Hickman catheters, Broviac catheters, and port-a-caths), an initial attempt is usually made to treat without line removal, unless there is a clear indication for removal as described following. Nontunneled catheters should be removed empirically in patients with erythema or purulence over the exit site or who have signs of unexplained sepsis. In those with culture-proven catheter-related infection, if the device is easily removable, it should be removed unless the organism is a coagulase-negative staphylococcus and there is no evidence of persistent bloodstream infection. In those with tunneled or implanted devices, removal is still considered optimal management; however, if catheter salvage is of utmost importance, it may be attempted by combining antibiotic lock with systemic antibiotics. If the patient's condition deteriorates, local infection develops, or the bacteremia

BOX 10-2 ■ Management of Fever in a Child with a Central Venous Catheter

1. If the CVC has multiple lumens, obtain a blood culture from each one separately. If possible, obtain blood cultures from a peripheral vein also, using time-to-positivity or quantitative cultures (if available).

2. For immunocompromised hosts, begin an antipseudomonal cephalosporin empirically.[187] Vancomycin should be added if the patient is a neonate, is seriously ill, or if there are risk factors for MRSA or cephalosporin-resistant viridans streptococci. Gentamicin may also be added for the immunocompromised host who is severely ill.

3. For hosts with normal immune systems who do not appear particularly ill, it may be reasonable to withhold antibiotics pending culture results. For patients judged too ill for the "wait and watch" approach, a regimen that covers both gram-positive and gram-negative organisms is appropriate. Such a regimen might be oxacillin and an antipseudomonal cephalosporin or an aminoglycoside. In areas where MRSA is prevalent, vancomycin may be used instead of oxacillin.

4. For CVCs with multiple lumens, rotate the administration of antibiotics so that antibiotic is given through each lumen. Obtain repeat blood cultures daily to document clearance.

5. In the nonneutropenic patient, if blood cultures are negative at 48 hours, stop antibiotics unless there is evidence of nonbacteremic focus of infection (adjust choice of antibiotics).

6. If blood cultures are positive, adjust choice of antibiotics and treat for 10–14 days from the day of the first negative culture (if well) or longer if patient has not recovered.

7. Infected non-tunneled catheters should generally be removed. Tunneled, long-term catheters should be removed if the patient has severe sepsis and there is no other source of infection, if the patient does not respond clinically despite therapy, if there are persistently positive blood cultures for > 48 hours despite adequate therapy, if recrudescence of infection occurs despite adequate treatment, or if the infection is caused by *Candida* or certain difficult-to-treat resistant organisms (such as vancomycin-resistant enterococcus or multidrug-resistant gram-negative rods).

8. Other indications for removal of the catheter are infections of the subcutaneous track of a tunneled catheter (tunnel infection) and infection in the subcutaneous pocket containing an implanted catheter (pocket infection). Infections at the site where the catheter exits the skin (exit-site infections) can often be treated with a combination of local and systemic therapy, but may necessitate catheter removal if they are severe (especially in an immunocompromised host).

9. In neonates, early line removal may be prudent for organisms other than *S. epidermidis*. In neonates, CVCs are unlikely to be salvageable if cultures have been positive for 3 or more consecutive days, even when they are infected with relatively avirulent organisms such as *S. epidermidis*.[192,193]

10. If cultures are positive for *S. aureus*, especially if cultures remain positive after line removal and appropriate antistaphylococcal antibiotics, the clinician should actively seek a focus of infection such as endocarditis, infected thrombus (endocarditis equivalent), bone or joint infection, or intra-abdominal abscess.

11. If blood cultures obtained 48 hours after stopping antibiotics are negative, the CVC can be left in place.

12. In the nonneonatal population, if the patient is well despite persistently positive blood cultures, an attempt at antibiotic lock therapy may be made.

13. If the catheter is removed, the duration of therapy can often be shortened to 5–7 days after removal of nonimplantable catheters and 7–10 days after removal of implantable catheters. More virulent organisms may require longer therapy.

does not clear rapidly, the line should be removed.[183] Catheter salvage should not be attempted in patients whose blood cultures grow any species of *Candida*.

The risk of serious disease or death resulting from attempted catheter salvage depends on the identity of the infecting organism and on the patient population. Neonates may be at particularly high risk for complications of line infections. A retrospective cohort study of CVC infections in neonates suggested that *Staphylococcus epidermidis* and enterococci were more likely to be successfully treated without line removal. In contrast, enteric and non-enteric gram-negative rods, *S. aureus*, and fungi of any type were less likely to be successfully treated without line removal.[192] Adverse outcomes, including seeding of a secondary site and death, were more likely when treatment of these pathogens was attempted through the CVC. The chances of line salvage decreased with repeated recovery of the same organism from cultures drawn through the CVC. Even with coagulase-negative staphylococci, lines were not salvageable if line cultures were positive on three consecutive days.[192] Another study in neonates demonstrated similar findings.[193] Premature neonates may be particularly prone to adverse outcomes from line infections treated with the line in situ.

Reinsertion of a New CVC

If possible, a new CVC should not be placed until repeat blood cultures have been negative for at least 48 hours. Delaying reinsertion of a CVC should especially be considered in cases where the organism is known to be difficult to eradicate (e.g., *Candida* spp. and *S. aureus*).

Exit-Site Infections

Antibiotics alone can generally cure exit-site infections, although in neutropenic patients the catheter may need to be removed. Increasing the frequency of dressing changes is important in being able to monitor response to therapy. This also allows for more frequent local site care with povidone-iodine and alcohol, which may speed resolution of infection.

Tunnel or Pocket Infections

Tunnel infections of Hickman-type catheters and pocket infections of subcutaneously implanted ports nearly always require removal of the catheter.[176]

Contaminated IV Solutions or Tubing

Although quality control of manufactured products has improved since the initial major outbreaks of infection, these sources are still a potential problem and should be cultured if polymicrobial infection or two or more cases occur.[194,195] Lipid-containing solutions have special importance because they can support the growth of the superficial skin fungus *Malassezia furfur* (the cause of tinea versicolor and seborrheic dermatitis), which cannot be cultured in the laboratory without special techniques.

Difficult Microorganisms

M. furfur does not grow on conventional media. Consider it if high-lipid fluids have been given by CVC and fever occurs with negative blood cultures and there is no other site of infection. This pathogen is especially likely to be found in premature neonates and in patients with extreme immune-suppressive states. It might be seen as budding yeasts on Gram stain of a buffy coat smear from the patient.[196] Subculture of blood culture broth onto Sabouraud dextrose agar overlaid with sterile olive oil has also helped in diagnosis.[197] Other microorganisms difficult to cure without removal of the catheter include *Candida* species, *S. aureus*, glucose non-fermenting gram-negative rods, and *Bacillus* species.[177]

Septic Phlebitis

Peripheral Vein Phlebitis

Catheter-associated phlebitis often occurs more than 24 hours after withdrawal of the catheter in adults.[198] Incision and drainage of any purulent material in a peripheral septic phlebitis may be necessary, along with appropriate antibiotics.

Central Vein Phlebitis

Septic atrial thrombosis requires open heart surgery to remove the thrombus.[199] Urokinase, especially without antibiotic therapy, does not appear to resolve septic phlebitis in children.[200] Antibiotic therapy and anticoagulation can be effective for deep vein septic thrombophlebitis in adults, although incision and drainage of an abscess may be needed.[201] Consider septic thrombophlebitis to be a diagnostic possibility when removal of an infected catheter coupled with appropriate antimicrobial chemotherapy fails to clear a bloodstream infection.

Prevention of CVC Infections

Antibiotic-Impregnated Catheters

Multiple studies have shown that catheters impregnated with antibiotics (especially minocycline/rifampin or chlorhexidine/silver sulfadiazine) decrease the risk of both catheter colonization and catheter-related bacteremia.[202] Minocycline/rifampin appears to be the best combination thus far.[203]

Heparin-Bonding

Heparin-bonded CVCs were much less likely to become infected than were normal CVCs in one prospective study in a pediatric intensive care unit setting. Only 4 (4%) of 97 heparin-bonded catheters versus 34 (33%) of 103 normal CVCs became infected, yielding a relative risk of 0.34.[204] Thrombotic complications were also reduced.

"Antibiotic Lock" and Antibiotic Flush Techniques

A prospective trial of antibiotic lock versus heparin lock in children with cancer and neutropenia clearly delineated the benefits of antibiotic locking: 16% of catheters in the control group became colonized with bacteria, and 7% of these children developed bloodstream infections during the course of the trial; none of the children in the treatment group developed either adverse outcome.[205] The technique used in this trial was to place 25 micrograms of vancomycin in 10 units heparin per mL of solution, and to allow the solution to dwell in the catheter lumen for one hour every two days. This is a very small and infrequent dose of vancomycin. There is at least a theoretical risk of the development of vancomycin resistance when the antibiotic is used in this way. The authors of this study did not design the study to evaluate this potential outcome.

Another prospective, randomized clinical trial carried out in pediatric oncology patients used a vancomycin/heparin/ciprofloxacin flush in one group, a vancomycin/heparin flush in a second group, and a plain heparin flush in a third group.[206] A total of 153 CVCs in 126 patients were evaluated for the incidence of infection and occlusive episodes. There were 40 line infections, 31 of which

occurred in the heparin only control group. Occlusive episodes were also reduced by either antibiotic-containing flush solution. No measurable amount of any antibiotic was detected in the systemic circulation in any group, and no adverse outcomes were noted. The authors of this study also assayed for vancomycin resistance in enterococcal isolates, and found none in any group.

Vancomycin lock, which is usually accomplished by making the heparin solution have a concentration of 1–5 mg/mL of vancomycin, instilling just enough to fill the catheter lumen, and allowing it to sit in the lumen of the catheter for 8–12 hours a day, is sometimes successful at eradicating CVC-associated infections that are not amenable to therapy through the line. Despite a lack of controlled clinical trials, vancomycin locking has become a popular technique and was recommended by an expert panel.[183]

Scheduled Replacement of Catheters

About half of all intensivists report that they replace CVCs on a scheduled, routine basis. However, it appears as though the daily risk of catheter infections is a constant. Therefore, if you change lines on a scheduled basis, you will succeed in reducing the rate of infections *per catheter,* but the overall rate of infections per catheter-day will not change.[207] A study looking at the utility of replacement of peripheral IVs every three days, as recommended by the CDC, reported that there was no increased risk of infection or thrombosis after catheter day 3. In fact, the day-specific risk indicated a linear function for all outcome variables.[208] Thus it appears that there is neither an experimental nor a pathophysiologic basis for the routine replacement of bloodstream catheters of any kind. There is utility in replacing catheters that are no longer functioning properly. Obviously, catheters should be removed as soon as they are no longer needed.

Education About Sterile Catheter Placement and Maintenance Techniques

A simple study showed that educating students and residents to use a full-size sterile drape rather than a small drape at the time of catheter insertion procedures successfully decreased the rate of catheter infections from 4.5 per 1000 catheter-days to 2.9 per 1000 catheter-days. The sum total of the educational process was a one-day course on infection control practices and procedures that was given in

June of 1996 and repeated in July of 1997. This 28% decrease in catheter infection rate saved the hospital approximately $70,000 over the course of 18 months.[209] In another study involving intensive care unit nurses, a self-study module combined with verbal instructions and fact sheets decreased catheter-related infections from 10.8 per 1000 catheter-days to 3.7 per 1000 catheter-days, resulting in an 18-months' savings of well over $185,000.[210]

■ SEPSIS AND BACTEREMIA

Sepsis, septicemia, and bacteremia all refer to bacteria in the blood. As used in the United States, sepsis and septicemia are equivalent terms and usually imply an overwhelming infection and the patient's inflammatory response. However, surgeons and the British also use the word *sepsis* to refer to wound infections or any purulent drainage, as in *wound sepsis*. As explained following, this is an imprecise use of the term *sepsis*. This chapter will follow the common practice of using *sepsis* to mean *probable septicemia*.

Bacteremia is defined as a positive blood culture. Probable sepsis is best defined as a clinical diagnosis of probable bacteremia with a serious clinical status. Thus, sepsis is usually a clinical diagnosis and bacteremia a laboratory finding. The working diagnosis is phrased as probable sepsis, especially for the newborn or for patients who appear seriously ill. The diagnostic terminology suggested by the Society of Critical Care Medicine includes "systemic inflammatory response syndrome (SIRS)," which describes a condition of hyper- or hypothermia in the presence of elevated heart and/or respiratory rate and an abnormal peripheral WBC count and differential. This condition is usually, but not always, caused by bacterial infection. In this scheme, *sepsis* refers to SIRS caused by an infection. *Severe sepsis* is used to mean sepsis plus evidence of organ dysfunction, hypotension, or hypoperfusion. *Septic shock* is severe sepsis (i.e., sepsis plus hypotension) despite fluid resuscitation. Finally, *multiple organ dysfunction syndrome* is altered organ function that requires intervention.[211]

Clinical Patterns

Presumed Sepsis (Systemic Inflammatory Response Syndrome)

The clinical diagnosis of presumed sepsis should usually be made on the basis of one or more of the following clinical findings: fever, "toxicity," septic shock, disseminated intravascular coagulation, and often, a source of infection or a predisposing host defect. In addition to the seriously ill appearance of the patient, the number of bacteria found in the blood by quantitative methods is often much higher than with other bacteremias such as subacute bacterial endocarditis, as discussed later.

Fulminating Bacteremia (Severe Sepsis or Septic Shock)

Like presumed sepsis, this clinical pattern has clinically serious findings such as rapid course, shock, and often, a predisposing factor such as a nonfunctioning spleen or neutropenia. In addition there is confirmed bacteremia, often in larger numbers than in other forms of bacteremia. One study that utilized quantitative cultures to study 43 children with meningococcal bacteremia showed that petechial/purpuric disease or meningitis occurred in those with more than 500 bacteria/mL, whereas all 13 with occult (unsuspected) bacteremia had fewer than 500 bacteria/mL.[212]

Bacteremia with Focal Infection

Bacterial meningitis, septic arthritis, buccal cellulitis, and severe wound infections are examples of focal infections clearly related to the bacteremia that have the same bacteria readily culturable from the focal source. Many series of bacteremias start with the bacteriology laboratory and report the total numbers and percentages of various bacteria without separating the clinical situations as outlined in this classification.

Bacteremia from Intravascular Cannulas (Line-Associated Infection)

The more frequent use of plastic tubing for long-term antibiotic or antineoplastic chemotherapy, for monitoring, or for parenteral nutrition has resulted in these transcutaneous catheters becoming the most common source of bacteremia for compromised patients and an increasingly common source in immunologically normal patients who need intravenous therapy for even a short time. Management of this category of bacteremia was discussed in the previous section.

Occult Bacteremia

This category consists of patients thought to be at risk of bacteremia because of young age, usually with a high fever and high white blood count, who are not hospitalized but rather observed as outpatients after laboratory studies including a blood culture have been done. The management of this group was discussed in detail in the preceding section on fever in infants and toddlers.

Neonatal Bacteremia

Because the bacteria are different and the prognosis so much worse than for other age groups, neonatal bacteremia is considered as a special category. It is also discussed in chapter 19.

Contaminated Blood Cultures

In infants and children, contamination of blood cultures is frequent and variable, occurring in about 10–40%. An emergency room study reported a contamination rate of 25%,[64] but more recent pediatric studies report rates of 2–3% if the blood is drawn by venipuncture and 3–9% if drawn through a catheter.[213,214] *Bacillus* species, *Propionibacterium acnes,* and *Corynebacterium* species are almost always contaminants, but may occasionally cause bacteremia in the certain populations (e.g., a neutropenic patient with a CVC). In the nonneonate, *S. epidermidis* can be considered a contaminant if there is no intravascular line. Enterococci and the viridans group of streptococci can be considered probable contaminants in immunocompetent children with no indwelling catheter, heart disease, urinary infection, or bowel disease. Separating a true-positive blood culture from a contaminant is made easier if the patient has no risk factors for infection with relatively avirulent organisms and appears well. Of course, such a patient is not usually a candidate for a blood culture in the first place. The reason for the recommendation that blood cultures usually be obtained in duplicate (i.e., two separate venipunctures) is that if both cultures grow the same organism, contamination is an unlikely explanation. From a practical standpoint, this policy is easier to adhere to in adults than in children. If the patient has underlying risks or appears seriously ill, a repeat set of blood cultures should be obtained and appropriate antibiotics started. If the patient appears well, it is simple enough to repeat the blood culture and withhold antibiotics. Any patient with a persistently positive blood culture should be investigated for the possibility of an occult focus of infection, especially endocarditis (Chapter 18).

Age Frequency of Bacteremia

Initial antibiotic therapy for suspected sepsis is based on results of past studies. Age and underlying disease influence the bacteria found (Tables 10-6 and 10-7) and hence the choice of initial therapy (Table 10-8). Table 10-6 lists the commonest causes of bacteremia in normal children by age groups to show the major changes by age, although obviously many other causes of bacteremia are possible, especially with unrecognized predisposing conditions.[213,214]

In addition, other life-threatening conditions can mimic bacterial sepsis. One example is RMSF, which requires therapy with an antimicrobial (doxycycline) that is not normally used in the empiric therapy for sepsis. Another is neonatal HSV infection, for which prompt therapy with acyclovir may be life saving.

Group B streptococci and enteric bacteria cease

TABLE 10-6. BACTEREMIA IN NORMAL CHILDREN BY AGE

AGE	MOST COMMON BACTERIA
0 to 30 days	Group B streptococci, *E. coli*, other enteric bacteria, *Listeria monocytogenes*, *S. aureus*
1 to 3 months	*S. pneumoniae*, the preceding bacteria, *N. meningitidis*
3 to 24 months	*S. pneumoniae*, *N. meningitidis*, *Salmonella* spp., Group A streptococci, *S. aureus*, *H. influenzae* type b (unimmunized), *H. influenzae* non type b
2 to 5 years	Same as 3 to 24 months
> 5 years	*N. meningitidis*, *S. aureus*, *S. pneumoniae*

TABLE 10-7. PREDISPOSING FACTORS ASSOCIATED WITH BACTEREMIA IN CHILDREN

PREDISPOSING FACTOR	MOST COMMON BACTERIA
Intravascular device	*S. epidermidis*, *S. aureus*, *C. albicans*, other *Candida* spp., enterococci, *Corynebacteria*
Hematologic malignancy; neutropenia	Same as preceding plus: Enterobacteriaciae (*E. coli*, *Klebsiella*, others), *Pseudomonas aeruginosa*, other nonenteric GNRs
Prior therapy with broad-spectrum antibiotics	Resistant enteric and nonenteric GNRs, *Candida* spp.
Splenic dysfunction	Encapsulated bacteria (*S. pneumoniae*, *N. meningitidis*, *Klebsiella*, *H. influenzae*)
Immunologic disorders	Pyogenic bacteria (antibody deficiency); *N. meningitidis* (terminal complement deficiency; properdin deficiency); *Salmonella* spp., GNRs (chronic granulomatous disease)

to be common after 3 months of age and *S. aureus* becomes more common after 6 years of age. In vaccinated children, *H. influenzae* type b bacteremia is uncommon. Predisposing factors are shown in Table 10-7 with most common bacteria found. In general, the age frequency in Table 10-6 is an added factor. Often, several predisposing factors are present in the same patient. For special exposures not listed in Table 10-7, see Chapter 21.

Empiric Therapy of Suspected Sepsis

Some suggested initial regimens for suspected sepsis are listed in Table 10-8. The actual choice of therapy will depend both on local epidemiologic factors (most common organisms, current resistance patterns) and on patient-specific considerations. For example, in some locations, a high percentage of penicillin-resistant *S. pneumoniae* or

TABLE 10-8. SOME CHOICES FOR EMPIRIC THERAPY OF SUSPECTED SEPSIS IN CHILDREN

AGE OR SITUATION	EMPIRIC THERAPY
0 to 12 weeks old,* previously healthy	Ampicillin plus gentamicin OR Ampicillin plus cefotaxime
0 to 12 weeks old,* suspicion of bowel perforation	Ampicillin plus gentamicin plus metronidazole (plus fluconazole or amphotericin B in selected patients)
1 to 12 weeks old,* residence in neonatal intensive care unit and presence of an intravenous line	Ceftazidime plus vancomycin (plus fluconazole or amphotericin B in selected patients)
3 months to 5 years, previously healthy	Cefotaxime† OR Cefotaxime† plus vancomycin
> 5 years, previously healthy	Cefotaxime† OR Cefotaxime† plus nafcillin OR Cefotaxime† plus vancomycin
Malignancy, neutropenia or other immunosuppression	Cefepime plus vancomycin (plus gentamicin and/or amphotericin B in selected patients)

*In the first month of life, consideration should be given to testing for herpes simplex virus infection and for empiric acyclovir therapy (see Chapter 19)
†Or ceftriaxone

methicillin-resistant *S. aureus* may require empiric therapy with vancomycin, whereas in other geographic areas it may be unnecessary. A neutropenic patient who is only mildly ill may require treatment with cefepime alone. However, one whose condition is unstable might require therapy with cefepime, vancomycin, gentamicin, and an antifungal agent. Early consultation with an infectious diseases specialist is recommended. Once the susceptibility pattern of the organism is known, therapy can be changed if necessary.

Specific Bacteria

Staphylococcus aureus

S. aureus bacteremia often has an underlying focus such as osteomyelitis, septic arthritis, intraabdominal abscess, endocarditis, or skin infection.[215,216] In a child without a malignancy or intravenous device, the preliminary report of a blood culture showing gram-positive cocci can be regarded as a *S. epidermidis* contaminant provided the patient's clinical picture is consistent. Recovery of *S. aureus* from the blood of an ill child almost always prompts an evaluation for an underlying focus, usually including careful physical examination, echocardiography, and bone scan.

In certain children with malignancy, intravascular catheters, or hospital-acquired presumed sepsis, vancomycin is used in initial therapy because of the risk of methicillin-resistant (and hence nafcillin- and cephalosporin-resistant) *S. aureus* or *S. epidermidis.*[217,218] As mentioned earlier, failure to remove CVCs infected with *S. aureus* is associated with a higher risk of secondary sites of infection.

Staphylococcus epidermidis

Coagulase-negative staphylococci are usually reported as *S. epidermidis,* but some laboratories do further speciation studies and report *S. haemolyticus* and other such species. *S. epidermidis* has become the most frequent cause of nosocomial bacteremia because of the extensive use of intravascular catheters.

Most strains have the capacity to etch and erode the plastic and cover themselves with their cell-wall glycocalyx (slime). Perhaps antibiotic therapy has helped select these strains. Although fatalities from *S. epidermidis* are rare, many strains are methicillin resistant. Thus, if blood cultures reveal *S. epidermidis* and skin contamination is thought to be un-

likely, vancomycin is used pending susceptibility results. Beyond the neonatal period, most cases can be treated with retention of the catheter, although this results in a threefold increased risk for recurrent infection compared with patients whose catheters are removed.[219]

Group A Streptococcal Sepsis

Bacteremia due to Group A streptococcus typically occurs as a complication of cellulitis, bone or joint infection, chickenpox, pneumonia, or a wound infection. Of 60 children with Group A streptococcal bacteremia, 48 (80%) had an identifiable underlying source.[220] Rarely, a primary bacteremia without an obvious focus and with overwhelming sepsis can occur, with embolization and secondary foci in the lungs, meninges, or skin.[221] Disseminated intravascular coagulation can also occur.[222]

Fulminant Meningococcemia

Meningococcemia is the prototype of fulminating bacteremia in a clinically normal individual. Typically, there is high fever and a petechial or purpuric rash (purpura fulminans). Meningitis is variable, and the prognosis is slightly better if there has been time for a spinal fluid pleocytosis to develop. Obtaining a secure intravenous route for fluid therapy takes precedence over lumbar puncture. Arthritis or arthralgia is not unusual. Vomiting and diarrhea occasionally occur. Shock, disseminated intravascular coagulation, and myocarditis are common mechanisms of death. Myocardial dysfunction is due to a circulating meningococcal endotoxin.[223]

Measurement of left-ventricular shortening fraction appears to have some prognostic significance in children with meningococcal septic shock. In one study of 26 children with fulminant meningococcemia, 7 died; all 7 had shortening fractions of less than 0.30 as compared with 10 (50%) of 20 survivors (positive predictive value 41%).[223]

Treatment may require enormous volumes of fluid. Some patients have such fulminant disease that they die regardless of prompt diagnosis and treatment. The incidence of congenital or acquired complement deficiency in patients with meningococcal infection is much higher in those with recurrent disease.[224] Properdin deficiency also predisposes to recurrent meningococcal disease.

Fulminating Pneumococcemia

Typically, fulminating pneumococcemia occurs in a patient with an absent or nonfunctioning spleen, as in sickle cell anemia or after splenectomy.[225] The classic presentation is that of fever, chills, hypotension, and symmetric peripheral gangrene.[226] Because other encapsulated bacteria such as *H. influenzae* type b can also produce this pattern and can be ampicillin- or penicillin-resistant, initial therapy for presumed sepsis in a patient without a spleen should consist of ceftriaxone or its equivalent. This drug is also usually effective against encapsulated *Klebsiella* (rare), and the dog-saliva bacterium *Capnocytophaga canimorsus* (formerly called DF-2), which can cause fulminating sepsis after a dog bite.[226]

Fulminant H. influenzae *Sepsis*

Rarely, *H. influenzae* can resemble fulminant meningococcemia, with petechiae and purpura. As described in the section on petechial rashes, antibiotic therapy for suspected meningococcal sepsis (for example, ceftriaxone) should be effective against ampicillin-resistant *H. influenzae*.

Children with absent or nonfunctional spleens are susceptible to fulminating septicemia with these encapsulated bacteria, just as in fulminating pneumococcemia. Severe sepsis occasionally occurs in normal infants, with later foci of metastatic infection, but this represents a very small proportion of *H. influenzae* bacteremias.[228] Children who have not been immunized are at higher risk, especially if they live in a community of largely unimmunized children, as, for example, in a tight-knit community that refuses vaccinations for religious reasons.

With widespread use of Hib vaccine in the United States, invasive disease caused by non–type b strains of *H. influenzae* is now 10 times more common than that caused by Hib.[228a] Type f is currently the most common cause of invasive disease. In a population-based study conducted from 1989 to 1994, the incidence of invasive disease due to type f increased nearly fourfold.[228b] Of the 19 cases in children, 13 (68%) were younger than 12 months old. The case-fatality rate among children was 21%. In contrast, a case-report and literature review described 15 cases in children, none of whom died.[228c]

Uncommon Causes of Fulminant Septicemia

Few bacteria cause fulminant sepsis other than those described. *Pseudomonas aeruginosa* is a rare cause of bacteremia without a focal infection (pre-

sumably from bowel flora) in a normal infant,[230] but is the most common cause of fulminant septicemia in fragile premature infants in neonatal intensive care units. *Salmonella* species can cause bacteremia in association with diarrhea, but the illness is often no more severe than in normal children with nonbacteremic diarrhea.[231] In infancy, however, bacteremia with *Salmonella* sometimes seeds the meninges, causing a gram-negative meningitis.

Fulminating bacteremias caused by bacteria not mentioned previously can occur when there is an anatomic or immunologic defect that is unrecognized. None of the antibiotic regimens in Table 10-8 contains enough antibiotics to cover all unlikely possibilities. If bowel disease or malignancy is suspected but unproved, the appropriate regimen can be chosen.

Oral Therapy After Intravenous Therapy

Children who have received IV antibiotics for bacteremia in the hospital can be changed to oral therapy and discharged at some appropriate point. Criteria are best established for bone and joint infections and are discussed in Chapter 16.

Guidelines have not been established for occult bacteremia or for bacteremia secondary to a focal infection. The principal disadvantage to an oral regimen is that its success depends on absorption from the gastrointestinal tract. Additionally, these regimens are dependent on strict adherence to a prescribed regimen, which can seldom be ensured. Measurement of peak and trough serum levels after oral administration of an antibiotic and comparison of those levels with the minimum inhibitory concentration (MIC) of the patient's organism can be performed. Dosage adjustments can then be made, if necessary. Alternatively, the patient's serum can be serially diluted and tested against a culture of his own organism in the laboratory ("serum bactericidal titers"). For serious infections such as osteomyelitis, such measurements can provide some reassurance about the possible efficacy of an oral antibiotic regimen. However, these methods are costly and time consuming. Accurate bactericidal titers are also dependent on expertly trained laboratory personnel. Most clinicians favor the simpler approach of giving large dosages of antibiotics that are known to be well absorbed and scheduling close outpatient follow-up.

Possible criteria for changing from IV to oral

therapy include highly sensitive bacteria (e.g., group A streptococci, penicillin-sensitive pneumococci), bacteremias likely to be low grade (e.g., occult), absence of meningitis, early treatment after onset of fever, child and parents reliable for taking oral medication, and perhaps age more than 6 months. A major guideline should be documentation of negative blood cultures on therapy. Patients should generally be afebrile for 24–48 hours before switching to oral antibiotics. C-reactive protein is an acute phase reactant that usually returns to normal when an infection is being adequately treated; a normal C-reactive protein bodes well for successful oral completion of antibiotic therapy.

■ SEPTIC SHOCK

Definition

Shock is impaired tissue perfusion or failure to meet the metabolic demands of the body, which may be secondary to hypovolemia, cardiac failure, circulatory obstruction, or maldistribution of the circulation (distributive shock).[231] Poor tissue perfusion usually precedes shock, with cool extremities and poor refill of capillaries in the nail beds, and can be conveniently regarded as a preshock situation. When the potential for shock is not appreciated, the first recognized sign of shock may be falling blood pressure; this emphasizes the importance of taking the blood pressure in a febrile patient. Other signs of impending shock reflect the sympathetic nervous system's reactions to compensate for the inadequate tissue perfusion (e.g., tachycardia and anxiety).

In a broad sense, microorganisms other than bacteria can produce septic shock. Presumably, the mechanisms for other infecting organisms are much the same, with altered cellular metabolism and maldistribution of the circulation. *Rickettsiae* (RMSF), fungi (candidiasis), protozoans (malaria), and viruses (hemorrhagic fevers) can all produce septic shock.

Classification

Generally, shock is classified as either compensated or uncompensated. The other terms discussed following are used only for descriptive purposes.

Compensated Shock

This is shock in which blood pressure is preserved. Poor capillary refill in nail beds and cool extremities often precede shock of any kind.

Warm Shock

This is also called low-resistance shock, because the small blood vessels are dilated, producing little peripheral vascular resistance, and the skin feels warm. It usually signals early septic shock, as it characteristically occurs early in sepsis. The concept of warm shock is especially important for children, because it emphasizes the need to take the blood pressure in all febrile children.

Septic shock, as in meningococcemia, sometimes begins as warm shock and later, as compensatory vasoconstriction occurs, is manifested as cold shock (see following).[232] Septic shock can be associated with low, normal, or high cardiac output.

Cold Shock

Cold shock is also called high-resistance shock, because there is peripheral vasoconstriction, and the skin feels cold and clammy. It often occurs with hypovolemic shock because it characteristically occurs in hemorrhage, burns, diarrhea, or other conditions associated with low blood volume, including intussusception. However, cold shock is also characteristic of cardiogenic shock (primary pump failure) and obstructive shock (as in pericardial tamponade). Cold shock can follow warm shock as part of a continuum as septic shock evolves.

Cardiogenic Shock

Cardiogenic shock is also called congestive shock, because there is circulatory congestion secondary to reduced cardiac output. This is usually the principal mechanism of shock in acute myocardial infarction but it also may occur in myocarditis of infectious etiology.

More than one type of shock may occur simultaneously, as in meningococcemia, which usually is associated early with low-resistance (warm) shock but may also have a cardiogenic basis because of myocarditis.

Toxic Shock

The staphylococcal toxic shock syndrome typically resembles either hypovolemic shock after diarrhea or septic shock secondary to pyelonephritis or gastroenteritis. It is discussed as a separate section later in this chapter.

Mechanisms

The mechanisms of septic shock are multifactorial and include the effects of endotoxin on the cardiovascular system, including poor cardiac contractility, venous pooling, arteriolar vasodilation, and arteriovenous shunting, and increased capillary permeability in the lungs as well as the rest of the body. Endotoxin stimulates the release of inflammatory mediators. Tumor necrosis factor-alpha (TNF-alpha) is thought to be the most important of these in terms of production of septic shock or systemic inflammatory response syndrome.[233]

Meningococci produce immense amounts of endotoxin and can be regarded as the prototypic bacteria. Other bacteria such as *Escherichia coli*, *P. aeruginosa*, and *Klebsiella* are also good endotoxin producers and can produce septic shock. *H. influenzae* can produce septic shock, but it is usually much less severe than that produced by gram-negative enteric bacteria.[234]

Predisposing Factors

The predisposing factors for septic shock are the same as those for bacteremia (see Table 10-7).

Antibiotic Treatment

Initial antibiotic therapy for septic shock is based on the therapy for suspected sepsis. It should consist of broad-spectrum coverage, especially for patients who develop septic shock nosocomially. Outcomes of bloodstream infections have been linked to the appropriateness of the initial antimicrobial therapy in a large retrospective study (*n* = 341).[235] This turned out to be especially true for pediatric patients, those with abdominal infections, and those infected with *Klebsiella pneumoniae*.[235]

The clinical situation dictates which combination of antimicrobial agents should be used. The combination of a third-generation cephalosporin, an aminoglycoside (gentamicin or tobramycin), and vancomycin may be reasonable initially. If the patient is immunocompromised or a nosocomial infection is suspected, an antipseudomonal cephalosporin (such as ceftazidime), or a semisynthetic penicillin (such as ticarcillin or piperacillin) or a carbapenem (such as micropenem) in combination with an aminoglycoside should be used. If toxic shock syndrome is suspected, clindamycin can be added, as discussed following. If rickettsial disease is a possibility, doxycycline should be added. In the patient with nosocomial infection, antifungal coverage with amphotericin B is sometimes appropriate.

Nonantibiotic Treatment

The first priority (after the ABC's of airway, breathing, circulation) is to secure adequate intravenous access to support circulating blood volume, as well as for delivering medications. Femoral venous catheter insertion may be the most expedient route when the usual veins are not available because of vasoconstriction.[231] Intraosseous infusion should be considered if intravenous access is unattainable.

Doses for drugs on the basis of body weight should be available on cards or tables in the office, emergency room, or intensive care unit. The sequence of supportive therapy depends on monitoring.

In the most oversimplified terms, the circulatory system can be compared to a pump and a circulating duct system. The usual treatment sequence is

1. Fill up the circulation.
2. Help the pump work.
3. Direct the circulation to vital areas.
4. Prevent or repair leaks.

Some of the functions that ideally are monitored (such as pulmonary capillary wedge pressure) cannot be done without the availability of an intensive care unit and skilled personnel. The central venous pressure measured through a catheter from a peripheral vein to a large central vein may be a helpful guide to fluid replacement but is not as accurate as more invasive monitoring, as with a pulmonary artery catheter.

It has been well noted that many guidelines for the treatment of patients with septic shock are being developed by consensus rather than by science.[237] The initial therapy for hypoperfusion is establishing adequate intravascular volume and left ventricular preload. This is especially true in children. Most children with fluid-refractory septic shock respond to inotrope and/or vasodilator therapy. Hemodynamic states must be carefully monitored because they change over time. An incorrect cardiovascular regimen should be suspected in children with persistent shock who have sufficient intravenous fluids.[238] The amount of fluid required to resuscitate a child in shock is often underestimeted.

Corticosteroids

Although early studies suggested that corticosteroids may be beneficial for the treatment of septic shock,[239] this was not confirmed by subsequent studies.[240] Two meta-analyses of the literature have concluded that there is no evidence to support the use of steroids in patients with sepsis.[241,242]

Intravenous Immune Globulin (IVIG)

Polyclonal preparations of IVIG contain antibodies to a variety of endotoxins. Additionally, modulation of exuberant immune responses is effected by the administration of IVIG in many disease states. Therefore, it seems logical that IVIG may be of potential benefit as an adjunct in the treatment of bacterial sepsis and septic shock. IVIG is not widely used at present. However, a recent Cochrane database review has been published. The authors of this review included 27 of 55 published studies evaluating either polyclonal or monoclonal IVIG preparations versus placebo in a prospective fashion. Overall mortality was reduced in patients who received IVIG. Relative risk of death was 0.60, with 95% confidence intervals of 0.47–0.76. The authors concluded that the evidence suggests that IVIG significantly reduces mortality in sepsis and septic shock and can be used as adjunctive therapy.[243] These findings are tempered by the results of a recent multicenter trial comparing polyclonal IVIG with placebo in adults with sepsis. This study enrolled 653 patients (in comparison, the trials of polyclonal IVIG in the Cochrane review included a total of 492 patients) and showed, unfortunately, that 28-day mortality was not reduced among patients in the IVIG arm.[244]

Monoclonal Antibodies

Monoclonal antibodies to a variety of inflammatory mediators have been tried, either in human studies or in animal models. In general, no monoclonal antibody has consistently proven to be of value. This makes sense in light of the tremendous redundancy of the immune system and the complexity of the response to infection that leads to sepsis. In addition, the response to anti-inflammatory agents may depend on the infecting organism; the pathogenesis of sepsis from gram-positive organisms may differ in fundamental ways from the pathogenesis of sepsis due to infection with gram-negative organisms.[245]

Activated Protein C

The inflammatory cascade in sepsis includes a procoagulant response, and activated protein C has been shown to inhibit thrombosis and inflammation in patients with sepsis. A multicenter, randomized controlled trial comparing recombinant human activated protein C with placebo among 1690 adults with sepsis has been published.[246]

The 28-day mortality rate was 31% in the placebo group and 25% in the group receiving activated protein C ($p = 0.005$). Patients receiving activated protein C had a higher incidence of serious bleeding episodes (3.5% versus 2.0%, $p = 0.06$).

The experience using activated protein C in children is largely limited to those with meningococcemia. One group reported giving protein C to 12 patients with severe meningococcal sepsis; there was no control group. Based on the severity of their illness, the predicted mortality of the group was greater than 50%, but all patients survived. Both patients who received protein C more than 24 hours after admission required limb amputation as compared with none of those who received it sooner. Patients in this trial were also treated with hemofiltration, so the exact contribution of protein C is difficult to assess.[247] However, the use of protein C appears to be more promising than other adjunctive therapies for sepsis and deserves further study.[248]

Leukocytes, Plasma, and Complement

Newborns, the age group with the highest frequency of sepsis, have been studied to determine the efficacy of blood or its components in the treatment of sepsis.[249,250] The value of neutrophils (buffy coat transfusions) remains unclear. Complement or other plasma components such as opsonizing antibodies have theoretical but unproven value for treatment of the bacterial source of septic shock.

Other Adjunctive Therapies

Multiple other agents have been studied, including pentoxifylline, nitrous oxide synthesis inhibitors, platelet activating receptor antagonists, and plasma filtration with polymyxin B immobilized fiber, but none has been demonstrated unequivocally to be effective.[251–255]

A trial of human growth hormone in adults increased mortality from 9 to 20% ($p = 0.001$).[256]

Complications

Disseminated Intravascular Coagulation

This problem often occurs with shock. It can be anticipated, or it may be first suspected when oozing occurs at venipuncture sites. The diagnosis can be confirmed by coagulation studies and smear (low platelet count and fibrinogen concentration, increased activated partial thromboplastin time, fibrin split products, and prothrombin time).

Acute Respiratory Distress Syndrome (ARDS)

When pulmonary capillary leakage is severe in septic shock, and the chest roentgenogram is opaque in most areas, the complication is called ARDS or shock lung.[257]

Acute Renal Failure

Acute renal failure occurs in approximately 20–25% of patients, with moderate to severe sepsis and in 50% of patients with septic shock when blood cultures are positive.[257a]

■ TOXIC SHOCK SYNDROME (TSS)

This syndrome was originally described in 1978 by Todd and associates as a cluster of findings in children including fever, hypotension, *S. aureus* infection, and other findings attributable to a staphylococcal exotoxin.[258] The presentation of classic toxic shock syndrome included rash, injected bulbar conjunctivae, toxicity, and confusion, as these were present in the seven children originally described. Originally, Group A streptococcal infection was excluded by culture or serology. Staphylococcal TSS came to prominence with an outbreak of cases in the late 1970s and early 1980s in menstruating women that was associated with the use of super-absorbent tampons.

Currently, about half of cases of staphylococcal TSS are associated with neither tampons nor menstruation. Additionally, it is now known that invasive group A streptococcal infection can produce a clinical syndrome very similar to classic staphylococcal TSS. With cases caused by group A streptococcus, the onset is somewhat more insidious, the rash is more likely to be scarlatiniform, diarrhea and vomiting are less likely to be present, severe hyperesthesia is more common, and the mortality rate is much higher (about 50%). In addition, a focal source of infection is more often found in cases caused by group A streptococcus.

Upon initial presentation, the working diagnosis should generally be toxic shock syndrome, most likely due to *S. aureus* (or group A streptococcus).

Once the etiology is confirmed, the diagnosis is either staphylococcal TSS or streptococcal TSS.

Staphylococcal TSS

The Centers for Disease Control and Prevention has established strict guidelines for establishing the diagnosis of staphylococcal TSS. These guidelines may be remembered by using this mnemonic: "FDR Had three organs." The F stands for fever, the D for desquamation, the R for rash, the H for hypotension, and the remainder reminds the clinician that at least three organ systems must be involved. The diagnostic criteria for staphylococcal TSS are shown in Box 10-3. Serologic tests for leptospirosis, RMSF, and measles, if these diseases are suspected and blood work is drawn, are negative. Blood cultures are almost always negative, but sometimes grow *S. aureus*.

Subgroups

The syndrome is sometimes subdivided into menstrual and nonmenstrual subgroups based on the

---

BOX 10-3 ■ Definition of Staphylococcal Toxic Shock Syndrome

Major criteria (all required)
1. **Fever** ≥ 38.8°C (102°F)
2. **Hypotension** (orthostatic or shock)
3. **Rash** (erythroderma early and desquamation later)

Minor criteria (any three required)
1. **Gastrointestinal.** Vomiting or diarrhea
2. **Muscular.** Severe myalgia or creatinine phosphokinase ≥ 2x the upper limit of normal
3. **Mucous membranes.** Vaginal, oropharyngeal, or conjunctival hyperemia
4. **Renal.** BUN or serum creatinine ≥ 2 the upper limit of normal or urinalysis with >5 WBC per high-power field
5. **Hepatic.** Total bilirubin, AST or ALT ≥ 2 the upper limit of normal
6. **Hematologic.** Platelet count <100,000/μL
7. **Central nervous system.** Disorientation or alteration in level of consciousness without focality, noted when fever and hypotension are absent

Exclusion criteria
1. Absence of other explanations
2. Blood cultures negative (except for *S. aureus*)

source of the *S. aureus*. The epidemic of menstrual-associated toxic shock peaked in the early 1980s and has waned since the recognition of the role of tampons. These cases had the onset of illness within the first 5 days of menstruation, and tampons had been used.

Nonmenstrual toxic shock syndrome can be secondary to a staphylococcal infection in many possible locations, including wound infections, acute endocarditis, dental infections, and lymphadenitis.

Toxins

Toxic shock syndrome toxin-1 (TSST-1) is the most common enterotoxin responsible for producing the syndrome. Many isolates of *S. aureus* associated with TSS, however, do not produce TSST-1, or produce TSST-1 in association with another enterotoxin. Staphylococcal enterotoxins A, B, and C have also been associated with TSS-like illness.

Clinical Manifestations

Typical Presentation

The earliest symptoms are fever, myalgias, weakness, headache, vomiting, and abdominal pain soon followed by mucous membrane hyperemia, diffuse erythroderma, dizziness (postural hypotension), diarrhea, and confusion (Fig. 10-4).[259,260] Almost all organ systems are involved with clinical or laboratory findings attributable to the toxin. Herpes stomatitis or genital herpes may occur.

Early Differential Diagnosis

Scarlet fever may be suspected because of the fever, rash, injected conjunctivae, strawberry tongue, fever, and leukocytosis with a predominance of neutrophils. Acute diarrhea may be suspected as the primary disease because of diarrhea and abdominal pain and distension, although the degree and persistence of shock exceeds that expected from the amount of the diarrhea. Acute pyelonephritis with septic shock may be suspected because of the shock and pyuria, although bacteria are not prominent on urine microscopic examination and the urine culture does not confirm an infection. In children under 8 years of age, Kawasaki disease may be considered because of the fever, rash, and conjunctival injection.

Laboratory Findings

Typical early studies include a high WBC count with immature neurophils, pyuria, elevated blood

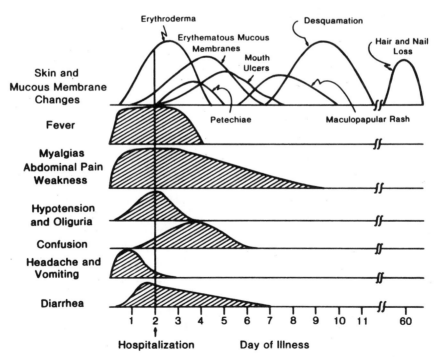

■ **FIGURE 10-4** Sequence of clinical findings in staphylococcal toxic shock syndrome. (Chesney PJ et al: JAMA 1981;246:741; copyright 1981, American Medical Association)

urea nitrogen (BUN) or creatinine, and slightly decreased platelet count. There may be a profound lymphopenia.

A chemistry panel typically shows that the levels of serum calcium, phosphorus, iron, total protein, and albumin are very low. Transaminase levels are elevated, especially the fraction from cardiac muscle, and the level of creatinine phosphokinase is very high, suggesting generalized muscle involvement. Cultures of the blood are usually negative, but cultures of body orifices, especially the vagina, rectum, or nares, or the site of a purulent infection, may reveal *S. aureus*. The chest roentgenogram may show transient infiltrates.

Treatment

If possible, identification and drainage of the site of infection is an important aspect of management. Foreign bodies, such as tampons, need to be removed. Wounds need to be drained and/or irrigated. Antistaphylococcal antibiotic therapy, usually with a semisynthetic penicillin such as nafcillin or oxacillin, is initiated. Because toxic shock syndrome is a toxin-mediated illness, the concomitant use of a protein-synthesis inhibiting antibiotic such as clindamycin has been recommended. In vitro, subinhibitory concentrations of clindamycin greatly decrease the production of TSST-1. In contrast, subinhibitory concentrations of nafcillin tend to cause levels of TSST-1 in culture supernatants to increase. This effect is blocked by the addition of a protein-synthesis inhibitor. Therefore, the combination of nafcillin and clindamycin seems advisable. In some geographic areas, the use of vancomycin may be appropriate. Optimal duration of therapy has not been clearly established. In the past, antistaphylococcal therapy was thought to be of minor importance in the care of TSS; inadequate antibiotic therapy, however, clearly leads to a higher incidence of recurrence. Most experts recommend antibiotic therapy for 10–14 days.

Although there are no randomized, placebo-controlled trials of IVIG in the treatment of TSS, anecdotal evidence favors its use in severe cases. The absence of a protective antitoxin antibody is one of the prerequisites to the development of staphylococcal TSS. This is in contrast to the general population, most of which has measurable levels, even if they lack a history of staphylococcal disease. Therefore, all lots of IVIG contain antibody directed against the toxins that are perpetuating the illness.

In animal models of TSS, administration of IVIG prior to infection is protective against the syndrome, and survival is enhanced even when IVIG is administered up to 29 hours after infection is established.[261] Case reports confirm rapid improvement following administration of IVIG in some patients with TSS. A dose of 400 mg/kg infused over several hours results in serum antibody titers that are sufficient to block the action of TSST-1.[262]

Intravenous fluids are usually effective in maintaining a low to low-normal blood pressure with adequate urine output, but occasionally pressor agents such as dopamine are necessary. Maintenance of adequate blood pressures and monitoring of patients for the development of adult respiratory distress syndrome, renal failure, cardiac arrhythmias, and other adverse events comprises the remainder of the important management points.

Complications

Renal insufficiency may occur, sometimes making the illness resemble hemolytic-uremic syndrome, especially with the burr cells, anemia, and low platelets. Disseminated intravascular coagulation and adult-type respiratory distress syndrome (ARDS or "shock lung") have been observed. Dysrhythmia, possibly related to electrolyte imbalances, and cardiac failure, possibly due to toxic cardiomyopathy, may occur. Rarely, fatal dysrhythmia develops. Death is rare and may be due to adult respiratory distress syndrome or myocardial failure.

Desquamation of the palms and soles in thick sheets occurs 7–10 days after the onset. At about this time, edema or a pruritic rash also may be noted. Damage or loss of hair or nails can occur 2–3 months later.

Recurrences

Adequate antistaphylococcal therapy of the first episode and discontinuing use of tampons are significant factors in decreasing the risk of recurrences.[263] Davis et al. showed that after an episode of menstrual TSS, two-thirds of women who were not treated with an antibiotic and who continued to use tampons developed recurrent TSS during the next 5 months.[260] Recurrences have also been reported in cases of nonmenstrual TSS.[264] Most patients do not develop protective levels of antistaphylococcal toxin antibodies following an episode of TSS; this is likely related to recurrences.

Recalcitrant, Erythematous Desquamating Disorder (REDD)

This unusual variant, in which redness, desquamation, and other symptoms of TSS occur in a milder form for a prolonged time, has been seen mostly in patients with AIDS. Recurrences are frequent, and sometimes the disorder is fatal. A single case of this clinical syndrome in a patient with no known immunodeficiency has been reported.[264]

Streptococcal Toxic Shock Syndrome

Clinical Manifestations and Epidemiology

Group A streptococci produce several toxins that can produce a confusing multisystem disease similar in some ways to staphylococcal toxic shock syndrome.[266,267] There is usually a focus of Group A streptococcal infection such as the sinuses, skin, or lungs. Blood cultures are positive more frequently than in staphylococcal TSS. However, the multisystem involvement (CNS, liver, lungs, kidney, cardiovascular system, and skin) is probably related to toxemia. Group A streptococci produce three pyrogenic (erythrogenic) toxins (called A, B, and C), which may cause renal insufficiency and an erythematous rash with subsequent desquamation. Fever, sterile pyuria, and sometimes hypotension are found. Superinfection of varicella lesions is a common predisposing factor for streptococcal TSS.[268] The incidence of invasive group A streptococcal infection among children with varicella is 12-fold higher than among children without varicella.[269] Invasive disease with group A streptococci is on the rise, and about 15% of invasive Group A streptococcal infection in childhood is related to primary varicella infection.[270] Streptococcal toxic shock syndrome accounted for 7% of pediatric cases of invasive Group A streptococcal disease in one large study.[269]

Diagnosis

The diagnostic criteria for streptococcal toxic shock syndrome are listed in Box 10-4.[267] Note that, unlike with staphylococcal TSS, a rash is not required for the diagnosis. Thus, severe cases of necrotizing fasciitis may meet the case definition of streptococcal TSS. A definite case requires isolation of Group A streptococci from a normally sterile body site.

BOX 10-4 ■ Definition of Streptococcal Toxic Shock Syndrome

Hypotension or shock, plus any two of the following:
1. Scarlet fever rash
2. Hepatic abnormalities
3. Renal insufficiency
4. Disseminated intravascular coagulopathy
5. Adult respiratory distress syndrome
6. Soft-tissue necrosis

Definite case: preceding requirements plus isolation of group A streptococcus from a normally sterile body site

Probable case: preceding requirements plus isolation of group A streptococcus from a nonsterile body site

---

Treatment

Penicillin is the drug of choice for documented infections with group A streptococci. Analogous to the discussion with staphylococcal TSS, clindamycin is often added because of its ability to halt toxin production.[270] Similarly, IVIG is often given to patients with streptococcal TSS based on theoretical considerations[271] and studies using historical controls,[272] but randomized controlled trials are lacking. Massive amounts of fluids may be needed to maintain adequate blood pressure. Pressors are sometimes used but can result in peripheral gangrene with loss of digits.[273] In general, the hypotension associated with streptococcal TSS is much more difficult to manage than that associated with staphylococcal TSS, resulting in substantially greater morbidity and mortality.

■ REFERENCES

1. Schmitt BD. Fever in childhood. Pediatrics 1984; 74(suppl):S929–36.
2. Mackowiak PA, Bartlett JG, Borden EC, et al. Concepts of fever: recent advances and lingering dogma. Clin Infect Dis 1997;25:119–38.
3. Saper CB, Breder CD. The neurologic basis of fever. N Engl J Med 1994;330:1880–6.
4. Mackowiak PA, Boulant JA. Fever's glass ceiling. Clin Infect Dis 1996;22:525–36.
5. Kresch MJ. Axillary temperature as a screening test for fever in children. J Pediatr 1984;104:596–9.
6. Tanberg D, Sklar D. Effect of tachypnea on the estimation of body temperature by an oral thermometer. N Engl J Med 1983;308:945–6.

7. Banco L, Veltri D. Ability of mothers to subjectively assess the presence of fever in their children. Am J Dis Child 1984;138:976–8.

8. Bonadio WA, Hegenbarth M, Zachariason M. Correlating reported fever in young infants with subsequent temperature patterns and rate of serious bacterial infections. Pediatr Infect Dis J 1990;9:158–60.

9. Cross KW, Hey EN, Kennaird DL, et al. Lack of temperature control in infants with abnormalities of central nervous system. Arch Dis Child 1971;46:437–43.

10. Musher DM, Fainstain V, Young EJ, et al. Fever patterns. Arch Intern Med 1979;139:1225–8.

11. Flatauer FE, Ballou SP, Wolinsky E. Comparative response of fever to corticosteroids in tuberculosis and in connective tissue disease. Am J Med Sci 1981;281:111–5.

12. Kramer MS, Naimark L, Leduc DG. Parental fever phobia and its correlates. Pediatrics 1985;75:1110–3.

13. Schmitt BD. Fever phobia: misconceptions of parents about fevers. Am J Dis Child 1980;134:176–81.

14. Van Stuijvenberg M, DeVos S, Tjiang GC, et al. Parents' fear regarding fever and febrile seizures. Acta Paediatr 1999;88:618–22.

15. Poirier MP, Davis PH, Gonzalez-del Rey JA, Monroe KW. Pediatric emergency department nurses' perspectives on fever in children. Pediatr Emerg Care 2000;16:9–12.

16. Aksoylar S, Aksit S, Caglayan S, et al. Evaluation of sponging and antipyretic medications to reduce body temperature in febrile children. Acta Paediatr Jpn 1997;39:215–7.

17. O'Donnell J, Axelrod P, Fisher C, Lorber B. Use and effectiveness of hypothermia blankets for febrile patients in the intensive care unit. Clin Infect Dis 1997;24:1208–13.

18. Mackowiak PA. Assaulting a physiological response. Clin Infect Dis 1997;24:1214–6.

19. Newman J. Evaluation of sponging to reduce body temperature in febrile children. Can Med Assoc J 1985;132:641–2.

20. Watson PD, Galletta G, Braden NJ, Alexander L. Ibuprofen, acetaminophen, and placebo treatment of febrile children. Clin Pharmacol Ther 1989;46:9–17.

21. VanEsch A, VanSteensel-Moll HA, Steyerberg EW, et al. Antipyretic efficacy of ibuprofen and acetaminophen in children with febrile seizures. Arch Pediatr Adolesc Med 1995;149:632–7.

22. Vauzelle-Kervroedan F, d'Athis P, Pariente-Khayat A, Debregeas S, Olive G, Pons G. Equivalent antipyretic activity of ibuprofen and paracetamol in febrile children. J Pediatr 1997;131:683–7.

23. Mayoral CE, Marino RV, Rosenfeld W, Greensher J. Alternating antipyretics: is this an alternative? Pediatrics 2000;105:1009–12.

24. Rumack BH. Aspirin and acetaminophen. Pediatrics 1978;62(suppl):S865–946.

25. Moghal NE, Hulton SA, Milford DV. Care in the use of ibuprofen as an antipyretic in children. Clin Nephrol 1998;49:293–5.

26. Zerr DM, Alexander ER, Duchin JS, et al. A case-control study of necrotizing fasciitis during primary varicella. Pediatrics 1999;103:783–90.

27. Hellewell PG, Young SK, Henson PM, Worthen GS. Paradoxic effect of ibuprofen on neutrophil accumulation in pulmonary and cutaneous inflammation. Am J Resp Crit Care Med 1995;151:1218–27.

28. Choo PW, Donahue JG, Platt R. Ibuprofen and skin and soft tissue superinfections in children with varicella. Ann Epidemiol 1997;7:440–5.

29. Moss MH. Alcohol-induced hypoglycemia and coma caused by alcohol sponging. Pediatrics 1970;46:445–7.

30. Arditi M, Killner MS. Coma following use of rubbing alcohol for fever control. Am J Dis Child 1987;141:237–8.

31. Dechovitz AB, Moffet HL. Classification of acute febrile illnesses in childhood. Clin Pediatr 1968;7:649–53.

32. Moffet HL, Cramblett HG, Smith A. Group A streptococcal infections in a children's home. II: clinical and epidemiologic patterns of illness. Pediatrics 1964;33:11–7.

33. Sanford JP, Sulkin SE. The clinical spectrum of ECHOvirus infection. N Engl J Med 1959;261:1113–22.

34. Konerding K, Moffet HL. New episodes of fever in hospitalized patients. Am J Dis Child 1970;120:515–9.

35. Schultz I, Gundelfinger B, Rosenbaum M, et al. Comparison of clinical manifestations of respiratory illnesses due to Asian strain influenza, adenovirus and unknown cause. J Lab Clin Med 1960;55:497–509.

36. Biggar RJ, Wood JP, Walter PD, et al. Lymphocytic choriomeningitis outbreak associated with pet hamsters. JAMA 1975;232:494–500.

37. Goodpasture HC, Poland JD, Francy DB, et al. Colorado tick fever: clinical, epidemiologic, and laboratory aspects of 228 cases in Colorado in 1973–1974. Ann Intern Med 1978;88:303–10.

38. Horton JM, Blaser NU. The spectrum of relapsing fever in the Rocky Mountains. Arch Intern Med 1985;145:871–5.

39. Maeda K, Markowitz N, Hawley RC, et al. Human infection with *Ehrlichia canis*, a leukocytic rickettsia. N Engl J Med 1987;316:853–6.

40. Fishbein DB, Sawyer LA, Holland CJ, et al. Unexplained febrile illnesses after exposure to ticks: infection with *Ehrlichia*? JAMA 1987;257:3100–4.

41. Schutze GE, Jacobs RF. Human monocytic ehrlichiosis in children. Pediatrics 1997;100:e10.

42. Brouqi P, Raoult D. In vitro antibiotic susceptibility of the newly recognized agent of ehrlichiosis in humans, *Ehrlichia chaffeensis*. Antimicrob Agents Chemother 1992;36:2799–803.

43. Dumler JS, Dey C, Meier F, Lewis LL. Human monocytic ehrlichiosis: a potentially severe disease in children. Arch Pediatr Adolesc Med 2000;154:847–9.

43a. Felek S. Unver A. Stich RW. Rikihisa Y. Sensitive detection of *Ehrlichia chaffeensis* in cell culture, blood, and tick specimens by reverse transcription-PCR. J Clin Microbiol 2001;39:460–3.

43b. Dumler JS, Barbet AF, Bekker CP, et al. Reorganization of genera in the families Rickettsiaceae and Anaplasmataceae in the order Rickettsiales: unification of some species of *Ehrlichia* with *Anaplasma*, *Cowdria* with *Ehrlichia* and *Ehrlichia* with *Neorickettsia*, descriptions of six new species combinations and designation of *Ehrlichia equi* and "HGE agent" as subjective synonyms of *Ehrlichia phagocytophilia*. Int J Syst Evol Microbiol 2001;51:2145–65.

43c. Moss WJ. Dumler JS. Simultaneous infection with *Borrelia burgdorferi* and human granulocytic ehrlichiosis. Pediatr Infect Dis J 2003;22:91–2.

44. Bauchner H, Philipp B, Dashefsky B, et al. Prevalence of bacteriuria in febrile children. Pediatr Infect Dis J 1987; 6:239–42.

45. Roberts KB. Management of young, febrile infants [editorial]. Am J Dis Child 1983;137:1143–4.

46. McCarthy PL, Dolan TF. The serious implications of high fever in infants during their first three months. Clin Pediatr 1976;15:794–6.

47. Pantell RH, Naber M, Lamar R, et al. Fever in the first six months of life: risks of underlying infection. Clin Pediatr 1980;19:77–82.

48. Press S, Fawcett NP. Association of temperature greater than 41.1°C (106°F) with serious illness. Clin Pediatr 1985;24:21–5.

49. Krober MS, Bass JW, Powell JM, et al. Bacterial and viral pathogens causing fever in infants less than 3 months old. Am J Dis Child 1985;139:889–92.

50. Murray DL, Zonana J, Seidel JS, et al. Relative importance of bacteremia and viremia in the course of acute fevers of unknown origin in outpatient children. Pediatrics 1981;68:157–60.

51. Dagan R, Hall CB. Influenza A virus infection imitating bacterial infection in early infancy. Pediatr Infect Dis 1984;3:218–21.

52. Meurman O. Fever in respiratory virus infection. Am J Dis Child 1986;140:1159–63.

53. Crain EF, Shelov SP. Febrile infants: predictors of bacteremia. J Pediatr 1982;101:686–9.

54. Burke JP, Mein JO, Gezon HM, et al. Pneumococcal bacteremia: review of 111 cases, 1957–1969, with special reference to cases with undetermined focus. Am J Dis Child 1971;121:353–9.

55. Torphy DE, Ray CG. Occult pneumococcal bacteremia. Am J Dis Child 1970;119:336–8.

56. Heldich FJ Jr. *Diplococcus pneumoniae* bacteremia. Am J Dis Child 1970;119:12–7.

57. Alpern ER, Alessandrini EA, Bell LM, et al. Occult bacteremia from a pediatric emergency department: current prevalence, time to detection, and outcome. Pediatrics 2000;106:505–11.

58. Bass JW, Steele RW, Wittler RR, et al. Antimicrobial treatment of occult bacteremia: a multicenter cooperative study. Pediatr Infect Dis J 1993;12:466–73.

59. Lorin MI, Feigin RD. Fever without source and fever of unknown origin. In: Feigin RD, Cherry JD, Demmler GJ, Kaplan SL, eds. Textbook of Pediatric Infectious Diseases. 5th ed. Philadelphia: Saunders, 2004: 827.

60. Baraff LJ, Oslung S, Prather M. Effect of antibiotic therapy and etiologic microorganism on the risk of bacterial meningitis in children with occult bacteremia. Pediatrics 1993;92:140–3.

61. Shapiro ED, Aaron NH, Wald ER, Chiponis D. Risk factors for development of bacterial meningitis in children with occult bacteremia. J Pediatr 1986;109:15–9.

62. Lee GM, Harper MB. Risk of bacteremia in young children in the post-*Haemophilus influenzae* type b era. Arch Pediatr Adolesc Med 1998;152:624–8.

63. Teele DW, Pelton SI, Grant MJA, et al. Bacteremia in febrile children under 2 years of age: results of cultures of blood of 600 consecutive febrile children seen in a "walk in" clinic. J Pediatr 1975;87:227–30.

64. Crocker PJ, Quick G, McCombs W. Occult bacteremia

in the emergency department: diagnostic criteria for the young febrile child. Ann Emerg Med 1985;14:1172–7.

65. Dashefsky B, Teele DW, Klein JO. Unsuspected meningococcemia. J Pediatr 1983;102:69–72.

66. McCarthy PL, Lembo RM, Fink H, et al. Observation, history and physical examination in diagnosis of serious illnesses in febrile children < 24 months. J Pediatr 1987; 110:26–30.

67. McCarthy PL, Lembo RM, Baron MA, et al. Predictive value of abnormal physical examination findings in ill-appearing and well-appearing febrile children. Pediatrics 1985;76:167–71.

68. McCarthy PL, Sharpe MR, Spiegel SZ. Observation scales to identify serious illnesses in febrile children. Pediatrics 1982;70:802–9.

69. McCarthy PL, Jekel JF, Stashwick CA, et al. History and observation variables in assessing febrile children. Pediatrics 1980;65:1090–5.

70. McCarthy PL, Cicchetti DV, Stashwick CA, et al. Diagnostic styles of attending pediatricians, residents, and nurses in evaluating febrile children. Clin Pediatr 1982;21: 534–7.

71. Teach SJ, Fleisher GR. Duration of fever and its relationship to bacteremia in febrile outpatients 3 to 36 months old. Pediatr Emerg Care 1997;13:317–9.

72. Mine MW, Lorin MI. Bacteremia in children afebrile at presentation to an emergency room. Pediatr Infect Dis J 1987;6:197–8.

73. Baker MD, Fosarelli PD, Carpenter RO. Childhood fever: correlation of diagnosis with temperature response to acetaminophen. Pediatrics 1987;80:315–8.

74. Baker RC, Tiller T, Bausher JC, et al. Severity of disease correlated with fever reduction in febrile infants. Pediatrics 1989;83:1016–9.

75. McCarthy PL, Jekel JF, Dolan TF Jr. Temperature greater than or equal to 40°C in children less than 24 months of age: a prospective study. Pediatrics 1977;59:663–8.

76. Ruuskanen O, Meurman O, Sarkkinnen H. Adenoviral diseases in children: a study of 105 hospital cases. Pediatrics 1985;76:79–83.

77. Baron MA, Fink HD. Bacteremia in pediatric private practice. Pediatrics 1980;66:171–6.

78. Caspe WB, Chamudes O, Louie. The evaluation and treatment of the febrile infant. Pediatr Infect Dis 1983;2: 131–5.

79. Dagan R, Powell KR, Hall CB, et al. Identification of infants unlikely to have serious bacterial infection although hospitalized for suspected sepsis. J Pediatr 1985;107: 855–60.

80. Liu CH, Lehan C, Speer ME, et al. Early detection of bacteremia in an outpatient clinic. Pediatrics 1985;75: 827–31.

81. Adams RC, Dixon JH, Eichner ER. Clinical usefulness of polymorphonuclear leukocyte vacuolization in predicting septicemia in febrile children. Pediatrics 1978;62: 67–70.

82. Clyne B, Olshaker JS. The C-reactive protein. J Emerg Med 1999;17:1019–25.

83. Isaacman DJ, Burke BL. Utility of the serum C-reactive protein for detection of occult bacterial infection in children. Arch Pediatr Adolesc Med 2002;156:905–9.

84. Chirouze C, Schuhmacher H, Rabaud C, et al. Low serum

procalcitonin level accurately predicts the absence of bacteremia in adult patients with acute fever. Clin Infect Dis 2002;35:156–61.

85. Hausfater P, Garric S, Ayed SB, et al. Usefulness of procalcitonin as a marker of systemic infection in emergency department patients: a prospective study. Clin Infect Dis 2002;34:895–901.

86. Shapiro ED, Aaron NH, Wald ER, et al. Risk factors for development of bacterial meningitis among children with occult bacteremia. J Pediatr 1986;109:15–9.

87. Roberts KB, Charney E, Sweren RJ, et al. Urinary tract infection in infants with unexplained fever: a collaborative study. J Pediatr 1983;103:864–7.

88. Hoekelman R, Lewin EB, Shapira MB, et al. Potential bacteremia in pediatric practice. Am J Dis Child 1979; 133:1017–9.

89. Korones DN, Marshall GS, Shapiro ED. Outcome of children with occult bacteremia caused by *Haemophilus influenzae* type b. Pediatr Infect Dis J 1992;11:516–20.

90. Roberts KB. Blood cultures in pediatric practice. Am J Dis Child 1979;133:996–8.

91. Todd JK. High fever and diagnostic expenses [letter]. Pediatrics 1978;62:618–9.

92. Segal GS, Chamberlain JM. Resource utilization and contaminated blood cultures in children at risk for occult bacteremia. Arch Pediatr Adolesc Med 2000;154; 469–73.

93. Bratton L, Teele DW, Klein JO. Outcome of unsuspected pneumococcemia in children not initially admitted to the hospital. J Pediatr 1977;90:703–6.

94. Carroll WL, Farrell MK, Singer JI, et al. Treatment of occult bacteremia: a prospective randomized clinical trial. Pediatrics 1983;72:608–12.

95. Jaffe DM, Tanz RR, Davis AT, et al. Antibiotic administration to treat possible occult bacteremia in febrile children. N Engl J Med 1987;317:1175–80.

96. Rothrock SG, Harper MB, Green SM, et al. Do oral antibiotics prevent meningitis and serious bacterial infections in children with *Streptococcus pneumoniae* occult bacteremia? A meta-analysis. Pediatrics 1997;99:438–44.

97. Ros SP, Herman BE, Beissel TJ. Occult bacteremia: is there a standard of care? Pediatr Emerg Care 1994;10:264–7.

97a. Baraff LJ, Oslund S, Prather M. Effect of antibiotic therapy and etiologic microorganism on the risk of bacterial meningitis in children with occult bacteremia. Pediatrics 1993;92:140–3.

98. Fleisher GR, Rosenberg N, Vinci R, et al. Intramuscular versus oral antibiotic therapy for the prevention of meningitis and other bacterial sequelae in young, febrile children at risk for occult bacteremia. J Pediatr 1994;124: 504–12.

98a. Long SS. Antibiotic therapy in febrile children: "best-laid schemes... " [editorial]. J Pediatr 1994;124:585–8.

98b. Rothrock SG, Green SM, Harper MB, et al. Parenteral vs oral antibiotics in the prevention of serious bacterial infections in children with *Streptococcus pneumoniae* occult bacteremia: a meta-analysis. Acad Emerg Med 1998; 5:599–606.

99. Bulloch B, Craig WR, Klassen TP. The use of antibiotics to prevent serious sequelae in children at risk for occult bacteremia: a meta-analysis. Acad Emerg Med 1997;4: 679–83.

100. Baraff LJ, Bass JW, Fleisher GR, et al. Practice guideline for the management of infants and children 0 to 36 months of age with fever without source. Ann Emerg Med 1993;22:1198–210.

101. DeAngelis C, Joffe A, Wilson M, et al. Iatrogenic risks and financial costs of hospitalizing febrile infants. Am J Dis Child 1983;137:1146–9.

102. Baker MD, Bell LM, Avner JR. The efficacy of routine outpatient management without antibiotics of fever in selected infants. Pediatrics 1999;103:627–31.

103. Jaskiewicz JA, McCarthy CA, Richardson AC, et al. Febrile infants at low risk for serious bacterial infection—an appraisal of the Rochester criteria and implications for management. Pediatrics 1994;94:390–6.

104. Chiu CH, Lin TY, Bullard MJ. Identification of febrile neonates unlikely to have bacterial infections. Pediatr Infect Dis J 1997;16:59–63.

105. Petersdorf RG, Beeson PB. Fever of unexplained origin: report on 100 cases. Medicine 1961;40:1–30.

106. Feigin Rd, Shearer WT. Fever of unknown origin in children. Curr Probl Pediatr 1976;6:1–65.

107. Kleiman MB. The complaint of persistent fever: recognition and management of pseudo fever of unknown origin. Pediatr Clin North Am 1982;29:201–8.

108. Pizzo PA, Lovejoy FH Jr, Smith DH. Prolonged fever in children: review of 100 cases. Pediatrics 1975;55: 468–73.

109. Lohr JA, Hendley JO. Prolonged fever of unknown origin: a record of experiences with 54 childhood patients. Clin Pediatr 1977;16:768–74.

110. Blau EB, Morris RF, Yunis EJ. Polyarteritis nodosa in children. Pediatrics 1977;60:227–34.

111. Picus D, Siegel MJ, Balfe DM. Abdominal computed tomography in children with unexplained prolonged fever. J Comput Assist Tomogr 1984;8:851–6.

112. Listernick R, Shulman S. Tuberculous mesenteric lymphadenitis in children. Pediatr Infect Dis 1983;2:237–9.

113. Broughton RA, Edwards MS, Taber LH, et al. Systemic *Haemophilus influenzae* type b infection presenting as fever of unknown origin. J Pediatr 1981;98:925–8.

114. Memish ZA, Balkhy HH. Brucellosis and international travel. J Travel Med 2004;11:49–55.

115. Buchanan TM, Faber LC, Feldman RA. Brucellosis in the United States: an abattoir-associated disease. Medicine 1974;53:403–14.

116. Noble JT. Mark EJ. Case Records of the Massachusetts General Hospital. Weekly clinicopathological exercises. Case 22-2002. A 37-year-old man with unexplained fever after a long trip through South America. N Engl J Med 2002;347(3):200–6.

117. Young EJ. Serologic diagnosis of human brucellosis: analysis of 214 cases by agglutination tests and review of the literature. Rev Infect Dis 1991;13:359–72.

118. Jacobs RF, Schutze GE. *Bartonella henselae* as a cause of prolonged fever and fever of unknown origin in children. Clin Infect Dis 1998;26:80–4.

119. Dunn MW, Berkowitz FE, Miller JJ, Snitzer JA. Hepatosplenic cat-scratch disease and abdominal pain. Pediatr Infect Dis J 1997;16:269–72.

120. Ventura A, Massei F, Not T, et al. Systemic *Bartonella henselae* infection with hepatosplenic involvement. J Pediatr Gastroenterol Nutr 1999;29:52–6.

121. Kain KC, Harrington MA, Tennyson S, Keystone JS. Imported malaria: prospective analysis of problems in diagnosis and management. Clin Infect Dis 1998;27:142–9.

122. Centers for Disease Control and Prevention. Probable locally acquired mosquito-transmitted *Plasmodium vivax* infection—Suffolk County, New York, 1999. MMWR 2000;49:495–8.

123. White NJ. The treatment of malaria. New Engl J Med 1996;335(11):800–6.

124. Spach DH, Liles WC, Campbell GL, et al. Quick RE. Anderson et al. Tick-borne diseases in the United States. New Engl J Med 1993;329:936–47.

125. Lam K, Bayer AS. *Mycoplasma pneumoniae* as a cause of the "fever of unknown origin" syndrome. Arch Intern Med 1982;142:2312–3.

126. Hearey CD Jr, Daley TJ, Shaw EB. Prolonged fever from unusual cause (retinoblastoma). Am J Dis Child 1972; 123:51–2.

127. Miller JS, Miller D III. Benign giant lymph node hyperplasia presenting as fever of unknown origin. J Pediatr 1975; 87:237–9.

128. Edwards MS, Butler KM. "Hyperthermia of trickery" in an adolescent. Pediatr Infect Dis J 1987;64:411–4.

129. Mackowiak PA, LeMaistre CF. Drug fever: a critical appraisal of conventional concepts. Ann Intern Med 1987; 106:728–33.

130. Tsai MJ, Lin SC, Wang JK, Chou CC, Chiang BL. A patient with familial Takayasu's arteritis presenting with fever of unknown origin. J Formos Med Assoc 1998;97:351–3.

131. Gedalia A, Shetty AK, Ward KJ, Correa H, Heinrich S. Role of MRI in diagnosis of childhood sarcoidosis with fever of unknown origin. J Pediatr Orthop 1997;17: 460–2.

132. Lien CH, Yang W, Tsai YC, Huang PH. Kikuchi's disease (histiocytic necrotizing lymphadenitis): report of one case. Chung Hua Min Kuo Hsiao Erh Ko I Hsueh Hui Tsa Chih 1999;40:344–7.

133. Boyce TG, Moffet HL, Roh SK, Desouky SS. Pathological cases of the month. Kikuchi's disease (histiocytic necrotizing lymphadenitis). Arch Pediatr Adolesc Med 1994; 148:427–8.

134. Fisher RG, Wright PF, Johnson JE. Inflammatory pseudotumor presenting as fever of unknown origin. Clin Infect Dis 1995;21:1492–4.

135. Gratz S, Behr TM, Herrmann A, et al. Immunoscintigraphy in neonates and infants with fever of unknown origin. Nucl Med Commun 1998;19:1037–45.

136. Buonomo C, Treves ST. Gallium scanning in children with fever of unknown origin. Pediatr Radiol 1993;23: 307–10.

137. Calabro JJ, Marchesano JM. Fever associated with juvenile rheumatoid arthritis. N Engl J Med 1967;276:11–8.

138. Brewer EJ Jr. Manifestations of disease: juvenile rheumatoid arthritis. Major Probl Clin Pediatr 1970;6:1–47.

139. Schaller J, Wedgwood RJ. Juvenile rheumatoid arthritis: a review. Pediatrics 1973;50:940–53.

140. Calabro JJ, Marchesano JM. Rash associated with juvenile rheumatoid arthritis. J Pediatr 1968;72:611–9.

141. Ansell BM, Bywaters EGL. Diagnosis of "probable" Still's disease and its outcome. Ann Rheumat Dis 1962;21: 253–62.

142. Schlesinger B. Rheumatoid arthritis in the young. Br Med J 1949;2:197–201.

143. Schaller J, Beckwith B, Wedgwood RJ. Hepatic involvement in juvenile rheumatoid arthritis. J Pediatr 1970;77: 203–10.

144. Pelkonen P, Swanljung K, Siimes MA. Ferritinemia as an indicator of systemic disease activity in children with systemic juvenile rheumatoid arthritis. Acta Paediatr Scand 1986;75:64–8.

145. Marin-Garcia J, Sheridan R, Hanissian AS. Echocardiographic detection of early cardiac involvement in juvenile rheumatoid arthritis. Pediatrics 1984;73:394–7.

146. Doughty RA, Giesecke L, Athreya B. Salicylate therapy in juvenile rheumatoid arthritis: dose, serum level, and toxicity. Am J Dis Child 1980;134:461–3.

147. Lietman PS, Bywaters EGL. Pericarditis in juvenile rheumatoid arthritis. Pediatrics 1963;32:856–60.

148. Yancey CL, Doughty RA, Cohlan BA, et al. Pericarditis and cardiac tamponade in juvenile rheumatoid arthritis. Pediatrics 1981;68:369–73.

149. Lovell D, Lindsley C, Langston C. Lymphoid interstitial pneumonia in juvenile rheumatoid arthritis. J Pediatr 1984;105;947–50.

150. Holland P, Holland NH. Histoplasmosis in early infancy: hematologic, histochemical, and immunologic observations. Am J Dis Child 1966;112:412–21.

151. Wilson ER, Malluh A, Stagno S, et al. Fatal Epstein-Barr virus-associated hemophagocytic syndrome. J Pediatr 1981;98:260–2.

152. Miller DR. Familial reticuloendotheliosis: concurrence of disease in five siblings. Pediatrics 1966;38:986–95.

153. Persing DH, Herwaldt BL, Glaser C, et al. Infection with a babesia-like organism in northern California. N Engl J Med 1995;332:298–303.

154. Hughes WT. Leukemia monitoring with fungal bone marrow cultures. JAMA 1971;218:441–3.

154a. John CC, Gilsdorf JR. Recurrent fever in children. Pediatr Infect Dis J 2002;21:1071–7.

155. Thompson RS, Burgdorfer W, Russell A, et al. Outbreak of tickborne relapsing fever in Spokane County, Washington. JAMA 1969;210:1045–50.

156. Southern PM Jr, Sanford JP. Relapsing fever: a clinical and microbiological review. Medicine 1969;48:129–49.

157. Cross KW, Hey EN, Kennaird DL, et al. Lack of temperature control in infants with abnormalities of central nervous system. Arch Dis Child 1971;46:437–43.

158. Ramchander V, Jankey N, Ramkissoon R, et al. Anhidrotic ectodermal dysplasia in an infant presenting with pyrexia of unknown origin. Clin Pediatr 1978;17:51–4.

159. Riley CM. Familial dysautonomia. Adv Pediatr 1957;9: 157–90.

160. Smith A, Forbman A, Dancis J. Absence of tastebud papillae in familial dysautonomia. Science 1965;147:1040–1.

161. Thomas KT, Feder HM Jr, Lawton AR, Edwards KM. Periodic fever syndrome in children. J Pediatr 1999;135: 15–21.

162. Galanakis E, Papadakis LE, Giannoussi E, et al. PFAPA syndrome in children evaluated for tonsillectomy. Arch Dis Child 2002;86:434–5.

163. Feder HM Jr. Cimetidine treatment for periodic fever associated with aphthous stomatitis, pharyngitis and cervical adenitis. Pediat Infect Dis J 1992;11:318–21.

164. Samuels J, Aksentijevich I, Torosyan Y, et al. Familial Mediterranean fever at the millennium: clinical spectrum, ancient mutations, and a survey of 100 American referrals to the National Institutes of Health. Medicine 1998;77: 268–97.

165. Lehman TJA, Peters RH, Hanson V, et al. Long-term colchicine therapy of familial Mediterranean fever. J Pediatr 1978;93:876–8.

166. Saatci U, Ozen S, Ozdemir S, et al. Familial Mediterranean fever in children: report of a large series and discussion of the risk and prognostic factors of amyloidosis. Eur J Pediatr 1997;156:619–23.

167. Palmer SE, Dale DC, Livingston RJ. Autosomal dominant cyclic hematopoiesis: exclusion of linkage to the major hematopoietic regulatory gene cluster on chromosome 5. Hum Genetics 1994; 93:195–7.

168. Hammond WPT, Price TH, Souza LM, Dale DC. Treatment of cyclic neutropenia with granulocyte colony-stimulating factor. N Engl J Med 1989;320:1306–11.

169. Bar-Joseph G, Halberthal M, Sweed Y, et al. *Clostridium septicum* infection in children with cyclic neutropenia. J Pediatr 1997;131:317–9.

170. Drenth JP, van der Meer JW. Hereditary periodic fever. N Engl J Med 2001;345:1748–57.

171. Toro JR, Aksentijevich I, Hull K, et al. Tumor necrosis factor receptor-associated periodic syndrome: a novel syndrome with cutaneous manifestations. Arch Dermatol 2000;136:1487–94.

172. Moffet HL. Pediatric nosocomial infections in the community hospital. Pediatr Infect Dis 1982;1:430–42.

173. Staheli LT. Fever following trauma in childhood. JAMA 1967;503–4.

174. Sessler DI. Malignant hyperthermia. J Pediatr 1986;109: 9–14.

175. Halloran LL, Bernard DW. Management of drug-induced hyperthermia. Curr Opin Pediatr 2004; 16:211–5.

176. Press OW, Ramsey PG, Larson EB, et al. Hickman catheter infections in patients with malignancies. Medicine 1984;63:189–200.

177. Hiemenz J, Skelton J, Pizzo P. Perspective on the management of catheter-related infections in cancer patients. Pediatr Infect Dis 1986;5:6–11.

178. Adamkiewicz TV, Lorenzana A, Doyle J, Richardson S. Periperheral vs. central blood cultures in patients admitted to a pediatric oncology ward. Pediatr Infect Dis J 1999;18:556–7.

179. Blot F, Nittenberg G, Brun-Buisson C. New tools in diagnosing catheter-related infections. Support Care Cancer 2000;8:287–92.

180. Malgrange VB, Escande MC, Theobald S. Validity of earlier positivity of central venous blood cultures in comparison with peripheral blood cultures for diagnosing catheter-related bacteremia in cancer patients. J Clin Microbiol 2001;39:274–8.

181. Pelletier SJ, Crabtree TD, Gleason TG, et al. Bacteremia associated with central venous catheter infection is not an independent predictor of outcomes. J Am Coll Surg 2000;190:671–80.

182. Brun-Buisson C, Abrouk F, Legrand P. Diagnosis of central venous catheter-related sepsis: critical level of quantitative tip cultures. Arch Intern Med 1987;147:873–7.

183. Mermel LA, Farr BM, Sherertz RJ, et al. Guidelines for the management of intravascular catheter-related infections. Clin Infect Dis 2001;32:1249–72.

184. Whimbey E, Wong B, Kiehn TE, et al. Clinical correlations of serial quantitative blood culture determined by lysis-centrifugation in patients with persistent septicemia. J Clin Microbiol 1984;19:766–71.

185. Raucher HS, Hyatt AC, Barzilai A, et al. Quantitative blood cultures in the evaluation of septicemia in children with Broviac catheters. J Pediatr 1984;104:29–33.

186. Flynn PM, Shenep JL, Stokes DC, et al. In situ management of confirmed central venous catheter-related bacteremia. Pediatr Infect Dis J 1987;6:729–34.

187. Prince A, Heller B, Levy J, et al. Management of fever in patients with central vein catheters. Pediatr Infect Dis 1986;5:20–4.

188. Shapiro ED, Wald ER, Nelson KA, et al. Broviac catheter-related bacteremia in oncology patients. Am J Dis Child 1982;136:679–81.

189. Wang EEL, Prober CG, Ford Jones L, et al. The management of central intravenous catheter infections. Pediatr Infect Dis 1984;3:110–3.

190. Johnson PR, Decker MD, Edwards KM, et al. Frequency of Broviac catheter infections in pediatric oncology patients. J Infect Dis 1986;154:570–8.

191. Donnelly JP, Cohen J, Marcus R, et al. Bacteremia and Hickman catheters [letter]. Lancet 1985;2:48.

192. Benjamin DK Jr, Miller W, Garges H, et al. Bacteremia, central catheters, and neonates: when to pull the line. Pediatrics 2001;107:1272–6.

193. Karlowicz MG, Furigay PJ, Croitoru DP, Buescher ES. Central venous catheter removal versus in situ treatment in neonates with coagulase-negative staphylococcal bacteremia. Pediatr Infect Dis J 2002;21:22–7.

194. Jarvis WR, Highsmith AK, Allen JR, et al. Polymicrobial bacteremia associated with lipid emulsion in a neonatal intensive care unit. Pediatr Infect Dis 1983;2:203–8.

195. Fleer A, Senders RC, Visser MR, et al. Septicemia due to coagulase-negative staphylococci in a neonatal intensive care unit: clinical and bacteriological features and contaminated parenteral fluids as a source of sepsis. Pediatr Infect Dis 1983;2:426–31.

196. Long JG, Keyserling HL. Catheter-related infection in infants due to an unusual lipophilic yeast *Malessezia furfur*. Pediatrics 1985;76:896–900.

197. Powell DA, Aungst J, Snedden S, et al. Broviac catheter-related *Malessezia furfur* sepsis in five infants receiving intravenous fat emulsions. J Pediatr 1984;105:987–90.

198. Hershey CO, Tomford JW, McLaren CE, et al. The natural history of intravenous catheter-associated phlebitis. Arch Intern Med 1984;144:1373–5.

199. Haddad W, Idowu J, Georgeson K, et al. Septic atrial thrombosis: a potentially lethal complication of Broviac catheters in infants. Am J Dis Child 1986;140:778–80.

200. Haffar AAM, Rench MA, Ferry GD, et al. Failure of urokinase to resolve Broviac catheter-related bacteremia in children. J Pediatr 1984;104:256–8.

201. Verghese A, Widrich WC, Arbeit RD. Central venous septic thrombophlebitis: the role of medical therapy. Medicine 1985;64:394–400.

202. Veenstra DL, Saint S, Saha S, et al. Efficacy of antibiotic-impregnated central venous catheters in preventing cath-

eter-related bloodstream infection: a meta-analysis. JAMA 1999;281:261–7.

203. Darouiche RO, Raad II, Heard SO, et al. A comparison of two antimicrobial-impregnated central venous catheters. N Engl J Med 1999;340:1–8.

204. Pierce CM, Wade A, Mok Q. Heparin-bonded central venous lines reduce thrombotic and infective complications in critically ill children. Intensive Care Med 2000; 26:967–72.

205. Carratala J, Niubo J, Fernandez-Sevilla A, et al. Randomized, double-blinded trial of an antibiotic-lock technique for prevention of gram-positive central venous catheter-related infection in neutropenic patients with cancer. Antimicrob Agents Chemother 1999;43:2200–4.

206. Henrickson KJ, Axtell RA, Hoover SM, et al. Prevention of central venous catheter-related infections and thrombotic events in immunocompromised children by the use of vancomycin/ciprofloxacin/heparin flush solution: a randomized, multicenter, double-blind trial. J Clin Oncol 2000;18:1269–78.

207. Timsit JF. Scheduled replacement of central venous catheters is not necessary. Infect Control Hosp Epidemiol 2000;21:371–4.

208. Bregenzer T, Conen D, Sakmann P, Widmer AF. Is routine replacement of peripheral intravenous catheters necessary? Arch Intern Med 1998;26:151–6.

209. Sherertz RJ, Ely EW, Westbrook DM, et al. Education of physicians-in-training can decrease the risk for vascular catheter infection. Ann Intern Med 2000;18:641–8.

210. Coopersmith CM, Rebmann TL, Zack JE, et al. Effect of an education program on decreasing catheter-related bloodstream infections in the surgical intensive care unit. Crit Care Med 2002;30:59–64.

211. Bone RC, Belk RA, Cerra FB, et al. Definitions for sepsis and organ failure and guidelines for the use of innovative therapies in sepsis: the ACCP/SCCM Consensus Conference Committee. Chest 1992;101:1644–55.

212. Sullivan TD, La Scolea LJ Jr. *Neisseria meningitidis* bacteremia in children: quantitation of bacteremia and spontaneous clinical recovery without antibiotic therapy. Pediatrics 1987;80:63–7.

213. Norberg A, Christopher NC, Ramundo ML, Bower JR, Berman SA. Contamination rates of blood cultures obtained by dedicated phlebotomy vs intravenous catheter. JAMA 2003; 289:726–9.

214. Ramsook C, Childers K, Cron SG, Nirken M. Comparison of blood-culture contamination rates in a pediatric emergency room: newly inserted intraverious catheters versus venipuncture. Infect Control Hosp Epidemiol 2000; 21: 649–51.

215. Shulman ST, Ayoub EM. Severe staphylococcal sepsis in adolescents. Pediatrics 1976;58:59–66.

216. Hieber JP, Nelson AJ, McCracken GH Jr. Acute disseminated staphylococcal disease in childhood. Am J Dis Child 1977;131:181–5.

217. Storch GA, Rajogapalan L. Methicillin-resistant *Staphylococcus aureus* bacteremia in children. Pediatr Infect Dis 1986;5:59–67.

218. Friedman LE, Brown AE, Miller PR, et al. *Staphylococcus epidermidis* septicemia in children with leukemia and lymphoma. Am J Dis Child 1984;138:715–9.

219. Raad I, Davis S, Khan A, Tarrand J, Elting L, Bodey GP.

Impact of central venous catheter removal on the recurrence of catheter-related coagulase-negative staphylococcal bacteremia. Infect Control Hosp Epidemiol 1992;13: 215–21.

220. Christie CD, Havens PL, Shapiro ED. Bacteremia with group A streptococci in childhood. Am J Dis Child 1988; 142:559–61.

221. Burech DL, Koranyi KI, Haynes RE. Serious Group A streptococcal diseases in children. J Pediatr 1976;88: 972–4.

222. Cannaday P, McNitt T, Horn K, et al. A family outbreak of serious streptococcal infection. JAMA 1976;236:585–7.

223. Hagmolen of ten Have W, Wiegman A, Van den Hoek GJ, Vreede WB, Derkx HH. Life-threatening heart failure in meningococcal septic shock in children: non-invasive measurement of cardiac parameters is of important prognostic value. Eur J Pediatr 2000;159:277–82.

224. Ellison RT, Kohler PF, Curd JG, et al. Prevalence of congenital or acquired complement deficiency in patients with sporadic meningococcal disease. N Engl J Med 1983; 308:913–6.

225. Chiloote RR, Dampier C. Overwhelming pneumococcal septicemia in a patient with HbSC disease and splenic dysfunction. J Pediatr 1984;104:734–5.

226. Berrey MM. van Burik JA. Images in clinical medicine. Symmetric peripheral gangrene. N Engl J Med 2001;344: 1593.

227. Martone WJ, Zuehl RW, Minson GE, et al. Postsplenectomy sepsis with DF2: report of a case with isolation of the organism from the patient's dog. Ann Intern Med 1980;93:457–8.

228. Dajani AS, Asmar BI, Thirumoorth MC. Systemic *Haemophilus influenzae* disease: an overview. J Pediatr 1979;94: 305–364.

228a. Centers for Disease Control and Prevention. *Haemophilus influenzae* invasive disease among children aged < 5 years—California, 1990–1996. MMWR 1998;47: 737–40.

228b. Urwin G, Krohn JA, Deaver-Robinson K, Wenger JD, Farley MM. Invasive disease due to *Haemophilus influenzae* serotype f: clinical and epidemiologic characteristics in the *H. influenzae* serotype b vaccine era. Clin Infect Dis 1996;22:1069–76.

228c. Nitta DM, Jackson MA, Burry VF, Olson LC. Invasive *Haemophilus influenzae* type f disease. Pediatr Infect Dis J 1995;14:157–60.

229. Chusid MJ, Hillmann SM. Community-acquired *Pseudomonas* sepsis in previously healthy infants. Pediatr Infect Dis J 1987;6:681–4.

230. Meadow WL, Schneider H, Beem MO. *Salmonella enteritidis* bacteremia in childhood. J Infect Dis 1985;152: 185–9.

231. Zimmerman JJ, Dietrich KA. Current perspectives on septic shock. Pediatr Clin North Am 1987;34:131–63.

232. Forgacs P. Treatment of septic shock. Med Clin North Am 1979;63:465–71.

233. Dunzendorfer S, Schratzberger P, Reinisch N, Kahler CM, Wiedermann CJ. Pentoxifylline differentially regulates migration and respiratory burst activity of the neutrophil. Ann NY Acad Sci 1997;832:330–40.

234. Naqvi SH, Chundu KR, Friedman AD. Shock in children

with gram-negative bacillary sepsis and *Haemophilus influenzae* type b sepsis. Pediatr Infect Dis 1986;5:512–5.

235. Leibovici L, Shraga I, Drucker M, Konigsberger H, Samra Z, Pitlik SD. The benefit of appropriate empirical antibiotic treatment in patients with bloodstream infection. J Intern Med 1998;244:379–86.

236. Kanter RK, Zimmerman JJ, Strauss RH, et al. Central venous catheter insertion by femoral vein: safety and effectiveness for the pediatric patient. Pediatrics 1986;77: 842–7.

237. Dellinger RP. Current therapy for sepsis. Infect Dis Clin North Am 1999;13:495–509.

238. Ceneviva G, Paschall JA, Maffei F, Carcillo JA. Hemodynamic support in fluid-refractory pediatric septic shock. Pediatrics 1998;102:e19.

239. Schumer W. Steroids in the treatment of clinical septic shock. Ann Surg 1976;184:333–41.

240. Bone RC, Fisher CJ, Clemmer TP, et al. A controlled clinical trial of high-dose methylprednisolone in the treatment of severe sepsis and septic shock. N Engl J Med 1987;317:653–8.

241. Cronin L, Cook DJ, Carlet J, et al. Corticosteroid treatment for sepsis: a critical appraisal and meta-analysis of the literature. Crit Care Med 1995;23:1430–9.

242. Lefering R, Neugebauer EA. Steroid controversy in sepsis and septic shock: a meta-analysis. Crit Care Med 1995; 23:1294–303.

243. Alejandria MM, Lansang MA, Dans LF, Mantaring JB. Intravenous immunoglobulin for treating sepsis and septic shock. Cochrane Database Syst Rev 2000;CD001090.

244. Werdan K. Intravenous immunoglobulin for prophylaxis and therapy of sepsis. Curr Opin Crit Care 2001;7: 354–61.

245. Opal SM, Cohen J. Clinical gram-positive sepsis: does it fundamentally differ from gram-negative bacterial sepsis? Crit Care Med 1999;27:1608–16.

246. Bernard GR, Vincent JL, Laterre PF, et al. Efficacy and safety of recombinant human activated protein C for severe sepsis. N Engl J Med 2001;344:699–709.

247. Smith OP, White B, Vaughan D, et al. Use of protein C concentrate, heparin, and haemodiafiltration in meningococcus-induced purpura fulminans. Lancet 1997;350: 1590–3.

248. Alberio L, Lammle B, Esmon CT. Protein C replacement in severe meningococcemia: rationale and clinical experience. Clin Infect Dis 2001;32:1338–46.

249. Wheeler JG, Chauvenet AR, Johnson CA, et al. Buffy coat transfusions in neonates with sepsis and neutrophile storage pool depletion. Pediatrics 1987;79:422–5.

250. Cairo MS, Worcester C, Rucker R, et al. Role of circulating complement and polymorphonuclear leukocyte transfusion in treatment and outcome in critically ill neonates with sepsis. J Pediatr 1987;110:935–41.

251. Staubach KH, Schroder J, Stuber F, Gehrke K, Traumann E, Zabel P. Effect of pentoxifylline in severe sepsis: results of a randomized, double-blind, placebo-controlled study. Arch Surg 1998;133:94–100.

252. Avontuur JA, Tutein-Nolthenius RP, van Bodegom JW, Bruining HA. Prolonged inhibition of nitric oxide synthesis in severe septic shock: a clinical study. Crit Care Med 1998;26:660–7.

253. Suputtamongkol Y, Intaranongpai S, Smith MD, et al. A double-blind placebo-controlled study of an infusion of lexipafant (platelet-activating factor receptor antagonist) in patients with severe sepsis. Antimicrob Agents Chemother 2000:44:693–6.

254. Nakamura T, Ebihara I, Shoji H, Ushiyama C, Suzuki S, Koide H. Treatment with polymyxin B-immobilized fiber reduces platelet activation in septic shock patients: decrease in plasma levels of soluble P-selectin, platelet factor 4 and beta-thromboglobulin. Inflamm Res 1999;48: 171–5.

255. Reeves JH, Butt WW, Shann F, et al. Continuous plasmafiltration in sepsis syndrome. Crit Care Med 1999;27: 2287–9.

256. Takala J, Ruokonene E, Webster NR. Increased mortality associated with growth hormone treatment in critically ill adults. N Engl J Med 1999;341:785–92.

257. Rogall JA, Levin DL. Adult respiratory distress syndrome in pediatric patients. I. Clinical aspects, pathophysiology, pathology, and mechanisms of lung injury. II. Management. J Pediatr 1988;112:169–180, 335–347.

257a. Schrier RW, Wang W. Acute renal failure and sepsis. N Engl J Med 2004; 351:159–69.

258. Todd J, Fishant M, Kapral F, et al. Toxic shock syndrome associated with phage group I staphylococci. Lancet 1978;2:1116–8.

259. Chesney PJ, Davis JP, Purdy WK, et al. The clinical manifestations of toxic shock syndrome in women. JAMA 1981;246:741–8.

260. Davis JP, Osterholm MT, Helms CM, et al. Tri-state toxic-shock syndrome study. II. Clinical and laboratory findings. J Infect Dis 1982;145:441–8.

261. Melish ME, Murata S, Fukunaga C, et al. Corticosteroid and immunoglobulin therapy in TSS. Rev Infect Dis 1989;11(suppl):S332–3.

262. Parsonnet J. Nonmenstrual toxic shock syndrome: new insights into diagnosis, pathogenesis and treatment. Curr Clin Top Infect Dis 1996;16:1–20.

263. Helgerson SD, Mallery BL, Foster LR. Toxic shock syndrome in Oregon: risk of recurrence. JAMA 1984;252: 3402–4.

264. Andrews M-M, Parent EM, Barry M, Parsonnet J. Recurrent nonmenstrual toxic shock syndrome: clinical manifestations, diagnosis, and treatment. Clin Infect Dis 2001; 32:1470–9.

265. Verbon A, Fisher CJ Jr. Severe recalcitrant erythematous desquamating disorder associated with fatal recurrent toxic shock syndrome in a patient without AIDS. Clin Infect Dis. 1997;24:1274–5.

266. Bartter T, Dascal A, Carroll K, et al. "Toxic Strep Syndrome": a manifestation of Group A streptococcal infection. Arch Intern Med 1988;148:1421–4.

267. Working Group. Defining the group A streptococcal toxic shock syndrome. JAMA 1993;269:390–1.

268. Sztajnbok, J, Lovgren M, Brandileone MC, et al. Fatal group A streptococcal toxic shock-like syndrome in a child with varicella: report of the first well documented case with detection of the genetic sequences that code for exotoxins spe A and B, in Sao Paulo, Brazil. Rev Inst Med Trop Sao Paulo 1999;41:63–5.

269. Zurawski CA, Bardsley M, Beall B, et al. Invasive group A streptococcal disease in metropolitan Atlanta: a popula-

tion-based assessment. Clin Infect Dis 1998;27(1):150–7.

270. Laupland KB, Davies HD, Low DE, et al. Invasive group A streptococcal disease in children and association with varicella-zoster virus infection. Pediatrics 2000;105:e60.

271. Stevens DL, Gibbons AE, Bergstrom R, Winn V. The Eagle effect revisited: efficacy of clindamycin, erythromycin, and penicillin in the treatment of streptococcal myositis. J Infect Dis 1988;158:23–8.

272. Norrby-Teglund A, Low DE, McGeer A, Kotb M. Super-antigenic activity produced by group A streptococcal isolates is neutralized by plasma from IVIG-treated streptococcal toxic shock syndrome patients. Adv Exp Med Biol 1997;418:563–6.

273. Kaul R, McGeer A, Norrby-Teglund A, et al. Intravenous immunoglobulin therapy for streptococcal toxic shock syndrome—a comparative observational study. Clin Infect Dis 1999;28(4):800–7.

274. Stevens DL. Streptococcal toxic-shock syndrome: spectrum of disease, pathogenesis, and new concepts in treatment. Emerging Infect Dis 1995;1:69–78.

CHAPTER 11

Rash Syndromes

■ INTRODUCTION

Rashes in children are often caused by a systemic infection and are frequently associated with fever. The same pathologic process that is producing the skin eruption can involve other parts of the body as well, such as the lungs, liver, and spleen. Infections of the skin are covered in Chapter 17.

Definitions

Exanthem is a term sometimes used to describe a rash associated with a systemic illness, especially with fever. The word *exanthem* comes from Latin and means a "breaking out" or "blossoming out" and implies a generalized illness accompanied by a rash. The word is less useful than "fever and rash" as a broad preliminary problem-oriented diagnosis.

Enanthem is sometimes used to describe an eruption on the oral mucosa. It usually represents the same pathologic process as the rash but occurring in the mouth.

Most viral exanthems are more prominent in areas exposed to the sun, especially if there is a sunburn.[1]

Classification

Rashes can be classified according to either the appearance of the rash itself (maculopapular, petechial, pustular) or the total illness pattern (rubella-like illness or scarlet fever-like illness). In this chapter, both forms of classification will be used. Within each category of rash, the principal specific causes will be described. It is a better and more specific problem-oriented diagnosis to say "scarlet fever-like illness" and reserve the broader diagnosis of "erythematous rash" for cases with few, if any, features of scarlet fever present.

■ ERYTHEMATOUS RASHES

Erythematous rashes (Box 11-1) usually are generalized and extensive but may involve only part of the body. They may resemble sunburn, with redness that blanches when pressed with the fingers but involving areas not exposed to the sun. They may be slightly papular or perfectly flat (macular).

Possible Etiologies

Scarlet Fever

The scarlet fever rash is produced by an erythrogenic toxin of Group A streptococci. Multiple toxins can produce the syndrome. One study demonstrated that strains of Group A streptococcus (GAS) that produced two or three different toxins caused a more intense rash. Those that produced erythrogenic toxin B caused illness with a higher fever.[2] Scarlet fever can occur more than once in a single individual. Other than the rash, scarlet fever is no different from streptococcal pharyngitis. Therefore, the child typically will have clinical manifestations of streptococcal pharyngitis, as discussed in Chapter 2. Typically, these include headache, abdominal complaints, and a sore throat. Actual pharyngeal findings may be minimal. Suppurative and nonsuppurative complications may also occur. A study from Japan suggested that scarlet fever was associated more frequently with GAS serotype T4, which, in their study, was more difficult to eradicate from the pharynx than the other T types.[3]

Scarlet fever (scarlatina) is characterized by very small, often confluent, fine red papules and typically occurs on the trunk and extremities. In dark-skinned individuals, it is sometimes easier to diagnose by palpation than by vision. Patients often complain that the rash itches. There is increased redness in the folds of the skin, especially in the inguinal or antecubital creases, producing lines of redness called Pastia's lines (Fig. 11-1). The face is typically flushed, and there is circumoral pallor. A "strawberry tongue" (rough and red), sometimes with a white coating, may be present. The skin typically feels slightly rough, like fine sandpaper. The rash of scarlet fever also involves areas of the body usually covered by clothing, thus distinguishing it from ordinary sunburn. After about 7–10 days, the superficial layers of the skin may peel (desquamation), especially on the hands and feet. Occasionally, a localized area of streptococcal cellulitis is overlooked because of the generalized scarlet fever rash. Jaundice secondary to hepatocellular damage can complicate scarlet fever and may cause some diagnostic confusion if the physician is unaware of this possibility.[4] Rare reports of autoimmune diseases such as guttate psoriasis occurring after scarlet fever suggest the possibility that, in some patients, superantigenic toxin stimulation of the immune system may lead to immune dysregulation.[5]

When there is no clinical evidence of a streptococcal pharyngitis, cellulitis, or other infection, other possible causes of scarlet fever-like (scarlatiniform) rashes should be considered.

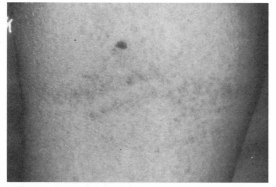

■ **FIGURE 11-1** Pastia's lines in the antecubital fossa, a useful aid in the diagnosis of scarlet fever (Photo from Dr. Charles Kallick).

Staphylococcal Scarlet Fever

Some strains of *Staphylococcus aureus* can produce a scarlet fever-like rash that has been called staphylococcal scarlet fever.[6] Enterotoxins G and I seem to be involved in the pathogenesis of this syndrome.[7] Unlike streptococcal scarlet fever, there is usually no circumoral pallor or strawberry tongue, and the erythematous skin is often painful or tender. As in streptococcal scarlet fever, desquamation of the superficial epidermis may occur after about a week. If the superficial skin separates and sloughs after only a few days, the patient should be classified as having scalded skin syndrome. This syndrome includes a group of illnesses, of which staphylococcal scarlet fever is a mild form, and is described further in Chapter 17.

Toxic Shock Syndrome (TSS)

This condition may be caused by Group A streptococcus or *S. aureus*. In toxic shock syndrome (TSS), the skin is flushed, and a scarlet fever-like rash may be noted. Fever, mild diarrhea, dizziness, and hypotension are common. Headache, sore throat, and severe myalgia are often present. Sometimes, confusion ensues. Misleading clinical features that may be present include a red swollen tongue; a generalized scarlet fever-like rash; nonpurulent conjunctivitis, sometimes with a subconjunctival hemorrhage; and mild subcutaneous edema. These clinical features may resemble Kawasaki disease, described later in this chapter. Herpes stomatitis or genital herpes may occur. All mucous membranes are typically very red. The focus of staphylococcal infection may be quite subtle, such as a mildly inflamed cervical lymph node. Tampon use is still a risk factor for staphylococcal TSS. Although cases associated with tampon use are less common today, they still comprise about half of all cases.

The white blood cell count (WBC) is typically greater than 15,000/mcL[3] with many immature neutrophils. The hemoglobin may fall several grams, suggesting hemolysis. The sedimentation rate is very high. Urinalysis reveals proteinuria, pyuria, and mild hematuria, but there are few or no bacteria in the sediment. Other findings are described in more detail in Chapter 10. Diagnostic criteria are listed in Boxes 10-3 and 10-4.

Penicillin can be given without waiting for throat culture results in a patient with pharyngitis and a scarlet fever-like rash. If a wound infection is present and the patient appears seriously ill or if TSS is suspected, intravenous nafcillin (or vancomylin) and clindamycin should be used (see Chapter 10).

Arcanobacterial Scarlet Fever

Arcanobacterium haemolyticum has been recognized as a cause of pharyngitis and a scarlet fever rash, particularly in teenagers and young adults.[8,9] An urticarial or erythema multiforme-like rash has been observed in some patients. Detection requires incubating sheep blood agar for at least 72 hours and observing for small alpha-hemolytic colonies; alternatively, human or rabbit blood agar can be used for more rapid detection. *A. haemolyticum* is generally susceptible to penicillin, the cephalosporins, and the macrolides. Whether antibiotic therapy speeds recovery from this self-limited illness is unknown. Rheumatic fever has not been reported in association with *A. haemolyticum* infection.[9]

The terms *streptococcal, staphylococcal,* and *arcanobacterial* should be used as adjectives to further define scarlet fever when possible.

Erythema infectiosum ("Fifth Disease")

Usually a mild disease, erythema infectiosum is caused by human parvovirus B19. The rash has been aptly described to occur in three phases. Early in the illness, there is an erythematous rash on the cheeks ("slapped cheeks"), resembling that seen in scarlet fever. Later, there is a macular or maculopapular, variably pruritic red rash that favors the extensor surfaces of the limbs; it starts as solid red areas, but as it progresses the middle parts clear in a seemingly random fashion, leading to the classic lacy, reticular appearance (Fig. 11-2), which typically lasts 2–5 days. The third phase of the rash is recurrence. Patients and their families should be informed that the rash may reappear after it is seemingly gone. Recurrences are sometimes associated with environmental triggers such as hot water or sunlight.

Typically, the patient with erythema infectiosum is not sick and seeks medical attention only because of the rash. Arthralgia may occur but is much more common in adults. Outbreaks are common. Complications such as encephalitis are rare.[10] Other clinical conditions that have been reported to occur in association with erythema infectiosum include acute cerebellar ataxia,[11] Guillain-Barré syndrome,[12] hepatitis[13] or fulminant liver failure,[14] and chronic fatigue syndrome.[15] Proof of causality is lacking for most of these conditions, although

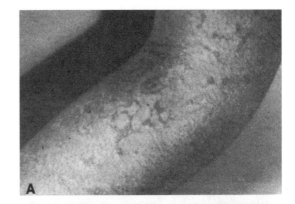
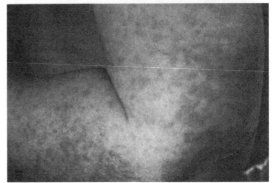
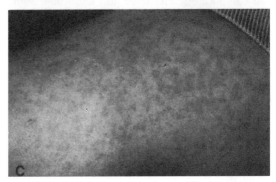

■ **FIGURE 11-2** Erythema infectiosum (fifth disease) showing typical gyrate rash in **A** and other appearances of the rash in **B** and **C**. (Balfour HH Jr. Clin Pediatr. (Phila) 1969;8: 721–7).

parvovirus B19 DNA was found by polymerase chain reaction (PCR) in the serum of some patients with idiopathic hepatitis and was found in liver biopsy specimens of some patients with fulminant hepatic failure.

The historical background of fifth disease is of some interest. About 1900, there was a controversy over the number of rash diseases that might occur in epidemics. At a boys' school in Rugby, England, Dukes observed what he thought were two different rash diseases and wrote an article entitled "Confusion of Two Diseases under the Name of Rubella (Rose-Rash)." Another physician questioned Dukes's observations in an article entitled, "Scarlet Fever, Measles, and German Measles—Is there a Fourth Disease?"[16] Dukes claimed there was a fourth disease on the basis of the absence of repeated attacks at the boys' school. In the modern era, medical history scholars have concluded that this "fourth disease" described by Dr. Dukes probably never existed. Rather, these were likely to have been cases of misdiagnosed rubella and scarlet fever.[17] Nevertheless, Dukes's article led to the naming of various exanthems as "fifth disease," "sixth disease," and "seventh disease." Of these numbered diseases, only the term *fifth disease* is still sometimes used as a synonym for erythema infectiosum. Sixth disease probably was roseola infantum, described later in this chapter.

The etiology of the disease was in doubt for some time, but parvovirus B19 has been clearly established as the etiologic agent of erythema infectiosum. Serologic studies of outbreaks were the first to support causality.[18] Subsequently, PCR studies demonstrated viral DNA in plasma samples of patients with erythema infectiosum.

Erythema infectiosum had an incubation period of 4–12 days in a Canadian outbreak[18] and of 13–18 days in a 1985 New York state cluster.[19] In the Canadian outbreak, respiratory and systemic symptoms were more prominent, the rash occurred on the palms and soles, and facial erythema and a lacy rash were less prominent than in previously published cases.[18]

The rash appears to be preceded by a viremic phase, with the virus present later in respiratory secretions. The contagious period is not clearly established, but patients are generally not contagious by the time the rash is obvious. In a small but thorough study in Canada, the attack rate in adults was only 14%.[18] The epidemiology is somewhat confusing in that there appear to be peaks of disease that last 3 years and occur every 6 years. The frequency of infection in susceptible adult household contacts is about 50%.[20]

Erythema infectiosum has always been regarded as a benign illness in normal children. The virus attachment protein is erythrocyte antigen P (globoside). This protein is expressed in largest amounts on erythrocyte precursor cells. Hence, infection with parvovirus B19 shuts down the production of red cells in the bone marrow and reduces the reticulocyte count to near zero. This transient shut-

down of red cell production is not a problem for patients with normal hemoglobin. However, patients with sickle cell anemia or other hemoglobinopathies, who are dependent on maintaining a high reticulocyte count, can experience aplastic crises when infected with parvovirus. These crises can be severe and even life threatening. Patients with aplastic crises should be considered to be contagious. Polyarthritis can occur in adults during outbreaks of the rash in children, and laboratory results also support a role for parvovirus in arthritis.[21] Chronic bone marrow failure with persistence of parvovirus B19 in the marrow has been reported in patients with organ or bone marrow transplants,[21a] malignancies,[21] combined immunodeficiency,[22] and humoral immunodeficiencies.[23] This condition may respond to intravenous immunoglobulin (IVIG) therapy.[21a] Transient acute pancytopenia may occur in normal individuals.

Parvovirus infection during pregnancy is one of the most common causes of nonimmune hydrops fetalis (see chapter 19). Hydrops is more likely to occur when maternal infection occurs during the second trimester.[24] Seropositivity rates in women of childbearing age range from 35%[25] to 65%[26]; annual seroconversion rates are about 1.5%, but may be as high as 13% in epidemics.[26] The risk of seroconverting during pregnancy is higher with increasing numbers of children in the home; nursery school teachers have about a three-fold increased risk of acquiring infection during pregnancy.[26] When primary maternal infection does occur, the fetus is often infected. However, most cases are asymptomatic. One prospective study of 43 women who were infected during pregnancy documented that 51% of the fetuses became infected; however, all the babies were carried to term and were born healthy.[27] In another prospective study of 1,610 women, 60 became infected during pregnancy (3.7%); only one fetus was aborted secondary to parvovirus infection, yielding a risk of fetal loss of 1.7% in known infection.[25] The following calculations are helpful in counseling pregnant women who are exposed to parvovirus B19: approximately 50% of women of childbearing age are susceptible, approximately 30% of susceptible hosts become infected, approximately 25% of exposed fetuses become infected, and approximately 10% of infected fetuses die. Thus, the risk of fetal death in a woman exposed to parvovirus B19 is about $0.5 \times 0.3 \times 0.25 \times 0.1 = 0.4\%$.

Human parvovirus B19 is not the same parvovirus that infects dogs; that virus is species specific and poses no risk to humans.

Other Causes

Drug reactions occasionally produce an erythematous rash; for example, the pharmacologic effect of atropine, rapid vancomycin infusion, or a reaction to ampicillin. Chickenpox may have a transient erythematous appearance before the vesicular eruption. Many allergic reactions result in erythematous rashes.

Erythromelalgia is a rare episodic disease of unknown cause manifested by attacks of redness and pain in the hands and feet that is relieved by immersion in ice water or by aspirin.[28] Contact dermatitis, such as from plants, can produce erythematous rashes often associated with itching and papules or vesicles.[29] Kawasaki disease (KD) should be included in the differential diagnosis of scarlet fever-like rashes but is given its own section because of its importance.

■ KAWASAKI DISEASE

This disease was named in honor of Tokyo physician Tomisaku Kawasaki, who first reported it in the United States' literature in 1974.[30] Most of the children came to his attention during first 7 years of the 1960s. He called the syndrome the mucocutaneous lymph node syndrome because of the erythema of the eyes and mouth and either generalized or focal lymph node enlargement. The first cases in the United States were observed in 1971 in Hawaii, and it was first reported in the continental United States in 1976. Now that the disease is well described and known, it is not an uncommon diagnosis.

Epidemiology

The disease occurs almost exclusively in children, usually those less than 4 years of age, and is more severe in Asian children, who may have a fatality rate of 1–2% in severe cases. Sporadic case reports of a similar disease in adults have been appearing. There are over 6,000 cases per year in Japan, for an average annual incidence of 105 cases per 100,000 children under 5 years of age.[31] In San Diego, the disease was found to have a higher incidence in the coldest and rainiest months. Incidence was also seen to be higher in those of Asian or Pacific Island descent.[32] The disease in Japanese children is significantly more frequent in those with HLA antigen BW22. A recent case-control study suggested that the incidence was higher in the children of health care workers.[33] This finding is interesting but requires confirmation.

Etiology

Despite a resolute effort, the etiology of the disease remains elusive. Because the disease resembles toxin-mediated diseases such as scarlet fever and toxic shock syndrome, some researchers have assumed a bacterial cause; some have demonstrated staphylococci that overproduce enterotoxin B[34] or protein A[35] and have suggested, therefore, that staphylococci with mutations in the accessory gene regulation locus are responsible for the disease.[36] Unfortunately, it has not been easy to find staphylococcal infection in all cases of KD. Others have claimed streptococci as the cause, but a series of children with a history of KD had no antibodies to streptococcal superantigens.[37] A link to *Chlamydia pneumoniae* infection was sought but not established. Features of the disease resemble superantigen-mediated illness, but this has not been clearly established; even if it were, delineating the exact source and nature of the superantigen would require much more work.

At present, it is not entirely clear that KD is actually an infectious disease. Clustering of cases, however, suggests that it probably is. It may be that the disease is a final common pathway of multiple infectious insults, rather than being attributable to any one etiologic agent.

Pathophysiology

The clinical findings of KD are the result of the release of multiple inflammatory mediators. In the acute phase of the illness, vascular endothelial growth factor (VGEF),[38] monocyte chemotactic protein 1 (MCP-1),[39] and soluble CD4 levels[40] are increased in patients with KD. Some of these mediators have been linked to specific manifestations of the disease. For example, VGEF levels are highest in children who develop coronary artery abnormalities[38] and MCP-1 has been found in cardiac tissues of children who died of KD.[41] It is possible that there is a genetic predisposition to the disease. Peripheral blood mononuclear cells from patients who long ago recovered from KD overexpress TNF-alpha in vitro compared with cells from patients without disease history.[42] Anticardiac myosin antibodies have also been demonstrated in the sera of patients suffering from acute KD,[43] which may help explain the propensity of the disease to damage vessels and specifically to damage the arteries that feed the heart.

Clinical Presentation

Kawasaki disease may resemble scarlet fever because of the fever, the generalized erythematous rash, the red oral mucosa and tongue, a marked leukocytosis with a shift to the left, and later, the desquamation of the fingertips and toes. Nonsuppurative cervical adenitis may be prominent, but is the most frequently absent of the classic findings. The fever lasts 5–14 days and does not respond to penicillin or other antibiotics.

The Centers for Disease Control and Prevention (CDC) has defined criteria for the case definition Box 11-2.[44] It is important to remember that this case definition was created for epidemiologic purposes, not clinical ones. Epidemiologic case definitions are meant to be specific (strict), so that patients with other diseases do not end up being incorrectly classified as having the disease of interest. The trade-off is that such definitions may lack sensitivity. Such is the case with KD. If only patients meeting the CDC criteria are diagnosed with KD, cases will be missed. Often, only three or four of the characteristics of KD are found, causing a great diagnostic difficulty. Swelling of hands and feet is a very helpful diagnostic point and may sometimes be discovered only by the history. The rash is usually nonspecific, generalized, and maculopapular, but may take almost any form, including one that resembles erythema multiforme. The rash tends to be most intense in the diaper area. Involvement of the conjunctivae is one of the most constant features of the disease. The sclerae tend to be injected with many bright red vessels. The limbus is spared. There is almost never a purulent discharge. Clinical experience teaches that children (especially toddlers) with KD are usually extremely irritable. The fever is normally quite high and responds poorly, if at all, to antipyretic administration.

A mild myocarditis is common at the time of presentation, and careful auscultation will reveal gallop rhythms in some patients. Despite this, fluid tolerance is normally good, and even patients with gallops tolerate the fluid load associated with IVIG administration. Hydrops of the gallbladder is less frequently seen (about 10% of cases), but its presence suggests KD in the appropriate clinical setting.[45,46] Abdominal ultrasound, therefore, is sometimes helpful is paring down the differential diagnosis. Similarly, anterior uveitis (iritis) can be detected on slit lamp examination in > 50% of patients, and its presence is supportive of KD in the child with features consistent with the diagnosis.[47] If the diagnosis of KD is clinically obvious, lumbar puncture is not necessary. A retrospective review of patients eventually shown to have KD who underwent spinal tap at presentation in the ER showed that almost 40% of them had a mild cerebrospinal fluid (CSF) pleocytosis (mean of 23 WBC, 6% neutrophils). About 17% had an elevated protein, but hypoglycorrhachia was not associated with the disease.[48] In several different cases, children with KD presented with a peritonsillar phlegmon or abscess.[49] Children from other countries who received BCG in the newborn period occasionally develop granulomatous inflammation at the site of the BCG during acute KD.[50]

Differential Diagnosis

KD may be mistaken for Stevens-Johnson syndrome (see following) because of the rash; conjunctivitis; red oral mucosa with red, dry, fissured lips; and failure to respond to antibiotics. The rash also can resemble erythema multiforme, with central clearing and iris lesions.[51] However, the conjunctivitis in KD is nonpurulent.

Other diseases resembling KD include Rocky Mountain spotted fever (more common during the summer months)[52] and leptospirosis.[53] Toxic

---

BOX 11-2 ■ Case Definition of Kawasaki Disease

Fever for 5 or more days
Plus four of the following five clinical findings:
- Bilateral injection of the conjunctivae
- Fissuring of the lips, strawberry tongue, or erythema of the oropharynx
- Early erythema of the palms and soles with edema of dorsum of the hands and feet with later desquamation
- Polymorphous erythematous rash
- Acute nonsuppurative enlargement of a cervical lymph node (≥ 1.5 cm)
Plus exclusion of other causes

shock syndrome (Chapter 10) caused by either *S. aureus* or *S. pyogenes* may also resemble KD. Systemic onset juvenile rheumatoid arthritis (Chapter 10) may mimic KD, as may adenoviral infection.

Laboratory Studies

Typically, there is a marked leukocytosis with a shift to the left, slight anemia, thrombocytosis (a useful later finding), elevated C-reactive protein (CRP), increased alpha2-globulin, and a markedly increased erythrocyte sedimentation rate (ESR). The serum IgM and IgE are typically elevated.[54] The serum IgE often is persistently elevated if arthritis or cardiac complications occur. Mild jaundice or slightly increased serum amino-transferases occur.

Additional Findings and Complications

Often, the patient will have or develop prominent findings other than those in the case definition. These include diarrhea, focal ileus, myositis, malabsorption, arthralgia or arthritis, uveitis, hemolytic-uremic syndrome, hyponatremia, proteinuria, sterile pyuria, and others listed in Box 11-3.[55–59]

BOX 11-3 ■ Kawasaki Disease: Additional Findings and Complications

Cardiac
Acute myocarditis
Acute mitral insufficiency
Coronary artery aneurysm or thrombosis (later)
Pericardial effusion

Other
Nonpurulent meningitis
Hydrops of gallbladder
Obstructive jaundice
Diarrhea, abdominal pain, ileus
Pancreatitis (later)
Arthralgia, arthritis
Sterile pyuria, urethritis
Uveitis, frequent and mild
Parotitis
Coombs-positive hemolytic anemia
Hemolytic-uremic syndrome
Retropharyngeal lymphoid mass
Myositis, weakness due to hypokalemia
Aseptic necrosis of bone (later)
Hyponatremia
Psoriatic skin lesions
Distal limb ischemia
Facial nerve palsy

Aneurysm or thrombosis of the coronary arteries (resembling, but different from, infantile polyarteritis nodosa) is the most frequent of the severe complications.[60] Myocardial infarction and sudden death can occur.

Echocardiography may be useful to detect coronary artery aneurysms. However, the timing of a cardiac evaluation can be a source of uncertainty to the physician. In the great majority of patients who will develop coronary artery aneurysms, early echocardiographic signs are present by 10–14 days after illness onset.[61] Consequently, the American Heart Association (AHA) recommends an initial echocardiogram at 10–14 days. The initial appearance of aneurysms more than 6 weeks after onset is very uncommon.[62] Thus, the AHA guidelines call for a second echocardiogram 6–8 weeks after illness onset.[61] A third echocardiogram is sometimes performed 6–12 months after illness onset if there is any concern about the previous studies.

Facial nerve palsy is an extremely rare complication of KD, but is of importance because of a possible association with coronary artery aneurysms; of 25 cases reported in the literature, more than half also had coronary artery aneurysms.[63]

Complications of treatment occasionally develop. One patient who developed aseptic meningitis in response to IVIG therapy has been reported.[64] We have also cared for a patient who developed an infusion reaction that resulted in a fever spike to 105°F and a febrile seizure. The theoretical possibility of the development of Reye's syndrome exists because of long-term aspirin therapy during the months when both varicella and influenza infection are common. However, this has never been reported. When feasible, influenza vaccination should be administered. Varicella vaccination can also be given but may not be effective for several months after receipt of IVIG. The recommended time interval between IVIG and varicella or measles vaccination is 11 months in the United States and 6–7 months in Japan. A recent study suggests that even for patients who require repeat dosing (i.e., a total of 4g/kg), 9 months was a sufficient interval.[64a]

Treatment

High-dose IVIG is the most effective treatment, both in ameliorating the signs and symptoms and in preventing the cardiac consequences of the disease. The incidence of coronary artery abnormalities following KD has been shown to be inversely related to the dose of IVIG received.[65] For this reason, dosages less than 2 gm/kg are not recommended. The physician should attempt to make the diagnosis and start appropriate therapy as expeditiously as possible. Prospective studies of IVIG therapy for KD have included only those patients diagnosed within 10 days of the onset of fever. However, retrospective data suggest that for patients who are diagnosed later, IVIG therapy is still beneficial after the 10th day of illness.[66] Most experts recommend administering IVIG to such patients if there are signs of ongoing inflammation.[67]

High-dose aspirin (80–100 mg/kg/day divided in four doses) has been advocated for the acute part of the illness, which is variously interpreted as a duration of 2 weeks, until the patient is afebrile, or until the CRP normalizes. In the study of outcomes by IVIG dosage cited earlier, coronary artery abnormalities were shown to be unrelated to the dosage of aspirin.[65] Japanese physicians use 30–50 mg/kg/day as their high-dose standard. In the past, serum levels of aspirin were monitored, and a level of 20 mg/dL or greater was targeted; reaching those levels often required as much as 100–180 mg/kg/day. There is no evidence that serum aspirin levels predict outcome. Consequently, frequent aspirin level measurements and dosage adjustments seem unwarranted.

After the acute period of the disease, low-dose aspirin is used to reduce the risk of coronary artery thrombosis. Most American physicians use 3–5 mg/kg/day in a single dose. Low-dose aspirin is continued until the ESR normalizes, which usually takes 1–3 months. Some believe that even if the ESR normalizes sooner, low-dose aspirin therapy should be continued no less than 8 weeks.[68] Alternatively, the most practical approach is probably to discontinue the aspirin if the echocardiogram done 6–8 weeks after the illness is negative.

The use of corticosteroids has never been studied in a controlled fashion, but there is some suggestion that they are associated with an increased risk of coronary artery aneurysm. On the other hand, they are sometimes used in the patient who fails to respond to two doses of IVIG.[69]

Surgical correction of coronary artery damage from Kawasaki disease is difficult but sometimes possible.[70,71]

Prognosis

The most important predictor of outcome is whether the patient receives IVIG or not. The rate of coronary artery aneurysms at 7 weeks in patients who do not receive IVIG is 15%.[71a] In contrast, if IVIG is administered within 10 days of illness onset, the rate is 2.4%.[71b]

If coronary artery aneurysms do not occur, the prognosis is excellent. Most patients respond quite dramatically to the infusion of IVIG. In some cases, parents will describe how they watched the conjunctival injection disappear right before their eyes as the infusion progressed. However, there is a significant minority of patients who do not respond promptly to IVIG therapy. Many of them respond to a second administration. Investigators have sought clinical or laboratory parameters that would be predictive of a poor response to the first dose of IVIG. Results have been mixed. Some have found that a CRP greater than 10 mg/dL, an LDH greater than 590, and a hemoglobin of less than 10 g/dL were predictive both of poor response to therapy and of high risk for the development of coronary artery aneurysms.[72] Others have not been able to identify any features of either the disease pattern or laboratory values that reliably predict response to therapy.

The following have been identified as placing the patient at high-risk for coronary artery aneurysms: duration of fever greater than 9 days prior to IVIG therapy,[73] age less than 1 year or greater than 8 years,[74] highly elevated CRP level, presence of pericardial effusions or ventricular dysfunction at presentation, and a recurrent case.[75] A poor response to the first dose of IVIG, including failure to become afebrile within 48 hours or recrudescence of fever after becoming afebrile,[76] elevated WBC count, absolute neutrophil count, or CRP level after IVIG infusion have also been associated with the development of coronary artery aneurysms.

About half of all coronary artery abnormalities that are discovered within the first few days of treatment regress and never reform.[77]

Incomplete Kawasaki Disease

The disease is harder to recognize in patients less than 6 months or greater than 8 years of age, in the former because it tends to occur in an incomplete form and in the latter largely because it is unexpected in that age group. In either case, the prognosis is worse than in children of the ages in between, who have a more readily recognizable form of the disease. Children who have incomplete or atypical KD, therefore, are at higher risk of developing coronary artery disease.[78] Echocardiography has therefore been recommended for children who have a long unexplained febrile illness with subsequent desquamation.[79,80] Because delayed in diagnosis and treatment may be at least partially responsible for the increased incidence of coronary artery aneurysms in infants with incomplete KD, the diagnosis should be considered in patients with clinical and/or laboratory findings noted in Box 11-4.

■ MEASLES-LIKE ILLNESSES

Measles-like illness has been defined for use in epidemic control by the CDC as a very broad syndrome:

1. Fever of 101°F or higher
2. Rash lasting 3 or more days
3. One or more of the following: cough, conjunctivitis, or coryza

The preceding definition is useful in measles vaccination campaigns in areas of the world where measles is common. In the United States, the vast majority of children with symptoms meeting this definition will not have measles. The spectrum of measles virus infection is described in this section

---

BOX 11-4 ■ Clinical and Laboratory Findings Suggestive of Possible Incomplete Kawasaki Disease

Clinical findings

Daily high spiking fevers for 5 days or longer without evidence of bacterial infection, with either:

1. One or more diagnostic criteria for KD, especially conjunctival injection, oral mucosal changes, and/or rash, OR
2. Anterior uveitis by slit-lamp examination

Laboratory findings

1. Markedly elevated ESR or CRP
2. Elevated peripheral WBC count or normal WBC count with > 60% neutrophils
3. Thrombocytosis after 7th day of fever, with or without:
4. Sterile pyuria
5. Elevated alanine aminotransferase
6. Aseptic meningitis
7. Anemia
8. Hypoalbuminemia
9. Echocardiogram showing pericardial effusion

From Rowley AH. Incomplete (atypical) Kawasaki disease. Pediatr Infect Dis J 2002;21:563–5.

---

using the terms *classic, vaccine-modified,* and *immunoglobulin-modified.* Other maculopapular rashes that may resemble measles are described in the next section. Rubeola is an older name for measles that one hopes will become obsolete, because it is easily confused with "rubella" (which is unfortunately sometimes referred to as German measles).

Classic Measles

Epidemiology

Measles was once a very common childhood disease in the United States; an average of 500,000 cases a year were reported in this country before widespread vaccination took place. Serologic surveys in military recruits in the late 1960s found that almost all were measles antibody positive. Disease occurred in epidemics every 2–5 years. Epidemics lasted from 2–4 months. In temperate climates, measles was a disease of the late winter and spring. In the prevaccine era, elementary school children were most often infected. Measles is a highly contagious disease. The virus spreads very rapidly through a population, infecting all susceptible individuals. In the developing world, measles remains a leading cause of preventable illness; it causes 800,000 deaths each year in children < 5 years old.[81]

Killed virus vaccine was introduced first, and then attenuated live virus vaccine was introduced. The vaccine is highly effective, inducing durable protection in approximately 95% of vaccinees with a single dose. Widespread use of measles vaccine caused the incidence of epidemic measles to drop rapidly. By 1968 the number of cases of measles reported to the CDC had decreased by more than 90% compared with the number reported in 1964. However, over a 3-year period from 1988–1991 the incidence of measles jumped up again; there were 27,786 reported cases in 1990. This resurgence of measles cases prompted the recommendation for two doses of live, attenuated measles virus vaccine. The principal purpose of the second dose of vaccine is to produce immunity in subjects who failed to make a response to the first dose of vaccine, rather than to "boost" immunity in those who responded; however, there is some evidence that protection against disease is better in those who have received two doses of vaccine.[82] Additionally, avidity studies of antibodies in vaccinees show that in outbreak situations, some symptomatic measles infections occur in patients who were vaccinated years prior to the epidemic.[83] This effect was most pronounced among those who received vaccine prior to their first birthday. The two-dose measles vaccine schedule appears to be working: the number of reported measles cases in the United States during both 2001–2003 was 216, which is an all-time low and represents an incidence of less than 0.3 cases per one million population.[84]

Clinical Presentation

Classic measles is a moderate to severe illness with fever of 39.5–40.6°C (103–105°F) and severe cough and conjunctivitis for several days before the appearance of the rash. The early problem-oriented diagnoses (before the rash appears) are likely to be febrile bronchitis and nonpurulent conjunctivitis. The incubation period between the exposure and the first symptoms is 8–12 days, averaging about 10 days. The rash typically begins on the face and neck and spreads downward to involve the entire body. The rash is extensive and confluent and lasts about 7 days. It tends to be more confluent in the areas first affected and less so in the extremities. A small amount of desquamation may occur as the rash clears. Fever persists for several days after the onset of the rash and then breaks abruptly. An enanthem (Koplik spots) often precedes the rash by a day and consists of white papules the size of a small pinhead on an erythematous base on the buccal mucosa. Koplik's spots are diagnostic of measles. A generalized enanthem is often found during the peak of the rash. Cough, rhinitis, and conjunctivitis are prominent (Fig. 11-3). The conjunctivitis usually produces a copious, watery discharge, and older patients sometimes describe photophobia. Lymphadenopathy may be prominent, especially in head and neck. Mortality is higher in developing countries with crowded conditions or with more than one case in a household.

Modified Measles

This is a technical term defined as measles virus infection made milder by previous antibodies. The term was commonly used when immunoglobulin (IG) was given to exposed susceptible siblings before measles vaccine was available, from about 1950 to 1967. Mild to moderate measles-like illness can have several causes, but in an endemic area measles virus infection modified by antibodies is the commonest. These antibodies may be transplacental maternal antibodies, which are present in the first year of life, or be derived from recently administered serum immune globulin. A modifying dose of IG (0.05 ml/kg) prolongs the incubation period and makes the illness milder. The traditional view was that transplacental antibodies prevented disease in the infant in the first 6 months of life and allowed a *modified* measles illness between 6 and 12 months of life. The term *modified measles* has also been used to describe mild measles confirmed by serologic testing in individuals who have received one or another form of measles vaccine (Table 11-1).[85]

Revised Terminology

Because of the difficulty of using traditional terminology to describe the live-vaccine alteration of measles virus infections, a very useful classification has been proposed.[86] In this classification, "classic measles" is infection with wild measles virus. Vaccine-modified measles is then subdivided into killed or live vaccine modification, which seem to have different patterns, the former with a more severe course and an atypical rash and the latter with a milder course much like immune globulin-modified measles. The term *modified measles* as used earlier is then changed to "immunoglobulin-modified measles" (see Table 11-1).

Killed Vaccine Modified Measles ("Atypical Measles")

Contracting measles after receipt of the killed virus vaccine caused a variant form of measles that was difficult to diagnose because it often lacked classic features such as conjunctivitis, coryza, and Koplik's spots. The rash was also altered, sometimes being vesicular or urticarial. Killed measles vaccine has not been used in over three decades, so atypical measles is no longer seen.

Live-Vaccine Modified Measles

After a person who has been immunized with live attenuated measles vaccine is exposed to the wild virus, there are three possible results. In at least 90% of exposures, the individual will be completely protected and get no illness at all. Rarely, the individual will get classic measles, indicative of a "vaccine failure," sometimes attributable to improper storage of vaccine, use in children younger than 12 months, or use with immune globulin, as was sometimes done in the 1960s. Finally, a live-vaccine-modified measles can occur, with a shorter,

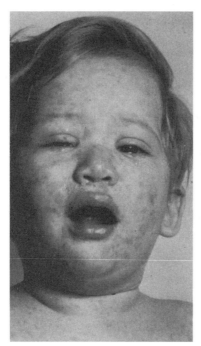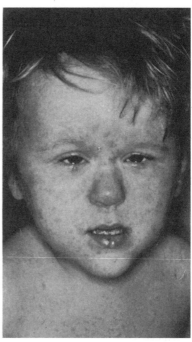

■ **FIGURE 11-3** Faces of two children with classic measles. Note eye swelling, nasal discharge and obstruction, mouth breathing, and rash (Photos from Dr. Robert Lawson).

TABLE 11-1. FORMS OF MEASLES

	CLASSIC	KILLED VACCINE-MODIFIED	IMMUNOGLUBLIN OR LIVE-VACCINE-MODIFIED
Incubation (days)	10	10	14–20
Fever (°F[C])	104 (40)	104 (40)	<102 (38.8)
Cough	Prominent	Prominent	Mild or absent
Nasal discharge	Prominent	Variable	Mild
Koplik spots	Present near onset of rash	Absent	Absent
Rash			
Duration (days)	10 (until faded)	3–6	1–3
Kind	Moves downward from head; maculopapular; confluent	Can begin in extremities; changing or variable, possibly petechial, vesicular, or maculopapular	Sparse, discreet
Other	Lymphadenopathy, esp. head and neck, rare encephalitis	Headache, abdominal pain; peripheral edema	None
Laboratory findings	Leukopenia	Leukopenia Possible eosinophilia, focal pneumonia or pleural effusions	Not remarkable; virtually never any complications
Antibody titer	Usual rise	Exaggerated	Usual
Contagiousness	Very	Rarely, if ever	Not

milder measles-like illness. This pattern resembles the killed vaccine-modified pattern ("atypical measles") but does not seem to have any focal pneumonia or atypical rash attributable to an antigen–antibody reaction. Live-vaccine-modified measles more nearly resembles immunoglobulin-modified measles; that is, with all the features of classic measles made shorter and milder.

Diagnosis of Classic Measles

The diagnosis is usually a clinical one. In the setting of an outbreak, diagnosis is relatively easy. Because many currently practicing physicians have never seen a case of measles, this disease, once fairly reliably diagnosed by parents, may escape diagnosis in some cases. Serologic studies are available when the diagnosis is suspected, but in doubt; hemagglutinin-inhibition methods are the most reliable. IgM is usually detectable for about a month after the rash begins. Acute and convalescent titers that show a fourfold or greater rise in the setting of clinical measles may be considered diagnostic. Nasopharyngeal swab specimens or urine may be sent off for viral culture. The physician should contact their state laboratory before collecting specimens.

Treatment of Classic Measles

Specific antiviral therapy directed against measles virus has not been shown to be efficacious in the treatment of measles. Ribavirin is active against measles virus in vitro and is used in the treatment of severe measles virus disease in immune-compromised hosts. Anecdotal, uncontrolled reports of cure in patients with severe measles virus pneumonia treated with ribavirin[87] or the combination of ribavirin and IVIG[88] have been published. Experimental antiviral agents that show greater activity against measles virus in vitro[89] and in the cotton rat model[90] are not yet available, nor are they recommended.

Acute measles virus infection takes a more serious course in patients who have vitamin A deficiency, and vitamin A levels are depressed during disease even in patients of normal nutritional status.[91] Severity of clinical illness correlates inversely with vitamin A levels. Supplementation of vitamin A during acute disease hastens recovery. A large, retrospective study from South Africa is revealing: The authors reviewed 1,061 cases of measles prior to their use of vitamin A and compared these cases

with 651 seen after the institution of vitamin A therapy for measles. Length of hospital stay (10 vs. 13 days), requirement for intensive care (4.3% vs. 10.5%) and mortality (1.6% vs. 5%) were all significantly reduced in patients who received vitamin A.[92] The current recommendation is for patients between the ages of 6 months and 2 years of age who are hospitalized with measles to receive one dose of vitamin A (100,000 units for children 6 months to 1 year of age, and 200,000 units for children older than 12 months). Children who have eye findings suggestive of a preexisting vitamin A deficiency should get another dose the next day and another one at 4 weeks.

Complications of Classic Measles

Common Respiratory Complications

Croup may complicate measles and is sometimes severe and occasionally fatal. Cervical lymphadenitis and bacterial pharyngitis are common. Otitis media may occur and is usually nonbacterial, being related to lymphoid hyperplasia obstructing the eustachian tube.

Interstitial Pneumonia

Radiographic interstitial pneumonia is common during measles virus infection. Sometimes, it is complicated by secondary bacterial pneumonia. In an outbreak in St. Louis in 1970, pneumonia necessitating hospitalization was about ten times as frequent as encephalitis and had a 10% mortality rate.

Acute Measles Encephalitis

This complication occurred in about 1 of 1,000 to 10,000 reported cases of measles during an outbreak when measles was common. It is associated with a mortality rate of about 10%. Some degree of neurologic damage, such as convulsive disorder or mental retardation, follows in about 50% of cases. Cell-mediated immunity is probably most important in protection from the development of encephalitis. In a mouse model, CD8 cytotoxicity correlates with protection.[93] Laboratory studies of a patient who was immunosuppressed because of therapy for ankylosing spondylitis and who eventually died of measles encephalitis revealed intact humoral immunity but virtually no cell-mediated immunity.[94] Patients with pure humoral immune deficiency syndromes such as Bruton's agammaglobulinemia almost always recover from measles uneventfully. This makes sense given that measles is an enveloped virus, and therefore infected cells can produce progeny virions without being lysed. Ultimately, clearance of these infections usually requires active lysis by the host's immune system. Measles encephalitis typically begins sometime during the period when the rash is present. About half of the children with measles encephalitis in the 1970 St. Louis outbreak eventually required custodial care.

Fatal Giant-Cell Pneumonia

In immunocompromised patients, such as those with leukemia, there may be a fatal progressive bilateral pneumonia. In such cases, giant cells are typically found at autopsy. The measles may occur without a rash. In one report of four immunocompromised patients who developed giant cell pneumonia during acute measles virus infection, autopsy revealed the concomitant occurrence of pancreatitis, sialoadenitis, and thyroiditis.[95] Occasionally, this pneumonia occurs in otherwise-normal hosts.

Dissemination of Tuberculosis or Fungal Infections

During measles, the virus may impair cell-mediated immunity, and unrecognized tuberculosis or pulmonary infection with fungi may disseminate. This dissemination is typical in countries where unrecognized tuberculosis is common.

Acute measles virus infection and vaccination with measles-mumps-rubella (MMR) vaccine can temporarily suppress tuberculin reactivity. A TST can be given during the same visit that MMR is given. However, if tuberculin testing is indicated and cannot be performed at the same time as MMR immunization, tuberculin testing should be deferred for 4–6 weeks.[96]

Subacute Sclerosing Panencephalitis (SSPE)

This condition occurs about 2 to 10 years after the initial infection and represents a latent measles virus infection in the brain. The incidence of SSPE following wild-type measles infection is somewhere between 0.5 and 2.0 per 100,000 cases. Attempts to define risk factors for the development of SSPE have been difficult; most experts believe that earlier acquisition of measles virus infection leads to higher risk.[97] Usually, the disease begins with subtle men-

tal changes and poorer performance in school and progresses to an intractable convulsive disorder. Rare presentations include chorioretinitis[98] and optic neuritis.[99] The condition progresses inexorably to death within a year or two.

Whether SSPE can occur after vaccination with MMR vaccine is controversial. If it does, it is extremely rare.

Encephalopathy in Children with Malignancies

Children with leukemia or neuroblastoma can develop a chronic progressive encephalopathy, apparently caused by the measles virus, during the period of acute measles infection.

■ OTHER MACULOPAPULAR RASHES

Many infectious and noninfectious illnesses can produce a rash resembling measles. In such a case, it is called morbilliform or measles-like. A maculopapular rash has elevated red bumps (papules) and red flat areas (macules). The individual macules and papules may become confluent after a day or so.

Papular rashes are described in a later section of this chapter.

Causes and Manifestations

Severe Rubella

Rubella virus infection can produce a moderately severe measles-like illness in adolescents and young adults. Prodromal respiratory symptoms, cough, rhinitis, conjunctivitis, pharyngitis, palatal petechiae, and a rash lasting longer than 5 days have been observed in laboratory-confirmed rubella virus infections in this age group.[100] Pain on motion of the eyes, chills, and fever have been observed in young adults with proven rubella virus infection.[101]

Unknown Agents

In communities where live measles vaccine has been used extensively, measles-like illnesses are sporadic and should be studied serologically to determine if measles virus is the cause. In one study, measles virus infection could not be demonstrated serologically in 22 of 32 illnesses clinically compatible with measles, and it was suggested that other unidentified agents, presumably viruses, produced the illnesses, including some with an enanthem thought to be Koplik spots.[102]

Rubella-like Illness

This condition is defined as a mild illness with minimal fever or respiratory symptoms. Generalized lymphadenopathy and a generalized rash that lasts about 3 days are essential to the clinical diagnosis. Laboratory studies are extremely important if exposure of a pregnant woman is involved, as described in Chapter 19.

Rubella virus is the most important cause of rubella-like illness. Classical rubella virus infection is usually a mild disease with little fever. The rash appears about 14–21 days after the exposure, is nonconfluent and maculopapular, and lasts about 3 days. Generalized lymphadenopathy, particularly behind the ears (postauricular) and at the back of the head (occipital), is usually present. Mild splenomegaly may also be present. Rubella virus can be cultured from skin biopsies taken from the rash or a nonrash area.

Other viruses or allergies can cause a rubella-like illness, and there has been confusion and controversy over the clinical diagnosis of rubella for more than 100 years.[103,104] Serologic studies have shown the lack of reliability of the clinical diagnosis of rubella by a physician or of the patient's history of having had rubella. This is even more likely to be true today, when fewer and fewer physicians have personal experience caring for patients with the disease. Rubella virus infection also can occur without a rash.[105] Therefore, it is essential to do specific serologic studies of a patient with the clinical diagnosis of rubella if the prevention of congenital rubella infection is involved.

Infection with wild-type rubella virus produces lifelong immunity against rubella virus-induced disease. In the prerubella vaccine era, when wild-type rubella virus was in wide circulation, asymptomatic reinfection with rubella virus, as defined by a rise in rubella antibody titer, was not unusual. Reinfection with a second clinical illness has been reported, although this presumably is exceedingly rare.[106] There are no recent serologic surveys that examine the rate of asymptomatic rubella virus reinfection, but it would presumably be much less prevalent than it was in years past.

Arthritis is an occasional complication of rubella, especially in women. Testicular pain is not uncommon in postpubertal males.[107] Other complications, such as encephalitis, are rare.[108,109]

Rubella immunization and congenital rubella syndrome are discussed in Chapter 19.

As noted, many viruses other than rubella can produce a rubella-like illness. Postauricular and occipital node enlargement have, in the past, been regarded as very useful in the diagnosis of rubella. However, this clinical pattern can be duplicated by infection with adenoviruses, echoviruses, or coxsackieviruses.[103]

Febrile Maculopapular Exanthem

This is a noncommittal descriptive diagnosis that can be made when the patient has fever, a maculopapular rash, and none of the typical associated findings of measles, roseola, or rubella.[110,111] Typically, such illnesses occur more frequently in the summer and in outbreaks involving enough patients to make the physician recognize that this is the rash disease that is "going around." Coxsackie viruses are the best-recognized causes of this type of rash and should be suspected when the rash appears within about 24 hours of the fever.[112] Erythema infectiosum also may produce this type of rash but typically has little or no fever (see Fig. 11-2B, C).

Drug Rashes

Drugs, particularly ampicillin, can cause maculopapular exanthems (Fig. 11-4). Often, the patient is receiving ampicillin for a febrile illness, so that the rash appears to be a febrile exanthem.

Other Causes

In 1951, a maculopapular exanthem that occurred after the patient's fever had subsided and principally involved the face was observed in Boston. For

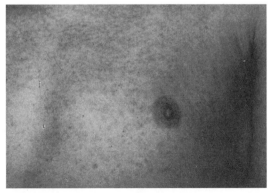

■ FIGURE 11-4 Ampicillin rash, a maculopapular rash often confused with viral exanthems (Photo from Dr. Norman Fost).

a time, the phrase "Boston exanthem" was used to describe this particular pattern. This Boston outbreak was caused by type 16 echovirus.[111,113,114] Other outbreaks of exanthems occurred in Boston in 1959 and 1961 and were reported to be caused by different echovirus types or by coxsackieviruses and had a somewhat different clinical pattern. Based on this experience, some physicians felt that they could differentiate the viral etiology of an exanthematous disease based on the clinical pattern and rash distribution alone. However, there was always a fair amount of variability even in the patterns observed in a single outbreak. Thus, it is difficult if not impossible to predict the type of echovirus or coxsackievirus on clinical grounds.

Respiratory syncytial virus infection has rarely been associated with a maculopapular rash, along with the more usual lower respiratory disease.[115]

Meningococcal bacteremia is a rare cause of maculopapular rash with high fever. A blanching blotchy rash has often been noted before the appearance of petechiae and probably is a vascular phenomenon. Maculopapular rashes may also be seen in Rocky Mountain spotted fever and, especially, ehrlichiosis.

Scarlet fever should always be considered in patients with maculopapular exanthems, because the rash is sometimes atypical. Other signs usually associated with scarlet fever may not yet have appeared. Lyme disease is a possible cause of a maculopapular rash, although the rash is usually macular. As discussed earlier, KD is usually associated with a maculopapular rash.

Diagnostic Approach

Throat cultures to exclude Group A streptococcal pharyngitis may be indicated in some maculopapular exanthems because scarlet fever is sometimes atypical.

If rubella is suspected and an exposure of a pregnant woman is involved, serum should be obtained as soon as possible during the first week of the illness for use as an acute-phase serum. This specimen can be held until a second serum is obtained 2–3 weeks later (convalescent-phase serum). Testing of paired sera is especially important for laboratory confirmation of rubella virus infection, but it also can be used for demonstration of measles virus infection in difficult cases.

Viral cultures can be obtained for recognition of infections caused by adenoviruses, echoviruses, or coxsackie B viruses. Recovery of one of these viruses is sometimes useful, along with negative serologic studies for rubella, to demonstrate that a rubella-like illness was *not* caused by rubella virus.

Treatment

Antibiotic therapy is not indicated before a specific diagnosis such as streptococci pharyngitis is confirmed unless the patient appears so seriously ill as to suggest possible septicemia or otitis media, pneumonia, or a similar complication is present.

■ PETECHIAL-PURPURIC RASHES AND VASCULITIS

Petechial rashes have been given special importance because they may be caused by bacteremia, particularly meningococcemia (Box 11-5). Petechiae typically are circular flat lesions 1 mm or less in diameter. At first, they are pink but change over the course of 1–12 hours to dark red and then to purple or brown. Unlike other exanthems, petechiae do not blanch with pressure. Petechiae can be seen in normal children after compression of an arm by a tourniquet or a blood pressure cuff or on the chest, face, or arms after prolonged coughing, crying, sneezing, forceful vomiting, or other Valsalva maneuvers. Petechiae also can be a result of thrombocytopenia, which can be produced by several noninfectious diseases, but the patient is usually not febrile or acutely ill.

Prospective studies on children hospitalized with fever and petechiae have generally documented approximately an 7% rate of meningococcemia.[116] Interestingly, a more recent, larger prospective trial that enrolled all children under age 18 who presented to the emergency department with a temperature over 38°C and petechiae found that only 8 (2%) of 411 had bacteremia or clinical sepsis.[117] All studies to date have shown that an approximation of the risk of serious disease in children with fever and petechiae can be refined by clinical and laboratory parameters, especially "ill appearance" of the child, the location of the petechiae, whether or not a mechanical factor known to produce petechiae exists, and peripheral WBC counts. In the largest study, the lack of ill appearance had a negative predictive value of 1.0, as did a WBC count between 5000 and 15,000/mL. A prothrombin time less than 13.5 seconds, a partial thromboplastin time of less than 30 seconds, and

Common

"Viral syndrome" (no specific etiologic agent
recovered)
Valsalva effect of cough or vomiting
Trauma of blood pressure cuff or tourniquet
Streptococcal pharyngitis with petechiae

Uncommon

Meningococcemia
Pneumococcal bacteremia
H. influenzae bacteremia
Rocky Mountain spotted fever
Ehrlichiosis
Toxic shock syndrome
Infective endocarditis
Bacterial septic emboli (S. aureus, Pseudomonas,
gonococcus)
Disseminated intravascular coagulation (any
cause)
Infectious mononucleosis
Adenovirus
Cytomegalovirus, especially in newborn
Rubella virus
Coxsackie or echoviruses
Parvovirus B19 (papular-purpuric gloves and socks
syndrome)
RSV
Influenza or parainfluenza viruses
HIV
Anaphylactoid purpura
Thrombocytopenia from noninfectious causes

Rare

Murine typhus
Disseminated histoplasmosis
Brucellosis
Salmonellosis
Q fever
Dengue hemorrhagic fever
Brazilian purpuric fever (H. aegyptius infection)
Hantavirus
Collagen-vascular diseases

the absence of purpura had negative predictive values of 0.99.[117] Both studies were in agreement that if the petechiae were located only above the nipple line, or if an obvious mechanical factor caused the petechiae, the risk of serious infection is minimal. The incidence of serious infection in children with fever who had petechiae only above the nipple line was zero in both studies (total $n = 601$).

The blood pressure should be obtained immediately in any febrile patient with a petechial rash (see Chapter 10).

Purpura resembles traumatic bruising. Generally speaking, children who present with fever and purpura are at higher risk of having serious bacterial infections than are children with fever and petechiae. In Mandl's study, the sensitivity of the finding of a purpuric rash in predicting serious disease was 83%, and the positive predictive value was 0.31, despite the very low incidence of invasive disease in their cohort.[117] Children presenting with purpura and sepsis generally have other physical findings and laboratory values suggestive of sepsis.

Noninfectious diseases with signs resembling purpura include cutaneous vasculitis. In children, a relatively common form of cutaneous vasculitis is called anaphylactoid purpura (Henoch-Schönlein purpura), which occurs predominately below the waist except in infants.[118] Purpura in children may also result from immune thrombocytopenic purpura, hemolytic-uremic syndrome or thrombotic thrombocytopenic purpura, thrombocytopenia due to HIV or other infectious agents, or thrombocyte dysfunction secondary to drug therapy. Rarely, aspirin in therapeutic dosages has been reported to cause thrombocytopenia[119]; this condition is rarer still now that most children never receive aspirin therapy.

Thrombocytopenia occurs commonly during bacterial septicemia as part of the syndrome of disseminated intravascular coagulation (DIC). This syndrome can also be caused by severe viral, fungal, or parasitic infections and is discussed further in Chapter 10.

Possible Infectious Etiologies

Meningococcemia

This is the most important cause to be considered in a patient with a petechial or purpuric rash, because the disease is rapidly fatal if untreated. Patients with a purpuric rash often develop septic shock or DIC, as described in chapter 10. Patients with a macular or petechial rash are likely to have a better prognosis than those with purpuric lesions.[120] Meningeal signs may be present, but meningococcemia can occur without meningitis and carries a worse prognosis. Early in the course of meningococcemia, the rash may be absent. In order to detect the possibility of occult meningococcemia, careful measurement of blood pressure and serial physical examinations are indicated in the child with high fever.

Haemophilus Influenzae

In a study of 129 children hospitalized for fever and petechiae, 13 (10%) had *Neisseria meningitidis,* 8 (6%) had *H. influenzae* type b (Hib), and the majority had a viral illness.[121] Septicemia secondary to Hib is now a rarity in the United States because of the routine use of the conjugated Hib vaccine.

Management of contacts exposed to the meningococcus or *H. influenzae* is discussed in Chapter 21.

Streptococcal Pharyngitis

A common cause of petechiae and fever is streptococcal pharyngitis.[122] The child does not appear septic, and there is usually an exudative pharyngitis, especially in school-aged children. In children younger than age 3, Group A streptococcal infection causing fever and petechiae in the absence of any signs or symptoms of pharyngitis has been described.[117]

Rocky Mountain Spotted Fever (RMSF)

The typical clinical pattern here includes exposure to wood ticks or dog ticks and headache, myalgia, chills, and high fever.[123] The headache of RMSF is relentless and intractable to pain relievers. Abdominal pain is not uncommon and can be severe. Typically, myalgia is extreme, and tenderness of the muscles, especially of the calf and thigh, can be elicited on physical examination. An explicit exposure history is often not obtainable. Most patients, however, live in areas or participate in activities where exposure to ticks might be expected. Prevalence of the disease is widely disparate. North Carolina, Oklahoma, Texas, and South Carolina accounted for almost half the cases in the United States between 1981 and 1992.[124] Disease occurs during the warmer months; 90% of cases occur between April and September.[124] RMSF is almost unheard of in the dead of winter.

The incubation period is about 3–12 days. The rash begins on about the fourth day of illness and is first noted on the extremities, especially around the ankles or the wrists. It usually begins as a macular rash but progresses to include petechiae. It sometimes involves the palms and soles (Fig. 11-5). Edema of the eyelids and extremities is common. Photophobia may be present. Shock, neurologic or pulmonary involvement, or renal failure may occur in severe cases. The cerebrospinal fluid often reveals a pleocytosis of less than 300 WBC/mL, predominantly lymphocytes, with normal glucose and elevated protein. Usually, there is a moderate thrombocytopenia. The peripheral WBC count is often elevated, with mostly neutrophils. The finding of hyponatremia, though not specific for RMSF, supports the diagnosis.

RMSF carries a fairly high morbidity and mortality; bad outcomes are related to the duration of time between onset of symptoms and receipt of appropriate antimicrobial therapy. Mortality increases by almost fourfold if therapy is not started by the fifth day of illness.[125] Therefore, a high index of suspicion must be maintained. A helpful adage to remember is that "summertime influenza" should be considered RMSF until proven otherwise. Thus, in highly endemic areas during the appropriate season, it is reasonable to treat patients who present with fever, headache, and myalgia with an empiric course of doxycycline. Diagnosis is usually made (retrospectively) by acute and convalescent serology, although immunofluorescence or immunoperoxidase staining of biopsied skin is available.[126] For patients with suspected RMSF, therapy must not be withheld pending definitive diagnosis. Treatment with doxycycline is most reliably curative. This drug should be given to all patients with suspected or proven RMSF, without regard to the fear of staining the teeth in young children. Long-term follow-up study of patients treated with short courses of doxycycline during early childhood shows no appreciable staining of the teeth.[127] Early therapy can be life saving. Chloramphenicol is sometimes used but is associated with a higher mortality than treatment with doxycycline.[124]

Prevention is best accomplished by measures directed at minimizing tick exposure and at removing attached ticks promptly. It is thought that approximately 6 hours of attachment is necessary to transmit the infection. A vaccine, although thought to be regionally needed,[128] is not yet available. Several candidate vaccines have been successful in protection against disease in animal models. A formalin-killed vaccine produced measurable immune responses, but only protected 4 of 16 subjects from developing RMSF when challenged.[129]

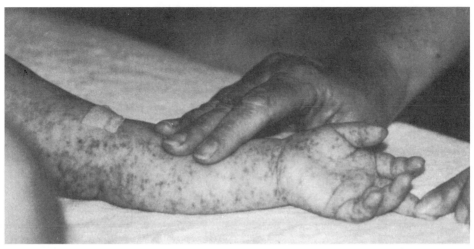

■ **FIGURE 11-5** Rocky Mountain spotted fever, showing edema of the hand (Photo from Dr. Arnold Benardette).

Ehrlichiosis

Ehrlichiosis is a disease that is related to RMSF. It is also transmitted by ticks. Patients with ehrlichiosis present with some of the same features as patients with RMSF. Rash is present in about two-thirds of children; it can be macular, maculopapular, or petechial.[130]

Thrombocytopenia and leukopenia are frequent. Depression of two cell lines often raises the diagnostic possibility of malignancy. Serum aminotransfer-

ase levels are increased in nearly 90% of patients.[130] Treatment is with doxycycline as in RMSF.

Thrombocytopenia of Disseminated Intravascular Coagulation (DIC)

Thrombocytopenia and DIC (discussed in Chapter 10) can produce a petechial or purpuric rash, regardless of the cause. It can occur in any of the infections mentioned in this section. Disseminated histoplasmosis or other disseminated fungal infec-

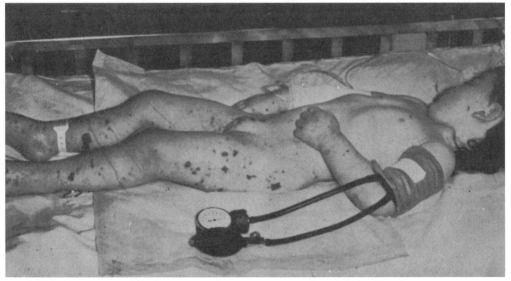

■ **FIGURE 11-6** Purpuric rash in meningococcemia. Blood pressure and circulation perfusion should be monitored carefully (Photo from Dr. Norman Fost).

tions can involve the liver, spleen, and bone marrow, with resultant fever and petechiae, as well as hepatosplenomegaly and lymphopenia.

Infective Endocarditis

This diagnosis is considered when a patient with heart disease develops fever (see Chapters 10 and 18). Typically, the petechiae are about 1 mm in diameter and are accompanied by other manifestations, particularly splenomegaly and a history of heart disease.

Septic Emboli (Pustular Purpura)

Staphylococcal septicemia can produce a pustular purpura that may be mistaken for meningococcal lesions.[131] *Pseudomonas* septicemia also may be associated with skin lesions that sometimes appear purpuric. The characteristic evolution is from a red macule to a purple hemorrhagic bullous lesion.[132] The lesion is called ecthyma gangrenosum and is seen most frequently in neutropenic hosts (see Chapter 22). Other organisms, such as *Aeromonas,* can cause ecthyma gangrenosum as well.

Disseminated gonococcemia, occasionally seen in sexually active adolescents, also has characteristic lesions that evolve from petechiae to papule to pustule to central necrosis or hemorrhagic vesicles.[133]

Thus, the typical evolution of septic skin lesions begins with the early lesions of petechiae, small erythematous macules, or small papules on an erythematous base (Fig. 11-6).[131,132] Later lesions can be pustules or bullae, which can be hemorrhagic and may contain purple or black necrotic areas of skin infarction.

Many infected insect bites or scabies can sometimes resemble pustules of septicemia, but the child is typically afebrile.

Chronic Congenital Infections

In the newborn infant, congenital rubella, cytomegalovirus, syphilis, parvovirus B19, or toxoplasmosis may be associated with petechiae or purpura (Chapter 19). The lesions can be due to thrombocytopenia, but sometimes lesions that are thought to be hemorrhagic are actually areas of dermal erythropoiesis.

Infectious Mononucleosis

Occasionally, thrombocytopenia with petechial or purpuric lesions occurs in infectious mononucleosis.

Adenoviruses

Fever and a petechial rash are occasionally associated with adenovirus infection.[134]

Murine Typhus

Caused by infection with *Rickettsia typhi*, this disease occurs rarely in the United States, but 47 cases were reported from Hawaii in 2002.[135] There may be a known exposure to rodents or cat fleas. Fever lasts several days before the appearance of a macular or petechial rash, which begins on the trunk, in contrast to that of RMSF. The disease resembles a mild case of epidemic louse-borne typhus, in which high fever and delirium are usually severe.

Brazilian Purpuric Fever

This is a syndrome not yet seen in the United States in which children develop purulent conjunctivitis, high fever, prostration, and purpura. Blood cultures are positive for a particular clone of *Haemophilus aegyptius* that tends to be resistant to the bactericidal activity of human serum.[136]

Dengue Hemorrhagic Fever

This disease, spread by the bite of the mosquito, is a reasonably common cause of petechiae/purpura in South America and Asia. Most cases seen in the United States are imported (diagnosed in people recently returned from areas of endemicity). A review of 130 hospitalized patients in Singapore revealed that the majority of patients were between 15 and 30 years of age. Petechiae developed in half of this cohort. Seventy-five percent of those with petechiae had a platelet count of less than 100,000/mL. The petechiae developed about 6 days into the illness and lasted approximately 3.5 days. Nineteen (15%) of the 130 patients developed bleeding; the gums were the most common site. All patients recovered.[137]

Other Infectious Causes

Several viral infections can cause petechial rashes via thrombocytopenia. Acquired cytomegalovirus infection has been associated with thrombocytopenia.[138] Acquired rubella virus infection can cause thrombocytopenic purpura.[139] *Mycoplasma pneumoniae* can produce a rash that can be petechial and purpuric and that is associated with fever and leukocytosis. Usually, there is at least a mild pneumonia.[140] Petechiae in infants infected with RSV has been described. Influenza virus or parainfluenza virus was isolated from 11 (17%) of 63 children with an etiologic diagnosis of fever and petechiae in one study.[116] A variety of echoviruses and coxsackievir uses have been recovered from children with petechiae and fever.

Papular-pupuric gloves and socks syndrome is an interesting manifestation of a viral infection. It is usually attributed to infection with parvovirus B 19.[140a] One report suggests that in young children this condition may also be associated with EBV or CMV infection.[140b]

Other infections causing fever and petechiae may include *Escherichia coli* urinary infections, KD, salmonellosis, brucellosis, Q fever, reaction to MMR immunization, and herpangina.[121] Pertussis is commonly associated with petechiae on the trunk and face because of the forceful coughing.

Noninfectious Causes

Petechiae can also be caused by thrombocytopenia secondary to immune thrombocytopenic purpura, leukemia/lymphoma, or Langham's cell histiocytosis. In the latter condition, the infant usually has an enlarged spleen, fever, anemia, and other skin lesions, which usually resemble eczema.[141] Thrombocytopenia may follow acute poststreptococcal glomerulonephritis or be part of the hemolytic-uremic syndrome.[142]

Cutaneous Vasculitis

This phrase is used to describe skin lesions caused by inflammatory and necrotizing changes in the blood vessels of the skin attributable to an immunopathogenic mechanism.[143] In adults, the underlying vasculitides are usually polyarteritis nodosa, Wegener's granulomatosis, or a hypersensitivity reaction; but in children, the most frequent diagnosis is anaphylactoid (Henoch-Schönlein) purpura.[143] Children with anaphylactoid purpura often have dermal and glomerular deposition of IgA and alterations of their complement system. The diagnosis of cutaneous vasculitis is confirmed in the laboratory only by histologic examination. However, the cutaneous lesion is suspected to be secondary to vasculitis because of the patient's underlying disease and its clinical features of palpable, purpuric lesions on an erythematous or necrotic base and in the absence of thrombocytopenia. The lesions also may be indurated, purpuric macules and are typically found below the waist, especially on the legs and buttocks.

Anaphylactoid purpura sometimes has an additional resemblance to meningococcemia when there are neurologic complications such as hemiparesis or focal weakness, seizures, or mental changes.[144] Anaphylactoid purpura may occur without the rash and resemble acute glomerulonephritis, in which case it is called Berger's disease.[145]

Vasculitis can involve various sizes of veins or arteries.[146,147] This accounts for the variability of the clinical presentation of vasculitis, which may appear urticarial or nodular.[146] Usually, vasculitis is recognized as palpable purpura but it may be papules, nodules, plaques, vesicles or hemorrhagic bullae.[147] Corticosteroids and other immune modulators are used in an attempt to interfere with immune complex formation.[147]

Meningococcemia is usually more fulminant but milder cases can mimic anaphylactoid purpura, with fever, arthritis, and gastrointestinal symptoms, especially if there is concurrent therapy with oral antibacterials and antipyretics.[148] Cytomegalovirus can cause cutaneous vasculitis, especially in the immunosuppressed host.[149]

Purpura with Eosinophilia

A syndrome of nonthrombocytopenic purpura with eosinophilia has been noted in children and young adults in Southeast Asia and immigrants from this area.[150] The cause of this spontaneous bruising of limbs, trunk, and face is unknown. Laboratory abnormalities include a prolonged bleeding time and platelet function abnormalities with a normal platelet count. The duration of the illness is 5–12 months.

Acute Febrile Neutropenic Dermatosis (Sweet Syndrome)

This rare skin disease can produce a fever and rash illness in infants and children.[151] There is often a peripheral leukocytosis. The rash consists of waxy erythematous to violaceous papules at sites of trauma. The papules enlarge over several days to become raised plaques and may heal with an atrophic scar. Biopsy reveals infiltration with mature neutrophils. The cause is unknown. It is most commonly seen in association with underlying malignancy, but it can be idiopathic.

Diagnostic Plan

In the past, because of the specter of possible meningococcemia, which can be rapidly fatal, all children presenting with fever and petechiae were down evaluated and treated as though they had meningococcemia. At present there is not a clear consensus as to the scope of the evaluation required or as to whether a patient requires hospitalization and empiric antimicrobial therapy. Infectious diseases clinicians tend to be more conservative than community general pediatricians, perhaps because their view is skewed by the experience of caring for the sickest of this group of patients.[152] Prospective studies on fever and petechiae, however, suggest that not all children with this condition are at the same risk of serious disease. Risk factors for invasive disease reported by Mandl and colleagues were mentioned earlier. Principally, they included ill appearance, the presence of purpura, and a prothrombin time of greater than 13.5 seconds. A group in England published a similar, albeit much smaller, experience in children with fever and petechiae. They reached similar conclusions (i.e., risk of serious disease in children with fever and petechiae can be semiquantitated). They used the acronym "ILL," (irritable, lethargic, low capillary refill) and added abnormal WBC count ($< 5,000$ or $> 15,000$ per/mL) and an elevated CRP as indications of higher risk.

If a child does not appear ill, and petechiae are located only in areas of mechanical trauma or are above the nipple line and associated with forceful coughing or vomiting, the chance that the petechiae signal severe or life-threatening infection is vanishingly small. WBC from between 5,000–15,000 per/mL is also reassuring. The predictive value of CRP in this setting has not yet been clearly established. Perhaps a period of observation to document that deterioration does not occur would allow a less aggressive workup. A normal blood pressure should be documented. Follow-up evaluation would have to be readily available.

If the child is irritable or lethargic, or has signs of dehydration or shock, workup and treatment as though the child has meningococcemia may be life saving. During the warm months, doxycycline can be added to treat RMSF, particularly in endemic areas. WBC count and a peripheral blood smear may show thrombocytopenia, blast forms, or other evidence of a hematologic explanation of the petechial or purpuric rash.

Throat cultures for Group A streptococci and a blood culture are usually indicated. In many patients with fever and a petechial or purpuric rash, ceftriaxone therapy for possible meningococcemia or ampicillin-resistant *H. influenzae* is indicated immediately after obtaining these cultures without awaiting their results. Lumbar puncture may be indicated to detect meningitis, and careful observation for signs of shock should certainly be done, as discussed in Chapter 10. Gram stain of a scraping or puncture of a petechia is helpful if gram-negative diplococci (meningococci) are seen.

An acute serum specimen for measurement of antibodies for infectious mononucleosis, RMSF, ehrlichiosis, or murine typhus may be indicated. If available, ehrlichia PCR can be done on whole blood. In contrast, PCR for the agent of RMSF (*Rickettsia rickettsiae*) is insensitive, because the target organ is the endothelial cell, not the WBC. If RMSF is suspected on clinical grounds, treatment with doxycycline should not be delayed while awaiting serologic confirmation of this disease.[153]

If anaphylactoid purpura is considered, examination for fecal occult blood and microscopic hematuria may be helpful.

Children with deficiencies of one of the late components of complement are at higher risk of acquiring meningococcemia, as are those with properdin deficiency. Many experts recommend a CH50 to screen for complement problems in patients admitted with meningococcemia or meningococcal meningitis. These deficiencies are more common in African Americans. A family history of meningococcal disease also increases the chances of finding such a deficiency. A second episode of infection with *N. meningitidis* is highly suggestive of late complement deficiency or a barrier breach such as a basilar skull fracture.

■ CHICKENPOX-LIKE RASHES

Chickenpox-like rashes have a characteristic evolution from papule (bump) to vesicle (blister) to pustule (small boil) to ulcer with a crust (scab or eschar) (Fig. 11-7). Chickenpox is the most familiar example of this type of rash. Bullous rashes are characterized by large blisters that undergo a similar evolution. Sometimes these two types of rash are classified together as vesiculobullous eruptions (Box 11-6). However, it is useful to separate bullous rashes, which are discussed in a later section. Pus-

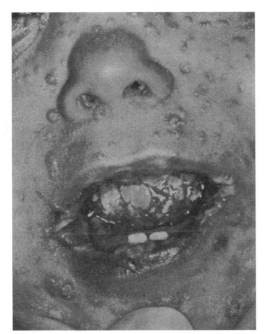

■ **FIGURE 11-7** This child with moderately severe chickenpox has most skin lesions in the pustular stage, some of which are umbilicated, and mucosal lesions in the mouth.

tules, boils, and abscesses are also discussed in Chapter 17.

Possible Etiologies

Chickenpox

Chickenpox is caused by primary infection with varicella zoster virus (VZV). Usually a mild disease in children, chickenpox produces minimal respiratory symptoms and mild to moderate fever. The parent usually knows the exposure, or the disease is known to be present in the community. The rash occurs 10–21 days after the exposure, with an average of 14 days. The characteristic lesions are clear vesicles on an erythematous base, small pustules, and small crusted ulcers (see Fig. 11-7). The pox lesions appear in crops, and if several stages of the lesion are present at the same time the diagnosis is assured. Itching is prominent, and physicians are often consulted only because of the itching. Lymphadenopathy also is prominent, particularly in the nodes draining the scalp or areas of scratched lesions. A brief generalized erythematous rash may precede the vesicular lesions. Mucosal lesions can occur. Occasionally, the lesions are larger than the usual 1 or 2 mm in diameter. Large bullae may occur, which may resemble (or be due to) scalded

skin syndrome.[154] Secondary infection of the pustules with *S. aureus* or Group A streptococci occasionally occurs, which can be relatively benign, or herald severe, necrotizing infection. Other complications are discussed later in this section.

Chickenpox can occur in children or adults with malignancy, such as Hodgkin's disease or leukemia.[155] In such cases, there is a high mortality rate without acyclovir therapy, as discussed in Chapter 22.

Other skin diseases that may resemble chickenpox are discussed later in this chapter in the sections on bullous rashes and bitelike rashes.

Zoster

Zoster (shingles) is a disease that increases in frequency with advancing age, but it can be seen at any age, including neonates. It represents reactivation of

---

BOX 11-6 ■ Vesicular and Bullous Rashes

Vesicular
Chickenpox
Zoster
Herpes simplex virus infection
Hand-foot-mouth syndrome
Poison ivy
Scabies
Insect bites
Smallpox
Mastocytosis
Urticaria pigmentosa
Incontinentia pigmenti
Miliaria crystallina
Acropustulosis of infancy
Hyper IgE syndrome
Acrodermatitis enteropathica
Langerhans' cell histiocytosis
Pityriasis lichenoides et varioliformis acuta
  (PLEVA)

Bullous
Stevens-Johnson syndrome
Congenital syphilis
Bullous impetigo
Bullous tinea
Dermatitis herpetiformis
Bullous pemphigoid
Pemphigus
Chronic bullous dermatosis of childhood (linear
  IgA bullous dermatosis)
Epidermolysis bullosa

latent VZV from dorsal root ganglia. The disease is three times more common among adolescents than it is in preschoolers. Zoster is at least three times more common among children who contract primary varicella in the first year of life.[156]

A vesiculopustular rash in a sensory nerve dermatome distribution is the typical appearance of herpes zoster, although herpes simplex can also sometimes produce this pattern (Fig. 11-8). It is convenient to omit the term *herpes* in reference to zoster to lessen the confusion with herpes simplex. Zoster often occurs on the trunk and is unilateral, ending abruptly at the midline or in the distribution of the fifth cranial nerve. It is usually less painful in children than in adults.[157]

Zoster-like distribution of vesicles in a sensory dermatome is observed rarely with other viruses, such as echoviruses.[158]

Zoster is contagious by direct contact with a pustular lesion, whereas chickenpox is contagious by respiratory spread as well. Patients with disseminated zoster may spread VZV infection by both routes.

Infants who present with zoster must be presumed to have experienced varicella infection in the womb. It is probably reasonable to have these babies undergo chorioretinal examination by an ophthalmologist, as retinitis may be the only sign of congenital varicella syndrome. Some patients with HIV infection (Chapter 20) or with a primary immunodeficiency syndrome (Chapter 23) experience recurrent or severe cases of zoster. Zoster is rarely the presenting symptom of malignancy.

Herpes Simplex Infections

The skin lesions of herpes simplex virus (HSV) typically present as groups of vesicles, which evolve into pustules and crusts (Fig. 11-9). However, in unusual locations, in patients with underlying diseases, or at a certain stage of the evolution, the lesions are easily misdiagnosed. When located at a fingertip the deep vesicles may resemble a bacterial paronychia or felon and are referred to as herpetic whitlow.[159] Children who suck a thumb or finger may also get a herpetic whitlow, which appears yellow and pustular. Occasionally, a herpetic whitlow occurs in a baby whose mother trims the baby's fingernails with her teeth. When located in the genital area, the superficial circular ulceration might be mistaken for a chancre. Wrestlers may infect each other in unusual locations during their body contact in areas of superficial trauma (herpes gladiatorum).[160]

Infection of abnormal skin by HSV can be confusing. Eczematous skin can become infected (Kaposi's varicelliform eruption), producing a severe purulent condition that is often mistaken for a bacterial infection. Burns can become infected with HSV, as described in Chapter 17. Patients with leukemia can develop large herpetic bullae, which rupture and leave shallow ulcerations.[161] Ulcerations

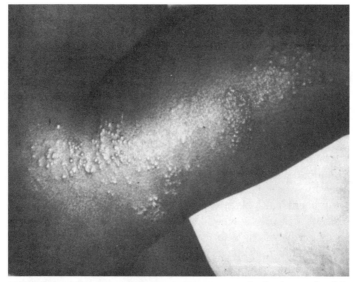

■ **FIGURE 11-8** Zoster, showing typical dermatome distribution on the right lateral thigh (Photo from Dr. Norman Fost).

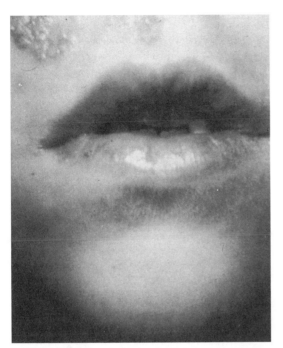

■ **FIGURE 11-9** Herpes simplex virus lesion near nose, showing groups of vesicles (Photo from Dr. Gordon Tuffli).

from HSV can be chronic in immunosuppressed patients.

Vesicles on a newborn infant may be a manifestation of life-threatening HSV infection, as the virus can be transmitted from the mother's cervix to the skin of the infant. Perinatal herpesvirus infections are discussed in Chapter 19.

Hand-Foot-Mouth Syndrome

This syndrome typically occurs in the summer or fall. It is characterized by shallow ulcers in the mouth and papular or vesicular lesions on the hands and feet. Vesicular or papular lesions are also frequently found on the buttocks (Fig. 11-10). Coxsackie A virus is the usual cause.[162,163] Echoviruses and coxsackieviruses can also produce the typical papular or vesicular lesions of the hands, feet, and buttocks without accompanying mouth lesions.

The prognosis is typically benign, but a few patients develop the nonpurulent meningitis syndrome (see Chapter 9). Patients with antibody deficiencies have a particularly hard time with nonenveloped viruses like those that cause hand-foot-mouth disease; a case of three recurrent episodes of typical hand-foot-mouth syndrome in a patient with common variable immune deficiency

has been reported.[164] Fatal carditis and pneumonia also have been reported.[165]

Mycoplasma pneumoniae

Mycoplasma pneumoniae can produce a rash that resembles chickenpox and may be associated with arthralgia.[166]

Smallpox

Smallpox is a systemic disease with fever and high mortality. Although the disease has been eradicated, there is concern that hidden supplies of virus could be used as a weapon of bioterrorism.[167]

Like varicella, smallpox lesions go through various stages of evolution. However, the rash of smallpox may be distinguished from varicella by its initial appearance on the face and extremities, the presence of umbilicated pustules, and the fact that the lesions are generally all at the same stage of development at any one point in time.[168] In addition, the prodrome of smallpox is typically much more severe, with 1–4 days of high fever and myalgias prior to development of the rash.

Any patient who is suspected of having smallpox should be placed in airborne precautions. Infection control and public health officials should be contacted immediately.

Vaccination against smallpox involves the use of a live-attenuated vaccine (vaccinia virus). Because smallpox vaccination has been almost entirely abandoned, vaccinia virus disease is now rare. Laboratory workers are still vaccinated. Accidental transmission of vaccine virus to the broken skin of another individual can produce the same stages as deliberate vaccination, from papule to pustule to crusted ulcer and finally scar. The pustules can be mistaken for bacterial pustules. Fever up to 39°C (104°F) may occur at the peak of the local reaction. These days, most vaccinia-like illness (for example, near the eye, as in Fig. 3-5) is likely to be caused by herpes simplex virus. However, for reasons cited earlier, the use of smallpox vaccine is likely to increase, and physicians should be aware of the possible side effects of the vaccine. These include encephalitis (four per million), eczema vaccinatum in patients with atopic dermatitis (40 per million), and progressive vaccinia or vaccinia gangrenosa in immunocompromised hosts (2 per million).[169] Except in dire circumstances, the vaccine is contraindicated in patients with atopic dermatitis or immunodeficiency and in persons who have household con-

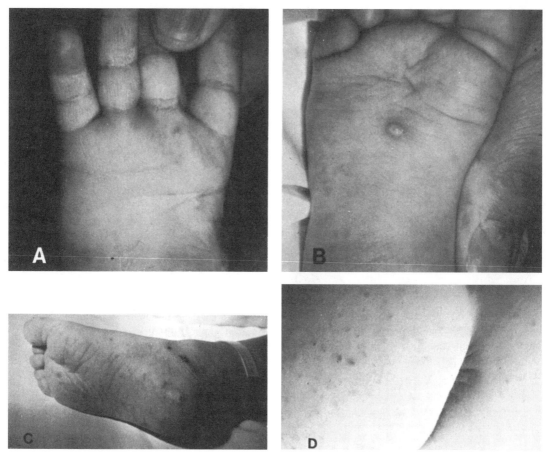

■ **FIGURE 11-10** Hand-foot-mouth syndrome showing typical rash: (**A**) hand; (**B**) foot; (**C**) foot; (**D**) buttocks (**A** and **B** from Dr. Gordon Tuffli).

tact with such individuals. Accidental inoculation of the eye with live vaccinia virus should be less frequent in any future vaccine campaigns because of improved materials for covering the vaccine site.

Monkeypox

Previously not reported in the Western Hemisphere, an outbreak of 72 cases of monkeypox virus infections occurred in the midwest United States in the summer of 2003.[169a] Patients, including several children, developed symptoms after exposure to ill prairie dogs that were imported from West Africa. Patients with monkeypox present with a short prodrome of high fever, sweats, and headache before rash and lymphadenopathy occur. The skin lesions evolve from papules to vesiculopustules and then to serous or hemorrhagic crusts before detaching. Several patients in the U.S. outbreak were hospitalized, but there were no deaths. In African out-

breaks, case-fatality rates have ranged from 4–22%.[169a]

Noninfectious Diseases

Ulcerative colitis may be associated with pustular lesions that resemble chickenpox, but these lesions are chronic.[170]

A noninfectious disease that resembles scabies or atopic dermatitis to some extent is infantile acropustulosis.[171–173] Typically, the itching pustules appear on the palms and soles in early infancy. The individual lesions last from 7–10 days, and new crops appear every 2 or 3 weeks.[171] The lesions may also occur on the extremities, trunk, or face. The cause is unknown. A high percentage of patients have a history of a clinical diagnosis of scabies, but the relationship between the two conditions is unclear.[174] Relapses may occur. Dapsone is sometimes effective, as are topical corticosteroids.[174] The disease usually has disappeared by the age of 2 or 3 years.

Dermatitis herpetiformis is now thought to be the cutaneous manifestation of gluten sensitivity.[175] IgA is deposited in the skin, producing itching, burning papules, and vesicles or bullae. It is usually bilateral and symmetrical.[176] It is rare in children but is important to identify because it often responds to treatment with a gluten-free diet. Other immunobullous disorders of childhood may also mimic varicella or HSV infection. These include bullous pemphigoid, linear IgA bullous dermatosis, pemphigus, and epidermolysis bullosa.[177] Diagnosis is by skin biopsy.

Pityriasis lichenoides et varioliformis acuta (PLEVA) is a disorder of T-cell proliferation that is characterized by the development of maculopapular lesions that evolve into vesicles, followed by crusting, much like varicella. However, the rash recurs for several months, and the patient is not systemically ill. In addition, the lesions are not pruritic.[178]

Patients with Langerhans cell histiocytosis may present with a rash that is easily confused with varicella or HSV infection.

Stevens-Johnson syndrome often is mistaken for bullous chickenpox or HSV and is discussed both later in this chapter and in the section on stomatitis in Chapter 2.

Diagnostic Approach

Viral cultures of pustular lesions may be useful if laboratory confirmation of infection with herpes simplex or varicella virus is needed. Coxsackie A viruses are usually not recovered unless mouse inoculations are done, and this is not practical.

Gram stain and culture of pustular or bullous lesions is indicated if secondary bacterial infection is suspected. Unfortunately, in immunocompromised children, where it is important to detect chickenpox or zoster, the clinical appearance is often atypical, and the Tzanck preparation is often falsely negative. Some laboratories have fluorescent antibody or PCR tests that are accurate. Serology is not useful for diagnosis. Airborne precautions should be instituted until the clinical appearance or laboratory studies are diagnostic.

Complications of Chickenpox

Secondary Bacterial Infections of the Skin

Secondary bacterial infection of lesions is the most common complication of chickenpox. A clue is new onset of fever after an initial defervescence. Prompt use of antibiotics is justified in suspected secondary bacterial infections of chickenpox, particularly when there is unusually high fever or an unusual amount of erythema, tenderness, or purulent discharge. Beta-hemolytic streptococci can produce potentially serious complications, such as varicella gangrenosa,[179] septic arthritis, or osteomyelitis. Pain out of proportion to the clinical findings, hyponatremia, and hypocalcemia suggest necrotizing fasciitis.[180] Management of necrotizing fasciitis requires prompt surgical assistance and is discussed in Chapter 17.

Central Nervous System (CNS) Complications

Nervous system manifestations are the second most commonly encountered complication of varicella infection. Of these, cerebellar ataxia is by far the most frequent, occurring in approximately 1 of every 4,000 cases of chickenpox. The onset is acute and usually follows resolution of the skin disease. The prognosis is excellent. Reye's syndrome (see Chapter 9) is a rare but serious complication of chickenpox. Encephalitis that occurs prior to the onset of the rash[181] is thought to be secondary to direct viral invasion of the CNS, whereas the far more common postinfectious encephalitis is thought to be strictly immune mediated. There are two clinical syndromes of encephalitis. The more common one has a gradual onset of symptoms of lethargy, ataxia, and change in mental status. Rarer is an acute disease heralded by high fever, seizures, and sometimes paralysis. CSF pleocytosis is seen in either form. The mortality rate of acute varicella encephalitis is from 5–20% and 15% of survivors have neurologic sequelae. The incidence of encephalitis is approximately 2.5 per 10,000 cases of varicella.[182]

Pneumonia and Hepatitis

Varicella zoster virus (VZV) has a predilection for the lungs and the liver. Patients with compromised immunity are most likely to suffer from pneumonia or hepatitis. The pneumonia usually has an interstitial pattern and can be severe, sometimes necessitating mechanical ventilation and even extracorporeal membrane oxygenation (ECMO) or nitric oxide therapy. Women who experience primary varicella during pregnancy seem to have a particularly poor prognosis. Acyclovir is the drug of choice. Recovery, if it occurs, typically takes 6–10 days. Hepatitis is less common than pneumonia and is usually not life threatening, although severe cases with associated disseminated intravascular coagulation have been reported.[183]

Miscellaneous Complications

Hemorrhagic varicella has several forms. Hemorrhage at the site of pox lesions does not always indicate a more severe course, but some patients develop "malignant chickenpox" with purpura, which carries a high mortality. Thrombocytopenia is common in any form of hemorrhagic varicella. Postinfectious purpura can also occur, which is associated with a prolonged thrombocytopenia that lasts weeks. Mono- or polyarticular arthritis occasionally occurs with VZV infection. It is often due to secondary bacterial infections, but sometimes the virus is either recovered from joint fluid by culture or proven to be present by the use of PCR.[184] Myocarditis with VZV infection has been reported, as has intractable ventricular tachycardia.[185] Transverse myelitis, neuromyelitis optica, post-varicella bacterial meningitis, facial palsy, vasculitis with stroke, acute retinal necrosis, hemolysis in patients with congenital hemoglobinopathy, paroxysmal cold hemoglobinuria, glomerulonephritis, and Guillain-Barré syndrome are additional reported complications.[186–188] (Box 11-7). A temporal association between primary varicella infection and meningococcal disease was noted in three children.[189] Oddly, acute varicella seemed to greatly improve the symptoms of juvenile rheumatoid arthritis in two children with refractory joint disease.[190] There are two reports of children developing KD during the course of varicella.[191,192]

We have cared for a girl who developed high fever 3 days into her illness with otherwise uncomplicated varicella. Her fever persisted, and the diagnosis of KD was suspected when she developed peeling around her fingers 14 days later. Echocardiogram showed coronary artery ectasia, and abdominal ultrasound showed a hydropic gallbladder, suggesting the diagnosis of KD. It is likely that these cases represent mere temporal coincidence of two relatively common diseases in childhood.

Treatment

Nonspecific Therapy

Therapy for uncomplicated chickenpox focuses mainly on treatment of pruritus and includes appli-

---

BOX 11-7 ■ Complications of Chickenpox

Secondary bacterial infection, especially with staphylococci and streptococci
Interstitial pneumonia
Encephalitis (CSF pleocytosis)
Reye's syndrome (no CSF pleocytosis)
Cerebellar ataxia or transverse myelitis
Labyrinthitis or vertigo
Septic arthritis or varicella arthritis
Glomerulonephritis (unrecognized secondary streptococcal infection?)
Purpura fulminans
Progressive disseminated chickenpox (in immunosuppressed)
Fatal transplacental chickenpox when mother has onset of rash 1 week before or after delivery (Chapter 19)
Congenital skin scarring and hypoplastic limbs from prenatal infection (Chapter 19)
Myocarditis with dysrhythmias
Acute retinal necrosis
Acute hemolysis in a patient with hereditary spherocytosis
Facial palsy
Guillain-Barré syndrome
Group A streptococcal epiglottitis
Paroxysmal cold hemoglobinuria

---

cation of lotions such as calamine. Absorption of the diphenhydramine from excessively used Caladryl lotion has been reported to cause delirium and hallucinations masquerading as an encephalitis or Reye's syndrome in a child with extensive skin lesions.[193] The physician should be especially cautious not to administer oral diphenhydramine at the same time a child is receiving topical treatment with a diphenhydramine-containing lotion. Oatmeal baths or cool compresses are benign forms of therapy that are sometimes effective. Oral antihistamines may be indicated for patients with severe itching. Aspirin should not be given to patients with chickenpox because it increases the risk of Reye's syndrome (Chapter 9). The use of ibuprofen for antipyresis during acute chickenpox has been associated with the development of necrotizing fasciitis in some case-control studies but not in others, as discussed in Chapters 10 and 17. If pain control or antipyresis is needed in children with chickenpox, acetaminophen would appear to be the best choice.

Specific Antiviral Therapy

Acyclovir is a pro-drug that must be phosphorylated three times to become active. The first phosphorylation step is catalyzed by a viral enzyme. Acyclovir is poorly absorbed from the gastrointestinal tract. Therefore, serious or life-threatening VZV infections should be treated with the intravenous form. Oral therapy for primary chickenpox has been shown to decrease both the total number of lesions and the total duration of the illness, but the benefit is incremental. For this reason, and the inconvenience of taking the drug four times a day, it is not recommended for uncomplicated chickenpox except in certain circumstances, such as for treatment of chickenpox in adolescents, adults, or secondary household cases, all situations in which the primary infection might reasonably be expected to be severe. The dose is 80 mg/kg/day in 4 divided doses for 5 days.

In immunosuppressed patients, intravenous acyclovir is potentially lifesaving therapy for chickenpox, zoster, and herpes simplex virus infections. Treatment is mandatory for immunocompromised children and for patients thought to be immune competent but in whom varicella pneumonia develops. Most experts would also recommend therapy for varicella encephalitis, despite the fact that this condition is usually immune mediated and not typically caused by ongoing viral replication. The dose is 30 mg/kg/day in infants and 1,500 mg/m²/day in older children, given in three divided doses and administered over the course of an hour. Maintenance of good hydration is important to prevent the principal adverse event of acyclovir; namely, precipitation in the urinary tract and subsequent renal impairment. Once it has been decided that therapy is necessary, treatment is generally continued for a minimum of 7 days or until 24 hours after all lesions are crusted over.

Acyclovir has been used in normal adults with zoster, who often have painful disease. It is probably not necessary in normal children unless there is a complication, such as facial paralysis or ophthalmic zoster. Oral acyclovir may be useful for some children with zoster managed as outpatients. The dose is 600 mg/m² per dose five times a day for 7–10 days,[194] or 4000 mg/day in 5 divided doses for children over 12 years of age. However, all trials show benefit only if treatment is begun within 3 days of the onset of rash. In the immunocompromised host, intravenous acyclovir is indicated if zoster is severe, involves more than one dermatome or the trigeminal nerve, is disseminated, or is not responding to oral therapy.

Prevention

Varicella-Zoster Immune Globulin

Immunosuppressed children who have not had chickenpox and are exposed to the disease should be given varicella-zoster immune globulin (VZIG). They must be isolated if they are in a hospital, as they still may get chickenpox despite the VZIG and may transmit the disease to others. They should be placed in airborne precautions (negative pressure room) from 8 to 28 days after exposure. Newborn infants whose mothers have onset of chickenpox within 5 days before or 2 days after delivery should also be given VZIG, as discussed in Chapter 19. Premature infants born at or before 28 weeks gestation, or who weighed less than 1000 grams at birth, or hospitalized premature infants born at greater than 28 weeks gestation but whose mothers lack a reliable history of chickenpox, are also candidates for VZIG on exposure to VZV. Because of the stated predilection toward a more severe disease course, varicella-susceptible pregnant women should also be given VZIG when exposed. VZIG should be given as soon as possible after exposure and not more than 96 hours thereafter.

Varicella Vaccine

Live-attenuated varicella vaccine was licensed for use in the United States in 1995. It is recommended as part of the routine childhood immunization schedule and is required for day care attendance and kindergarten entry in many states. The vaccine works quite well, providing almost 100% protection against severe chickenpox and approximately 80–90% protection against any form of chickenpox.[195] Breakthrough infections that do occur are almost always much milder than unmodified chickenpox.

The vaccine has been very well tolerated; most reactions are local and mild. About one-fifth of recipients develop local redness and swelling. Approximately 5% develop skin lesions. These lesions may never develop a vesicular appearance. A very small percentage of vaccinees develop a more generalized vesicular rash after being vaccinated with varicella vaccine; counterintuitively, studies show that such rashes that occur within the first 2 weeks of vaccination are more likely to be caused by wild-type virus, whereas those that occur a month or later after vaccination are more likely to contain the Oka (vaccine) strain. Regardless, any child with vesicular lesions should be considered contagious until the vesicles crust. Transmission of vaccine virus from vaccinees to susceptibles has been documented but is uncommon.[196]

Several concerns about and objections to varicella vaccination have been widely discussed; some physicians are still not routinely recommending the vaccine because of them. For the most part, these objections stem from misunderstandings about vaccinology and virologic pathology. The most common objections and their fallacies follow:

Q. The immunity produced by the vaccine will probably wane, and chickenpox is a more severe disease in older persons. Aren't we just going to produce a nation full of susceptible adolescents and young adults? A. The earliest recipients in Japan got the vaccine over 20 years ago. To date, no waning of protection has been observed. There are several possible reasons for the durability of immunity. First, this is a pattern commonly seen when using other attenuated live-virus vaccines against viral diseases that include a systemic (viremic) component, such as measles, mumps, and rubella. Second, it has been well documented that people who are immune to varicella undergo boosting of their antibody titers when they are in contact with an active case of varicella, for example, mothers with prior immunity whose children develop chickenpox.[197] This implies that local replication in the nasopharynx (i.e., varicella *infection*) occurs, even though varicella *disease* does not. Vaccinees may periodically boost their immunity when they come in contact with the virus in the community. Third, there is a suggestion that asymptomatic endogenous reactivation of the Oka vaccine strain may occur in some vaccine recipients; this is most likely to occur in those who mounted borderline responses to the vaccine initially.[198] This endogenous reactivation serves the same purpose as a booster vaccination. The upshot of all this is that waning immunity is unlikely to be a significant problem. However, in the future it is certainly possible that, as with MMR vaccine, a second vaccination will be recommended to provide coverage for the 5–10% of the population who do not respond to the first vaccination.

Q. Is it really wise to immunize a healthy person with a live, replication-competent virus that establishes latency in the dorsal root of sensory ganglia? Do we want to give these well children a lifelong infection? A. On the face of it, this seems like a logical question. It would be a reasonable concern if it weren't for the fact that almost all these children are eventually going to have a virus of one type or another residing in their sensory ganglia. In other words, we have a choice of having the child's sensory ganglia occupied by an attenuated (weakened) virus, or by a wild-type (virulent) virus. There *is* no third choice. If you were a landlord and had an apartment to rent, would you rather rent it to a choirboy or to the leader of the local hell's angels motorcycle club? Data from clinical studies support the logic, as vaccine recipients have a lower incidence of zoster than do people who were infected with wild-type virus.[199]

Q. Why do we need to vaccinate against chickenpox at all? The disease is self-limited and benign. A. Although it is true that the disease is mild in the vast majority of children, it does have serious consequences to some. Prior to its licensure, varicella was responsible for 4 million cases, 11,000 hospitalizations, and 100 deaths each year in the United States.[182,200] The majority of deaths occurred in previously healthy persons. In areas with active surveillance, hospitalizations and deaths have decreased 80% since implementation of vaccination.[201] However, until vaccine coverage increases further, varicella will continue to be responsible for more U.S. deaths than any other vaccine-preventable illness. Given that an immunogenic, well-tolerated vaccine is available, the deaths, neurologic diseases, and severe secondary infections can and should be prevented.

■ BULLOUS RASHES

A bulla is a large vesicle, a centimeter or more in size. Bullae may occur as part of an acute infectious illness or as part of a chronic and recurrent skin disease.[202]

Possible Infectious Etiologies

Staphylococci

Bullous impetigo, which is typically caused by *S. aureus*, should be excluded by culture of the bullous fluid and is discussed further in Chapter 17.

Streptococci

Group A streptococci can cause a large vesicle, especially at the fingertips, where this infection can produce blistering distal dactylitis.[203]

Herpes Simplex Virus

This virus can produce bullae, especially in children with a malignancy or who are otherwise immunosuppressed.[204]

Congenital Syphilis

This is a rare cause of a vesicular or bullous rash in the newborn period but should be considered because it is essential to recognize and treat.

Chickenpox

The pustules of chickenpox are occasionally large and bullous, which should make the physician consider secondary infection with *S. aureus* or Group A streptococci.

Bacteremia

Bullous skin lesions may occur in association with bacteremia caused by almost any bacterium but are more frequently associated with gram-negative bacteremia, such as from *Pseudomonas*, *E. coli*, *Aeromonas*, *Vibrio vulnificus*, or *Yersinia*.

Skin Fungi

Occasionally, tinea lesions can take on a bullous appearance.[205] In such cases, fungi can be visualized on potassium hydroxide preparations or grown in culture of fluid obtained from bullous lesions.[206]

Noninfectious Etiologies

Chronic or Recurrent Bullous Diseases

Possible causes of this condition include chronic bullous dermatosis of childhood, bullous pemphigoid,[207] dermatitis herpetiformis, and epidermolysis bullosa.[202,208] Each of these conditions can be distinguished on the basis of direct and indirect immunofluorescence staining patterns. Chronic bullous dermatosis is caused by the linear deposition of IgA in the skin.[209] Hence, it is also called linear IgA bullous dermatosis of childhood. It is treated with immune modulating agents such as dapsone or sulfapyridine. Systemic steroids are reserved for severe or refractory cases. The prognosis is good; the disease usually remits after a few months to 3 years of activity.

Stevens-Johnson Syndrome

This condition is characterized by bullae formation and shallow ulcerations of mucosa of the mouth, conjunctivae, urethra, anus, or vagina. In Stevens-Johnson syndrome, one of the most constant features is erosion of the lips, often with thick hemorrhagic crusting. It is discussed in Chapter 2 and later in this chapter.

Pemphigoid Gestationis (Herpes Gestationis)

This is a rare bullous disease that typically first develops in early pregnancy, flares at the time of delivery, and subsides during the postpartum period.[210] It can also be seen in the babies born to mothers who suffer with this disorder.[211] Its importance is that it might be mistaken for HSV infection in a pregnant woman. The fact that the disease has been referred to as "herpes gestationis" only adds to the confusion.

Chemical Irritations

Contact-type diaper rash and poison ivy should be considered in the differential diagnosis of small bullous lesions.

Burns

Bullae may be the result of a second-degree burn. Child abuse with cigarette burns is occasionally manifested as isolated bullae.

Mucha-Habermann's Disease

This is a rare, chronic papulovesicular disease with few symptoms except for crops of papules that evolve into hemorrhagic or necrotic ulcers.[212] It may be improved by erythromycin. The initial presentation may resemble scabies or chickenpox. Rarely, patients may present with fever and ulceronecrotic lesions. This form of the disease can be severe and may require methotrexate therapy.[213]

"Bug Bites"

Spider or insect bites can cause vesicular or bullous lesions.

■ URTICARIAL-MULTIFORME-ANNULAR RASHES

Urticarial-multiforme-annular rashes resemble each other and may sometimes change from one category to another (Box 11-8).

Types

Urticaria

This term is a synonym for hives and is characterized by pale red, elevated, intradermal edematous plaques, often around joints. Biopsy of typical urticarial lesions reveals no evidence of vasculitis.[214]

Erythema Multiforme (EM)

This general descriptive diagnosis pertains to a group of rashes including circular macules, often

---

BOX 11-8 ■ Urticarial-Multiforme-Annular Rashes

Stevens-Johnson Syndrome
Drugs, especially sulfonamides (frequent)
M. pneumoniae (uncommon)
Herpes simplex, enteroviruses, or other viruses (rare)
Often unknown

Erythema Multiforme
Herpes simplex (frequent)
M. pneumoniae, enteroviruses, other viruses (occasional)
Any hypersensitivity
Juvenile rheumatoid arthritis

Annular Rashes
Erythema migrans (Lyme disease)
Erythema marginatum (rheumatic fever)
Erythema annulare centrifugum
Tinea
Creeping eruption (cutaneous larva migrans)
Larva currens (*Strongyloides* infection)
Neonatal lupus
Congenital Lyme disease
Annular erythema of infancy
Familial annular erythema
Urticarial bullous pemphigoid
Granuloma annulare
Erythema gyratum perstans

Urticaria
Any allergy: drugs, foods, infections (especially parasites and systemic fungi, hepatitis B, enteroviruses, group A streptococci), and hot or cold temperature

---

with target shapes with a 'bull's-eye.[215] Small papules, often with a dusky, bullous top or urticarial components, may be present. Bullae may develop. There is a recurrent oral form of erythema multiforme described in the section on stomatitis. EM is most commonly triggered by an infection, such as HSV.

Stevens-Johnson Syndrome (SJS)

Once thought to be simply a more severe form of EM, it is now clear that EM and SJS are distinct entities.[216] The clinical picture of SJS is one of much more severe, widely distributed macules and blisters, with involvement of the mucous membranes (eyes, nose, and/or mouth). It has a more severe course than EM and carries a mortality rate of around 15%. It is probably more closely related to toxic epidermal necrolysis than it is to EM. Most cases are due to adverse reactions to drugs. Of infectious causes, *M. pneumoniae* infection is probably the most common.

"Erythema multiforme-like rash" is a general descriptive diagnosis that is useful when a more accurate diagnosis is not certain. "Urticaria" or a "multiforme-like rash" may be as precise a diagnosis as the clinician can make in many cases. These rashes often are the presentation of systemic diseases such as an enteroviral infection or Kawasaki disease.

Erythema Migrans

This rash is usually the initial manifestation of Lyme disease and consists of circular or curved bands of a widening red macular rash, which occasionally has central clearing.[217] The disease is caused by a spirochete (*Borrelia burgdorferi*) transmitted by the bite of a tick (*Ixodes* spp) and most often occurs in the summer. The rash typically begins as a red macule at the site of the tick bite and expands outward with central clearing. It also can have an expanding triangular shape as a flat erythematous rash. Occasionally, there is a central pustule at the bite site that ulcerates and crusts.[217] At the time of the rash, most patients also will have fever and fatigue, and some will have arthralgia and headache. Multiple lesions occur as a result of hematogenous dissemination in about one-quarter of patients.[218]

This rash was thought to be pathognomonic for Lyme disease. However, a similar rash can be caused by a related, but distinct, pathogen known as *Borrelia lonestari*, which is carried by the Lone Star tick (*Amblyomma americanum*) in areas of the southeastern United States (where the presence of true Lyme disease has not been convincingly documented).[219] The rash develops around a tick bite, exactly identical to erythema migrans associated with *Borrelia burgdorferi* infection. The distinction is that *B. lonestari* does not cause any of the other, later symptoms associated with Lyme disease, such as arthritis, carditis, facial palsies, and encephalitis.

For treatment of childhood Lyme disease, amoxicillin is adequate when given for 2–3 weeks.[220] Doxycycline is preferred for children older than 8 years of age. For patients unable to take amoxicillin or doxycycline, cefuroxime axetil is recommended. Macrolide antibiotics are not recommended as first-line therapy of Lyme disease but may be used in the patient unable to take any of the three drugs mentioned earlier. Patients with arthritis or Bell's palsy are treated for 4 weeks. If neurologic involvement is present (aseptic meningitis or polyneuritis), intravenous ceftriaxone for 14 to 31 days is usually recommended.

Erythema Marginatum

This rash is rarely seen but is important to recognize because it is associated with acute rheumatic fever, almost exclusively with recurrences. It is a rapidly expanding erythematous macular rash, which typically develops a pale center as it enlarges. It is called "marginatum" because the margins are sometimes elevated. The flat form of this rash is also called erythema annulare.

Possible Etiologies

Herpes Simplex Virus

HSV is the most common cause of erythema multiforme. A history of clinically obvious antecedent herpes infection is not necessary; in one study, 8 (80%) of 10 children without preceding HSV infection had HSV DNA detected in lesional skin by PCR techniques.[221] Molecular study shows that the pathogenesis of HSV-associated erythema multiforme is different from that of cases that are induced by medications; lesional skin in HSV-associated cases is full of cells that express interferon-gamma, whereas tumor necrosis factor-alpha is found in drug-induced cases.[222] HSV can also cause recurrent attacks of SJS,[223] although most cases of SJS are due to drug reactions.

Other Viruses

Coxsackie or echovirus infections appear to be causes of urticaria.[224] Hepatitis B virus infection should always be considered, as urticaria and fever can precede jaundice; in such cases, aminotransferase elevation should be present.[225] Arthralgia may also be present, resulting in a serum sickness-like illness (see Chapter 13).[226] A case in which erythema multiforme developed 3 days prior to a classic chickenpox eruption has been described.[227]

Mycoplasma pneumoniae

Urticaria and erythema multiforme are sometimes seen in patients with *Mycoplasma* infection,[228] but the association between *Mycoplasma* and SJS appears to be the strongest.[229]

Giardiasis

Urticaria can be associated with giardiasis, although this is rare.[230]

Syphilis

The diagnosis of syphilis should be considered in adolescents or newborns with any puzzling rash. Secondary syphilis in the adolescent may be multiforme-like, papular, or papulo-squamous and may involve the palms and soles. In the newborn, congenital syphilis may be vesicular or bullous.

Collagen-Vascular Diseases

An erythema multiforme-like rash is often seen in patients with juvenile rheumatoid arthritis with an acute systemic onset (see chapter 10).[231] This rash is sometimes quite typical, with salmon-pink, large papules or nodules, and is then called erythema multiforme rheumatoides. However, these patients often have rashes that are not typical except for their brief duration.

Systemic lupus erythematosus is sometimes associated with urticaria and multiforme lesions (as well as papular, bullous, ulcerative, or nodular lesions). These lesions (erythema multiforme with bullae especially) have been called urticarial vasculitis.[232] Deposits of immunoglobulins, chronic hypocomplementemia, and circulating immune complexes are found.

At the onset, the rash of anaphylactoid purpura (Henoch-Schönlein purpura) often resembles an urticarial rash. It is discussed further in a preceding section of this chapter.

Bacterial Infections

Infection with Group A streptococcus is occasionally associated with acute urticaria.[233] Antibiotic therapy is usually discontinued because of concern for drug allergy, which may not be the cause of the urticaria.[233]

Bacterial Endotoxin

Intradermal injection of heat-killed gram-negative bacteria or their endotoxin can produce typical erythema multiforme, indicating that a variety of bacterial infections may be capable of producing erythema multiforme.[234] *Vibrio parahaemolyticus* septicemia, for example, has been reported with generalized erythema multiforme.

Allergy

Most urticarial rashes and some erythema multiforme-like rashes are probably caused by an allergic reaction, although most such rashes never have the etiology conclusively proven.[235] Penicillin is a common cause of hives. The rash due to ampicillin typically is maculopapular and resembles measles, but it can be urticarial. Cold temperature is also a cause.

Treatment

For urticaria, diphenhydramine has been the traditional therapy. Hydroxyzine is also currently used. If treatment is discontinued too soon, the frequency of recurrence is higher. Known precipitating causes, such as heat or cold, should be avoided if possible.[233] Subcutaneously administered epinephrine 1:1000, 0.01 mL/kg (maximum 0.3 mL) will result in rapid relief of severe urticaria. This is sometimes helpful diagnostically as well.

For SJS, one retrospective analysis suggested that IVIG may be helpful,[236] but its use is not routine. Corticosteroids are not advisable, as they not only do not increase the speed of recovery, but they increase the frequency of complications.

For erythema multiforme, a search for the underlying etiology may yield a potentially treatable cause, such as HSV infection. Most cases self-resolve.

■ ITCHING BITE-LIKE RASHES

Insect Bites

The typical bite-like rash is a papule that itches intensely, often with surrounding erythema or urticaria. Often, the top is scratched off and becomes crusted and may resemble a pox-like rash. Such rashes are occasionally confused with chickenpox, which is the most frequent itching pox-like rash. This type of itching papule occurs with mosquito, spider, chigger, kissing bug, or flea bites; scabies; and schistosomal cercarial infestation (swimmer's itch).

Infections

Scabies

Human scabies is caused by infestation with *Sarcoptes scabiei*. These mites burrow under the skin and produce intense itching, which is the hallmark of scabies.[237] The itching is caused by sensitization to the mite which takes 2–4 weeks after primary infection and a much shorter period after reinfestation. Visible burrows are present in less than 25% of affected infants.[238] Typically, the fingerwebs and the abdomen have the most characteristic lesions. Blisters, ruptured bullae, and excoriation may make the diagnosis more difficult. Scabies complicating atopic dermatitis can be more severe and extensive. Rarely, the source of scabies is contact with an animal (such as a dog) that has extensive sarcoptic mange. The papules occur in areas that have come in contact with the animal.

Hyperkeratotic crusted scabies of the hands and feet, called Norwegian scabies, is usually seen only in patients with immune suppression.[239] This form of the infestation sometimes leads to large outbreaks because (1) it is often not recognized and properly diagnosed in a timely fashion, (2) it usually does not itch, which also hampers diagnosis, (3) the lesions contain large numbers of mites, and (4) it is more difficult to eradicate. The mite can be seen under the microscope in a scraping from a burrow. A burrow can be well seen by applying a small amount of ink, which flows readily into the burrow.[240]

Permethrin 5% cream is the topical drug of choice for scabies. It is applied to the entire body (including head, scalp, and neck in infants and young children) and washed off 8–14 hours later. Some experts recommend repeat application in 7 days to kill any newly hatched mites. Lindane 1%

lotion (gamma benzene hexachloride) (Kwell; Gammene) is an alternate treatment that is applied in a similar manner. It is effective but can be toxic, as it is absorbed. It should generally be avoided in infants, preschoolers, and pregnant or nursing women. Precipitated 5% sulfur in petrolatum and crotamiton 10% have considerably lower cure rates.[241]

A single dose of 150–200 micrograms/kg of oral ivermectin is usually curative[242] except in Norwegian scabies, where multiple doses are sometimes required.[243] Ivermectin, along with strict isolation and infection control procedures, has been used for recalcitrant cases in outbreak settings.[239,244] In Colombia, 12 adults and 20 children were treated topically with a 1% ivermectin in propylene glycol solution at a dose of 400 micrograms/kg, repeated once the following week. No side effects were observed, and all patients were cured.[245] The drug has not been approved by the FDA for this indication, and questions remain about its safety profile.

The rash of scabies is largely due to a hypersensitivity response to the mites; therefore, even after the mites are all dead, some of the symptoms may persist for a few weeks. Children who have been treated with an effective scabicide should be allowed to return to school or day care despite persistence of symptoms. Sometimes topical steroids or oral antihistamines are helpful for controlling itching in this resolution stage.

The patient's clothing, towels, and bedding should be washed in hot water to prevent reinfestation or transmission to another person. Alternatively, they can be placed in a sealed plastic bag for 3 days.

Molluscum Contagiosum

This condition is caused by infection with the molluscipox virus. It is manifested by 1- to 2-mm flesh-colored to white or yellowish nodules, often umbilicated, which can be scratched or curetted out, leaving a shallow ulcer. When the top has been scratched off, the lesions may resemble those of scabies. Uncommonly, the lesions may be surrounded by a small to moderate-sized halo of eczema-like erythema.[246] Treatment with curettage, light, or a blistering agent is helpful but not essential, as the disease abates over a period of several months to 3 years.[247] We are aware of one unfortunate child whose early varicella lesions were confused for molluscum contagiosum. The physician

described the curetting procedure to the mother, who mistakenly attempted to curette the lesions as they appeared. The child ended up in the intensive care unit with extensive staphylococcal cellulitis and sepsis.

Chronic molluscum is a common problem in children with HIV infection and AIDS (Chapter 20).

Schistosomal Cercariae

Swimmers in U.S. lakes and oceans can get intensely itching papules caused by the larval state (cercariae) of wild duck schistosomes. In vitro, cercariae activate the release of histamine from rat peritoneal mast cells, even without direct physical attachment of the cercariae to the mast cells.[248] The release of histamine may be part of the pathogenesis of the pruritus associated with the condition. Antihistamines and lotions may help relieve the itching, which can last 2 weeks. Prevention is difficult but is facilitated by limiting the time spent in the water and by toweling off thoroughly as soon as possible after exiting the water.

Other Causes

Infantile pustular acrodermatitis is also intensely pruritic and is described in a previous section on chickenpox-like rashes. Papular urticaria is a result of hypersensitivity to insect bites, with intensely itching urticarial papules.

■ MISCELLANEOUS RASHES

Roseola Syndrome (Exanthem Subitum)

This syndrome typically occurs in an infant 6 months to 2 years of age and is one of the most common rash illnesses of young childhood. It is manifested by high fever, often to 105°F, for 2–5 days, sometimes with irritability, but the child does not appear "toxic" or seriously ill. When the rash abates, a pink macular to maculopapular rash appears. The rash consists of discrete lesions rather than large areas of confluence. The difficulty posed by this illness is that during the febrile period, there are no specific signs or symptoms that suggest the diagnosis to the clinician. Palpebral edema ("droopy eyelids") sometimes can be noted on the first or second day of the fever.[249] Erythema of the tympanic membranes, without frank otitis media, is frequently found. Otherwise, the physical examination is usually normal. The physician may suspect the diagnosis of roseola on the basis of the lack of toxicity and lack of convincing physical evidence of another diagnosis and advise observation without antibiotic therapy. Of course, the parents and physicians must continue to watch for signs of illness other than fever (i.e., a change in consciousness, difficulty breathing, or any area of pain or tenderness) because the diagnosis of roseola cannot be made with certainty until the rash appears.

The most common cause of roseola is human herpesvirus type 6 (HHV-6). Roseola caused by HHV-6 does not have a seasonal occurrence pattern, and does not usually occur in outbreaks. HHV-6 is ubiquitous, and infection with HHV-6 is common; most infections do not lead to the clinical features of roseola. In one study, HHV-6 was sought in 243 consecutive children who presented to an emergency room with a nonspecific febrile illness; 34 of these (14%) had evidence of HHV-6 infection. Children viremic with HHV-6 tended to be highly febrile and irritable, but had few other physical findings. Only 3 (approximately 10%) went on to develop roseola (that is, rash that appeared at the time of defervescence).[250] Seroprevalence is somewhat variable, but in all studies it is common. It is generally high at birth (secondary to the presence of maternal antibody), declines during the first 6 months, and then increases between 6 and 24 months of life, which corresponds to the peak age of clinical roseola.[251–253]

In children with roseola secondary to HHV-6 infection, viremia is common in the first 3 days of illness;[254] the titer of viremia correlates with the severity of symptoms.[255] Virus can be found by PCR in the saliva and stool intermittently both during and after the acute phase of the illness. HHV-7 is a less-frequent cause of roseola. Roseola-like illness caused by respiratory isolates of coxsackie A23 virus or echovirus 16 can occur in epidemics and tends to occur during the summer months.[256]

The most common complication of roseola is a febrile seizure. This is not surprising, given that the virus causes high fevers, and infection occurs most commonly in children of the age most likely to experience seizures with fever. A case-control study compared the incidence of HHV-6 infection in children with febrile seizures versus those with high fever but no seizures and found that HHV-6 was implicated in about 45% of illness in both groups.[257] This study suggests that the reason children get febrile seizures with HHV-6 infection is because of high fever, rather than because of some special neurotropism of the virus or neuropathology caused by the virus. However, one study showed that patients with febrile seizures in association with acute HHV-6 infection are more likely to have complicated (i.e., focal, prolonged, or recurrent) febrile seizures than are matched controls with febrile seizures but no HHV-6 infection.[258] Additionally, occasional cases of encephalitis have been reported; in some, evidence of virus replication within the CNS was found.[259,260] Other uncommon complications include thrombocytopenia, elevation of liver enzymes, and inappropriate secretion of antidiuretic hormone.[261,262]

Papulosquamous Rashes

Papulosquamous rashes are characterized by red or pink papules and a scaling surface. In children, the most common rash of this kind is pityriasis rosea.[263] Occasionally, parapsoriasis and guttate psoriasis occur in older children or teenagers[263] or even in infants[264] but are uncommon in children compared with pityriasis rosea. Tinea corporis and tinea versicolor are possible causes of a papulosquamous rash and are discussed in Chapter 17.

Pityriasis rosea produces a papulosquamous rash, particularly on the trunk. The rash may have a "Christmas tree" distribution on the back, because the rash follows a symmetric diagonal pattern slanting downward from the spine along the ribs. It is preceded for a few days by a herald patch, a larger (2–10 cm) patch, usually on the trunk.

This condition is common in children and tends to last from 4–12 weeks. The onset may be mistaken for a viral exanthem, but the characteristic scaling or squamous feature of the rash makes the physician recognize that it belongs in the category of papulosquamous rashes. Occasionally, oral lesions occur on the tongue, lip, or palate.[265] The oral lesions tend to improve at about the same time as the rash.

Outbreaks of pityriasis rosea have occurred. This has been reported in terms of approximately 100 cases over a period of 2 years in a small area in England. The etiology is unknown. Although some believe that HHV-7 is the cause, evidence of infection with this virus is found no more frequently in patients with pityriasis rosea than in controls.[266] No treatment is necessary.

Papular Rashes

Papular acrodermatitis of childhood (Gianotti-Crosti syndrome) was first recognized as a complication of hepatitis B virus infection and was described in 1955 as erythematous flat papules occurring primarily on the cheeks, arms, and legs, often associated with mild hepatitis, arthritis or arthralgia, and generalized lymphadenopathy. The usual age is approximately 1–4 years.[267]

Other causes of papular acrodermatitis include infection with Epstein-Barr virus,[268] cytomegalovirus,[269] coxsackieviruses, and parainfluenza viruses.[270] Additional findings include fever, periorbital edema, and generalized lymphadenopathy. The hepatitis may not be associated with any jaundice.[271]

Outbreaks have been observed in Japan, Italy, and the United States. In some cases, the condition may be related to an antigen–antibody reaction, with the antigen being the surface antigen of hepatitis B (HBsAg).

Other Rashes

Pseudomonas Folliculitis

Exposure to heated swimming pools or hot tubs is the typical predisposing factor in *Pseudomonas aeruginosa* folliculitis.[272] The rash may be papular or pustular and is variably pruritic. It tends to be worst in the areas covered by the swimsuit. No antibiotic therapy is needed.

Leptospirosis

This infection is occasionally associated with sparse generalized macular or papular rash.[273] Sometimes the rash is predominately over the skin of the lower legs in a form of leptospirosis called pretibial fever.

Pustulosis Palmaris et Plantaris

This rash occurs in all age groups, including children under the age of 10, although the peak frequency is in adults aged 30–60. The disease is characterized by a chronic recurring disorder of the palms and soles that appears pustular and may contain deep-seated eczematous vesicles.[274]

Rose Spots

This descriptive diagnosis can be made when there are rosetted macules 1–4 mm in diameter. The classic cause of rose spots is typhoid fever,[275] in which the spots characteristically occur on the trunk during the period of fever and blanch on pressure. Rose spots are reported in 5%–30% of patients with typhoid fever.[276]

They may appear in crops but usually are not numerous (6–12 spots),[275] and they are very difficult to detect in dark-skinned patients. A few diseases other than typhoid, such as shigellosis, can produce this rash.[277] Hemangioma-like lesions associated with echovirus infections bear some resemblance to rose spots because they are sparse and blanch on pressure.[278]

Sarcoidosis

Sarcoidosis is a rare cause of a chronic nonpruritic maculopapular or follicular skin rash in children.[279] Arthritis and uveitis are typical accompanying features.[280,281]

Secondary Syphilis

The rash of secondary syphilis can be papulosquamous, papular, or macular. It can occur on the palms and soles and is sometimes associated with lymphadenopathy.[282] Pruritus, headaches, myalgias, fever, and loss of scalp hair may also occur.

Hypersensitivity Rashes

Hypersensitivity to an antibiotic (e.g., ampicillin) often produces a rash at a time the patient is receiving the drug for another febrile illness. The rash is generally diffuse and maculopapular, with small bumps. Sometimes the combination of a respiratory viral illness (which does not require treatment with antibiotics) and the administration of an antibiotic seems to conspire to produce a rash. These rashes do not necessarily imply that the child is allergic to the antibiotic, nor do they necessarily predict a recurrence of rash at a subsequent exposure to the same drug. Skin testing for IgE-mediated hypersensitivity is usually negative.

■ RASHES IN NEWBORNS

Pustule-like Rashes

Erythema Toxicum Neonatorum

The name of this rash is a misnomer, because the word *toxicum* seems to imply that the disease is serious. Rather, this is a benign, self-limited papular rash occurring in approximately 50% of newborns during the first few days of life, sometimes appearing at birth and possibly present as late as the 10th day of life.[283] The rash often appears macular at first but generally is papular and sometimes pustular. The appearance of the pustules should alert the examiner who is unsure to do a simple Gram stain or Wright stain of a broken pustule. If the condition is erythema toxicum neonatorum, eosinophils will be seen, with few neutrophils and no gram-positive cocci, as would be present in a staphylococcal pustule. The cause is unknown. No treatment is necessary.

Infectious Pustules

The most common cause of ordinary pustules in a newborn, particularly after a day or two of life, is *S. aureus*.[283] The bacteria can be seen on Gram stain of the pustule and are readily cultured. Characteristically, staphylococcal pustules appear in areas of irritation, particularly in the inguinal area, especially in boys. Hemorrhagic pustules that are scattered and generalized may represent septic emboli in a sick baby and should be Gram stained. If septic pustules are suspected, immediate intravenous antibiotic therapy for septicemia is indicated (see Chapter 10).

Herpes Simplex Virus

These pustules are characteristically surrounded by an area of erythema and appear in groups of two to six or more confluent vesicles that quickly evolve into pustules. Gram staining of grouped HSV pustules may reveal some neutrophils but rarely reveals any organisms. A histologic examination with Giemsa staining may reveal characteristic multinucleated giant cells. HSV grouped pustules appear particularly in areas that may have been traumatized, such as where scalp electrodes have been placed. A history of HSV in the mother is not necessarily found, as most babies with disseminated HSV are born to mothers who are unaware of having had genital herpes. The virus is readily cultured out of the base of a lanced pustule or vesicle, usually requiring only a day or two to produce its characteristic cytopathic effect in cell culture. In our experience, even pustules that look like they are full of purulent fluid are essentially dry when opened with a lancet. Tzanck smears are both insensitive and nonspecific and should never be a substitute for viral culture. Rapid testing with direct fluorescent antibodies or with PCR is available in many centers; both tests are sensitive and specific. If the diagnosis

is suspected, treatment with acyclovir should not await laboratory confirmation (Chapter 19).

Candida albicans

Pustules may occur in congenital candidiasis or in an acquired candidal infection that may appear after birth (about 2 weeks) when the baby has acquired infection during vaginal delivery.[283]

Transient Neonatal Pustular Melanosis

This disease is characterized by hyperpigmented macules and pustules in a newborn infant. Typically, there is a collarette of scale surrounding the pigmented macules. The frequency in black babies is estimated to be approximately 4% and that in other babies about 1%.[284] Examination of these pustular-like lesions rarely shows any eosinophils but does show a moderate number of neutrophils. In most cases, the pustules are present at birth. They usually last about 24–48 hours, but the hyperpigmented macules may take a number of weeks to fade completely.

Acropustulosis of Infancy

Described in the section on chickenpox-like rashes, this pustular disease of the extremities occasionally occurs in the newborn period.[283]

Neonatal Scabies

In newborns, scabies tends to form pustules early in the course and consistently involves the face, neck, axilla, scalp, palms, and soles.[285] Laboratory confirmation and treatment of scabies are described under bite-like rashes.

Bullous Rashes

Staphylococcal Scalded Skin Syndrome

Staphylococcal scalded skin syndrome (SSSS) occurs as a bullous disease, usually of the newborn, and is caused by infection with an epidermolytic toxin-producing strain of *S. aureus*. The disease usually begins with a diffuse erythroderma, but then progresses to bullae formation. The bullae may be small and localized, or they may cover almost the entire body surface area (see Fig. 17-3). The bullae tend to rupture easily and leave a tender, erythematous base that dries quickly. Nikolsky's sign (i.e., easy sloughing of superficial layers of skin with slight finger pressure) is usually present. The formation of bullae is mediated by the toxin, which is usually released systemically from a distant, often inconsequential local infection such as an infected skin abrasion or conjunctivitis. Therefore, cultures of the lesional fluid or the base of the lesions are usually sterile (or they may be positive because of bacteria colonizing adjacent skin). The disease was originally described by Ritter and so is occasionally called Ritter's disease.

Cultures of the blood and the bullae should be obtained. Some experts recommend also culturing the nasopharynx, because the antibiotic susceptibility pattern of a staphylococcal isolate obtained from any site might be helpful in guiding antibiotic choice.[286] If a patient outside the neonatal period presents with a localized exfoliative rash and is otherwise well, and the rash is consistent with SSSS, cultures may be obtained, and oral anti-staphylococcal antibiotics begun, with close follow-up. If the patient is a neonate, appears systemically ill, or has diffuse skin involvement, hospitalization for intravenous antibiotics is warranted. There is no literature to guide the duration of therapy, which is considered on a case-by-case basis but is usually 7–14 days.

Bullous Impetigo

Bullous impetigo is essentially a localized form of SSSS, the pathophysiologic difference being that the condition is caused by a localized infection of the superficial skin. The bullae, however, are caused by locally produced and locally acting epidermolytic toxin. In contrast to classic SSSS, described earlier, cultures of the lesions of bullous impetigo will almost always yield the pathogen. There is a report in the literature of a family outbreak of staphylococcal disease in which the first patient had SSSS, and subsequent family members developed bullous impetigo with the same bacterium.[287]

Epidermolysis Bullosa

Epidermolysis bullosa describes a group of genetic disorders characterized by blistering after minor trauma. Sometimes, a newborn infant presents with no family history of the blistering disorder.[283,288]

Chronic Bullous Dermatosis of Childhood

This disease, also called linear IgA bullous dermatosis, resembles or is the same as transient bullous dermolysis of the newborn.[283,289] It is characterized by multiple blisters or bullae and is occasionally confused with neonatal HSV infection. It can be distinguished from more severe congenital bullous diseases by immunofluorescence staining of a skin biopsy.

Localized Epidermolysis Bullosa (Bart Syndrome)

This autosomal dominant disorder has a favorable prognosis but may resemble a bullous infection.[290] Nail deformities and bullae on the medial surfaces of the upper legs, where the thighs can rub together, may be present.

Congenital Bullous Urticaria Pigmentosa

This is a rare disease associated with bullae and hyperpigmented macules seen shortly after delivery.[291] There is a positive Darier sign, meaning that after the skin has been lightly scratched, there will be hyperemia and a wheal.

Urticarial Papules and Plaques

The occurrence of urticarial papules and plaques in pregnancy is a rare disorder that has also been observed in the newborn infant.[292] The lesions in the mother are pruritic, papular, vesicular, or urticarial plaques that typically involve the trunk and proximal limbs in the third trimester. The lesions in the newborn are multiple red papules that blanch on pressure.[292]

Incontinentia Pigmenti

The vesicular rash from incontinentia pigmenti in the newborn can be mistaken for the vesicles of herpes simplex, and biopsy and viral culture are usually indicated.[293] After the vesicles resolve, the patient is left with a darkly pigmented, swirling rash.

Tinea

Superficial fungal infections can occur in the newborn period and are discussed in Chapters 17 and 19.

Neonatal Lupus Erythematosus

Newborn infants of mothers with lupus erythematosus (LE) can develop sharply marginated erythematous plaques with a fine scale, telangiectasia, or atrophic lesions, usually beginning within the first 3 months of life but occasionally occurring during the newborn period.[294] The LE preparation is often positive, and there may be leukopenia. The infant may be photosensitive and may develop a first-degree heart block later in infancy. Ro (SSA) antibody is typically found in the baby, representing transplacental passage of antibody. No treatment is needed.

Cellulitis and Fasciitis

Necrotizing Fasciitis

Circumcision can be a predisposing factor for necrotizing fasciitis.[295] When the scrotum is involved, necrotizing fasciitis is also called Fournier's disease,[296] described in Chapter 17. An infant whose Plastibell circumcision ended up diverting his urinary stream into a potential space in the abdomen, producing a condition that mimicked necrotizing fasciitis, has been described.[297]

Streptococcal Cellulitis

Either Group A or Group B streptococci can cause neonatal cellulitis.[298] Group B cellulitis in the newborn typically involves the head, face, and neck.[298]

■ REFERENCES

1. Gilchrest B, Baden HP. Photodistribution of viral exanthems. Pediatrics 1974;54:136–8.
2. Knoll H, Sramek J, Vrbova K, et al. Scarlet fever and types of erythrogenic toxins produced by the infecting streptococcal stains. Zentralbl Bakteriol 1991;276: 94–106.
3. Ohga S, Okada K, Mitsui K, et al. Outbreaks of group A beta-hemolytic streptococcal pharyngitis in children: correlation of serotype T4 with scarlet fever. Scand J Infect Dis 1992;24:599–605.
4. Fishbein WN. Jaundice as an early manifestation of scarlet fever. Ann Intern Med 1962;57:60–72.
5. Pacifico L, Renzi AM, Chiesa C. Acute guttate psoriasis after streptococcal scarlet fever. Pediatr Dermatol 1993; 10:388–9.
6. Feldman CA. Staphylococcal scarlet fever. N Engl J Med 1963;267:877–8.
7. Jarraud S, Cozon G, Vandenesch F, et al. Involvement of enterotoxins G and I in staphylococcal toxic shock syndrome and staphylococcal scarlet fever. J Clin Microbiol 1999;37:2446–9.
8. Miller RA, Brancato F, Holmes KK. *Corynebacterium haemolyticum* as a cause of pharyngitis and scarlatiniform rash in young adults. Ann Intern Med 1986;105:867–72.
9. Banek G, Nyman M. Tonsillitis and rash associated with *Corynebacterium haemolyticum*. J Infect Dis 1986;154: 1037–40.
10. Hall CB, Horner FA. Encephalopathy with erythema infectiosum. Am J Dis Child 1977;131:65–7.
11. Shimizu Y, Ueno T, Komatsu H, et al. Acute cerebellar ataxia with human parvovirus B19 infection. Arch Dis Child 1999;80:72–3.
12. Minohara Y, Koitabashi Y, Kato T, et al. A case of Guillain-Barré syndrome associated with parvovirus B19 infection. J Infect 1998;36:327–8.
13. Yoto Y, Kudoh T, Haseyama K, et al. Human parvovirus B19 infection associated with acute hepatitis. Lancet 1996;347:868–9.
14. Langnas AN, Markin RS, Cattral MS, Naides SJ. Parvovirus B19 as a possible causative agent of fulminant liver failure and associated aplastic anemia. Hepatology 1995; 22:1661–5.
15. Jacobson SK, Daly JS, Thorne GM, McIntosh K. Chronic parvovirus B19 infection resulting in chronic fatigue syndrome: case history and review. Clin Infect Dis 1997;24: 1048–51.
16. Ker CB. Scarlet fever, measles, and German measles: is there a fourth disease? Practitioner 1902;68:139–56.
17. Morens DM, Katz AR. The "fourth disease" of childhood: reevaluation of a nonexistent disease. Am J Epidemiol 1991;134:628–40.
18. Plummer FA, Hammond GW, Forward K, et al. An erythema infectiosum-like illness caused by human parvovirus infection. N Engl J Med 1985;313:74–9.
19. Joseph PR. Incubation period of fifth disease. Lancet 1986;2:1390–1.
20. Chorba T, Coccia P, Holman RC, et al. The role of parvovirus B19 in aplastic crisis and erythema infectiosum (fifth disease). J Infect Dis 1986;154:383–93.
21. Reid DM, Reid TMS, Brown T, et al. Human parvovirus-associated arthritis: a clinical and laboratory description. Lancet 1985;1:422–5.
21a. Liefeldt L, Buhl M, Schweickert B, et al. Eradication of parvovirus B19 infection after renal transplantation requires reduction of immunosuppression and high-dose immunoglobulin therapy. Nephrol Dial Transplant 2002; 17:1840–2.
21b. Fattet S, Cassinotti P, Popovic MB. Persistent human parvovirus B19 infection in children under maintenance chemotherapy for acute lymphocytic leukemia. J Pediatr Hematol Oncol 2004;26:497–503.
22. Kurtzman GJ, Ozawa K, Cohen B, et al. Chronic bone marrow failure due to persistent B19 parvovirus infection. N Engl J Med 1987;317:287–94.
23. Hasle H, Kerndrup G, Jacobsen BB, et al. Chronic parvovirus infection mimicking myelodysplastic syndrome in a child with subclinical immunodeficiency. Am J Pediatr Hematol Oncol 1994;16:329–33.
24. Yaegashi N, Okamura K, Tsunoda A, et al. A study by means of a new assay of the relationship between an outbreak of erythema infectiosum and non-immune hydrops fetalis caused by human parvovirus B19. J Infect 1995; 31:195–200.
25. Gratacos E, Torres PJ, Vidal J, et al. The incidence of human parvovirus B19 infection during pregnancy and its impact on perinatal outcome. J Infect Dis 1995;171: 1360–3.
26. Valeur-Jensen AK, Pedersen CB, Westergaard T, et al.

Risk factors for parvovirus B19 infection in pregnancy. JAMA 1999;281:1099–105.

27. Koch WC, Harger JH, Barnstein B, Adler SP. Serologic and virologic evidence for frequent intrauterine transmission of human parvovirus B19 with a primary maternal infection during pregnancy. Pediatr Infect Dis J 1998;17:489–94.

28. Mandel F, Folkman J, Matsumoto S. Erythromelalgia. Pediatrics 1977;59:45–58..

29. Spoerke DG, Temple AR. Dermatitis after exposure to a garden plant (*Euphorbia myrsinites*). Am J Dis Child 1979;133:28–9.

30. Kawasaki T, Kosaki F, Okawa S, et al. A new infantile acute febrile mucocutaneous lymph node syndrome (MLNS) prevailing in Japan. Pediatrics 1974;54:271–6.

31. Yanagawa H, Nakamura Y, Yashiro M, et al. Results of the nationwide epidemiologic survey of Kawasaki disease in 1995 and 1996 in Japan. Pediatrics 1998;102:e65.

32. Bronstein DE, Dille AN, Austin JP, et al. Relationship of climate, ethnicity and socioeconomic status to Kawasaki disease in San Diego County, 1994 through 1998. Pediatr Infect Dis J 2000;19:1087–91.

33. Fujiwara M, Matsubara T, Furukawa S. Is Kawasaki disease frequent in the children of parents engaged in medical work? Pediatr Infect Dis J 2000;19:769–70.

34. Hall M, Hoyt L, Ferrieri P, et al. Kawasaki syndrome-like illness associated with infection caused by enterotoxin B-secreting *Staphylococcus aureus*. Clin Infect Dis 1999;29:586–9.

35. Wann ER, Fehringer AP, Ezepchuk YV, et al. *Staphylococcus aureus* isolates from patients with Kawasaki disease express high levels of protein A. Infect Immun 1999;67:4737–43.

36. Ezepchuk YV, Fehringer AP, Harbeck R, et al. *Staphylococcus aureus* isolated from Kawasaki disease patients hyper-releases extracellular protein A. Mol Gen Mikrobiol Virusol 1999;2:29–34.

37. Morita A, Imada Y, Igarashi H, Yutsudo T. Serologic evidence that streptococcal superantigens are not involved in the pathogenesis of Kawasaki disease. Microbiol Immunol 1997;41:895–900.

38. Hamamuchi Y, Ichida F, Yu X, et al. Neutrophils and mononuclear cells express vascular endothelial growth factor in acute Kawasaki disease: its possible role in progression of coronary artery lesions. Pediatri Res 2001;49:74–80.

39. Asano T, Ogawa S. Expression of monocyte chemoattractant protein-1 in Kawasaki disease: the anti-inflammatory effect of gamma globulin therapy. Scand J Immunol 2000;51:98–103.

40. Takeshita S, Nakatani K, Tsujimoto H, et al. Increased levels of circulating soluble CD14 in Kawasaki disease. Clin Exp Immunol 2000;119:376–81.

41. Schiller B, Elinder G. Inflammatory parameters and soluble cell adhesion molecules in Swedish children with Kawasaki disease: relationship to cardiac lesions and intravenous immunoglobulin treatment. Acta Pediatr 1999;88:844–8.

42. Kamizono S, Yamada A, Higuchi T, Kato H, Itoh K. Analysis of tumor necrosis factor-alpha production and polymorphisms of the tumor necrosis factor-alpha gene in individuals with a history of Kawasaki disease. Pediatr Int 1999;41:341–5.

43. Cunningham MW, Meissner HC, Heuser JS, et al. Anti-human cardiac myosin autoantibodies in Kawasaki syndrome. J Immunol 1999;163:1060–5.

44. Morens DM, Anderson LJ, Hurwitz ES. National surveillance of Kawasaki disease. Pediatrics 1980;65:21–5.

45. Tizard EJ, Suzuki A, Levin M, Dillon MJ. Clinical aspects of 100 patients with Kawasaki disease. Arch Dis Child 1991;66:185–8.

46. Crankson S, Nazer H, Jacobsson B. Acute hydrops of the gallbladder in childhood. Eur J Pediatr 1992;151:318–20.

47. Burke MJ, Rennebohm RM. Eye involvement in Kawasaki disease. J Pediatr Ophthalmol Strabismus 1981;18:7–11.

48. Dengler LD, Capparelli EV, Bastian JF, et al. Cerebrospinal fluid profile in patients with acute Kawasaki disease. Pediatr Infect Dis J 1998;17:478–81.

49. Ravi KV, Brooks JR. Peritonsillar abscess—an unusual presentation of Kawasaki disease. J Laryngol Otol 1997;111:73–4.

50. Kuniyuki S, Asada M. An ulcerated lesion at the BCG vaccination site during the course of Kawasaki disease. J Am Acad Dermatol 1997;37:303–4.

51. Bitter JJ, Friedman SA, Paltzils RL, et al. Kawasaki's disease appearing as erythema multiforme. Arch Dermatol 1979;115:71–72.

52. Bergeson PS, Schoenike SL. Mucocutaneous lymph node syndrome: a case masquerading as Rocky Mountain spotted fever. JAMA 1977;237:2299–302.

53. Wong ML, Kaplan S, Dunkle LM, et al. Leptospirosis: a childhood disease. J Pediatr 1977;90:532–7.

54. Goldsmith RW, Gribetz D, Strauss L. Mucocutaneous lymph node syndrome (MLNS) in the continental United States. Pediatrics 1976;57:431–5.

55. Ferriero DM, Wolfsdorf JI. Hemolytic uremic syndrome associated with Kawasaki disease. Pediatrics 1981;68:405–6.

56. Germain BF, Moroney JD, Guggino GS, et al. Anterior uveitis in Kawasaki disease. J Pediatr 1980;97:780–1.

57. Koutras A. Myositis with Kawasaki's disease. Am J Dis Child 1982;136:78–9.

58. Bradley MK, Crowder TH. Retropharyngeal mass in a child with mucocutaneous lymph node syndrome. Clin Pediatr 1983;22:444–5.

59. Stoler J, Biller JA, Grand RJ. Pancreatitis in Kawasaki disease. Am J Dis Child 1987;141:306–8.

60. Fujiwara H, Hamashima Y. Pathology of the heart in Kawasaki disease. Pediatrics 1978;61:100–7.

61. Dajani AS, Taubert KA, Takahashi M, et al. Guidelines for long-term management of patients with Kawasaki disease. Report from the Committee on Rheumatic Fever, Endocarditis, and Kawasaki Disease, Council on Cardiovascular Disease in the Young, American Heart Association. Circulation 1994;89:916–22.

62. Dajani AS, Taubert KA, Gerber MA, et al. Diagnosis and therapy of Kawasaki disease in children. Circulation 1993;87:1776–80.

63. Bushara K, Wilson A, Rust RS. Facial palsy in Kawasaki syndrome. Pediatr Neurol 1997;17:362–4.

64. Boyce TG, Spearman P. Acute aseptic meningitis second-

ary to intravenous immunoglobulin in a patient with Kawasaki syndrome. Pediatr Infect Dis J 1998;17:1054–6.

64a. Miura M, Katada Y, Ishihara J. Time interval of measles vaccination in patients with Kawasaki disease treated with additional intravenous immune globulin. Eur J Pediatr 2004;163:25–9.

65. Terai M, Shulman ST. Prevalence of coronary artery abnormalities in Kawasaki disease is highly dependent on gamma globulin dose but independent of salicylate dose. J Pediatr 1997;131:888–93.

66. Marasini M, Pongiglone G, Gassolo D, Campelli A, Ribaldone D, Caponnetto S. Late intravenous gamma globulin treatment in infants and children with Kawasaki disease and coronary artery abnormalities. Am J Cardiol 1991;68:796–7.

67. Curtis A. Kawasaki disease. Br Med J 1997;315:322–3.

68. Bierman FZ, Gersony WM. Kawasaki disease: clinical perspective. J Pediatr 1987;111:789–93.

69. Wright DA, Newburger JW, Baker A, Sundel RP. Treatment of immune globulin-resistant Kawasaki disease with pulsed doses of corticosteroids. J Pediatr 1996;128:146–9.

70. Mains C, Wiggins J, Groves B, et al. Surgical therapy for a complication of Kawasaki's disease. Ann Thorac Surg 1983;35:197–200.

71. American Heart Association Subcommittee of Cardiovascular Sequelae, Subcommittee of Surgical Treatment, Kawasaki Research Committee. Guidelines for treatment and management of cardiovascular sequelae in Kawasaki disease. Heart Vessels 1987;3:50–4.

71a. Newberger JW, Takahashi M, Burns JC, et al. The treatment of Kawasaki syndrome with intravenous gamma globulin. N Engl J Med 1986;315:341–7.

71b. Newberger JW, Takahashi M, Beiser AS, et al. A single intravenous infusion of gamma globulin as compared with four infusions in the treatment of acute Kawasaki syndrome. N Engl J Med 1991;324:1633–9.

72. Fukunishi M, Kikkawa M, Hamana K, et al. Prediction of non-responsiveness to intravenous high-dose gamma-globulin therapy in patients with Kawasaki disease at onset. J Pediatr 2000;137:172–6.

73. Yanagawa H, Nakamura Y, Sakata K, Yashiro M. Use of intravenous gamma-globulin for Kawasaki disease: effects on cardiac sequelae. Pediatr Cardiol 1997;18:19–23.

74. Stockheim JA, Innocentini N, Shulman ST. Kawasaki disease in older children and adolescents. J Pediatr 2000;137:250–2.

75. Nakamura Y, Oki I, Tanihara S, et al. Cardiac sequelae in recurrent cases of Kawasaki disease: a comparison between the initial episode of the disease and a recurrence in the same patients. Pediatrics 1998;102:e66.

76. Burns JC, Capparelli EV, Brown JA, et al. Intravenous gamma-globulin treatment and retreatment in Kawasaki disease. Pediatr Infect Dis J 1998;17:1144–8.

77. Kato H, Sugimura T, Akagi T, et al. Long-term consequences of Kawasaki disease: a 10- to 21-year follow-up study of 594 patients. Circulation 1996;94:1379–85.

78. Witt MT, Minich LL, Bohnsack JF, Young PC. Kawasaki disease: more patients are being diagnosed who do not meet American Heart Association criteria. Pediatrics 1999;104:e10.

79. Rowley AH, Gonzalez-Crussi F, Gidding SS, et al. Incom-

plete Kawasaki disease with coronary artery involvement. J Pediatr 1987;110:409–13.

80. Rowley AH. Incomplete (atypical) Kawasaki disease. Pediatr Infect Dis J 2002;21:563–5.

81. World Health Report 2000. Health systems: improving performance. Geneva: WHO, 2000.

82. Vitek CR, Aduddell M, Brinton MJ, et al. Increased protection during a measles outbreak of children previously vaccinated with a second dose of measles-mumps-rubella vaccine. Pediatr Infect Dis J 1999;18:620–3.

83. Paunio M, Hedman K, Davidkin I, et al. Secondary measles vaccine failures identified by measurement of IgG avidity: high occurrence among teenagers vaccinated at a young age. Epidemiol Infect 2000;124:263–71.

84. Centers for Disease Control and Prevention. Epidemiology of Measles—United States, 2001–2003. MMWR 2004;53:713–6.

85. Welliver RC, Cherry JD, Holtzman AE. Typical, modified, and atypical measles: an emerging problem in the adolescent and adult. Arch Intern Med 1977;137:39–41.

86. Spirer Z, Shalit I. Problem of nonclassical measles in the immunization era and the terminology of the various forms of measles [letter]. Pediatr Infect Dis 1986;5:276–7.

87. Gururangan S, Stevens RF, Morris DJ. Ribavirin response in measles pneumonia. J Infect 1990;20:219–21.

88. Stogner SW, King JW, Black-Payne C, Bocchini J. Ribavirin and intravenous immune globulin therapy for measles pneumonia in HIV infection. South Med J 1993;86:1415–8.

89. Shigeta S, Mori S, Baba M, et al. Antiviral activities of ribavirin, 5-ethynyl-1-beta-D-ribofuranosylimidazole-4-carboxamide, and 6'-(R)-6'-C-methylneplanocin A against several ortho- and paramyxoviruses. Antimicrob Agents Chemother 1992;36:435–9.

90. Wyde PR, Moore-Poveda DK, DeClercq E, et al. Use of cotton rats to evaluate the efficacy of antivirals in treatment of measles virus infections. Antimicrob Agents Chemother 2000;44:1146–52.

91. Butler JC, Havens PL, Sowell AL, et al. Measles severity and serum retinol (vitamin A) concentration among children in the United States. Pediatrics 1993;91:1176–81.

92. Hussey GD, Klein M. Routine high-dose vitamin A therapy for children hospitalized with measles. J Trop Pediatr 1993;39:342–5.

93. Weidinger G, Czub S, Neumeister C, et al. Role of CD4(+) and CD8(+) T cells in the prevention of measles virus-induced encephalitis in mice. J Gen Virol 2000;81:2707–13.

94. Gazzola P, Cocito L, Capello E, et al. Subacute measles encephalitis in a young man immunosuppressed for ankylosing spondylitis. Neurology 1999;52:1074–7.

95. Vargas PA, Bernardi FD, Alves VA, et al. Uncommon histopathologic findings in fatal measles infection: pancreatitis, sialoadenitis and thyroiditis. Histopathology 2000;37:141–6..

96. American Academy of Pediatrics Tuberculosis In: Pickering LK, ed. Red Book: 2003 Report of the Committee on Infectious Diseases, 26th ed. Elk Grove Village, IL: American Academy of Pediatrics, 2003:642–60.

97. Zilber N, Kahana E. Environmental risk factors for sub-

acute sclerosing panencephalitis (SSPE). Acta Neurol Scand 1998;98:49–54.

98. Caruso JM, Robbin-Tien D, Brown WD, Antony JH, Gascon GG. Atypical chorioretinitis as an early presentation of subacute sclerosing panencephalitis. J Pediatr Ophthalmol Strabismus 2000;37:119–22.

99. Tandon R, Khanna S, Sharma MC, Seshadri S, Menon V. Subacute sclerosing panencephalitis presenting as optic neuritis. Indian J Ophthalmol 1999;47:250–2.

100. Gross PA, Portnoy B, Mathies AW Jr, et al. A rubella outbreak among adolescent boys. Am J Dis Child 1970; 119:326–31.

101. Finklea JF, Sandifer SH, Moore GT, Jr. Epidemic rubella at The Citadel. Am J Epidemiol 1968;87:367–72.

102. Schaffner W, Schluederberg AES, Byrne EB. Clinical epidemiology of sporadic measles in a highly immunized population. N Engl J Med 1968;279:783–9.

103. Kibrick S. Rubella and rubelliform rash. Bacteriol Rev 1964;28:452–7.

104. Forbes JA. Rubella: historical aspects. Am J Dis Child 1969;118:5–11.

105. Brody JA, Sever JL, McAlister R, et al. Rubella epidemic on St. Paul Island in the Pribilofs, 1963. I: epidemiologic, clinical, and serologic findings. JAMA 1965;191:619–23.

106. Wilkins J, Leedom JM, Salvatore MA, et al. Clinical rubella with arthritis resulting from reinfection. Ann Intern Med 1972;77:930–2.

107. Schlossberg D, Topolosky MK. Military rubella. JAMA 1977;238:1273–4.

108. Sherman FE, Michaels RH, Kenny FM. Acute encephalopathy (encephalitis) complicating rubella. JAMA 1965; 192:675–81.

109. Naveh Y, Friedman A. Rubella encephalitis successfully treated with corticosteroids. Clin Pediatr 1975;14:286–7.

110. Cherry JD, Lerner AM, Klein JO, et al. Coxsackie B5 infections with exanthems. Pediatrics 1963;31:455–62.

111. Lerner AM, Klein JO, Cherry JD, et al. New viral exanthems. N Engl J Med 1963;269:678–85 and 736–40.

112. Lepow ML, Carver DH, Robbins RC. Clinical and epidemiologic observations on enterovirus infection in a circumscribed community during an epidemic of ECHO 9 infection. Pediatrics 1960;26:12–26.

113. Neva FA, Feemster RF, Borbach IJ. Clinical and epidemiologic features of an unusual epidemic exanthem. JAMA 1954;155:544–8.

114. Hall CB, Cherry JD, Halch MH, et al. The return of Boston exanthem: echovirus 16 infections in 1974. Am J Dis Child 1977;131:323–6.

115. Berkovich S, Kibrick S. Exanthem associated with respiratory syncytial virus infection. J Pediatr 1964;65:368–70.

116. Baker RC, Seguin JH, Leslie N, Gilchrist MJ, Myers MG. Fever and petechiae in children. Pediatrics 1989;84: 1051–5.

117. Mandl KD, Stack AM, Fleisher GR. Incidence of bacteremia in infants and children with fever and petechiae. J Pediatr 1997;131:398–404.

118. Allen DM, Diamond LK, Howell DA. Anaphylactoid purpura in children (Schönlein-Henoch syndrome). Am J Dis Child 1960;99:833–54.

119. Casteelsvan Daele M, DeGaetano G. Purpura and acetylsalicylic acid therapy. Acta Paediatr Scand 1971;60: 203–8.

120. Toews WH, Bass JW. Skin manifestations of meningococcal infection: an immediate indicator of prognosis. Am J Dis Child 1974;127:173–6.

121. Nguyen QV, Nguyen EA, Weiner LB. Incidence of invasive bacterial disease in children with fever and petechiae. Pediatrics 1984;74:77–80.

122. Strong WB. Petechiae and streptococcal pharyngitis. Am J Dis Child 1969;117:156–60.

123. Haynes RE, Sanders DY, Cramblett HG. Rocky Mountain spotted fever in children. J Pediatr 1970;76:685–93.

124. Dalton MJ, Clarke MJ, Holdman RC, et al. National surveillance for Rocky Mountain spotted fever, 1981–1992: epidemiologic summary and evaluation of risk factors for fatal outcome. Am J Trop Med Hyg 1995;52:405–13.

125. Kirkland KB, Wilkinson WE, Sexton DJ. Therapeutic delay and mortality in cases of Rocky Mountain spotted fever. Clin Infect Dis 1995;20:1118–21.

126. Procop GW, Burchette JL Jr, Howell DN, Sexton DJ. Immunoperoxidase and immunofluorescent staining of *Rickettsia rickettsii* in skin biopsies: a comparative study. Arch Pathol Lab Med 1997;121:894–9.

127. Lochary ME, Lockhart PB, Williams WT Jr. Doxycycline and staining of permanent teeth. Pediatr Infect Dis J 1998; 17:429–31.

128. Walker DH, Montenegro MR, Hegarty BC, Tringali GR. Rocky Mountain spotted fever vaccine: a regional need. South Med J 1984;77:447–9.

129. Dumler S, Wisseman CL Jr, Fiset P, Clements ML. Cell-mediated immune responses of adults to vaccination, challenge with *Rickettsia rickettsii*, or both. Am J Trop Med Hyg 1992;46:105–15.

130. Jacobs RF, Schutze GE. Ehrlichiosis in children. J Pediatr 1997;131:184–92.

131. Plaut ME. Staphylococcal septicemia and pustular purpura. Arch Dermatol 1969;99:82–5.

132. Dorff GJ, Geimer NF, Rosenthal DR, et al. Pseudomonas septicemia: illustrated evolution of its skin lesion. Arch Intern Med 1971;128:591–5.

133. Holmes KK, Counts GW, Beatty HN. Disseminated gonococcal infection. Ann Intern Med 1971;74:979–93.

134. Sahler OJZ, Wilfert CM. Fever and petechiae with adenovirus type 7 infection. Pediatrics 1974;53:233–5.

135. Centers for Disease Control and Prevention. Murine typhus-Hawaii, 2002. MMWR 2003;52:1224–6.

136. Porto MH, Noel GJ, Edelson PJ. Resistance to serum bactericidal activity distinguishes Brazilian purpuric fever (BPF) case strains of *Haemophilus influenzae* biogroup *aegyptius* (*H. aegyptius*) from non-BPF strains. J Clin Microbiol 1989;27:792–4.

137. Tai DY, Chee YC, Chan KW. The natural history of dengue illness based on a study of hospitalised patients in Singapore. Singapore Med J 1999;40:238–42.

138. Sahud MA, Bachelor MM. Cytomegalovirus-induced thrombocytopenia: an unusual case report. Arch Intern Med 1978;138:1573–7.

139. Ozsoylu S, Kanra G, Savas G. Thrombocytopenia purpura related to rubella infection. Pediatrics 1978;62:567–9.

140. Ramilo AC, Jackson MR, Wise RD, et al. *Mycoplasma* infection simulating acute meningococcemia. Arch Dermatol 1983;119:786–8.

140a. Harel L, Strqussberg I, Zeharia A, Praiss D, Amir J. Papular purpuric rash due to parvovirus B19 with distribution on the distal extremities and the face. Clin Infect Dis 2002;15:1558–61.

140b. Hsieh MY, Huang PH. The juvenile variant of Papular-purpuric gloves and socks syndrome and its association with viral infections. Br J Dermatol 2004;151:201–6.

141. Scully RE, Mark EJ, McNealey BU. Case records of the Massachusetts General Hospital: Litterer-Siwe disease. N Engl J Med 1985;313:874–83.

142. Kaplan BS, Esseltine D. Thrombocytopenia in patients with acute poststreptococcal glomerulonephritis. J Pediatr 1978;93:974–6.

143. Fauci AS, Haynes BF, Katz P. The spectrum of vasculitis. Ann Intern Med 1978;89:660–6.

144. Lesgold Belman A, Leicher CR, Moshe SL, et al. Neurologic manifestations of Schönlein-Henoch syndrome purpura: report of three cases and review of the literature. Pediatrics 1985;75:687–92.

145. Meadow SR, Scott DG. Berger disease: Henoch-Schönlein syndrome without the rash. J Pediatr 1985;106:27–32.

146. Sanchez NP, Van Hale HM, Su WPD. Clinical and histopathologic spectrum of necrotizing vasculitis. Arch Dermatol 1985;121:220–4.

147. Mackel SE. Treatment of vasculitis. Med Clin North Am 1982;66:941–54.

148. Rosenberg H. Rash resembling anaphylactoid purpura as meningococcemia. Can Med Assoc J 1981;125:179–80.

149. Sandler A, Snedeker JD. Cytomegalovirus infection in an infant presenting with cutaneous vasculitis. Pediatr Infect Dis J 1987;6:422–3.

150. Bayever E, Rosove MH, Lenarsky C. Nonthrombocytopenic purpura with eosinophilia. J Pediatr 1984;105:277–8.

151. Hazen PG, Kark EC, Davis BR, et al. Acute febrile neutrophilic dermatosis in children. Arch Dermatol 1983;119:998–1002.

152. Nelson DG, Leake J, Bradley J, Kupperman N. Evaluation of febrile children with petechial rashes: is there consensus among pediatricians? Pediatr Infect Dis J 1998;17:1135–40.

152a. Brogan PA, Raffles A. The management of fever and petechiae: making sense of rash decisions. Arch Dis Child 2000;83:506–7.

153. Woodward TE. Rocky Mountain spotted fever: epidemiological and early clinical signs are keys to treatment and reduced mortality. J Infect Dis 1984;150:465–8.

154. Saslaw S, Prior JA. Varicella bullosa. JAMA 1960;173:1214–7.

155. Feldman S, Hughes WT, Daniel CB. Varicella in children with cancer: seventy-seven cases. Pediatrics 1975;56:388–97.

156. Guess HA, Broughton DD, Melton LJ 3rd, Kurland LT. Epidemiology of herpes zoster in children and adolescents: a population-based study. Pediatrics 1985;76:512–7.

157. Brunnell PA, Miller LH, Lovejoy F. Zoster in children. Am J Dis Child 1968;115:432–7.

158. Meade RH III, Chang TW. Zoster-like eruption due to echovirus 6. Am J Dis Child 1979:133:283–4.

159. Stern H, Elek SD, Millar DM, et al. Herpetic whitlow: a form of cross-infection in hospitals. Lancet 1959;2:871–4.

160. Selling B, Kibrick S. An outbreak of herpes simplex among wrestlers (herpes gladiatorum). N Engl J Med 1964;270:979–82.

161. Nishimura K, Nagamoto A, Igarashi M. Extensive skin manifestations of herpesvirus infection in an acute leukemia child. Pediatrics 1972;49:294–7.

162. Cherry JD, Jahn CL. Hand, foot, and mouth syndrome: report of six cases due to Coxsackie virus, Group A, Type 16. Pediatrics 1966;37:637–43.

163. Tindall JP, Callaway JL. Hand, foot, and mouth disease: it's more common than you think. Am J Dis Child 1972;124:372–5.

164. LeCleach L, Benchikhi H, Liedman D, et al. Hand-foot-mouth syndrome recurring during common variable deficiency [French]. Ann Dermatol Venereol 1999;126:251–3.

165. Baker DA, Phillips CA. Fatal hand-foot-and-mouth disease in an adult caused by coxsackievirus A7. JAMA 1979;242:1065.

166. Sequeira W, Jones E, Bronson DM. *Mycoplasma pneumoniae* infection with arthritis and a varicella-like eruption. JAMA 1981;246:1936–7.

167. Henderson DA, Inglesby TV, Bartlett JG, et al. Smallpox as a biological weapon: medical and public health management. JAMA 1999;281:2127–37.

168. Breman JG, Henderson DA. Diagnosis and management of smallpox. N Engl J Med 2002;346:1300–8.

169. Baltimore RS, McMillan JA. Smallpox and the smallpox vaccine controversy. Pediatr Infect Dis J 2002;21:789–90.

169a. Reed KD, Melski JW, Graham MB. The detection of monkeypox in humans in the Western Hemisphere. NEJM 2004;350:342–50.

170. Fenske NA, Gern JE, Pierce D, et al. Vesiculopustular eruption of ulcerative colitis. Arch Dermatol 1983;119:664–9.

171. Lucky AW, McGuire JS. Infantile acropustulosis with eosinophilic pustules. J Pediatr 1982;100:428–9.

172. Hayden GF, Quackenbush K. Infantile acropustulosis: a "new" vesiculopustular eruption of infants and children. J Fam Pract 1984;18:925–32.

173. Findlay RF, Odom RB. Infantile acropustulosis. Am J Dis Child 1983;137:455–7.

174. Mancini AJ, Frieden IJ, Paller AS. Infantile acropustulosis revisited: history of scabies and response to topical corticosteroids. Pediatr Dermatol 1998;15:337–41.

175. Hervonen K, Karell K, Holopainen P, Collin P, Partanen J, Reunala T. Concordance of dermatitis herpetiformis and celiac disease in monozygous twins. J Invest Dermatol 2000;115:990–3.

176. Soter NA. Dermatitis herpetiformis [editorial]. N Engl J Med 1973;288:1020–1.

177. Eichenfield LF, Honig P. Blistering disorders of childhood. Pediatr Clin North Am 1991;38:959–76.

178. Magro C, Crowson AN, Kovatich A, Burns F. Pityriasis lichenoides: a clonal T-cell lymphoproliferative disorder. Human Pathol 2002;33:788–95.

179. Smith EWP, Garson A Jr, Boyleston JA, et al. Varicella gangrenosa due to Group A beta-hemolytic streptococcus. Pediatrics 1976;57:306–10.

180. Wilson GJ, Talkington DF, Gruber W, Edwards K, Dermody TS. Group A streptococcal necrotizing fasciitis fol-

lowing varicella in children: case reports and review. Clin Infect Dis 1995;20:1333–8.

181. Wagner HJ, Seidel A, Grande-Nagel I, Kruse K, Sperner J. Pre-eruptive varicella encephalitis: case report and review of the literature. Eur J Pediatr1998;157:814–5.

182. Galil K, Brown C, Lin F, Seward J. Hospitalizations for varicella in the United States, 1988 to 1999. Pediatr Infect Dis J 2002;21:931–5.

183. Yuki T, Nakajima Y, Tanaka T, et al. A case of acute hepatitis (severe type) due to varicella-zoster virus with DIC [Japanese]. Nippon Shokakubyo Gakkai Zasshi 1998;95:33–6.

184. Chen MK, Wang CC, Lu JJ, Perng CL, Chu ML. Varicella arthritis diagnosed by polymerase chain reaction. J Formos Med Assoc 1999;98:519–21.

185. Dwivedi S, Suresh K. Unusual complications of varicella infection: myocarditis, incessant ventricular tachycardia and transverse myelitis. J Assoc Physicians India 1998; 46:831.

186. McCarthy JT, Amer J. Postvaricella acute transverse myelitis: a case presentation and review of the literature. Pediatrics 1978;62:202–4.

187. Singer J. Postvaricella suppurative meningitis: case reports and review of the literature. Am J Dis Child 1979; 133:934–5.

188. Priest JR, Urick JJ, Groth KE, et al. Varicella arthritis documented by isolation of virus from joint fluid. J Pediatr 1978;93:990–2.

189. Maitland K. Temporal association of chickenpox and meningococcal disease in children: a report of three cases [letter]. Acta Paediatr 2000;89:744–5.

190. Saulsbury FT. Remission of juvenile rheumatoid arthritis with varicella infection. J Rheumatol 1999;26:1606–8.

191. Kuijpers TW, Tjia KL, de Jager F, Peters M, Lam J. A boy with chickenpox whose fingers peeled. Lancet 1998;351: 1782.

192. Ogboli MI, Parslew R, Verbov J, Smyth R. Kawasaki disease associated with varicella: a rare association. Br J Dermatol 1999;141:1145–6.

193. Filloux F. Toxic encephalopathy caused by topically applied diphenhydramine. J Pediatr 1986;108:1018–20.

194. Novelli VM, Marshall WC, Yeo J, et al. High-dose oral acyclovir for children at risk of disseminated herpesvirus infections. J Infect Dis 1985;151:372.

195. Gershon AA. Live-attenuated varicella vaccine. Infect Dis Clin North Am 2001;15:65–81.

196. Sharrar RG, LaRussa P, Galea SA, et al. The postmarketing safety profile of varicella vaccine. Vaccine 2000;19: 916–23.

197. Arvin AM, Koropchak CM, Wittek AE. Immunologic evidence of reinfection with varicella zoster virus. J Infect Dis 1983;148:200–5.

198. Krause PR, Klinman DM. Varicella vaccination: evidence for frequent reactivation of the vaccine strain in healthy children. Nat Med 2000;6:451–4.

199. Hardy I, Gershon AA, Steinberg SP, LaRussa P. The incidence of zoster after immunization with line attenuated varicella vaccine: a study in children with leukemia. N Engl J Med 1991;325:1545–50.

200. Meyer PA, Seward JF, Jumaan AO, Wharton M. Varicella mortality: trends before vaccine licensure in the United States, 1970–1994. J Infect Dis 2000;182:383–90.

201. Centers for Disease Control and Prevention. Varicella-related deaths—United States, 2002. MMWR 2003;52: 545–7.

202. Ramsdell W, Jarratt M, Fuerst J, et al. Bullous disease of childhood. Am J Dis Child 1979;133:791–4.

203. Hays GC, Mullard JE. Blistering distal dactylitis: a clinically recognizable streptococcal infection. Pediatrics 1975;56:129–31.

204. Lopygan L, Young AW Jr, Menyus M. Generalized acute herpes simplex type 2 with fatal outcome. Arch Dermatol 1977;113:816–8.

205. Terragni L, Marelli MA, Oriani A, Cecca E. Tinea corporis bullosa. Mycoses 1993;36:135–7.

206. Yeraldi S, Scarabelli G, Oriani A, Vigo GP. Tinea corporis bullosa anularis. Dermatology 1996;192:349–50.

207. Gould WM, Zlotnick DA. Bullous pemphigoid in infancy: a case report. Pediatrics 1977;59:942–5.

208. Hertz KC, Katz WI, Aaronson C. Juvenile dermatitis herpetiformis: an immunological proven case. Pediatrics 1977;59:945–8.

209. Kanitakis J, Mauduit G, Cozzani E, et al. Linear IgA bullous dermatosis of childhood with autoantibodies to a 230 kDa epidermal antigen. Pediatr Dermatol 1994;11: 139–44.

210. Fine JD, Omura EF. Herpes gestationis: persistent disease activity 11 years postpartum. Arch Dermatol 1985;121: 924–6.

211. Chen SH, Chopra K, Evans TY, et al. Herpes gestationis in a mother and child. J Am Acad Dermatol 1999;40: 847–9.

212. Shavin JS, Jones TM, Aton JK. Mucha-Habermann's disease in children: treatment with erythromycin. Arch Dermatol 1978;114:1679–80.

213. Suarez J, Lopez B, Villalba R, Perera A. Febrile ulceronecrotic Mucha-Habermann disease: a case report and review of the literature. Dermatology 1996;192:277–9.

214. Synkowski DR, Levine MI, Rabin BS, Yunis EJ. Urticaria: an immunofluorescence and histopathology study. Arch Dermatol 1979;115:1192–4.

215. Edmond BJ, Huff JC, Weston WL. Erythema multiforme. Pediatr Clin North Am 1983;30:631–40.

216. Roujeau JC, Stern RS. Severe adverse cutaneous reactions to drugs. N Engl J Med 1994;331:1272–85.

217. Berger BW. Erythema chronicum migrans of Lyme disease. Arch Dermatol 1984;120:1017–21.

218. Gerber MA, Shapiro ED, Burke GS, et al. Lyme disease in children in southeastern Connecticut. N Engl J Med 1996;335:1270–4.

219. Kirkland KB, Klimko TB, Meriwether RA, et al. Erythema migrans-like rash at a camp in North Carolina: a new tick-borne disease? Arch Intern Med 1998;158:2162–5.

220. Wormser GP, Nadelman RB, Dattwyler RJ, et al. Practice guidelines for the treatment of Lyme disease. Clin Infect Dis 2000;31:1–14.

221. Weston WL, Brice SL, Jester JD, et al. Herpes simplex virus in childhood erythema multiforme. Pediatrics 1992; 89:32–4.

222. Kokuba H, Aurelian L, Burnett J. Herpes simplex virus associated erythema multiforme (HAEM) is mechanistically distinct from drug-induced erythema multiforme: interferon-gamma is expressed in HAEM lesions and

tumor necrosis factor-alpha in drug-induced erythema multiforme lesions. J Invest Dermatol 1999;113:808–15.

223. Major PP, Morisset R, Kurstak C. Isolation of herpes simplex virus type 1 from lesions of erythema multiforme. Can Med Assoc J 1978;118:821–2.

224. Forman ML, Cherry JD. Exanthems associated with uncommon viral syndromes. Pediatrics 1968;41:873–82.

225. Dienstag JL, Rhodes AR, Bhan AK, et al. Urticaria associated with acute viral hepatitis B. Ann Intern Med 1978; 89:34–40.

226. Segool RA, Lejtenyi C, Taussig LM. Articular and cutaneous prodromal manifestations of viral hepatitis. J Pediatr 1975;87:709–12.

227. Prais D, Grisuru-Soen G, Barzilai A, Amir J. Varicella zoster virus infection associated with erythema multiforme in children. Infection 2001;29:37–9.

228. Villiger RM, von Vigier RO, Ramelli GP, Hassink RI, Bianchetti MG. Precipitants in 42 cases of erythema multiforme. Eur J Pediatr 1999;158:929–32.

229. Tay YK, Huff JC, Weston WL. *Mycoplasma pneumoniae* infection is associated with Stevens-Johnson syndrome, not erythema multiforme (von Hebra). J Amer Acad Dermatol 1996;35:757–60.

230. Hamrick HJ, Moore GW. Giardiasis causing urticaria in a child. Am J Dis Child 1983;137:761–3.

231. Calabro JJ, Marchesano JM. Rash associated with juvenile rheumatoid arthritis. J Pediatr 1968;72:611–9.

232. Gammon WR, Wheeler CE Jr. Urticarial vasculitis: case report and a review of the literature. Arch Dermatol 1979; 115:76–80.

233. Schuller DE, Elvey SM. Acute urticaria associated with streptococcal infection. Pediatrics 1980;65:592–6.

234. Shelley WB. Bacterial endotoxin (lipopolysaccharide) as a cause of erythema multiforme. JAMA 1980;243:58–60.

235. Biachine JR, Macaraeg PV Jr, Lasagna L, et al. Drugs as etiologic factors in the Stevens-Johnson syndrome. Am J Med 1968;44:390–405.

236. Morici MV, Galen WK, Shetty AK, et al. Intravenous immunoglobulin therapy for children with Stevens-Johnson syndrome. J Rheumatol 2000;27:2494–7.

237. Orkin M, Maibach HI. Scabies in children. Pediatr Clin North Am 1978;25:371–85.

238. Ginsburg CM. Scabies. Pediatr Infect Dis 1984;3:133–4.

239. Obasanjo OO, Wu P, Conlon N, et al. An outbreak of scabies in a teaching hospital: lessons learned. Infect Control Hosp Epidemiol 2001:22:13–8.

240. Woodley D, Sauret JH. The burrow ink test and the scabies mite. J Am Acad Dermatol 1981;4:715–22.

241. Taplin D, Meinking TL, Chen JA, Sanchez R. Comparison of crotamiton 10% cream (Eurax) and permethrin 5% cream (Elimite) for the treatment of scabies in children. Pediatr Dermatol 1990;7:67–73.

242. Nnoruka EN, Agu CE. Successful treatment of scabies with oral ivermectin in Nigeria. Trop Doct 2001;31: 15–8.

243. Cestari SC, Petri V, Rotta O, Alchorne MM. Oral treatment of crusted scabies with ivermectin: report of two cases. Pediatr Dermatol 2000;17:410–4.

244. Leppard B, Naburi AE. The use of ivermectin in controlling an outbreak of scabies in a prison. Br J Dermatol 2000;143:520–3.

245. Victoria J, Trujillo R. Topical ivermectin: a new successful treatment for scabies. Pediatr Dermatol 2001;18:63–5.

246. Rockoff AS. Molluscum dermatitis. J Pediatr 1978;92: 945–7.

247. Weston WL, Lane AT. Should molluscum be treated [letter]? Pediatrics 1980;65:865.

248. Catto BA, Lewis FA, Ottesen EA. Cercaria-induced histamine release: a factor in the pathogenesis of schistosome dermatitis? Am J Trop Med Hyg. 1980;29:886–9.

249. Berliner BC. A physical sign useful in diagnosis of roseola infantum before rash. Pediatrics 1960;25:1034.

250. Pruksananonda P, Hall CB, Insel RA, et al. Primary human herpesvirus 6 infection in young children. N Engl J Med 1992;327:1099–100.

251. Kositanont U, Wasi C, Ekpatcha N, et al. Seroprevalence of human herpesvirus 6 and 7 infections in the Thai population. Asian Pacific J Allergy Immunol 1995;13:151–7.

252. Ward KN, Gray JJ, Fotheringham MW, Sheldon MJ. IgG antibodies to human herpesvirus-6 in young children: changes in avidity of antibody correlate with time after infection. J Med Virol 1993;39:131–8.

253. Hall CB, Long CE, Schnabel KC, et al. Human herpesvirus-6 infection in children: a prospective study of complications and reactivation. N Engl J Med 1994;331:432–8.

254. Asano Y, Yoshikawa T, Suga S, et al. Viremia and neutralizing antibody response in infants with exanthem subitum. J Pediatr 1989;114:535–9.

255. Asano Y, Nakashima T, Yoshikawa T, Suga S, Yazaki T. Severity of human herpesvirus-6 viremia and clinical findings in infants with exanthem subitum. J Pediatr 1991;118:891–5.

256. Takos MJ, Weil M, Sigel MM. Outbreak of ECHO 9 exanthemata traced to a children's party. Am J Dis Child 1960; 100:360–4.

257. Hukin J, Farrell K, MacWilliam LM, et al. Case-control study of primary human herpesvirus 6 infection in children with febrile seizures. Pediatrics 1998;101:e3.

258. Suga S, Suzuki K, Ihira M, et al. Clinical characteristics of febrile convulsions during primary HHV-6 infection. Arch Dis Child 2000;82:62–6.

259. Yoshikawa T, Nakashima T, Suga S, et al. Human herpesvirus-6 DNA in cerebrospinal fluid of a child with exanthem subitum and meningoencephalitis. Pediatrics 1992; 89:888–90.

260. McCullers JA, Lakeman FD, Whitley RJ. Human herpesvirus 6 is associated with focal encephalitis. Clin Infect Dis 1995;21:571–6.

261. Yoshikawa T, Morooka M, Suga S. Five cases of thrombocytopenia induced by primary human herpesvirus 6 infection. Acta Paediatr Jpn 1998;40:278–81.

262. Okafuji T, Uchiyama H, Okabe N, Akatsuka J, Maekawa K. Syndrome of inappropriate secretion of antidiuretic hormone associated with exanthem subitum. Pediatr Infect Dis J 1997;16:532–3.

263. Watson W, Farber EM. Psoriasis in childhood. Pediatr Clin North Am 1971;18:875–95.

264. Farber EM, Jacobs AH. Infantile psoriasis. Am J Dis Child 1977;131:1266–9.

265. Kay MH, Rapini RP, Fritz KA. Oral lesions in pityriasis rosea. Arch Dermatol 1985;121:1449–51.

266. Kosuge H, Tanaka-Taya K, Miyoshi H, et al. Epidemio-

logic study of human herpesvirus-6 and human herpesvirus-7 in pityriasis rosea. Br J Dermatol 2000;143:795–8.

267. San Joaquin VH, Ward KE, Marks MI. Gianotti disease in a child and acute hepatitis B in mother. JAMA 1981; 246:2191–2.

268. Iosub S, Santos C, Gromisch DS. Papular acrodermatitis with Epstein-Barr virus infection. Clin Pediatr 1984;23: 33–4.

269. Berant M, Naveh Y, Weissman I. Papular acrodermatitis with cytomegalovirus hepatitis. Arch Dis Child 1983;58: 1024–5.

270. Spear KL, Winkelmann RK. Gianotti-Crosti syndrome: a review of ten cases not associated with hepatitis B. Arch Dermatol 1984;120:891–6.

271. Konno M, Klkuta H, Ishikawa N, et al. A possible association between hepatitis B antigen-negative infantile papular acrodermatitis and Epstein-Barr virus infection. J Pédiatr 1982;101:222–4.

272. Sausker WF, Aeling JL, Fitzpatrick JE, et al. *Pseudomonas* folliculitis acquired from a health spa whirlpool. JAMA 1978;239:2362–5.

273. Peter G. Leptospirosis: a zoonosis of protean manifestations. Pediatr Infect Dis 1982;1:282–8.

274. Nehara M. Pustulosis palmaris et plantaris: a review of clinical features and aggravating factors. Acta Otolaryngol 1983;(Supp)1401:7–11.

275. Litwack KD, Hoke AW, Borchardt KA. Rose spots in typhoid fever. Arch Dermatol 1972;105:252–5.

276. Parry CM, Hien TT, Dougan G, White NJ, Farrar JJ. Typhoid fever. N Engl J Med 2002; 347:1770–82.

277. Goscienski PJ, Haltalin KC. Rose spots associated with shigellosis. Am J Dis Child 1970;119:152–4.

278. Cherry JD, Bobinski JE, Horvath FL, et al. Acute hemangioma-like lesions associated with ECHO viral infections. Pediatrics 1969;44:498–502.

279. Waldman DJ, Stiehm ER. Cutaneous sarcoidosis of children. J Pediatr 1977;91:271–3.

280. Lindsley CB, Petty RE. Overview and report on international registry of sarcoid arthritis in childhood. Curr Rheumatol Rep 2000;2:343–8.

281. Shetty AK, Gedalia A. Sarcoidosis: a pediatric perspective. Clin Pediatr 1998;37:707–17.

282. Chapel TA. The signs and symptoms of secondary syphilis. Sex Transm Dis 1980;7:161–4.

283. Schachner L, Press S. Vesicular, bullous and pustular disorders in infancy and childhood. Pediatr Clin North Am 1982;30:609–29.

284. Ramamurthy RS, Reveri M, Esterly NB, et al. Transient neonatal pustular melanosis. J Pediatr 1976;88:831–5.

285. Burns BR, Lampe RM, Hansen GH. Neonatal scabies. Am J Dis Child 1979;133:1031–4.

286. Ladhani S, Joannou C. Difficulties in diagnosis and management of the staphylococcal scalded skin syndrome. Pediatr Infect Dis J 2000;19:819–21.

287. Ladhani S, Newson T. Familial outbreak of staphylococcal scalded skin syndrome. Pediatr Infect Dis J. 2000;19: 578–9.

288. Buchbinder LH, Lucky AW, Ballard E, et al. Severe infantile epidermolysis bullosa simplex. Arch Dermatol 1987; 122:190–8.

289. Hashimoto K, Matsumoto M, Iacobelli D. Transient bullous dermolysis of the newborn. Arch Dermatol 1985; 121:1429–38.

290. Sirota L, Dulitzky F, Metzker A. Bart's syndrome: a mechanobullous disease of the newborn. Clin Pediatr 1986; 25:252–4.

291. Fenske NA, Lober CW, Pautler SE. Congenital bullous urticaria pigmentosa: treatment with concomitant use of H1-H2 receptor antagonists. Arch Dermatol 1985;121: 115–8.

292. Uhlin SR. Pruritic urticarial papules and plaques of pregnancy: involvement in mother and infant. Arch Dermatol 1981;117:238–9.

293. Barson WJ, Reiner CB. Coxsackievirus B2 infection in a neonate with incontinentia pigmenti. Pediatrics 1986;77: 897–900.

294. Lane AT, Watson RM. Neonatal lupus erythematosus. Am J Dis Child 1984;138:663–6.

295. Woodside JR. Necrotizing fasciitis after neonatal circumcision. Am J Dis Child 1980;130:301–2.

296. Sussman SJ, Schiller RP, Shashikumar VL. Fournier's syndrome: report of three cases and review of the literature. Am J Dis Child 1978;132:1189–91.

297. Fisher RG. A novel complication of Plastibell circumcision. J Pediatr 1998;13:469.

298. Pathak A, Hsinhui H. Group B streptococcal cellulitis. South Med J 1985;78:67–8.

CHAPTER 12

Gastrointestinal Syndromes

■ GENERAL CONSIDERATIONS

Classification

The principal symptoms of infections involving the gastrointestinal tract are diarrhea, vomiting, acute abdominal pain, and jaundice. Often, these symptoms occur in combinations, but the clinician can usually make a preliminary diagnosis based on which of these symptoms is predominant.

Gastrointestinal infections are discussed in this chapter under the following syndromes: acute diarrhea, chronic diarrhea, vomiting, acute abdominal pain, and abdominal abscesses. Hepatitis syndromes are discussed in Chapter 13.

Overall Frequency

Acute diarrhea (acute gastroenteritis) was the third most frequent syndrome seen in general practice by Hodgkin.[1] Among children younger than 5 years old who are hospitalized, 13% have a discharge diagnosis of diarrhea.[1a] The Centers for Disease Control and Prevention (CDC) estimates that foodborne illness is responsible for 76 million illnesses, 325,000 hospitalizations, and 5,200 deaths each year in the United States.

Frequency of Various Pathogens

On the basis of reviews of studies done in the United States, including projections and estimates, it is clear that most diarrhea in children is caused by noncultivatable viral pathogens. Usually, diarrhea acquired in the United States is noninvasive (nonbloody), no specific etiologic diagnosis is made, and the child responds to symptomatic treatment. In contrast, bloody diarrhea in children usually has a bacterial cause, and the child may benefit from appropriate antibiotic therapy, depending on the cause.

The frequency also varies with the age of the patient and special exposure situations such as child-care centers, where several pathogen-frequency studies have been done.[2–4] An increasing percentage of children are enrolled in child-care centers, with an estimated 75% of mothers working outside the home in the year 2000.[5] The rate of diarrheal disease in children cared for outside the home is two- to threefold higher than for children who stay at home.[6] Outbreaks of diarrheal disease occur at a rate of approximately 1–2 per year for centers that house children who are still in diapers.[7]

■ ACUTE DIARRHEA

Diarrhea can be defined as excessively liquid feces. Most epidemiologic studies require at least three loose stools in a 24-hour period for inclusion as a case. Hyperactive bowel sounds and slight abdominal tenderness are usually present. Vomiting may occur briefly at the onset but usually is not persistent in patients who should be classified as having acute diarrhea. Colicky (cramping) abdominal pain may occur.

If the patient does not have vomiting, diarrhea is a better term to use as a preliminary diagnosis than is gastroenteritis, because "gastroenteritis" implies an inflammatory or infectious disease. Although acute diarrhea is usually caused by an infectious agent, it also can be caused by poisoning or have a number of other noninfectious etiologies. Patients with vomiting and diarrhea may reasonably be classified as having gastroenteritis.

Clinical Patterns

Acute diarrhea syndromes can be classified on the basis of the severity of the illness, the appearance of the stool, and the history of contact with others with a similar illness. A secondary classification can be made on the basis of possible etiologic agents (Table 12-1).

Acute Inflammatory Diarrhea

Also called dysentery-like diarrhea, acute inflammatory diarrhea is characterized by mucosal invasion and usually involves the large intestine. The

TABLE 12-1. CLASSIFICATION AND COMMON CAUSES OF ACUTE DIARRHEA

DIARRHEA PATTERN	POSSIBLE CAUSES
Bloody	*Campylobacter; Shigella*
	Salmonella
	Yersinia (rare)
	Ulcerative colitis; Crohn's disease
	Postantibiotic pseudomembranous colitis
	E. coli hemorrhagic colitis
	Other invasive *E. coli*
	V. parahaemolyticus
	Aeromonas; Pleisomonas
	Acute amebiasis
	Sexually transmitted pathogens producing proctitis
Watery	Diarrheagenic viruses
	Enterotoxigenic *E. coli*
	Giardiasis; cryptosporidiosis
	V. cholera; noncholeral vibrios
Commmon-source (food, water)	Salmonellosis; *Campylobacter*
	Diarrheagenic viruses
	C. perfringens; Bacillus cereus
Neonatal	Necrotizing enterocolitis
	Any of the above
Traveler's	Enterotoxigenic *E. coli*
	Giardiasis, *Salmonella, Shigella*
	Diarrheagenic viruses
Acute, not classifiable above	Any of the above infectious agents

stools may contain blood, pus, or mucus, and fecal leukocytes may be seen microscopically. Fever, crampy abdominal pain, and urgency of defecation occur frequently. The most common causes are bacteria, which may or may not produce toxins. The most common causes are *Salmonella, Shigella, Campylobacter,* and Shiga toxin–producing *Escherichia coli* (especially *E. coli* O157:H7). In addition to the infectious causes listed in Table 12-1, noninfectious causes, such as inflammatory bowel disease, intussusception, and cow's milk allergy, should be considered.

Acute Noninflammatory Diarrhea

This type is characterized by mucosal hypersecretion or decreased absorption without mucosal invasion. It is sometimes referred to as secretory diarrhea, but this implies that the mechanism is known, which is not usually the case. Acute noninflammatory diarrhea usually involves the small intestine. Vomiting and abdominal pain is common, but fever is variable. Stools are watery (without blood or mucus), and fecal leukocytes, if present, are infrequent (< 5 per high-powered field). The most common causes are viruses, such as rotavirus, caliciviruses (which include noroviruses and sapoviruses), enteric adenoviruses (serotypes 40 and 41), and astrovirus. Enteroviruses are so-named because of replication in and recovery from the enteric tract; however, they are not a common cause of diarrhea. Certain toxin-producing bacteria (*Clostridium perfringens, Bacillus cereus*) also cause noninflammatory diarrhea. The classic cause of severe secretory diarrhea, *Vibrio cholerae*, is rare in the United States, even among returning travelers.[8]

Traveler's Diarrhea

In areas of poor sanitation, newly arrived individuals often suffer an attack of acute diarrhea, whereas residents of the area are apparently immune because of past infection. Although this may in part be true, it is important to remember that diarrhea is a common cause of morbidity and mortality among residents of the developing world, particularly children younger than 5 years old. Each year, more than 2 million children die of diarrheal diseases, the vast majority in the developing world.[9]

Traveler's diarrhea is common, particularly in young children. In a study of 363 children spending at least 14 days in the developing world, the attack rate was 40% for children younger than 2 years old, 9% for children 3–6 years, 22% for children 7–14 years, and 36% in persons 15-20 years old.[10]

The majority of episodes of traveler's diarrhea are caused by enterotoxigenic *E. coli* (ETEC). Other common pathogens are *Campylobacter jejuni*, *Salmonella* spp., *Shigella* spp., rotavirus, caliciviruses, and *Giardia lamblia*.[11]

Common-Source Diarrhea

When many individuals develop diarrhea at about the same time, the clinician should suspect a common source of infection, such as food or water. This pattern also can be called diarrheal food poisoning, sewage poisoning, or waterborne diarrhea, but it is useful to use the term *common source* until the source is identified. *Salmonella* and *C. perfringens* are the most common causes of diarrheal food poisoning, whereas *Staphylococcus aureus* typically produces food poisoning with predominately vomiting and retching. Causes of common-source vomiting are discussed later in this chapter in the section on vomiting syndromes.

Neonatal Diarrhea

Diarrhea occurring in the first month of life is a special case and should be sorted out with the diagnosis of neonatal diarrhea. In the past, enteropathogenic *E. coli* (EPEC) was a common cause of newborn nursery outbreaks, but this is rarely reported now. *Salmonella* and *Yersinia* can cause diarrhea in young infants, but other bacteria rarely do so. Viruses are probably the most common cause. Neonatal diarrhea raises the possibility of necrotizing enterocolitis or of septicemia and its differential diagnosis.

■ CAUSES OF ACUTE NONINFLAMMATORY DIARRHEA

Diarrheagenic Viruses

The majority of acute diarrheal illnesses in the United States studied before 1975 did not have any recognized pathogen recovered when conventional bacterial and viral cultures were done.[12] Most of these illnesses were believed to have an infectious etiology on the basis of concurrent findings, such as acute onset, fever, and apparent contagiousness to contacts, rather than on the basis of the ability to demonstrate an infectious agent known to cause diarrhea. This clinical pattern has been called "infectious nonbacterial gastroenteritis" or "viral gastroenteritis," but "acute diarrhea, probably viral" (without etiologic guesses) is a more accurate problem-oriented diagnosis.

Rotavirus

First recognized by electron microscopy,[13] much of the acute diarrhea in infants in the United States is now known to be caused by rotaviruses.[14] Rotavirus is the most common cause of diarrheal syndromes severe enough to require hospitalization for intravenous fluid rehydration therapy. Worldwide, dehydration due to rotavirus is estimated to cause more than 800,000 deaths a year.[15]

Mortality from rotavirus infection is rare in the United States, but it is a common cause of hospitalization.[14] Rotavirus is also a common nosocomial pathogen. Rarely, rotavirus infection causes seizures or other central nervous system (CNS) symptoms not related to electrolyte disturbances; rotavirus antigens have been found in cerebrospinal fluid (CSF) using molecular techniques.[16]

In the late 1990s, a rhesus-reassortant, live-attenuated rotavirus vaccine was briefly placed on the market and recommended as a part of the routine childhood vaccination schedule. The vaccine virus was replication competent and produced protection against severe rotavirus disease (although it did not protect against infection). During the clinical trials, the vaccine was well tolerated, with the major adverse event being fever, which was reported in approximately 15–20% of recipients.[17]

However, after being placed into routine clinical use, a rare complication of the vaccine was discovered. Some vaccine recipients developed intussusception in temporal association with receipt of the vaccine.[18] Case-control studies estimated that, compared with controls, the odds ratio for intussusception among vaccine recipients was between 16 and 22. It was estimated that approximately 1 in every 5,000–10,000 vaccinees would develop intussusception if routine use continued. There is a biologically plausible explanation for the occurrence of intussusception in vaccine recipients; vaccine virus replication in the gut could produce local inflammation and lymph node hypertrophy. This, in turn, could serve as a lead point for the development of intussusception. The vaccine was eventually pulled from the market,[19] not because the risk of intussusception was high, but because the morbidity from this rare complication was unacceptable, considering that rotavirus infection in the United States is generally self-limited.

Two new investigational, live-attenuated rotaviruses are currently undergoing large-scale trials. One is a multivalent reassortant vaccine based on a bovine rotavirus genome (Rotateq),[19a] and the other is a monovalent human rotavirus strain that has been attenuated by serial passage in cell culture (Rotarix).[19b]

Caliciviruses

These viruses, the prototype of which is norovirus (previously referred to as Norwalk-like virus), most commonly infect older children and adults. Infections occur year-round, but there is an increase in outbreaks during the winter months.[20] These viruses are the principal cause of epidemic viral gastroenteritis in all age groups, what is frequently referred to inaccurately as the "stomach flu." Respiratory symptoms occur in about one-third of children, and the extreme contagiousness suggests possible respiratory transmission, although this has not been proved. Fever and myalgias are common. The incubation period is 12–48 hours. Some patients, especially young children, tend to have more vomiting, whereas adults usually have more diarrhea. Detection in stools by electron microscopy is specific but relatively insensitive. In addition, this test is generally available only in research laboratories.

Astrovirus

Astroviruses are small, double-stranded RNA viruses that are named for their appearance under electron microscopy, which is rather like a star. Infection with astrovirus produces principally a self-limited, watery diarrhea. Illness is generally much milder than that caused by rotavirus. In a prospective study of 214 children from Mexico, the mean duration of illness was 3 days, 20% of the patients reported emesis, and only 7% had fever. Severe illness was not seen.[21] A study from Finland characterized the disease in 102 children who had astrovirus detected in diarrheal stools. In this study, 72% had watery diarrhea, 59% had vomiting, and 26% had fever; however, only 5% required oral rehydration, and 3% were hospitalized.[22] In both studies, disease peaked in the winter and was most common in toddlers from 13–18 months. Different serotypes co-circulate during the same season.[23]

Enteric Adenovirus

Adenovirus serotypes 40 and 41 are the fourth most common cause of childhood viral gastroenteritis in most series.[24,25] Infections occur year-round, with a slight increase in summer. Children younger than 2 are primarily affected, and transmission occurs from person to person by the fecal–oral route. Respiratory symptoms occur in more than half of patients.[26] The incubation period is 3–10 days. The duration of symptoms is typically longer than with other viruses, occasionally lasting as long as 2 weeks.[26] In one study, the mean duration of symptoms was 5.4 days.[27] An enzyme-linked immunosorbent assay for detection of adenovirus serotypes 40 and 41 in stool is commercially available but not widely used.

Other Possible Causes

Other viruses, such as coronavirus, have been postulated to cause diarrhea, but their etiologic role has not been confirmed. Diarrhea sometimes occurs as a nonspecific finding in children with systemic infections. For example, although influenza virus does not infect the gastrointestinal tract, infants with documented influenza occasionally have diarrhea.[28] In the immunocompromised host, cytomegalovirus and some enteroviruses are a possible cause of diarrhea (see Chapter 22).

Other Causes of Acute Noninflammatory Diarrhea

In addition to the diarrheagenic viruses discussed earlier, bacteria can cause noninflammatory diarrhea as well. This occasionally occurs with the classic causes of bacterial gastroenteritis (*Shigella, Salmonella, Campylobacter,* and Shiga toxin–producing *E. coli*). However, it is the usual presentation with a few bacterial causes, such as *V. cholerae, S. aureus, C. perfringens, B. cereus,* and enterotoxigenic *E. coli* (ETEC). ETEC is discussed in the section on traveler's diarrhea. *S. aureus* is discussed in the section on vomiting syndromes.

Vibrio cholerae

Cholera is the classic cause of secretory diarrhea. Mild illness is similar to that of ETEC infection. However, severe cholera is distinctive, with massive fluid loss (> 1 L per hour) and rapid death in the absence of rehydration. Cholera toxin activates adenylate cyclase in the small intestinal mucosa. The increased intracellular concentration of cAMP stimulates secretion of sodium and chloride into the gut lumen, and water follows passively. The diarrhea is usually watery and flecked with mucus ("rice-water" stools). Vomiting is very common, but fever and abdominal cramps are unusual. In areas with poor sanitation, such as refugee camps, the potential for epidemic spread is devastating. Rapid rehydration with oral rehydration solution (or intravenous Ringer's lactate for severe cases) can be life saving. Definitive diagnosis requires recovering the organism from stool culture, which is best accomplished by plating the stool on thiosulfate citrate bile-salts sucrose (TCBS) agar. If cholera is suspected, the microbiology laboratory should be notified so that this special culture medium can be used.

Vibrio parahaemolyticus

This is a common cause of diarrheal food poisoning in Japan and has also been recognized in the United States.[29] Steamed crabs, boiled shrimp, and clams have been sources of infection with this organism, presumably after inadequate cooking. About 12 hours after ingestion, moderately severe abdominal cramps, diarrhea, some vomiting, headache, chills, and mild fever have been observed. Bloody diarrhea occurs in about 5% of persons.[29]

Several other species of vibrio can produce a similar illness after ingestion of contaminated and undercooked seafood.

Clostridium perfringens

This organism produces toxins that are elaborated in vivo and can cause diarrheal food poisoning. These heat-labile toxins typically produce an illness about 12 hours after the meal or experimental exposure. Typically, the source is meat or gravy that has been adequately cooked but inadequately refrigerated and served without cooking again.[30]

The predominant symptoms are watery diarrhea and abdominal cramps. Vomiting and fever are uncommon. Symptoms last 1 to 2 days.

Bacillus cereus

This organism can cause two different syndromes, depending on which of two toxins it elaborates. The strains elaborating preformed enterotoxin produce a syndrome indistinguishable from that of *S. aureus* food poisoning and are discussed in the section on vomiting syndromes. Other strains produce a heat-labile toxin that is elaborated in vivo and causes a syndrome indistinguishable from that of *C. perfringens.* As with *C. perfringens,* meats and gravies are common vehicles.

Enterotoxigenic E. coli (ETEC)

A classification of diarrhea-causing *E. coli* is shown in Box 12-1. The first four types on the list primarily cause watery diarrhea among persons in the developing world. In contrast, EHEC cause bloody diarrhea and are discussed in the section on acute inflammatory diarrhea.

ETEC are now recognized as a common cause of diarrhea in developing countries and the most common cause of traveler's diarrhea. A large inoculum (approximately 10^8 organisms) is required to produce disease. Risk factors for traveler's diarrhea include eating raw fruits or vegetables (especially salads), ingesting foods or beverages sold by street vendors, and drinking tap water. ETEC are also a cause of acute gastroenteritis in the United States. These pathogens are distinguished by their ability to make toxins. The heat-stable toxin (called ST) causes fluid and electrolyte secretion and is responsible for the watery diarrhea typical of infection with

---

BOX 12-1 ■ Classification of *E. coli*

Enterotoxigenic (ETEC) (heat-labile toxin or
  heat-stable toxin or both)
Enteropathogenic (EPEC)
Enteroinvasive (EIEC)
Enteroaggregative[79,80] (EaggEC)
Enterohemorrhagic (EHEC) (Shiga toxin
  producers)

these bacteria. The heat-labile (LT) toxin is similar to cholera toxin. Adhesion is also necessary for pathogenesis.

Enteropathogenic E. coli (EPEC)

Although EPEC can infect people of all ages, they are generally thought of as pathogens of the very young. The incidence is highest in infants under the age of 6 months who are not breast-fed. Once a common cause of diarrhea outbreaks in nurseries, this subtype is now rare in the United States. In vitro, they adhere to cells either diffusely or in localized areas; those that adhere locally are the pathogenic strains.

Enteroinvasive E. coli (EIEC)

EIEC display a pattern of enterocyte invasion that is indistinguishable from that of *Shigellae*. Despite the pathogenetic similarity, disease caused by enteroinvasive *E. coli* is usually marked by watery, rather than bloody, diarrhea and low-grade fevers. EIEC are primarily a concern in the developing world. A large inoculum of bacteria is required to produce disease. In experimental studies, the disease is made more severe by prior ingestion of sodium bicarbonate, which decreases gastric acidity and thus increases the viability of the ingested bacteria.[31]

Enteroaggregative E. coli (EAggEC)

EAggEC stick to one another in a "stacked brick" pattern in cell culture. Disease caused by these organisms tends to be of lower severity and longer duration. Diarrhea for 2 weeks or more is not uncommon. However, in careful studies, these organisms are commonly identified in asymptomatic individuals. Like the other types of *E. coli* listed earlier, they are primarily a concern in developing countries and can be a cause of traveler's diarrhea.

None of the types of *E. coli* causing noninflammatory diarrhea can be detected in the clinical microbiology laboratory using routine techniques. Thus, their true incidence is unknown.

Aeromonas Species

Aeromonas species are a possible cause of diarrhea.[32] Most studies have demonstrated a higher rate of recovery of the organism in children with diarrhea than without diarrhea.[33]

The organism is a normal inhabitant of fresh or brackish waters. Young children in the developing world are most commonly affected. It can produce a heat-labile enterotoxin. The diarrhea is usually watery but dysentery occurs occasionally.[34] Most infections are self-limited, but persistent or severe infections may respond to trimethoprim-sulfamethoxazole therapy.[34]

Yersinia enterocolitica

Yersinia enterocolitica is a cause of acute gastroenteritis[4,35] that seems to be more common in colder climates of the United States and in Scandinavia. The bacterium grows well at room temperature, and growth is enhanced after storage at refrigerator temperature. *Yersinia* species have also been incriminated as a possible cause of mesenteric adenitis, as discussed in the section on abdominal pain. About 65% of patients have abdominal pain,[36] and in one outbreak from contaminated chocolate milk in Oneida County, New York, 16 (44%) of 36 hospitalized children with yersiniosis had unnecessary appendectomies. The organism can cause bloody stools[37] (especially in children)[38] or chronic diarrhea but more typically causes watery diarrhea.[35] Reactive arthritis can occur as a complication, particularly in adults.[35,37,38]

The main risk factors are consumption of undercooked pork or unpasteurized milk. Infants may be infected indirectly via the hands of caregivers who prepare chitterlings (pig intestines, "chitlins").[39]

Plesiomonas shigelloides

Plesiomonas shigelloides is a member of the vibrio family that appears to be an uncommon cause of diarrhea in the United States, typically related to eating insufficiently cooked shellfish.[40] Travel to Mexico and other areas of the developing world is also a risk factor for disease. More common in adults than children, disease caused by this pathogen tends to last longer than disease caused by other enteropathogenic bacteria; in one study, 76% of patients were sick for longer than 2 weeks and 32% for over a month.[41] Whether antimicrobial therapy shortens the duration of diarrhea is unclear.[42]

Most isolates are susceptible to trimethoprim-sulfamethoxazole and to the fluoroquinolones.[42]

■ CAUSES OF ACUTE INFLAMMATORY DIARRHEA

Bacteria

Shigella

Until the discovery of the importance of *Campylobacter*, shigellosis was accepted as the usual cause of dysentery-like diarrhea in the United States. There are four species of *Shigella*: *S. sonnei, S. boydii, S. flexneri,* and *S. dysenteriae. S. sonnei* causes the mildest symptoms and is by far the most common species found in the United States. *S. dysenteriae* causes the most severe illness; it occurs in Africa and India but is not endemic in the United States. Among *Shigella* species, only *S. dysenteriae* type I is capable of producing Shiga toxin and is thus associated with the hemolytic-uremic syndrome.

Classically, shigellosis presents with high fever, abdominal pain, and cramping, which may precede the diarrhea by a day or two (Fig. 12-1). This is consistent with observations of experimental shigellosis in human volunteers, in which fever preceded the diarrhea by about 2 days on the average.[43] Shigellosis caused by food-borne transmission tends to be with a high inoculum and thus severe symptoms, as listed earlier. However, in toddlers who acquire it via person-to-person transmission, the inoculum is much lower, and the symptoms tend to be milder. This is particularly true with *S. sonnei*.

In a study of adult prisoners, the infectious dose of *Shigella* was as few as 200 organisms.[43] The mean incubation period to fever was 2 days; to diarrhea, 4 days. The duration of excretion of *Shigella* without antibiotic therapy was as long as 78 days, with a mean of 27 days. A more recent study confirmed the extremely low infectious dose and high acid-tolerance of this organism; as few as 100 bacteria were sufficient to induce disease.[44]

In addition to food-borne and waterborne transmission, *Shigella* infection is spread by the fecal–oral route. Spread within households and day-care settings is common, probably because of the low inoculum required to produce disease[45]. Antacid use increases the risk of infection, because it enhances the ability of the organism to survive transit through the stomach. Outbreaks in association with innumerable vehicles have been reported. Common sources include salads touched by infected food workers and raw produce such as fresh parsley, lettuce, and green onions.[46–48] Recreational water fountains and pools have served as a point source for other outbreaks.[49]

The signs and symptoms of *Shigella* infection may vary considerably based on the serotype of the infecting organism and the size of the inoculum. In

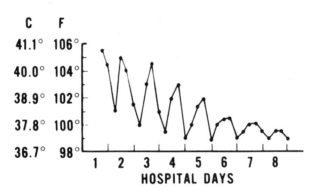

	C	F
	41.1°	106°
	40.0°	104°
	38.9°	102°
	37.8°	100°
	36.7°	98°

HOSPITAL DAYS 1 2 3 4 5 6 7 8

Convulsion	brief							
CSF	normal							
Vomiting	+	±						
Number of Stools	5	20	15	15	10	8	7	5
Toxicity	2+	1+						
Dehydration	1+							
Gross Blood in Stools	+							
Diarrhea in Family	+							
W.B.C.	13.2	10.0						
% Band Forms	35%	15%						

■ **FIGURE 12-1** Typical clinical course of severe shigellosis in a child.

the United States, most cases are due to *S. sonnei,* and disease is often acquired by low-inoculum means, resulting in less-severe disease that may be self-limited even without therapy (treatment is still indicated for prevention of spread). Severe cases are typified by sudden onset of high fever and dysentery. There may be other members of the family suffering from diarrheal disease. In rare cases, there is loss of anal sphincter tone. A study of dysentery in Bolivia found that crying during defecation, fever, greater than five loose stools a day, and the finding of more than 50 white blood cells (WBCs) per high power field were associated with the isolation of *Shigella* from stool cultures.[50]

Vomiting may be present early. Appendicitis is occasionally suspected because of the severity of the abdominal pain. Generally speaking, exploratory laparotomy is not indicated in patients with severe abdominal pain in whom the diagnosis of shigellosis has been clearly established. However, surgical complications of *Shigella* infection occasionally occur, including appendicitis, peritonitis, and intestinal obstruction.[51] Lumbar puncture is sometimes done in patients with shigellosis when the diarrhea does not begin until after fever and convulsions. The spinal fluid is usually normal.

The key pathophysiologic event in *Shigella* dysentery is invasion of the intestinal mucosa. Intense local inflammation is incited by a cytokine cascade. *Shigellae* that are ingested by macrophages can induce apoptosis in those cells. Once the organism gets into the cytoplasm, it can then spread from cell to cell.[52] Although local inflammation and mucosal ulceration can be severe, *Shigellae* rarely penetrate the lamina propria; therefore, bacteremia is uncommon.[53] The components of innate immunity are probably important both in protection from disease and in recovery; high levels of lactoferrin, myeloperoxidase, and leukotriene B4 are found in the stools of patients suffering from *Shigella* infection,[54] and in animal models, lack of natural killer cells predisposes to more severe and progressive disease.[55] The pathophysiology behind the CNS effects of shigellosis is not well understood.

Campylobacter

This organism was formerly included in the genus *Vibrio*. The species associated with diarrhea is *C. jejuni*.[56–60] The species *C. intestinalis* typically causes bacteremia in humans who are immunocompromised or have a malignancy. *C. jejuni* was not recognized as a cause of diarrhea before the mid 1970s because special culture techniques are needed to isolate the organism. The frequency of this pathogen as a cause of diarrhea has been underestimated because of the broad spectrum of disease and the difficulty in its isolation. However, it is now known to be more common than shigellosis in the United States. Rates of *Campylobacter* infection are highest in the state of Hawaii. A case-control study there found two historical events that were significantly associated with the acquisition of disease: (1) consumption of chicken prepared by a commercial food establishment in the 7 days prior to illness, and (2) antibiotic use within 28 days of infection.[61] There is a bimodal distribution of *Campylobacter* illness, with the first peak in infancy and the second in young adulthood.[62]

The clinical illness typically produced by *Campylobacter* can mimic shigellosis in its various degrees of severity, including diarrhea with convulsions at the onset of the fever.[60] Probably campylobacteriosis was the real cause of most of the past clinical illnesses called "shigellosis" in which no *Shigella* were cultured. In children, the diarrheal illness is typically associated with mild vomiting, fever with moderate abdominal pain, and frankly bloody stools that begin about 2–4 days after the onset of the other symptoms.[58] The diarrhea and abdominal pain last an average of 7 days. Fever has an average duration of about 2 days. The illness may be confused with acute idiopathic ulcerative colitis, especially when it occurs in young adults. Disease is typically milder than that seen with *Shigella* infection, although severe cases, including two associated with colonic perforation, have been reported.[63]

Comparatively little is known about the pathogenesis of *Campylobacter* enteritis. Attachment and invasion are thought to be important. Rarely, asymptomatic individuals can shed *Campylobacter* organisms in their stool. Molecular comparison of these isolates with those recovered from individuals with illness revealed that there is an identifiable marker found on disease-associated strains.[64] This locus has been named the invasion-associated marker. The exact protein encoded and its function have yet to be elucidated.

Waterborne outbreaks of *Campylobacter* diarrhea have been observed. It is normal flora of domestic livestock, and it can be acquired from ingestion of unpasteurized milk. Multiple studies have documented that the vast majority of commercial chicken is contaminated with *Campylobacter*.[65]

Much of the disease caused by *Campylobacter* in the United States comes from eating improperly cooked or handled chicken. Backyard barbecues are a particular risk, as the organisms can be spread from raw meat to other foods that will not be cooked, such as salads. Unfortunately, one study of 60 "domestic kitchens" showed that many surfaces are contaminated with *Campylobacter* after preparation of a chicken-containing meal, and that washing with soap and water did not change the rate of recovery of the organisms from surfaces. The situation was improved when hypochlorite was added to the cleaning solution.[66] *C. jejuni* is also found as a cause of diarrhea in puppies and kittens. In one case report, an infant developed *Campylobacter* bacteremia, and the organism was traced to a puppy in the home. Person-to-person transmission occurs but is uncommon.

Salmonella

Salmonellosis is the most frequent cause of diarrheal food poisoning in the United States.[67] Salmonellosis was on the increase in the United States for approximately 40 years; however, recent data support a decrease in the incidence of this disease in the years from 1987 to 1997.[68] The highest incidence is seen in infancy, with a rate of approximately 159 cases per 100,000 at the age of 2 months.[68] Infection with some serotypes is on the rise despite a global downward trend; all such serotypes are associated with exposure to reptiles and amphibians.[68a]

Because *Salmonella* spp are commensals in many animals used for food, consumption of contaminated foodstuffs is the usual route of infection. Inadequately cooked poultry and raw or undercooked eggs or egg products are usually impugned. Outbreaks due to alfalfa sprouts, chopped lettuce and tomato, fresh cilantro, and even peanut butter have been reported. These outbreaks are probably secondary to cross contamination from infected workers or irrigation systems. All of these vehicles have been experimentally proven to support the growth of *Salmonellae*.[69,70] Many *Salmonella* species are remarkably resistant to acid pH, explaining their survival in chopped tomatoes and fresh salsa,[71] which naturally have a pH of around 4.3. Interestingly, the serotypes that most often cause human disease are not the same as the serotypes that are found in highest frequency in food animals after slaughter.[72]

Salmonella species are normal flora in all reptiles and many amphibians. *Salmonella* is commonly transmitted from pet reptiles (such as turtles, snakes, iguanas, and lizards). Even without direct contact with the reptile, infants can still acquire salmonellosis when a caregiver prepares a bottle after handling a reptile or touching its cage.[73] Person-to-person transmission also occurs but is uncommon.

Studies in adult volunteers have demonstrated that, compared with *Shigella* spp, a much larger number of organisms needs to be ingested to cause disease; infection of children is probably more easily accomplished. The pathogenesis of the disease involves internalization of the bacteria into the epithelial cells of the gut. This has been shown to be a complex sequence of events that terminates with an actin-dependent rearrangement of the cellular cytoskeleton.[74] A series of virulence factors that allows the bacterium to survive inside macrophages and resist the bactericidal activity of complement has been described.

In diarrhea caused by *Salmonella* species, fever is often present, and occasionally blood or mucus is present in the stool (dysentery-like diarrhea). Often, however, the clinical pattern is that of a subacute diarrhea, which does not have an explosive onset but is somewhat persistent and may lead to moderate dehydration after several days. It is most severe in infants, young children, and debilitated elderly adults. Bacteremia may occur without greater severity of illness.[75] However, the risk of bacteremia is sufficient that antibiotic therapy has been recommended for infants younger than 3 months old with *Salmonella* gastroenteritis.[75] Young infants may develop meningitis if there is bacteremic seeding of the meninges.

In one outbreak, a healthy child who ingested the largest dose (as quantitated by the amount of ice cream ingested) died, indicating that severity is likely to be proportional to dose.[76] In a study of children with leukemia or solid cancers, there were no deaths, and the severity of illness was similar to that in children without cancer.[77] However, splenectomized children are at risk for more severe illness (Chapter 22).

Typhoid Fever

Infection with *Salmonella typhi* causes a systemic illness with bacteremia that is distinct from other salmonelloses. It is uncommon in the United States but is occasionally seen in returning travelers.

Transmission is from food or water that is contaminated by a human carrier. The incubation period is longer than in other *Salmonella* infections; it is usually about 14 days (range 3–60 days).

Initially, influenza-like symptoms develop with fever, malaise, headache, dry cough, and myalgia. Poorly localized abdominal discomfort and nausea are common. Children may develop diarrhea, but constipation is more common in adults. Young children may present with seizures. Fever rises progressively, until by the second week it is high grade and sustained. On physical examination, abdominal tenderness and hepatosplenomegaly are common. Occasionally, there is a faint maculopapular truncal rash (referred to as rose spots). Complications, such as gastrointestinal bleeding, intestinal perforation, and typhoid encephalopathy, occur in 10–15% of patients.[78]

Diagnosis is made by culture of blood (60–80% sensitive) or bone marrow (80–95% sensitive). Stool cultures are only positive in about 30% of patients.

For persons traveling to endemic areas, two vaccines are available, each with approximately 80% efficacy.[79] The oral, live-attenuated vaccine (Ty21a) is approved for use in immunocompetent persons older than 6 years of age, and the intramuscularly administered subunit vaccine (ViCPS) is approved for persons older than 2 years old. Both have good safety profile.[80]

Enterohemorrhagic E. coli (EHEC)

The classification of *E. coli* is shown in Box 12-1. Only EHEC are a cause of inflammatory diarrhea and are discussed here. EHEC are also referred to as Shiga toxin–producing *E. coli* (STEC).

Enterohemorrhagic *E. coli* can cause severe, hemorrhagic colitis. These organisms are of special interest because of the propensity of infection with these pathogens to cause a microangiopathic hemolytic anemia. This may lead to a condition known as the hemolytic-uremic syndrome (HUS). Although more than 100 Shiga toxin–producing serotypes of *E. coli* have been isolated from humans, not all such serotypes have been shown to cause diarrhea or HUS. Non-O157 EHEC appear less likely than *E. coli* O157:H7 to cause bloody diarrhea. It is likely that some non-O157 EHEC tend to produce bloody diarrhea, others produce nonbloody diarrhea, and others are not human pathogens.[81]

In the United States, more than 80% of all post-diarrheal HUS is caused by *E. coli* O157:H7.[82] In some European countries, non-O157 serotypes are relatively more common.[83] *E. coli* O157:H7 is estimated to cause more than 70,000 infections, more than 2,000 hospitalizations, and approximately 60 deaths each year in the United States.[84] The infectious dose is on the order of several hundred organisms. Children between the ages of 2 and 10 and the elderly are at highest risk.

E. coli O157:H7 is normal intestinal flora in about 1% of healthy cattle,[85] and most infections are due to consumption of undercooked ground beef. However, numerous other vehicles have been implicated. Unpasteurized apple cider has been a common vehicle.[86,87] Interestingly, in separate outbreaks in the Northwest United States that were traced to steak restaurants, careful epidemiologic investigation revealed that the consumption of meat was not a risk factor for infection; rather, cases were traced to items in the salad bar.[88] The largest outbreak occurred in Sakai, Japan, in 1996. In it, approximately 10,000 children were infected by consuming white radish sprouts in their school lunches.[89] Houseflies were incriminated as possible vectors in one nursery school outbreak in Japan.[90] An experimental study showed that when houseflies were fed *E. coli* O157:H7, large numbers of bacteria adhered to the mouthparts and proliferated in the "minute spaces of the labellum." The bacteria were excreted in the flies' feces for 3 days.[90]

Well-documented routes of transmission include unchlorinated municipal drinking water and swimming in fecally contaminated lakes or waterparks.[91–93] Person-to-person transmission is common, especially in the day-care setting, where secondary attack rates as high as 22% have been reported.[94]

Less than 10% of children symptomatically infected with *E. coli* O157:H7 develop HUS, which manifests a median of 6 days (range, 2–14 days) after the onset of diarrhea.[85] Several retrospective studies have attempted to enumerate risk factors for the development of HUS among patients infected with *E. coli* O157:H7. One study of 252 children involved in the Japanese outbreak found that an elevated C-reactive protein (CRP) (defined as greater than 1.2 mg/dL), an elevated WBC count (defined as greater than 11,000/mcL), and an elevated body temperature (defined as greater than 38°C) were risk factors, or perhaps more precisely, clinical and laboratory markers of a high risk of HUS.[95] Another study, this one involving 221 children, found that young age was protective, and that a duration of prodromal illness less than 3 days and an elevated WBC count at presentation were predictive of progression to HUS.[96]

Among children with HUS, risk factors for more severe disease include age younger than 2 years, anuria before admission, and elevated WBC count.[96a] A prospective study of 71 children, 10 of whom developed HUS, found that a high initial WBC count carried a relative risk of 1.3 for progression to HUS. The major finding of this study, however, was that antibiotic treatment of hemorrhagic colitis due to E. coli O157:H7 was the most important risk factor for the development of HUS, with a relative risk of 14. Antibiotic therapy remained an independent risk factor in the multivariate analysis, with a relative risk of 17 (95% confidence interval, 2.2–137).[97] This clinical finding is not surprising, given that in vitro studies show that production of Shiga toxin is increased by subinhibitory concentrations of several different classes of antibiotics.[85]

When ordering a bacterial stool culture, it is important to recognize that not all laboratories screen stool specimens for the presence of E. coli O157:H7.[98] The clinician may need to specifically request that stools be plated on sorbitol-MacConkey agar for detection of the organism. An enzyme immunoassay for direct detection of Shiga toxin in stool has been developed. It has a sensitivity of approximately 90% compared with culture for detection of E. coli O157:H7. Its greatest benefit is in detecting non-O157 serotypes. If used, it should be performed in addition to—not in place of—culture on sorbitol-MacConkey agar.[99]

Clostridium difficile

This organism is the most common cause of antibiotic-associated diarrhea for which an etiology can be determined. Diarrhea as a side effect of either oral or intravenous antibiotic administration is common, occurring in 5–10% of antibiotic courses.[100]

C. difficile is responsible for 10–20% of antibiotic-associated diarrhea; the remainder are idiopathic. C. difficile is especially likely to be the cause if it is an inflammatory diarrhea with fever, cramps, and bloody stools. The major risk factors are advanced age, hospitalization, and exposure to antibiotics.[100] The severity of disease caused by C. difficile is quite variable, from mild diarrhea to extensive pseudomembranous colitis, which has a character-istic endoscopic appearance with gray or yellow plaques.

Diagnosis of C. difficile is usually by enzyme immunoassays that detect either toxin A or both toxins A and B. Particularly in children, tests that detect both toxins are preferred to avoid missing cases.[101] A positive test in a young infant with diarrhea does not automatically prove a causal relation.[4,102–104] The bacteria, with or without the toxins, can be found in from 40–80% of healthy neonates and is recovered from about 3% of older outpatients without diarrhea.[105] Therefore, treatment (discussed later) is not automatically indicated. First, any antibiotic should be stopped if possible, as the antibiotic may itself be a cause of diarrhea or may alter bowel flora and so produce diarrhea.

Children with Hirschsprung's disease can develop an enterocolitis, which may be caused by C. difficile.[106] Because C. difficile may be spread from one patient to another via personnel, hospitalized patients should be kept in contact isolation, as should patients with diarrhea of unidentified cause.

Parasites

Entamoeba histolytica

E. histolytica is a rare cause of acute dysentery in the United States. It occurs in warmer climates in the South and in Mexican immigrants. Amebiasis can cause bloody diarrhea even in young infants and can be fulminant with perforations, peritonitis, and hepatic abscesses.[107–109]

■ CHRONIC DIARRHEA

Diarrhea can be defined as chronic when it persists for more than 2 weeks. In the United States, noninfectious causes are at least as common as infectious ones, particularly if the diarrhea persists for longer than 4 weeks. The noninfectious causes of chronic diarrhea are numerous and vary depending on the child's age. In the infant, common causes include disaccharidase deficiency, cow or soy milk protein intolerance, cystic fibrosis, or immunodeficiency. In toddlers, chronic nonspecific diarrhea (toddler's diarrhea) and celiac disease should be considered. In the older child, inflammatory bowel disease, lactose intolerance, and irritable bowel syndrome are common causes.[110] Several excellent reviews on the approach to the patient with chronic diarrhea are available.[110–113]

The rest of this discussion focuses on infectious

causes only. The infectious causes of chronic diarrhea can be divided into parasitic and nonparasitic. Parasites are far more common as agents of chronic diarrhea than are viruses or bacteria. However, any of the common causes of acute diarrhea can occasionally cause persistent symptoms, especially *Salmonella, Campylobacter,* and enteric adenovirus. *C. difficile* sometimes causes recurrent episodes of diarrhea. Oral vancomycin appears to be superior to metronidazole in treatment of recurrent disease.[114] One study suggested that the use of a probiotic agent (*Saccharomyces boulardii*) provided added benefit.[115]

Parasitic Causes of Chronic Diarrhea

Amebiasis

The term *amebiasis* is usually understood to mean infection with *Entamoeba histolytica*. This infection is uncommon in the United States but is an occasional cause of chronic diarrhea after infancy.[116,117] Often, there is a history of travel to a foreign country, such as Mexico. "Histolytica" refers to the invasive power of this species, which secretes a lytic substance that allows tissue invasion. Other species of amoebae (e.g., *Entamoeba coli, E. hartmanni,* and *E. dispar*) may be found in human feces as normal flora.

The motile trophozoite of *E. histolytica* survives only briefly after defecation. It is destroyed by gastric acid and so is usually not contagious. The cyst is the usual form seen and is the infective form. It also is the usual form recovered from the patient with chronic diarrhea.

Chronic or recurrent diarrhea secondary to amebiasis may be associated with episodes of abdominal pain.[116] Mild diarrhea may alternate with constipation. Weakness, weight loss, and anemia may occur. Eosinophilia is unusual and is not striking when present. Fever is usually absent or low-grade (less than 38.4°C [101°F]).

Chronic amebiasis is often considered in the differential diagnosis of ulcerative colitis. There may be blood passed with the stool without much diarrhea.[117] Hepatomegaly may be present, as may hepatic abscess.[118]

E. histolytica is morphologically indistinguishable from the nonpathogenic (and much more common) *E. dispar*. A commercially available EIA performed on stool is the best means of distinguishing the two.[119]

Giardiasis

Giardia lamblia is a flagellated protozoan that is the most common gastrointestinal parasitic infection in the United States. It is a relatively frequent cause of diarrhea, especially among those attending day-care centers.[120,121] Its usual mode of spread is fecal-oral. Disease in adolescents and adults is related to diaper changing.[122] Outbreaks in day-care centers, therefore, are most frequent in classrooms of diapered children.[123] It has been transmitted by contaminated water, although the risk of acquiring giardiasis from backcountry water has not been well quantified.[124] Dogs can be a source of human infection.[121] The incubation period is usually about 1 week but may be as short as 3 days or as long as 3 weeks.

At least two different clinical syndromes are associated with *Giardia* infection. The acute form features bulky, loose, foul-smelling stools, flatulence, and sometimes abdominal cramping. Fever is uncommon. The chronic form of the disease is insidious; it is marked by waxing and waning symptoms. Long-term bulky diarrhea, belching, flatulence, and poor weight gain are the principal symptoms. Malabsorption and failure to thrive may be the only symptoms. Rarely, vomiting may be associated. Hypogammaglobulinemia is a predisposing factor, with great difficulty eradicating the parasite in these patients.[125]

The pathophysiology of giardiasis is not completely understood. The trophozoites in the duodenum reach large numbers. They are not invasive, but rather attach themselves to the outside of the endothelial cells. Some experts believe that the cause of the diarrhea and malabsorption is the actual physical obstruction caused by multitudinous trophozoites attached to the absorptive layer of the bowel wall.

The diagnosis can be made by visualizing the cysts in stool. One stool sample provides at least 66% sensitivity for the diagnosis; two samples must be evaluated to elevate the sensitivity to 90% or greater.[126,127] Enzyme immunoassays that test for giardial antigens in stool have been developed and are somewhat more sensitive than microscopy.[126] Neither test attains 100% sensitivity, because some patients with giardiasis shed the cysts intermittently. If the suspicion of giardiasis is high, a repeat stool sample should be sent. The string test, in which a weighted string is swallowed and allowed to pass through the duodenum, is an older test that was generally reserved for patients in whom the diagnosis could not be otherwise established. However, the test is quite unpleasant and there is no scientific evidence that it is more sensitive than microscopy or antigen testing. Rarely, diagnosis will be established by esophagogastroduodenoscopy (EGD) with biopsy. Invasive procedures such as EGD, however, are almost never required.

Cryptosporidiosis

This protozoan belongs to the same suborder of parasites as does Toxoplasma.[128] Prior to 1976 it was not known to be a cause of gastrointestinal disease. However, it clearly can cause diarrhea outbreaks in day-care centers.[129] It is a cause of diarrhea in domestic animals, which can be a source of human infections. A food-borne outbreak in which the source was traced to raw produce in a restaurant has been reported; one of the food handlers at the restaurant was excreting oocysts in the stool.[130]

Cryptosporidia were also found to be the cause of the largest outbreak of waterborne diarrhea in the history of the United States, when over 400,000 people in Milwaukee became ill from cryptosporidial contamination of the municipal water supply.[131] Control of waterborne outbreaks is difficult; the oocysts manage to elude municipal water purification systems and are remarkably resistant to chlorination. In outbreak situations, residents are usually asked to boil water for at least 1 minute prior to consumption. Post-outbreak surveys indicate that the majority of people comply with this request; however, 20% admitted to washing produce with tap water prior to consumption, and 57% used tap water for toothbrushing.[132] These exposures are likely to pose significant risk, especially for immunocompromised hosts. The importance of boiling water for *all* uses needs to be emphasized in outbreak situations. Submicron point-of-use water filters proved to be protective against disease during the Milwaukee outbreak, reducing the infection rate from 50–80% to 18%.[133] Filters with pores larger than one micron don't do anything but provide a false sense of security.

Recreational water exposures such as swimming pools and waterparks are also a common source of infection.[93,134,135] Because the infectious dose is as small as 30 oocysts,[136] person-to-person transmission is also common, especially in day-care centers.[137]

After an incubation period of about a week (range, 2–14 days), the illness is marked by watery diarrhea in immunocompetent hosts. Study of the Milwaukee outbreak showed the median duration of illness to be 9 days. Ninety-three percent of patients with proven cryptosporidiosis had watery diarrhea, 84% reported abdominal cramping, 57% experienced low-grade fever, and about half had at least one episode of vomiting.[131] In immunocompromised hosts, the disease tends to be more insidious and lasts indefinitely. Patients with advanced HIV disease are particularly prone to problematic cryptosporidiosis. Over time, weight loss progresses to cachexia. Involvement of the biliary tract can cause acalculous cholecystitis. Infection of the respiratory tract can also occur in immunosuppressed hosts. The virulence of cryptosporidia varies by serotype,[138] and even within a serotype.

Degree of illness, duration of symptoms, and duration of oocyst shedding vary widely. In a study of traveler's diarrhea in normal adults, the mean incubation period was 1 week, the mean duration of illness was 12 days, and the majority of patients stopped excreting oocysts about 1 week after the end of symptoms.[139] In an outbreak associated with a day-care center, symptoms lasted 1 day to 4 weeks, and oocyst excretion lasted as long as 48 days after the onset of symptoms.[129] Interferon-gamma seems to be important in protection against severe cryptosporidiosis.[140] The importance of cell-mediated immunity in resolution of infection is attested to by the inability of patients with advanced HIV disease to clear the parasite. Many of these patients mount aggressive antibody responses but are still unable to resolve the disease. Antibodies are not entirely unimportant, however, as witnessed by the fact that patients with antibody-deficiency states tend to suffer more severe disease when infected with cryptosporidia.

Clinicians should be aware that routine ova and parasite examination of stool does not detect the presence of *Cryptosporidium*—testing for the organism needs to be specifically requested.[141] Special stains are required, and most laboratories do not perform them routinely.[142] When they do test for *Cryptosporidium,* three-fourths of laboratories use modified acid-fast staining. The sensitivity of this stain for *Cryptosporidium* is relatively low, 41–76%, particularly in cases in which the diarrheal illness is mild.[141] Auramine-rhodamine staining may be more sensitive but lacks specificity.[143] Enzyme-linked immunosorbent and monoclonal antibody techniques appear to be have the best sensitivity and specificity but tend to be more costly.[143,144]

Cyclospora cayetanensis

Infection with this protozoan causes a watery diarrhea that can last for several weeks. Disease was originally found in returning travelers from areas of endemicity. In one study of traveler's diarrhea, *Cyclospora* was found to be the cause in about 2–4% of cases. More than two-thirds of patients had symptoms for greater than 2 weeks, and about 40% had a greater than 3-kg weight loss.[145]

In the 1990s, several outbreaks were reported in the United States.[146] Most outbreaks were due to the consumption of imported produce from Latin America, the largest implicating raspberries from Guatemala.[147] Other implicated vehicles include mixed greens and fresh basil.[146] In one outbreak, traced to a fruit dessert at a wedding reception, the incubation period averaged 7 days. All those who were infected had watery diarrhea, 93% had weight loss, 91% felt fatigued, and 90% had a loss of appetite. In almost 90% of patients, the symptoms waxed and waned, and in 61% of patients, symptoms lasted longer than 3 weeks.[148] In immunocompromised patients, the disease is similar but lasts even longer. One report of cholecystitis from cyclosporiasis in a patient with AIDS has been published.[149]

Cyclospora oocysts in freshly excreted stool are noninfectious; they require days to weeks in the environment to sporulate into the infectious form. Thus, in contrast to *Cryptosporidium*, person-to-person transmission has not been documented.

As with *Cryptosporidium*, routine ova and parasite testing will not detect *Cyclospora*, and the physician should request that it be looked for when there is a suspicion of cyclosporiasis.[146] Safranin is the best stain for demonstrating the oocysts.[150] The disease may be underdiagnosed; in one study in Great Britain, only 58% of laboratories were able to correctly identify this pathogen.[151] Treatment with trimethoprim-sulfamethoxazole (TMP-SMX) alleviates symptoms and decreases the duration of oocyst shedding.[152]

Isospora belli

This protozoan is very similar to *C. cayetanensis*, except that large food-borne outbreaks have not been reported. Infection is more common in tropical and subtropical areas of the world. Disease in immunocompetent patients is marked by watery diarrhea that resolves over several weeks. This pathogen is particularly problematic for patients with immune deficiencies, especially AIDS, in whom it causes massive secretory diarrhea with weight loss and cachexia, which can last for 6–10 months. When HIV infection is aggressively treated, isosporiasis tends to resolve.[153] It can be diagnosed by fluorescence microscopy of concentrated feces in a wet mount preparation.[154] Alternatively, acid-fast or safranin stains can be used.[155] Treatment with TMP-SMX is effective, but relapses are common.[156]

Microsporidia

Microsporidia is the name given to a group of protozoan parasites. Over 1,200 species have been identified, but only a few have been demonstrated to cause disease in humans. Two species, *Enterocytozoon bieneusi* and *Encephalitozoon intestinalis*, primarily cause gastrointestinal infection.[157]

These pathogens are apparently rare in people with normal immunity, although one report of returning travelers with diarrhea found microsporidiosis in 5 (3%) of 148 of them.[158] Aside from this report, however, almost all reported cases are in patients with AIDS. Diagnosis is accomplished by microscopy using a chromotrope-based or fluorescent stain.[159,160]

Patients with AIDS who are treated with effective antiretroviral regimens respond much more favorably to treatment for microsporidiosis.[153] Albendazole is effective against some species (including *E. intestinalis*),[161] but not others (such as *E. bieneusi*). Cases where cure of *E. bieneusi* infection was effected with nitazoxanide have been reported but controlled data are lacking.[162] Despite reports of thalidomide treatment, this drug should not be used. In vitro, thalidomide does not suppress the growth of any species of microsporidia.[163]

Dientamebiasis

Dientamoeba fragilis is closely related to the flagellates, such as *Trichomonas*. It is a rare cause of chronic diarrhea and abdominal pain and sometimes causes acute diarrhea.[164] Peripheral eosinophilia is common. The symptoms respond to metronidazole.

Strongyloidiasis

This intestinal nematode can cause chronic diarrhea associated with eosinophilia, weight loss, and steatorrhea.[165] Patients usually come from Puerto Rico, Mexico, or the rural southern United States.[165]

Balantidium coli

Infection with this protozoan pathogen is usually asymptomatic but can result in acute or chronic diarrhea. Infection is most frequent in areas of the developing world in which contact with pigs is common. Diagnosis is by direct visualization of fresh stool, and treatment is with tetracycline or metronidazole.[166]

Probable Nonpathogenic Protozoa

Several organisms are occasionally reported by the microbiology laboratory when found in stool submitted for routine ova and parasite testing.[167] They include Blastocystis hominis, Endolimax nana, and nonpathogenic species of Entamoeba (E. dispar, E. coli, and E. hartmanni). These organisms are detected more frequently in children than adults and may predict the presence of other (pathogenic) protozoa. However, conclusive evidence that they are a cause of gastrointestinal symptoms is lacking.

Postinfectious Lactase Intolerance

The concept that lactose malabsorption is common in the recovery phase of acute bacterial or viral diarrheal illnesses, and that in some children this results in a significant persistence of the diarrhea,[168] was a popular notion. Many physicians still prescribe a period of lactose restriction following an acute diarrheal episode. Lactose-free formula has even been developed to fill this clinical niche. Although this concept may still hold true for individual children, in population-based studies the time to recovery from acute diarrheal illness is similar between groups receiving lactose-containing formula or breast milk and those receiving lactose-free milk.[169]

Thus, routine use of non-lactose-containing formulas is not recommended for children with *acute* diarrhea. However, the contribution of lactase deficiency in young children with *chronic* diarrhea in the developing world is thought to be substantial.[170] Risk factors for lactose intolerance in this population include age younger than 6 months, low socioeconomic class, and severe dehydration.

Bowel Bacteria Overgrowth

Bacteria such as *Proteus* or *Pseudomonas*, which normally are found in the bowel in small numbers, often become the predominant species in a patient with diarrhea. These organisms should not be assumed to be the cause of the diarrhea but probably are a "result" of the diarrhea. *Klebsiella, Pseudomonas,* and other enteric gram-negative rods occasionally contain plasmids that encode for toxins or invasiveness, much as *E. coli* do. Therefore, these organisms may occasionally be the cause of diarrhea.[171] However, causation is difficult to prove unless isolates are studied for virulence factors in a research laboratory.

Unknown Agents

In surveys of diarrhea using all available techniques to detect the frequency of various agents, there is a moderate percentage of cases with no cause found. Clearly, some agents that cause diarrhea remain to be discovered.

■ DIARRHEA IN COMPROMISED HOSTS

Hirschsprung's disease (aganglionic megacolon) is associated with severe enterocolitis in some children, sometimes attributable to *C. difficile* infection.[172]

Bone marrow transplant recipients can have diarrhea, especially from adenoviruses, rotaviruses, enteroviruses, and *C. difficile* (Chapter 22).[173] Chronic enterovirus infection and giardiasis are common in children with agammaglobulinemia (Chapter 23).

Diarrhea may be a prominent feature of disseminated histoplasmosis in infants. Despite the presence of massive hepatosplenomegaly, disseminated histoplasmosis is sometimes initially misdiagnosed as infantile inflammatory bowel disease.

Rotaviral infection, giardiasis, cryptosporidiosis, cyclosporiasis, isosporiasis, and microsporidiosis can cause persistent diarrhea in immunocompromised children, such as those with AIDS (Chapter 20). All of these agents can also infect the immunologically normal host as well and were discussed earlier. Disease in immunocompromised hosts tends to be of longer duration. In addition, complications, such as cholecystitis or disseminated infection with protozoan parasites, are more likely to occur.

■ LABORATORY APPROACH

Several thoughtful reviews are available about the clinical analysis and laboratory approach to children with diarrhea.[174–177] A variety of tests is available, but many of these are nonspecific. Even the most important test—bacterial stool culture—needs to be used selectively. As with any test that is ordered, careful consideration should be given to whether the results of the test will influence the care of the patient or be of public health significance. For example, rapid testing for rotavirus is widely available, but the management of the young child with rotavirus diarrhea is identical to that of a child with watery diarrhea of any cause. In addition, there are no specific public health implications of detecting a child with rotaviral diarrhea.

Bacterial Cultures

Indications for this test include

1. Diarrhea with blood or mucus
2. Patients sick enough to be hospitalized
3. Special circumstances: day-care outbreaks, foreign travel, or suggestive exposure history

In acute-inflammatory diarrhea, stool culture is usually the best laboratory procedure and often can influence antibiotic therapy. In acute noninflammatory diarrhea, no laboratory test is of much value in determining the etiology or specific antibiotic therapy, although culture should be done to exclude a treatable bacterial cause when the illness is moderately severe or necessitates hospitalization. In chronic diarrhea, testing for specific parasitic causes (*Giardia, Cryptosporidium,* and *Cyclospora*) is reasonable. Patients with severe diarrhea and recent antibiotic exposure should be tested for *C. difficile* infection. A positive test in a young infant may represent colonization, but in an older child it is usually indicative of a causal relationship.

Bacterial Stool Cultures in Hospitalized Patients

Studies in both adults and children have demonstrated the extremely low yield of stool cultures in the hospitalized patient. In a study of all 14,125 stool cultures from inpatients at Children's Hospital in Boston over a 5-year period, 174 (1%) were positive. Of 9,378 cultures from patients hospitalized for more than 3 days, only 13 (0.1%) were positive. Most of these were sent to document clearance in a patient known to be infected with an enteric pathogen.[178] Many hospital laboratories reject requests for stool cultures in patients hospitalized more than 3 days, with substantial savings in costs.

Rectal Swab Cultures

Rectal swabbings may be taken directly from a patient or by swabbing the stool after it has been passed, trying to swab any visible areas of pus or mucus.

When a rectal swabbing is taken from a patient who has watery stools, the swab sometimes will not appear stool-colored. This does not mean that the sample is inadequate, because the swab absorbs much fecal water, which contains many organisms. Weighing of swabs before and after swabbing indicates that the swab collects about 50 mg of fecal liquid, even when not discolored,[12] and this is sufficient for detecting bacterial pathogens, as the organism is present in large numbers. Whole-stool specimens are necessary only to detect a carrier state, where a large sample is needed to detect the small numbers of organisms (< 1000 per gram of stool) that may be found in carriers.[179]

Rectal swabbings may be streaked directly onto a culture plate at the bedside at the time they are obtained. Alternatively, the swab can be transported in broth or on a culturette and then plated at the laboratory, a procedure of equal sensitivity.

Number of Cultures

Usually, one culture is sufficient to exclude the common bacterial pathogens, but a second culture should be done if the diarrhea persists. The main disadvantage of a single culture is not so much that the pathogen is irregularly excreted, but that an error may occur in the collection or transportation of a single specimen.

A presumptive laboratory identification of *Shigella, Salmonella, E. coli* O157:H7, or *Campylobacter* should be available 48 hours after the culture is taken.

Fecal Leukocyte Smear

Smears for fecal leukocytes are occasionally done to narrow the differential diagnosis. However, they are generally unhelpful for several reasons. First, the presence of fecal leukocytes is not specific for infection; they can be seen with inflammatory bowel disease as well as other non-infectious causes. Second, even if the presence of fecal leukocytes were specific for bacterial infection, testing for their presence would not guide therapy, because some bacterial causes of diarrhea require antibiotics and others do not. Finally, if the stool has gross blood, it is not necessary to see fecal leukocytes to recognize the disease as invasive. Studies that claim a diagnostic value for leukocyte smears usually have not analyzed the data after excluding grossly bloody stools and include cases of *Salmonella* (which usually do not require treatment) and enterohemorrhagic *E. coli* (for which treatment is contraindicated). Testing the stool for lactoferrin (a product of WBCs), if the test is available, may be a slightly more sensitive way of showing the presence of WBCs in the stool. A meta-analysis of all studies published to date suggests that lactoferrin is the single most accurate laboratory predictor of a bacterial etiology of diarrheal illness.[180] Again, however, none of these studies excluded cases of bacterial enteritis due to organisms that should not be treated with antibiotics.

Peripheral Blood Smear

If the differential smear has more band forms than segmented neutrophils, *Shigella* is much more likely than other etiologies.[181]

Parasites

If two bacterial cultures are presumptively negative for enteric pathogens in persistent nonbloody diarrhea, or if there is a predisposing situation (such as foreign travel or a day-care or institutional outbreak), then microscopic stool examination for parasites is appropriate. Nonimported amebiasis is rare in the United States, so giardiasis and cryptosporidiosis are the principal parasitic diseases to exclude. Specific antigen detection in the stool is probably the most sensitive means of detecting these two organisms. *Giardia* is usually also visualized on routine stool microscopy (ova and parasite testing). *Cryptosporidium* requires specials stains.

Follow-up examination to detect asymptomatic carriers or study of asymptomatic family members is not necessary.

Viral Cultures

Because almost all diarrheagenic viruses can be detected only by electron microscopy, cell cultures are not useful.

Viral Antigen Detection

Rapid antigen detection is available in many laboratories for rotavirus and in fewer laboratories for enteric adenovirus. Whether detecting these organisms saves the expense of further testing is doubtful.

Enterohemorrhagic *E. coli* Tests

In patients with hemorrhagic colitis, the laboratory should be requested to culture for *E. coli* O157:H7. This serotype is detected by its lack of sorbitol fermentation plus serologic testing with O157 antisera. Rapid detection of Shiga toxin in stool has a sensitivity of about 90% compared with culture of *E. coli* O157:H7. It is most useful in detection of non-O157 strains of enterohemorrhagic *E. coli*.

Serology

Serum antibodies are rarely studied, either because they are not reliably produced or because their production is too delayed to be helpful in acute infection. One study reported that a rapid method of detecting serum IgM antibodies to *Salmonella* was 93% sensitive and 95% specific compared with culture.[182]

■ PHYSIOLOGIC DISTURBANCES

The early recognition and treatment of the physiologic disturbances of acute diarrhea is usually more important than antibiotic therapy directed at possible bacterial pathogens. The three principal physiologic disturbances that are most likely to occur in acute diarrhea are dehydration, hypernatremia, and metabolic acidosis (Fig. 12-2). Other possible disturbances are hypokalemia, hypocalcemia, hypomagnesemia, hypoglycemia, and hypochloremic alkalosis.

■ MANAGEMENT

Fluids and Symptomatic Therapy

Since the World Health Organization adopted oral rehydration therapy (ORT) in 1978 as its primary tool to fight diarrhea, the number of deaths among children suffering from acute diarrhea has fallen from 4.6 million to 1.5 million annually.[183] Despite this dramatic success, ORT remains woefully underutilized, particularly in the United States, where more expensive intravenous therapy is often used instead.[184] Practical guidelines for the outpatient management of acute gastroenteritis in children have been published[185] and are summarized in Box 12-2.

The practice of "bowel rest" for infants with diar-

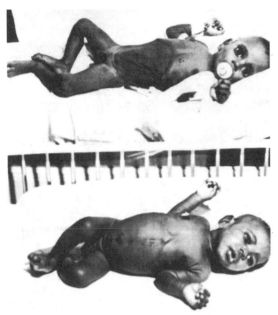

■ **FIGURE 12-2** Dehydration in infants is often associated with poor tissue turgor recognized by the failure of pinched skin to snap back to normal. Top: Dehydrated baby with poor turgor (demonstrated by pinching skin on the abdomen) and sunken eyes. Bottom: Same infant 48 hours later after intravenous fluids (Moffet HL: Clinical Microbiology. Philadelphia: JB Lippincott, 1980).

BOX 12-2 ■ Practical Guidelines for the Management of Acute Diarrhea in Young Children

1. Use of "clear fluids" is inappropriate because they lack adequate sodium.
2. Use of juices, carbonated beverages, and sports drinks can worsen diarrhea because of the osmolar load.
3. Use commercially available oral rehydration solutions.
4. Calculate the fluid deficit and replace over 4 hours. For example, in a 10-kg child with 5% dehydration, the deficit is 5% of 10,000 g = 500 mL. Therefore give 125 mL of ORT per hour for 4 hours.
5. If the child is breast-fed, continue breast-feeding.
6. Reassess at 4 hours.
7. If rehydrated, start normal feeding, including maintenance fluids.
8. Continue to supplement with ORT 10 mL/kg for each watery stool or vomitus until child recovers.

---

rhea, with all its conventions (clear liquids for a day, then half-strength formula for a day, etc.) has no basis in science. Studies have clearly shown that continuing to give formula or breast milk to infants suffering from acute diarrheal illnesses hastens recovery and does not worsen the severity of the disease.[169]

Drug Therapy

Antimotility Agents

Studies of Lomotil (diphenoxylate and atropine) in humans indicate that it makes experimental shigellosis worse.[187] In general, Lomotil or similar antidiarrheal preparations such as loperamide (Imodium) that inhibit intestinal motility should not be used in infants or children under 5 years old.[188]

Kaolin-Pectin Suspension

Kaolin (a clay), pectin (found in apples), and a combination of the two do not decrease the frequency of defecation or the water content or the weight of the stools[189] but may decrease the urgency to defecate and self-soiling. Use of these preparations is unnecessary.

Lactobacilli

Commercial lactobacillus preparations often do not survive in the intestine when administered to humans; a study comparing the incidence of diarrhea in children attending a day-care center who were given yogurt, lactobacillus-fermented milk, cultures of *Lactobacilli casei*, or a control preparation for one month at a time showed no difference in the number of diarrheal episodes.[190] There is likely no potential benefit to be gained by eating yogurt or drinking lactobacillus-fermented milk as an aid to recovery from acute diarrheal episodes or as a preventive against antibiotic-associated diarrhea.

However, a strain of lactobacillus known as lactobacillus GG (LGG) does appear to have some salutory effect in certain circumstances, although there are some inconsistencies in the data. For example, in one study, LGG or placebo was given to 119 children being treated with antibiotics for respiratory infections; although the severity and duration of diarrheal episodes were identical, the incidence of diarrhea was 5% in the LGG group and 16% in controls.[191] In a very similar study, 188 children were randomized to receive either LGG or placebo as prophylaxis against diarrhea while being treated with antibiotics for other indications; in this study, not only was the incidence of diarrhea decreased, but there was also a decrease in stool frequency and an increase in stool consistency.[192] A reduction in nosocomial diarrhea[193] and hastened recovery from acute diarrheal episodes in children given oral rehydration fluids plus lactobacilli[194] have been demonstrated. In the latter study, a significant difference between groups was found, even though the lactobacilli that were administered had been heat-killed. Finally, the duration of viral shedding in children suffering from rotavirus infection seems to be decreased by LGG administration.[195]

A meta-analysis of 10 randomized, double-blind placebo controlled trials suggested a benefit of probiotics in the treatment of acute diarrhea in children (pooled estimate risk 0.43, 95% confidence interval 0.34–0.53).[196]

Complications

A list of possible complications of diarrhea is shown in Table 12-2.

Convulsions were observed in 11% of children with diarrhea caused by *Shigella,* compared with 5% of those with diarrhea caused by *Salmonella* and 4% with diarrhea of undiagnosed etiology.[197] The pathophysiology of seizures in shigellosis has not been clearly defined; in one animal model, an increase in the production of TNF-alpha and interferon-beta 1b was found within the CNS very early in infection.[198]

This is a difficult area of study, because high fever, severe dehydration, hypoglycemia, and hyponatremia, all clinical features known to be associated with seizures, may be present in patients with dysentery. However, in many cases, seizures that occur in association with *Shigella* infection actually antedate the gastrointestinal symptoms. A recent study of 863 patients in Bangladesh found that the incidence of seizures in children with shigellosis varied by age; of the children younger than age 15 years, 9% were unconscious at presentation, and 8% had seizures either by direct observation or by history.[199] No patient over the age of 15 had seizures in association with *Shigella* infection. The spinal fluid is almost always normal, but a few patients with convulsions associated with shigellosis have been found to have 10–400 WBCs per mcL.[197,200] For the usual generalized convulsions

TABLE 12-2. COMPLICATIONS OF ACUTE DIARRHEA

COMPLICATIONS	USUAL AGENTS
Bacteremia	*Salmonella, Yersinia*
Convulsions and fever	*Shigella, Campylobacter, Salmonella*
Encephalopathy	*Shigella* (more common) or *Salmonella*
Extraintestinal infections	*Salmonella* (more common); other bacteria occasionally
Guillain-Barré syndrome	*Campylobacter jejuni*
Hemolytic-uremic syndrome	*E. coli* O157: H7
Meningitis	*Salmonella* (neonates/young infants)
Reactive arthritis	*Salmonella, Shigella, Campylobacter, Yersinia*
Bowel perforation, toxic megacolon, secondary bacteremia	Invasive (bloody) diarrhea group
Dural sinus thrombosis, renal vein thrombosis, transient methemoglobinemia, urinary infection	Any severe diarrhea
Convulsions/altered mental status	Severe diarrhea producing electrolyte imbalances
Subdural effusions	Any hypernatremic diarrhea

lasting less than 10 minutes, neither drug therapy nor diagnostic procedures were recommended in one large study.[201] Focal, continuing, or recurrent seizures were observed in 20% of the children in this series from Israel.[201]

Bacteremia is not unusual in diarrhea caused by some species of *Salmonella* but is rare in shigellosis.[202] Bacteremia with a different enteric organism, such as *Enterobacter,* has been reported 5 or 6 days after the onset of shigellosis in association with new clinical findings, particularly high fever, leukocytosis, and toxicity.[203] Secondary bacteremia with enteric organisms is not surprising given the extent of local mucosal destruction seen in shigellosis.

Perforation of the bowel and toxic megacolon are rare complications of salmonellosis. Encephalopathy has been reported in children with salmonellosis or shigellosis but also appears to be rare.[204,205] Extraintestinal infections that can occur with *Shigella* include conjunctivitis, urinary tract infection, vaginitis, pneumonia, and arthritis.[206] Bacteremia and meningitis may complicate salmonellosis in the newborn period.[207] Subdural effusions may occur because of brain shrinkage secondary to hypernatremia. These are usually small and require no therapy.[200] The odd case of subdural empyema[208] or brain abscess[209] due to *Salmonella* species has been reported.

Urinary tract infection occasionally complicates or causes acute diarrhea. Collection of a noncontaminated specimen from a female infant with diarrhea is difficult, but urinalysis reports in such patients should not be ignored. A specimen obtained by catheter or bladder puncture may be needed for a definitive diagnosis.

Secondary disease, presumably due to the immune system's response to the pathogen, can occur, especially after *Campylobacter* infections. The association of Guillain-Barré syndrome and campylobacteriosis is discussed in Chapter 9. There seems to be a component of molecular mimicry in its pathogenesis. The incidence is less than 1 in 1,000 cases of *Campylobacter* infection.[62]

Hemolytic-uremic syndrome complicates about 5–10% of cases of *E. coli* O157:H7 infection, as discussed previously.

Reactive arthritis is an occasional complication of bacterial enteritis (see Chapter 16). The joints are painful and swollen, but, if aspirated, no organisms are recovered. The patient usually remains afebrile. Over a course of days to weeks or even months, the condition resolves, and no sequelae are usually seen. In one study of 52 adults with reactive arthritis, a definite etiologic cause could be found in 56% if appropriate studies were done.[210] *Salmonella* spp were the most commonly identified agents and were the causative infections in 33% of cases in which the cause could be elucidated. In another 74 adults with "undifferentiated oligoarthritis" who lacked a preceding illness history, 35 (47%) were found to have an identifiable cause. *Salmonella* caused 12% of these cases and *Yersinia* spp, 19%. *Shigella* and *Campylobacter* can also cause a reactive arthritis; *C. difficile* and *Giardia* have been implicated less frequently.

Acquired steatorrhea or acquired lactose intolerance may follow mild infectious diarrhea in infancy and may be the first step toward chronic diarrhea and malnutrition, especially in developing countries.[211,212]

Management of Exposed Persons

Outbreaks of diarrhea in newborn nurseries may present many problems in control, requiring adherence to strict contact precautions. Careful hand hygiene in newborn nurseries may decrease exposure, as indirect evidence indicates that hands are an important means of colonization by diarrheagenic *E. coli* in the nursery.[213] If an obstetric patient has diarrhea, her infant should be isolated from other newborn infants.

Isolation of hospitalized patients with diarrhea is important. All caretakers should wear a gown and gloves if contact with the patient or the patient's environment is expected.

Antibiotic Therapy

Before Culture Results

As discussed earlier, only some of the causes of bacterial enteritis require therapy (Table 12-3). In addition, antimicrobial therapy is contraindicated for diarrhea caused by *E. coli* O157:H7. Because of the difficulty in distinguishing the various causes of acute inflammatory diarrhea on a clinical basis, empiric therapy is generally discouraged. One exception is the situation in which the patient is a contact of a known case of shigellosis, in which case the likelihood of infection with the same organism is great.

Shigellosis

Ampicillin or TMP-SMX were long considered the drugs of choice for hospitalized children with shig-

TABLE 12-3. SPECIFIC CHEMOTHERAPY FOR ACUTE DIARRHEA

PATHOGEN	FIRST-LINE CHEMOTHERAPY (ALTERNATIVES)
Unknown (before culture results)	None
Amebiasis	Metronidazole followed by paromomycin or iodoquinol
Campylobacteriosis	None (erythromycin, if severe)
Clostridium difficile	Stop offending agent; Metronidazole (vancomycin)
Cryptosporidium	Nitasoxanide
Cyclospora	TMP-SMX
E. coli O157:H7	None (antibiotics increase risk of HUS)
Enterotoxigenic *E. coli*	Azithromycin (a fluoroquinolone)
Giardiasis	Metronidazole (furazolidone)
Salmonellosis	None (ampicillin, ceftriaxone, TMP-SMX)
Shigellosis	Cefixime (TMP-SMX, a fluoroquinolone)
Typhoid fever	A fluoroquinolone (ceftriaxone)
Vibrio parahaemolyticus	None (doxycycline)
Yersiniosis	None (ceftriaxone, doxycycline)

TMP-SMX = trimethoprim-sulfamethoxazole
HUS = hemolytic-uremic syndrome

ellosis. The existence of many ampicillin- and TMP-SMX-resistant strains in third-world countries has been well reported. Until recently it was thought that most U.S. strains remained sensitive to either ampicillin or TMP-SMX. However, a report from Oregon that looked at 369 isolates found that 63% were resistant to ampicillin, and 59% were resistant to TMP-SMX.[214] A prospective, randomized trial of 2-day versus 5-day cefixime therapy for children with shigellosis showed that all patients were either improved or completely better by day 3, but that bacteriologic failure 1 week later was much less frequent in patients who received the 5-day course.[215] About 20% of patients in each group experienced a relapse. Cefixime resistance was rare (3%) in the Oregon study cited earlier.[214] A study comparing 5 days of cefixime with 5 days of ampicillin-sulbactam also found that recovery was much quicker in the cefixime-treated group.[216]

Patients who require antibiotic therapy for shigellosis probably should be empirically treated with cefixime (or a similar oral third-generation cephalosporin) rather than ampicillin or TMP-SMX. Most shigellae are also sensitive to fluoroquinolones. An-

tibiotic susceptibility testing of isolates should be used to guide therapy. Patients with severe shigellosis who are infected with a strain sensitive only to the fluoroquinolones should be treated with a fluoroquinolone, regardless of age.

Individuals who have recovered from their diarrhea by the time the laboratory report of *Shigella* is received need not be treated with antibiotics, unless the patient may be exposing others because he or she is not toilet trained. A convalescent carrier state (carriage for < 1 month) may occur, but a more chronic carrier state is extremely unusual in shigellosis.[217]

Salmonellosis

There is no indication that duration of symptoms in uncomplicated salmonellosis is shortened by antibiotic therapy. Because of the risk of dissemination to the bloodstream and CNS, salmonellosis in infants 3 months of age or younger is generally treated with ampicillin or a third-generation cephalosporin. Susceptibility studies should guide therapy. This area is somewhat controversial, because the benefit of this approach has not been demonstrated.

Salmonella Carriers

Family members or contacts of a patient with salmonellosis may be found to be excreting the same serotype, but it is likely that they were infected by the same food source as the patient, rather than being a source themselves. Such carrier contacts should be regarded as convalescent carriers and usually should not be treated.

Carriers of *Salmonella* species other than *S. typhi* are a possible source of infection to others, but unlike the case in typhoid fever, other sources, such as food, are more likely. In one study, severely debilitated individuals who were carriers of *S. derby* for 2–11 months apparently had no complications related to the carrier state.[218] When the carrier state must be eradicated for admission to an institution, parenteral ampicillin or oral amoxicillin combined with probenecid may be effective.

Typhoid Fever

Ampicillin and TMP-SMX resistance among *S. typhi* is now common. Fluoroquinolones are the most effective drugs for the treatment of typhoid fever; they should generally be used, even in young children. Several trials have shown that they are associated with the most rapid resolution of symptoms and with the lowest rates of clinical and microbiological failure. In areas where fluoroquinolone resistance has emerged, ceftriaxone, cefixime, or azithromycin may be used and are usually very effective also.[78]

In patients with chronic carriage, attempts at eradication should be made. If susceptible, amoxicillin 100 mg/kg/day with probenecid (30 mg/kg/day) can be given for 3 months. Other regimens may be tried, depending on the susceptibility of the organism. Some carriers have chronic infection of the gallbladder, in which case cholecystectomy may be necessary to eradicate the organism.

Campylobacter

Mild cases probably do not require therapy. Children with severe symptoms, grossly bloody diarrhea, fever, or suspected immune deficiencies should be treated with oral erythromycin.[219] There is some controversy as to whether patients actually benefit from erythromycin therapy; studies in children seem to show some shortening of the duration of illness and of fecal shedding. Clarithromycin and azithromycin are likely to be effective and may be better tolerated.[220] Fluoroquinolones are often used in the empiric treatment of dysentery in third-world countries. However, resistance of *Campylobacter* to fluoroquinolones ranges from 11–29% in studies done in the mid-1990s.[221] Resistance rates seem to be rapidly increasing,[62] probably secondary to extensive quinolone use in the farm industry.[222]

Giardiasis

Furazolidone suspension is useful for young children, given for 10 days at 9 mg per kg per day (maximum 400 mg per day) divided in three or four doses.[121] Metronidazole is probably the most commonly used drug for giardiasis, although it has not been approved by the FDA for this indication. Metronidazole carries a warning label that it is carcinogenic in mice and rats, and a pediatric usage label that "safety and effectiveness in children have not been established, except in amebiasis." After noting this, textbook and journal articles proceed to give a dose of metronidazole for giardiasis in children. Metronidazole can be used at 15 mg/kg/day (maximum 750 mg) in three divided doses for 5 days. It should not be given to pregnant women because of possible adverse effects on the fetus. The bitter taste can be disguised somewhat with jam or chocolate syrup. It has a powerful Antabuse-like effect, so it should not be used concurrently with any medication in an elixir form.

Nitazoxanide is available in a liquid formulation and has recently been approved by the FDA for treatment of giardiasis in children ages 1–11 years old.[223] In a clinical trial among Peruvian children with *Giardia* infection, nitazoxanide was as effective as metronidazole; both drugs had a cure rate of 80–85%.[224] The dose in children 1–3 years old is 100-mg po BID for 3 days; children 4–11 years old are given 200-mg po BID for 3 days. Quinacrine is an effective drug, but it is no longer readily available. The dose is 6 mg/kg/day (maximum 300 mg) for 7 days in three divided doses.[225] The drug can be obtained by calling Panoroma Pharmacy in Panaroma City, CA, at 1-800-487-7113.

Enterohemorrhagic E. coli (EHEC)

In the case of *E. coli* O157:H7 infection, antibiotics increase the risk of hemolytic-uremic syndrome and should be avoided.[97] Whether this is true for the non-O157 EHEC is not clear, but it would be prudent to avoid antibiotics in those cases as well.

Enterotoxigenic E. coli (ETEC)

Traditionally, TMP-SMX was the preferred agent for treatment of traveler's diarrhea, the most common cause of which is ETEC. However, antimicrobial resistance to TMP-SMX has become common. In one study from Thailand, more than 90% of *Shigella* isolates and 40% of ETEC isolates were resistant to TMP-SMX.[226] Thus, fluoroquinolones have replaced TMP-SMX as the empiric therapy of choice for adult travelers with diarrhea.[220]

Azithromycin is a reasonable alternative in young children for whom fluoroquinolones are relatively contraindicated. In the Thailand study, azithromycin resistance was found in 15% of ETEC.[226] In addition, for children older than 5 years old, loperamide may be considered in conjunction with an antibiotic for treatment of traveler's diarrhea.[220] For children, the main early treatment for traveler's diarrhea is oral rehydration. The use of prophylactic antibiotics for travelers is generally not advised.

Cryptosporidiosis

In the past, no therapy had been shown to be effective in treating cryptosporidiosis. However, more recent studies have shown efficacy of a new drug, nitazoxanide, and in 2003 the FDA approved it for treatment of *Cryptosporidium* infection in children 1–11 years old.[223] A study in Egypt compared a 3-day course of nitazoxanide with placebo. After 7 days, 21 (88%) of 24 children receiving nitazoxanide were cured of diarrhea compared with 9 (38%) of 24 children receiving placebo.[227] Nitazoxanide also decreased the duration of oocyte shedding in the stool. A similar study in Zambia also demonstrated effectiveness in immunocompetent children; however, among children with HIV infection, the drug was no more effective than placebo.[228]

Several other agents, including spiramycin, paromomycin, and azithromycin have been reported to be effective in uncontrolled trials in immunocompromised patients, who may have diarrhea for months. Unfortunately, none has been shown to be effective in placebo-controlled trials.[229,230] In patients with AIDS, the best treatment for *Cryptosporidium* is improvement of immune function with highly active antiretroviral therapy.[231,232]

Clostridium Difficile

If possible, the offending antibiotic should be stopped. If symptoms are mild, this may be all that is needed. In more severe cases, or if the antibiotic therapy cannot be discontinued, both oral metronidazole and oral vancomycin are effective, with response rates greater than 90%. Metronidazole is preferred because it is less expensive and does not promote the development of vancomycin-resistant enterococci.[100] If intravenous therapy is required, metronidazole (but not vancomycin) may be used.- Because of its enterohepatic circulation, sufficient concentrations of metronidazole may reach the colon, although this is not reliable.

Yersinia Diarrhea

Yersinia species can produce mesenteric adenitis with abdominal pain severe enough to lead to appendectomy.[223] *Yersinia* species also can produce dysentery-like diarrhea. Usually, the organism is not detected by conventional bacteriologic methods. Most *Yersinia* species are resistant to penicillins but are sensitive in vitro to TMP-SMX tetracycline, ceftriaxone, and gentamicin. In one clinical trial of TMP-SMX, there was no benefit compared with placebo.[234] Patients with severe immunocompromise or who have extraintestinal sites of infection other than the mesenteric nodes may benefit from antibiotic therapy.

Staphylococcus

S. aureus is found in about 15% of rectal cultures of normal children. The physician should not treat on the basis of the laboratory report of *S. aureus* in the stool unless the Gram stain of the feces and the clinical illness are compatible with staphylococcal enterocolitis.

Cholera

Replacement of fluids and electrolytes is the mainstay of cholera therapy.[235] Therapy with tetracycline or doxycycline eradicates *V. cholerae*, reduces contagion, and shortens the duration of diarrhea, and should be considered for patients with moderate to severe illness. TMP-SMX may be used in children younger than 8 years old.

Questionable Pathogens

Pseudomonas, Proteus, Enterobacter, and *Citrobacter* may be recovered in pure culture or as the predominant aerobic bacteria from the stool of a patient with diarrhea, but there is no reasonable statistical or experimental evidence that the dominance of these organisms is anything other than a result of changed flora secondary to diarrhea or selective growth during antibiotic therapy.

■ VOMITING SYNDROMES

Vomiting can be defined as the forceful ejection of gastric contents. Regurgitation can be defined as passive spitting up of stomach contents with relatively little effort, especially after eructation.

Diagnoses to Avoid

Stomach (or intestinal) flu, gastritis, and gastroenteritis should be avoided as preliminary diagnoses, because they are usually not a precise enough description of the degree of vomiting or diarrhea and imply an inflammatory etiology. *Stomach flu* is a lay term that is not adequately defined but usually implies an outbreak. Caliciviruses are a common cause. However, in some human volunteer experiments, ingesting caliciviruses produced predominantly vomiting in some subjects and predominantly diarrhea in others.

"Gastritis" implies that stomach inflammation is involved in a vomiting illness, but this is rarely testable and is often not the principal factor. "Gastroenteritis" should not be used if vomiting rather than diarrhea is the major manifestation. Keep in mind that, in children, vomiting is often a nonspecific symptom of systemic illness and does not necessarily imply a gastrointestinal or even an abdominal source. "Vomiting" or "vomiting with fever" may be a more accurate problem-oriented diagnosis than "gastroenteritis." As discussed later, pharyngitis, cystitis, meningitis, pneumonia, myocarditis, and sepsis may all present initially with vomiting.

Classification

To aid the classification of a vomiting syndrome, it is important to find out the frequency and severity of the vomiting, the appearance of the vomitus, and any exposure to other persons who are vomiting. If diarrhea is more prominent, the patient should be classified into one of the diarrheal syndromes. If the patient has severe abdominal pain, signs of intestinal obstruction, or signs of increased intracranial pressure, the preliminary syndrome diagnosis should be in one of these areas. When vomiting is the principal clinical finding, the preliminary diagnosis should be based on whether the patient has

exposure to, or association with, other persons who are also vomiting, as described later.

Clinical Syndromes

Epidemic Vomiting Syndrome

Epidemic vomiting syndrome is characterized by repeated episodes of nausea and vomiting, often with heaving, gagging, and retching.[236,237] In the typical case, vomiting occurs frequently over a period of approximately 8 hours, with a gradual decrease in frequency over the next several days. In order to define an illness as epidemic vomiting syndrome, it is necessary to know that the patient has been exposed to another person with the same general illness or that an outbreak of vomiting is occurring in the community. Contacts may be friends or others in the family or neighborhood who have had similar illnesses. Alternatively, a point-source outbreak may be responsible in which multiple people have ingested a contaminated item.

Winter Vomiting Disease

Winter vomiting disease[237,238] was a term originally applied to a form of sequential-onset vomiting illness that occurred more commonly in the winter. As the epidemiology of caliciviruses has been more clearly elucidated, it has been suggested that this syndrome is just another name for epidemic calicivirus outbreaks (discussed in more detail later). Thus, the term *winter* adds nothing and should be abandoned. Although epidemiologically it is useful to contrast sequential onset vomiting from simultaneous onset vomiting, both syndromes are frequently caused by caliciviruses.

Common-Source Vomiting

This syndrome also could be called emetic food poisoning or simultaneous onset vomiting, which is cumbersome but more precise. It can be defined as the occurrence of vomiting in more than one individual with the onset at approximately the same time (within only a few hours of each other). The vomiting pattern and other associated symptoms may resemble those of epidemic vomiting syndrome. Some diarrhea may also be present. The usual cause is staphylococcal enterotoxin produced in food contaminated by a pustule from a food handler, or caliciviruses shed by a food worker who is either in the prodromal stages or is just recovering from acute epidemic vomiting illness.[238]

Food poisoning should not be used as a preliminary syndrome diagnosis without further description, such as emetic food poisoning. Food poisoning is usually defined as any illness transmitted by food. Many anatomic syndromes can be produced by the variety of microorganisms or toxins that can be transmitted by food. Examples of such syndromes and the usual etiology of the syndrome are simultaneous onset vomiting, typically caused by staphylococcal enterotoxin or caliciviruses; acute diarrhea, typically caused by *Salmonella, Campylobacter, C. perfringens,* or *B. cereus;* febrile exudative pharyngitis, caused by Group A streptococci; cranial nerve paralysis, caused by *Clostridium botulinum;* and histamine effects (headache, flushing, and diarrhea) caused by scombroid (tuna family) fish poisoning (Table 12-4). The existence of the so-called Chinese restaurant syndrome, which was thought to be secondary to monosodium glutamate ingestion, has been called into question.[240] The syndrome is not reproducible even in self-proclaimed sufferers if monosodium glutamate is given with food and an appropriate placebo is used.[241]

Mushroom poisoning may affect only a few members of a family but is especially important to identify, as specific therapies may reduce the mortality rate.[242]

Possible Etiologies

Onset of an Acute Infection

Other signs of the infection besides vomiting become more prominent with time and are discussed in the sections on these diseases. *Mumps virus infection* can cause persistent vomiting without parotitis. *Reye's syndrome* usually begins with severe vomiting followed by signs of acute encephalopathy. *Shigellosis* may be manifested by vomiting at the onset, although vomiting is usually not persistent, and diarrhea quickly becomes the predominant symptom. A brief episode of vomiting precedes diarrhea, as a general rule, in experimental *Shigella* infections. *Meningitis* is often associated with vomiting at the onset, probably because of increased intracranial pressure. Young children with Group A streptococcal pharyngitis often experience vomiting in association with headache and abdominal pain. At the time of the first clinic visit, these symptoms may even predominate. Infants with urinary tract infections often present with vomiting and fever as the principal symptoms. Other possibilities to keep in mind are pneumonia, sepsis, and myocarditis.

Caliciviruses

Caliciviruses (noroviruses and sapoviruses) are the most common causes of epidemic vomiting syndrome. Because these viruses are not cultivatable in the laboratory, progress in virologic and epidemiologic studies has been slow. These viruses were first seen using immunoelectron microscopy. All these viruses were first called "small round-structured viruses" (SRSV) because of their appearance on electron microscopy. They are all now classified as types of calicivirus. These viruses are extremely small and relatively simple. Norwalk virus was named for Norwalk, Ohio, where an outbreak of epidemic vomiting syndrome occurred in 116 students and teachers in an elementary school in 1968. Nausea and vomiting occurred in 95%, abdominal cramps in 60%, and diarrhea in 40% of the primary cases. The secondary attack rate in families of the primary cases was about 30%, indicating a contagious agent. In an outbreak of Norwalk-related disease in a boys' camp, the majority had nausea and vomiting, whereas 9% of the campers (younger) had diarrhea, and 55% of the staff (older) had diarrhea.[243]

Other similar viruses, all classified as caliciviruses, resemble Norwalk virus morphologically and can cause gastroenteritis.[244] They are being named for the locations or patients where they were first recovered: Hawaii agent, MC (Montgomery County) virus, W agent (Britain), Snow Mountain agent (Colorado), Otofuke agent (Japan), and Marin (County) agent. Collectively, these viruses are known as noroviruses (formerly Norwalk-like viruses). Sapporo virus is another calicivirus that causes epidemic vomiting syndrome. It is distributed worldwide. It is structurally different enough that it and similar viruses are now classified in the genus Sapovirus (formerly Sapporo-like viruses).

It is believed that the fecal–oral route is the main mechanism of transmission of noroviruses. However, outbreaks in which airborne transmission has appeared to play a major role have been described.[245] The secondary household infection rate is higher than might be expected were fecal–oral transmission the only mechanism of spread.

Immunity to noroviruses is type specific.[246] Therefore, infection with one serotype is not protective against infection with a related virus. Additionally, it appears that homotypic protection is not long lived; therefore, after a couple of years, infection with the exact same serotype can occur.[247] Virus is shed in the feces prior to the onset of symp-

TABLE 12-4. FOOD POISONING SYNDROMES AND THEIR COMMON CAUSES

SYNDROME	COMMON CAUSES
Gastrointestinal	
Primarily vomiting	S. aureus, B. cereus (emetic toxin), caliciviruses, heavy metals
Diarrhea (with or without vomiting)	C. perfringens, B. cereus (diarrheal toxin), Salmonella, Shigella, Campylobacter, enterohemorrhagic E. coli, enterotoxigenic E. coli, Caliciviruses, Vibrio parahaemolyticus, Cryptosporidium, Cyclospora
Persistent diarrhea (≥ 14 days)	Cyclospora, Cryptosporidium, Entamoeba histolytica, Giardia lambia
Central nervous system	
Cranial nerve palsies (descending paralysis)	Botulism
Ascending paralysis and sensory deficits	Guillain-Barré syndrome secondary to C. jejuni infection
Paresthesias, numbness, weakness	Ciguatera fish poisoning, shellfish toxins, puffer fish, scombroid, thallium, mercury, nitrites
Seizures	Organophosphates, carbamates
Respiratory symptoms	
Febrile exudative pharyngitis	Group A streptococcus, possibly other streptococci
Systemic illness	
Anemia, thrombocytopenia, renal failure	Hemolytic-uremic syndrome secondary to enterohemorrhagic E. coli infection
Flu-like illness, cervical adenopathy	Toxoplasma gondii
Diarrhea, fever, myalgia, periorbital edema	Trichinella spiralis
Flu-like illness, bacteremia, meningitis	Listeria monocytogenes
Fever, abdominal pain, jaundice	Hepatitis A
Headache, fever, myalgia, arthralgia	Brucellosis
Special situations	
Mushroom poisoning (short acting, < 2 h)	Vomiting, diarrhea, confusion, visual disturbance, salivation, diaphoresis, confusion
Mushroom poisoning (long acting, 4–8 h)	Diarrhea, abdominal cramps, hepatic and renal failure
Mass hysteria	Occasionally seen in schools or other close contact situations; common complaints include hyperventilation, dyspnea, headache, nausea, and abdominal pain

toms, and for several days (even up to a week) after the symptomatic phase of the disease is over.[248] The virus has also been found in vomitus.

Staphylococcal enterotoxin

Staphylococcal enterotoxin is probably the most frequent cause of simultaneous onset vomiting. In a large outbreak in Japan, the incubation period was able to be determined for 2975 cases. Most patients developed symptoms between 3 and 4 hours after ingesting the contaminated milk; 85% of patients developed illness within 6 hours, and 96% developed illness within 12 hours.[249] Symptoms reported were nausea or vomiting (75%), diarrhea (75%), abdominal cramps (50%), and low-grade fever (12%).[249] Staphylococcal food poisoning can cause severe illness or even be fatal in older or immunocompromised individuals.[250]

In outbreaks of staphylococcal food poisoning, the source can usually be suspected on the basis of the food history, usually a previously cooked high-protein food, and is confirmed by testing the items for enterotoxin.[251,252] A food worker usually has contaminated the food. Typically, it has been stored without refrigeration at temperatures sufficient to allow staphylococcal growth.[253] The enterotoxin is heat stable; therefore, reheating foods stored at incorrect temperatures can kill the bacteria, but the toxin is not inactivated.

At least five serologically different types, labeled A through E, have been identified. The most frequent and most severe disease is caused by type A enterotoxin. Enterotoxin-producing *S. aureus* can cause osteomyelitis and other staphylococcal diseases but such infections are typically not associated with vomiting.[254] They are also occasionally responsible for staphylococcal toxic shock syndrome, although strains producing TSST-1 are a more common cause.

Bacillus cereus

Those strains of *B. cereus* that elaborate emetic toxin cause an illness indistinguishable from that of *S. aureus*. Sudden onset of severe vomiting occurs 1–6 hours after ingestion of the preformed toxin. Fried rice is the most common vehicle. This is because many cooks allow the boiled rice to cool to room temperature to avoid clumping. The bacteria replicate in the rice and produce the heat-stabile toxin, which is not inactivated by frying the rice.

Botulism

Occasionally, vomiting is prominent in botulism and may divert attention from the usual neurologic findings.[255,256] In type E botulism, the expected pupillary dilatation and extraocular paralysis may be absent, but the mouth is usually dry (see Fig. 9-8).

The CDC advises that suspected food be saved, that stool and serum specimens be obtained from the patient, that CSF be examined, that an electromyogram be done, and that the patient's vital capacity be monitored preferably in an intensive care unit.[257] As described in Chapter 9 (paralysis and weakness section), artificial ventilation may be required for the paralysis. An equine polyvalent antiserum is available 24 hours a day through the CDC and is obtained by contacting the appropriate state health department.

Heavy Metals

Ingestion of certain heavy metals (e.g., antimony, arsenic, copper, thallium, tin, and zinc) may cause vomiting. The incubation period is characteristically very short (a few hours). Eating foods stored in a metallic container may be a clue. Treatment is supportive.[258]

Noninfectious Causes

Vomiting can be a result of many noninfectious conditions. These include ingestion of toxins; intestinal obstruction; increased intracranial pressure; metabolic causes, including diabetic acidosis and adrenal insufficiency; and pregnancy.

Physiologic Disturbances

Dehydration, metabolic alkalosis from loss of gastric acid, and later acidosis secondary to dehydration may occur.

Prevention

In theory, many cases of epidemic vomiting syndrome or food poisoning are preventable. Good kitchen hygiene and refrigeration practices should decrease the number of cases of food-borne disease from home-cooked meals. Health inspection services attempt to keep commercial food-borne disease at bay with frequent inspections and education, but it is impossible to prevent all such cases.

Secondary household cases of vomiting illness due to caliciviruses are, at least in theory, minimizable by careful hand washing and cleaning, although airborne spread may still occur.

Regarding future calicivirus vaccine prospects, it is known that the second open-reading frame of the calicivirus genome encodes the entire structure of the virus; this portion of the genome can be expressed in baculovirus to produce "empty virions."[259] These resemble caliciviruses in every way, but are only the outer structure. In animal models, oral administration of these empty viruses is successful at producing antibodies to the most important outer membrane proteins. These empty virions may prove to be viable vaccine candidates.

Management

Withhold Oral Feeding

Usually, no treatment is necessary except withholding oral feedings for a few hours before trying clear fluids.[260] In the absence of diarrhea, dehydration will usually not be severe in an older child who has no fluid for a 24-hour period, and infants generally do reasonably well without fluid for 12 hours. A useful guide to dehydration is documentation of weight loss, which can be done by the family or in the physician's office.

Cautious Oral Fluids

Once the frequency of the vomiting decreases, small feedings are begun with oral rehydration solution (ORS) every 15 minutes (see Box 12–2). Even if the child continues to vomit, some of the ORS will still be absorbed. Intravenous therapy is seldom necessary except when there is an underlying disease such as diabetes or if the patient is a very young infant. If diarrhea is also present, intravenous fluids may be necessary in the infant.

Drug Therapy

In general, to avoid masking serious disease and because the ordinary bout of epidemic vomiting is benign and self-limited, antiemetics should not be used in vomiting patients. The phenothiazine drugs such as prochlor perazine (Compazine™) probably are not indicated because of the rare occurrence of neurologic complications resembling tetanus (discussed in Chapter 9), particularly spasms of the neck muscles, which have been reported as a cause of death.[261] Promethazine (Phenergan™) is commonly used as an antiemetic but lacks proof of efficacy. Trimethobenzamide (Tigan™) has been associated with extrapyramidal toxicity. A small, prospective, randomized, placebo-controlled study showed that intravenous ondansetron (Zofran™) decreased subsequent bouts of emesis, and, in the subset of children with serum carbon dioxide levels greater than or equal to 15 mEq/L, decreased hospital admission for fluid therapy.[262]

■ FOOD-BORNE DISEASE

An estimated 76 million persons contract food-borne illnesses each year in the United States.[67,84] Formal surveillance is collected for only some of the causes of food-borne illness. Nearly all of the organisms discussed earlier as a cause of diarrhea or vomiting can be acquired by food-borne transmission, although some are more commonly transmitted from person to person (e.g., rotavirus)[263] or via contaminated water (e.g., *Giardia*).[264] In addition, some organisms are transmitted via the food-borne route but typically are not associated with either vomiting or diarrhea (e.g., *Listeria*).[258] Common causes of food-borne illness are listed in Table 12-4.

■ WATERBORNE ILLNESS

The causes of waterborne illness are somewhat different from those of food-borne illness, although there is overlap. Waterborne illness may be caused by exposure to contaminated drinking water or recreational water (e.g., swimming or wave pools). The most common causes of gastroenteritis caused by contaminated drinking water are *Giardia*, *Shigella*, *Salmonella*, *E. coli* O157:H7, caliciviruses, *Cryptosporidium*, and chemical agents.[266]

The most common causes of gastroenteritis caused by contaminated recreational water are *Cryptosporidium*, *E. coli* O157:H7, and *Shigella*.[266] This is intuitive because each of these three agents has a low infectious dose.

■ PEPTIC ULCER DISEASE

Definitions

An *erosion* is a mucosal break that does not penetrate the muscularis mucosa. An *ulcer* is deeper and extends through the muscularis into the submucosa. *Peptic ulcer disease* refers to erosions or ulcers of the stomach or duodenum. They may be *primary* (the most common cause of which is *Helicobacter pylori* infection) or they may be *secondary*. The causes of secondary ulcers are numerous and include sepsis, autoimmune disease, and multiple drugs (such as nonsteroidal anti-inflammatory drugs and steroids).[267] If there is histologic evidence of inflammation in a biopsy specimen, the terms *gastritis* or *duodenitis* are appropriate.

Helicobacter pylori

H. pylori is a gram-negative rod initially classified as a *Campylobacter*. During the past decade, it has become accepted that chronic infection with *H. pylori* is the major factor in the pathogenesis of primary peptic ulcer disease.[268]

Although peptic ulcer disease is less common in children than adults, the diagnosis should be considered in the child with periumbilical or epigastric abdominal pain, particularly if accompanied by vomiting, blood in the stools (which may be occult), and anemia. A family history of ulcers is also often elicited.

In addition to causing most duodenal and gastric ulcers, *H. pylori* infection is a strong risk factor for the development of gastric carcinoma and gastric lymphoma. Eradication of *H. pylori* infection dramatically decreases the subsequent risk of gastric cancer.[269]

The diagnosis of *H. pylori* infection can be made endoscopically or with noninvasive tests. However, documentation of an ulcer can only be made endoscopically. There is much controversy regarding whether nonulcer dyspepsia in a patient who tests positive for *H. pylori* infection requires treatment. A recent systematic review reported that eradication *of H. pylori* improves symptoms in only about 10% of patients with nonulcer dyspepsia.[270] However, given the long-term benefit of eradication, it is possible that treatment for confirmed *H. pylori* nonulcer dyspepsia will become accepted practice in the future.

Noninvasive tests include serology, urea breath test, and stool antigen detection. Serologic testing in children is much less sensitive than in adults.[271] In addition, serology cannot be used as a test of cure, because antibody levels tend to remain elevated despite eradication of the organism. The urea breath test has sensitivity and specificity of approximately 95% compared with endoscopic biopsy and can be used to determine eradication.[272] However, the test needs further validation in children < 6 years old.[273]

H. pylori antigen detection in stool has a sensitivity and specificity of about 93%, performs well in children of all ages, and is probably the most convenient test.[268,272] It can be used for follow-up testing starting 8 weeks after completion of therapy.

Combination therapy is required for successful eradication of *H. pylori*. Several regimens are FDA-approved in adults.[268] However, treatment of *H. pylori* infection in children is less well studied.[267] The most commonly used regimen includes omeprazole (1 mg/kg/day divided BID) plus clarithromycin (15 mg/kg/day divided BID) plus either amoxicillin (50 mg/kg/day divided BID) or metronidazole (30 mg/kg/day divided BID). A treatment course of 14 days is recommended.[267]

■ APPENDICITIS AND ABDOMINAL PAIN SYNDROMES

Appendicitis is the most important and most frequent of the severe, treatable, acute abdominal pain syndromes. It is therefore the first diagnosis the clinician should consider in a child with acute abdominal pain. This section goes into considerable detail about appendicitis and its differential diagnosis, with some information of use primarily to the surgeon. However, this material is often a source of discussion between the primary care physician and the surgeon and is not readily available in nonsurgical textbooks.

Appendicitis can be defined in terms of the gross appearance of the appendix as observed at operation or by the microscopic appearance of the appendix as visualized by the pathologist. However, the clinician usually makes a presumptive preoperative diagnosis of appendicitis primarily on the basis of acute abdominal pain with right lower quadrant pain and tenderness, especially with tenderness lateralized to the right on rectal examination.

Appendicitis is relatively common; the lifetime risk is estimated to be between 7% and 9%. The peak incidence occurs between ages 12 and 20 years. In one series, during a 12-month period in Britain, about 1 of every 200 children under 12 years of age in the general population was hospitalized because of abdominal pain.[274] Approximately half of these children had a laparotomy, and most had an appendectomy.[274] In England and Wales in the 1960s, about 1 in every 800 children with appendicitis died, and the mortality rate was eight times higher for children under 5 years of age.[275]

In one study, appendicitis occurred most frequently between 6 and 16 years of age, and the percentage of perforations rose sharply from 20–30% in the 8- to 18-year-olds to 60–80% for children younger than 5 years of age.[276]

Clinical Patterns

Classic Appendicitis

Typically, abdominal pain is the principal symptom. At first, the pain is periumbilical; later, it is localized to the right lower quadrant. Fever is usually slight to moderate, usually less than 38.9°C (102°F). Rectal examination usually confirms tenderness on the right. Generalized abdominal tenderness is not present unless there is perforation and peritonitis, in which case gentle percussion of the abdomen usually reveals exquisite tenderness. In the earlier stages, a moderate tap on the heel of the patient who is lying on the examination table may elicit abdominal pain. Young children can be asked to hop down off the exam table; this maneuver produces pain in patients with peritonitis, but is tolerated by children with nonspecific abdominal pain.

The WBC count is usually 10,000–20,000/mcL. High fever (above 38°C) or leukocytosis greater than 20,000/mcL, if found early in the illness, should make the physician consider another source of infection. Perforation usually induces a profound left shift, causing a bandemia, although the WBC count may be similar to that seen in patients with appendicitis without rupture.[277] Urinalysis may show pyuria secondary to the appendicitis.

Atypical Appendicitis

The clinical diagnosis is much easier to make in older children and adults than in young children and infants, in whom signs and symptoms may be somewhat atypical. In this patient population, pediatricians are likely to misdiagnose acute appendicitis as acute gastroenteritis. Young children are more likely to: (1) have nonlocalizing abdominal symptoms, (2) have misleading signs to another, unrelated illness, and (3) receive antibiotics prior to receiving the diagnosis of appendicitis. The fact that younger children cannot adequately express the extent and character of the abdominal pain also hampers early diagnosis. In preschool children, fever and toxicity may be greater, rectal examination may not be helpful, and perforation occurs earlier.[278,279] In adolescents receiving tetracycline for acne, the clinical manifestations of appendicitis might be milder.[280]

In the newborn with appendicitis, failure to eat well, vomiting, and abdominal distension are usually present, early perforation is common, and the mortality rate is high.[281,282] Involuntary muscle spasm may be found, particularly on the right, or a right-lower-quadrant mass (abscess) may be felt.

Another atypical presentation is a predominance of diarrhea.[283] In this case, the patient is almost always misdiagnosed as having gastroenteritis. However, a careful history will reveal that the amount of diarrhea is not sufficient to account for the degree of toxicity, tachycardia, or hypotension. In one study, one-third of young children had a diarrheal presentation, and a history of diarrhea was independently correlated with a longer hospital stay.[284]

Ruptured Appendix

In reviews of appendicitis in which the appendices had ruptured, the most prominent clinical manifestations, found in more than 75% of the children, were cramping pain, vomiting, nausea, loss of appetite, diffuse abdominal tenderness, guarding, and rebound tenderness.[276,278,279] Rectal tenderness was found in about half of the group. About 5–10% had diarrhea or dysuria.

Diagnostic delay and young age are probably interrelated, because the young child is less likely to have typical symptoms of appendicitis. Of 120 children under the age of 5 in one series, rate of rupture was inversely related to age; all of 10 children under 12 months of age had undergone perforation before the diagnosis of appendicitis was established.[285] The overall rate of perforation was an astounding 74%. Another study showed that the rate of perforated appendicitis was lower in children who were admitted from an emergency department versus from any outlying facility (including general pediatricians' offices).[286] This may also be a result of diagnostic delay; of children who went to their general pediatrician's office first, half were erroneously assigned a diagnosis of acute gastroenteritis.[287]

Predisposing Infections

Any viral disease that produces lymphoid hyperplasia could theoretically produce obstruction of the appendiceal lumen. Influenza, measles, and adenovirus infection can produce lymphoid hyperplasia, and there is a reasonable suspicion that these viruses predispose to appendicitis, although no clear etiologic relationship has been demonstrated statistically. There is some epidemiologic evidence suggesting that common infectious agents may have a part in the development of appendicitis, as some spatiotemporal clustering of cases has been demonstrated.[288] Using fluorescent antibody techniques, adenovirus and coxsackievirus B antigen have been demonstrated in appendices removed at operation.[289]

The most clear-cut relation of a predisposing infection is pinworm infestation, in which the worm may obstruct the appendiceal lumen. Other roundworms can also do this.

Several bacterial species have been found in pure culture in the appendix, but it is not clear that they have any specific causal role. They are probably coincidental findings, although possibly capable of producing inflammatory changes predisposing to obstruction.

There is a slight familial tendency toward having appendicitis, especially if a sibling has had it.[290] Some studies demonstrate an approximately twofold higher risk for Caucasians as compared with African Americans.

It is important to consider appendicitis as a new diagnosis or complication, even if the child is already known to have a disease that can cause abdominal pain.

Infectious Causes of Abdominal Pain

Many infectious diseases can resemble appendicitis and should be included in the differential diagnosis.

Pneumonia

Lower-lobe pneumonia can produce pain that may be mistaken for abdominal pain, and the presence of high fever and leukocytosis may lead the physician to suspect a ruptured appendix.[291] Pleurodynia secondary to coxsackievirus B also may produce pain that may resemble the abdominal pain of appendicitis.[292]

Acute Mesenteric Lymphadenitis

The syndrome of acute mesenteric lymphadenitis is characterized by abdominal pain, tenderness, fever, and vomiting, which leads the surgeon to operate on the patient for possible appendicitis.[293–296] The appendix is normal, but large mesenteric nodes are found. Cultures of these nodes have revealed a variety of pathogens, including beta-hemolytic streptococci, the meningococcus, *Yersinia enterocolitica,* and *Yersinia pseudotuberculosis.*[295–296] This syndrome has also been temporally associated with EBV[297] and adenoviruses.

Acute Salpingitis

A pelvic examination should be done in sexually active adolescent girls with lower abdominal pain. Acute salpingitis can often be diagnosed clinically on the basis of an enlarged tender fallopian tube. Purulent discharge may be present in the cervical os, and a culture for gonococcus should be done. Culture, antigen, or DNA-based testing for *Chlamydia trachomatis* should be done as well. A ruptured tubal pregnancy is typically associated with vaginal bleeding and can usually be excluded by a pregnancy test. Ultrasound examination may be helpful to detect these conditions in sexually active adolescent girls.[298]

Gastroenteritis

Acute viral or bacterial gastroenteritis can be mistaken for appendicitis, particularly early in the illness, before diarrhea is prominent. However, the pain and tenderness are typically generalized rather than localized to the right lower quadrant. *Y. enterocolitica,* described earlier under mesenteric adenitis, is probably the most common cause of gastroenteritis to mimic the symptoms of appendicitis.

Urinary Tract Infection

Urinalysis and culture of a carefully collected urine specimen should be done (see Chapter 14).

Rare Infectious Causes

Hepatitis and Perihepatitis

Abdominal pain caused by liver infection is usually associated with right upper quadrant tenderness (see Chapter 13). Perihepatitis is also called Fitz-Hugh-Curtis syndrome and is principally a disease of sexually active adolescent females (Chapter 15).

Cholecystitis and Cholangitis

Inflammation of the gallbladder with associated infection of the bile ducts is rare in children, but it does occur.[299] Obesity, gallstones, prior pregnancy, a hemolytic disease, leukemia, Crohn's disease, cystic fibrosis, and congenital stenosis of the biliary tract are possible predisposing causes of cholecystitis in children and adolescents. In childhood, cholecystitis appears to be divisible into two distinct syndromes: acute (symptoms for less than 1 month) and chronic (greater than 1 month). In one review of 25 children with cholecystitis, 13 had acute disease. Of the 13 children with *acute* acalculous cholecystitis, 10 (75%) were male, 6 (46%) developed symptoms in an immediate postoperative period, 5 (38%) had an associated systemic illness, and 2 (15%) had *Salmonella* infection.[300] All patients had fever, right-upper-quadrant pain, and emesis. Five (38%) of the 13 had jaundice, and three (23%) had a palpable right-upper-quadrant mass. Most of the patients had leukocytosis, and 8 (62%) had abnormal liver function tests. Ultrasound demonstrated inflammation of the gallbladder wall. By contrast, of 12 children with *chronic* acalculous cholecystitis, 8 (67%) were female. WBC counts and liver function tests were normal in all patients. Symptoms consisted of chronic right-upper-quadrant pain with nausea or vomiting. Cholecystography or HIDA scanning demonstrated gallbladder dysfunction in 9 patients (75%).[300]

Cholangitis can be defined as sepsis in association with biliary tract disease. The condition is rare in children, in whom it is usually a late complication of biliary atresia. However, it can complicate biliary cirrhosis or cholecystitis from any cause,[301] including gallstones or biliary parasites. In children with biliary atresia, recurrent episodes of bacterial cholangitis are common after portoenterostomy (Kasai procedure) and may also occur after liver transplantation.[302] Only 70% of children display all three components—fever, right-upper-quadrant pain, and jaundice—of Charcot's classic triad. In cholangitis in adults, the serum alkaline phosphatase (a sensitive indicator of biliary obstruction) is almost always elevated, but this study is much less useful in children, in whom the alkaline phosphatase usually reflects active bone growth. In children, gamma glutamyl transferase (GGT) is much more useful than alkaline phosphatase as a sensitive indicator of biliary obstruction. The most common organisms causing suppurative cholangitis are *E. coli*, *Enterococcus* spp, *Klebsiella* spp, and gut anaerobes; infections are usually polymicrobial.[303] Blood culture will yield the organism in about half of cases. In one series, percutaneous liver aspirate culture produced an etiologic diagnosis in 40% of the children whose blood cultures were sterile.[304] Treatment involves antimicrobial therapy (e.g., piperacillin/tazobactam or ampicillin/sulbactam or cefotaxime) with drainage of the obstructed biliary tract in severe cases.[305] In patients who develop cholangitis after transplantation, the antimicrobial regimen should include coverage for *P. aeruginosa*.

Ultrasound or computed tomography (CT) scan to exclude hepatic abscess is usually indicated. Operative relief of biliary obstruction is indicated if the response to antibiotic therapy is poor.

Kawasaki disease may be complicated by hydrops of the gallbladder. In some cases, this condition produces extreme abdominal pain and even a "surgical abdomen," although emergency cholecystectomy is rarely, if ever, required. In leukemia, primary gallbladder infections can occur, although they are uncommon. In the largest published report, 5 (1.7%) of 302 children with leukemia were diagnosed with acute acalculous cholecystitis.[306]

Acute Pancreatitis

Acute pancreatitis is much more common in adults than in children. The abdominal pain is intense, of rapid onset, and usually localized to the midline. Vomiting may be severe, and shock may be present. Only about a third of patients are febrile at the time of presentation. The patient may lie on the examination table with knees flexed. Epigastric tenderness and decreased bowel sounds are commonly found. An elevated serum amylase is useful to support the diagnosis provided parotitis is not present, as discussed in the section on parotitis in Chapter 6. Amylase levels correlate poorly with disease severity. Additionally, they may normalize over the first 1–2 days of illness, causing false-negative results. Lipase is more specific for the pancreas, but may be normal over the first day or two of illness. Judicious interpretation of laboratory tests results in correct diagnosis. Although nonspecific, CRP is relatively sensitive in detecting acute pancreatitis; in addition, the CRP value at 48 hours is currently the best available laboratory marker of severity.[306a]

In adults, pancreatitis is usually secondary to alcoholism or biliary disease, whereas in children the causes are more diverse. In one series of 54 children, drugs (such as steroids, thiazides, azathioprine, and tetracycline), trauma, and biliary anomalieswere the most common causes.[307] Antimicrobial agents, especially sulfonamides, erythromycin, rifampin, nitrofurantoin, and metronidazole, occasionally cause acute pancreatitis. Two drugs employed in the care of children with HIVinfection deserve special mention: didanosine (ddI) is a relatively frequent cause of pancreatitis, and pentamidine, used in both prevention and treatment of *Pneumocystis jiroveci* (old name, *carinii*) infection, has been linked to severe and sometimes life-threatening cases. In both children and adults, steroid therapy and postoperative pancreatic duct obstruction may be the cause of acute pancreatitis. Hereditary pancreatitis and cystic fibrosis are rare causes. Children with metabolic diseases may have repeated episodes. Acute pancreatitis may be part of multisystemic vasculitic diseases such as Kawasaki disease, Henoch-Schönlein purpura, and systemic lupus erythematosus. In two series of children with hemolytic-uremic syndrome, 20% of patients developed pancreatitis.[308,309] In many cases of pancreatitis, the cause is not found.[307,310]

When pancreatitis is due to an infectious agent, a virus is almost always to blame. Mumps virus has been thought to be the most common viral cause, based on the fact that about 15% of patients with mumps virus infection suffer from abdominal pain and vomiting, and serum amylase is elevated. The difficulty lies in the fact that serum amylase concentrations are also elevated by parotid inflammation, which is the most obvious symptom of mumps virus infection. Sometimes the abdominal pain antedates the parotid swelling, but the source of the amylase may still be the parotid. It is likely that the importance of pancreatitis as a complication of mumps is overestimated. However, acute necrotizing pancreatitis has been documented at operation in association with unsuspected mumps virus infection.[311] Very few patients have been reported with unsuspected pancreatitis proved by surgery who were later discovered to have mumps virus infection.[311] Because the presence of parotid enlargement or a history of recent mumps exposure is often overlooked, one might expect this to have occurred more often if pancreatitis were really a frequent complication of mumps. A study of serum total amylase, pancreatic isoamylase, and lipase in patients suspected of having pancreatitis indicated that almost all discordant results were due to elevation of the serum total amylase by *salivary* amylase.[312]

Coxsackievirus B has been clearly established as a cause of pancreatitis. The abdominal findings may be accompanied by nonpurulent meningitis, rash, myocarditis, or other symptoms suggestive of coxsackievirus infection. In one study, one-third of patients with nonpurulent meningitis had elevations of serum amylase concentration.[313]

Hepatitis A virus infection is rarely accompanied by pancreatitis. Several viruses of the herpesvirus group have been associated with pancreatic inflammation. Pancreatitis is a rare complication of infectious mononucleosis.[314] One case of pancreatitis occurring with acute varicella zoster virus infection in an apparently immunocompetent child has been reported.[315] In immunocompromised patients, cytomegalovirus can be a cause, as can the antiviral agents used to treat it, including ganciclovir and foscarnet. Adenovirus is a rare cause, especially in bone marrow transplant recipients.

Especially in developing countries, ascariasis is a cause of obstructive pancreatitis. In severely immunocompromised patients, *Cryptosporidium parvum* can be associated with pancreatic disease.

Mycoplasma pneumoniae appears to be a cause of pancreatitis in children,[316] usually in concert with an atypical pneumonia syndrome. The fact that some pancreatic cellular antigenic components may cross react with *Mycoplasma* in serologic tests has caused some confusion about how often *Mycoplasma* infection truly causes pancreatitis.[317]

Exploratory abdominal operation should be avoided if pancreatitis is suspected. Antibiotics or anticholinergic drugs do not appear to alter the course of acute nonnecrotizing pancreatitis.[307] Treatment, therefore, consists of pain control, fluid support, and bowel rest and/or nasogastric suction. Surgery may be required if obstruction is present. This is in contrast to acute necrotizing pancreatitis (diagnosed by CT scan), which has a higher mortality rate and which should be treated with intravenous antibiotics.[318]

Primary Peritonitis

This condition, also referred to as spontaneous bacterial peritonitis, is very uncommon. Children with nephrotic syndrome or ascites for any reason are more susceptible to primary peritonitis, probably because (1) the presence of decreased serum immunoglobulins allows organisms entry to the peritoneal space and (2) the ascitic fluid acts as a culture medium for such bacteria. Primary (spontaneous) peritonitis in children not receiving antibiotics is usually pneumococcal or streptococcal. However, primary peritonitis can be caused by gram-negative enteric bacteria, meningococci, anaerobic bacteria, or *H. influenzae*.[319–321] Tuberculous peritonitis is very rare and can be difficult to diagnose. A history of exposure is usually present.[322]

Therapy of peritonitis should be guided by results of a Gram stain of paracentesis fluid.[319] If no organisms are seen, the initial therapy should be the same as for bowel perforation until culture results are definitive. Exploration of an abdominal perforation may be indicated.[319]

Perirectal Abscess

Rectal tenderness, fever, and leukocytosis may be caused by perirectal abscess.[323] This is rarely mistaken for appendicitis except during the first two years of life, when most cases in childhood occur and the diagnosis of appendicitis is especially difficult. In the older child or adolescent, such perianal disease should alert the physician to consider Crohn's disease and the possibility of necrotizing fasciitis. Treatment includes operative drainage and initial antibiotic therapy such as ticarcillin-clavulanate or piperacillin-tazobactam until culture results are available.

Spinal Infections

Abdominal pain can be produced or simulated by disease of the spine, intervertebral disks, or nerve roots. For example, intravertebral disk infection has produced abdominal pain sufficient to result in operation for appendicitis.[324]

Psoas Abscess

Characteristically, a psoas abscess produces signs and symptoms referable to the hip joint and is discussed in the differential diagnosis of septic arthritis in Chapter 16.

Acute Rheumatic Fever

In rheumatic fever, abdominal pain may be prominent, and the patient may be operated on for suspected appendicitis.[325]

Pharyngitis and Abdominal Pain

Occasionally, streptococcal or nonstreptococcal pharyngitis is associated with abdominal pain. The abdominal pain may be accompanied by vomiting or headache. Ordinarily, the clinical picture is not that of an acute abdomen, and the pharyngitis is readily apparent to the clinician. This association was described by Brenneman in the 1920s,[326] but it has not been adequately studied using modern laboratory methods. Perhaps the mechanism is the concurrence of mesenteric adenitis and pharyngitis due to the same cause, such as an adenovirus or a Group A *Streptococcus*.

Influenza Virus Infection

Outbreaks of influenza infection occasionally include individual children in whom abdominal pain is a prominent symptom.[327,328] This seems to be much more common in infection with influenza B virus.[327] Physicians wish to discourage the use of the lay term *flu* for gastrointestinal diseases, but abdominal pain, vomiting, and diarrhea do occur in some children during influenza virus outbreaks (see Chapter 7).[329]

Abdominal Pain from Other Infections

Pyogenic sacroiliitis,[330] pyomyositis of the rectus abdominis muscle,[331] Rocky Mountain spotted fever,[332] and an infected urachal cyst can cause abdominal pain.[333]

Noninfectious Causes

Intussusception, torsion of the ovary, rupture of a corpus luteal cyst, Henoch-Schönlein purpura, Mittelschmerz, abdominal migraine (cyclic vomiting syndrome), torsion of the greater omentum, juvenile rheumatoid arthritis with systemic onset, abdominal epilepsy, and porphyria are some of the noninfectious causes of acute abdominal pain. Sickle cell anemia can be associated with a sickle cell "crisis" manifested by abdominal pain.

Abdominal myalgia can produce tenderness without prominent myalgia in the muscles of the extremities, as may occur in children who have done strenuous or unusual exercises.

Laboratory Approach

WBC Count and Differential

Nonspecific information is provided by a white cell count, but it is sometimes useful nevertheless. A leukocytosis of more than 20,000/mcL suggests peritonitis, abscess, severe urinary infection, or pneumonia. A WBC count less than 10,000/mcL would raise the question of a viral infection as a cause of the abdominal pain. As mentioned earlier, bandemia is suggestive of perforated appendicitis.[277]

Urinalysis

Urinalysis (and usually culture) should be done in the patient with significant acute abdominal pain.

Abdominal Radiograph

Radiologic findings that are suggestive of appendicitis include a calcified fecalith in the right lower quadrant (rare), an increase in the thickness of the lateral abdominal wall on the right, scoliosis secondary to pain, paucity of bowel gas in the right lower abdomen, dilated transverse colon, and obscuration of the psoas shadow. The film might reveal a lower-lobe pneumonia if part of the chest is included. In actual clinical practice, the abdominal plain film suffers from a lack of sensitivity and specificity. In one large study, 268 (51%) of 525 patients with acute appendicitis had an abnormal abdominal x-ray; however, so did 139 (47%) of 296 patients without appendicitis. Additionally, in 82 (10%) of patients, the x-ray suggested a diagnosis, but in 47 (57%) of these cases, the diagnosis turned out to be incorrect. Ultimately, at a cost of $67 per film, the cost of one correct diagnosis of appendicitis made by plain film exceeded $1500.[334] Thus, in a patient with a classic presentation of appendicitis, proceeding directly to appendectomy is reasonable; if the diagnosis is in doubt, CT is probably the most reliable imaging study.

Barium Enema

A barium enema was advocated in the 1970s as a radiologic aid to the diagnosis of acute appendicitis. However, ultrasound and CT scanning have generally replaced this procedure for patients with a higher risk of having an operation, such as those with a bleeding problem.

Ultrasound and CT Scans

Graded compression ultrasound is now widely used to establish the diagnosis of appendicitis. The technique is so named because the examiner gradually adds increasing amounts of pressure with the transducer, which moves gas and fluid out of overlying bowel loops, maximizing the diagnostic utility of the procedure. This imaging modality has a sensitivity of 75% or above and a specificity of above 85% for establishing the diagnosis of acute appendicitis.[335] Non-contrasted helical CT scanning is another excellent test for visualizing acute appendiceal abnormalities. In one study of 443 patients who underwent CT scanning when acute appendicitis was suspected, the false-positive rate of CT was only 5%. Additionally, 243 (93%) of 260 patients with negative CT scanning were able to be discharged home. In 20%, the scan not only ruled out appendicitis, but also established an alternate diagnosis.[336] In a head-to-head comparison of graded compression ultrasound with helical CT scanning, the sensitivity of CT was 95% versus 78% for ultrasound. The specificity was 93% for both. Of 82 patients who underwent both ultrasound and CT scanning, the results were discordant in 20; the CT scan established the correct diagnosis in 17 (85%) of these.[337]

Appendicitis Management

Fluids

Intravenous fluid therapy for correction of dehydration has a high priority before operation and should be begun early in the evaluation of a child with suspected appendicitis. This is an important role for the primary care physician, who should obtain surgical consultation at an appropriately early time. The primary care physician is likely to be familiar with abdominal pain patterns in preschool children, can observe the patient through the early part of the illness, and can help recognize the atypical presentation described in young children.

Surgery

The surgeon will determine the techniques in the operation, but the primary care physician can dose the preoperative and postoperative antibiotics. The laparoscopic approach to patients with uncomplicated acute appendicitis has been used successfully in adult patients for quite a few years; its use in children was less popular because of a perception that operative complication risk would be higher. A prospective study compared the complication rate of 362 children who underwent conventional open laparotomy with 138 who underwent the laparoscopic procedure: the incidence of major complications was 3% in open and zero in laparoscopic,

and of minor complications was 20% in open and 15% in laparoscopic patients.[338] Unfortunately, without good randomization, selection bias is likely to affect the outcomes, because sicker patients would be relegated to the open appendectomy group.

There is considerable controversy about whether drains should be left in place after surgery for a ruptured appendix. Studies seem to indicate that drains may be beneficial in certain situations but harmful in others. One study showed that placement of a drain decreased postoperative complications only if symptoms had been present for at least 5 days prior to surgery.[339] In a prospective, randomized study, however, peritoneal lavage proved to be superior to tube drainage in length of hospitalization, duration of fever, and the duration of fasting required after surgery.[340] The number of postoperative wound infections was also higher in the tube drainage group.

Nonoperative Management ("Interval Appendectomy")

The practice of delaying surgery (treating with bed rest, intravenous antibiotics, and fluids and then performing "elective appendectomy" 4–8 weeks later) for children in whom the appendix has already ruptured has been a source of controversy. One study found that percutaneous drainages of an appendiceal abscess with interval appendectomy resulted in a lower complication rate and a shorter hospital stay.[341] Another study found that outcomes with interval appendectomy for perforated appendicitis were comparable to that of immediate appendectomy in a select group of children.[342] The authors recommend interval appendectomy for patients who present with little or no signs of peritonitis, only slightly elevated temperature, and a WBC count that falls by at least 25% within 3–4 days.

In contrast to the situation in which the appendix has already rupture, a patient with appendicitis in which the appendix has not rupture should be taking to operating room immediately. There is no role for 24–48 hours of antibiotics to "cool down" the appendix; such delay only leads to an increased risk of perforation or peritonitis.

Antibiotic Therapy

Preoperative antibiotics should be added to the intravenous fluids when the operating room is scheduled. If the appendix is not perforated, the antibiot-

TABLE 12-5. GUIDELINES FOR INITIATION AND DURATION OF ANTIBIOTIC THERAPY OF APPENDICITIS

CLINICAL SITUATION	RECOMMENDED TREATMENT
Abdominal pain; being observed for appendicitis	No antibiotics
In operating room, awaiting appendectomy	Begin IV antibiotics
Appendix visualized; nongangrenous, not perforated	24–48 hours of IV antibiotics
Gangrenous appendix, without perforation	48–72 hours of IV antibiotics; discontinue when patient is afebrile and able to eat
Perforated appendix	Minimum of 5 days of IV antibiotics and until normalization of temperature and WBC count and return of gastrointestinal function

ics can be stopped at 24–48 hours.[343] If the appendix is perforated, antibiotic therapy should be continued 5–10 days, depending on the patient's clinical course (see Table 12-5).[344]

For preoperative therapy, a single agent with activity against anaerobes (e.g., ampicillin-sulbactam or ticarcillin-clavulanate) may be used. If the appendix is ruptured, many surgeons use ampicillin, gentamicin, and clindamycin (or metronidazole) and may use this combination for initial therapy.[276,342–345] Prospective studies have shown that either ticarcillin-clavulanate plus gentamicin[346] or ticarcillin-clavulanate as a single agent is at least as effective as triple therapy.[347] The antibiotic regimen can be adjusted according to the sensitivities of organisms from peritoneal, abscess, or drainage cultures.

Intraperitoneal Antibiotics

Most antibiotics penetrate the peritoneal space, so that they need not be added to the irrigation fluid at operation. Indeed, some antibiotics can be absorbed and reach toxic concentrations if large doses are given intraperitoneally. Currently, most surgeons irrigate with saline.

Appendicitis Complications

Perforation occurs more frequently in preschool children. Peritonitis usually occurs early after perforation. Appendiceal abscess is more likely to be present if the illness has been modified by previous antibiotics. Diagnostic ultrasound or CT scan may be useful in detecting appendiceal or other intraabdominal abscesses.

Chronic or Recurrent Appendicitis

This diagnosis was used excessively in the past, so that its use is typically regarded now with great suspicion and skepticism. Nevertheless, chronic or recurrent appendicitis occasionally occurs.[348,349] If the recurrent pain localizes to the right lower quadrant, imaging studies should be obtained.

■ ABDOMINAL ABSCESSES

Abdominal abscesses can occur in a variety of locations, usually detected now by ultrasonography or CT scanning. The special features and treatment will be discussed for each location. Perirectal abscess is discussed in the preceding section on abdominal pain and in the section on abscesses in Chapter 17.

Predisposing Situations

Abdominal abscess is suspected in many situations where there is fever, leukocytosis, abdominal tenderness or mass, and a predisposing situation such as perforated gut, penetrating abdominal trauma, or bacteremia.

Radiographic Studies

CT scanning and ultrasonography are the usual way abdominal abscesses are localized, except for postoperative appendiceal abscess. CT appears to be more sensitive than ultrasonography in most situations, except perhaps for diagnosis of tuboovarian abscesses.[350]

Percutaneous Aspiration

Using CT or ultrasonography, many intraabdominal abscesses can be drained percutaneously, even in children.[351] Most abscesses should be drained using either an open procedure or percutaneously, although some surgeons prefer to administer antibiotic therapy for a day or two first to "cool off" the process.

Liver Abscesses

Liver abscess is rare in children compared with adults. In children, it generally occurs in the compromised host who has a malignancy, has had previous surgery, or has a bacteremia.[352] Fever, abdominal pain, and hepatomegaly are typically found.[353] Liver abscesses can be classified as pyogenic, amebic, or fungal.

Pyogenic Liver Abscess

In nonimmunocompromised children, the most frequent organism is *S. aureus*, but enteric aerobic and anaerobic bacteria may be found.[354,355] Typically, there is a marked leukocytosis and elevation of the erythrocyte sedimentation rate.

Liver abscess can occur in the newborn infant, especially as a complication of umbilical vein catheterization.[356] Sickle cell disease can present with a pyogenic liver abscess.[357] Liver abscess may also be associated with Crohn's disease.[358] In developing countries, helminthic infections are a common comorbidity.[359] Immunologic changes caused by the parasitic infection may make patients prone to develop abscesses during episodes of bacteremia.[360] Diabetes mellitus is a risk factor for liver abscess due to *Klebsiella pneumoniae*.[361]

Antibiotic therapy to cover the preceding possible causes (and also amebae) may be appropriate before drainage in some cases (e.g., in the patient with fever, toxicity, and possible bacteremia). Ceftriaxone with metronidazole is one reasonable regimen. For newborns, ampicillin and cefotaxime is reasonable, as anaerobes and amebiasis are unlikely. Ultimately, ultrasound-guided percutaneous drainage and intravenous antibiotics, reserving surgical resection for those failing to respond, is the treatment of choice.[362] Large, solitary, left-sided abscesses are more likely to require surgical drainage.[363]

Amebic Liver Abscess

Usually, amebic disease is known to be present in the geographic area or subpopulation.[364] In a review of 124 reported children with amebic liver abscess, 113 (91%) were less than 3 years old, and most had hepatomegaly, leukocytosis, and anemia.[365] A series of 48 children with amebic liver abscess confirmed that anemia is common by demonstrating that 45 (94%) of the patients had a hemoglobin level less than 10 g/dL. Growth failure (defined as below the 5th percentile for both height and weight) was found in 37 (77%).[366] Amebae often are not found in the stool, but serologic tests (usually available in endemic areas) may be positive.[367] Newer diagnostic tests such as PCR[368] and an ELISA for detecting salivary antibody[369] are being studied.

Treatment consists of metronidazole first, followed by aspiration if indicated for large abscesses or those that fail to improve after 72 hours of metronidazole.[370] Open operation is rarely indicated.[365,371] Rupture of the abscess can occur into the chest or abdomen, and surgery should be required only for secondary bacterial complications.[371] In 5 (33%) of 15 cases of rupture in one series, the patient was thought to have a ruptured appendix.[371]

After the abscess is cured, eradication of bowel parasites with paromomycin or iodoquinol is recommended.[365]

Fungal Liver Abscess

Usually, the child has been treated with many courses of antibiotics because of possible septicemia and has underlying problems of prematurity, an immunosuppressive disease, and a central venous catheter. *Candida albicans* is the most common organism, especially in premature infants, but *Aspergillus* or another fungus may occur in the immunosuppressed patient.

Nonhepatic Abscesses

Pancreatic Abscess

Most pancreatic abscesses are infections in a pancreas damaged by pancreatitis.[372]

Splenic Abscess

The usual predisposing causes in splenic abscesses are trauma or embolization from a septic focus, such as an infected intravenous line. Multiple small splenic abscesses may occur in immunodeficient hosts.[373] In severely immunocompromised hosts, splenic abscesses are usually considered fungal until proven otherwise, especially if they are multiple and widespread. In patients with fever and neutropenia, an underlying diagnosis of relapsed leukemia and positive surveillance ("colonization") cultures for *Candida* are risk factors for the development of splenic abscesses (usually in association (see Chapter 22).[374] Splenic abscess can also occur following nonoperative management of splenic trauma.[375] Splenic abscess rarely follows colonic perforation secondary to dysentery.[376]

When multiple small abscesses are found in previously well patients with fever or other nonspecific signs as the primary clinical manifestations, cat-scratch disease is a likely diagnosis in areas endemic for this infection.[377]

Subphrenic Abscess

This may occur as a complication of any contaminated intraabdominal operation. It may also be a result of gallstones "spilled" into the abdomen during laparoscopic cholecystectomy.[378] The chest roentgenogram typically shows unilateral pleural effusion, elevated hemidiaphragm, and atelectasis. Fluoroscopy of the diaphragm is the best screening procedure and typically shows decreased excursion on the involved side.[379] In the past, the usual predisposing cause was appendicitis, but recently, surgery of the colon and trauma have become the most important risk factors.

A 22-month-old child who presented with signs and symptoms suggestive of pneumonia but who proved to have a subphrenic abscess has been reported.[380] No obvious predisposing condition could be found.

Suprarenal Abscess

This location for an abscess will raise concern about a possible suprarenal malignancy. Preoperatively, CT scanning will define whether the abscess is perinephric or adrenal. Adrenal abscesses can occur in newborn and young infants, and may be due to Group B streptococcus.[381,382]

■ REFERENCES

1. Hodgkin K. Towards earlier diagnosis: a family doctor's approach. Baltimore: Williams & Wilkins, 1963.
1a. Chang HH, Glass RI, Smith PF, et al. Disease burden and risk factors for hospitalizations associated with rotavirus infection among children in New York State, 1989 through 2000. Pediatr Infect Dis J 2003;22:808–14
1b. Allos BM, Moore MR, Griffin PM, Tauxe RV. Surveillance for sporadic foodborne disease in the 21st century: the FoodNet perspective. Clin Infect Dis 2004;38S115–20.
2. Pickering LK, Evans DG, DuPont HL, et al. Diarrhea caused by *Shigella*, rotavirus, and *Giardia* in daycare centers: prospective study. Pediatrics 1981;99:51–6.
3. Guerrant RL, Lohr JA, Williams EK. Acute infectious diarrhea I: epidemiology, etiology and pathogenesis. Pediatr Infect Dis 1986;5:353–9.
4. San Joaquin VH, Marks MI. New agents in diarrhea. Pediatr Infect Dis 1982;1:53–65.
5. Thacker SB, Addiss DG, Goodman RA, Holloway BR, Spencer HC. Infectious diseases and injuries in a child day care: opportunities for healthier children. JAMA 1992;268:1720–6
6. Reves RR, Morrow AL, Bartlett AV, et al. Child day care increases the risk of clinic visits for acute diarrhea and diarrhea due to rotavirus. Am J Epidemiol 1993;137:97–107.
7. Churchill RB, Pickering LK. Infection control challenges in child-care centers. Infect Dis Clin North Am 1997;11:347–65.
8. Steinberg EB, Greene KD, Bopp CA, et al. Cholera in the United States, 1995–2000: trends at the end of the twentieth century. J Infect Dis 2001;184:799–802.
9. World Health Organization. World Health Report 2000. Health systems: improving performance. Geneva, WHO, 2000:164.
10. Pitzinger B, Steffen R, Tschopp A. Incidence and clinical features of traveler's diarrhea in infants and children. Pediatr Infect Dis J 1991;10:719–23.
11. Hostetter MK. Epidemiology of travel-related morbidity and mortality in children. Pediatr Rev 1999;20:228–33.
12. Moffet HL, Doyle HS, Burkholder EG. The epidemiology and etiology of acute infantile diarrhea. J Pediatr 1968;72:1–14.
13. Bishop RF, Davidson GP, Holmes IH, Ruck BJ. Virus particles in epithelial cells of duodenal mucosa from children with acute non-bacterial gastroenteritis. Lancet 1973;2:1281–3.
14. Glass RI, Kilgore PE, Holman RC, et al. The epidemiology of rotavirus diarrhea in the United States: surveillance and estimates of disease burden. J Infect Dis 1996;174 Suppl 1:S5–11.
15. Katyal R, Rana SV, Singh K. Rotavirus infections. Acta Virol 2000;44:283–8.
16. Pager C, Steele D, Gwamanda P, Driessen M. A neonatal death associated with rotavirus infection—detection of rotavirus dsRNA in the cerebrospinal fluid. S Afr Med J 2000;90:364–5.
17. Pérez-Schael I, Guntiñas MJ, Pérez M, et al. Efficacy of the rhesus rotavirus-based quadrivalent vaccine in infants and young children in Venezuela. N Engl J Med 1997;337:1181–7.

18. Murphy TV, Gargiullo PM, Massoudi MS, et al. Intussusception among infants given an oral rotavirus vaccine. N Engl J Med 2001;344:564–72.

19. Centers for Disease Control and Prevention. Withdrawal of rotavirus vaccine recommendation. JAMA 1999;282:2113–4.

19a. Clark HF, Berstein DI, Dennehy PH, et al. Safety efficacy, and immunogenicity of a live, quadrivalent human-bovine reassortantrotavirus vaccine in healthy infants. J Pediatr 2004;144:184–90

19b. Bernstein DI, Sack, DA, Rothstein E, et al. Efficacy of live, attenuated, human rotavirus vaccine 89–12 in infants: a randomized placebo-controlled trial. Lancet 1999;354–287–90.

20. Mounts AW, Ando T, Koopmans M, et al. Cold weather seasonality of gastroenteritis associated with Norwalk-like viruses. J Infect Dis 2000;181:S284–7.

21. Guerrero ML, Noel JS, Mitchell DK, et al. A prospective study of astrovirus diarrhea of infancy in Mexico City. Pediatr Infect Dis J 1998;17:723–7.

22. Pang XL, Vesikari T. Human astrovirus-associated gastroenteritis in children under 2 years of age followed prospectively during a rotavirus vaccine trial. Acta Pediatr 1999;88:532–6.

23. Walter JE, Mitchell DK, Guerrero ML. Molecular epidemiology of human astrovirus diarrhea among children from a periurban community of Mexico City. J Infect Dis 2001;183:681–6.

24. Rodriguez-Baez N, O'Brien R, Qiu SQ, Bass DM. Astrovirus, adenovirus, and rotavirus in hospitalized children: prevalence and association with gastroenteritis. J Pediatr Gastroenterol Nutr 2002;35:64–8.

25. Marie-Cardine A, Gourlain K, Mouterde O, et al. Epidemiology of acute viral gastroenteritis in children hospitalized in Rouen, France. Clin Infect Dis 2002;34:1170–8.

26. Uhnoo I, Wadell G, Svensson L, Johansson ME. Importance of enteric adenoviruses 40 and 41 in acute gastroenteritis in infants and young children. J Clin Microbiol 1984;20:365–72.

27. Kotloff KL, Losonsky GA, Morris JG Jr, et al. Enteric adenovirus infection and childhood diarrhea: an epidemiologic study in three clinical settings. Pediatrics 1989;84:219–25.

28. Wright PF, Ross KB, Thompson J, Karzon DT. Influenza A infections in young children. Primary natural infection and protective efficacy of live-vaccine-induced or naturally acquired immunity. N Engl J Med 1977;296:829–34.

29. Lawrence DN, Blake PA, Yashuk JC, et al. Vibrio parahaemolyticus gastroenteritis outbreaks aboard two cruise ships. Am J Epidemiol 1979;109:71–80.

30. Lowenstein MS. Epidemiology of Clostridium perfringens food poisoning. N Engl J Med 1972;286:1026–8.

31. DuPont HL, Hornick SB, Dawkins AT, et al. Pathogenesis of Escherichia coli diarrhea. N Engl J Med 1971;285:1–9.

32. Nazer H, Prince EH, Hunt GH, et al. Clinical associations of Aeromonas spp. in fecal specimens from children. Clin Pediatr 1986;25:516–9.

33. Challapalli M, Tess BR, Cunningham DG, Chopra AK, Houston CW. Aeromonas-associated diarrhea in children. Pediatr Infect Dis J 1988;7:693–8.

34. Rahman AFMS, Willoughby JMT. Dysentery-like syndrome associated with Aeromonas hydrophila. Br Med J 1982;218:976.

35. Rodriquez WJ, Controni G, Cohen GJ, et al. Yersinia enterocolitica enteritis in children. JAMA 1979;242:1978–80.

36. Marks MI, Pai CH, Lafleur L, et al. Yersinia enterocolitica gastroenteritis: a prospective study of clinical, bacteriologic, and epidemiologic features. J Pediatr 1980;96:26–31.

37. Kohl S. Yersinia enterocolitica infections in children. Pediatr Clin North Am 1979;26:433–43.

38. Ostroff SM, Kapperud G, Lassen J, et al. Clinical features of sporadic Yersinia enterocolitica infections in Norway. J Infect Dis 1992;166:812–7.

39. Lee LA, Gerber AR, Lonsway DR, et al. Yersinia enterocolitica O:3 infections in infants and children associated with the household preparation of chitterlings. N Engl J Med 1990;322:984–7.

40. Holmberg SD, Wachsmuth IK, Hickman-Brenner FW, et al. Pleisiomonas enteric infections in the United States. Ann Intern Med 1986;105:690–4.

41. Kain KC, Kelly MT. Clinical features, epidemiology, and treatment of Plesiomonas shigelloides diarrhea. J Clin Microbiol 1989;27:998–1001.

42. Visitsunthorn N, Komolpis P. Antimicrobial therapy in Plesiomonas shigelloides-associated diarrhea in Thai children. Southeast Asian J Trop Med Public Health 1995;26:86–90.

43. DuPont HL, Hornick RB, Dawkins AT, et al. The response of man to virulent Shigella flexneri 2a. J Infect Dis 1969;199:296–9.

44. Gorden J, Small PLC. Acid resistance in enteric bacteria. Infect Immun 1993;61:364–7.

45. Centers for Disease Control and Prevention. Day care-related outbreaks for rhamnose-negative Shigella sonnei—six states, June 2001–March 2003. MMWR 2004;53:60–3.

46. Davis H, Taylor JP, Perdue JN, et al. A shigellosis outbreak traced to commercially distributed shredded lettuce. Am J Epidemiol 1988;128:1312–21.

47. Martin DL, Gustafson TL, Pelosi JW, et al. Contaminated produce—a common source for two outbreaks of Shigella gastroenteritis. Am J Epidemiol 1986;124:299–305.

48. Naimi TS, Wicklund JH, Olsen SJ, et al. Concurrent outbreaks of Shigella sonnei and enterotoxigenic Escherichia coli infections associated with parsley: implications for surveillance and control of foodborne illness. J Food Prot 2003;66:535–41.

49. Centers for Disease Control and Prevention. Shigellosis outbreak associated with an unchlorinated fill-and-drain wading pool—Iowa, 2001. MMWR 2001;50:797–800.

50. Townes JM, Quick R, Gonzales OY, et al. Etiology of bloody diarrhea in Bolivian children: implications for empiric therapy. J Infect Dis 1997;175:1527–30.

51. Miron D, Sochotnick I, Yardeni D, et al. Surgical complications of shigellosis in children. Pediatr Infect Dis J 2000;19:898–900.

52. Sansonetti PJ, Tran Van Nhieu G, Egile C. Rupture of the intestinal epithelial barrier and mucosal invasion by Shigella flexneri. Clin Infect Dis 1999;28:466–75.

53. Duncan B, Fulginiti VA, Sieber OF, et al. Shigella sepsis. Am J Dis Child 1981;135:151–4.

54. Raqib R, Mia SM, Qadri F, et al. Innate immune responses

in children and adults with shigellosis. Infect Immun 2000;68:3620–9.

55. Way SS, Borezuk AC, Dominitz R, Goldberg MB. An essential role for gamma interferon in innate resistance to *Shigella flexneri* infection. Infect Immun 1998;66: 1342–8.

56. Rettig PJ. *Campylobacter* infections in human beings. J Pediatr 1979;94:855–64.

57. Torphy D, Bond WW. *Campylobacter fetus* infections in children. Pediatrics 1979;46:898–903.

58. Karmali MR, Fleming PC. *Campylobacter* enteritis in children. J Pediatr 1979;94:527–33.

59. Solomon NH, Lavie S, Teeney BL, et al. *Campylobacter* enteritis presenting with convulsions. Clin Pediatr 1982; 21:118–9.

60. Melamed I, Bujanover Y, Igra YS, et al. *Campylobacter* enteritis in normal and immunodeficient children. Am J Dis Child 1983;137:752–3.

61. Effler P, Ieong MC, Kimura A, et al. Sporadic *Campylobacter jejuni* infections in Hawaii: associations with prior antibiotic use and commercially prepared chicken. J Infect Dis 2001;183:1152–5.

62. Allos BM. *Campylobacter jejuni* infections: update on emerging issues and trends. Clin Infect Dis 2001;32: 1201–6.

63. Fang SB, Lee HC, Chang PY, Wang NL. Colonic perforation in two children with *Campylobacter* enterocolitis. Eur J Pediatr 2000;159:714–5.

64. Carvalho AC, Ruiz-Palacios GM, Romaos-Cervantes P, et al. Molecular characterization of invasive and non-invasive *Campylobacter jejuni* and *Campylobacter coli* isolates. J Clin Microbiol 2001;39:1353–9.

65. Kramer JM, Frost JA, Bolton FJ, Wareing DR. *Campylobacter* contamination of raw meat and poultry at retail sale: identification of multiple types and comparison with isolates from human infection. J Food Prot 2000;63: 1654–9.

66. Cogan TA, Bloomfield SF, Humphrey TJ. The effectiveness of hygiene procedures for prevention of cross-contamination from chicken carcasses in the domestic kitchen. Lett Appl Microbiol 1999;29:354–8.

67. Centers for Disease Control and Prevention. Preliminary FoodNet data on the incidence of infection with pathogens transmitted commonly through food–selected sites, United States, 2003. MMWR 2004;53:338–43.

68. Olson SJ, Bishop R, Brenner FW, et al. The changing epidemiology of *Salmonella*: trends in serotypes isolated from humans in the United States, 1987–1997. J Infect Dis 2001;183:753–61.

68a. Mermin J. Hutwagner L, Vugia D, et al. Reptiles, amphibians, and human *Salmonella* infection: a population-based, case-control study. Clin Infect Dis 2004;38: S253–61.

69. Campbell JV, Mohle-Boetani J, Reporter R, et al. An outbreak of *Salmonella* serotype Thompson associated with fresh cilantro. J Infect Dis 2001;183:984–7.

70. Burnett SL, Gehm ER, Weissinger WR, Beuchat LR. Survival of *Salmonella* in peanut butter and peanut butter spread. J Appl Microbiol 2000;89:472–7.

71. Weissinger WR, Chantarapanont W, Beuchat LR. Survival and growth of *Salmonella baildon* in shredded lettuce and diced tomatoes, and effectiveness of chlorinated water as a sanitizer. Int J Food Microbiol 2000;62: 123–31.

72. Sarwari AR, Magder LS, Levine P, et al. Serotype distribution of *Salmonella* isolates from food animals after slaughter differs from that of isolates found in humans. J Infect Dis 2001;183:1295–9.

73. Mermin J, Hoar B, Angulo FJ. Iguanas and *Salmonella marina* infection in children: a reflection of the increasing incidence of reptile-associated salmonellosis in the United States. Pediatrics 1997; 99:399–402.

74. Zhou D, Chen LM, Hernandez L, et al. A *Salmonella* inositol polyphosphatase acts in conjunction with other bacterial effectors to promote host cell actin cytoskeleton rearrangements and bacterial internalization. Mol Microbiol 2001;39:248–59.

75. Torrey S, Fleisher G, Jaffe D. Incidence of *Salmonella* bacteremia in infants with *Salmonella* gastroenteritis. J Pediatr 1986;108:718–21.

76. Taylor DN, Bopp C, Birkness K, et al. An outbreak of salmonellosis associated with a fatality in a healthy child: a large dose and severe illness. Am J Epidemiol 1984; 119:907–12.

77. Novak R, Feldman S. Salmonellosis in children with cancer. Am J Dis Child 1979;133:298–300.

78. Parry CM, Hien TT, Dougan G, White NJ, Farrar JJ. Typhoid fever. N Engl J Med 2002;347:1770–82.

79. Lo Re V III, Gluckman SJ. Travel immunizations. Am Fam Physician 2004;70:89–99.

80. Begier EM, Burwen DR, Haber P, Ball R. Postmarketing safety surveillance for typhoid fever vaccines from the Vaccine Adverse Event Reporting System. July 1990 through June 2002. Clin Infect Dis 2004;38:77–9.

81. Boyce TG, Swerdlow DL, Griffin PM. Shiga toxin–producing *Escherichia coli* infections and the hemolytic uremic syndrome. Semin Pediatr Infect Dis 1996;7:258–64.

82. Griffin PM, Boyce TG. *Escherichia coli* O157:H7. In Scheld WM, Armstrong D, Hughes JM, eds. Emerging infections I. Washington, DC: American Society for Microbiology, 1998:137–45.

83. Gerber A, Karch H, Allerberger F, Verweyen HM, Zimmerhackl LB. Clinical course and the role of shiga toxin-producing *Escherichia coli* infection in the hemolytic-uremic syndrome in pediatric patients, 1997–2000, in Germany and Austria: a prospective study. J Infect Dis 2002; 186:493–500.

84. Mead PS, Slutsker L, Dietz V, et al. Food-related illness and death in the United States. Emerg Infect Dis 1999; 5:607–25.

85. Boyce TG, Swerdlow DL, Griffin PM. *Escherichia coli* O157:H7 and the hemolytic-uremic syndrome. N Engl J Med 1995;333:364–8.

86. Hilborn ED, Mshar PA, Fiorentino TR, et al. An outbreak of *Escherichia coli* O157:H7 infections and hemolytic uremic syndrome associated with consumption of unpasteurized apple cider. Epidemiol Infect 2000;124:31–6.

87. Dingman DW. Prevalence of *Escherichia coli* in apple cider manufactured in Connecticut. J Food Prot 1999;62: 567–73.

88. Jackson LA, Keene WE, McAnulty JM, et al. Where's the beef? The role of cross-contamination in 4 chain-restaurant-associated outbreaks of *Escherichia coli* O157:H7 in

the Pacific Northwest. Arch Intern Med 2000;160: 2380–5.

89. Michino H, Araki K, Minami S, et al. Massive outbreak of Escherichia coli O157:H7 infection in schoolchildren in Sakai City, Japan, associated with consumption of white radish sprouts. Am J Epidemiol 1999;150:787–96.

90. Kobayashi M, Sasaki T, Saito N, et al. Houseflies: not simple mechanical vectors of enterohemorrhagic Escherichia coli O157:H7. Am J Trop Med Hyg 1999;61:625–9.

91. Swerdlow DL, Woodruff BA, Brady RC, et al. A waterborne outbreak in Missouri of Escherichia coli O157:H7 associated with bloody diarrhea and death. Ann Int Med 1992;117:812–9.

92. Keene WE, McAnulty JM, Hoesly FC, et al. A swimming-associated outbreak of hemorrhagic colitis caused by Escherichia coli O157:H7 and Shigella sonnei. N Engl J Med 1994;331:579–84.

93. Centers for Disease Control and Prevention. Surveillance for waterborne-disease outbreaks—United States, 1999–2000. MMWR 2002;51(no. SS-8).

94. Belongia EA, Osterholm MT, Soler JT, et al. Transmission of Escherichia coli O157:H7 infection in Minnesota child day-care facilities. JAMA 1993;269:883–8.

95. Ikeda K, Ida O, Kimoto K, et al. Predictors for the development of hemolytic uremic syndrome with Escherichia coli O157:H7 infections: with focus on the day of illness. Epidemiol Infect 2000;124:343–9.

96. Buteau C, Proulx F, Chaibou M, et al. Leukocytosis in children with Escherichia coli O157:H7 enteritis developing the hemolytic-uremic syndrome. Pediatr Infect Dis J 2000;19:642–7.

96a. Siegler RL, Pavia AT, Christofferson RD, Milligan MK. A 20-year population-based study of postdiarrheal hemolytic uremic syndrome in Utah. Pediatrics 1994;94: 35–40.

97. Wong CS, Jelacic S, Habeeb RL, et al. The risk of hemolytic-uremic syndrome after antibiotic treatment of Escherichia coli O157:H7 infections. N Engl J Med 2000;342: 1930–6.

98. Boyce TG, Pemberton AG, Wells JG, Griffin PM. Screening for Escherichia coli O157:H7—a nationwide survey of clinical laboratories. J Clin Microbiol 1995;33:3275–7.

99. Klein EJ, Stapp JR, Clausen CR, et al. Shiga toxin-producing Escherichia coli in children with diarrhea: a prospective point-of-care study. J Pediatr 2002;141:172–7.

100. Bartlett JG. Antibiotic-associated diarrhea. N Engl J Med 2002;346:334–9.

101. Kader HA, Piccoli DA, Jawad AF, et al. Single toxin detection is inadequate to diagnose Clostridium difficile diarrhea in pediatric patients. Gastroenterology 1998;115: 1329–34.

102. Elstner CL, Lindsay AN, Book LS, et al. Lack of relationship of Clostridium difficile to antibiotic-associated diarrhea in children. Pediatr Infect Dis 1983;2:364–6.

103. Jarvis WR, Feldman RA. Clostridium difficile and gastroenteritis: how strong is the association in children? Pediatr Infect Dis 1984;3:4–6.

104. Boenning DA, Fleisher GR, Campos JM, et al. Clostridium difficile in a pediatric outpatient population. Pediatr Infect Dis 1982;1:336–8.

105. Viscidi R, Willey S, Bartlett JG. Isolation rates and toxigenic potential of Clostridium difficile isolates from various patient populations. Gastroenterology 1981;81:5–9.

106. Thomas DF, Fernie DS, Malone M, et al. Association between Clostridium difficile and enterocolitis in Hirschsprung's disease. Lancet 1982;1:78–9.

107. Dykes AC, Ruebush TK II, Gorelkin L, et al. Extraintestinal amebiasis in infancy: report of three patients and epidemiologic investigations of their families. Pediatrics 1980;65:799–803.

108. Brooks JL, Kozarek RM. Amebic colitis: preventing morbidity and mortality from fulminant disease. Postgrad Med 1985;78:267–74.

109. Haque R, Huston CD, Hughes M, Houpt E, Petri WA Jr. Amebiasis. N Engl J Med 2003;348:1565–73.

110. Leung AK, Robson WL. Evaluating the child with chronic diarrhea. Am Fam Physician 1996;53:635–43.

111. Branski D, Lerner A, Lebenthal E. Chronic diarrhea and malabsorption. Pediatr Clin North Am 1996;43:307–31.

112. Donowitz M, Kokke FT, Saidi R. Evaluation of patients with chronic diarrhea. N Engl J Med 1995;332:725–9.

113. Baldassano RN, Liacouras CA. Chronic diarrhea: a practical approach for the pediatrician. Pediatr Clin North Am 1991;38:667–86.

114. McFarland LV, Elmer GW, Surawicz CM. Breaking the cycle: treatment strategies for 163 cases of recurrent Clostridium difficile disease. Am J Gastroenterol 2002;97: 1769–75.

115. Surawicz CM, McFarland LV, Greenberg RN, et al. The search for a better treatment for recurrent Clostridium difficile disease: use of high-dose vancomycin combined with Saccharomyces boulardii. Clin Infect Dis 2000;31: 1012–7.

116. Krogstad DJ, Spencer HC Jr, Healy GR. Amebiasis. N Engl J Med 1978;298:262–5.

117. Merritt RJ, Coughlin E, Thomas DW, et al. Spectrum of amebiasis in children. Am J Dis Child 1982;136:785–9.

118. Patterson M, Schoppe LE. The presentation of amoebiasis. Med Clin North Am 1982;66:689–705.

119. Haque R, Mollah NU, Ali IK, et al. Diagnosis of amebic liver abscess and intestinal infection with the TechLab Entamoeba histolytica II antigen detection and antibody tests. Clin Microbiol 2000;38:3235–9.

120. DuPont HL, Sullivan PS. Giardiasis: the clinical spectrum, diagnosis and therapy. Pediatr Infect Dis 1986;5:S131–8.

121. Craft JC. Giardia and giardiasis in children. Pediatr Infect Dis 1982;1:196–211.

122. Hoque ME, Hope VT, Scragg R, Kjellstrom T, Lay-Yee R. Nappy handling and risk of giardiasis. Lancet 2001;357: 1017–8.

123. An LH. Outbreak of giardiasis in a daycare nursery. Commun Dis Public Health 2000;3:212–3.

124. Welch TP. Risk of giardiasis from consumption of wilderness water in North America: a systematic review of epidemiologic data. Int J Infect Dis 2000;4:100–3.

125. LoGalbo PR, Sampson HA, Buckley RH. Symptomatic giardiasis in three patients with X-linked agammaglobulinemia. J Pediatr 1982;101:78–80.

126. Hanson KL, Cartwright CP. Use of an enzyme immunoassay does not eliminate the need to analyze multiple stool specimens for sensitive detection of Giardia lamblia. J Clin Microbiol 2001;39:474–7.

127. Maraha B, Buiting AG. Evaluation of four enzyme immu-

noassays for the detection of *Giardia lamblia* antigen in stool specimens. Eur J Clin Microbiol Infect Dis 2000; 19:485–7.

128. Janoff EN, Reller LB. *Cryptosporidium* species, a protean protozoan. J Clin Microbiol 1987;25:967–75.

129. Combee CL, Collinge ML, Britt EM. Cryptosporidiosis in a hospital-associated day care center. Pediatr Infect Dis 1986;5:528–32.

130. Quiroz ES, Bern C, MacArthur JR, et al. An outbreak of cryptosporidiosis linked to a foodhandler. J Infect Dis 2000;181:695–700.

131. MacKenzie WR, Hoxie NJ, Proctor ME, et al. A massive outbreak in Milwaukee of *Cryptosporidium* infection transmitted through the public water supply. N Engl J Med 1994;331:11–7.

132. Willcocks LJ, Sufi F, Wall R, et al. Compliance with advice to boil drinking water during an outbreak of cryptosporidiosis. Commun Dis Public Health 2000;3:137–8.

133. Addiss DG, Pond RS, Remshak M, et al. Reduction of risk of watery diarrhea with point-of-use water filters during a massive outbreak of waterborne *Cryptosporidium* infection in Milwaukee, Wisconsin, 1993. Am J Trop Med Hyg 1996;54:549–53.

134. Louis K, Gustafson L, Fyfe M, et al. An outbreak of Crytosporidium parvum in a Surrey pool with detection in pool water sampling. Can Commun Dis Rep 2004;30: 60–6.

135. MacKenzie WR, Kazmierczak JJ, Davis JP. An outbreak of cryptosporidiosis associated with a resort swimming pool. Epidemiol Infect 1995;115:545–53.

136. DuPont HL, Chappell CL, Sterling CR, et al. The infectivity of *Cryptosporidium parvum* in healthy volunteers. N Engl J Med 1995;332:855–9.

137. Cordell RL, Addiss DG. Cryptosporidiosis in child care settings: a review of the literature and recommendations for prevention and control. Pediatr Infect Dis J 1994;13: 310–17.

138. Okhuysen PC, Chappell CL, Crabb JH, et al. Virulence of three distinct *Cryptosporidium parvum* isolates for healthy adults. J Infect Dis 1999;180:1275–81.

139. Jokipii L, Jokipii AMM. Timing of symptoms and oocyst excretion in human cryptosporidiosis. N Engl J Med 1986;315:1643–7.

140. Pollock RC, Farthing MJ, Bajaj-Elliot M, et al. Interferon gamma induces enterocyte resistance against infection by the intracellular pathogen *Cryptosporidium parvum*. Gastroenterol 2001;120:99–107.

141. MacPherson DW, McQueen R. Cryptosporidiosis: multiattribute evaluation of six diagnostic methods. J Clin Microbiol 1993;31:198–202.

142. Boyce TG, Pemberton AG, Addiss DG. *Cryptosporidium* testing practices among clinical laboratories in the United States. Pediatr Infect Dis J 1996;15:87–8.

143. Arrowood MJ, Sterling CR. Comparison of conventional staining methods and monoclonal antibody-based methods for *Cryptosporidium* oocyst detection. J Clin Microbiol 1989;27:1490–5.

144. Rosenblatt JE, Sloan LM. Evaluation of an enzyme-linked immunosorbent assay for detection of *Cryptosporidium* spp. in stool specimens. J Clin Microbiol 1993;31: 1468–71.

145. Gascon J, Alvarez M, Eugenia VM, et al. Cyclosporiasis: a clinical and epidemiological study in travellers with imported *Cyclospora cayetanensis* infection. Med Clin (Barc) 2001;116:461–4.

146. Herwaldt BL. *Cyclospora cayetanensis*: a review, focusing on the outbreaks of cyclosporiasis in the 1990s. Clin Infect Dis 2000;31:1040–57.

147. Herwaldt BL, Ackers ML. An outbreak in 1996 of cyclosporiasis associated with imported raspberries. N Engl J Med 1997;336:1548–56.

148. Fleming CA, Caron D, Gunn JE, Barry MA. A foodborne outbreak of *Cyclospora cayetanensis* at a wedding: clinical features and risk factors for illness. Arch Intern Med 1998;158:1121–5.

149. De Gorgolas M, Fortes J, Fernandez Guerrero ML. *Cyclospora cayetanensis* cholecystitis in a patient with AIDS. Ann Intern Med 2001;134:166.

150. Negm AY. Identification of *Cyclospora cayetanensis* in stool using different stains. J Egypt Soc Parasitol 1998; 28:429–36.

151. Cann KJ, Chalmers RM, Nichols G, O'Brien SJ. *Cyclospora* infections in England and Wales: 1993 to 1998. Commun Dis Public Health 2000;3:46–9.

152. Verdier RI, Fitzgerald DW, Johnson WD Jr, Pape JW. Trimethoprim-sulfamethoxazole compared with ciprofloxacin for treatment and prophylaxis of *Isospora belli* and *Cyclospora cayetanensis* infection in HIV-infected patients: a randomized, controlled trial. Ann Intern Med 2000;132:885–8.

153. Maggi P, Larocca AM, Quarto M, et al. Effect of antiretroviral therapy on cryptosporidiosis and microsporidiosis in patients infected with human immunodeficiency virus type 1. Eur J Clin Microbiol Infect Dis 2000;19:213–7.

154. Bialek R, Binder N, Dietz K, et al. Comparison of autofluorescence and iodine staining for detection of *Isospora belli* in feces. Am J Trop Med Hyg 2002;67:304–5.

155. Goodgame RW. Understanding intestinal spore-forming protozoa: *Cryptosporidia*, microsporidia*, Isospora*, and *Cyclospora*. Ann Int Med 1996;124:429–41.

156. DeHovitz JA, Pape JW, Boncy M, Johnson WD Jr. Clinical manifestations and therapy of *Isospora belli* infection in patients with the acquired immunodeficiency syndrome. N Engl J Med 1986;15:87–90.

157. Mathis A. Microsporidia: emerging advances in understanding the basic biology of these unique organisms. Int J Parasitol 2000;30:795–804.

158. Muller A, Bialek R, Kamper A, et al. Detection of microsporidia in travelers with diarrhea. J Clin Microbiol 2001; 39:1630–2.

159. Weber R, Bryan RT, Owen RL, et al. Improved lightmicroscopical detection of microsporidia spores in stool and duodenal aspirates. N Engl J Med 1992;326:161–6.

160. van Gool T, Snijders F, Reiss P, et al. Diagnosis of intestinal and disseminated microsporidial infections in patients with HIV by a new rapid fluorescence technique. J Clin Pathol 1993;46:694–9.

161. Molina JM, Oksenhendler E, Beauvais B, et al. Disseminated microsporidiosis due to *Septata (Encephalitozoon) intestinalis* in patients with AIDS: clinical features and response to albendazole therapy. J Infect Dis 1995;171: 245–9.

162. Bicart-See A, Massip P, Linas MD, Datry A. Successful treatment with nitazoxanide of *Enterocytozoon bieneusi*

microsporidiosis in a patient with AIDS. Antimicrob Agents Chemother 2000;44:167–8.

163. Ridoux O, Drancourt M. Lack of in vitro antimicrosporidian activity of thalidomide. Antimicrob Agents Chemother 1999;43:2305–6.

164. Spencer MJ, Garcia LS, Chapin MR. *Dientamoeba fragilis*: an intestinal pathogen in children? Am J Dis Child 1979; 133:390–3.

165. Burke JA. Strongyloidiasis in childhood. Am J Dis Child 1978;132:1130–6.

166. Anonymous. Drugs for parasitic infections. Med Lett Drugs Ther 2002;April:1–12 (accessed at www.medletter.com).

167. Kappus KK, Juranek DD, Roberts JM. Results of testing for intestinal parasites by state diagnostic laboratories, United States, 1987. MMWR CDC Surveill Summ 1991; 40:25–45.

168. Davidson GP, Goodwin D, Robb TA. Incidence and duration of lactose malabsorption in children hospitalized with acute enteritis: study in a well-nourished urban population. J Pediatr 1984;105:587–90.

169. Brown KH, Peerson JM, Fontaine O. Use of nonhuman milks in the dietary management of young children with acute diarrhea: a meta-analysis of clinical trials. Pediatrics 1994;93:17–27.

170. Walker-Smith J, Barnard J, Bhutta Z, et al. Chronic diarrhea and malabsorption (including short gut syndrome): Working Group Report of the First World Congress of Pediatric Gastroenterology, Hepatology, and Nutrition. J Pediatr Gastroenterol Nutr 2002;35:S98–110.

171. Panigrahi D, Roy P, Chakrabarti A. Enterotoxigenic *Klebsiella pneumoniae* in acute childhood diarrhoea. Indian J Med Res 1991;93:293–6.

172. Brearly S, Armstrong GR, Nairn R, et al. Pseudomembranous colitis: a lethal complication of Hirschsprung's disease unrelated to antibiotic usage. J Pediatr Surg 1987; 22:257–9.

173. Yolken RH, Bishop CA, Townsend TR, et al. Infectious gastroenteritis in bone marrow transplant recipients. N Engl J Med 1982;306:1009–12.

174. DeWitt TG, Humphrey KF, McCarthy P. Clinical predictors of acute bacterial diarrhea in young children. Pediatrics 1985;76:551–6.

175. Radetsky M. Laboratory evaluation of acute diarrhea. Pediatr Infect Dis 1986;5:230–8.

176. Pickering LK. Evaluation of patients with acute infectious diarrhea. Pediatr Infect Dis 1985;4:13–9.

177. Williams EK, Lohr JA, Guerrant RL. Acute infectious diarrhea II: diagnosis, treatment and prevention. Pediatr Infect Dis 1986;5:458–65.

178. Zaidi AK, Macone A, Goldmann AD. Impact of simple screening criteria on utilization of low-yield bacterial stool cultures in a Children's Hospital. Pediatrics 1999; 103:1189–92.

179. McCall CE, Martin WT, Boring JR. Efficiency of cultures of rectal swabs and fecal specimens: correlation with numbers of *Salmonella* excreted. J Hyg 1966;64:261–9.

180. Huicho L, Campos M, Rivera J, Guerrant RL. Fecal screening tests in the approach to acute infectious diarrhea: a scientific overview. Pediatr Infect Dis J 1996;15: 486–94.

181. Ashkenazi S, Amir Y, Dinari G, et al. Differential leuko-

cyte count in acute gastroenteritis. Clin Pediatr 1983;22: 356–8.

182. Oracz G, Feleszko W, Golicka D, et al. Rapid diagnosis of acute *Salmonella* gastrointestinal infection. Clin Infect Dis 2003;36:112–5.

183. Victora CG, Bryce J, Fontaine O, Monasch R. Reducing deaths from diarrhoea through oral rehydration therapy. Bull World Health Organ 2000; 78:1246–55.

184. Atherly-John YC, Cunningham SJ, Crain EF. A randomized trial of oral vs intravenous rehydration in a pediatric emergency department. Arch Pediatr Adolesc Med 2002; 156:1240–3.

185. Sandhu BK. Practical guidelines for the management of gastroenteritis in children. J Pediatr Gastroenterol Nutr 2001;33 Suppl 2:S36–39.

186. Grunenberg N. Is gradual introduction of feeding better than immediate normal feeding in children with gastroenteritis? Arch Dis Child 2003;88:445–7.

187. DuPont HL, Hornick RB. Adverse effect of Lomotil therapy in shigellosis. JAMA 1973;226:1525–8.

188. Rosenstein G, Freeman M, Standard AL, et al. Warning: the use of Lomotil in children. Pediatrics 1973;51:132–4.

189. Portnoy BL, DuPont HL, Pruit D, et al. Antidiarrheal agents in the treatment of acute diarrhea in children. JAMA 1976;236:844–6.

190. Pedone CA, Bernabeu AO, Postaire ER, et al. The effect of supplementation with milk fermented by *Lactobacillus casei* (strain DN-114 001) on acute diarrhea in children attending day care centers. Int J Clin Pract 1999;53: 179–84.

191. Arvola T, Laiho K, Torkkeli S. Prophylactic *Lactobacillus* GG reduces antibiotic-associated diarrhea in children with respiratory infections: a randomized study. Pediatrics 1999:104;e64.

192. Vanderhoof JA, Whitney DB, Antonson DL, et al. *Lactobacillus* GG in the prevention of antibiotic-associated diarrhea in children. J Pediatr 1999;135:535–7.

193. Szajewska H, Kotowska M, Mrukowicz JZ, et al. Efficacy of *Lactobacillus* GG in prevention of nosocomial diarrhea in infants. J Pediatr 2001;138:361–5..

194. Simakachorn N, Pichaipat V, Rithipornpaisarn P, et al. Clinical evaluation of the addition of a lyophilized, heat-killed *Lactobacillus acidophilus* LB to oral rehydration therapy in the treatment of acute diarrhea in children. J Pediatr Gastroenterol Nutr 2000;30:68–72.

195. Guarino A, Canani RB, Spagnuolo MI, et al. Oral bacterial therapy reduces the duration of symptoms and of viral excretion in children with mild diarrhea. J Pediatr Gastroenterol Nutr 1997;25:516–9.

196. Szajewska H, Mrukowicz JZ. Probiotics in the treatment and prevention of acute infectious diarrhea in infants and children: a systematic review of published randomized, double-blind, placebo-controlled trials. J Pediatr Gastroenterol Nutr 2001;33:17–25.

197. Rosenstein BJ. *Shigella* and *Salmonella* in infants and children: an analysis of 492 cases. Johns Hopkins Hosp Bull 1964;115:407–15.

198. Nofech-Mozes Y, Yuhas Y, Kaminsky E, et al. Induction of mRNA for tumor necrosis factor-alpha and interleukin-1-beta in mice brain, spleen, and liver in an animal model of *Shigella*-related seizures. Isr Med Assoc J 2000;2: 86–90.

199. Khan WA, Dhar U, Salam MA, et al. Central nervous system manifestations of childhood shigellosis: prevalence, risk factors, and outcome. Pediatrics 1999;103: e18.

200. Kowlessar M, Forbes GH. The febrile convulsions in shigellosis. N Engl J Med 1958;258:520–6.

201. Ashkenazi S, Dinari G, Zevulunov A, et al. Convulsions in childhood shigellosis: clinical and laboratory features in 153 children. Am J Dis Child 1987;141:208–10.

202. Martin T, Habbick BF, Nyssen J. Shigellosis with bacteremia: a report of two cases and a review of the literature. Pediatr Infect Dis 1983;2:21–6.

203. Haltalin KC, Nelson JD. Coliform septicemia complicating shigellosis with children. JAMA 1965;192:441–3.

204. Sandyk R, Brennan MJ. Fulminating encephalopathy associated with Shigella flexneri infection. Arch Dis Child 1983;58:70–1.

205. Avital A, Maayan C, Goitein KJ. Incidence of convulsions and encephalopathy in childhood Shigella infections: survey of 117 hospitalized patients. Clin Pediatr 1982;21: 645–8.

206. Barrett CE, Connor JD. Extraintestinal manifestations of shigellosis. Am J Gastroenterol 1970;53:234–45.

207. Rabinowitz SG, MacLeod NR. Salmonella meningitis: a report of three cases and review of the literature. Am J Dis Child 1972;123:259–62.

208. Chandy MJ. Subdural Salmonella empyema in an adult. Neurol India 2000;48:297.

209. Sarria JC, Vidal AM, Kimbrough RC 3rd. Salmonella enteritidis brain abscess: case report and review. Clin Neurol Neurosurg 2000;102:236–9.

210. Fendler C, Laitko S, Sorensen H, et al. Frequency of triggering bacteria in patients with reactive arthritis and undifferentiated oligoarthritis and the relative importance of the tests used for diagnosis. Ann Rheum Dis 2001;60: 337–43.

211. MacLean WC Jr, Klein GL, Lopez DE, et al. Transient steatorrhea following episodes of mild diarrhea in early infancy. J Pediatr 1978;93:562–5.

212. Kumar V, Chandrasekaran R, Bhaskar R. Carbohydrate intolerance associated with acute gastroenteritis: a prospective study of 90 well-nourished Indian infants. Clin Pediatr 1977;16:1123–7.

213. Balassanian N, Wolinsky E. Epidemiologic and seriologic studies of E. coli O4:H5 in a premature nursery. Pediatrics 1968;41:463–72.

214. Repogle ML, Fleming DW, Cieslak PR. Emergence of antimicrobial-resistant shigellosis in Oregon. Clin Infect Dis 2000;30:515–9.

215. Martin JM, Pitetti R, Maffei F, et al. Treatment of shigellosis with cefixime: two days vs. five days. Pediatr Infect Dis J 2000;19:522–6.

216. Helvaci M, Bektaslar D, Ozkaya B, et al. Comparative efficacy of cefixime and ampicillin-sulbactam in shigellosis in children. Acta Pediatr Jpn 1998;40:131–4.

217. Levine MM, DuPont HL, Khodabandelou M, et al. Long-term Shigella-carrier state. N Engl J Med 1973;288: 1169–71.

218. McCall CE, Sanders WE, Boring JR, et al. Delineation of chronic carriers of Salmonella derby within an institution for uncurables. Antimicrob Agents Chemother 1964;4: 717–21.

219. Salazar-Lindo E, Sack RB, Chea-Woo, E, et al. Early treatment with erythromycin of Campylobacter jejuni-associated dysentery in children. J Pediatr 1986;109:355–60.

220. Adachi JA, Ostrosky-Zeichner L, DuPont HL, Ericcson CD. Empirical antimicrobial therapy of traveler's diarrhea. Clin Infect Dis 2000;31:1079–83.

221. Talsma E, Goettsch WG, Nieste HL, et al. Resistance in Campylobacter species: increased resistance to fluoroquinolones and seasonal variation. Clin Infect Dis 1999;29: 845–8.

222. Aarestrup FM, Wegener HC. The effect of antibiotic usage in food animals on the development of antimicrobial resistance of importance for humans in Campylobacter and Escherichia coli. Microbes Infect 1999;1:639–44.

223. Anonymous. Nitazoxanide (Alinia)—a new anti-protozoal agent. Med Lett Drugs Ther 2003;45:29–31.

224. Ortiz JJ, Ayoub A, Gargala G, et al. Randomized clinical study of nitazoxanide compared to metronidazole in the treatment of symptomatic giardiasis in children from Northern Peru. Aliment Pharmacol Ther 2001;15: 1409–15.

225. Turner JA. Giardiasis and infections with Dientamoeba fragilis. Pediatr Clin North Am 1985;32:865–80.

226. Hoge CW, Gambel JM, Srijan A, et al. Trends in antibiotic resistance among diarrheal pathogens isolated in Thailand over 15 years. Clin Infect Dis 1998;26:341–5.

227. Rossignol JF, Ayoub A, Ayers MS. Treatment of diarrhea caused by Cryptosporidium parvum: a prospective randomized, double-blind, placebo-controlled study of nitazoxanide. J Infect Dis 2001;184:103–6.

228. Amadi B, Mwiya M, Musuku J, et al. Effect of nitazoxanide on morbidity and mortality in Zambian children with cryptosporidiosis: a randomised controlled trial. Lancet 2002;360:1375–80.

229. Wittenburg DF, Miller NM, Van den Ende J. Spiramycin is not effective in treating Cryptosporidium diarrhea in infants: results of a double-blind randomized trial. J Infect Dis 1989;159:131–2.

230. Hewitt RG, Yiannoutsos CT, Higgs ES, et al. Paromomycin: no more effective than placebo for treatment of cryptosporidiosis in patients with advanced human immunodeficiency virus infection. Clin Infect Dis 2000;31: 1084–92.

231. Hommer V, Eichholz J, Petry F. Effect of antiretroviral protease inhibitors alone, and in combination with paromomycin, on the excystation, invastion and in vivo development of Cryptorsporidium parvum. J Antimicrob Chemother 2003;52:359–64.

232. Chen XM, Keithly JS, Paya CV, LaRusso NF. Cryptosporidiosis. N Engl J Med 2002;346:1723–31.

233. Sakellaris G, Kakavelakis K, Stathapoulos E, et al. A palpable right lower abdominal mass due to Yersinia mesenteric lymphadenitis. Pediatr Surg 2004;20:155–7.

234. Pai CH, Gillis F, Tuomanen E, et al. Placebo-controlled double-blind evaluation of trimethoprim-sulfamethoxazole treatment of Yersinia enterocolitica gastroenteritis. J Pediatr 1984;104:308–12.

235. Sack DA, Islam S, Rabbani H, et al. Single dose doxycycline for cholera. Antimicrob Agents Chemother 1978; 14:462–4.

236. Webb CH, Wallace WM. Diagnosis and treatment: epi-

demic gastroenteritis, presumably viral. Pediatrics 1966; 38:494–8.

237. Adler JL, Zick R. Winter vomiting disease. J Infect Dis 1969;119:668–73.

238. Winter vomiting disease [editorial]. Br Med J 1980;1: 506–7.

239. Johansson PJ, Torven M, Hammarlund, et al. Food-borne outbreak of gastroenteritis associated with genogroup I calicivirus. J Clin Microbiol 2002;40:794–8.

240. Tarasoff L, Kelly MF. Monosodium L-glutamate: a double-blind study and review. Food Chem Toxicol 1993; 12:1019–35.

241. Geha RS, Beiser A, Ren C, et al. Review of alleged reaction to monosodium glutamate and outcome of a multicenter double-blind placebo-controlled study. J Nutr 2000; 130(4S Suppl):S1058–62.

242. Hanrahan JP, Gordon MA. Mushroom poisoning: case reports and a review of therapy. JAMA 1984;251: 1057–61.

243. Jenkins S, Horman YT, Israel E, et al. An outbreak of Norwalk-related gastroenteritis at a boys' camp. Am J Dis Child 1985;139:787–9.

244. Guest C, Spitalny KC, Madore HP, et al. Foodborne Snow Mountain agent gastroenteritis in a school cafeteria. Pediatrics 1987;79:559–63.

245. Marks PJ, Vipond IB, Carlisle D, et al. Evidence for airborne transmission of Norwalk-like virus (NLV) in a hotel restaurant. Epidemiol Infect 2000;124:481–7.

246. Parrino TA, Schreiber DS, Trier JS, et al. Clinical immunity in acute gastroenteritis caused by Norwalk agent. N Engl J Med 1977;297:86–9.

247. Graham DY, Jiang X, Tanaka T, et al. Norwalk virus infection of volunteers: new insights based on improved assays. J Infect Dis 1994;170:34–43.

248. Okhuysen PC, Jiang X, Ye L, et al. Viral shedding and fecal IgA response after Norwalk virus infection. J Infect Dis 1995;171:566–9.

249. Asao T, Kumeda Y, Kawai T, et al. An extensive outbreak of staphylococcal food poisoning due to low-fat milk in Japan: estimation of enterotoxin A in the incriminated milk and powered skim milk. Epidemiol Infect 2033; 130:33–40.

250. Currier RWI, Taylor A Jr, Wolf FS. Fatal staphylococcal food poisoning. South Med J 1973;66:703–5.

251. Holmberg SD, Blake PA. Staphylococcal food poisoning in the United States: new facts and old misconceptions. JAMA 1984;251:487–9.

252. Merrill, GA, Werner SB, Bryant RG, et al. Staphylococcal food poisoning associated with an Easter egg hunt. JAMA 1984;252:1019–22.

253. Hodge B. Control of staphylococcal food poisoning. Publ Health Rep 1960;75:353–61.

254. Sourek J, Vymola F, Trojanová M, et al. Enterotoxin production by Staphylococcus aureus strains isolated from cases of chronic osteomyelitis. J Clin Microbiol 1979;9: 266–8.

255. Armstrong RW, Stenn F, Dowell VR Jr, et al. Type E botulism from home-canned gefilte fish: report of three cases. JAMA 1969;210:303–5.

256. Terranova W, Breman JG, Locey RP. Botulism type B: epidemiologic aspects of an extensive outbreak. Am J Epidemiol 1978;108:150–6.

257. Shapiro RL, Hathway C, Swerdlow DL. Botulism in the United States: a clinical and epidemiologic review. Ann Intern Med 1998;129:221–8.

258. Centers for Disease Control and Prevention. Diagnosis and management of foodborne illnesses: a primer for physicians. MMWR Recomm Rep 2001;RR50:1–69.

259. Jiang X, Zhong WM, Farkas T, et al. Baculovirus expression and antigenic characterization of the capsid proteins of three Norwalk-like viruses. Arch Virol 2002;147: 119–30.

260. Book LS. Vomiting and diarrhea. Pediatrics 1984; 74(Suppl):S950–4.

261. Feldman V. Serious reactions to phenothiazines [letter]. J Pediatr 1976;89:163–4.

262. Reeves JJ, Shannon MW, Fleisher GR. Ondansetron decreases vomiting associated with acute gastroenteritis: a randomized, controlled trial. Pediatrics 2002;109:e62.

263. Mikami T, Nakagomi T, Tsutsui R, et al. An outbreak of gastroenteritis during school trip caused by serotype G2 group A rotavirus. J Med Virol 2004;73:460–4.

264. Meyer EA. The epidemiology of giardiasis. Parasitol Today 1985;1:101–5.

265. Lim LS, Varkey P, Giesen P, Edmonson L. Cryptosporidiosis outbreak in a recreational swimming pool in Minnesota. J Environ Health 2004;67:16–20.

266. Lee SH, Levy DA, Craun GF, et al. Surveillance for waterborne-disease outbreaks—United States, 1999–2000. MMWR Surveill Summ 2002;51:1–47.

267. Hassall E. Peptic ulcer disease and current approaches to *Helicobacter pylori*. J Pediatr 2001;138:462–8.

268. Suerbaum S, Michetti P. *Helicobacter pylori* infection. N Engl J Med 2002; 347:1175–86.

269. Uemura N, Okamoto S, Yamamoto S, et al. *Helicobacter pylori* infection and the development of gastric cancer. N Engl J Med 2001;345:784–9.

270. Moayyedi P, Soo S, Deeks J, et al. Eradication of *Helicobacter pylori* for non-ulcer dyspepsia. Cochrane Database Syst Rev 2003:CD002096.

271. Koletzko S, Feydt-Schmidt A. Infants differ from teenagers: use of non-invasive tests for detection of *Helicobacter pylori* infection in children. Eur J Gastroenterol Hepatol 2001;13:1047–52.

272. Vaira D, Vakil N. Blood, urine, stool, breath, money, and *Helicobacter pylori*. Gut 2001;48:287–9.

273. Drumm B, Koletzko S, Oderda G. *Helicobacter pylori* infection in children: a consensus statement. European Paediatric Task Force on *Helicobacter pylori*. J Pediatr Gastroenterol Nutr 2000;30:207–13.

274. Winsey HS, Jones PF. Acute abdominal pain in childhood: analysis of a year's admissions. Br Med J 1967;1: 653–5.

275. Pledger HG, Buchan R. Deaths in children with acute appendicitis. Br Med J 1969;4:466–70.

276. Gilbert SR, Emmens RW, Putnam TC. Appendicitis in children. Surg Gynecol Obstet 1985;161:261–5.

277. Nelson DS, Bateman B, Bolte RG. Appendiceal perforation in children diagnosed in a pediatric emergency department. Pediatr Emerg Care 2000;16:233–7.

278. Graham JM, Pokorny WJ, Harberg FJ. Acute appendicitis in preschool age children. Am J Surg 1980;139:247–50.

279. Brender JD, Marcuse EK, Koepsell TD, et al. Childhood

appendicitis: factors associated with perforation. Pediatrics 1985;76:301–6.

280. Landes RG, Mullen P, Robbins P. Acute appendicitis in patients on antibiotics [letter]. N Engl J Med 1976;294:674.

281. Parsons JM, Miscall BG, McSherry CK. Appendicitis in the newborn infant. Surgery 1970;67:841–3.

282. Shaul WL. Clues to the early diagnosis of neonatal appendicitis. J Pediatr 1981;98:473–6.

283. Picus D, Shackelford GD. Perforated appendix presenting with severe diarrhea. Radiology 1983;149:141–3.

284. Horwitz JR. Importance of diarrhea as a presenting symptom of appendicitis in very young children. Am J Surg 1997;173:80–2.

285. Nance ML, Adamson WT, Hedrick HL. Appendicitis in the young child: a continuing diagnostic challenge. Pediatr Emerg Care 2000;16:160–2.

286. Buckley RG, Distefan J, Gubler KD, Slymen D. The risk of appendiceal rupture based on hospital admission source. Acad Emerg Med 1999;6:596–601.

287. Cappendijk VC, Hazebroek FW. The impact of diagnostic delay on the course of acute appendicitis. Arch Dis Child 2000;83:64–6.

288. Anderrson R, Hugander A, Thulin A, Nystrom PO, Olaison G. Clusters of acute appendicitis: further evidence for an infectious etiology. Int J Epidemiol 1995;24:829–33.

289. Tobe T. Inapparent virus infection as a trigger of appendicitis. Lancet 1965;1:1343–6.

290. Brender JD, Marcuse EK, Weiss NS, et al. Is childhood appendicitis familial? Am J Dis Child 1985;139:338–40.

291. Jona JZ, Belin RP. Basilar pneumonia simulating acute appendicitis in children. Arch Surg 1976:111:552–3.

292. Bain HW, McLean DM, Walker SJ. Epidemic pleurodynia (Bornholm disease) due to Coxsackie B5 virus. Pediatrics 1961;27:889–903.

293. Artwood SEA, Mealy K, Cafferkey MT, et al. *Yersinia* infection and acute abdominal pain. Lancet 1987;1:529–33.

294. Pai CH, Gillis F, Marks MI. Infection due to *Yersinia enterocolitica* in children with abdominal pain. J Infect Dis 1982;146:705.

295. Saebø A. The *Yersinia enterocolitica* infection in acute abdominal surgery. Ann Surg 1983;198:760–5.

296. Kunkel MJ, Brown LG, Bauta H, et al. Meningococcal mesenteric adenitis and peritonitis in a child. Pediatr Infect Dis 1984;3:327–8.

297. O'Brien A, O'Briain DS. Infectious mononucleosis. Arch Pathol Lab Med 1985;109:680–2.

298. Swayne LC, Love MB, Karasick SR. Pelvic inflammatory disease: sonographic pathologic correlation. Radiology 1984;151:751–5.

299. Takiff H, Fonkalsrud EW. Gallbladder disease in childhood. Am J Dis Child 1984;138:565–8.

300. Tsakayannis DE, Kozakewich HP, Lillehei CW. Acalculous cholecystitis in children. J Pediatr Surg 1996;31:127–30.

301. Rogers CA, Isenberg JN, Leonard AS, et al. Ascending cholangitis diagnosed by percutaneous hepatic aspiration. J Pediatr 1976;88:83–6.

302. Ecoffey C, Rothman E, Bernard O, Hadchouel M, Valayer J, Alagille D. Bacterial cholangitis after surgery for biliary atresia. J Pediatr 1987;111:824–9.

303. Brook I. Aerobic and anaerobic microbiology of biliary tract disease. J Clin Microbiol 1989;27:2373–5.

304. Thompson JE Jr, Tompkins RK, Longmire WP Jr. Factors in the management of acute cholangitis. Ann Surg 1982;95:137–45.

305. Van den Hazel SJ, Speelman P, Tytgat GN, Dankert J, van Leeuwen DJ. Role of antibiotics in the treatment and prevention of acute and recurrent cholangitis. Clin Infect Dis 1994;19:279–86.

306. Buyukasik Y, Kosar A, Demiroglu H, Altinok G, Ozcebe OI, Dundar S. Acalculous cholecystitis in leukemia. J Clin Gastroenterol 1998;27:146–8.

306a. Yadav D, Agarwal N, Pitchumoni CS. A critical evaluation of laboratory tests in acute pancreatitis. Am J Gastroenterol 2002;97:1309–18.

307. Jordan SC, Ament ME. Pancreatitis in children and adolescents. J Pediatr 1977;91:211–6.

308. Brandt JR, Fouser LS, Watkins SL, et al. *Escherichia coli* O157:H7-associated hemolytic-uremic syndrome after ingestion of contaminated hamburgers. J Pediatr 1994;125:519–26.

309. Grodinsky S, Telmesani A, Robson WL, Fick G, Scott RB. Gastrointestinal manifestations of hemolytic uremic syndrome: recognition of pancreatitis. J Pediatr Gastroenterol Nutr 1990;11:518–24.

310. Blumenstock DA, Mithoefer J, Santulli TV. Acute pancreatitis in children. Pediatrics 1957;19:1002–10.

311. Witte CL, Schanzer EB. Pancreatitis due to mumps. JAMA 1968;203:1068–9.

312. Eckfeldt JH, Kolars JC, Elson MK, et al. Serum tests for pancreatitis in patients with abdominal pain. Arch Pathol Lab Med 1985;109:316–9.

313. Nakao T, Nitta T, Miura R, et al. Clinical and epidemiological studies on an outbreak of aseptic meningitis caused by Coxsackie B5 and A9 viruses in Aomori in 1961. Tohoku J Exp Med 1964;83:94–102.

314. Koutras A. Epstein-Barr virus infection with pancreatitis, hepatitis and proctitis. Pediatr Infect Dis 1983;2:312–3.

315. Torre JA, Martin JJ, Garcia CB, Polo ER. Varicella infection as a cause of acute pancreatitis in an immunocompetent child. Pediatr Infect Dis J 2000;19:1218–9.

316. Oderda G, Kraut JR. Rising antibody titer to *Mycoplasma pneumoniae* in acute pancreatitis. Pediatrics 1980;66:305–6.

317. Leinikki PO, Panzar P, Tykka H. Immunoglobulin M antibody response against *Mycoplasma pneumoniae* lipid antigen in patients with acute pancreatitis. J Clin Microbiol 1978;8:113–8.

318. Baron TH, Morgan DE. Acute necrotizing pancreatitis. N Engl J Med 1999;340:1412–17.

319. Clark JH, Fitzgerald JF, Kleiman MB. Spontaneous bacterial peritonitis. J Pediatr 1984;104:495–500.

320. Freij BJ, Votteler TP, McCracken GH Jr. Primary peritonitis in previously healthy children. Am J Dis Child 1984;138:1058–61.

321. Matthews P. Primary anaerobic peritonitis. Br Med J 1979;2:903–4.

322. Woolf A, Christie D, Wilson CB. Tuberculous peritonitis in an infant. Pediatr Infect Dis 1985;4:684–6.

323. Krieger RW, Chusid MJ. Perirectal abscess in childhood: a review of 29 cases. Am J Dis Child 1979;133:411–2.

324. Leahy AL, Fogarty EE, Fitzgerald RJ, et al. Discitis as a

cause of abdominal pain in children. Surgery 1984;95: 412–4.

325. Lin JS, Rodriquez-Torres R. Appendectomy in children with acute rheumatic fever. Pediatrics 1969;43:573–7.

326. Brenneman J. The abdominal pain of throat infections. Am J Dis Child 1922;22:493–9.

327. Kerr AA, McQuillin J, Downham M, et al. Gastric flu: influenza B causing abdominal symptoms in children. Lancet 1975;1:291–5.

328. Moffet HL, Cramblett HG, Dobbins J. Outbreak of influenza A2 among immunized children. JAMA 1964;190: 806–10.

329. Wang YH, Huang YC, Chang LY. Clinical characteristics of children with influenza A virus infections requiring hospitalization. J Microbiol Immunol Infect 2003;36: 111–6.

330. Cohn SM, Schoetz DJ Jr. Pyogenic sacroiliitis: another imitator of the acute abdomen. Surgery 1987;100:95–8.

331. Beck W, Grose C. Pyomyositis presenting as acute abdominal pain. Pediatr Infect Dis 1984;3:445–8.

332. Davis AE, Bradford WD. Abdominal pain resembling acute appendicitis in Rocky Mountain spotted fever. JAMA 1982;247:2811–2.

333. Newman BM, Karp MP, Jewett TC, et al. Advances in the management of infected urachal cysts. J Pediatr Surg 1986;21:1051–4.

334. Rao PM, Rhea JT, Rao JA, Conn AK. Plain abdominal radiography in clinically suspected appendicitis: diagnostic yield, resource use, and comparison with CT. Am J Emerg Med 1999;17:325–8.

335. Paulson EK, Kalady MF, Pappas TN. Suspected appendicitis. N Engl J Med 2003;348:236–42.

336. Peck J, Peck A, Peck C, Peck J. The clinical role of noncontrast helical computed tomography in the diagnosis of acute appendicitis. Am J Surg 2000;180:133–6.

337. Sivit CJ, Applegate KE, Stallion A, et al. Imaging evaluation of suspected appendicitis in a pediatric population: effectiveness of sonography versus CT. Am J Roentgenol 2000;175:977–80.

338. Paya K, Fakhari M, Rauhofer U, et al. Open versus laparoscopic appendectomy in children: a comparison of complications. J Soc Laparoendosc Surg 2000;4:121–4.

339. Koloska ER, Silen ML, Tracy TF Jr, et al. Perforated appendicitis in children: risk factors for the development of complications. Surgery 1998;124:619–25.

340. Toki A, Ogura K, Horimi T, et al. Peritoneal lavage versus drainage for perforated appendicitis in children. Surg Today 1995;25:207–10.

341. Brown CV, Abrishami M, Muller M, Velmahos GC. Appendiceal abscess: immediate operation or percutaneous drainage? Am Surg 2003;69:829–32.

342. Bratzler DW, Houck PM. Antimicrobial prophylaxis for surgery: an advisory statement from the National Surgical Infection Prevention Project. Clin Infect Dis 2004;38: 1706–15.

344. Solomkin JS, Mazuski JE, Baron EJ, et al. Guidelines for the selection of anti-infective agents for complicated intra-abdominal infections. Clin Dis 2003;37:997–1005.

345. David IB, Buck JR, Filler RM. Rational use of antibiotics for perforated appendicitis in childhood. J Pediatr Surg 1982;17:494–500.

346. Rodriguez JC, Buckner D, Schoenike S, et al. Comparison

347. Fishman SJ, Pelosi L, Klavon SL, O'Rourke EJ. Perforated appendicitis: prospective outcome analysis for 150 children. J Pediatr Surg 2000;35:923–6.

348. Savrin RA, Clausen K, Martin EW Jr. Chronic and recurrent appendicitis. Am J Surg 1979;137:355–7.

349. Grossman EB Jr. Chronic appendicitis. Surgery 1978; 146:596–8.

350. Dobrin PB, Gully PH, Greenlee HB, et al. Radiologic diagnosis of an intraabdominal abscess: do multiple tests help? Arch Surg 1986;121:41–6.

351. Diament NU, Stanley P, Kangarloo H, et al. Percutaneous aspiration and catheter drainage of abscesses. J Pediatr 1986;108:204–8.

352. Kaplan S, Feigin RD. Pyogenic liver abscess in normal children with fever of unknown origin. Pediatrics 1976; 58:614–6.

353. Chusid NV. Pyogenic hepatic abscess in infancy and childhood. Pediatrics 1978;62:554–9.

354. Bilfinger TV, Hayden CK, Oldham KT, et al. Pyogenic liver abscess in nonimmunocompromised children. South Med J 1986;79:37–40.

355. Goldenring JM, Flores M. Primary liver abscesses in children and adolescents: review of 12 years' clinical experience. Clin Pediatr 1986;25:153–8.

356. Moss TJ, Pysher TJ. Hepatic abscess in neonates. Am J Dis Child 1981;135:726–8.

357. Shulman ST, Beem MO. An unique presentation of sickle cell disease: pyogenic hepatic abscess. Pediatrics 1971; 47:1019–22.

358. Goletti O, Angrisano C, Lippolis PV, et al. Percutaneous management of multiple bilateral liver abscesses complicating Crohn's disease. Surg Laparosc Endosc Percutan Tech 2001;11:131–3.

359. Pereira FE, Musso C, Castelo JS. Pathology of pyogenic liver abscess in children. Pediatr Dev Pathol 1999;2: 537–43.

360. Lambertucci JR, Rayes AA, Serufo JC, Nobre V. Pyogenic abscesses and parasitic diseases. Rev Inst Trop Sao Paulo 2001;43:67–74.

361. Chang FY, Chou ROC. Comparison of pyogenic liver abscesses caused by *Klebsiella pneumoniae* and non-*K. pneumoniae* pathogens. J Formos Med Assoc 1995;94:232–7.

362. Olivera MA, Kershenobich D. Pyogenic liver abscess. Curr Treat Options Gastroenterol 1999;2:86–90.

363. Moore SW, Millar AJ, Cywes S. Conservative initial treatment for liver abscesses in children. Br J Surg 1994;81: 872–4.

364. Harrison HR, Crowe CP, Fulginiti VA. Amebic liver abscess in children: clinical and epidemiologic features. Pediatrics 1979;64:923–8.

365. Haffar A, Boland FJ, Edwards MS. Amebic liver abscess in children. Pediatr Infect Dis 1982;1:322–7.

366. Moazam F, Nazir Z. Amebic liver abscess: spare the knife but save the child. J Pediatr Surg 1998;33:119–22.

367. Cushing AH, O'Keefe P, Florman A. Metronidazole concentrations in a hepatic abscess. Pediatr Infect Dis 1985; 4:697–8.

368. Zindrou S, Orozco E, Linder E, Tellez A, Bjorkman A.

Specific detection of *Entamoeba histolytica* DNA by hemolysin gene-targeted PCR. Acta Trop 2001;78:117–25.

369. Abd-Alla MD, Jackson TF, Reddy S, Ravdin JI. Diagnosis of invasive amebiasis by enzyme-linked immunosorbent assay of saliva to detect amebic lectin antigen and antilectin immunoglobulin G antibodies. J Clin Microbiol 2000;38:2344–7.

370. Thompson JE, Forlenza S, Verma R. Amebic liver abscess: a therapeutic approach. Rev Infect Dis 1985;7:171–9.

371. Greaney GC, Reynolds TB, Donovan AJ. Ruptured amebic liver abscess. Arch Surg 1985;120:555–61.

372. Katz S, Rivkind A, Cohen O. Pancreatic abscess: an unusual complication of pancreatitis in infancy. J Pediatr Surg 1983;18:306–7.

373. Chulay JD, Lankerani MR. Splenic abscess: report of 10 cases and a review of the literature. Am J Med 1976;61:513–21.

374. Chubachi A, Miura I, Ohshima A, et al. Risk factors for hepato splenic abscesses in patients with acute leukemia receiving empiric azole treatment. Am J Med Sci 1994;308:309–12.

375. Sands M, Page D, Brown RB. Splenic abscess following nonoperative management of splenic rupture. J Pediatr Surg 1986;21:900–1.

376. Squires RH, Keating JP, Rosenblum JL, et al. Splenic abscess and hepatic dysfunction caused by *Shigella flexneri*. J Pediatr 1981;98:429–30.

377. Mehanna D, Peck N, Arnot R, Solano T, Sheldon D. Cat scratch disease presenting as splenic abscess. Aust N Z J Surg 2000;70:622–4.

378. Patterson EJ, Nagy AG. Don't cry over spilled stones? Complications of gallstones spilled during laparoscopic cholecystectomy: case report and literature review. Can J Surg 1997;40:300–4.

379. Sherman NJ, Davis JR, Jesseph JE. Subphrenic abscess. Am J Surg 1969;117:123.

380. Schwab J, Gerber S, Benya E. A subphrenic abscess in a previously healthy child. Pediatrics 1997;99:621–3.

381. Atkinson GO, Kodroff MB, Gay BB, et al. Adrenal abscess in the neonate. Radiology 1985;155:101–4.

382. Walker KM, Coyer WF. Suprarenal abscess due to group B streptococcus. J Pediatr 1979;94:970–1.

CHAPTER 13

Hepatitis Syndromes

Hepatitis is injury to the liver, with or without hepatocyte necrosis, which results in an influx of acute or chronic inflammatory cells. Damage to the liver cell membrane results in release of liver enzymes into the bloodstream. Thus, from a practical standpoint, hepatitis can be broadly defined as the presumptive diagnosis when the serum aminotransferase levels are elevated. This definition remains useful, despite the following limitations. First, mild elevations are present in a small percentage of healthy persons, causing some experts to consider aminotransferase levels elevated only if they are persistently twice the upper limit of normal, especially in asymptomatic persons.[1] Second, although predominantly found in hepatocytes, aspartate aminotransferase (AST) and, to a lesser extent, alanine aminotransferase (ALT) are found in other tissues as well. Congestive heart failure, severe myositis, and celiac disease are some of the conditions that may cause elevation of serum aminotransferases in the absence of liver disease.[2] Third, some patients with viral hepatitis do not have elevated liver enzymes, despite histologic evidence of chronic hepatitis.[3,4]

Although the term *hepatitis* is sometimes used to mean infection caused by one of the lettered hepatitis viruses, it is more useful to regard hepatitis as a syndrome of many possible etiologies.

■ CLASSIFICATION

A number of syndromes of hepatitis can be defined on the basis of the onset, severity, and course. No specific etiology should be inferred from these terms.

Acute Icteric Hepatitis

Acute icteric hepatitis is best defined as the abrupt onset of hepatocellular—not obstructive or hemolytic—jaundice. The degree of hyperbilirubinemia is variable, and fractionation is of little clinical value. The early detection of urobilinogen is helpful because it usually precedes jaundice. Fever, malaise, anorexia, and vomiting are often prodromes but are not essential to the definition. On physical examination, the liver is usually enlarged and may be tender. Typically improvement begins within a week or two. It is useful to use the etiologically neutral syndrome diagnosis of "acute hepatitis" as a preliminary diagnosis rather than "infectious hepatitis," in order to remain alert to the possible noninfectious causes of this syndrome.

Anicteric Hepatitis

This is the most frequent form of hepatitis, especially in children, and is detected primarily by serial measurement of serum aminotransferase levels in a patient with a known exposure. The child may be entirely asymptomatic or may have only nonspecific symptoms such as fever and malaise, often leading to the diagnosis of an influenza-like illness.

Fulminant Hepatitis

Fulminant hepatitis is characterized by rapid progression to liver failure, manifested primarily by a change in consciousness progressing to coma over the course of a few days. Bleeding often occurs secondary to hepatocellular failure and disseminated intravascular coagulopathy. Although some children recover spontaneously, emergency liver transplantation is usually required for survival. The cause of most cases of fulminant hepatitis remains unknown, although viral infections, toxins, drugs, and autoimmune diseases are occasionally implicated.

Chronic Hepatitis

Chronic hepatitis is defined arbitrarily as hepatic injury that persists for at least 6 months, with persistently elevated bilirubin or liver enzymes in the serum.[5] In the past, terms such as *chronic persistent hepatitis* or *chronic active hepatitis* were used as descriptors. However, it is most useful to specify the etiology and histologic status, if known (e.g., chronic hepatitis B with mild fibrosis).

Recrudescent (Relapsing) Hepatitis

A small percentage of patients with acute viral hepatitis develop an increase in aminotransferase levels after an initial period of recovery. In one study of patients with hepatitis A virus infection, nearly 10% developed this biphasic pattern, some of whom were symptomatic during the second phase.[6] In hepatitis C virus infection, repeated episodes of recrudescence are usually a harbinger of chronic infection.[7] Occasionally, an apparent recrudescence in a high-risk patient is the result of new infection with a different hepatitis virus.

Hepatitis During Pregnancy

Hepatitis occurring during pregnancy is important because of increased severity (particularly with hepatitis E virus infection) and because of the risk of transmission of infection to the fetus (especially with hepatitis B virus infection and to a lesser extent with hepatitis C virus infection).[8] Maternal–fetal transmission is discussed in the section on prevention.

Neonatal Hepatitis

In the first month of life, hepatitis with an infectious cause is often a congenital infection and is discussed in Chapter 19.

Perihepatitis

The Fitz-Hugh-Curtis syndrome complicating gonorrhea or *Chlamydia trachomatis* infection is associated with liver tenderness but not with significant elevation of liver enzymes. Therefore, it does not meet this chapter's definition of hepatitis.

Granulomatous Hepatitis

Many systemic disorders, infectious and noninfectious, can produce hepatic granulomas,[9] which is a more appropriate term than granulomatous hepatitis because the liver enzymes are usually normal. Patients often present with fever of unknown origin, and the granulomas are usually diagnosed by ultrasound or computed tomography (CT) of the liver. In children from an area of high endemicity, cat-scratch disease is now recognized as a relatively

common cause of hepatic granulomas.[10] There may be splenic involvement as well, and abdominal pain may be a presenting symptom.[11] Other causes of hepatic granulomas include tuberculosis, histoplasmosis, sarcoidosis, chronic granulomatous disease, and reactions to certain drugs.

Reactive Hepatitis

Many systemic infections are associated with focal liver injury and elevated serum aminotransferase levels. These are discussed in the subsequent section on Other Infectious Causes. Because it is often clinically difficult to differentiate between a reactive hepatitis and hepatitis caused by a hepatotropic virus, the distinction is not usually made until an etiologic diagnosis is apparent. When encountering a patient with hepatitis and systemic findings, it is best to describe them both (e.g., acute icteric hepatitis in a patient with exudative pharyngitis).

■ LETTERED CAUSES OF HEPATITIS

Although many infections can cause hepatitis, the lettered hepatitis viruses have particular tropism for the liver and are discussed separately. Table 13-1 gives an explanation of common abbreviations associated with these viruses, and Table 13-2 summarizes their major characteristics.

Hepatitis A Virus

Most cases of hepatitis A result from person-to-person transmission by the fecal-oral route during prolonged communitywide outbreaks.[12] Children in day-care centers play an important role in transmitting infection to adult contacts.[13] Infection may also be acquired during foreign travel or as part of a common-source food borne outbreak.[14] About half of cases have no recognized source.

The spectrum of clinical illnesses produced by hepatitis A virus has been well described on the basis of experimental volunteer studies and outbreaks. A landmark article describing the differences between hepatitis A and B was published in 1967.[15] In children younger than 6 years of age, most infections are asymptomatic. If illness does occur, jaundice is usually absent. In contrast, older children and adults usually present with acute icteric hepatitis. About 1 month after exposure, the patient with this form of hepatitis A develops high fever, sweating, shaking chills, myalgia, severe anorexia, nausea, and possibly vomiting. Occasion-

TABLE 13-1. TERMINOLOGY OF LETTERED HEPATITIS VIRUSES

ABBREVIATION	TERM	COMMENTS
Hepatitis A		
HAV	Hepatitis A virus	Picornavirus (RNA genome).
Anti-HAV	Total (IgM and IgG) antibody to HAV	Detectable at onset of symptoms; lifetime persistence following infection or vaccination.
IgM anti-HAV	IgM class antibody to HAV	Indicates recent infection with hepatitis A; positive up to 6–12 mo after infection.
Hepatitis B		
HBV	Hepatitis B virus	Hepadnavirus (DNA genome). Can be measured with quantitative PCR.
HBsAg	HBV surface antigen	Envelope proteins of HBV made in excess and detectable in large quantity in serum.
HBcAg	HBV core antigen	Nucleocapsid that encloses the viral DNA; no commercial test available.
HBeAg	HBV e antigen	Circulating peptide derived from core gene; correlates with HBV replication and infectivity of serum.
Anti-HBs	Antibody to HBsAg	Indicates recovery from past infection with and immunity to HBV, passive antibody from HBIG, or immunity from HBV vaccine.
Anti-HBc	Antibody to HBcAg	Indicates current or past infection with HBV; unlike anti-HBs, this antibody is not protective.
IgM anti-HBc	IgM class antibody to HBcAg	Indicates recent (4–6 mo) infection with HBV.
Anti-HBe	Antibody to HBeAg	Indicates clearance of e antigen; virus is no longer replicating.
HBIG	Hepatitis B immune globulin	Contains high-titer antibodies to HBV for passive immunization.
Hepatitis C		
HCV	Hepatitis C virus	Flavivirus (RNA genome) Can be measured with quantitative PCR (a positive result indicates ongoing infection); multiple subtypes.
Anti-HCV	IgG antibody to HCV	Indicates either acute, chronic, or resolved infection with HCV.
Hepatitis D		
HDV	Hepatitis D virus (delta agent)	Defective RNA virus; requires presence of HBV to replicate.
Anti-HDV	Antibody to HDV	Indicates past or present infection with HDV.
Hepatitis E		
HEV	Hepatitis E virus	Unclassified (RNA genome); cause of endemic and epidemic hepatitis in some developing areas.
IgM anti-HEV	IgM class antibody to HEV	Indicates recent infection (assay not widely available).
IgG anti-HEV	IgG class antibody to HEV	Indicates recent or past infection (assay not widely available).
Hepatitis G		
HGV (HGBV-C)	Hepatitis G virus	Flavivirus (RNA genome); no serologic test available; detected by RNA PCR in research laboratories.

TABLE 13-2. FEATURES OF LETTERED HEPATITIS VIRUSES

	HAV	HBV	HCV	HDV	HEV	HGV
Major routes of transmission	Fecal–oral, foodborne	Blood, sexual, perinatal	Blood, sexual, perinatal	Blood, especially injection-drug use	Fecal–oral, waterborne	Unknown
Incubation	2–7 wk	6–25 wk	3–16 wk	3–20 wk	8–10 wk	Unknown
Diagnosis	IgM anti-HAV	HBsAg	Anti-HCV	Anti-HDV	Anti-HEV	HGV PCR (research)
Epidemics	Yes	No	No	No	Yes	Unknown
Chronic Infection	No	Yes	Yes	Yes	No	Yes
Liver cancer	No	Yes	Yes	Yes	No	Unknown
Vaccine	Yes	Yes	No	No	No	No

ally, a mono-like illness with or without atypical lymphocytes may occur.[16] An enlarged, tender liver is palpable, but jaundice and bile in the urine may not be noted for several days. The maximum serum aminotransferase concentration usually occurs about 2 days after the onset of illness. Symptoms usually resolve by 2 months, but some patients have one or more relapses. Fulminant hepatic failure is very uncommon.[17,18]

Patients are most contagious during the 2-week period before the onset of jaundice or elevation of liver enzymes, when the concentration of virus in the stool is highest.[19] Viral excretion then declines and is usually absent within 1 week after jaundice appears.[20] Occasionally, the virus may be shed for several months, especially in infants and young children.[21] Viral shedding can also recur in patients with relapsing illness.[22]

Hepatitis B Virus

Unlike hepatitis A virus, hepatitis B virus (HBV) is not transmitted fecal-orally and is not associated with common-source outbreaks. In areas of the world with a high prevalence of hepatitis B infection, such as Asia and Africa, most infections are acquired vertically at the time of birth. In contrast, the majority of hepatitis B infections in developed countries result from sexual activity, injection-drug use, or occupational exposure.[4] Because of donor screening, the risk of hepatitis B infection from a single blood transfusion is estimated to be 1 in 63,000.[23] Importantly, no clear risk factors for infection are found in 20–30% of patients.[4]

Clinical symptoms and course depend on the age of the patient. Hepatitis B virus is not cytopathic; the host immune response is the cause of the liver injury.[23a] A vigorous immune response, as seen in older children and adults, results in symptomatic infection and high likelihood of viral clearance. In contrast, because of their immature immune system, more than 90% of infected neonates have an asymptomatic infection followed by chronic hepatitis. Up to 25% of persons with chronic infection eventually die of end-stage liver disease or hepatocellular carcinoma.[24]

In the older child, hepatitis B infection clinically resembles hepatitis A, although symptoms are usually milder. Occasionally, an acute polyarthritis and urticarial rash may precede the jaundice. Gianotti-Crosti syndrome, also called papular acrodermatitis of childhood, is an erythematous papular rash sometimes seen in the child with acute hepatitis B infection. It is thought to result from deposition of immune complexes. Other viral infections such as Epstein-Barr virus, coxsackievirus, and parainfluenza virus can produce an identical rash (see Chapter 11).[25,26]

Hepatitis C Virus

This virus was identified in the late 1980s as the cause of most transfusion-associated "non-A, non-B" hepatitis. Currently, nearly 2% of the U.S. population is chronically infected with hepatitis C virus (HCV), leading to its label as the "silent epidemic."[27] HCV-associated end-stage liver disease is the most frequent indication for liver transplantation in adults. With the widespread implementation of blood product screening in 1992, the current risk of transfusion-associated hepatitis C is estimated at 1 in 100,000 units.[23] The virus can also be transmitted perinatally, sexually, and by injection drug use. Approximately 5% of neonates born to HCV-positive mothers become infected; if the mother also has HIV infection, the risk is 2–3 times higher.[28] Sexual activity appears to be a relatively inefficient means of transmission. Long-term spouses of patients with chronic HCV infection have a prevalence of infection of less than 5%.[29,30] In approximately 10% of people with hepatitis C infection, no source can be identified.[28]

Most acute infections with HCV are inapparent; fewer than a third of patients will have jaundice, which may be accompanied by anorexia, malaise, or abdominal pain. As with hepatitis A and B infection, a fulminant presentation with acute hepatitis C infection is rare but has been reported in children.[31] The hallmark of hepatitis C infection is its chronicity; approximately 80% of infected people develop chronic infection, which is often asymptomatic and without abnormalities in liver enzymes. For this reason, the Centers for Disease Control and Prevention (CDC) has made recommendations for routine screening of people in high-risk categories.[28] These include people with a history of injection-drug use, long-term hemodialysis, persistently elevated ALT levels, and those who received blood products or an organ transplant prior to July 1992.[28] In addition, children born to women known to be HCV-positive should be tested for the presence of HCV antibody at 15–18 months of age, when passively transferred maternal antibody is no longer detectable.

The natural history of hepatitis C infection in children is largely unknown. Of 67 infants with transfusion-acquired infection, only 55% had evidence of chronic infection 20 years later, a figure substantially lower than is usually seen in adults.[32] In addition, only three patients had histologic evidence of progressive liver disease. The majority of neonates who acquire hepatitis C perinatally develop chronic infection with only mild liver disease during childhood, although long-term follow-up data are lacking.[33] In adults with chronic hepatitis C infection, 15–20% eventually develop end-stage liver disease.[34] Once cirrhosis is established, the risk of hepatocellular carcinoma is approximately 1% to 4% per year.[35]

Hepatitis D Virus

Also called delta virus, this is a defective RNA virus that needs the help of the hepatitis B virus to replicate. Thus, it is seen exclusively in patients acutely or chronically infected with hepatitis B. Most infections occur in injection-drug users. Coinfection with hepatitis D virus (HDV) considerably worsens the prognosis of HBV infection. Therefore, hepatitis D coinfection is an important consideration when the condition of a patient with chronic hepatitis B infection worsens or when a test for HBeAg is negative but active liver disease persists.[4]

Hepatitis E Virus

Previously known as enterically transmitted "non-A, non-B" hepatitis, hepatitis E virus (HEV) shares many similarities with hepatitis A, including route of transmission, epidemic potential, increased incidence in the developing world, and lack of a chronic carrier state. The disease was first recognized in the early 1980s when sera from persons affected during a 1955 waterborne epidemic of hepatitis in Delhi, India, were found to lack serological markers of acute hepatitis A and B.[36] The genome was cloned and sequenced in the early 1990s.[37,38]

Large, waterborne outbreaks have been reported from southeast and central Asia, Africa, the Middle East, and Mexico.[39] In contrast to hepatitis A, person-to-person transmission is uncommon. Women infected with HEV during the third trimester of pregnancy may transmit infection to their fetuses, with significant perinatal morbidity and mortality.[40] The majority of clinically apparent infections occur in young adults; most infected children are probably asymptomatic.[41] Symptomatic infection is indistinguishable from acute icteric hepatitis of other causes. A notable exception is that infection in pregnant women often causes fulminant hepatic failure, with mortality rates of 15–25%.[42]

Hepatitis G Virus

This virus, also referred to as hepatitis GB virus C, has been detected in the serum of 1–2% of healthy blood donors and can be transmitted by transfusion.[43] However, there is no evidence that it causes hepatitis.[44] As with the elusive hepatitis F virus,[45] its inclusion in the group of lettered hepatitis viruses was probably premature.

■ FREQUENCY IN CHILDREN

Of the lettered hepatitis viruses, hepatitis A virus is the most frequent cause of hepatitis in children in the United States.[45a] The incidence varies by race and ethnicity, with the highest rates occurring among American Indians/Alaskan Natives and Hispanics.[46] Hepatitis B virus infection is much less common and is usually secondary to transmission during delivery. With the implementation of routine screening of pregnant women and postexposure prophylaxis of newborns with hepatitis B vaccine and hepatitis B immune globulin (see section on Prevention), the incidence of hepatitis B in children continues to decline.[47] Among all age groups, the prevalence of chronic hepatitis C infection in the United States is approximately twice that of hepatitis B.[35] In children, the seroprevalence of hepatitis C virus infection is 0.2% for those younger than 12 years of age and 0.4% for those 12–19 years of age,[48] although rates are highly variable among population subgroups. Hepatitis in children in the United States is frequently caused by agents other than the lettered hepatitis viruses.

■ OTHER INFECTIOUS CAUSES

Many viruses can produce hepatitis in children, especially Epstein-Barr virus (EBV) (see Chapter 3). Nonviral infections can also cause hepatitis (Box 13-1). Most of these infections are discussed in other chapters and so are only mentioned here.

Bacterial sepsis can cause jaundice (especially in the newborn) by several mechanisms, including hemolysis and liver cell destruction, and the serum aminotransferase concentrations can be significantly elevated at the onset of jaundice.[49] Hepatitis with jaundice is an occasional complication of urinary infection,[50] scarlet fever,[51] or Kawasaki disease.[52,53] Acute suppurative cholangitis and, less frequently, acute cholecystitis may be associated with elevated bilirubin and aminotransferase levels in the serum.[54]

Common Viruses

EBV can present with hyperbilirubinemia[55] or as anicteric hepatitis.[56] Fulminant hepatitis is rare.[57] There is some evidence to suggest that EBV infection can induce autoimmune hepatitis in suscepti-

---

BOX 13-1 ■ Some Infectious Causes of Hepatitis in Children Other than the Lettered Hepatitis Viruses

Viruses
Epstein-Barr virus[56]
Enteroviruses (coxsackieviruses, echoviruses)[70]
Human immunodeficiency virus[65]
Adenoviruses (immunocompromised host)[76]
Disseminated herpes simplex,[59] varicella,[61] cytomegalovirus[63]

Bacterial infections
Scarlet fever[51]
Urinary tract infections, especially in neonates[50]
Liver abscesses[132]
Cholangitis[54]

Uncommon infections
Psittacosis (pneumonia)[133]
Leptospirosis[79]
Brucellosis (FUO)[134]
Rocky Mountain spotted fever (rash)[135]
Ehrlichiosis (cytopenia)[136]
Early syphilis[137]
Cat-scratch disease (FUO)[10]
Mycoplasma (pneumonia)[138]
Lyme disease[139]
Visceral larva migrans[140]

Usually acquired outside the United States
Yellow fever (and other viral hemorrhagic fevers)[141,142]
Amebic liver abscess[143]
Schistosomiasis[144]
Liver flukes[145]
Hydatid disease[146]
Malaria[147]
Typhoid fever[148]
Dengue fever[149]

---

ble individuals.[58] In addition to EBV, disseminated infection by other members of the herpes virus family (herpes simplex virus, varicella zoster virus, cytomegalovirus, human herpes virus 6) typically involves the liver, with the severity primarily dependent on the immune status of the patient.[59–64] Hepatic involvement in patients with primary HIV infection is not uncommon; 20% of patients with the acute retroviral syndrome will have elevated liver enzymes.[65]

Neonates with disseminated disease due to herpes simplex virus,[66,67] enterovirus,[68] or adenovirus[69] infection commonly have elevated aminotransferase levels and may present with a picture of fulminant hepatitis (see Chapter 19). Common viruses that may on rare occasions produce hepatitis after the neonatal period include coxsackieviruses A and B[70] and parvovirus B19.[71] Measles in teenagers and young adults can be associated with mild hepatocellular jaundice.[72] Adenovirus infection is a cause of severe hepatitis in the immunocompromised host.[73–76]

■ LEPTOSPIRA SPECIES

These spirochetes are usually encountered by exposure to animal urine (Chapter 21). Outbreaks may occur in persons exposed to contaminated water.[77,78] Leptospirosis is typically a biphasic illness, with fever, chills, headache, and myalgia for 4–7 days in the first (septicemic) phase.[79] Vomiting and abdominal pain may be prominent, and nonpurulent conjunctival injection is a common physical finding. After an asymptomatic period of 1–3 days, the second (immune) phase is heralded by return of fever and headache. The patient usually has nonpurulent meningitis with a cerebrospinal fluid (CSF) cell count less than 500/mcL, normal to elevated protein and normal glucose (see Chapter 9 for discussion of nonpurulent meningitis). About 10% of patients develop a severe, icteric form of leptospirosis known as Weil's syndrome. These patients present with hemorrhage, renal failure, and jaundice and have a case fatality rate of 5–10%. The separation between the two phases may be indistinct.

The diagnosis of leptospirosis requires a high index of suspicion and is made by culture of the organism from blood or CSF during the first 10 days of illness or from urine between 10–30 days after onset. Special media are required, so the laboratory must be notified that you suspect leptospirosis. Several serologic tests are also available.[79] Examination of urine by darkfield microscopy may reveal the presence of the causative spirochete. However, this method of diagnosis is insensitive and requires a trained and experienced observer. Penicillin G is the treatment of choice.

Disseminated Mycobacterial, Fungal, or Parasitic Infections

As discussed in the section on granulomatous hepatitis, these agents may occasionally cause hepatic granulomas. Although tuberculosis is a more frequent cause, nontuberculous mycobacteria may be associated with liver involvement, especially in patients with AIDS. Disseminated histoplasmosis is the most common fungal etiology of hepatic granulomas in the United States, although other fungal infections are occasionally implicated.[9] Hepatosplenic candidiasis is a well-described cause of hepatic granulomas in the neutropenic cancer patient.[80] Parasitic infections associated with hepatic granulomas include schistosomiasis, amebiasis, and visceral larva migrans (see Chapter 21).[9]

Hepatitis in the Returning Traveler

The causes of liver disease in the developing world are numerous (Box 13-1), and a careful travel history should be obtained in the patient with hepatitis.

■ NONINFECTIOUS HEPATITIS

Many noninfectious diseases can cause elevated liver enzymes and be confused with infectious hepatitis (Table 13-3). Reye's syndrome, which has become rare, resembles a fulminant hepatitis (Chapter 9). Almost any medication can cause an elevation in liver enzymes.[81] Common culprits include nonsteroidal antiinflammatory drugs, antibiotics, and antiepileptic drugs.[1] Some drug reactions can produce hepatic injury as part of a multisystem illness including fever and rash, such as with Stevens-Johnson syndrome or toxic epidermal necrolysis.[82] Early recognition of the association and withdrawal of the offending drug can be lifesaving. The physician should also inquire about the patient's use of herbal preparations, illicit drugs, and recreational sniffing of chemicals. For patients with autoimmune hepatitis, it is especially important to make the diagnosis in a timely fashion, because the treatment for this disorder—immunosuppression—is different from that for other causes of hepatitis, and without treatment the prognosis is poor.[83] Some cases of aplastic anemia are preceded by a clinical hepatitis.[84] The cause is unknown, and it does not appear to be caused by any of the known hepatitis viruses.

■ DIAGNOSTIC APPROACH

Tests for Infectious Mononucleosis

Laboratory studies should be selected on the basis of the clinical findings. A complete blood count and examination of a peripheral smear should be performed. Atypical lymphocytes are most commonly associated with EBV infection but can be

TABLE 13-3. NONINFECTIOUS DISEASES THAT MAY RESEMBLE HEPATITIS

CAUSE OF ELEVATED LIVER ENZYMES	SUPPORTIVE FINDINGS
Medications (including prescription, over-the-counter, and herbal)	History
Halothane anesthesia	History
Chemicals and toxins	History; toxicology testing
Wilson's disease	Decreased ceruloplasmin levels; increased urinary copper excretion
Autoimmune hepatitis	Hypergammaglobulinemia; autoantibodies
Nonalcoholic steatohepatitis	Obesity; fatty infiltration of the liver on ultrasound
Reye syndrome	Encephalopathy; recent aspirin use
Severe congestive heart failure	History and physical examination
Parenteral hyperalimentation (mostly cholestatic)	History
Hereditary muscular disorders	Elevated serum creatinine kinase and aldolase levels
Celiac disease	Elevated serum antiendomysial and antigliadin antibodies
Hereditary primary hemochromatosis	Elevated serum iron; transferrin saturation > 45%
Inflammatory bowel disease	Occult blood in the stool; imaging and endoscopic findings of Crohn's disease or ulcerative colitis
Alpha$_1$-antitrypsin deficiency	Decreased serum alpha$_1$-antitrypsin levels

seen with other viral infections, including hepatitis A. A rapid slide test for heterophile antibody may be done, but this test is insensitive, especially in young children, and it is expected to be negative in CMV-induced mononucleosis. Thus, a complete serologic profile for both EBV and CMV should usually be performed (Chapter 3). IgM antibody to the EBV viral capsid antigen is the best test to detect recent or current EBV infection. However, false-positive results can occasionally occur in patients with CMV, hepatitis A, parvovirus B19, and leptospirosis.[85,86] It is helpful to remember that patients with primary EBV infection usually have elevated specific IgG antibodies and the absence of antibodies to Epstein-Barr nuclear antigen.

Serologic Tests for Lettered Hepatitis Viruses

Hepatitis A

If there are no risk factors for hepatitis B or C, it may be more direct and less expensive to obtain serum for measurement of IgM antibody to hepatitis A virus. If this study is negative, tests for hepatitis B and C can be done. Some laboratories test for antibodies to all three viruses in a panel for a single charge. Hepatitis A IgM antibody is usually gone within 6 months of the onset of jaundice, but may persist for more than a year.[87,88] Persons who have received the hepatitis A vaccine will have anti-HAV total antibody. In addition, IgM anti-HAV can sometimes be detected transiently about 2 weeks after vaccination.[89]

Hepatitis B

A peculiar feature of hepatitis B virus infection is the great excess of envelope material produced. Thus, detection of surface antigen (HBsAg) in the blood is the usual means of making the diagnosis of acute HBV infection. In the rare patient with a negative assay for HBsAg, the presence of IgM to core antigen establishes the diagnosis. To determine past infection, obtaining surface antibody and core antibody (anti-HBs and anti-HBc) can be done. Theoretically, both should be present after infection, but sometimes only one antibody is found. Core antibody is usually regarded as the best indicator of past infection. After immunization with hepatitis B vaccine, only surface antibody is produced, as the vaccine contains only purified HBsAg.

The most confusing pattern, which can occur shortly after hepatitis B infection, is the presence of core antibody for several weeks before surface antibody is produced (so-called window period). During this time, an IgM core-antibody titer should be obtained. If the IgM anti-HBc is positive, this indicates a recent hepatitis B infection and possible infectivity. If the IgM anti-HBc is negative with a positive anti-HBc and negative anti-HBs, the result is usually interpreted as evidence of a loss of anti-HBs after an infection in the distant past.

The e antigen of HBV serves as a marker of active viral replication and correlates with infectivity. However, any time a patient is positive for surface antigen, there is a risk of infectivity, even if the e antigen is absent. Therefore, the precautions are the same regardless of the presence of the e antigen.

All pregnant women should be routinely tested for HBsAg during an early prenatal visit in each pregnancy.[90] Tests for other hepatitis B markers are not necessary for the purpose of maternal screening. However, HBsAg-positive women identified during screening may have HBV-related liver disease and should be evaluated.

Hepatitis C

Currently available serologic tests for this virus measure IgG antibody to hepatitis C infection and do not distinguish between acute, chronic, or resolved infection. Because approximately 80% of patients with hepatitis C infection develop chronic infection, most true-positive tests represent chronic infection. Both enzyme immunoassay (EIA) and recombinant immunoblot assay (RIBA) techniques are more than 97% sensitive, but the latter is more specific (fewer false-positives). Thus, the EIA is usually performed first and, if positive, confirmed with the RIBA. To determine whether the patient has an active infection, polymerase chain reaction (PCR) is used to detect hepatitis C RNA in serum or plasma. More than 95% of persons with acute or chronic hepatitis C will test positive for HCV RNA.[28]

In infants born to HCV-positive mothers, sero-

logic testing for perinatally acquired HCV infection is confounded by the presence of maternal antibody. In > 95% of uninfected children, maternal antibody will be absent by 15 months of age,[91] and testing is usually deferred until then. After the first month of life, PCR is highly sensitive and specific for diagnosing HCV infection.[91] However, unlike the situation with perinatal HIV infection, early diagnosis does not affect management and thus it is reasonable to omit PCR testing.

Hepatitis D

Patients with severe or rapidly progressing HBV infection may be coinfected with HDV. ELISA is used to demonstrate antibodies to HDV. Serial testing may be necessary.

Hepatitis E

Serologic testing for hepatitis E is available in some reference laboratories. IgM anti-HEV appears early during acute infection and disappears over 4–5 months. IgG anti-HEV is detectable a few days after IgM and remains elevated at least for a few years; the exact duration of its persistence is not known.[39]

Other Studies

Enteroviruses, cytomegalovirus, and adenoviruses can be recovered by conventional cell culture techniques, although PCR is rapidly replacing culture in many laboratories. In the patient with hepatitis, it is usually helpful to measure alkaline phosphatase and bilirubin to look for evidence of cholestasis and biliary obstruction. If elevated, ultrasonography of the right upper quadrant can be done to assess the hepatic parenchyma and bile ducts. Measuring the prothrombin time and serum albumin assesses hepatic synthetic function. The preceding tests are not necessary in the patient with uncomplicated viral hepatitis of known cause, but should be performed in patients with severe hepatitis or hepatitis of uncertain etiology. Liver biopsy is often useful for determining the prognosis of fulminant or chronic hepatitis and is occasionally helpful in determining the etiology of liver disease.[92]

■ TREATMENT

Acute Hepatitis

In mild acute hepatitis A, no special treatment or restrictions are necessary. In moderate to severe hepatitis of any cause, the patient should be hospitalized and liver function monitored daily. Drugs metabolized by the liver should be avoided if possible. If their use is necessary, the dose should be reduced and serum levels monitored. If a specific cause for the hepatitis is found, therapy should be directed to the underlying condition. For the most common viral causes of hepatitis in the immunocompetent host (EBV, CMV, and the lettered hepatitis viruses), no specific therapy is necessary in the acute stage.

Chronic Hepatitis

The treatment of chronic infection with hepatitis B or C virus is complex and should be undertaken in concert with a gastroenterologist or an infectious diseases specialist familiar with the currently available therapies. In the past, the mainstay of therapy for both forms of chronic hepatitis has been interferon alfa.[93] Unfortunately, the side effects (e.g., headache, fatigue, myalgia, depression, and cytopenias) prompt discontinuation of therapy in approximately 10% of patients.

Among patients with HBV infection, those who are HBeAg-positive are at increased risk of progression to cirrhosis, and thus they should generally be treated. Response to therapy (defined as loss of HBeAg and decline at ALT and HBV DNA levels) occurs in about 30% of patients treated with interferon alfa and in about 40% of patients treated with lamivudine.[23a,94,95] Development of resistance of lamivudine is common, but the clinical significance of this is uncertain. Recently, a third drug (adefovir), was approved for the treatment of HBV infection.[23a]

For patients with chronic HCV infection, treatment is recommended for those with detectable HCV RNA and at least moderate inflammation with bridging or portal fibrosis on biopsy.[96] Treatment is usually with a combination of interferon alfa and vibavirin for 12 months. A sustained viral response to therapy is defined as absence of serum HCV RNA 6 months after completion of therapy. Although data in children are limited, one small study reported a response rate of 40% with this regimen.[97] Attaching polyethylene glycol to interferon alfa provides a longer half-life and possible a higher rate of response.[98]

For patients with end-stage liver disease due to either hepatitis B or C, liver transplantation is required. In the case of hepatitis C, recurrence of infection in the transplanted liver is nearly universal. In contrast, recurrences in patients receiving liver transplants for hepatitis B infection can largely be prevented by the use of hepatitis B immune globulin (HBIG) and lamivudine.[99]

■ COMPLICATIONS

Acute hepatic failure (also called fulminant hepatitis) is defined as that occurring within 8 weeks of onset and fortunately is rare in children.[100,101] It can result from hepatitis of any cause. Signs of impending acute liver failure include persistent vomiting, progressive lethargy, increasing serum bilirubin and liver enzymes, and prolonged prothrombin time. Intensive medical care is required. Depending on the stability of the patient and the availability of a donor organ, a liver transplant may be performed.

Other complications that have been reported in children with hepatitis A infection include urticaria,[102] acute pancreatitis,[103] encephalitis,[104] transverse myelitis,[105] cerebella ataxia,[106] seizures,[107] acute renal failure,[108] ascites,[109] pleural effusion,[110] and subsequent development of autoimmune hepatitis.[111] Hepatitis B virus infection is occasionally complicated by immune complex formation, which may manifest as pleuritis, arthritis, vasculitis, or glomerulonephritis.[4] A number of parainfectious phenomena have been associated with chronic hepatitis C infection. In a multicenter trial of 321 patients, 38% had at least one extrahepatic manifestation, including cutaneous findings, arthralgia, and neuropathy.[112] Immunologic abnormalities, such as the presence of mixed cryoglobulins, rheumatoid factor, antinuclear antibodies, and thrombocytopenia, were also common.

■ PREVENTION

Hepatitis A

Guidelines for preventing hepatitis A infection are updated regularly by the Advisory Committee on Immunization Practices (ACIP).[46] The two means of preventing hepatitis A are vaccination and immune globulin (IG). In contrast to IG administration, hepatitis A vaccination provides long-term protection and thus is generally preferred. However, hepatitis A vaccine is not approved for use in children younger than 2 years, and its effectiveness in the patient who has had a recent exposure to hepatitis A is unknown (i.e., for postexposure prophylaxis).

Immune Globulin

A single intramuscular dose of IG (0.02 mL/kg, maximum 2 mL) should be administered to all previously unvaccinated household or day-care contacts of a person with serologically confirmed hepatitis A infection. It should be given as soon as possible and not more than 2 weeks after the exposure. If given within this time frame, it is more than 85% effective in preventing hepatitis A. It is reasonable to also administer hepatitis A vaccine at the same time to provide long-term protection from future exposures. (IG does not interfere with the immune response to inactivated vaccines.) For preexposure prophylaxis in children younger than 2 years old traveling to endemic areas, the dose of IG depends on the length of stay: 0.02 mL/kg for stays less than 2 months and 0.06 mL/kg for stays of 3 to 5 months.

Hepatitis A Vaccine

Two inactivated hepatitis A vaccines are approved for use in children in the United States. Both are administered in two-dose schedules, and both are highly immunogenic and effective in children older than 2 years old. Physicians should consult the current Red Book or the package insert for doses, as there are dosing differences between the two vaccines.

Currently, the ACIP recommends that children living in areas where rates of hepatitis A are at least twice the national average (primarily the western United States) should be routinely vaccinated.[46] Because children often have unrecognized infections, they play an important role in hepatitis A virus transmission in families and in the community.[113] It is hoped that more widespread immunization of children will significantly lower the incidence of hepatitis A in the United States. Persons at increased risk for infection with hepatitis A should also be vaccinated. This includes homosexual males, illegal drug users, persons with clotting-factor disorders, and those traveling to countries with high rates of hepatitis A. Although two doses are recommended, most travelers present for advice only shortly before their trip. Thus, a single dose is given, and the traveler is instructed to return in 6 months to complete the series. No data are available regarding the timing of appearance of protective antibody in children. In adults, over 95% of vaccinees develop anti-HAV antibodies within a month after receipt of a single dose, and up to 80% may have antibodies within 2 weeks.[114] The booster dose given 6 to 12 months later results in higher antibody titers and extends the duration of protection. Children with chronic liver disease, including those who are awaiting or who have received liver transplants, should receive hepatitis A vaccine. Finally, public health authorities may institute a widespread vaccination campaign during certain communitywide epidemics.

Hepatitis B

Two hepatitis B vaccines, which contain purified HBsAg produced by recombinant DNA technology, are approved for use in the United States. They are highly immunogenic and effective in all age groups, including newborns. Despite some claims espoused by the media, they are also very safe; a recent study demonstrated no association between hepatitis B vaccination and the development of multiple sclerosis.[115] Universal hepatitis B vaccination has been shown to decrease the incidence of chronic hepatitis in children by more than 90%[116] and to decrease the incidence of hepatocellular carcinoma.[117]

Routine Immunization

Hepatitis B vaccine is recommended for routine immunization of all infants. Initial attempts to implement a vaccine program targeted at high-risk groups did not result in decreased HBV infection rates. Universal infant vaccination is appropriate because it is not possible to predict which children will subsequently engage in high-risk behaviors and because nearly one-third of people with HBV infection have no known risk factors. Giving the first dose during the birth hospitalization increases the likelihood of completing the three-dose series.[118] It may also be associated with timely receipt of other routine vaccinations in infancy.[119] Theoretical concerns about the use of thimerosal, a mercury-based compound used as a preservative, caused a decrease in newborn vaccination rates.[120] However, thimerosal is no longer used as a preservative in any of the pediatric hepatitis B vaccines licensed in the United States.[121] The most efficient way to assure high immunization rates in this setting is for hospitals to have standing orders for routine hepatitis B vaccination of newborns.

Older children who have not previously received the hepatitis B vaccine series should be vaccinated at 11–12 years of age.[122] An alternate two-dose schedule for adolescents aged 11–15 years using a higher titer of vaccine has recently been approved and should lead to higher vaccination rates in this age group.[123]

Premature Infants

Preterm infants weighing less than 2 kg have a decreased immune response to the vaccine. For these children, initiation of immunization should be delayed until just before hospital discharge if the infant weighs 2 kg or more, or until approximately 2 months of age when other routine immunizations are given.[124]

High-risk Groups

In addition to routine vaccination of the age groups outlined previously, children at high risk for hepatitis B infection should be vaccinated at any age. These include the following groups: Alaskan Native/Pacific Islanders, children in households of first-generation immigrants from countries where HBV infection is endemic, adoptees from HBV-endemic areas, children in households with a known hepatitis B carrier, and children receiving hemodialysis or clotting-factor concentrates. Adolescents who are sexually active (heterosexual or homosex-

ual) or injecting drug users should be vaccinated.[90] Children who are awaiting or have received a liver transplant should also receive hepatitis B vaccine.[125]

Screening Pregnant Women

Because screening only high-risk pregnant women failed to identify more than half of HBV-infected mothers,[126] prenatal HBsAg testing of all pregnant women is now recommended.[90]

Newborn of Hepatitis B Carrier

Children, including preterm infants, who are born to HBsAg-positive mothers should receive hepatitis B vaccine and HBIG (0.5 mL) at different sites within 12 hours of birth. This regimen reduces the risk of hepatitis B infection in the newborn from approximately 80% to 5%.[127] Breast-feeding is not contraindicated for babies who have received these prophylactic measures. For infants born to mothers whose HBsAg status is unknown, hepatitis B vaccine should be given within 12 hours of birth. If the newborn is a premature baby weighing less than 2 kg, HBIG (0.5 mL) is also given.

TABLE 13-4. POSTEXPOSURE PROPHYLAXIS AFTER PERCUTANEOUS OR MUCOSAL EXPOSURE TO HEPATITIS B VIRUS[128]

VACCINATION HISTORY AND ANTIBODY RESPONSE STATUS OF EXPOSED PERSON	TREATMENT		
	SOURCE HBsAg-POSITIVE	SOURCE HBsAg-NEGATIVE	SOURCE STATUS UNKNOWN
Unvaccinated	HBIG* × 1; initiate HBV vaccine series	Initiate HBV vaccine series	Initiate HBV vaccine series
Previously vaccinated:			
Known responder†	No treatment	No treatment	No treatment
Known nonresponder†	HBIG × 2 or HBIG × 1 and initiate revaccination	No treatment	If known high-risk source, treat as if source were HBsAg positive
Antibody response unknown	Test exposed person for anti-HBs:	No treatment	Test exposed person for anti-HBs:
	1. If adequate†, no treatment		1. If adequate†, no treatment
	2. If inadequate, HBIG × 1 and vaccine booster		2. If inadequate, give vaccine booster and recheck titer in 1–2 months

* Dose of HBIG is 0.06 mL/kg intramuscularly.
† Responder is defined as person with serum antibody to HBsAg ≥ 10 mIU/mL.

Postexposure Prophylaxis

A rough estimate of the comparative risks of viral transmission through a contaminated needlestick is provided by the rule of threes: HBV is transmitted in approximately 30% of exposures, HCV in 3%, and HIV in 0.3%.[35] The CDC's recommendations for accidental percutaneous or mucosal exposure are given in Table 13-4.[128] Although such exposures usually occur in a medical setting, hepatitis B can also be transmitted by a human bite.[129] It has also been transmitted by a needlestick from a syringe that was discarded in a public place.[130] Previously unvaccinated children with such exposures should receive the hepatitis B vaccine as outlined in Table 13-4. The effectiveness of postexposure prophylaxis against HBV infection is > 75%.[128]

Combined Hepatitis A and B Vaccine

A combination vaccine was recently approved as a three-dose series for adults older than 18 years. It appears to be immunogenic in children as well.[131] If approved for use in children, it would decrease the number of injections for those requiring both hepatitis A and B vaccination.

Hepatitis C

No vaccine is available for hepatitis C. In addition, because immune globulin is manufactured from plasma documented to lack antibodies to hepatitis C, postexposure prophylaxis with this product is not effective. Cesarean delivery does not decrease perinatal transmission. Breast-feeding by mothers with hepatitis C infection has not been documented to transmit infection and may be permitted. Whether body piercing or tattooing are risk factors for hepatitis C infection is unclear. Currently, the primary means of prevention is to avoid high-risk drug and sexual practices.[28]

Hepatitis E

Travelers to areas endemic for hepatitis E can avoid infection by drinking only boiled or bottled water. Immune globulin is not effective, as most plasma donors in the United States lack antibodies to hepatitis E.

■ REFERENCES

1. Pratt DS, Kaplan MM. Evaluation of abnormal liver-enzyme results in asymptomatic patients. N Engl J Med 2000;342:1266–71.

2. Bardella MT, Vecchi M, Conte D, et al. Chronic unexplained hypertransaminasemia may be caused by occult celiac disease. Hepatology 1999;29:654–7.

3. Zylberberg H, Pol S, Thiers V, et al. Significance of repeatedly normal aminotransferase activities in HCV-infected patients. J Clin Gastroenterol 1999;29:71–5.

4. Lee WM. Hepatitis B virus infection. N Engl J Med 1997; 337:1733–45.

5. Desmet VJ, Gerber M, Hoofnagle JH, et al. Classification of chronic hepatitis: diagnosis, grading and staging. Hepatology 1994;19:1513–20.

6. Tanno H, Fay OH, Rojman JA, Palazzi J. Biphasic form of hepatitis A virus infection: a frequent variant in Argentina. Liver 1988;8:53–7.

7. Tateda A, Kikuchi K, Numazaki Y, Shirachi R, Ishida N. Non-B hepatitis in Japanese recipients of blood transfusions: clinical and serologic studies after the introduction of laboratory screening of donor blood for hepatitis B surface antigen. J Infect Dis 1979;139:511–8.

8. Duff P. Hepatitis in pregnancy. Semin Perinatol 1998;22: 277–83.

9. Harrington PT, Gutierrez JJ, Ramirez-Ronda CH, et al. Granulomatous hepatitis. Rev Infect Dis 1982;4:638–55.

10. Estrada B, Silio M, Begue RE, Van Dyke RB. Unsuspected hepatosplenic involvement in patients hospitalized with cat-scratch disease. Pediatr Infect Dis J 1996;15:720–1.

11. Dunn MW, Berkowitz FE, Miller JJ, Snitzer JA. Hepatosplenic cat-scratch disease and abdominal pain. Pediatr Infect Dis J 1997;16:269–72.

12. Bell BP, Shapiro CN, Alter MJ, et al. The diverse patterns of hepatitis A epidemiology in the United States—implications for vaccination strategies. J Infect Dis 1998;178: 1579–84.

13. Hadler SC, Webster HM, Erben JJ, et al. Hepatitis A in day-care centers. A community-wide assessment. N Engl J Med 1980;302:1222–7.

14. Hutin YJ, Pool V, Cramer EH, et al. A multistate, foodborne outbreak of hepatitis A. National Hepatitis A Investigation Team. N Engl J Med 1999;340:595–602.

15. Krugman S, Giles JP, Hammond J. Infectious hepatitis. Evidence for two distinctive clinical, epidemiological, and immunological types of infection. JAMA 1967;200: 365–73.

16. Garcia-Erce JA, Salvador-Osuna C, Seoane A, et al. [Mononucleosis syndrome caused by hepatitis A virus]. Rev Clin Esp 1999;199:777.

17. Willner IR, Uhl MD, Howard SC, et al. Serious hepatitis A: an analysis of patients hospitalized during an urban epidemic in the United States. Ann Intern Med 1998; 128:111–4.

18. Rodriguez MJ, Schiff ER, Tzakis AG. Hepatitis A: a potentially serious disease. Ann Intern Med 1998;129:506.

19. Rakela J, Mosley JW. Fecal excretion of hepatitis A virus in humans. J Infect Dis 1977;135:933–8.

20. Dienstag JL, Feinstone SM, Kapikian AZ, Purcell RH. Faecal shedding of hepatitis-A antigen. Lancet 1975;1: 765–7.

21. Rosenblum LS, Villarino ME, Nainan OV, et al. Hepatitis A outbreak in a neonatal intensive care unit: risk factors for transmission and evidence of prolonged viral excretion among preterm infants. J Infect Dis 1991;164: 476–82.

22. Sjogren MH, Tanno H, Fay O, et al. Hepatitis A virus in stool during clinical relapse. Ann Intern Med 1987;106: 221–6.

23. Schreiber GB, Busch MP, Kleinman SH, Korelitz JJ. The risk of transfusion-transmitted viral infections. The Retrovirus Epidemiology Donor Study. N Engl J Med 1996; 334:1685–90.

23a. Ganem D, Prince AM. Hepatitis B virus infection: natural history and clinical consequences. N Engl J Med 2004; 350:1118–29.

24. Hsieh CC, Tzonou A, Zavitsanos X, et al. Age at first establishment of chronic hepatitis B virus infection and hepatocellular carcinoma risk. A birth order study. Am J Epidemiol 1992;136:1115–21.

25. Spear KL, Winkelmann RK. Gianotti-Crosti syndrome. A review of ten cases not associated with hepatitis B. Arch Dermatol 1984;120:891–6.

26. Caputo R, Gelmetti C, Ermacora E, et al. Gianotti-Crosti syndrome: a retrospective analysis of 308 cases. J Am Acad Dermatol 1992;26:207–10.

27. Lee WM. The silent epidemic of hepatitis C. Gastroenterology 1993;104:661–2.

28. Recommendations for prevention and control of hepatitis C virus (HCV) infection and HCV-related chronic disease. Centers for Disease Control and Prevention. MMWR Morb Mortal Wkly Rep 1998;47:1–39.

29. Eyster ME, Alter HJ, Aledort LM, et al. Heterosexual co-transmission of hepatitis C virus (HCV) and human immunodeficiency virus (HIV). Ann Intern Med 1991;115: 764–8.

30. Brettler DB, Mannucci PM, Gringeri A, et al. The low risk of hepatitis C virus transmission among sexual partners of hepatitis C-infected hemophilic males: an international, multicenter study. Blood 1992;80:540–3.

31. Taga T, Ikeda M, Suzuki K, et al. Fulminant hepatitis caused by hepatitis C virus. Pediatr Infect Dis J 1998;17: 1174–6.

32. Vogt M, Lang T, Frosner G, et al. Prevalence and clinical outcome of hepatitis C infection in children who underwent cardiac surgery before the implementation of blood-donor screening. N Engl J Med 1999;341:866–70.

33. Bortolotti F, Resti M, Giacchino R, et al. Hepatitis C virus infection and related liver disease in children of mothers with antibodies to the virus. J Pediatr 1997;130:990–3.

34. Liang TJ, Rehermann B, Seeff LB, Hoofnagle JH. Pathogenesis, natural history, treatment, and prevention of hepatitis C. Ann Intern Med 2000;132:296–305.

35. Lauer GM, Walker BD. Hepatitis C virus infection. N Engl J Med 2001;345:41–52.

36. Wong DC, Purcell RH, Sreenivasan MA, Prasad SR, Pavri KM. Epidemic and endemic hepatitis in India: evidence for a non-A, non-B hepatitis virus aetiology. Lancet 1980; 2:876–9.

37. Reyes GR, Purdy MA, Kim JP, et al. Isolation of a cDNA from the virus responsible for enterically transmitted non-A, non-B hepatitis. Science 1990;247:1335–9.

38. Tam AW, Smith MM, Guerra ME, et al. Hepatitis E virus (HEV): molecular cloning and sequencing of the full-length viral genome. Virology 1991;185:120–31.

39. Aggarwal R, Krawczynski K. Hepatitis E: an overview and recent advances in clinical and laboratory research. J Gastroenterol Hepatol 2000;15:9–20.

40. Khuroo MS, Kamili S, Jameel S. Vertical transmission of hepatitis E virus. Lancet 1995;345:1025–6.

41. Aggarwal R, Shahi H, Naik S, et al. Evidence in favour of high infection rate with hepatitis E virus among young children in India. J Hepatol 1997;26:1425–6.

42. Tsega E, Hansson BG, Krawczynski K, Nordenfelt E. Acute sporadic viral hepatitis in Ethiopia: causes, risk factors, and effects on pregnancy. Clin Infect Dis 1992; 14:961–5.

43. Alter HJ, Nakatsuji Y, Melpolder J, et al. The incidence of transfusion-associated hepatitis G virus infection and its relation to liver disease. N Engl J Med 1997;336: 747–54.

44. Alter MJ, Gallagher M, Morris TT, et al. Acute non-A-E hepatitis in the United States and the role of hepatitis G virus infection. Sentinel Counties Viral Hepatitis Study Team. N Engl J Med 1997;336:741–6.

45. Fagan EA, Ellis DS, Tovey GM, et al. Toga-like virus as a cause of fulminant hepatitis attributed to sporadic non-A, non-B. J Med Virol 1989;28:150–5.

45a. Leach CT. Hepatitis A in the United States. Pediatr Infect Dis J 2004; 23:551–2.

46. Prevention of hepatitis A through active or passive immunization: Recommendations of the Advisory Committee on Immunization Practices (ACIP). MMWR Morb Mortal Wkly Rep 1999;48:1–37.

47. Program to prevent perinatal hepatitis B virus transmission in a health-maintenance organization—Northern California, 1990–1995. MMWR Morb Mortal Wkly Rep 1997;46:378–80.

48. Hepatitis C virus infection. American Academy of Pediatrics. Committee on Infectious Diseases. Pediatrics 1998; 101:481–5.

49. Miller DJ, Keeton DG, Webber BL, et al. Jaundice in severe bacterial infection. Gastroenterology 1976;71:94–7.

50. Hamdan JM, Rizk F. Jaundice complicating urinary tract infection in childhood. Pediatr Infect Dis 1985;4:418–9.

51. Kocak N, Ozsoylu S, Ertugrul M, Ozdol G. Liver damage in scarlet fever. Descriptions of two affected children. Clin Pediatr (Phila) 1976;15:462–4.

52. Kawasaki T, Kosaki F, Okawa S, et al. A new infantile acute febrile mucocutaneous lymph node syndrome (MLNS) prevailing in Japan. Pediatrics 1974;54:271–6.

53. Bader-Meunier B, Hadchouel M, Fabre M, et al. Intrahepatic bile duct damage in children with Kawasaki disease. J Pediatr 1992;120:750–2.

54. Carpenter HA. Bacterial and parasitic cholangitis. Mayo Clin Proc 1998;73:473–8.

55. Mahoney DJ Jr, Fernbach DJ, Starke JR, Reid BS. Profound hyperbilirubinemia: an unusual presentation of childhood infectious mononucleosis. Pediatr Infect Dis J 1987;6:73–4.

56. Markin RS. Manifestations of Epstein-Barr virus-associated disorders the in liver. Liver 1994;14:1–13.

57. Feranchak AP, Tyson RW, Narkewicz MR, et al. Fulminant Epstein-Barr viral hepatitis: orthotopic liver transplantation and review of the literature. Liver Transpl Surg 1998;4:469–76.

58. Vento S, Guella L, Mirandola F, et al. Epstein-Barr virus as a trigger for autoimmune hepatitis in susceptible individuals. Lancet 1995;346:608–9.

59. Barton LL, Weaver-Woodard S, Gutierrez JA, Lee DM.

Herpes simplex virus hepatitis in a child: case report and review. Pediatr Infect Dis J 1999;18:1026–8.

60. Kaufman B, Gandhi SA, Louie E, Rizzi R, Illei P. Herpes simplex virus hepatitis: case report and review. Clin Infect Dis 1997;24:334–8.

61. Feldman S, Crout JD, Andrew ME. Incidence and natural history of chemically defined varicella-zoster virus hepatitis in children and adolescents. Scand J Infect Dis 1997; 29:33–6.

62. Morgan ER, Smalley LA. Varicella in immunocompromised children. Incidence of abdominal pain and organ involvement. Am J Dis Child 1983;137:883–5.

63. Eddleston M, Peacock S, Juniper M, Warrell DA. Severe cytomegalovirus infection in immunocompetent patients. Clin Infect Dis 1997;24:52–6.

64. Steeper TA, Horwitz CA, Ablashi DV, et al. The spectrum of clinical and laboratory findings resulting from human herpesvirus-6 (HHV-6) in patients with mononucleosis-like illnesses not resulting from Epstein-Barr virus or cytomegalovirus. Am J Clin Pathol 1990;93:776–83.

65. Kahn JO, Walker BD. Acute human immunodeficiency virus type 1 infection. N Engl J Med 1998;339:33–9.

66. Whitley R, Arvin A, Prober C, et al. Predictors of morbidity and mortality in neonates with herpes simplex virus infections. The National Institute of Allergy and Infectious Diseases Collaborative Antiviral Study Group. N Engl J Med 1991;324:450–4.

67. Greenes DS, Rowitch D, Thorne GM, et al. Neonatal herpes simplex virus infection presenting as fulminant liver failure. Pediatr Infect Dis J 1995;14:242–4.

68. Verboon-Maciolek MA, Swanink CM, Krediet TG, et al. Severe neonatal echovirus 20 infection characterized by hepatic failure. Pediatr Infect Dis J 1997;16:524–7.

69. Abzug MJ, Levin MJ. Neonatal adenovirus infection: four patients and review of the literature. Pediatrics 1991;87: 890–6.

70. Lansky LL, Krugman S, Hug G. Anicteric Coxsackie B hepatitis. J Pediatr 1979;94:64–5.

71. Wiggers H, Rasmussen LH, Moller A. [Parvovirus B19 infection as the cause of hepatitis and neutrophil granulocytosis in a 20-year old woman]. Ugeskr Laeger 1995; 157:5994–5.

72. Gavish D, Kleinman Y, Morag A, Chajek-Shaul T. Hepatitis and jaundice associated with measles in young adults. An analysis of 65 cases. Arch Intern Med 1983;143: 674–7.

73. Krilov LR, Rubin LG, Frogel M, et al. Disseminated adenovirus infection with hepatic necrosis in patients with human immunodeficiency virus infection and other immunodeficiency states. Rev Infect Dis 1990;12:303–7.

74. Ohbu M, Sasaki K, Okudaira M, et al. Adenovirus hepatitis in a patient with severe combined immunodeficiency. Acta Pathol Jpn 1987;37:655–64.

75. Shields AF, Hackman RC, Fife KH, et al. Adenovirus infections in patients undergoing bone-marrow transplantation. N Engl J Med 1985;312:529–33.

76. Michaels MG, Green M, Wald ER, Starzl TE. Adenovirus infection in pediatric liver transplant recipients. J Infect Dis 1992;165:170–4.

77. From the Centers for Disease Control and Prevention. Outbreak of leptospirosis among white-water rafters—Costa Rica, 1996. JAMA 1997;278:808–9.

78. Update: leptospirosis and unexplained acute febrile illness among athletes participating in triathlons—Illinois and Wisconsin, 1998. MMWR Morb Mortal Wkly Rep 1998;47:673–6.

79. Farr RW. Leptospirosis. Clin Infect Dis 1995;21:1–6.

80. Kontoyiannis DP, Luna MA, Samuels BI, Bodey GP. Hepatosplenic candidiasis. A manifestation of chronic disseminated candidiasis. Infect Dis Clin North Am 2000; 14:721–39.

81. Lee WM. Drug-induced hepatotoxicity. N Engl J Med 1995;333:1118–27.

82. Roujeau JC, Stern RS. Severe adverse cutaneous reactions to drugs. N Engl J Med 1994;331:1272–85.

83. Obermayer-Straub P, Strassburg CP, Manns MP. Autoimmune hepatitis. J Hepatol 2000;32:181–97.

84. Brown KE, Tisdale J, Barrett AJ, et al. Hepatitis-associated aplastic anemia. N Engl J Med 1997;336:1059–64.

85. Gray JJ, Caldwell J, Sillis M. The rapid serological diagnosis of infectious mononucleosis. J Infect 1992;25:39–46.

86. Fikar CR, McKee C. False positivity of IGM antibody to Epstein-Barr viral capsid antigen during acute hepatitis A infection. Pediatr Infect Dis J 1994;13:413–4.

87. Kao HW, Ashcavai M, Redeker AG. The persistence of hepatitis A IgM antibody after acute clinical hepatitis A. Hepatology 1984;4:933–6.

88. Dollberg S, Kerem E, Klar A, Branski D. Disappearance of IgM antibodies to hepatitis A virus after an acute infection in children and adolescents. J Pediatr Gastroenterol Nutr 1990;10:307–9.

89. Sjogren MH, Hoke CH, Binn LN, et al. Immunogenicity of an inactivated hepatitis A vaccine. Ann Intern Med 1991;114:470–1.

90. Hepatitis B virus: a comprehensive strategy for eliminating transmission in the United States through universal childhood vaccination. Recommendations of the Immunization Practices Advisory Committee (ACIP). MMWR Morb Mortal Wkly Rep 1991;40:1–25.

91. Dunn DT, Gibb DM, Healy M, et al. Timing and interpretation of tests for diagnosing perinatally acquired hepatitis C virus infection. Pediatr Infect Dis J 2001;20:715–6.

92. Bravo AA, Sheth SG, Chopra S. Liver biopsy. N Engl J Med 2001;344:495–500.

93. Hoofnagle JH, di Bisceglie AM. The treatment of chronic viral hepatitis. N Engl J Med 1997;336:347–56.

94. Wong DK, Cheung AM, O'Rourke K, et al. Effect of alpha-interferon treatment in patients with hepatitis B e antigen-positive chronic hepatitis B. A meta-analysis. Ann Intern Med 1993;119:312–23.

95. Lai CL, Chien RN, Leung NW, et al. A one-year trial of lamivudine for chronic hepatitis B. Asia Hepatitis Lamivudine Study Group. N Engl J Med 1998;339:61–8.

96. Emerick K. Treatment of hepatitis C in children. Pediatr Infect dis J 2004 2004; 23: 257–8.

97. Shoglu DOD, Elkabes B, Sokucu S, Saner G. Does interferon and ribavirin combination therapy increase the rate of treatment response in children with hepatitis C? J Pediatr Gastroenterol Nutr 2002;34:199–206.

98. Zeuzem S, Feinman SV, Rasenack J, et al. Peginterferon alfa-2a in patients with chronic hepatitis C. N Engl J Med 2000;343:1666–72.

99. Rosen HR, Martin P. Viral hepatitis in the liver transplant recipient. Infect Dis Clin North Am 2000;14:761–84.

100. Williams R. Classification, etiology, and considerations of outcome in acute liver failure. Semin Liver Dis 1996; 16:343–8.

101. Russell GJ, Fitzgerald JF, Clark JH. Fulminant hepatic failure. J Pediatr 1987;111:313–9..

102. Dollberg S, Berkun Y, Gross-Kieselstein E. Urticaria in patients with hepatitis A virus infection. Pediatr Infect Dis J 1991;10:702–3.

103. Shrier LA, Karpen SJ, McEvoy C. Acute pancreatitis associated with acute hepatitis A in a young child. J Pediatr 1995;126:57–9.

104. Davis LE, Brown JE, Robertson BH, et al. Hepatitis A post-viral encephalitis. Acta Neurol Scand 1993;87: 67–9.

105. Breningstall GN, Belani KK. Acute transverse myelitis and brainstem encephalitis associated with hepatitis A infection. Pediatr Neurol 1995;12:169–71.

106. Tuthill D, Verrier Jones ER. Acute cerebellar ataxia after subclinical hepatitis A infection. Pediatr Infect Dis J 1996; 15:546–7.

107. Dollberg S, Hurvitz H, Reifen RM, et al. Seizures in the course of hepatitis A. Am J Dis Child 1990;144:140–1.

108. Martino R, Aebischer CC, Baehler P, Bianchetti MG. Acute renal failure complicating nonfulminant hepatitis A in childhood. Nephron 1996;74:490.

109. Dagan R, Yagupsky P, Barki Y. Acute ascites accompanying hepatitis A infection in a child. Infection 1988;16: 360–1.

110. Alhan E, Yildizdas D, Yapicioglu H, Necmi A. Pleural effusion associated with acute hepatitis A infection. Pediatr Infect Dis J 1999;18:1111–2.

111. Huppertz HI, Treichel U, Gassel AM, et al. Autoimmune hepatitis following hepatitis A virus infection. J Hepatol 1995;23:204–8.

112. Cacoub P, Renou C, Rosenthal E, et al. Extrahepatic manifestations associated with hepatitis C virus infection. A prospective multicenter study of 321 patients. Medicine (Baltimore) 2000;79:47–56.

113. Smith PF, Grabau JC, Werzberger A, et al. The role of young children in a community-wide outbreak of hepatitis A. Epidemiol Infect 1997;118:243–52.

114. Lemon SM, Thomas DL. Vaccines to prevent viral hepatitis. N Engl J Med 1997;336:196–204.

114a. Craig AS, Schaffner W. Prevention of hepatitis A with the hepatitis A vaccine. N Engl J Med 2004; 350:476–81.

115. Ascherio A, Zhang SM, Hernan MA, et al. Hepatitis B vaccination and the risk of multiple sclerosis. N Engl J Med 2001;344:327–32.

116. Durand AM, Sabino H, Jr., Mahoney F. Success of mass vaccination of infants against hepatitis B. JAMA 1996; 276:1802–3.

117. Chang MH, Chen CJ, Lai MS, et al. Universal hepatitis B vaccination in Taiwan and the incidence of hepatocellular carcinoma in children. Taiwan Childhood Hepatoma Study Group. N Engl J Med 1997;336:1855–9.

118. Yusuf HR, Daniels D, Smith P, et al. Association between administration of hepatitis B vaccine at birth and completion of the hepatitis B and 4:3:1:3 vaccine series. JAMA 2000;284:978–83.

119. Lauderdale DS, Oram RJ, Goldstein KP, Daum RS. Hepatitis B vaccination among children in inner-city public housing, 1991–1997. JAMA 1999;282:1725–30.

120. Oram RJ, Daum RS, Seal JB, Lauderdale DS. Impact of recommendations to suspend the birth dose of hepatitis B virus vaccine. JAMA 2001;285:1874–9.

121. Update: expanded availability of thimerosal preservative-free hepatitis B vaccine. MMWR Morb Mortal Wkly Rep 2000;49:642–51.

122. Update: recommendations to prevent hepatitis B virus transmission—United States. MMWR Morb Mortal Wkly Rep 1999;48:33–4.

123. Centers for Disease Control and Prevention. Alternate two-dose hepatitis B vaccination schedule for adolescents aged 11–15 years. MMWR Morb Mortal Wkly Rep 2000; 49:261.

124. Amarican Academy of Pediatrics. Hepatitis B. In: Pickering LK, ed. 2000 Red Book: Report of the Committee on Infectious Diseases. Elk Grove Village, IL: American Academy of Pediatrics, 2000:289–302.

125. Burroughs M, Moscona A. Immunization of pediatric solid organ transplant candidates and recipients. Clin Infect Dis 2000;30:857–69.

126. Cruz AC, Frentzen BH, Behnke M. Hepatitis B: a case for prenatal screening of all patients. Am J Obstet Gynecol 1987;156:1180–3.

127. Stevens CE, Taylor PE, Tong MJ, et al. Yeast-recombinant hepatitis B vaccine. Efficacy with hepatitis B immune globulin in prevention of perinatal hepatitis B virus transmission. JAMA 1987;257:2612–6.

128. Centers for Disease Control and Prevention. Updated U.S. public health service guidelines for the management of occupational exposures to HBV, HCV, and HIV and recommendations for postexposure prophylaxis. MMWR 2001;50:20–2.

129. Stornello C. Transmission of hepatitis B via human bite. Lancet 1991;338:1024–5.

130. Garcia-Algar O, Vall O. Hepatitis B virus infection from a needle stick. Pediatr Infect Dis J 1997;16:1099.

131. Van Der Wielen M, Van Damme P, Collard F. A two dose schedule for combined hepatitis A and hepatitis B vaccination in children ages one to eleven years. Pediatr Infect Dis J 2000;19:848–53.

132. Johannsen EC, Sifri CD, Madoff LC. Pyogenic liver abscesses. Infect Dis Clin North Am 2000;14:547–63

133. Samra Z, Pik A, Guidetti-Sharon A, Yona E, Weisman Y. Hepatitis in a family infected by *Chlamydia psittaci*. J R Soc Med. 1991;84:347–8.

134. Losurdo G, Timitilli A, Tasso L, et al. Acute hepatitis due to brucella in a 2 year old child. Arch Dis Child 1994; 71:387.

135. Walker DH. Rocky Mountain spotted fever: a seasonal alert. Clin Infect Dis 1995;20:1111–7.

136. Schutze GE, Jacobs RF. Human monocytic ehrlichiosis in children. Pediatrics 1997;100:E10.

137. Musher DM. Syphilis. Infect Dis Clin North Am 1987;1: 83–95.

138. Arav-Boger R, Assia A, Spirer Z, Bujanover Y, Reif S. Cholestatic hepatitis as a main manifestation of *Mycoplasma pneumoniae* infection. J Pediatr Gastroenterol Nutr 1995; 21:459–60.

139. Edwards KS, Kanengiser S, Li KI, Glassman M. Lyme disease presenting as hepatitis and jaundice in a child. Pediatr Infect Dis J 1990;9:592–3.

140. Kaushik SP, Hurwitz M, McDonald C, Pavli P. *Toxocara canis* infection and granulomatous hepatitis. Am J Gastroenterol 1997;92:1223–5.

141. Robertson SE, Hull BP, Tomori O, et al. Yellow fever: a decade of reemergence. JAMA 1996;276:1157–62.

142. Lacy MD, Smego RA. Viral hemorrhagic fevers. Adv Pediatr Infect Dis 1996;12:21–53.

143. Johnson JL, Baird JS, Hulbert TV, Opas LM. Amebic liver abscess in infancy: case report and review. Clin Infect Dis 1994;19:765–7.

144. Bica I, Hamer DH, Stadecker MJ. Hepatic schistosomiasis. Infect Dis Clin North Am 2000;14:583–604.

145. el-Shabrawi M, el-Karaksy H, Okasha S, et al. Human fascioliasis: clinical features and diagnostic difficulties in Egyptian children. J Trop Pediatr 1997;43:162–6.

146. Clarkson MJ. Hydatid disease. J Med Microbiol 1997;46: 24–6, 8–33.

147. Murthy GL, Sahay RK, Sreenivas DV, et al. Hepatitis in falciparum malaria. Trop Gastroenterol 1998;19:152–4.

148. Gurkan F, Derman O, Yaramis A, Ece A. Distinguishing features of *Salmonella and* viral hepatitis. Pediatr Infect Dis J 2000;19:587.

149. Hayes EB, Gubler DJ. Dengue and dengue hemorrhagic fever. Pediatr Infect Dis J 1992;11:311–7.

CHAPTER 14

Urinary Syndromes

Urinary tract infection (UTI) is one of the most common bacterial infections in children, affecting approximately 8% of girls and 2% of boys in the first 6 years of life.[1] The exact prevalence depends on multiple factors, including age, sex, race, presence of fever, and, for boys, whether the child is circumcised. Among febrile infants in the first 3 months of life, the likelihood of UTI is approximately 13% for girls, 2% for circumcised boys, and 19% for uncircumcised boys.[2] Among children less than 1 year old with fever, the prevalence is about 6% for girls and 3% for boys. Between 1 and 2 years of age, the prevalence in girls is 8%, and in boys it is 2%.[3]

The symptoms of UTI are commonly nonspecific, especially in infants and toddlers. Unfortunately, testing for UTI in the febrile child is often omitted. When testing is performed, results of urinalysis and culture may be misinterpreted. Despite its frequency, many controversies regarding the diagnosis and management of UTI persist. Most clinicians can agree on basic definitions.

■ DEFINITIONS

A presumptive diagnosis of UTI can be made on the basis of typical *clinical manifestations* and *pyuria*, but a laboratory-confirmed diagnosis depends on the demonstration of significant *bacteriuria*. These three characteristics need further definition.

Clinical Manifestations

The manifestations of UTI vary greatly depending on the patient's age. In adults and adolescents with a urinary infection, high fever (>103°F; 39.5°C) usually indicates renal involvement. Children may occasionally have high fever without renal involvement, although reflux with renal infection should be suspected.[4] Frequent or urgent urination implies urethral or bladder irritation. Cloudy urine may be caused by bacterial growth but may also result from precipitated solutes. Foul-smelling urine im-

plies bacterial growth, but occasionally the parent regards concentrated urine as foul smelling. Suprapubic pain or tenderness implies infection involving the bladder; flank pain or tenderness implies infection involving the kidney. Vomiting and other gastrointestinal symptoms not suggesting the urinary tract may be present.

In infants, symptoms are more likely to be absent, mild, or not referable to the urinary tract. Fever may be the only symptom. It is the infant group for whom it is most important, and also most difficult, to diagnose a UTI. The distinction between cystitis and pyelonephritis is particularly difficult in this age group. Among febrile children less than 24 months old with UTI, approximately 60% are found to have renal involvement by scintigraphy.[5–7]

Although peripheral white blood cell (WBC) count, erythrocyte sedimentation rate, and C-reactive protein tend to be higher in children with renal involvement,[8] these markers are not specific for pyelonephritis. Asymptomatic infections are also not rare in females and are detected in about 1% of school-aged girls. True asymptomatic bacteriuria is probably not a risk factor for adverse sequelae in this population.[9] However, in reality, some girls with recurrent UTI have subtle symptoms, often the same with each infection, which should not be considered "asymptomatic bacteriuria."

Pyuria

Generally, "pyuria" is defined as more than 5 (or 10) leukocytes per high-power field in the centrifuged sediment or as an elevated leukocyte count in the uncentrifuged urine, using a hemocytometer to determine the count rapidly.[10] Most authorities agree that 10 or more leukocytes per microliter, as counted on a hemocytometer, represents pyuria. (Centrifuging helps by concentrating the findings of dilute urine and adding the potential for observation of other formed elements.) There is no widely accepted definition of "pyuria," so that the upper limit of normal for leukocytes in the urine is defined by the laboratory or by the physician doing the examination and depends on the methods used. Usually, however, the number of leukocytes in the urine is clearly more than normal, and there is no question about the presence of pyuria. A recent meta-analysis of 48 studies defined "pyuria" as 10 WBC or greater per high-powered field of centrifuged urine or 10 WBC or greater per µl of unspun urine.[11]

Clumps or casts of WBCs also indicate pyuria. The detection of pyuria (or its absence) is extremely helpful in assessing the likelihood of UTI, with a sensitivity of 80–90% and a specificity of 90–95%.[8,12] This does not imply that a culture is unnecessary—it demonstrates that pyuria can help with interpretation of the culture results. In a population with an overall prevalence of UTI of 5% (e.g., infants and young children who have fever without localizing signs), the absence of pyuria predicts the absence of a UTI with greater than 99% accuracy (negative predictive value). The presence of pyuria in this population predicts the presence of UTI in approximately 50% (positive predictive value). The presence of pyuria and microscopic bacteriuria (discussed later) increases the positive predictive value to 85%.[8] The leukocyte esterase test is a surrogate for the presence of WBCs. Its sensitivity and specificity are both about 80%. In contrast, the nitrite reaction is highly specific (approx. 98%) but lacks sensitivity (approx. 50%).[3]

Bacteriuria

Microscopic

Microscopic examination for pyuria is also useful for immediate recognition of the presence of bacteria, which correlates well with the results of urine culture.[10,13] Although the absence of bacteria in the centrifuged sediment does not exclude urinary infection, especially with cocci, bacteria can usually be seen in the sediment if the culture is going to result in more than 100,000 bacteria/mL. Bacteria in casts indicate pyelonephritis. A methylene blue or Gram stain of a drop of uncentrifuged urine is a slightly more sensitive test for microscopic bacteriuria.[13]

Controlled studies have repeatedly demonstrated the usefulness of these methods, which have a sensitivity of 80–90% for unstained centrifuged urine, 85–94% for stained uncentrifuged urine, and 87–98% for stained centrifuged urine, depending on the number of bacteria designated significant in the microscopic study (1 or 5 or 10/hpf) and using 100,000 colonies/mL as the standard culture criterion for significance.[13] Obviously, some significant cultures are not predicted by these methods. Most experts regard any bacteria visualized as being significant, especially if a gram-negative rod is seen.[11,14]

Microscopic bacteriuria with a negative culture can have several possible explanations. Most frequently, the bacteria seen are contaminants that are not recovered by the usual bacteriologic media, for example, diphtheroids, vaginal lactobacilli, or *Haemophilus* spp.[15] However, artifacts and technical errors in collection and culture are much more likely explanations than failure to grow a fastidious pathogen.[16,17]

Significant Bacterial Growth

This term indicates that a properly collected urine culture has had a quantitative culture ("colony count"). Kass found that more than 100,000 bacteria/mL in a clean voided urine usually indicates urinary infection.[17a] The difficulties of this figure do not lie with the accuracy of the counting, which is well within the capabilities of office bacteriology, using a quantitative loop, but rather with the collection of the specimen. The value of more than 100,000 bacteria/mL should not be taken as absolutely reliable in itself, because it assumes a clean voided urine.

Specimens obtained by catheter or suprapubic puncture are significant for infection at a lower concentration. Many experts consider any pure growth from a suprapubic puncture to be significant. Specimens obtained by catheter are subject to a greater risk of contamination by periurethral skin flora (about 9% contamination rate) than suprapubic puncture, and a higher cutoff is appropriate. Hoberman et al.[14] obtained 3257 catheterized urine specimens from young febrile children and found that counts less than 50,000 per mL were most likely to be associated with nonpathogens, mixed flora, or the absence of pyuria. Accordingly, they recommend greater than 50,000 organisms per mL as the cutoff for significant growth from a catheterized specimen.

Interpretation of urine cultures requires that multiple factors be taken into consideration. For example, in a young febrile child without another apparent source for the fever, pure growth of a common urinary pathogen at less than 50,000 organisms per mL from a catheterized specimen may be significant, particularly if the urinalysis shows pyuria. On the other hand, growth of 50,000 to 100,000 organisms per mL is unlikely to indicate a UTI if there is another apparent cause of fever (such as a viral illness), if the organism does not commonly cause UTI (such as *Staphylococcus aureus*), if multiple organisms grow in culture (indicating a contaminated specimen), or if there is no pyuria.

Logical Classification

Using the three factors—clinical manifestations, pyuria, and significant bacteriuria—it is possible to classify any patient into one of eight logical possibilities of combinations (Table 14-1). The use of such a preliminary diagnostic category aids the clinician by giving a guide to an anatomic diagnosis. The logical preliminary diagnoses can have a number of possible etiologies. Typical urinary infection means that all three features (clinical findings, pyuria, and significant bacteriuria) are present.

Urinary symptoms without pyuria or bacteriuria should be the preliminary diagnosis when there are signs and symptoms suggesting a UTI but no pyuria or significant bacteriuria. There are several possible causes of this pattern. Urethritis or vaginitis, especially that caused by *Chlamydia* (discussed in Chapter 15), is a common cause. Infection with *Ureaplasma urealyticum* (and possibly *Mycoplasma hominis*) may cause these symptoms, especially in adults.[18]

Recent or current antibiotic therapy that has suppressed culture-confirmation of the infection is one of the most frequent causes. Overhydration, with rapid urine flow and frequent voiding before bacteria can reach high concentrations, is a rare cause.[19] Medications, such as atropine-like drugs, are an occasional cause of transient frequent urination. Unilateral pyelonephritis with complete ureteral obstruction can produce unusual or intermittent urinary abnormalities.

Urinary symptoms and pyuria without bacteriuria is probably most frequently caused by urethritis. The urethral syndrome (dysuria-pyuria syndrome) can do this and is discussed later in this chapter. Gonorrhea and nongonococcal urethritis are discussed in Chapter 15. Fastidious or anaerobic organisms causing a bladder or kidney infection are an uncommon cause of this pattern.[16] However, *Haemophilus influenzae* is an example of an organism that will not grow on the plating media usually used for urine and that should be regarded as a rare cause of this pattern, usually only in association with clinically suspected bacteremia.[17] Suppression of bacterial growth by contamination of the urine with the disinfectant used to prepare the urethral area is also a very unlikely cause.

Adenoviral cystitis is an uncommon cause of microscopic hematuria and pyuria without bacteriuria.[20]

M. hominis has been implicated in kidney infections in adults by antibody studies.[21] *Ureaplasma urealyticum* can cause a urethritis even in prepubertal children.[22] *Gardnerella vaginalis* is an uncommon urinary pathogen.[23]

Campylobacter jejuni, which requires special

TABLE 14-1. LOGICAL COMBINATIONS OF THREE MAJOR VARIABLES IN URINARY INFECTIONS*

DIAGNOSTIC CLASSIFICATION	SYMPTOMS	PYURIA	BACTERIURIA
Typical urinary infection	+	+	+
Urinary symptoms without pyuria or bacteriuria	+	0	0
Urinary symptoms and pyuria without bacteriuria	+	+	0
Urinary symptoms and bacteriuria without pyuria	+	0	+
Asymptomatic bacteriuria and pyuria	0	+	+
Asymptomatic bacteriuria without pyuria	0	0	+
Asymptomatic pyuria without bacteriuria	0	+	0
No bacterial urinary infection	0	0	0

* Modified from Moffet HL; Urinalysis and urine cultures in children. Urol Clin North Am 1974;1:387–396.

media and higher incubator temperatures to grow, can be missed if it is not suspected, as in a Gram stain. It has been reported as a cause of urinary infection in a girl who did not have any recent diarrhea, as might have been expected.[24]

Urinary symptoms and bacteriuria without pyuria is uncommon. The specimen may have been obtained very early on, before the development of an inflammatory response (as manifested by pyuria) could develop. Alternatively, symptoms may not occur until several days after the onset of an infection when pyuria has decreased. The urinalysis and culture should be repeated to clarify the situation, if an antibiotic has not been given that would be likely to eradicate the bacteriuria.

Asymptomatic bacteriuria and pyuria can be a manifestation of a urinary infection where signs and symptoms are suppressed by recent or current antibiotic therapy. It may also be attributable to poor technique in collecting voided urine when there is no true infection. This is especially likely if there is vaginitis, or if the patient is an uncircumcised male, or if there is a delay in inoculation of the culture media.

Asymptomatic bacteriuria without pyuria can have several causes. The most common reason is bacterial contamination of the urine specimen. Uncommonly, it may be seen early in an infection (before an inflammatory response occurs) or late in an infection (after the initial clinical manifestations and pyuria have disappeared). Rarely, it follows suppression of symptoms and pyuria by inadequate chemotherapy. Asymptomatic bacteriuria is not uncommon, especially in young girls, as discussed in the introduction section of this chapter.

Asymptomatic pyuria without bacteriuria has many possible causes, including several infectious ones.[25] A bacterial urinary infection suppressed by antimicrobial therapy may produce this pattern. Cystitis secondary to gram-positive bacteria is another possible cause. Urethritis can be gonococcal, nonspecific, or chemical, as discussed later. Renal tuberculosis should also be considered in the appropriate setting.

Poor urine collection, as mentioned previously, is a possible cause. Pyuria without infection often occurs after urethral instrumentation or bladder surgery.[26] Noninfectious subacute or chronic renal disease can be associated with pyuria, but proteinuria, casts, or hematuria are often present. Fever in a patient with chronic renal disease may stimulate pyuria. Pyuria is also observed during convalescence from acute glomerulonephritis or toxic nephritis, but some hematuria is also usually present. Kawasaki disease is frequently associated with a sterile pyuria. Extreme dehydration can also produce pyuria. Patients with medication-induced interstitial nephritis may have pyuria, especially with eosinophils.

No bacterial urinary infection is a secure diagnosis if all three variables are negative, provided that there has been no recent antibiotic therapy.

Risk Factors

The rate of UTI in uncircumcised males is approximately 5–10 times higher than in circumcised males.[27,28] The incidence of UTI is higher in white children than in black children. The likelihood of UTI increases with increased height and duration of fever. UTI is less likely if there is another possible explanation for the fever (such as a viral exanthem).[14,29]

Any anatomic or functional abnormality that inhibits the ability to empty the bladder completely will predispose to UTI. Examples include neurogenic bladder in patients with myelomeningocele; obstruction from stones, tumors, or constipation; congenital defects (such as ureteral stenosis or posterior urethral valves in boys); and purposefully infrequent voiding. Indwelling urinary catheters are also a risk for infection, as discussed later.

Vesicoureteral reflux (VUR) refers to the retrograde flow of urine from the bladder into the upper urinary tract. It is present in about 1% of children and is a predisposing factor for pyelonephritis in children with bladder infection.[30] VUR is present in 25–40% of children with acute pyelonephritis.[31] As mentioned, among young children with UTI, about 60% have evidence of renal involvement by scintigraphy; thus, about 15–25% of children with UTI will have VUR. The degree of reflux is graded from I to V based on results of voiding cystourethrogram (VCUG). Grade I indicates reflux to the proximal ureter, Grade II indicates reflux to the renal pelvis without dilation, and Grades III, IV, and V indicate mild, moderate, and severe ureteral and calyceal dilation, respectively. The management of VUR is discussed later in this chapter.

■ ROUTINE SCREENING OF HEALTHY CHILDREN

Although the American Academy of Pediatrics recommends a screening urinalysis at the age of 5 years,[32] the practice of obtaining urinalyses on children at well-child visits is controversial. Among preschool-aged children, the rate of asymptomatic bacteriuria is about 1% in girls and 0.03% in boys. There are currently no data to suggest that detection of and treatment of asymptomatic bacteriuria prevents subsequent pyelonephritis or renal scarring. Routine screening is costly and results in follow-up testing and imaging in a large percentage of healthy children with false-positive tests.[33]

Intermittent screening for UTI may be appropriate for the child at particular risk (such as those with neurogenic bladder). In addition, a low threshold for obtaining a urinalysis and culture should be maintained in the child with a previous history of UTI who has symptoms, however mild, that suggest the possibility of recurrent infection.

Some nephrologists believe that a screening urinalysis (without culture) by laboratory methods or even by "dipstick" at ages 5 and 12 years may be helpful in the early diagnosis of certain glomerulonephritides.

■ COLLECTION AND CULTURE OF URINE

Methods

The bacteriologic confirmation of urinary tract infection is only as accurate as the method of urine collection and several variables involved in its culture. In school-aged children, the physician should proceed from simple to more complicated methods of urine collection and use the least painful method appropriate for the clinical situation. In children who cannot cooperate well, or in infants or children who are not toilet trained and cannot produce a reliable specimen, the clinician should not proceed with antibiotic therapy without a specimen obtained for culture by a highly reliable method. Uncertainty about the validity of the diagnosis because of a poorly collected urine sample may lead to a decision for radiographic evaluations to avoid missing a correctable defect when there would have been no basis for expensive and uncomfortable procedures if the urine had been collected properly.

Random Voided Bag Specimens

This method may be used to obtain a urinalysis when looking for the presence of proteinuria, glycosuria, or pyuria. It may also be used to detect cytomegalovirus (CMV) infection in the young infant. However, it is of no value for performing a bacterial urine culture because of the high rate of contamination. A large study (7584 cultures) revealed a contamination rate of 63% when bag specimens were cultured versus only 9% in catheterized specimens. Uncertainty regarding culture results led to unnecessary recall, treatment, radiologic investigations, and even hospital admission for some infants.[34] The problem with bag specimens is that the culture generally reflects the bacteria present on the skin of the periurethral area. In one study of 98 children, a periurethral culture was obtained, followed immediately by a bag urine culture. In 20 (95%) of 21 urine cultures that contained a pathogen, the same organism was isolated from the periurethral swab culture.[35] Assuming a 5% prevalence of UTI, the positive predictive value of a bag urine specimen is 15% (that is, 85% of positive cultures are false-positive). If the prevalence of UTI is 2% (febrile boys), the false-positive rate is 93%; if the prevalence is 0.2% (circumcised boys), the false-positive rate is 99%.[3]

Bag specimens are only useful if they are culture-negative. Unfortunately, they are so often positive that it is hard to justify their use.

Midstream Specimens

Midstream specimens are readily obtainable from cooperative toilet-trained children.[36,37] In one study of girls 2–12 years of age, there was a 97% correlation between culture results of a midstream clean-voided specimen and a simultaneous catheter specimen.[36] In older girls, a plastic device to spread the labia may be useful.[38] However, in actual practice, unless the office or clinic staff is very experienced and supervises the urine collection, the "clean catch" midstream urine might more accurately be called the "dirty catch" specimen.[19]

The above comments apply to girls. For toilet-trained boys who produced a midstream specimen, 5–10% had low colony counts and obvious contaminants, but cleaning the meatus with soap actually resulted in a higher contamination rate (10%) than when the same boys were not cleaned before the collection (5%).[39] Similar studies in women have shown that the contamination rate is the same whether they are instructed to clean first, or whether they are simply told to urinate into a cup.[40]

So-called midstream, or clean-catch, specimens can also be obtained in infants or neonates, but the technique requires extreme patience. The infant is held over a sterile collection device and then given oral fluids. This results in fairly reliable specimens, even when performed by parents.[41] In a study of 50 circumcised males who served as their own controls, the midstream collection technique was just as reliable as suprapubic bladder aspiration.[42]

Catheterization

Young children who are not toilet trained and for whom the diagnosis of UTI is being considered should generally undergo bladder catheterization. In addition to culture results, catheterization can provide additional useful information. Bladder catheterization is essential to determine residual urine, which may be useful for evaluation of patients with recurrent urinary infection. Often, the determination of residual urine can be combined with obtaining a specimen for culture. The child should be allowed to void without anxiety under comfortable conditions, so maximum emptying is likely. Then, the catheterization is done. This catheterization can also be used in preparation for a voiding cystourethrogram (VCUG), thus doing only one catheterization for the three procedures.

For patients in whom a first UTI is suspected, the specificity of a catheterized specimen can be increased by discarding the first few drops of urine and then collecting the specimen for culture. Practically speaking, however, there is often not enough specimen to allow for any wastage, especially in neonates, who often urinate just as catheterization is about to be performed or who urinate "around" a too-small catheter. Anecdotally, if the person doing the catheterization is prepared to catch urine in a sterile cup in case the patient urinates prior to catheterization, the results are usually reliable.

When catheterization is done for relief of obstruction, the urine should be cultured. Likewise, when catheterization is done for severe acute illnesses, such as in a child hospitalized because of diabetic acidosis, the urine should be cultured.

Catheterization should not be regarded as a dangerous procedure; the risk of introducing infection is extremely low.[43] In one study of children with myelomeningocele, children who underwent clean intermittent catheterization starting in the first year of life (mean age of 7 months) had improved long-term renal function compared with children in whom catheterization was started after age 3 years (mean age 44 months).[44] Complications of urinary catheterization were not seen.

Suprapubic Aspiration (Bladder Puncture)

Still considered the gold standard by some physicians, suprapubic aspiration has generally fallen out of favor in clinical practice, mainly because of the desire to be as noninvasive as possible, but also because of the frequency of "dry taps." The following three conditions[45] are indications for bladder puncture:

1. Inability to get a clean-voided midstream specimen, usually related to the patient's inability to cooperate, as in a newborn, small child, or comatose patient;
2. Urgency of the specimen, as when a patient has a severe illness and information about urine must be obtained immediately (e.g., suspected septicemia); and
3. Urethral catheterization undesirable or impractical, as when vaginitis, urethritis, a tiny urethra, or meatal disease is present.

If these three conditions are not met, catheterization is the preferred method for obtaining urine for culture. Contraindications to suprapubic bladder aspiration include any bleeding problem and recent voiding that has resulted in an empty bladder. If the procedure is done on an infant or small child, the patient should be immobilized in a supine position. After cleaning and disinfecting the suprapubic area, the urethra is compressed with a gloved finger to prevent spontaneous voiding while a 10-mL syringe with a 22-gauge needle is quickly inserted perpendicular to the table (Fig. 14-1). Gentle suction should aspirate urine, although failure to obtain urine is not rare. In some studies, greater than 50% of aspirates failed to obtain urine.[3]

Success of the procedure depends upon the amount of urine in the bladder; therefore, it is least likely to be successful in a baby who is quite ill and, therefore, dehydrated. In one study, unsuccessful suprapubic aspirations were followed by successful catheterizations in all 27 cases.[46] Some gross hematuria occasionally is noted on the next spontaneous voiding. Puncture of the bowel is rare.

Considerations in Diagnosing UTI

Recent or Current Antimicrobial Therapy

Antimicrobial therapy can inhibit bacterial growth in the bladder, so that colony counts will be below 100,000/mL. No prospective studies have been done to define precisely the length of time antimi-

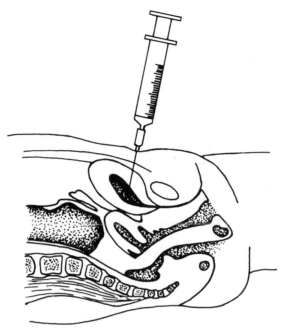

■ **FIGURE 14-1** Anatomic relations for bladder puncture of infant girl.

crobial therapy must be stopped in order to allow bacterial growth. In general, 48 hours appears to be reasonable on the basis of clinical experience with this interval,[37] although longer would, of course, be better.

Concentration of Urine and Frequency of Voiding

The lowest concentrations of bacteria in the urine occur in the late afternoon and the highest concentrations in the early morning, presumably because of concentration of the urine. However, this finding may also be a function of infrequent voiding through the night, because frequent voiding reduces bacterial concentrations in the urine.

Delay Before Inoculation

If there must be a delay in inoculation, refrigeration of the urine specimen is appropriate to inhibit multiplication of bacteria, but the value of this depends on urine pH and the species of the organism. For example, enterococci that are causing an infection may produce low colony counts (fewer than 40,000 organisms/mL) because they grow so poorly in acid urine.

Skin Flora

Staphylococcus epidermidis is a cause of urinary infection in children in rare cases, so it should not automatically be regarded as a contaminant when reported as a pure growth in concentrations exceeding 100,000/mL.

Staphylococcus saprophyticus is a coagulase-negative staphylococcus that is distinguished from *S. epidermidis* primarily by the former's resistance to the obsolete antibiotic novobiocin. *S. saprophyticus* is an important cause of UTI in adolescent girls and young women that is temporally related to sexual intercourse.[47]

Office Tests

A number of chemical screening tests have been studied for use in the physician's office for detection of urinary infections without the delay and problems of culture. Many of these have been found unsatisfactory after an initial period of enthusiasm. Two methods have been used to simplify culturing.

Quantitative Loop

This method is clearly the best for culture of the specimen; if the physician has facilities for office throat cultures for β-hemolytic streptococci, all that is necessary is the purchase of a quantitative loop for streaking the urine. This method is the one used by most clinical bacteriology laboratories and has an established record of practical utility in many physicians' offices.[19] It is probably the best method and can be combined with urine collection in Dixie cups, as described in the section on screening near the end of this chapter. Usually a 0.001 mL loop is used. The number of colonies of the same type are counted and then multiplied by 1000 to calculate the number of organisms per mL of urine.

Susceptibility testing of isolates should not be attempted in the office, because too much standardization and several controls are required.

Other Bacteriologic Culture Methods

Dip slides have an agar coating and are simply dipped in the urine and then incubated. The inoculum of urine is less accurately measured than with the quantitative loop. However, the screw-cap tubes with an agar slide attached to the cap are convenient for transport, especially from home to office, and are sufficiently accurate for screening or follow-up.[19,48,49]

■ ANATOMIC LOCALIZATION OF INFECTION

Once the general diagnosis of UTI is made, the physician should attempt to make a clinical diagnosis of the anatomic location of the infection. This determination is often more difficult than one might expect, because the exact location of the infection by laboratory methods depends on excluding infection higher in the urinary tract. The possible anatomic locations of a urinary infection are the kidney, bladder, urethra, and prostate.

Kidney

Pyelonephritis

The term "pyelonephritis" refers to infection of the kidney. The diagnosis may be based on several kinds of observations.

Clinical Pyelonephritis

The manifestations of pain and tenderness in the vicinity of the kidney, along with fever and significant bacteriuria, are sufficient for this as a presumptive diagnosis. In young children, in whom classic signs such as costovertebral angle tenderness or flank pain are often absent, the combination of an abnormal urinalysis and fever has been considered diagnostic. Recently, that clinical assumption has been proven to be valid; at least 60% of young children with fever and a positive urine culture will have pyelonephritis by DMSA scanning.[5,6]

Radiologic Pyelonephritis

Sometimes children present primarily with severe abdominal pain, and the initial study performed is an abdominal CT scan, which demonstrates multiple streaky areas of poor enhancement in a kidney. Alternatively, Doppler ultrasound may show increased echogenicity with poor vascular flow. Both of these studies would be highly suggestive of pyelonephritis. However, a catheterized urine specimen should still be obtained for culture and susceptibility testing.

Bacteriologic Pyelonephritis

Localization of a UTI to the kidney by culture methods is rarely done or needed. Culture of urine obtained at cystoscopy by ureteral catheterization is evidence for infection in the kidney, particularly if the bladder has been washed out before collecting urine coming from the kidney. Culture of kidney tissue obtained by biopsy or nephrectomy is definitive. Cultures obtained at autopsy are less reliable, if there is any postmortem delay.

Histologic Pyelonephritis

Kidney tissue showing evidence of infection is suggestive but not conclusive. Chronic pyelonephritis at autopsy diagnosed by histologic examination has formerly been presumed to be bacterial in origin. However, ascribing these findings at autopsy to past infections is unlikely to be accurate unless such renal infections have been documented.[50]

In most cases, the clinical diagnosis of pyelonephritis should be considered only presumptive unless the patient has reflux. An exception can be made for neonates, many of whom seed the kidney via bloodstream infection. The term "urinary tract infection" can be generally used when involvement of the kidney is unknown. Scintigraphy (DMSA scanning) has a sensitivity of about 90% in detecting acute pyelonephritis. However, its use rarely alters the management of UTI in the acute setting, and so it is not routinely employed.[7]

Renal Abscess

Renal abscesses can be subdivided into renal cortical abscess and renal corticomedullary abscess. The distinction is important because the pathophysiology and bacteriology of the two conditions differ markedly.

Renal Cortical Abscess

Most renal cortical abscesses are secondary to primary bacteremia. There may be a lag of weeks or even months between the primary bacteremic episode and the development of the abscess.[51] Alternatively, the patient may have an obvious primary focus, such as the skin or a lymph node. Ninety percent of these abscesses are caused by *S. aureus*.[52] Most cases occur in adults, in whom men outnumber women by about 3 to 1. They are almost all unilateral and solitary. A small number of these may rupture, producing a perinephric abscess. Signs and symptoms are usually nonspecific and include fever, chills, and back or abdominal pain. Urinary symptoms are uncommon, and the urinalysis is usually normal (most of these abscesses do not communicate with the collecting system).[53] Both ultrasound and CT scan are helpful in diagnosis, but CT is better at distinguishing these from renal tumors. If the abscess is large or very well walled

off, surgery may be required, but many patients recover with intravenous antistaphylococcal antibiotics for 10–14 days, followed by oral antistaphylococcal agents for several weeks.[51,52] Percutaneous drainage is sometimes both therapeutically and diagnostically helpful.

Renal Corticomedullary Abscess

In contrast to cortical abscesses, most of these lesions are precipitated by ascending infection and are thus associated with urinary tract abnormalities, such as stones, outflow obstruction, or vesicoureteral reflux (VUR). The bacteriology is concordant with the pathophysiology: *Escherichia coli, Klebsiella spp,* and *Proteus mirabilis* are the most common isolates.[51,52] Renal corticomedullary abscesses can be subdivided into acute focal bacterial nephritis and xanthogranulomatous pyelonephritis.

Acute Focal Bacterial Nephritis

Acute focal bacterial nephritis ("acute lobar nephronia" is an older term) occurs when pyelonephritis develops into a focal renal infection that resembles an abscess but has neither walled itself off nor gone on to liquefaction (Fig. 14-2). Presentation with fever, chills, and flank or abdominal pain, coupled with nausea and vomiting in two-thirds of patients

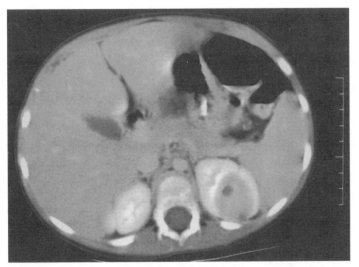

■ **FIGURE 14-2** Left renal corticomedullary abscess in a 4-year-old girl who presented with a 3-day history of high fever and vomiting. This CT scan with contrast shows a thin rim of enhancement surrounding the phlegmon, with only a very small area of liquefaction centrally. Urine cultures grew *E. coli.* Complete resolution of the infection was achieved with a prolonged course of intravenous antibiotics, without surgical drainage.

may suggest an intra-abdominal process. A flank mass, or even hepatomegaly, may be found on physical examination. The presence of a grossly abnormal urine clearly differentiates this entity from renal cortical abscess.[51,52] Ultrasound or computed tomography (CT) allow definition of this infection and exclusion of abscess or tumor. Antibiotic therapy without operative drainage is often successful.[54] However, pediatric patients with multifocal bacterial nephritis who have severe VUR often do not respond to antibiotic therapy alone.

Xanthogranulomatous Pyelonephritis (XGP)

This rare condition, more commonly seen in older adults or malnourished children, is associated with infection, urinary tract abnormalities, and stones.[55] The diffuse form of the disease is much more common than the focal form, especially in pediatrics.[56] XGP often mimics malignancy, especially when it is nonobstructive.[57] Radiographically, the lesions of XGP are less well demarcated than a Wilms' tumor.[57] Clinical presentation can be vague; fever of unknown origin or subacute fatigue are common.[58] There may be a palpable abdominal mass.[59] Recurrent or recalcitrant pyelonephritis is a more direct sign.[58] E. coli and P. mirabilis are the usual pathogens. The chronic renal infection is usually associated with obstruction, and the parenchyma is replaced by lipid-laden macrophages. Treatment consists of nephrectomy or resection of the diseased segment with antibiotic therapy directed at the bacteria found in the specimen. Occasionally, patients will recover with conservative management.[59]

Perinephric Abscess

By definition, a perinephric abscess involves the space between the renal capsule and Gerota's fascia. The pathophysiology is mixed; most cases are due to extension of a renal corticomedullary abscess (usually focal bacterial nephritis, described earlier). In these cases, the infection is usually due to gram-negative enteric bacteria and commonly associated with urinary tract abnormalities, abnormal urinalysis, and, typically, positive urine cultures. Occasionally, a renal cortical abscess may rupture into the perinephric space, producing a staphylococcal abscess. Case reports of children who developed a perinephric abscess due to a ruptured retrocecal appendicitis have been published.[60]

The onset is insidious. Fever is the most constant symptom and may be prolonged. A perinephric abscess should, therefore, be considered in the workup of patients with fever of unknown origin (see Chapter 10). Unilateral flank pain and dysuria are symptoms that may help the clinician to localize the infection. Symptoms that may be misleading include nausea and vomiting (seen in about 25% of patients) and pain that is referred to the hip, thigh, or knee. Careful physical examination may reveal costovertebral angle tenderness, splinting, pain on bending toward the contralateral side, or a slightly altered gait.[51,52]

An elevated white count with a "left shift" is common. Anemia is seen in 40% of patients. Urinalysis usually reveals pyuria and sometimes proteinuria. Urine cultures are positive in about 60% of patients, and blood cultures are positive in approximately 40% of patients.[52] CT scanning is the imaging modality of choice; MRI does not usually provide additional information.[61]

Unlike the other focal kidney infections described earlier, parenteral antibiotic therapy by itself is unlikely to result in cure for patients with perinephric abscesses. A drainage procedure is usually necessary.[60] Antibiotic therapy must cover both gram-negative enteric organisms and S. aureus; the combination of an antistaphylococcal penicillin and an aminoglycoside is a reasonable empiric choice. Definitive therapy should be guided by culture and susceptibility results. Nephrectomy is occasionally required.

Bladder

Cystitis

This term is used to mean infection of the bladder. Whether the kidney is also assumed to be involved is not clearly defined by common usage, so that for complete clarity, one of the following phrases should be used: cystitis without clinical pyelonephritis; cystitis, renal status unknown; or urinary tract infection. The term UTI indicates a lack of data with which to differentiate upper-tract infection (pyelonephritis) from lower-tract infection (cystitis).

Recurrent Cystitis

This is common in school-aged girls, and the diagnosis implies that vesicoureteral reflux and renal pain or tenderness are not present.

Hemorrhagic Cystitis

In otherwise healthy children, acute hemorrhagic cystitis is generally a benign, self-limited disease. Patients present with the abrupt onset of gross hematuria, dysuria, frequency, and urgency. Fever is distinctly uncommon. Adenoviruses are the most common cause. Adenovirus types 7, 11, and 21 have been most frequently associated with hemorrhagic cystitis. These serotypes are usually not co-circulating as respiratory pathogens. Occasionally, E. coli causes hemorrhagic cystitis, so culture of the urine is appropriate. No other bacteria have been definitively associated with hemorrhagic cystitis. In immunocompromised children, adenoviruses are still the most likely cause, but the disease is neither benign nor self-limited. Unusual viruses, such as BK virus, can also be causative in this subset of patients.[62,63]

Eosinophilic Cystitis

Hemorrhagic cystitis and an eosinophilic infiltration of the bladder is rare in children.[64] In some cases this condition mimics bladder tumor.[65] Peripheral eosinophilia is occasionally seen. A small percentage of patients present with urinary retention as the principal sign.[66] Otherwise, nonspecific signs, such as urgency, frequency, and abdominal pain, predominate.[66] The male to female ratio is approximately 2 to 1 in childhood.[66] The etiology is unknown. Although most cases are self-limited and require no therapy, many physicians give a trial of nonsteroidal anti-inflammatory agents. Two children with chronic granulomatous disease who presented with urinary signs and symptoms suggesting eosinophilic cystitis have been reported.[67]

Acute interstitial nephritis, which may be drug-induced or caused by various infections or autoimmune disorders, is sometimes accompanied by the presence of urine eosinophils.[67a] Hematuria, however, is uncommon in acute interstitial nephritis.

Schistosomiasis

Schistosoma haematobium infection of the bladder often presents as painless, gross hematuria.[68,69] It should be considered in any patient with hematuria who has a history of residence in or travel to an endemic area (primarily sub-Saharan Africa). Bacterial superinfection is common. Diagnosis is by cystoscopy with biopsy. Praziquantel is curative.

Urethra

Urethritis

Typically, the clinical symptoms of this condition are pain and burning on urination, but symptoms may be minimal if the urethritis is chronic. In the female, suprapubic aspiration may be useful to demonstrate that the bacteriuria does not have its origins in the bladder, although this is rarely necessary.

Urethritis can be caused by several sexually transmitted microorganisms, as discussed further in Chapter 15. Bacterial urethritis or cystitis is also associated with intercourse in sexually active women and teenagers.[70] As noted earlier, vaginitis and urethritis can mimic the symptoms of cystitis and produce the urethral syndrome (also called the dysuria-pyuria syndrome, discussed later).[71] In prepubertal children, especially girls, irritation by clothing, soaps, or other contact (including sexual abuse) should be considered.[45]

Urethral Syndrome (Dysuria-Pyuria Syndrome)

Urethral syndrome is the name given to the condition of recurrent or chronic urinary symptoms in the absence of demonstrable objective findings. Symptoms may include retropubic pressure, urinary frequency, dyspareunia, and dysuria. Cultures of urine are usually sterile. Some women with urethral syndrome have repeatable low counts of bacteria by bladder puncture, and some women have Chlamydia trachomatis recovered.[72] The gonococcus may be a cause of this syndrome in some cases. Anaerobes and low-virulence bacteria of the urethra have also been postulated as causes, but proof of causality is lacking.

The cause of the urethral syndrome is unknown. Many clinicians have assumed it to be a psychosomatic disease. One study of 58 patients and 21 controls found a clear relationship of flare-ups of urethral syndrome to stress events. These investigators also found a higher incidence of other psychopathologic symptoms in patients suffering from urethral syndrome.[73] Others have called the condition "irritable urethra syndrome" and have found higher mean scores on psychologic measures in patients versus controls. However, not all investigators have been able to replicate these findings.[74] Some investigators have postulated that these women have inflammation of the paraurethral glands, which are homologous to the male prostate, and have therefore called it "female prostatitis."[75] Finally, another study concluded that patients with urethral syndrome have poor control of the pelvic floor musculature.[76]

Prostate

Prostatitis can be broadly divided into three categories: acute, chronic, and prostatodynia. All three types are rare in children, even in sexually active teenagers. Acute prostatitis is a severe bacterial infection with systemic symptoms accompanying urinary tract symptoms, such as frequency, urgency, and urinary retention. The prostate is tender to palpation. The gland can be confirmed as the source of bacteriuria, which is often greater than 10,000 colonies/mL, by comparing culture results of the first-voided urine after prostatic massage with first-voided and midstream specimens obtained before prostatic massage. Chronic prostatitis is a slowly evolving condition that is usually associated with intermittent UTI and persistent urinary tract signs. Prostatodynia is the name given to chronic prostatitis when it has never been accompanied by bacterial infection. The cause is unknown. There may be a prominent psychosomatic component to prostatodynia.

■ INITIAL DIAGNOSIS AND MANAGEMENT OF UTI

A careful history should be taken for past symptoms related to urination, abdominal pain, or fever. History should be obtained for exposure of the urethra to bacteria by careless cleaning after bowel movements and for vaginitis or itching caused by pinworms, although these simple explanations are usually not the reason for infection. History should also be obtained for exposure to irritants, such as concentrated bubble-bath solutions that may produce urethritis. The physical examination should include deep palpation for kidney size as well as for renal or suprapubic tenderness. The blood pressure should always be taken and the optic fundi examined.

Possible Bacterial Etiologies

The types of bacteria usually recovered from the urine correlates with the perineal flora, with *E. coli* being the most frequent organism. *Enterobacter spp.,* *P. mirabilis,* and enterococci are occasionally recovered. Urinary infections by *Bacteroides* species

appear to be rare despite the fact that these organisms constitute more than 90% of the bacteria in the bowel. *S. aureus* and *Pseudomonas aeruginosa* rarely cause first urinary infections in normal children but are more likely to be recovered after antimicrobial therapy, instrumentation, or sitting in hot water tubs or whirlpool baths.[77] Coagulase-negative staphylococci are an uncommon cause of UTI but occasionally cause real disease, even resulting in prolonged fever in some children. Unusual organisms can be found with the first documented UTI in a child with an underlying anatomic defect, often after several episodes of treatment with antibiotics for questionable otitis media or other reasons without recognition of the UTI.

Laboratory Approach

Urinalysis

In most situations in a toilet-trained girl, the physician suspects a UTI because of typical clinical manifestations and does a urinalysis on a midstream voided specimen that reveals WBC and bacteria in the sediment.

In infants, great care should be taken to get a reliable specimen for urinalysis and culture, as described earlier, because false-positive results can lead to unnecessary radiologic investigation. An infant should not be started on antibiotic therapy for suspected sepsis without a catheter or bladder-puncture specimen. Likewise, an infant should not be treated with antibiotics for a UTI on the basis of results from a bagged urine specimen.

Urine Culture

Initial management usually consists of chemotherapy based on the likely bacterial etiology while the urine culture confirms the diagnosis and provides an organism for susceptibility testing, if necessary. The urine culture is the foundation upon which the diagnosis and evaluation of UTI is built. If the physician has bacteriologic facilities for throat cultures available in the office, quantitative urine culture can be done easily using a quantitative loop. Causes of negative cultures in suspected UTI are discussed earlier in this chapter.

■ MANAGEMENT OF UNCOMPLICATED INFECTIONS

The first UTI in a toilet-trained girl is the least complicated situation, and this section discusses only this situation. All other clinical circumstances, including infections in infancy, are regarded as more complicated problems and are discussed in the next section.

Chemotherapy

In most cases, the diagnosis is suspected based on symptoms and signs referable to the bladder and on microscopic examination of the urine that shows WBCs and bacteria. Although results need not be awaited before beginning therapy, a culture should always be obtained. Extremely convoluted clinical situations result when physicians treat patients as though they have a UTI but do not confirm the clinical impression with a urine culture. Uncomplicated infections can be treated for 7–10 days with an oral drug, such as trimethoprim-sulfamethoxazole (TMP-SMX) or cefixime.[49,78] Amoxicillin was the drug of choice for years, but resistance to amoxicillin among isolates of E. coli has been increasing over the past few years. It may be used if susceptibility results are favorable. Cefixime is a convenient antibiotic because of its once-daily dosing schedule and palatability in suspension. It has broad activity against most urinary tract pathogens and is excreted in the urine, so good levels at the site of infection can be obtained. Unfortunately, availability of cefixime is variable. A different third-generation oral cephalosporin (such as cefpodoxime or cefdinir) may be substituted for cefixime.

Nitrofurantoin is frequently associated with vomiting, and amoxicillin can be associated with diarrhea or a rash. Nitrofurantoin has been reported to cause pulmonary hypersensitivity (rarely in children) and is contraindicated in infants less than 1 month of age and in patients with glucose-6-phosphate dehydrogenase deficiency. It is a good choice for prophylaxis and can be used for treatment of cystitis. However, its use is discouraged if there is a possibility of pyelonephritis because it does not reach therapeutic levels in the bloodstream.

Short-Course Chemotherapy

The use of short-course antimicrobial therapy (usually defined as less than 5 days' duration) in children with uncomplicated cystitis is controversial. A recent meta-analysis based on data from 1279 patients suggests that resolution is better with longer-duration therapy.[79] For older adolescents and adults, a 3-day course of ciprofloxacin seems to be as effective as 7 days of TMP-SMX or nitrofurantoin, with a better side-effect profile.[80] A 3-day course of TMP-SMX is also effective, if the isolate is sensitive.

Relapse or Reinfection

It is useful to try to distinguish recurrent infections with different bacteria from a persistent or chronic infection with the same organism, a distinction based usually on analysis of serial culture results. If a second clinical infection or post-treatment culture can be demonstrated to involve the same organism as the first infection, it is defined as a relapse. If the species is different (e.g., first E. coli, then P. mirabilis), it is clearly a reinfection. If, however, E. coli is recovered on both occasions, reinfection and relapse can be distinguished only by serotyping, unless there is a significant difference between the antibiotic susceptibility patterns of the two isolates, and serotyping of E. coli is usually not available. In adult patients, if relapse occurs, it does so promptly, usually by 1 week after stopping antibiotic therapy, whereas reinfection is usually not noted until 1 month or later, after the completion of therapy.

Oral Fluids

Urging oral fluids is traditional therapy that has some theoretic basis. The mechanical factor of voiding is a major defense in eradicating infection, as demonstrated by experiments in humans and in mechanical models of bacterial growth, and increased fluid intake increases the frequency of voiding. Some children will not be able to comply and need not be pressured, although some children with low fluid intakes, by history, appear to benefit.

Correct Contributing Habits

Constipation has been suggested as a possible contributing factor to urinary infections. This possibility is probably rarely related to recurrent urinary infections, but if the constipation is severe, an ultrasound or CT done without prior laxatives might be considered to see whether distended bowel is producing urinary obstruction.

Poor toilet hygiene or pinworms with urethral itching may be important contributing causes. The role of self-manipulation of the urethral area has not been adequately evaluated. Infrequent or incomplete voiding may contribute to functional residual urine. A program of regular fluid ingestion throughout the day, with a more conscientious effort to be sure the bladder is fully emptied at urination, may be helpful.

Sexual intercourse increases the concentration of bacteria in the urine in young women, but the increase is transient. Whether post-coital voiding prevents UTIs in young women is unclear. In one small study, women who urinated less than 15 minutes after intercourse had a lower risk of UTI, but the results were not statistically significant.[81]

Residual Urine

Residual urine is determined by catheterization immediately after normal voiding. Normally, residual urine should be less than 10 mL. A child may not take time to empty the bladder and thus may have residual urine without any anatomic obstruction. Residual urine obtained by catheter should be sent for culture and microscopic examination.

■ INITIAL RADIOGRAPHIC EVALUATION

Some minor differences of opinion exist over the criteria for doing radiologic evaluation and which tests should be done first.[78,82] The most reasonable approach individualizes the decisions on the basis of the patient's age and the severity of infection.[50]

Criteria for Hospitalized Infants

Young infants, and older infants and children with renal tenderness and systemic findings or fever, should be hospitalized, undergo a reliable procedure to obtain a urine specimen, and should be initially treated with intravenous antibiotics. AAP guidelines recommend routine testing with ultrasound and VCUG after the first documented UTI.[3] However, evidence supporting these recommendations is lacking.[83]

Ultrasound is useful to demonstrate a dilated pelvis, pelvocaliectasis, hydronephrosis, ureteral dilatation, and urinary anomalies. It has replaced intravenous pyelography for this purpose. Whether ultrasound is necessary in a patient whose mother underwent prenatal ultrasound testing is unclear,[84] although one study has shown that postnatal ultrasound is superior to prenatal ultrasound for detection of congenital uropathies.[85]

In a recent study of 309 children 1–24 months old with UTI, the ultrasound was abnormal in 37 (12%) of patients. However, according to the authors, the findings did not affect management.[7] The percentage of children in the study whose mothers had prenatal ultrasound was not reported.

Voiding cystourethrogram (VCUG) has been recommended in children with a first UTI to detect reflux.[3] In the past, it was taught that inflammation associated with acute infection produced false-positive VCUG studies, and that VCUG should, therefore, be delayed for several weeks. Recent studies have demonstrated no difference in the rate of VUR among children who underwent VCUG within 7 days of diagnosis versus greater than 7 days after diagnosis.[86,87] Attempting to perform the VCUG later, on the other hand, resulted in about half the patients never receiving the study.[87] Additionally, patients were generally placed on prophylaxis with TMP-SMX pending the results of VCUG, which exposed many patients to unnecessary antibiotic therapy.

Most experts recommend radiologic investigation for all hospitalized patients as described earlier, all males of any age, and all children with a febrile UTI.[4] Girls less than 3 years of age should be evaluated after the first confirmed UTI because the danger of renal scarring is age related, with the younger infants being at the highest risk for renal scarring.[88] A recent cohort study of 309 children with UTI evaluated the utility of routine radiologic evaluation. All children underwent VCUG and 117 (39%) were found to have reflux. DMSA scans performed at 6 months showed renal scarring in 10% of patients.[7] However, the question of whether routine VCUG in children with UTI is beneficial cannot be answered by this study, because all the children with VUR received prophylactic antibiotics. Omitting the VCUG might be reasonable if it can be demonstrated that prophylactic antibiotics do not affect the rates of recurrent UTI and long-term sequelae (such as renal scarring and hypertension). Currently, good evidence to support or refute this practice is lacking.[89]

There are no randomized trials comparing prophylactic antibiotics with placebo for children with reflux. The basis for the widespread practice of prophylactic antibiotics in these children stems from two small studies of children greater than 2 years old with recurrent UTI and normal renal tracts (patients with VUR were excluded). Both studies demonstrated a decreased incidence of UTI during therapy, but other sequelae were not assessed.[90,91]

Criteria for Toilet-Trained Girls

Many authorities advocate waiting for the second episode of confirmed UTI before doing radiographic evaluation of a school-aged girl. However, other authors have concluded that a VCUG should be done after the first UTI.[92]

Abnormalities Detectable by VCUG

A voiding cystourethrogram primarily detects reflux from the bladder up one or both ureters and bladder diverticula. It may detect gross urethral obstruction but is not a reliable guide to urethral stenosis. If reflux is demonstrated during filling of the bladder, it is called low-pressure reflux; if reflux is demonstrable only when bladder pressure is high, as during voiding, it is called high-pressure reflux. Reflux is graded acccording to its severity, grade I being the mildest and grade V the most severe. Most evidence indicates that infection in the presence of reflux causes renal scarring.[48]

Abnormalities Detected by Ultrasound

Unsuspected abdominal masses may be detected with this method. The size of the kidneys, the patency of the renal veins, the site of any obstruction of the ureters, and grossly enlarged ureters or hydronephrosis can be detected.[93,94]

Radionuclide Cystography

Radionuclide cystography is a method involving less radiation than VCUG and is useful to monitor patients with reflux but does not show bladder or urethral abnormalities.[3]

Renal Cortical Scintigraphy (DMSA Scans)

These scans can be used acutely to demonstrate pyelonephritis or later in the patient's course to document the presence of renal scarring. However, the importance of documenting either of these conditions is unclear.[84]

■ MANAGEMENT OF COMPLICATED PROBLEMS

Treatment of Infants and Young Children

A randomized controlled trial comparing intravenous cefotaxime for 3 days followed by oral cefix-ime for 11 days versus oral cefixime for 14 days showed no difference in time to defervescence or in the rate of reinfection or renal scarring,[95] suggesting that infants and young children with UTIs who do not otherwise require hospitalization may be treated with oral antibiotics. This study has not yet been replicated. Many physicians continue to advocate hospitalization with intravenous antibiotics for a minimum of 48–72 hours for infants because of the high rate of true pyelonephritis in this population, and the potential long-term adverse outcome of improperly treated kidney infection.

Infants who are ill-appearing or vomiting should be hospitalized and treated with intravenous antibiotics initially. Cefotaxime or the combination of ampicillin and gentamicin is commonly used. The latter regimen has the advantage of activity against enterococcus, which is an occasional cause of UTI. Cefotaxime may be preferred if gram-negative rods are seen on Gram stain. Once a clinical response has been demonstrated and susceptibility results determined, antibiotics can be changed to an oral agent to complete a 10- to 14-day course. TMP-SMX or cefixime (or another oral third-generation cephalosporin) are commonly used. TMP-SMX is usually avoided in the first 6 weeks of life because of its ability to displace bilirubin and result in hyperbilirubinemia.

Delays in Treatment

In one study, children treated 24 hours after the onset of fever did not have an increased risk of renal scarring compared with those who were treated earlier.[95] In contrast, several studies have demonstrated that a prolonged delay (>4 days) in therapy is associated with increased renal scarring.

Need for Follow-Up Cultures

In general, routine follow-up cultures 48 hours into therapy are not necessary if the patient has had a good clinical response to therapy and the organism is determined to be susceptible to the antimicrobial agent used to treat it. If either of these two criteria is not met, a follow-up culture 48 hours into therapy is appropriate.[3]

In a study of 306 children ages 1–24 months with UTI, all had sterile urine cultures by 24 hours into therapy.[95] Similarly, follow-up cultures 2–7 days after completing a course of therapy are not usually necessary. However, if desired, a catheterized urine specimen can be obtained when the child undergoes VCUG. The value of such a specimen is even lower if the patient has already been placed on prophylactic antibiotics. Some experts recommend repeat follow-up cultures every few months for a couple of years after a UTI. However, the value of this approach has not been studied. It is probably more important to make sure that a catheterized urine specimen is obtained with each subsequent episode of fever without localizing signs and whenever the child develops symptoms that are localized to the urinary tract.

Reflux

Vesicoureteral Reflux

Reflux is usually congenital but may be acquired. It has many causes and degrees of severity and should not be discussed as a simple single entity. The management depends on its severity, whether it is unilateral or bilateral, the age of the child, the presence or absence of renal scarring, and whether it is complicated by other conditions (such as voiding dysfunction, neuropathic bladder, posterior urethral valves, or other anatomic abnormalities).[50,96–99]

The spontaneous resolution of nondilated reflux (grades I, II, and III) is high (75–90%), whereas resolution of dilated reflux (grades IV and V) is considerably lower (25–65%).[97]

The American Urological Association recommends medical management for all children with grades I to III reflux and for most with unilateral grade IV reflux. Children with bilateral grade IV reflux and with unilateral or bilateral grade V reflux should generally undergo ureteral reimplantation. Other indications include failure of conservative therapy and deterioration of renal function.[99]

As discussed earlier, despite a lack of compelling evidence of their effectiveness, prophylactic antibiotics are generally used for patients with VUR of any grade. Because of the increased risk of pyelonephritis in patients with VUR, this approach is reasonable until controlled trials demonstrate otherwise. Prophylaxis is discussed in the section on recurrent UTI.

Intrarenal Reflux

Renal scars are more likely to develop in areas of the kidney that contain the type of renal papillae that permit intrarenal reflux.[50] Because about one-third of kidneys are not predisposed to have intrarenal reflux, some children with reflux do not develop scars.[50]

Obstruction

If obstruction is present at the bladder neck, ureterovesicle junction, or renopelvic outlet, the infection typically does not respond to chemotherapy, and fever and symptoms may remain prominent. Usually, such obstruction must be relieved before the patient responds.

Other Problems

Indwelling Catheter

UTIs are the most common nosocomial infection in adults. They are somewhat less common in children, accounting for about 10% of all pediatric nosocomial infections.[100,101]

The main risk factor is the presence of an indwelling catheter. The longer the catheter remains in place, the greater the likelihood that a catheter-associated UTI will occur. The most common pathogens are E. coli, Enterococcus spp., P. aeruginosa, Klebsiella spp, and Candida albicans.[101,102]

Routine early removal of catheters (48–72 hours) can reduce the incidence of nosocomial UTI by 90%.[101]

Catheter-associated UTI should be suspected in any patient with fever and a urinary catheter. Other symptoms, such as dysuria or abdominal pain, are uncommon. Diagnosis is by quantitative culture obtained through the aspiration port or at the time of recatheterization (collection containers are often contaminated).

Asymptomatic bacteriuria or candiduria usually responds to catheter removal alone. Empiric therapy for nosocomial UTI should be tailored to the results of urine Gram stain; treatment for 7–10 days is usually adequate. Initially, therapy is usually given intravenously, but oral therapy may be used as well. If possible, the urinary catheter should be removed (if even for a short period of time).

Candidal Infections

Children with impaired host defenses may develop C. albicans urinary infections that are not a result of continued candidal dissemination but may come from a brief corrected episode of candidemia or from the ascending route. These patients can often be treated successfully with a short course of fluconazole or amphotericin B. However, blood cultures should be obtained to rule out candidemia. In catheter-related candiduria, the catheter must be removed. In a study of neonates in an intensive care unit, candiduria was accompanied by mycetoma (renal fungus ball) in up to 40% of patients.[103] In this study only half of patients with mycetoma had an abnormal renal ultrasound at the time of diagnosis of candiduria. The other half developed them between 1 and 6 weeks later.[103]

Premature infants with candiduria and renal mycetoma should be presumed to be candidemic, even if blood cultures fail to grow the organism.[104] The optimal therapy has not been defined. We usually treat initially with amphotericin B and switch to fluconazole, if the organism is sensitive, to complete at least a 14-day course.

Complications

Complications of urinary tract infections include renal and perirenal abscesses, discussed in a previous section. In the neonate in particular, secondary bacteremia or meningitis can be a complication of UTI. A rare complication of UTI is hyperammonemic encephalopathy. This can occur when the infection is caused by a urea-splitting organism (e.g., *P. mirabilis*, *Klebsiella* spp.) in a patient with obstructive uropathy.[104a] Renal scarring in patients with VUR is discussed in the section on prognosis.

Recurrences

Recurrent Cystitis in Teenagers

Recurrent cystitis in these cases may be related to sexual activity. Emptying the bladder after intercourse may be a practical therapeutic measure. Colonization of the introitus by enteric bacteria and hygiene of male sex partners also may be important.

Recurrent Cystitis in Immature Girls

If a complete diagnostic evaluation indicates no abnormality, as is the case with a large proportion of girls with recurrent urinary infections, operative procedures will be of no value. Patients with frequent recurrences (three or more per year) are usually placed on prophylactic antibiotics for at least 6 months, but the necessity of this approach has not been well evaluated. If the infections are highly symptomatic, this is certainly reasonable. Nitrofurantoin or TMP-SMX may be used.

Continuous Chemoprophylaxis

Continuous prophylaxis is of no value unless the infecting organism is eliminated by the initial therapy. In girls with recurrent infections, nitrofurantoin 1–2 mg/kg once daily or low-dose TMP-SMX (1–2 mg/kg per dose of TMP and 5–10 mg/kg per dose of SMX) given every other day,[105] or daily, may be helpful.[45] In adult women, TMP-SMX has been effective in preventing recurrences, but its safety has not yet been confirmed by long-term studies in children nor is it FDA-approved for this use.[49] As discussed in the section on reflux, prophylaxis is usually used for patients with reflux of any grade until it resolves.

■ UROLOGIC OR NEPHROLOGIC CONSULTATION

A urologist or a nephrologist with experience with children should be consulted by the primary physician when there is obstruction, significant reflux (grade III or greater), other renal anomalies, renal insufficiency, renal scarring, or hypertension.[50] Operative procedures may be necessary to correct obstruction at various locations. Cystoscopic examination is rarely necessary in patients with VUR because it does not aid in predicting whether reflux will resolve.[99] Urethral dilation and internal urethrotomy are not beneficial.[99]

■ PROGNOSIS

In the absence of VUR or other anatomic abnormalities, the long-term prognosis in school-aged girls with either recurrent cystitis or asymptomatic bacteriuria is excellent.[106,107] Among infants and young children with UTI, renal scarring develops in 10–40% of patients, and the best predictor of scarring is the presence and severity of VUR.[7,108–110]

The long-term outcome of childhood VUR was determined by studying 226 adults 10–41 years after initial presentation. The investigators found that reflux resolved in 134 (69%) of 193 children managed medically and in 29 (88%) of 33 children treated surgically. Seventeen (8%) of adults had hypertension or elevated creatinine and 16 (7%) had renal scarring. One patient (0.4%) died of renal disease and 2 (0.9%) required renal transplant. Development of sequelae was predictable based on extensive scarring, elevated creatinine, and/or at least borderline hypertension as children.[111]

■ PREVENTION

Other than prophylactic antibiotics for the child with a history of recurrent UTI or reflux, few preventive measures are available. Proper hygiene practices after defecation may prevent recurrent bladder infections in young girls. Infants with certain problems, such as failure to thrive, intractable diaper rash, and irritability or excessive crying should have urinary tract infection excluded.[112]

The AAP recommends obtaining blood pressure measurements on well children at yearly intervals, starting at age 3.[32]

■ REFERENCES

1. Marild S, Jodal U. Incidence rate of first-time symptomatic urinary tract infection in children under 6 years of age. Acta Paediatr 1998;87:549–52.
2. Newman TB, Bernzweig JA, Takayama JI, et al. Urine testing and urinary tract infections in febrile infants seen in office settings: the Pediatric Research in Office Settings' Febrile Infant Study. Arch Pediatr Adolesc Med 2002;156:44–54.
3. American Academy of Pediatrics. Committee on Quality Improvement. Subcommittee on Urinary Tract Infection. Practice parameter: the diagnosis, treatment, and evaluation of the initial urinary tract infection in febrile infants and young children. Pediatrics 1999;103:843–52.
4. Johnson CE, Shurin PA, Marchant CD, et al. Identification of children requiring radiologic evaluation for urinary infection. Pediatr Infect Dis 1985;4:656–63.
5. Melis K, Vandevivere J, Hoskens C, et al. Involvement of the renal parenchyma in acute urinary tract infection: the contribution of 99mTc dimercaptosuccinic acid scan. Eur J Pediatr 1992;151:536–9.
6. Rosenberg AR, Rossleigh MA, Brydon MP, et al. Evaluation of acute urinary tract infection in children by dimercaptosuccinic acid scintigraphy: a prospective study. J Urol 1992;148:1746–9.
7. Hoberman A, Charron M, Hickey RW, et al. Imaging studies after a first febrile urinary tract infection in young children. N Engl J Med 2003;348:195–202.
8. Hoberman A, Wald ER, Reynolds EA, et al. Is urine culture necessary to rule out urinary tract infection in young febrile children? Pediatr Infect Dis J 1996;15:304–9.
9. Aggarwal VK, Verrier Jones K, Asscher AW, et al. Covert bacteriuria: long term follow up. Arch Dis Child 1991;66:1284–6.
10. Corman LI, Foshee WS, Katchmar GS, et al. Simplified urinary microscopy to detect significant bacteriuria. Pediatrics 1982;133–5.
11. Huicho L, Campos-Sanchez M, Alamo C. Meta-analysis of urine screening tests for determining the risk of urinary tract infection in children. Pediatr Infect Dis J 2002;21:1–11.
12. Bachur R, Harper MB. Reliability of the urinalysis for predicting urinary tract infections in young febrile children. Arch Pediatr Adolesc Med 2001;155:60–5.
13. Jenkins RD, Fenn JP, Matsen JM. Review of urine microscopy for bacteriuria. JAMA 1986;255:3397–403.
14. Hoberman A, Wald ER. Urinary tract infections in young febrile children. Pediatr Infect Dis J 1997;16:11–7.
15. McGuckin MB, Tomasco J, MacGregor RR. Significance of bacteriuria with presumed nonpathogenic organisms. J Urol 1980;124:240–1.
16. Gargan RA, Brumfitt W, Hamilton-Miller JM. Do anaerobes cause urinary infection? Lancet 1980;1:37.
17. Schmit KE. Isolation of *Haemophilus* in urine cultures from children. J Pediatr 1979;95:565–6.
17a. Kass EH. Bacteriuria and the diagnosis of infections of the urinary tract. Arch Intern Med 1957;100:709.
18. Pedraza Aviles AG, Ortiz Zaragoza MC. Symptomatic bacteriuria due to *Ureaplasma* and *Mycoplasma* in adults. Rev Latinoam Microbiol 1998;40:9–13.
19. Todd JK. Diagnosis of urinary tract infections. Pediatr Infect Dis 1982;1:126–31.
20. Lee HJ, Pyo JW, Choi EH, et al. Isolation of adenovirus type 7 from the urine of children with acute hemorrhagic cystitis. Pediatr Infect Dis J 1996;15:633–4.
21. Thomsen AC, Lindskov HO. Diagnosis of *Mycoplasma hominis* pyelonephritis by demonstration of antibodies in urine. J Clin Microbiol 1979;9:681–7.
22. Shawn DH, Quinn PA, Prober C, et al. Recurrent urethritis associated with *Ureaplasma urealyticum* in a prepubertal boy. Pediatr Infect Dis J 1987;6:687–8.
23. Woolfrey BF, Ireland GK, Lally RT. Significance of *Gardnerella vaginalis* in urine cultures. Am J Clin Pathol 1986;86:324–9.
24. Feder HM Jr, Rasoulpour M, Rodriquez AJ. *Campylobacter* urinary tract infection: value of the urine Gram's stain. JAMA 1986;256:2389.
25. McGuckin MA, Cohen L, MacGregor RR. Significance of pyuria in urinary sediment. J Urol 1978;120:452–4.
26. Moffet HL. Urinalysis and urine cultures in children. Urol Clin North Am 1974;1:387–96.
27. Wiswell TE, Roscelli JD. Corroborative evidence for the decreased incidence of urinary tract infections in circumcised male infants. Pediatrics 1986;78:96–9.
28. Spach DH, Stapleton AE, Stamm WE. Lack of circumcision increases the risk of urinary tract infection in young men. JAMA 1992;267:679–81.
29. Grady R, Krieger J. Urinary tract infection in childhood. Curr Opin Urol 2001;11:61–5.
30. Elder JS, Peters CA, Arant BS Jr, et al. Report of the Management of Primary Vesicoureteral Reflux in Children. Baltimore, MD: American Urological Association, 1997.
31. Agarwal S. Vesicoureteral reflux and urinary tract infections. Curr Opin Urol 2000;10:587–92.
32. American Academy of Pediatrics. Committee on Practice and Ambulatory Medicine. Recommendations for preventive pediatric health care. Pediatrics 2000;105:645–6.
33. Kemper KJ, Avner ED. The case against screening urinalyses for asymptomatic bacteriuria in children. Am J Dis Child 1992;146:343–6.
34. Al-Orifi F, McGillivray D, Tange S, et al. Urine culture from bag specimens in young children: are the risks too high? J Pediatr 2000;137:221–6.
35. Schlager TA, Hendley JO, Dudley SM, et al. Explanation for false-positive urine cultured obtained by bag technique. Arch Pediatr Adolesc Med 1995;149:170–3.
36. Pryles CV, Steg NL. Specimens of urine obtained from young girls by catheter versus voiding: a comparative study

of bacterial cultures, Gram stains, and bacterial counts in paired specimens. Pediatrics 1969;23:441–2.

37. King LR, Moffet HL. The significance of equivocal bacteriuria in girls with recurrent urinary tract infection as determined by a new technique. J Urol 1969;102:518–20.

38. Cade R, Raulerson JD, Mahoney JJ, et al. New method for obtaining uncontaminated urine from women. South Med J 1978;71:1536–1539.

39. Lohr JA, Donowitz LG, Dudley SM. Bacterial contamination rate for non-clean-catch and clean-catch midstream urine collection in boys. J Pediatr 1986;109:659–60.

40. Lifshitz E, Kramer L. Outpatient urine culture: does collection technique matter? Arch Intern Med 2000;160: 2537–40.

41. Liaw LCT, Nayar DM, Coulthard MG. Home collection of urine for culture from infants by three methods: survey of parents' preferences and bacterial contamination rates. BMJ 2000;320:1312–3.

42. Amir J, Ginzburg M, Staussberg R, et al. The reliability of midstream urine culture from circumcised male infants. Am J Dis Child 1993;147:969–70.

43. Turck M, Goffe B, Petersdorf RG. The urethral catheter and urinary tract infection. J Urol 1962;88:834–7.

44. Kochakarn W, Ratana-Olarn K, Lertsithichai P, Roongreungsilp U. Follow-up of long-term treatment with clean intermittent catheterization for neurogenic bladder in children. Asian J Surg 2004;27:134–6.

45. Sidor TA, Resnick MI. Urinary tract infections in children. Pediatr Clin North Am 1983;30:323–32.

46. Pollack CV Jr, Pollack ES, Andrew ME. Suprapubic bladder aspiration versus urethral catheterization in ill infants: success, efficiency and complication rates. Ann Emerg Med 1994;23:225–30.

47. Latham RH, Running K, Stamm WE. Urinary tract infections in young adult women caused by *Staphylococcus saprophyticus*. JAMA 1983;250:3063–6.

48. Durbin WA Jr, Peter G. Management of urinary tract infections in infants and children. Pediatr Infect Dis 1984;3: 564–74.

49. Eichenwald HF. Some aspects of the diagnosis and management of urinary tract infection in children and adolescents. Pediatr Infect Dis 1986;5:760–5.

50. Hellerstein S. Recurrent urinary tract infections in children. Pediatr Infect Dis 1982;1:271–281.

51. Andriole VT. Renal carbuncle. Med Grand Rounds 1983; 2:250.

52. Dembry LM, Andriole VT. Renal and perirenal abscesses. Infect Dis Clin North Am 1997;11:663–80.

53. Taylor KJ, Wasson JF, DeGraaff C, et al. Accuracy of grey scale ultrasound diagnosis of abdominal and pelvic abscesses in 220 patients. Lancet 1978;1:83–84.

54. Lawson GR, White FE, Alexander FW. Acute focal bacterial nephritis. Arch Dis Child 1985;60:475–7.

55. Rasoulpour M, Banco L, Mackay IM, et al. Treatment of focal xanthogranulomatous pyelonephritis with antibiotics. J Pediatr 1984;105:423–5.

56. Marteinsson VT, Due J, Aagenaes I. Focal granulomatous pyelonephritis presenting as renal tumour in children: case report with a review of the literature. Scand J Urol Nephrol 1996;30:235–9.

57. Samuel M, Duffy P, Capps S, et al. Xanthogranulomatous

58. Takamizawa S, Yamataka A, Kaneko K, et al. Xanthogranulomatous pyelonephritis in childhood: a rare but important clinical entity. J Pediatr Surg 2000;35:1554–5.

59. Rodo J, Martin ME, Salarich J. Xanthogranulomatous pyelonephritis in children: conservative management. Eur Urol 1996;30:498–501.

60. Kao CT, Tsai JD, Lee HC, et al. Right perinephric abscess: a rare presentation of ruptured retrocecal appendicitis. Pediatr Nephrol 2002;17:177–80.

61. Haddad MC, Hawary MM, Khoury NJ, et al. Radiology of perinephric fluid collections. Clin Radiol 2002;57: 339–46.

62. Arthur RR, Shah KV, Baust SJ, et al. Association of BK viruria with hemorrhagic cystitis in recipients of bone marrow transplants. N Engl J Med 1986;315:230–4.

63. Lin PL, Vats AN, Green M. BK virus infection in renal transplant recipients. Pediatr Transplant 2001;5:398–405.

64. Sulphin M, Middleton AW Jr. Eosinophilic cystitis in children: a self-limited process. J Urol 1984;132:117–9.

65. Gerhartz EW, Grueber M, Melekos MD, et al. Tumor-forming eosinophilic cystitis in children: case report and review of literature. Eur Urol 1994;35:138–41.

66. Van den Ouden D. Diagnosis and management of eosinophilic cystitis: a pooled analysis of 135 cases. Eur Urol 2000;37:386–94.

67. Bauer SB, Kogan SJ. Vesical manifestations of chronic granulomatous disease in childhood: its relation to eosinophilic cystitis. Urology 1991;37:463–6.

67a. Kodner CM, Kudrimoti A. Diagnosis and management of acute interstitial nephritis. Am Fam Physician 2003;67; 2527–34.

68. Lischer GH, Sweat SD. 16-year-old boy with gross hematuria. Mayo Clin Proc 2002;77:475–8.

69. Ross AG, Bartley PB, Sleigh AC, et al. Schistosomiasis. N Engl J Med 2002;346:1212–20.

70. Nicolle LE, Harding GKM, Preiksaitis J, et al. The association of urinary tract infection with sexual intercourse. J Infect Dis 1982;146:579–83.

71. Demetriou E, Emans SJ, Masland RP Jr. Dysuria in adolescent girls: urinary tract infection or vaginitis? Pediatrics 1982;70:299–301.

72. Stamm WE, Wagner KF, Amsel R, et al. Causes of the acute urethral syndrome in women. N Engl J Med 1980; 303:409–15.

73. Baldoni F, Ercolani M, Baldaro B, et al. Stressful events and psychological symptoms in patients with functional urinary disorders. Percept Mot Skills 1995;80:605–606.

74. Sumners D, Kelsey M, Chait I. Psychological aspects of lower urinary tract infections in women. Br Med J 1992; 304:17–9.

75. Gittes RF, Nakamura RM. Female urethral syndrome: a female prostatitis? West J Med 1996;164:435–8.

76. Bernstein AM, Phillips HC, Linden W, et al. A psychophysiological evaluation of female urethral syndrome: evidence for a muscular abnormality. J Behav Med 1992;15: 299–312.

77. Salmen P, Dwyer DW, Vorse H, et al. Whirlpool-associated *Pseudomonas aeruginosa* urinary tract infections. JAMA 1983;250:2025–6.

78. McCracken GH Jr. Diagnosis and management of acute

pyelonephritis in childhood. J Pediatr Surg 2001;36: 598–601.

urinary tract infections in infants and children. Pediatr Infect Dis J 1987;6:107–12.

79. Tran D, Muchant DG, Aronoff SC. Short-course versus conventional length antimicrobial therapy for uncomplicated lower urinary tract infections in children: a meta-analysis of 1279 patients. J Pediatr 2001;139:93–9.

80. Iravani A, Klimberg I, Briefer C, et al. A trial comparing low-dose, short-course ciprofloxacin and standard 7-day therapy with co-trimoxazole or nitrofurantoin in the treatment of uncomplicated urinary tract infection. J Antimicrob Chemother 1999;43(suppl A):67–75.

81. Beisel B, Hale W, Graves RS, et al. Does postcoital voiding prevent urinary tract infections in young women? J Fam Pract 2002;51:977.

82. Hamburger EK. Urinary tract infections in infants and children. Postgrad Med 1986;80:235–8.

83. Dick PT, Feldman W. Routine diagnostic imaging for childhood urinary tract infections: a systematic overview. J Pediatr 1996;128:15–22.

84. Bjerklund Johansen TE. Diagnosis and imaging in urinary tract infections. Curr Opin Urol 2002;12:39–43.

85. Hohenfellner K, Seemayer S, Stolz G, et al. Pre- and postpartum ultrasound examinations for diagnosis of urogenital abnormalities German. Klin Padiatr 2000;212:320–5.

86. Mahant S, To T, Friedman J. Timing of voiding cystourethrogram in the investigation of urinary tract infections in children. J Pediatr 2001;139:568–71.

87. McDonald A, Scranton M, Gillespie R, et al. Voiding cystourethrograms and urinary tract infections: how long to wait? Pediatrics 2000;105:e50.

88. Winter AL, Hardy BE, Alton DJ, et al. Acquired renal scars in children. J Urol 1983;129:1190–4.

89. Williams G, Lee A, Craig J. Antibiotics for the prevention of urinary tract infection in children: a systematic review of randomized controlled trials. J Pediatr 2001;138:868–74.

90. Lohr JA, Nunley DH, Howards SS, et al. Prevention of recurrent urinary tract infections in girls. Pediatrics 1977;59:562–5.

91. Smellie JM, Katz G, Gruneberg RN. Controlled trial of prophylactic treatment in childhood urinary tract infection. Lancet 1978;2:175–8.

92. Drachman R, Valevici M, Vardy PA. Excretory urography and cystourethrography in the evaluation of children with urinary tract infection. Clin Pediatr 1984;23:265–7.

93. Alon U, Pery M, Davidai G, et al. Ultrasonography in the radiologic evaluation of children with urinary tract infection. Pediatrics 1986;75:58–64.

94. Johnson CE, DeBaz BP, Shurin PA, et al. Renal ultrasound evaluation of urinary tract infections in children. Pediatrics 1986;78:871–8.

95. Hoberman A, Wald ER, Hickey RW, et al. Oral versus initial intravenous therapy for urinary tract infections in young febrile children. Pediatrics 1999;104:79–86.

96. Hodson CJ. Reflux nephropathy: a personal historical review. AJR 1981;137:451–62.

97. Report of the International Reflux Study Committee. Medical versus surgical treatment of primary vesicoureteral reflux. Pediatrics 1981;67:392–400.

98. Aladjem M, Boichis H, Hertz M, et al. The conservative management of vesicoureteric reflux: a review of 121 children. Pediatrics 1980;65:78–80.

99. Elder JS, Peters CA, Arant BS Jr, et al. Pediatric Vesicoureteral Reflux Guidelines Panel summary report on the management of primary vesicoureteral reflux in children. J Urol 1997;157:1846–51.

100. Langley JM, Hanakowski M, Leblanc JC. Unique epidemiology of nosocomial urinary tract infection in children. Am J Infect Control 2001;29:94–8.

101. Davies HD, Jones EL, Sheng RY, et al. Nosocomial urinary tract infections at a pediatric hospital. Pediatr Infect Dis J 1992;11:349–54.

102. Emori TG, Gaynes RP. An overview of nosocomial infections, including the role of the microbiology laboratory. Clin Microbiol Rev 1993;6:428–42.

103. Bryant K, Maxfield C, Rabalais G. Renal candidiasis in neonates with candiduria. Pediatr Infect Dis J 1999;18:959–63.

104. Benjamin DK Jr, Fisher RG, Benjamin DK, et al. Candidal mycetoma in the neonatal kidney. Pediatrics 1999;104:1126–9.

104a. Laube GF, Superti-Furga A, Losa M, et al. Hyperammonaemic encephalopathy in a 13-year-old boy. Eur J Pediatr 2002;161:163–4.

105. McCracken GH Jr. Recurrent urinary tract infections in children. Pediatr Infect Dis 1984;4(suppl):S28–S30.

106. Welch TR, Forbes PA, Drummond KN, et al. Recurrent urinary tract infection in girls: group with lower tract findings and a benign course. Arch Dis Child 1976;51:114–9.

107. Davison JM, Sprott MS, Selkon JB. The effect of covert bacteriuria in schoolgirls on renal function at 18 years and during pregnancy. Lancet 1984;2:651–5.

108. Rushton HG, Majd M, Jantausch B, et al. Renal scarring following reflux and nonreflux pyelonephritis in children: evaluation with 99m technetium-dimercaptosuccinic acid scintigraphy. J Urol 1992;147:1327–32.

109. Stokland E, Hellstrom M, Jacobsson B, et al. Renal damage one year after first urinary tract infection: role of dimercaptosuccinic acid scintigraphy. J Pediatr 1996;129:815–20.

110. Jakobsson B, Berg U, Svensson L. Renal scarring after acute pyelonephritis. Arch Dis Child 1994;70:111–5.

111. Smellie JM, Prescod NP, Shaw PJ, et al. Childhood reflux and urinary infection: a follow-up of 10 to 41 years in 226 adults. Pediatr Nephrol 1998;12:727–36.

112. Poole SR. The infant with acute, unexplained, excessive crying. Pediatrics 1991;88:450–5.

CHAPTER 15

Genital Syndromes

■ DEFINITIONS

A genital infection can be defined as any infection involving the reproductive organs. "Venereal disease" is an older phrase for a disease usually spread by sexual contact, now referred to as a *sexually transmitted disease* (STD). Genital and sexually transmitted diseases have important differences: STDs may involve anatomic areas other than the genitalia, and many genital infections are not spread by sexual contact. Therefore, it is useful to keep the working diagnosis of a genital infection in terms of an anatomic syndrome, such as vaginitis, and record the etiologic diagnoses as probabilities or possibilities until confirmed by laboratory methods.

Children can acquire STDs as sexually active teenagers or by sexual abuse of either sex, particularly before complete sexual maturity and before the age when they can tell about the abuse.[1–4]

The "traditional" STDs are syphilis, gonorrhea, donovanosis (granuloma inguinale), lymphogranuloma venereum (LGV), and chancroid. Many other infections can be sexually transmitted, including chlamydia, human immunodeficiency virus (HIV), hepatitis B, hepatitis C, *Trichomonas* infections, nonspecific urethritis and Reiter's syndrome, genital herpes, venereal warts (condyloma accuminata), various types of vaginitis, and molluscum contagiosum. Infestations with lice ("crabs") and mites (scabies) can also be sexually transmitted. Cystitis in the sexually active female may be a result of sexual intercourse, as discussed in Chapter 14. The physician should remember that the presence of one of these diseases should suggest the possibility of others.

Human immunodeficiency virus (HIV) infection is discussed in Chapter 20. Hepatitis B and C infections are discussed in Chapter 13. Congenitally-acquired infections are discussed in Chapter 19.

■ IMPLICATIONS OF SEXUALLY TRANSMITTED DISEASES IN CHILDREN

Sexual abuse of children should always be considered when the cause of a genital infection has been found to be a sexually transmitted pathogen.[2–4] Implications of commonly encountered STDs in children with regard to the possibility of abuse have been developed by the American Academy of Pediatrics (AAP) and are shown in Table 15-1.

■ FREQUENCY

In the United States, STDs constitute an epidemic of tremendous magnitude, with an estimated 15 million persons acquiring a new STD each year.[5] In the 1980s, chlamydia surpassed gonorrhea as the most common STD. Currently, it is estimated that there are 3 million new cases of chlamydia in the United States each year, compared with 650,000 cases of gonorrhea. The incidence of syphilis has decreased steadily; currently, about 70,000 cases occur each year. However, there is extreme geographic clustering, with half of all new cases reported from only 22 U.S. counties.[6]

The incidence of herpes simplex virus (HSV) type 2 infections has risen to 1 million cases per year. Because herpes viruses cause persistent infection, currently 45 million people (22% of the U.S. adult population) are infected with HSV type 2.[7]

Each year in the United States, there are approximately 5 million new cases of human papilloma virus (HPV) infections and a similar number of trichomonas infections.[5]

■ PREVENTION OF SEXUALLY TRANSMITTED DISEASES

Prevention of STDs is based on five major concepts[8]:

- Education and counseling of persons at risk on ways to adopt safer sexual behavior
- Identification of asymptomatically infected persons and of symptomatic persons unlikely to seek treatment
- Effective diagnosis and treatment of infected persons
- Evaluation, treatment, and counseling of sex partners of persons who are infected with an STD, and

TABLE 15-1. IMPLICATIONS OF COMMONLY ENCOUNTERED STDS FOR THE DIAGNOSIS AND REPORTING OF SEXUAL ABUSE OF INFANTS AND PREPUBERTAL CHILDREN

STD CONFIRMED	EVIDENCE FOR SEXUAL ABUSE	SUGGESTED ACTION
Gonorrhea	Diagnostic*	Report†
Syphilis	Diagnostic*	Report†
HIV	Diagnostic‡	Report†
Chlamydia trachomatis	Diagnostic*	Report†
Trichomonas vaginalis	Highly suspicious	Report†
Condylomata acuminata	Suspicious*	Report†
Genital herpes	Suspicious*	Report†¶
Bacterial vaginosis	Inconclusive	Medical follow-up

Source: Adapted from Guidelines for the evaluation of sexual abuse of children: subject review. American Academy of Pediatrics Committee on Child Abuse and Neglect. Pediatrics 1999;103:186–191.
STD, sexually transmitted disease; HIV, human immunodeficiency virus.
* If not likely to be perinatally acquired.
† Report to agency in the community mandated to receive reports of suggested sexual abuse.
‡ If not likely to be acquired perinatally or through transfusion.
¶ Unless there is a clear history of autoinoculation.

- Preexposure vaccination of persons at risk for vaccine-preventable STDs (e.g., hepatitis B).

The correct use of male condoms is effective in preventing some STDs. Because condoms do not cover all exposed areas, they are more effective in preventing infections transmitted by fluids from mucosal surfaces (e.g., Gonorrhea, *Chlamydia*, *Trichomonas*, and HIV) than in preventing those transmitted by skin-to-skin contact (e.g., HSV, HPV, syphilis, and chancroid).[8] The most reliable way to avoid transmission of STDs is to abstain from sexual intercourse or to be in a long-term, mutually monogamous relationship with an uninfected partner.[8]

A recent study assessed the efficacy of valacyclovir in preventing transmission from an HIV-2 seropositive person to their HIV-2 seronegative partner. A total of 1,484 heterosexual, monogamous couples were followed. The HSV-2 seropositive person received once daily valacyclovir. The overall acquisition of HSV-2 among susceptible persons was 3.6% in the placebo group and 1.9% in the valacyclovir group- a 47% relative reduction (p = 0.04).[8a]

■ GENITAL INFECTIONS OF MALES AND FEMALES

Genital Ulcers

This category includes ulceration of the skin on or near the external genitalia or on the mucosa (Fig. 15-1). Clinical differentiation of the various causes of genital ulcer disease (GUD) is difficult, even if standardized, quantitative diagnostic techniques are used.[9] The sensitivity of clinical features in establishing the diagnosis of syphilis, HSV infection, and chancroid was 31–35% in a study of 220 patients with microbiologically established diagnoses.[9]

Genital ulcer disease (GUD) is important for several reasons. Early treatment of syphilis prevents progression to secondary and tertiary disease. The seroprevalence of HIV is higher in patients with GUD, and it continued to increase among these patients during a period of rapid decline in patients without GUD.[10] It is thought that HIV is more readily spread by those with genital ulcers. The causes of GUD are discussed briefly later.

Genital Herpes

HSV is by far the most common cause of genital ulcer disease in the United States. The seroprevalence of HSV has increased 30% over the past 20–25 years in this country.[11] Women are infected more readily than are men.[12] HSV infection is also the most common sexually transmitted cause of genital ulcers in children.[13] The classic description of the disease is that of painful, clustered genital ulcerative lesions. The spectrum of disease, however, is much wider. Longitudinal studies show that 60% of primary HSV-2 infections are asymptom-

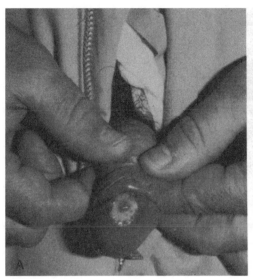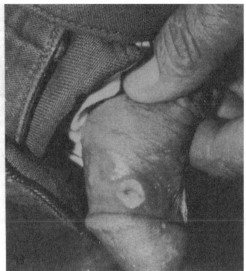

■ **FIGURE 15-1** (**A**) Syphilitic chancre; (**B**) chancroid (soft chancre), caused by *Haemophilus ducreyi*. (Photos from Dr. Larry Lantis.)

atic.[14] Of symptomatic patients, only 40% fit the classic clinical description; over a third have ulcerative lesions outside the genital area, approximately 10% have a single ulcer, about 5% have erosive lesions, and a few have crusting, fissuring, edema, and other atypical manifestations.[15] In addition to painful ulcerations, HSV can also produce vaginal discharge and dysuria.[16] Necrotizing ulceration of the glans penis (balanitis) has been described.[17] Occasionally, finger lesions (herpetic whitlow) are found in addition to the genital lesions.

Reactivation of latent infection occurs at varying frequency. Traditionally, it was believed that patients whose primary HSV infection was asymptomatic underwent very few recurrences, and thus presented a low risk of transmission of the infection to others; careful clinical studies have now shown that reactivation and viral shedding occurs with similar frequency in all patients, regardless of whether the primary infection caused noticeable disease.[18] Most patients eventually develop clinically apparent lesions. In the majority of patients, the frequency of reactivation declines over time.[19] Triggers for recurrence have not been carefully studied. One study concluded that short-term stressors did not increase the frequency of recurrence, but persistent stressors and "total anxiety level" were modestly associated with an increased number of reactivations.[20]

The gold standard for establishing the diagnosis is viral culture.[21] However, the sensitivity of culture depends on the stage of the lesions. About 95% of vesicular lesions will grow HSV, as compared with 70% of ulcerative lesions and 30% of crusted lesions.[21] PCR testing is about 30% more sensitive than conventional tissue culture methodology but is also considerably more expensive.[22,23] Vesicular fluid can be tested for the viral antigen, and although this may be useful if the result is positive, the test is not very sensitive. Similarly, a scraping of the base for microscopic examination for multinucleated giant cells (Tzanck test) is rapid but neither specific nor sensitive enough and may be painful.

Syphilis

Caused by infection with *Treponema pallidum* a syphilitic chancre is traditionally described as a solitary, painless, shallow ulcer about 1–2 cm in diameter with hard, elevated edges.[24,25] However, in one study of 64 men with primary syphilis proven by darkfield microscopy, 31 (47%) had two or more ulcers, 5 (8%) had nonindurated lesions, and in 5 (8%), the borders were irregular and slightly undermined (suggesting chancroid).[26] Thus, only 27 (43%) of the 64 patients had the classically described chancre of primary syphilis. Furthermore, although chancres are painless on the genitalia they may be painful if extra-genital. They are easily overlooked if on the cervix or rectum. In children younger than age 14 years, 95% of whom acquire syphilis by being victims of sexual abuse, the diagnosis is even more difficult. Chancres are rare. In 17 (81%) of 21 such patients, condylomata lata was the cutaneous feature of the disease.[27] These appear as multiple confluent moist gray-white papule. The incubation period is about 10–90 (usually about 21) days. Neither congenital nor acquired syphilis confers life-long immunity.

Chancroid

Soft chancre or chancroid is an ulcer produced by *Haemophilus ducreyi*. The organism is highly infectious; in experimental infection, inoculation of even one colony-forming unit (cfu) is enough to produce a papule in 50% of subjects. Pustule formation occurs in 50% of subjects at a dose of 27 cfu and in 90% with as few as 100 cfu.[28] The incubation period is 3–5 days. The pathogenesis is largely unknown, although it has been demonstrated that *H. ducreyi* releases a cytolethal distending toxin that arrests cells in the G2 phase.[29] Clinically, lesions begin as a papules or vesicles that later rupture to leave shallow, painful ulcers. Most patients have two or more soft lesions. Later, there are large ulcers in the genital area with beefy red granulation tissue and inguinal adenopathy. About 10% of persons who have chancroid acquired in the United States are coinfected with *Treponema pallidum* or HSV.[8]

Treatment failures are often related to the concomitant presence of HSV or to misdiagnosis of HSV-associated lesions as chancroid.[30] Patients with HIV infection are also less likely to be cured.[31] Culture of *H. ducreyi* requires special agar media. Newer diagnostic tests have been developed, including an enzyme immunoassay[32] and a PCR, but they are not widely available.[33]

Donovanosis (Granuloma Inguinale)

Donovanosis is endemic to Papua New Guinea, Southeast India, Southern Africa, the Caribbean, Brazil, and among the aborigines in Australia. This distribution of disease is unique among STDs.[34] Outbreaks in the United States have been described, predictably among travelers returning from areas of endemicity. Until recently, donovanosis has been attributed to infection with *Calymmatobacterium granulomatis,* a gram-negative bacillus.[1] However, the bacterium has been reclassified as a species of *Klebsiella*.[35] The condition is generally indolent, its pathogen is weakly infectious, and outcomes are excellent if antibiotic therapy is administered. Even

so, donovanosis causes substantial morbidity and mortality, mainly because it is often not correctly diagnosed. The incubation period is usually between 1 and 12 weeks but may extend out to a year.[36] Babies have presented at ages of up to 6 months with donovanosis acquired at birth.[37] The lesions begin as painless nodules that erode to leave beefy red, readily bleeding, exuberant patches of granulation tissue.[38] Primary lesions enlarge slowly. Secondary lesions may occur by autoinoculation. Not all cases follow the classic description; a more rapidly progressive, necrotic form has been well described. Extragenital lesions may also occur, even after the primary condition has apparently resolved. The mouth is the most commonly involved extragenital site.[36] Disseminated disease is often fatal. Bone infection may occur, usually in women, who may have an undiagnosed primary cervical infection. Cervical lesions are commonly misdiagnosed as carcinomatous.[39]

Donovanosis can be a difficult clinical diagnosis because of its rarity, the disparity of clinical presentations, and the fastidious nature of the organism. The diagnosis usually rests upon identifying Donovan bodies inside mononuclear cells obtained from active lesions by scraping or biopsy. Nonencapsulated forms of *Klebsiella granulomatis* comb. nov. have a "safety pin" appearance in tissue section because of polar chromatin densities. Recently, investigators have been able to cultivate the organism in cell culture systems.[40,41] PCR assays have been developed.[42,43] Studies show some utility of an indirect immunofluorescence assay.[44]

Doxycycline is the usual treatment, but comparative trials of antimicrobial agents are lacking. One gram of azithromycin once a week for 4 weeks produced apparent clinical cure in 11 patients.[45] However, relapses may occur a few months to 2 years after apparent clinical cure. Ceftriaxone, administered intramuscularly at a dose of 1 gram per day for 7–10 consecutive days, was successful at eradicating disease in a group of chronically infected aboriginal patients.[46]

Pemphigoid Gestationis

This bullous skin disease occurs during pregnancy. It may involve the trunk, extremities, groin, and buttocks. Previously, and regrettably still on occasion, the condition was referred to as "herpes gestationis." It is autoimmune in nature, and therefore has nothing to do with herpes simplex virus.[47] Histologically, there is deposition of C3 along basement membranes[48] and eosinophilic infiltration is prominent.[49] It is thought to be similar to bullous pemphigoid; sera from 79% of women with the condition recognize the antigenic domain of the bullous pemphigoid antigen.[50] There is a tendency for women with pemphigoid gestationis to develop other autoimmune conditions, especially Graves's disease.[51] Patients with this condition may also have chronic placental insufficiency, which leads to an increased frequency of preterm births and small for gestational age babies.[48]

Uncommon Causes

Cutaneous tuberculosis can present with ulcerative skin lesions in the inguinal or genital area. In childhood, however, cutaneous TB usually presents as condylomata lata rather than as a chancre.[52] In endemic areas, African trypanosomiasis causes genital ulcerative disease.[53] A chancre secondary to nodular mucocutaneous histiocytosis has been described.[54] In several patients, genital ulcerations have appeared coincidentally with infectious mononucleosis due to EBV. The ulcerations were described as having purple margins.[55] Obviously, genital ulcers from some other condition could occur coincidentally with EBV infection; however, laboratory tests for other causes were negative. Adding further support to the concept that EBV could be causally related to the genital ulcerations is a report from Thailand, in which 17 (57%) of 30 HSV culture-positive genital ulcerative lesions were also positive for EBV DNA by PCR.[56] Amebiasis of the glans penis is a rare cause of ulcerative disease; it should be suspected when ulcerative lesions are refractory to antibiotic therapy.[57]

Other possible causes of genital ulcers include moniliasis, psoriasis, scabies, molluscum contagiosum of the labia, erythema multiforme, and simple friction ulceration of the labia minora, penile shaft, or glans, which can be secondarily infected.[58,59]

Laboratory Approach

Culture of the lesions for HSV should be performed, but treatment for clinically suspected disease should not be delayed pending the culture result.[21] Darkfield microscopic examination of material from a chancre-like ulcer may reveal the spirochetes of syphilis, but darkfield facilities with experienced observers are usually available only in clinics where the disease is frequently seen. Gram stain of the smear of the chancre-like ulcer may reveal rows and chains of gram-negative rods, characteristic of *Haemophilus ducreyi. H. ducreyi* is difficult to culture because it is fastidious, but new media are being developed.

Special stains of a smear from crushed tissue preparations from donovanosis typically demonstrate oval Donovan bodies.

Serologic screening tests for syphilis, such as the VDRL test, are often not yet positive at the time the syphilitic chancre first appears but usually become positive within a few weeks thereafter. The VDRL should be obtained as soon as the chancre is seen and repeated in about 2 weeks. Antisyphilitic therapy should be given as soon as the physician suspects syphilis, without waiting for the VDRL results. Early treatment of the primary chancre usually results in a negative VDRL by 1 year, and treatment of secondary syphilis usually results in VDRL seronegativity by 24 months.[60]

All positive VDRL results should be confirmed by specific tests, such as the fluorescent treponemal antibody-absorbed test (FTA-ABS), because biologic false-positive VDRLs are common in adolescents. Even false-positive FTA-ABS tests can occur, so this test should not be used for screening purposes.

Treatment

Selected regimens from the 2002 Centers for Disease Control and Prevention (CDC) recommendations for treatment of STDs are shown in Table 15-2.[8] Not all of the CDC treatment regimens are shown. Fever, malaise, and intensification of skin lesions (Jarisch-Herxheimer reaction) occur in many patients within 12 hours of the start of parenteral penicillin therapy for syphilis.

Inguinal Lymphadenopathy

Enlargement of inguinal or femoral lymph nodes can have many causes unrelated to genital diseases and in children is usually due to infections of the lower extremities. However, tender or suppurative nodes in a postpubertal person should raise the question of a genital infection.

Lymphogranuloma Venereum (LGV)

Caused by the serovars L1, L2, or L3 of *Chlamydia trachomatis,* this STD is rare in the United States.[8] Its first manifestation is typically a tender inguinal

TABLE 15-2. TREATMENT OF SEXUALLY TRANSMITTED DISEASES (BASED ON 2002 CDC RECOMMENDATIONS# USING ADULT DOSAGES)

I. Gonorrhea, Uncomplicated (urethritis, endocervicitis, or proctitis; assuming possible coexisting chlamydial infection)

 1. Cefixime†, 400 mg p.o., one dose, OR

 2. Ceftriaxone, 125 mg IM, one dose, OR

 3. Ciprofloxacin, 500 mg p.o., one dose, OR

 4. Ofloxacin, 400 mg p.o., one dose, OR

 5. Levofloxacin, 250 mg p.o., one dose

AND, if Chlamydial coinfection is not ruled out:

 1. Doxycycline, 100 mg p.o. bid for 7 days, OR

 2. Azithromycin, 1 g p.o., one dose

Alternative Regimens

 1. Spectinomycin, 2 g IM, one dose

 2. Other single-dose cephalosporins (ceftizoxime 500 mg IM, cefoxitin 2 g IM with 1 g of p.o. probenecid, cefotaxime 500 mg IM)

 3. Other single-dose quinolones (gatifloxacin 400 mg p.o., norfloxacin 800 mg p.o., lomefloxacin 400 mg p.o.)

Gonococcal infection in pregnancy

 No quinolones or tetracyclines. Use cephalosporin regimen, as previously, or spectinomycin, 2 g IM PLUS antichlamydial regimen, as described later

II. Disseminated Gonococcal Infection

 1. Ceftriaxone, 1 g IV or IM q 24 hours; 24 to 48 hours after clinical improvement, may switch to cefixime†, 400 mg p.o. bid OR ciprofloxacin, 500 mg bid or ofloxacin, 400 mg bid

Alternate regimens

 1. Cefotaxime, 1 g IV q 8 hours

 2. Ceftizoxime, 1 g IV q 8 hours

For beta-lactam-allergic patients

 1. Ciprofloxacin, 500 mg IV q 12 hours

 2. Ofloxacin, 400 mg IV q 12 hours

III. Chlamydial Infection (urethritis, endocervicitis, or proctitis)

 1. Azithromycin, 1 g p.o., one dose

 2. Doxycycline, 100 mg p.o. bid for 7 days

Alternate regimens

 1. Erythromycin base, 500 mg p.o. qid for 7 days

 2. Erythromycin ethylsuccinate, 800 mg p.o. qid for 7 days

 3. Ofloxacin, 300 mg bid for 7 days

 4. Levofloxacin, 500 mg p.o. q day for 7 days

Chlamydial infection in pregnancy (repeat testing 3 weeks after therapy is recommended)

 1. Erythromycin base, 500 mg p.o. qid for 7 days

 2. Amoxicillin, 500 mg p.o. tid for 7 days

Alternate regimens

 1. Erythromycin ethylsuccinate, 800 mg p.o. qid for 7 days

 2. Erythromycin ethylsuccinate, 400 mg p.o. qid for 14 days

 3. Erythromycin base, 250 mg p.o. qid for 14 days

 4. Azithromycin, 1 g p.o., one dose

Recurrent or persistent urethritis

1. Metronidazole, 2 g p.o., one dose AND
   erythromycin base, 500 mg p.o. qid for 7 days, OR erythromycin ethylsuccinate, 800 p.o. qid for 7 days

IV. Nongonococcal Urethritis

Same as for chlamydia infection, earlier

V. Acute Pelvic Inflammatory Disease

Intravenous Regimens

1. Cefotetan, 2 g IV q 12 hours OR cefoxitin, 2 g IV q 6 hours PLUS doxycyline, 100 mg q 12 (oral is preferred)

2. Clindamycin, 900 mg IV q 8 hours PLUS gentamicin in standard dosages

Alternate regimens

1. Ofloxacin, 400 mg IV q 12 hours PLUS metronidazole, 500 mg IV q 8 hours

2. Ampicillin/sulbactam, 3 g IV q 6 hours PLUS doxycycline, 100 mg po q 12 hours

3. Ciprofloxacin, 200 mg IV q 12 hours PLUS doxycycline as previously, PLUS metronidazole, 500 mg IV q 8 hours

Other Regimens

1. Ofloxacin, 400 mg p.o. bid PLUS metronidazole, 500 mg bid

2. Ceftriaxone, 250 mg IM once PLUS doxycycline, 100 mg p.o. bid for 14 days

VI. Syphilis

Primary and Secondary Syphilis

Benzathine penicillin G, 2.4 million units IM once (pediatric dose, 50,000 units/kg IM, to maximum dose of 2.4 million units)

For penicillin-allergic patients

1. Doxycycline, 100 mg p.o. bid for 2 weeks

2. Tetracycline, 500 mg p.o. qid for 2 weeks

Less well-studied alternate therapies

1. Azithromycin, 2 g, one dose

2. Ceftriaxone, 1 g IM or IV q day for 8-10 days

Early latent syphilis

Benzathine penicillin G, 2.4 million units IM in a single dose (pediatric dose, 50,000 units/kg IM, to maximum dose of 2.4 million units)

Late latent syphilis, or syphilis of unknown duration

Benzathine penicillin G, 2.4 million units once weekly for three weeks (total dose 7.2 million units [pediatric dose, 50,000 units/kg/dose, given once a week for three weeks to maximum dose of 2.4 million units per dose])

Late latent syphilis, penicillin-allergic patients

1. Doxycycline, 100 mg p.o. bid for 4 weeks

2. Tetracycline, 500 mg p.o. qid for 4 weeks

Tertiary syphilis

Benzathine penicillin G, dosed as for late latent syphilis

Neurosyphilis

Aqueous penicillin G, 18–24 million units per day, given IV either in divided doses q 4 hours or as a continuous infusion, for a total of 10–14 days

Syphilis in pregnancy

Desensitization, followed by penicillin therapy appropriate to the stage of maternal disease

Congenital syphilis, proven or highly probable

Aqueous penicillin G, 100, 100,000–150,000 units/kg/day, given as 50,000 units/kg/dose IV q 12 hours for 7 days, then q 8 hours for 3 days (total duration of therapy is 10 days)

Congenital syphilis, intermediate risk

Same as previous for proven disease, OR benzathine penicillin G 50,000 units/kg IM in a single dose

VII. Chancroid (Test for HIV when this diagnosis is established)

1. Azithromycin, 1 g p.o., one dose

2. Ceftriaxone, 250 mg IM, one dose

3. Ciprofloxacin, 500 mg p.o. bid for 3 days (not for use in pregnant patients)

4. Erythromycin, 500 mg p.o. tid for 7 days

VIII. Bacterial Vaginosis

1. Metronidazole, 500 mg bid for 7 days

2. Clindamycin cream, 2%, 5 g intravaginally q hs for 7 days

3. Metronidazole gel, 0.75%, 5 g intravaginally q hs for 7 days

Alternate regimens

1. Metronidazole, 2 g p.o., one dose (less effective)

2. Clindamycin, 300 mg p.o. bid for 7 days

Bacterial vaginosis in pregnancy

1. Metronidazole, 250 mg p.o. tid for 7 days

2. Metronidazole, 2 g p.o., one dose

IX. Epididymo-orchitis in Sexually Active Males

1. Ceftriaxone, 250 mg IM one time, PLUS doxycycline, 100 mg p.o. bid for 10 days

2. Ofloxacin, 300 mg bid for 10 days (especially if enterics are suspected, or for patients with cephalosporin allergy)

X. Trichomonas Vaginitis

1. Metronidazole, 2 g orally once OR 500 mg p.o. bid for 7 days (effective alternatives are not available; desensitize, if necessary)

XI. Candidal Vaginitis

1. Many choices. Butoconazole 2% cream, 5 g a day intravaginally for 3 days, OR clotrimazole 1% cream, same dose, for 7–14 days, OR clotrimazole intravaginal tablets, 100 mg tablet once a day for 7 days, OR clotrimazole 100 mg tablets bid for 3 days, OR clotrimazole, 500 mg tablet for one application; many other topical options available.

2. Fluconazole, 150 mg p.o., one dose

Candidal vaginitis in pregnancy

Must use topicals only

XII. Genital Herpes Virus Infections

First clinical episode
Acyclovir, 400 mg tid for 7–10 days, OR 200 mg 5 times a day OR famciclovir, 250 mg tid for 7–10 days OR valacyclovir, 1 gm bid for 7–10 days (initiated within 6 days of onset of lesions).

Recurrent episodes
Acyclovir, 400 mg p.o. tid for 5 days, OR Acyclovir, 200 mg p.o. 5 times a day for 5 days, OR acyclovir, 800 mg p.o. bid for 5 days, OR famciclovir, 125 mg p.o. bid for 5 days, OR valacyclovir, 500 mg p.o. bid for 3–5 days, OR valacyclovir, 1 g p.o. q day for 5 days

Frequent recurrences
Acyclovir, 400 mg p.o. bid, OR famciclovir, 250 mg p.o. bid, OR valacyclovir, 500 mg p.o. a day (not as effective), OR valacyclovir, 1 g p.o. q day

Severe episodes requiring hospitalization
Acyclovir, 5–10 mg/kg IV q 8 hours for 5–7 days

Genital HSV in patients with HIV infection
Acyclovir, 400 mg p.o. tid for 5–10 days, OR acyclovir, 200 mg 5 times a day for 5–10 days, OR famciclovir, 500 mg p.o. bid for 5–10 days, OR valacyclovir, 1 g p.o. bid for 5–10 days

Suppressive therapy in patients with HIV infection
Acyclovir, 400–800 mg p.o. bid to tid, OR famciclovir, 500 mg p.o. bid, OR valacyclovir, 500 mg p.o. bid

XIII. Genital Warts (human papillomavirus infections)
1. Podofilox, 0.5% solution or gel bid times 3 days, off for 4 days, repeat for 4 cycles (maximum dose 0.5 mL/d)
2. Imiquimod 5% cream, 3 times a week for up to 16 weeks
3. Cryotherapy, q 1–2 weeks
4. Surgical removal
5. Laser therapy
Genital warts in pregnancy
Imiquimod, podophylline, and podofilox should not be used during pregnancy

Centers for Disease Control and Prevention. MMWR 2002;51:RR-6 : 1–84.

† Cefixime may not be commercially available.

* No prospective or comparative trials. Dose recommendation taken from: Augenbraun MH. Treatment of syphilis 2001: nonpregnant adults. Clin Infect Dis 2002;35(suppl 2):S187–S190.

node (bubo). Usually the primary lesion, a small papule or erosion that occurs 1–2 weeks after exposure, is not noticed or reported, and the bubo appears 2–4 weeks after exposure. The bubo may proceed to suppuration. Associated erythema nodosum (see Chapter 17) is common.[61] Its presentation may mimic psoas abscess,[62] carcinoma,[63] or incarcerated inguinal hernia.[64] Severe, untreated cases may lead to rectovaginal fistulae[65] or rectal strictures,[66] raising the specter of Crohn's disease.

Syphilis and chancroid also may produce inguinal adenopathy, with overlooked or denied primary lesions.[67] Occasionally, syphilitic inguinal adenitis, which is painless, resembles an incarcerated inguinal hernia.[68] In HIV-infected patients, *Mycobacterium chelonae* infection of an inguinal node may produce a bubo.[69]

Laboratory Diagnosis

The diagnosis of LGV can be difficult. The causative agent is difficult to culture, and the L1-L3 serovars of *C. trachomatis* may serologically cross-react with the more common varieties. In one study of 12 patients with LGV buboes, light microscopy demonstrated intracellular organisms whose morphology was consistent with *Chlamydia* spp in all 12.[70] A group of researchers made monoclonal antibodies against L1 and L3 serovars and developed an immunofluorescence assay for LGV. Using this test, they were able to diagnose LGV in 21 (84%) of 25 smear-negative patient samples.[71] Syphilis should be excluded by a VDRL test in sexually active teenagers with inguinal adenitis.

Treatment

Lymphogranuloma venereum can be effectively treated with a single dose of azithromycin or a 7-day course of doxycycline.[72] Aspiration of fluctuant nodes may also be helpful.[73]

Condylomata

Genital Warts (Condyloma Acuminata)

Caused by a papilloma virus similar to those causing common skin warts, these pointed warts can be transmitted by close contact, as well as by sexual contact.[74] Typically, the serotype of human papilloma virus (HPV) that causes skin lesions (type 2) is not the same as the serotypes that cause genital warts (types 6 and 11). However, in children, infection of the genitalia by type 2 can produce lesions indistinguishable from those caused by the "genital serotypes."[75] In one series of 25 children with genital condylomata, all children who had HPV type 2 infection in the genital area also had concomitant skin lesions.[75] However, in the same study, some children whose family members had common skin warts (type 2) were found to have typical genital serotypes (6 and 11). Therefore, the presence of a family member with skin lesions does not rule out sexual abuse.

In one series, 10 (91%) of 11 girls under age 12 with genital warts had historical or physical evidence other than the warts that confirmed sexual abuse.[76] Six of them had other infections, such as bacterial vaginosis, gonorrhea, or trichomonas vaginitis; all six had been abused by multiple perpetrators.[76] It is possible for these warts to be spread through close contact other than sexual abuse, and babies can acquire infection when passing through the birth canal. Experimentally, HPV DNA can be found on the fingertips of at least half of patients with active genital lesions.[77] However, epidemiologic evidence of spread of the virus through this mechanism is sparse. Adults with condyloma acuminata are likely to have other STDs as well. *Ureaplasma urealyticum* infection, in particular, has been associated with condylomata.[78]

The diagnosis is usually made by history and physical examination and can be confirmed by biopsy if necessary. Papilloma viruses cannot be grown in cell culture. A variety of treatment modalities exist, but all have drawbacks. Surgical resection is the least expensive form of therapy.[79] Electrodessication and laser treatments are somewhat more expensive. Topical podophyllin has been the favored first treatment for many years. However, its failure rate, coupled with a high incidence of side effects, has made some experts consider it an unfit form of therapy.[80] Imiquimod is a topical interferon and cytokine-inducing agent that is administered three times a week for 16 weeks. This regimen cures about two-thirds of females but only one-third of males.[81] More frequent application results in more side effects, without increasing the efficacy of the therapy.[81] Topical application of cidofovir has been effective in some cases.[82] Massive accumulations of these warts ("Buschke-Lowenstein tumors") can be very difficult to eradicate; some have used irradiation successfully.[83] In other cases, glansectomy or penectomy has been required.[84]

Malignant transformation of HPV-induced lesions sometimes occurs. A study in men with anal condylomata suggested an incidence of approximately 3.5%.[85] The HPV types most frequently associated with genital warts, however, are not typically associated with cervical carcinoma.[86] They do cause dysplasia, however, which may lead to considerable morbidity due to fear and over-treatment.[86] A pelvic examination and routine Pap smear should be offered as part of preventive health maintenance between the ages of 18 and 21 years.[87]

Condylomata latum are flat and may indicate secondary syphilis or papilloma virus infection.

Pink Pearly Papules

Resembling condylomata acuminata or ectopic sebaceous glands, these papules typically occur in rows surrounding the penile glans on the corona.[88] They seem to originate during adolescence and require no treatment.

Genital Edema

Edema can be secondary to friction injury and is usually attributable to repeated sexual activity, including masturbation. In one study, the causes included urethritis, infected penile lesions, gonorrhea, herpes simplex, and scabies.[89] Focal enlargement of areas of the external genitalia can be caused by lymphatic obstruction from LGV, but this is rare in children. A constricting hair or fine thread can produce distal swelling of the shaft of the penis or clitoris in infants. Crohn's disease may produce genital swelling in either sex.[90] Other symptoms suggestive of Crohn's disease may or may not be obvious, or may be remote in time.[91] Large pelvic tumors can compress pelvic and inguinal lymphatics and cause scrotal edema, but this is exceedingly rare.[92] Scrotal edema may accompany epididymal or testicular ailments; these are usually exquisitely painful. Occasionally, Henoch-Schönlein purpura (HSP) causes swelling of the genitals, but other stigmata of HSP accompany this finding. Donovanosis may be associated with massive genital edema, especially in women. Finally, there is a disorder known as idiopathic scrotal edema, which is a painless but slightly tender swelling of the scrotum that typically occurs in 4- to 6-year-old children. As the name suggests, the cause is unknown. The condition is self-limited and of a short duration.[93]

Urethritis

Strictly speaking, urethritis is defined by leukorrhea and physical examination findings suggestive of urethral inflammation. Operationally, it is often defined as redness of the urethra or pain in the urethra on voiding. Urethritis can be subdivided into purulent or nonpurulent, depending on the appearance of the discharge. As the presence of white cells in the discharge is part of the definition of the syndrome, even patients with "nonpurulent" urethritis have leukorrhea. Urethritis can also be classified as gonococcal or nongonococcal, according to the results of culture of the discharge, analogous to the classification of pharyngitis as streptococcal or nonstreptococcal. In prepubertal girls, urethritis is usually not sexually transmitted. It is most common in sexually active boys, where it can be regarded as the male counterpart of cervicitis.

HIV-positive men who have urethritis are more likely to transmit HIV infection than are those who do not have urethritis. Urethritis increases the number of HIV particles in the semen by at least eight-fold; this effect is strongest in patients with gonococcal infection.[94] The concentration of HIV in the semen decreases when the urethritis is appropriately treated with antibiotics. This makes identification and treatment of urethritis especially important in places where HIV infection is common.

Purulent Urethritis

This type typically occurs in the male and is usually due to the gonococcus. Symptoms commonly begin about 3–5 days after exposure but may take much longer. Urination is painful, and typically, there is a yellow discharge. Fever is usually absent. In females, findings of urethritis are often minimal or absent, and gonococcal infection is more likely to cause cervicitis, salpingitis, or prepubertal vaginitis, as described in a later section. As discussed in Chapter 14, gonorrhea is one of the possible causes of painful urination with negative urine culture for the usual urinary tract pathogens. Patients with culture-proven gonococcal infection may also be co-infected with other genitourinary tract pathogens. In one study, 12 (27%) of 45 patients were co-infected with *C. trachomatis* and 2 (4%) were co-infected with *Mycoplasma genitalium*.[95] Human papillomavirus may also be concomitantly present, especially in chronic cases.[96]

Bacteria other than the gonococcus are occasionally recovered from a purulent urethral discharge. Enteric bacteria, *Staphylococcus aureus,* or streptococci are sometimes found, but their etiologic significance is not easily proved. When sought, anaerobes can be found in about 60% of patients with urethritis, but are also found in a similar percentage of control patients.[97] Gram-negative anaerobes are more frequently found in those with symptoms of urethritis, but causality has not been proven.[97] Purulent urethritis may rarely be caused by *Acinetobacter iwoffi,* formerly *Mima polymorpha,* which was so named because of its ability to mimic the gonococcus by Gram stain and clinical illness. The causes of nonpurulent urethritis can also cause purulent urethritis.

Nonpurulent Urethritis

This may have a number of causes, including gonorrhea. Even with advanced molecular techniques,

an etiologic diagnosis is not established in about 35% of cases.[98] Nongonococcal nonpurulent urethritis is common in sexually active adolescents. In one retrospective case-control study, independent risk factors for acquisition of nongonococcal urethritis (NGU) were African-American race and having two or more sexual partners in the 2 months prior to diagnosis.[99] Condom use was negatively associated with development of NGU. Whereas spontaneous purulent discharge occurs frequently in gonococcal urethritis, either no discharge or a mucoid discharge after penile stripping is obtained in NGU. Dysuria is more common in chlamydial urethritis, but urethral discharge is more common in gonococcal urethritis.

There are several different infectious causes of nongonococcal urethritis (NGU). In the past, most cases were presumed to be due to *Chlamydia trachomatis.*[100] However, the majority of cases are not caused by *C. trachomatis*; it is now known to be responsible for only 19–31% of cases.[98] The diagnosis is generally established by enzyme immunoassays (Chlamydiazyme, for example). Ligase-chain reaction is equally sensitive and more specific than enzyme-based studies.[101] PCR is superior to either but is not widely available.[102]

Chlamydial urethritis and cervicitis tend to persist beyond the 2–3 months required for gonococcal urethritis to subside spontaneously. The sexual partner of a patient with chlamydial urethritis also should be treated with azithromycin or doxycycline (Table 15-2). The success rate of either regimen is 80–90%.[103]

Mycoplasma genitalium has been associated with NGU and is estimated to cause from 10–25% of cases.[98] Cases caused by *M. genitalium* infection tend to be more insidious, more difficult to eradicate, and more prone to relapse.[104] Causation is probable based on the low prevalence of *M. genitalium* in asymptomatic patients[105] and resolution of symptoms upon eradication of the organism.[104,106] Other species of mycoplasma do not cause urethral disease.[107]

Another possible cause of urethritis in sexually active teenagers is *U. urealyticum,* a member of the mycoplasma family. The exact role of ureaplasmas in NGU is not clear. On the one hand, ureaplasmas have been found in increased frequency in urethritis in male college students and in sexual partnerships, and a tetracycline-sensitive strain has been shown to produce urethritis in human volunteer experiments.[108] In other studies, evidence of *U. ure-*

alyticum has not been associated with *acute* NGU,[109] although it has convincingly been linked to chronic or recurrent disease.

Trichomonas vaginalis is a protozoan that can cause urethritis in the male or female. It is difficult to diagnose by smear in the male. It can be cultured from urethral swabs or urine sediment. In males, it is a more common cause in those older than 30 years.[110] In one small study, it spontaneously remitted in 36% of cases.[111] Of 21 men from whom *Trichomonas vaginalis* was isolated, 12 (57%) had signs and symptoms of urethritis. Only 2 of them remained symptomatic after infection was eradicated.[111] It is discussed further in the section on vaginitis.

Some investigators have found HSV to be a relatively important cause of NGU and suggest testing for the virus whenever more common causes have been ruled out.[112]

Allergy has been proposed as a cause of nonpurulent urethritis, but no evidence is available. Chemical or physical irritation of the urethra from soaps or masturbation is probably very common.

Rare causes of bacterial nongonococcal urethritis include *Staphylococcus saphrophyticus* and meningococci.[113,114] *Gardnerella vaginalis*, group B streptococci, and yeasts apparently do not cause urethritis in the male.

Reiter's Syndrome

Nongonococcal urethritis, arthritis, and conjunctivitis form a triad called Reiter's syndrome. The cause is unknown. Careful cultures do not recover the gonococcus.[115] The syndrome has been found at the same time as infection with chlamydia, other bacteria, or mycoplasmas, but the cause or mechanism remains unknown.[115] There is a high frequency of the HLA B27 histocompatibility antigen in children or adults with Reiter's syndrome: 96% of patients with Reiter's syndrome are HLA B27 positive, compared with an 8% rate of positivity in the general population.[115] The significance of this observation is not yet clear, but this test may be useful to support the diagnosis of Reiter's syndrome. Chlamydiae have been recovered from the joints of some patients with Reiter's syndrome.[115]

Urethritis is usually the initial complaint in Reiter's syndrome, with conjunctivitis and arthritis occurring later. Arthritis may be recurrent, suggesting that hypersensitivity may be involved.

Reiter's syndrome was probably the first described form of reactive arthritis, which is discussed in detail in Chapter 16.

Diagnostic Approach

A wet mount of the urethral discharge should be examined for *Trichomonas* and *Candida* in females with vaginitis. A Gram-stained smear of any discharge should also be examined, especially to look for gram-negative diplococci (gonococci). Culture for gonococci should always be done. Special cultures for *Trichomonas* may sometimes be available, as discussed in the section on vaginitis. Culture for *Ureaplasma* and culture and serologic studies for *Chlamydia* are available in some reference laboratories. *Chlamydia* may be detected by the use of enzyme immunoassays or ligase chain reaction tests, as mentioned previously. *Mycoplasma genitalium* is difficult to recover in the laboratory; PCR is the best test for its identification.

In 1998 the World Health Organization developed an algorithm for a clinical approach to the diagnosis and treatment of urethritis in men. Once a physician determines that a patient has a urethral discharge, the patient is treated with 500 mg of ciprofloxacin orally for one dose, and given doxycycline 100 mg twice a day for 7 days. This regimen is designed to eradicate both the gonococcus and *Chlamydia trachomatis*. This approach was field tested in Indonesia. Of 107 patients confirmed to have a urethral discharge, 104 (97%) were clinically cured, and 106 (99%) were microbiologically cured.[116] This method is microbiologically less cumbersome and considerably cheaper than the traditional approach; it is especially attractive for the developing world, where some tests are unavailable.

Treatment

Various regimens for treatment of urethritis are outlined in Table 15-2. If a person is treated for gonorrhea, that person's sexual contacts should be examined, cultured, and treated for gonorrhea without awaiting culture confirmation. Similar evaluation and treatment has been recommended for contacts of females with *Trichomonas* and other causes of nongonococcal urethritis.[8] Gonococcal isolates should be routinely tested for penicillin susceptibility using a β-lactamase test. Gonococci are generally sensitive to third-generation cephalosporins and fluoroquinolones. An increasing percentage of gonococcal isolates are becoming resistant to the fluoroquinolones, prompting recommendations against their use for certain patient groups in specefic geographics areas.[117] Early reports of cephalosporin-resistant gonococcal isolates from Japan are appearing.[118]

■ GENITAL INFECTIONS OF FEMALES

This section deals with infectious syndromes involving the female genitalia specifically. Urethritis, genital ulcers, and other syndromes common to both sexes have been discussed in preceding sections. The anatomic syndromes are analyzed by possible causes, whether the patient is sexually active or not. When the infecting agent should suggest sexual activity or abuse, that fact is indicated for each agent. In contrast to genital infections in males, infections in females are often clinically silent. Despite the paucity of symptoms, they can frequently lead to long-term problems with infertility, ectopic pregnancy, and chronic pelvic pain.

Vaginitis

Examination

Examination of a young girl's genitalia can be done in the knee-chest position or with the girl sitting on the mother's lap and may be aided by a veterinary otoscopic speculum.[119–121]

Definition

Vaginitis can be defined by redness and exudate of the vaginal mucosa.[122] Noninfectious causes predominate in young children and include poor perineal hygiene, foreign bodies, and chemical irritants.[123] Group A streptococcus is also a relatively common cause.

Normal Flora

The normal flora of the vagina in children includes predominantly diphtheroids, *S. epidermidis*, non-β-hemolytic streptococci, lactobacilli, and *E. coli*.[124] In one study, sexually active teenagers were much more likely than nonsexually active teenagers to have vaginal colonization with *U. urealyticum, Mycoplasma* species, and *Gardnerella vaginalis*.[125] *C. trachomatis, N. gonorrhea*, and *Trichomonas* were recovered only from sexually active teenagers in this study.

Gonorrhea

Gonorrhea is the most important cause of vaginitis to be excluded, because it can occur in infants and prepubertal girls. It should be considered especially if there is a possibility of sexual abuse.[126] Salpingitis can occur in preschool children as a complication of purulent gonococcal vaginitis.[127] The squamous epithelium of the postpubertal female is relatively resistant to infection by the gonococcus, so vaginitis is rarely gonococcal in women.

Bacterial Vaginosis (Nongonococcal Vaginitis)

Surprisingly little is known about the etiology, diagnosis, and treatment of bacterial vaginosis in adolescent and adult females, especially considering the prevalence of the disease. It can be thought of as an imbalance of the bacterial flora of the vagina.[128] When normal flora are overgrown by pathogenic bacteria, symptoms of bacterial vaginosis (BV) occur. The most likely bacterial causes of vaginitis in postpubertal females include *Gardnerella vaginalis, Mobiluncus* spp., and various anaerobes. In prepubertal girls, β-hemolytic streptococcus is also a possible cause. *Shigella* is an occasional cause of vaginitis, sometimes bloody, sometimes associated with diarrhea, in prepubertal girls.[129] *H. influenzae* is a rare cause.[130] Infection is generally polymicrobial. One study found anaerobes in 43 (91%) of 47 women with BV but in only 11 (18%) of 62 who did not have clinical evidence of disease.[131] In *Gardnerella* infection, the vaginal discharge is characteristically gray and malodorous, without trichomonads in the wet mount. *G. vaginalis* may have a reservoir in the male. A copious mucopurulent discharge is especially suggestive of *G. vaginalis* in women. Trichomonal vaginitis can rarely occur in newborns by acquisition from the mother.[131a]

G. vaginalis is often recovered from sexually active women without symptoms, so its presence does not automatically require treatment.[132] *U. urealyticum* is also recovered from so many sexually active young women that its presence does not call for treatment[132] unless there is a plan to eradicate it because of a history of repeated fetal loss.

Of the pathogens recovered from nonsexually active or prepubertal girls, the following should strongly raise the possibility of sexual activity, or possibly sexual abuse: *Trichomonas, C. trachomatis,* and *N. gonorrheae*.[133,134] The presence of *G. vagi-*

nalis may also signify abuse,[135] but it can sometimes be present in healthy controls as well (Table 15–1).

Bacterial vaginosis has been associated with premature rupture of the membranes and early delivery. Unfortunately, screening for and treating BV in early pregnancy did not alter pregnancy outcomes in a prospective study of 375 women. Treatment tended to be successful in the short term, but recurrences were common.[136] Women with recurrent or persistent BV were shown to have a higher rate of preterm deliveries.

Candidal Vaginitis

Common in postpubertal women,[137] candidiasis is uncommon in prepubertal girls unless there is some predisposing factor, such as antibiotic use or diabetes mellitus. Itching is prominent, and the discharge is slight and curdy.

Laboratory Diagnosis

A fresh wet mount and Gram stain should be examined. Recent douching or menstruation can interfere with these studies. In one study, the wet mount preparation was inadequate compared with culture for *Candida* or *Trichomonas.*[122] Some microbiology laboratories correctly report a minimal growth of *Candida* as "normal vaginal flora." "Clue cells," which are rounded epithelial cells with a granular-appearing cytoplasm, suggest *G. vaginalis.* Culture should be done to exclude the gonococcus in all cases. Special techniques are necessary for *Candida* and *Trichomonas,* so the laboratory should be informed if one of these organisms is suspected on the basis of clinical or microscopic evidence. Culture should be done if the wet mount is negative. Adding 10% KOH to the wet mount is not needed to destroy epithelial cells in a vaginal preparation but does liberate aromatic amines with the fishy odor associated with nonspecific vaginitis caused by *G. vaginalis.* This so-called "whiff test" may be helpful if it is positive, but it is frequently falsely negative.[138] Culture of *G. vaginalis* is not recommended, because it is not specific for BV.[8]

Diagnosis of BV is usually made clinically, when 3 of the following 4 criteria are met:

- a homogeneous, white, noninflammatory discharge that smoothly coats the vaginal walls;
- the presence of clue cells on microscopic examination;
- a pH of vaginal fluid >4.5; and

- a fishy odor of vaginal discharge before or after addition of 10% KOH (whiff test).[8]

The Pap smear is useful for detection of *Trichomonas* infections and is slightly more sensitive than the wet mount in detecting culture-positive patients. Culture is the most sensitive commercially available method of diagnosis.

Treatment

Therapy for STDs is shown in Table 15-2. In prepubertal children, nystatin suspension can be instilled with a dropper or a miconazole vaginal suppository cut to fit for candidiasis. Oral fluconazole is also a reasonable option. Pinworms, Group A streptococci, or other specific bacteria usually respond to standard oral therapy. CDC recommends the use of metronidazole in infants or children with trichomonas. Bacterial vaginosis can be treated with oral metronidazole or clindamycin, or topical preparations of clindamycin. A 3-day course of topical clindamycin delivered by an "ovule" system was preferred by most patients to a 7-day course of the cream form.[139]

Treatment is indicated for pregnant women with BV who are high risk for preterm delivery (i.e., those who previously delivered a premature infant). Metronidazole is more efficacious than clindamycin and should be first-line therapy in the high-risk pregnant woman.[8]

Cervicitis, Endometritis, Salpingitis, and Oophoritis

The syndromes of cervicitis, endometritis, salpingitis, and oophoritis are grouped together because a pelvic examination is usually necessary to identify them.

Acute cervicitis is defined by direct observation of the cervix, which is red or ulcerated or has adherent exudate at the os. The most common causes are *C. trachomatis* and *N. gonorrheae.* Herpes simplex virus is an important cause of disease of the cervix and may cause a necrotizing cervicitis.[140] Cytomegalovirus (CMV) may also be a cause of cervicitis. *Chlamydia trachomatis* may cause a mucopurulent cervicitis and also, like herpes simplex, an abnormal Pap smear.[141,142] It is the female counterpart of the male's nonspecific urethritis.[142] The presence of erythema, mucopus, and/or friability is more sensitive than endocervical Gram staining in establishing the diagnosis.[143] Mucopurulent cervicitis is an important clinical entity because it is a marker for endometritis, salpingitis, and adverse pregnancy outcomes.[144] It may be caused by *Neisseria gonorrheae*, *Trichomonas vaginalis*, *Ureaplasma urealyticum*, or *Mycoplasma genitalium*, in addition to *Chlamydia trachomatis*, HSV, and CMV.[144] Cervical infections with certain serovars of *Chlamydia trachomatis* (especially class C) can apparently persist for years.[145] In women with HIV infection, effective treatment of cervicitis reduced the number of HIV particles in cervical mucus about sevenfold.[146]

Acute endometritis is very rare in prepubertal girls, and in postmenarchal patients its symptoms are usually masked by those of cervicitis. The exception is postpartum endometritis, which occurs in less than 1%[147] to 20%[148] of women after delivery. Cesarean section delivery is the principal risk factor. The disease is manifested by fever and lower abdominal/pelvic tenderness, sometimes accompanied by leukocytosis and foul lochia. Uterine wiping,[149] intravaginal povidone-iodine,[150] and intrapartum cefoxitin[151] have all failed at preventing post-partum endometritis. Endometritis also occurs after abortion.

Acute salpingitis is an anatomic diagnosis that may be suspected based on tenderness on pelvic examination localized to the area of the Fallopian tubes. However, more frequently, localization of upper genital infection by physical examination is extremely difficult, and the diagnosis pelvic inflammatory disease (PID) is used for all cases of upper genital tract infection. PID is much more common in adolescents than in adult women. The diagnosis is suspected when lower abdominal pain, abdominal tenderness, cervical motion tenderness, and adnexal tenderness, in concert with fever, elevated white blood cell count, or elevated erythrocyte sedimentation rate (ESR) are found. The clinical diagnosis of PID, though, is fraught with difficulty; only about 65% of patients clinically suspected of having PID have the diagnosis confirmed when laparoscopy is performed. Additionally, signs of PID can be more subtle; in some cases mild pelvic pain may be the only sign.[152] The disease tends to be more acute and severe when it is caused by the gonococcus and more indolent and subtle when it is caused by *Chlamydia trachomatis*. Although the ESR has been better studied, a recent study of 50 patients with PID, 20 of whom had tubo-ovarian abscesses, showed that C-reactive protein was elevated in 96%, and returned to normal with appropriate therapy.[153]

The pathophysiology of salpingitis and PID usually involves ascending infection from the lower genital tract.[154] Seeding by bacteremia or adjacent infection is decidedly less common. Microorganisms that cause bacterial vaginosis are often recovered at laparoscopy from patients with PID, leading some to believe that BV may be an important co-factor in PID. The greatest predictors of PID, however, are previous genital tract infection with gonococcus or chlamydia. Physical examination is nonspecific and insensitive when it comes to determining the severity of the disease and the presence or absence of associated tubo-ovarian abscess.[155] Women with HIV infection are more likely to have associated tubo-ovarian abscesses, especially if they have advanced HIV disease.[156]

Most cases of PID are polymicrobial. The gonococcus and *Chlamydia trachomatis* are commonly involved. Cases of unilateral salpingitis due to *Enterobius vermicularis* have been reported.[157] PID is rare in prepubertal females, but cases caused by serotype 1 of *S. pneumoniae*[158] or Group A streptococcus[159] have been reported. Chronic salpingitis is usually caused by *Chlamydia trachomatis*, often with other pathogens.

PID has a high incidence of complications, including perihepatitis (known as Fitz-Hugh Curtis syndrome) in about 10–15%, tubo-ovarian abscess in approximately 20%, chronic abdominal pain secondary to adhesions in about 15%, and recurrence in 20–25%. Perihepatitis causes a tender, slightly enlarged liver and mildly elevated hepatic serum enzymes.[160] The condition may mimic gall bladder disease or other liver diseases. Either *N. gonorrheae* or *C. trachomatis* may cause perihepatitis. Late complications of PID include infertility, which is seen in up to a fifth of patients. Patients who recover from PID also have a sixfold increase in ectopic pregnancy. All of the complications of PID are minimized by early and effective treatment. Primary prevention is via the use of condoms or abstinence. Secondary prevention is thought to rest on routine screening for *Chlamydia* infection in asymptomatic women; this approach is especially effective in populations where the prevalence exceeds 5%.[161]

Acute oophoritis is difficult to diagnose, and its frequency thus may be underestimated. Abnormal tenderness of the ovary on pelvic examination is the essential criterion for diagnosis, and this may be overlooked. Many cases are likely to be autoimmune.[162] Mumps virus is one recognized infectious cause, as discussed in the section on mumps parotitis in Chapter 6. Abdominal actinomycosis may involve the ovary.[163] In some cases, oophoritis may have no localizing signs; one case of fever of unknown origin was traced, by gallium scanning, to ovarian infection.[164] In patients who are severely immunocompromised by AIDS[165] or bone marrow transplant,[166] necrotizing oophoritis due to CMV may develop; in reported cases, however, it was clinically silent and was discovered at autopsy.

Treatment

Selected regimens from the 2002 CDC recommendations for treatment of salpingitis and cervicitis are given in Table 15-2. Postpartum endometritis is best treated with intravenous clindamycin and gentamicin until patients are afebrile for 24 hours and tenderness abates.[167] No oral therapy is necessary.

■ GENITAL SYNDROMES OF MALES

This section deals with infectious syndromes of male genitalia. Urethritis and other syndromes common to both sexes have been discussed in an earlier section.

Epididymitis and Orchitis

In a review of 113 consecutive hospitalized boys less than 15 years of age with an acutely painful scrotum, 51 (45%) had testicular torsion, 40 (35%) had torsion of the appendix testis, and only 17 (15%) had acute epididymitis.[168] However, in a study of 65 children who presented to the emergency department with acute scrotum, 42 (65%) had epididymitis and only 12 (19%) had torsion. In a 20-year study of epididymitis in children less than 17 years old, thirty-one (89%) of 35 had been operated on.[169]

Ultrasound with Doppler studies has improved the accuracy of the diagnosis of testicular or appendix testis torsion to the point where emergency department physicians, properly trained, were able to correctly diagnose 35 (97%) of 36 patients at the bedside in the emergency department.[170] However, of the 36 patients, only 3 (8%) had testicular torsion and only 6 (17%) had epididymitis. It is very important to not delay surgery to correct torsion, because epididymitis is uncommon in prepubertal boys, and salvage of the testis depends on prompt operation.[171] Thus, early consultation with a urologist is strongly recommended for males with acute scrotal

pain. Clinically, most patients with acute testicular torsion lose the cremasteric reflex, versus only a small percentage of those with epididymitis.[172] Patients with epididymitis typically have relief of pain with gentle elevation of the testis (positive Prehn sign), whereas patients with torsion do not experience relief of pain with this procedure. The C-reactive protein may be a helpful laboratory test; in one study of 104 patients with scrotal pain, the C-reactive protein was highly elevated in 50 (96%) of 52 patients with acute epididymitis and was normal in 10 (91%) of 11 patients with torsion.[173]

Urinary tract anomalies may be the underlying reason for acute epididymitis in prepubertal boys,[174] and they should have urologic investigation to look for such anomalies. Polyarteritis nodosa,[175] Henoch-Schonlein purpura, and Kawasaki disease[176] are other conditions sometimes associated with epididymitis. Other findings of the syndromes are also often present. A primary inflammatory pseudotumor of the epididymis has been described.[177] Acute appendicitis can cause severe scrotal pain in a patient who has a patent processus vaginalis.[178] Leukemia and lymphoma rarely present with symptoms suggestive of epididymitis.[179,180]

In the United States, infectious causes of epididymitis other than sexually transmitted pathogens are uncommon. Tuberculosis can be a cause.[181] In endemic areas, brucellosis is a possible etiology. Between 1% and 2% of brucellosis cases in males are complicated by epididymitis.[182] Most patients are between 25 and 44 years of age. Rare infectious causes include *Pseudomonas aeruginosa*[183] and *E. coli*.[184] In patients with severe immune deficiencies, aspergillosis,[185] blastomycosis,[186] and CMV infection[187] have been reported. Drugs that cause epididymitis are seldom used in pediatrics, but up to 11% of adult patients on amiodarone develop sterile epididymitis. Cases in childhood have also been reported.[188]

After puberty, a urologic abnormality is an unlikely predisposing cause of epididymitis.[189] *C. trachomatis* is a frequent cause of epididymitis in sexually active males.[190] *C. trachomatis* may sometimes present as a solid, asymptomatic scrotal mass, simulating carcinoma.[191]

In preschool children, acute epididymo-orchitis can be the presenting symptoms of *H. influenzae* septicemia,[192] but systemic manifestations are prominent.

Coxsackievirus B has been recovered from a testicular biopsy of a patient with orchitis,[193] confirming the etiologic relation implied by the increased frequency of orchitis in patients with pleurodynia. Echoviruses and coxsackievirus A can also cause orchitis. Orchitis has also been seen in association with infection with other viruses such as varicella-zoster virus,[194] Epstein-Barr virus,[195] lymphocytic choriomeningitis virus,[196] and dengue fever virus, although in these cases causation has not been proven by testicular biopsy. A rubella outbreak in military recruits was associated with testicular pain in about 25% of the infected men.

Before mumps immunization was common in the United States, mumps virus was a relatively frequent cause of orchitis and a rare cause of isolated epididymitis.[197] Typically, the patient had parotitis and a known exposure to another individual with parotitis. In a controlled study, cortisone did not have any favorable effect on mumps orchitis in terms of acute symptoms or of testicular size 5 months later.[67]

In one case, bilateral granulomatous orchitis was attributed to sarcoidosis.[198]

Prostatitis

This disease is rare in adolescents. A very tender, soft prostate on rectal examination is sufficient evidence to make this diagnosis. It can be distinguished from proctitis, which is associated with generalized rectal tenderness. Infectious causes include the gonococcus, ureaplasmas and mycoplasmas, and, possibly, herpes simplex virus.[199,200]

"Prostatodynia" is a term used to describe a chronic syndrome of perianal pain and irritative voiding symptoms with negative cultures for bacteria. Prostatitis is discussed in more detail in Chapter 14.

■ REFERENCES

1. Neinstein LS, Goldenring J, Carpenter S. Nonsexual transmission of sexually transmitted disease: an infrequent occurrence. Pediatrics 1984;74:67–76.
2. Frau LM, Alexander ER. Public health implications of sexually transmitted diseases in pediatric practice. Pediatr Infect Dis 1985;4:453–67.
3. Emans SJ, Woods ER, Flagg NT, et al. Genital findings in sexually abused, symptomatic and asymptomatic, girls. Pediatrics 1987;79:778–85.
4. American Academy of Pediatrics Committee on Child Abuse and Neglect. Guidelines for the evaluation of sexual abuse of children: subject review. Pediatrics 1999; 103:186–91.
5. Cates W Jr. Estimates of the incidence and prevalence of sexually transmitted diseases in the United States. Sex Transm Dis 1999;26:S2–7.
6. Workowski KA, Levine WC, Wasserheit JN. Centers for Disease Control and Prevention guidelines for the treatment of sexually transmitted diseases: an opportunity to unify clinical and public health practice. Ann Intern Med 2002;137:255–62.
7. Fleming DT, McQuillan GM, Johnson RE, et al. Herpes simplex virus type 2 in the United States, 1976 to 1994. N Engl J Med 1997;337:1105–11.
8. Centers for Disease Control and Prevention. Sexually transmitted diseases treatment guidelines 2002. MMWR 2002;51:1–78.
8a. Corey L, Wald A, Patel R, et al. Once-daily valacyclovir to reduce the risk of transmission of genital herpes. N Engl J Med. 2004;350:11–20.
9. DiCarlo RP, Martin DH. The clinical diagnosis of genital ulcer disease in men. Clin Infect Dis 1997;25:299–300.
10. Torian LV, Weisfuse IB, Makki HA, et al. Increasing HIV-1 seroprevalence association with genital ulcer disease, New York City, 1990-1992. AIDS 1995;9:177–81.
11. Armstrong GL, Schillinger J, Markowitz L, et al. Incidence of herpes simplex virus type 2 infection in the United States. Am J Epidemiol 2001;153:912–20.
12. Wald A, Langenberg AG, Link K, et al. Effect of condoms on reducing the transmission of herpes simplex virus type 2 from men to women. JAMA 2001;27:3100–6.
13. Gardner M, Jones JG. Genital herpes acquired by sexual abuse of children. J Pediatr 1984;104:243–4.
14. Langenberg AG, Corel L, Ashley RL, et al. A prospective study of new infections with herpes simplex virus type 1 and type 2. N Engl J Med 1999;341:1432–8.
15. Lautenschlager S, Eichmann A. The heterogeneous clinical spectrum of genital herpes. Dermatology 2001;202: 211–9.
16. Nahmias AF, Dowdle WR, Naib ZM, et al. Genital infection with Herpesvirus hominis types 1 and 2 in children. Pediatrics 1968;42:659–66.
17. Powers RD, Rein MF, Hayden FG. Necrotizing balanitis due to herpes simplex type 1. JAMA 1982;248:215–6.
18. Wald A, Zeh J, Selke S, et al. Reactivation of genital herpes simplex virus type 2 infection in asymptomatic seropositive persons. N Engl J Med 2000;342:844–50.
19. Benedetti JK, Zeh J, Corey L. Clinical reactivation of genital herpes simplex virus infection decreases in frequency over time. Ann Intern Med 1999;131:14–20.
20. Cohen F, Kemeny ME, Kearney KA, et al. Persistent stress as a predictor of genital herpes recurrence. Arch Intern Med 1999;159:2430–6.
21. Kimberlin DW, Rouse DJ. Clinical practice. Genital herpes. N Engl J Med. 2004 May 6;350(19):1970–7.
22. Coyle PV, Desai A, Wyatt D, et al. A comparison of virus isolation, indirect immunofluorescence and nested multiplex polymerase chain reaction for the diagnosis of primary and recurrent herpes simplex type 1 and type 2 infections. J Virol Methods 1999;83:75–82.
23. Madhavan HN, Priya K, Anand AR, et al. Detection of herpes simplex virus (HSV) genome using polymerase chain reaction (PCR) in clinical samples comparison of PCR with standard laboratory methods for the detection of HSV. J Clin Virol 1999;14:145–51.

24. Ginsburg CM. Acquired syphilis in prepubertal children. Pediatr Infect Dis 1983;2:232–4.

25. Jaffe LR, Morgenthau JE. Syphilis and homosexuality in adolescents. J Pediatr 1979;95:1062–4.

26. Chapel TA. The variability of syphilitic chancres. Sex Transm Dis 1978;5:68–70.

27. Lowy G. Sexually transmitted diseases in children. Pediatric Dermatol 1992;9:329–34.

28. Al-Tawfiz JA, Harezlak J, Katz BP, et al. Cumulative experience with *Haemophilus ducreyi* 35000 in the human model of experimental infection. Sex Transm Dis 2000; 27:111–4.

29. Cortes-Bratti X, Chaves-Olarte E, Lagergard T, et al. Cellular internalization of cytolethal distending toxin from *Haemophilus ducreyi*. Infect Immun 2000;68:6903–11.

30. Malonza IM, Tydall MW, Ndinya-Achola JO, et al. A randomized, double-blind, placebo-controlled trial of single-dose ciprofloxacin versus erythromycin for the treatment of chancroid in Nairobi, Kenya. J Infect Dis 1999;180: 1886–93.

31. Schmid GP. Treatment of chancroid, 1997. Clin Infect Dis 1999;28(suppl 1):S14–20.

32. Elkins C, Yi K, Olsen B, et al. Development of a serological test for *Haemophilus ducreyi* for seroprevalence studies. J Clin Microbiol 2000;38:1520–6.

33. Roesel DJ, Gwanzura L, Mason PR, et al. Polymerase chain reaction detection of *Haemophilus ducreyi* DNA. Sex Transm Infect 1998;74:63–5.

34. O'Farrell N. Global eradication of donovanosis: an opportunity for limiting the spread of HIV-1 infection. Genitourin Med 1995;71:27–31.

35. Carter JS, Bowden FJ, Bastian I, et al. Phylogenetic evidence for reclassification of *Calymmatobacterium granulomatis* as *Klebsiella granulomatis* comb. nov. Int J Syst Bacteriol 1999;49:1695–1700.

36. Hart G. Donovanosis. Clin Infect Dis 1997;25:24–32.

37. Banerjee K. Donovanosis in a child of six months. J Indian Med Asssoc 1972;59:293.

38. Growdon WA, Lebgerz TB, Moore JG, et al. Granuloma inguinale in a white teenager: a diagnosis easily forgotten, poorly pursued. West J Med 1985;143:105–8.

39. Hoosen AA, Draper G, Moodley J, et al. Granuloma inguinale of the cervix: a carcinoma look-alike. Genitourin Med 1990;66:380–2.

40. Carter J, Hutton S, Sriprakash KS, et al. Culture of the causative organism of donovanosis (*Calymmatobacterium granulomatis*) in Hep-2 cells. J Clin Microbiol 1997;35: 2915–17.

41. Kharsany AB, Hoosen AA, Kiepiela P, et al. Growth and cultural characteristics of *Calymmatobacterium granulomatis*—the aetiological agent of granuloma inguinale (Donovanosis). J Med Microbiol 1997;46:579–85.

42. Carter JS, Kemp DJ. A colorimetric detection system for *Calymmatobacterium granulomatis*. Sex Transm Infect 2000;76:134–6.

43. Carter J, Bowden FJ, Sriprakash KS, et al. Diagnostic polymerase chain reaction for donovanosis. Clin Infect Dis 1999;28:1168–9.

44. Freinkel AL, Dangor Y, Koornhof JH, et al. A serological test for granuloma inguinale. Genitourin Med 1992;68: 269–72.

45. Bowden FJ, Mein J, Plunkett C, et al. Pilot study of azithromycin in the treatment of genital donovanosis. Genitourin Med 1996;72:17–9.

46. Merianos A, Gilles M, Chuah J. Ceftriaxone in the treatment of chronic donovanosis in central Australia. Genitourin Med 1994;70:84–9.

47. Lin MS, Gharia MA, Swartz SJ, et al. Identification and characterization of epitopes recognized by T lymphocytes and autoantibodies from patients with herpes gestationis. J Immunol 1999;15:4991–7.

48. Black MM. New observations on pemphigoid herpes gestationis. Dermatology 1994;189(suppl 1):50–1.

49. Borrego L, Peterson EA, Diez LI, et al. Polymorphic eruption of pregnancy and herpes gestationis: comparison of granulated cell proteins in tissue and serum. Clin Exp Dermatol 1999;24:213–5.

50. Matsumura K, Amagai M, Nishikawa T, et al. The majority of bullous pemphigoid and herpes gestationis serum samples react with the NC16a domain of the 180-kDa bullous pemphigoid antigen. Arch Dermatol Res 1996; 288:507–9.

51. Shornick JK, Black MM. Secondary autoimmune diseases in herpes gestationis (pemphigoid gestationis). J Am Acad Dermatol 1992;26:563–6.

52. Kumar B, Rai R, Kaur I, et al. Childhood cutaneous tuberculosis: a study over 25 years from northern India. Int J Dermatol 2000;40:26–32.

53. Malvy D, Djossou F, Weill FX, et al. Guess what! Human West African trypanosomiasis with chancre presentation. Eur J Dermatol 2000;10:561–2.

54. Caputo R, Gianotti R, Monti M. Nodular pure mucocutaneous histiocytosis X in an adult. Arch Dermatol 1987; 123:1274–5.

55. Taylor S, Drake SM, Dedicoat M, et al. Genital ulcers associated with acute Epstein-Barr virus infection. Sex Transm Infect 1998;74:296–7.

56. Kantakamalakul W, Naksawat P, Kanyok R, et al. Prevalence of type-specific Epstein-Barr virus in the genital tract of genital herpes suspected patients. J Med Assoc Thai 1999;82:263–7.

57. Hejase MJ, Bihrle R, Castillo G, et al. Amebiasis of the penis. Urology 1996;48:151–4.

58. Wilson JF. The nonvenereal diseases of the genitals: their differentiation from venereal lesions. Med Clin North Am 1964;48:787–809.

59. James WD. Cutaneous Group B streptococcal infection. Arch Dermatol 1984;120:85–6.

60. Fiumara NJ. Treatment of primary and secondary syphilis: serologic response. JAMA 1980;243:2500–2.

61. McClelland BA, Anderson PC. Lymphogranuloma venereum: outbreak on a university community. JAMA 1976; 235:56–7.

62. Speers D. Lymphogranuloma venereum presenting with psoas abscess. Aust NZ J Med 1999;29:563–4.

63. Kellock DJ, Barlow R, Suvarna SK, et al. Lymphogranuloma venereum: biopsy, serology, and molecular biology. Genitourin Med 1997;73:399–401.

64. Davies N, Crown LA. Lymphogranuloma venereum vs. incarcerated inguinal hernia: the Gordian knot unraveled. Tenn Med 1997;90:278–9.

65. Lynch CM, Felder TL, Schwandt RA, et al. Lymphogranuloma venereum presenting as a rectovaginal fistula. Infect Dis Obstet Gynecol 1999;7:199–201.

66. Papagrigoriadis S, Rennie JA. Lymphogranuloma venereum as a cause of rectal strictures. Postgrad Med J 1998; 74:168–9.

67. Farhi DC, Wells SJ, Siegel RJ. Syphilitic lyphadenopathy: histology and human immunodeficiency virus status. Am J Clin Pathol 1999;112:330–4.

68. Hartsock RJ, Halling LW, King FM. Luetic lymphadenitis: a clinical and histologic study of 20 cases. Am J Clin Pathol 1970;53:304–14.

69. Eichmann A, Huszar A, Bon A. *Mycobacterium chelonae* infection of lymph nodes in an HIV-infected patient. Dermatology 1993;187:299–300.

70. Hadfield TL, Lamy Y, Wear DJ. Demonstration of *Chlamydia trachomatis* in inguinal lymphadenitis of lymphogranuloma venereum: a light microscopy, electron microscopy and polymerase chain reaction study. Mod Pathol 1995;8:924–9.

71. Mittal A, Sachdeva KG. Monoclonal antibody for the diagnosis of lymphogranuloma venereum: a preliminary report. Br J Biomed Sci 1993;50:3–7.

72. Martin DH, Mroczkowski TF, Dalu ZA, et al. A controlled trial of a single dose of azithromycin for the treatment of chlamydial urethritis and cervicitis. N Engl J Med 1992; 24:921–5.

73. Abrams AJ. Lymphogranuloma venereum. JAMA 1968; 205:199–202.

74. De Jong AR, Weiss JC, Brent RL. Condyloma accuminata in children. Am J Dis Child 1982;136:704–6.

75. Obalek S, Misiewicz J, Jablonska S, et al. Childhood condyloma acuminatum: association with genital and cutaneous human papillomaviruses. Pediatr Dermatol 1993; 10:101–6.

76. Herman-Giddens ME, Gutman LT, Berson NL. Association of coexisting vaginal infections and multiple abusers in female children with genital warts. Sex Transm Dis 1988;15:63–7.

77. Sonnex C, Strauss S, Gray JJ. Detection of human papillomavirus DNA on the fingers of patients with genital warts. Sex Transm Infect 1999;75:317–9.

78. Zvulunov A, Medvedovsky E, Biton A, et al. Association of *Ureaplasma urealyticum* colonization in male urethra and condyloma acuminatum. Isr Med Assoc J 2000;2: 580–2.

79. Alam M, Stiller M. Direct medical costs for surgical and medical treatment of condylomata acuminata. Arch Dermatol 2001;137:337–41.

80. Longstaff E, von Krogh G. Condyloma eradication: self-therapy with 0.15-0.5% podophyllotoxin versus 20-25% podophyllin preparations—an integrated safety assessment. Regul Toxicol Pharmacol 2001;33:117–37.

81. Fife KH, Ferenczy A, Douglas JM Jr, et al. Treatment of external genital warts in men using 5% imiquimod cream applied three times a week, once daily, twice daily, or three times a day. Sex Transm Dis 2001;28:226–31.

82. Schurmann D, Bergmann F, Temmesfeld-Wollbruck B, et al. Topical cidofovir is effective in treating extensive penile condylomata acuminata. AIDS 2000;14:1075–6.

83. Sobrado CW, Mester M, Nadalin W, et al. Radiation-induced total regression of a highly recurrent giant perianal condyloma: report of a case. Dis Colon Rectum 2000; 43:257–60.

84. Hatzichristou DG, Apostolidis A, Tzortzis V, et al. Glansectomy: an alternative surgical treatment for Buschke-Lowenstein tumors of the penis. Urology 2001; 57:966–9.

85. Byars RW, Poole GV, Barber WH. Anal carcinoma arising from condyloma acuminata. Am Surg 2001;67:469–72.

86. Birley HD. Continuing medical ignorance: modern myths in the management of genital warts. Int J STD AIDS 2001; 12:71–4.

87. American Academy of Pediatrics Committee on Practice and Ambulatory Medicine. Recommendations for Preventive Pediatric Health Care. Pediatrics 2000;105:645. (Available at: http://www.aap.org/policy/RE9939.html)

88. Neinstein LS, Goldenring J. Pink pearly papules: an epidemiologic study. J Pediatr 1984;105:594–5.

89. Wright RA, Judson FN. Penile venereal edema. JAMA 1979;241:157–8.

90. Bel Pla S, Garcia-Patos Briones V, Garcia Fernandez D, et al. [Vulvar lymphedema: unusual manifestation of Crohn's disease.] Spanish. Gastroenterol Hepatol 2001; 24:297–9.

91. Case records of the Massachussetts General Hospital. Weekly clinicopathological exercises. Case 21-2000. A 13-year-old boy with genital edema and abdominal pain. N Engl J Med. 2000;343:127–33.

92. Palma L, Peterson MC, Ingelbrotsen R. Iliac vein compression syndrome from urinary bladder distention due to prostatism. South Med J 1995;88:959–60.

93. Evans JP, Snyder HM. Idiopathic scrotal edema. Urology 1977;9:549–51.

94. Cohen MS, Hoffman IF, Royce RA, et al. Reduction in concentration of HIV-1 in semen after treatment of urethritis: implications for prevention of sexual transmission of HIV-1. Lancet 1997;349:1868–73.

95. Uno M, Deguchi T, Komeda M, et al. Prevalence of *Mycoplasma genitalium* in men with gonococcal urethritis. Int J STD AIDS 1996;7:443–4.

96. Chiarini F, Pisani S, Gallinelli C, et al. Simultaneous detection of HPV and other sexually transmitted agents in chronic urethritis. Minerva Urol Nefrol 1998;50:225–31.

97. Mazuecos J, Aznar J, Rodriguez-Pichardo A, et al. Anaerobic bacteria in men with urethritis. J Eur Acad Dermatol Venereol 1998;10:237–42.

98. Burstein GR, Zenilman JM. Nongonococcal urethritis—a new paradigm. Clin Infect Dis 1999;28(suppl 1):S66–73.

99. Schwartz MA, Lafferty WE, Hughes JP, et al. Risk factors for urethritis in heterosexual men: the role of fellatio and other sexual practices. Sex Transm Dis 1997;24:449–55.

100. Chambers CV, Shafer MA, Adger H, et al. Microflora of the urethra in adolescent boys: relationships to sexual activity and nongonococcal urethritis. J Pediatr 1987; 110:314–21.

101. Deguchi T, Yasuda M, Uno M, et al. Comparison among performances of a ligase chain reaction-based assay and two enzyme immunoassays in detecting *Chlamydia trachomatis* in urine specimens from men with nongonococcal urethritis. J Clin Microbiol 1996;34:1708–10.

102. Stary A. Urethritis: diagnosis of nongonococcal urethritis. Dermatol Clin 1998;16:723–6.

103. Stamm WE, Hicks CB, Martin DH, et al. Azithromycin for empirical treatment of the nongonococcal urethritis syndrome in men: a randomized double-blind study. JAMA 1995;274:545–9.

104. Maeda SI, Tamaki M, Kojima K, et al. Association of *Mycoplasma genitalum* persistence in the urethra with recurrence of nongonococcal urethritis. Sex Transm Dis 2001; 28:472–6.

105. Totten PA, Schwartz MA, Sjostrom KE, et al. Association of *Mycoplasma genitalum* with nongonococcal urethritis in heterosexual men. J Infect Dis 2001;183:269–76.

106. Gambini D, Decleva I, Lupica L, et al. *Mycoplasma genitalium* in males with nongonococcal urethritis: prevalence and clinical efficacy of eradication. Sex Transm Dis 2000; 27:226–9.

107. Deguchi T, Gilroy CB, Taylor-Robinson D. Failure to detect *Mycoplasma fermentans*, *Mycoplasma penetrans*, or *Mycoplasma pirum* in the urethra of patients with acute nongonococcal urethritis. Eur J Clin Microbiol Infect Dis 1996;15:169–71.

108. Taylor-Robinson D, Csonka GW, Prentice MJ. Human intraurethral inoculation of ureaplasmas. Q J Med 1976; 46:309–26.

109. Horner P, Thomas B, Gilroy CB, et al. Role of *Mycoplasma genitalium* and *Ureaplasma urealyticum* in acute and chronic nongonococcal urethritis. Clin Infect Dis 2001; 32:995–1003.

110. Joyner JL, Douglas JM Jr, Ragsdale S, et al. Comparative prevalence of infection with *Trichomonas vaginalis* among men attending a sexually transmitted diseases clinic. Sex Transm Dis 2000;27:236–40.

111. Krieger JN, Verdon M, Siegel N, et al. Natural history of urogenital trichomoniasis in men. J Urol 1993;149: 1455–58.

112. Madev R, Nativ O, Benilevi D, et al. Need for diagnostic screening of herpes simplex virus in patients with nongonococcal urethritis. Clin Infect Dis 2000;30:982–3.

113. Hovelius B, Thelin I, Mårdh PA. *Staphylococcus saprophyticus* in the aetiology of nongonococcal urethritis. Br J Vener Dis 1979;55:369–74.

114. Miller MA, Millikin P, Griffin PA. *Neisseria meningitidis* urethritis: a case report. JAMA 1979;242:1656–57.

115. Rosenberg AM, Petty RE. Reiter's disease in children. Am J Dis Child 1979;133:394–8.

116. Djajakusumah T, Sudigdoadi S, Keersmackers K, et al. Evaluation of syndromic patient management algorithm for urethral discharge. Sex Transm Infect 1998;74(suppl 1):S29–33.

117. Centers for Disease Control and Prevention. Increases in fluoroquinone-resistant *Neisseria gonorrhea* among men who have sex with men- United States, 2003, and revised recommendations for gonorrhea treatment, 2004. MMWR 2004;53:335–8.

118. Akasaka S, Maratani T, Yamada Y, et al. Emergence of cephem- and aztreonam-high-resistant *Neisseria gonorrhoeae* that does not produce beta-lactamase. J Infect Chemother 2001;7:49–50.

119. Emans SF, Goldstein DP. The gynecologic examination of the prepubertal child with vulvovaginitis: use of the knee-chest position. Pediatrics 1980;65:758–60.

120. Redman JF, Bissada NK. How to make a good examination of the genitalia of young girls. Clin Pediatr 1976;15: 907–8.

121. Billmire ME, Farrell MK, Dine MS. A simplified procedure for pediatric vaginal examination: use of veterinary otoscope specula. Pediatrics 1980;65:823–5.

122. Singleton AF. Vaginal discharge in children and adolescents. Evolution and management: a review. Clin Pediatr 1980;19:799–804.

123. Huffman JW. Kindergarten gynecology. Postgrad Med 1970;47:121–6.

124. Hammerschlag MR, Alpert S, Rosner I, et al. Microbiology of the vagina in children: normal and potentially pathogenic organisms. Pediatrics 1978;62:57–62.

125. Shafer MA, Sweet RL, Ohm-Smith NU, et al. Microbiology of the lower genital tract in postmenarchal adolescent girls: differences by sexual activity, contraception, and presence of nonspecific vaginitis. J Pediatr 1985;107: 974–81.

126. Low RC, Cho CT, Duckling BA. Gonococcal infections in young children. Clin Pediatr 1977;16:623–6.

127. Anman GL, Waldenberg LM. Gonococcal periappendicitis and salpingitis in a prepubertal girl. Pediatrics 1976; 58:287–8.

128. Koumans EH, Markowitz LE, Hogan V, et al. CDC BV Working Group. Indications for therapy and treatment recommendations for bacterial vaginosis in nonpregnant and pregnant women: a synthesis of data. Clin Infect Dis 2002:35(suppl 2):S152–72.

129. Murphy TV, Nelson JD. *Shigella* vaginitis: report of 38 patients and review of the literature. Pediatrics 1979;63: 511–6.

130. Macfarlane DE, Sharma DP. *Haemophilus influenzae* and genital tract infections in children. Acta Paediatr Scand 1987;76:363–4.

131. Smayevsky J, Canigia LF, Lanza A, et al. Vaginal microflora associated with bacterial vaginosis in nonpregnant women: reliability of sialidase detection. Infect Dis Obstet Gynecol 2001;9:17–22.

131a. Danesh IS, Stephen JM, Gorbach J. Neonatal *Trichomonas vaginalis* infection. J Emerg Med 1995;13:51–4.

132. McCormack WM, Evrard JR, Laughlin CF, et al. Sexually transmitted conditions among women college students. Am J Obstet Gynecol 1981;139:130–33.

133. Jones JG, Yamauchi T, Lambert B. *Trichomonas vaginalis* infestation in sexually abused girls. Am J Dis Child 1985; 139:846–7.

134. Bump RC. *Chlamydia trachomatis* as a cause of prepubertal vaginitis. Obstet Gynecol 1985;65:384–8.

135. Hammerschlag MR, Cummings M, Doraiswamy B, et al. Nonspecific vaginitis following sexual abuse in children. Pediatrics 1985;75:1028–31.

136. Kekki M, Kurki T, Pelkonen J, et al. Vaginal clindamycin in preventing preterm birth and peripartal infections in asymptomatic women with bacterial vaginosis: a randomized, controlled trial. Obstet Gynecol 2001;97:643–8.

137. Anderson MR, Klink K, Cohrssen A. Evaluation of vaginal complaints. JAMA 2004;291:1368–79.

138. Bornstein J, Lakovsky Y, Lavi I, et al. The classic approach to the diagnosis of vulvovaginitis: a critical analysis. Infect Dis Obstet Gynecol 2001;9:105–11.

139. Broumas AG, Basara LA. Potential patient preference for 3-day treatment of bacterial vaginosis: responses to new suppository form of clindamycin. Adv Ther 2000;17: 159–66.

140. Willcox RR. Necrotic cervicitis due to primary infection with the virus of herpes simplex. Br Med J 1968;1:610–2.

141. Carr MC, Hanna L, Jawetz E. *Chlamydiae*, cervicitis, and

abnormal Papanicolaou smears. Obstet Gynecol 1979; 53:27–30.

142. Brunham RC, Paavonen J, Stevens CE, et al. Mucopurulent cervicitis—the ignored counterpart of urethritis in men. N Engl J Med 1984;311:1–6.

143. Myziuk L, Romanowski B, Brown M. Endocervical Gram stain smears and their usefulness in the diagnosis of Chlamydia trachomatis. Sex Transm Infect 2001;77:103–6.

144. Nyirjesy P. Nongonococcal and nonchlamydial cervicitis. Curr Infect Dis Rep 2001;3:540–5.

145. Dean D, Suchland RJ, Stamm WE. Evidence for long-term cervical persistence of Chlamydia trachomatis by omp1 genotyping. J Infect Dis 2001;183:1542–3.

146. McClelland RS, Wang CC, Mandaliya K, et al. Treatment of cervicitis is associated with decreased cervical shedding of HIV-1. AIDS 2001;15:105–110.

147. Chaim W, Bashiri A, Bar-David J, et al. Prevalence and clinical significance of postpartum endometritis and wound infection. Infect Dis Obstet Gynecol 2000;8:77–82.

148. Brumfield CG, Hauth JC, Andrews WW. Puerperal infection after cesarean delivery: evaluation of a standardized protocol. Am J Obstet Gynecol 2000;182:1147–51.

149. Magann EF, Chauhan SP, Martin JN Jr, et al. Does uterine wiping influence the rate of post-Cesarean endometritis? J Matern Fetal Med 2001;10:318–22.

150. Reid VC, Hartmann KE, McMahon M, et al. Vaginal preparation with povidone iodine and post-cesarean infectious morbidity: a randomized controlled trial. Obstet Gynecol 2001;97:147–52.

151. Bagratee JS, Moodley J, Kleinschmidt I, et al. A randomized controlled trial of antibiotic prophylaxis in elective caesarean delivery. Br J Obstet Gynecol 2001;108:143–8.

152. Henry-Suchet J. PID: clinical and laparoscopic aspects. Ann N Y Acad Sci 2000;900:301–8.

153. Reljic M, Gorisek B. C-reactive protein and the treatment of pelvic inflammatory disease. Int J Gynaecol Obstet 1998;60:142–50.

154. Soper DE, Brockwell NJ, Dalton HP, et al. Observations concerning the microbial etiology of acute salpingitis. Am J Obstet Gynecol 1994;170:1008–14.

155. Eschenbach DA, Wolner-Hannsen P, Hawes SE, et al. Acute pelvic inflammatory disease: associations of clinical and laboratory findings with laparoscopic findings. Obstet Gynecol 1997;89:184–92.

156. Cohen CR, Sinei S, Reilly M, et al. Effect of human immunodeficiency virus type 1 infection upon acute salpingitis: a laparoscopic study. J Infect Dis 1998;178:1352–8.

157. Erhan Y, Zekioglu O, Ozdemir N, et al. Unilateral salpingitis due to Enterobius vermicularis. Int J Gynecol Pathol 2000;19:188–9.

158. Sirotnak AP, Eppes SC, Klein JD. Tuboovarian abscess and peritonitis caused by Streptococcus pneumoniae serotype 1 in young girls. Clin Infect Dis 1996;22:993–6.

159. Brown-Harrison MC, Christenson JC, Harrison AM, et al. Group A streptococcal salpingitis in a prepubertal girl. Clin Pediatr (Phila) 1995;34:556–8.

160. Litt IF, Cohen MI. Perihepatitis associated with salpingitis in adolescents. JAMA 1978;240:1253–4.

161. Henry-Suchet J, Sluzhinska A, Serfaty D. Chlamydia trachomatis screening in family planning centers: a review of cost/benefit evaluations in different countries. Eur J Contracept Reprod Health Care 1996;1:301–9.

162. Garza KM, Lou YH, Tung KS. Mechanism of ovarian autoimmunity: induction of T cell and antibody responses by T cell epitope mimicry and epitope spreading. J Reprod Immunol 1998;37:87–101.

163. Theodoropoulos G, Haarmann W. Abdominal actinomycosis in tubo-ovarian abscess.[German] Zentralbl Gynakol 1995;117:494–7.

164. Shiomi S, Kuroki T, Kawabe J, et al. A case of oophoritis detected by gallium-67-citrate scintigraphy. Ann Nucl Med 1998;12:209–11.

165. Manfredi R, Alampi G, Talo S, et al. Silent oophoritis due to cytomegalovirus in a patient with advanced HIV disease. Int J STD AIDS 2000;11:410–2.

166. Nieto Y, Ross M, Gianani R, et al. Post-mortem incidental finding of cytomegalovirus oophoritis after an allogeneic stem cell transplant. Bone Marrow Transplant 1999;23:1323–4.

167. French LM, Smaill FM. Antibiotic regimens for endometritis after delivery. Cochrane Database Syst Rev 2002;(1):CD001067.

168. Anderson PAM, Giacomantonio JM. The acutely painful scrotum in children: review of 113 consecutive cases. Can Med Assoc J 1985;132:1153–5.

169. Lititnukul S, McCracken GH Jr, Nelson JD, et al. Epididymitis in children and adolescents. Am J Dis Child 1987;141:41–4.

170. Blaivas M, Sierzenski P, Lambert M. Emergency evaluation of patients presenting with acute scrotum using bedside ultrasonography. Acad Emerg Med 2001;8:90–3.

171. Haynes BE, Bessen HA, Haynes VE. The diagnosis of testicular torsion. JAMA 1983;249:2522–7.

172. Kadish HA, Bolte RG. A retrospective review of pediatric patients with epididymitis, testicular torsion, and torsion of testicular appendages. Pediatrics 1998;102:73–6.

173. Doehn C, Fornara P, Kausch I, et al. Value of acute-phase proteins in the differential diagnosis of acute scrotum. Eur Urol 2001;39:215–21.

174. Hermansen MC, Chusid MJ, Sty JR. Bacterial epididymoorchitis in children and adolescents. Clin Pediatr 1980;19:812–5.

175. de Vries M, van Der Horst I, van Der Kleij F, et al. Polyarteritis nodosa presenting as an acute bilateral epididymitis. Arch Intern Med 2001;161:1008.

176. Munden MM, Trautwein LM. Scrotal pathology in pediatrics with sonographic imaging. Curr Probl Diagn Radiol 2000;29:185–205.

177. Brauers A, Striepecke I, Mersdorf A, et al. Inflammatory pseudotumor of the epididymis. Eur Urol 1997;32:253–5.

178. Satchithananda K, Beese RC, Sidhu PS. Acute appendicitis presenting with a testicular mass: ultrasound appearances. Br J Radiol 2000;73:780–2.

179. Novella G, Porcaro AB, Righetti R, et al. Primary lymphoma of the epididymis: case report and review of the literature. Urol Int 2001;67:97–9.

180. Mehta HH, Thirumala S, Palestro CJ. Leukemic infiltration mimicking epididymo-orchitis on scrotal scintigraphy. Clin Nucl Med 1997;22:721–2.

181. Muttarak M, Peh WC, Lojanapiwat B, et al. Tuberculous epididymitis and epididymo-orchitis: sonographic appearances. AJR 2001;176:1459–66.

182. Memish ZA, Venkatesh S. Brucellar epididymo-orchitis in Saudi Arabia: a retrospective study of 26 cases and review of the literature. BJU Int 2001;88:72–6.

183. Kashiwage B, Okugi H, Morita T, et al. Acute epididymo-orchitis with abscess formation due to *Pseudomonas aeruginosa*: report of 3 cases. Hinyokika Kiyo 2000;46: 915–8.

184. Hsu CF, Wang CC, Chu CC, et al. Epididymo-orchitis in an infant resulting from *Escherichia coli* urinary tract infection. Zhonghua Min Guo Xiao Er Ke Yi Xue Hui Za Zhi 1996;37:48–51.

185. Hood SV, Bell D, McVey R, et al. Prostatitis and epididymo-orchitis due to *Aspergillus fumigatus* in a patient with AIDS. Clin Infect Dis 1998;26:229–31.

186. Seo R, Oyasu R, Schaeffer A. Blastomycosis of the epididymis and prostate. Urology 1997;50:980–2.

187. Kini U, Nirmala V. Post-transplantation epididymitis associated with cytomegalovirus. Indian J Pathol Microbiol 1996;39:151–3.

188. Hutcheson J, Peters CA, Diamond DA. Amiodarone induced epididymitis in children. J Urol 1998;160:515–7.

189. Gislason T, Noronha REX, Gregory JG. Acute epididymitis in boys: a 5-year retrospective study. J Urol 1980; 124:533–4.

190. Berger RE, Alexander ER, Monda GD, et al. *Chlamydia trachomatis* as a cause of acute idiopathic epididymitis. N Engl J Med 1978;298:301–4.

191. Ward AM, Rogers JH, Estcourt CS. *Chlamydia trachomatis* infection mimicking testicular malignancy in a young man. Sex Transm Infect 1999;75:270.

192. Waldman LS, Kosloske AM, Parson DW. Acute epididymoorchitis as the presenting manifestation of *Hemophilus influenzae* septicemia. J Pediatr 1977;90:87–9.

193. Craighead JE, Mahoney EM, Carver DH, et al. Orchitis due to Coxsackie virus Group B, type 5: report of a case with isolation of the virus from the testis. N Engl J Med 1962;267:498–501.

194. Turner RB. Orchitis as a complication of chickenpox. Pediatr Infect Dis 1987;6:489.

195. Ralston LS, Saiki AK, Powers WT. Orchitis as complication of infectious mononucleosis. JAMA 1960;173: 1348–9.

196. Riggs S, Sanford JP. Viral orchitis. N Engl J Med 1962; 266:990–3.

197. Coran AG, Perlmutter AD. Mumps epididymitis without orchitis. N Engl J Med 1965;272:735.

198. Evans SS, Fisher RG, Scott MA, et al. Sarcoidosis presenting as bilateral testicular masses. Pediatrics 1997;100: 392–4.

199. Morrisseau PM, Phillips CA, Leadbetter GW Jr. Viral prostatitis. J Urol 1970;103:767–9.

200. Brunner H, Weidner W, Schiefer HG. Studies on the role of *Ureaplasma urealyticum* and *Mycoplasma hominis* in prostatitis. J Infect Dis 1983;147:807–13.

CHAPTER 16

Orthopedic Syndromes

Orthopedic (bone and joint) infections can be classified into syndromes according to the anatomic area involved and the rate of onset.

Acute arthritis can be defined as a warm, swollen, erythematous joint. It is typically very painful and tender. *Purulent arthritis* (sometimes called *pyogenic arthritis* or *pyarthritis*) can be defined as cloudy, purulent fluid in a joint and is almost always secondary to a bacterial infection, although the culture is not always positive. The term *septic arthritis* implies a bacterial arthritis confirmed by culture. *Synovitis* can be defined as inflammation in a joint, with sterile fluid and no preceding antibiotics. Usually, the fluid is relatively clear and serous.

Osteomyelitis can be defined as infection in a bone. *Diskitis* (*spondylitis*) is an inflammatory process (with or without infection) of the intervertebral disk, often involving the adjacent vertebral bodies. *Chondritis* is infection of cartilage; adjacent bone may be infected as well, in which case the term *osteochondritis* is used.

Cellulitis (see Chapter 17) can be defined as inflammation (manifested as localized redness) of the skin and underlying soft tissue. Cellulitis over a bone or joint is often a sign of infection of the bone or joint.

■ CLASSIFICATION OF ACUTE ARTHRITIS

Acute Monarticular Arthritis

Acute monarticular arthritis is characterized by a rapid onset, usually with fever. The joint will typically be red, swollen, tender, and warm, with significant pain on motion of the joint. When a child has fever with a single hot and swollen joint, septic arthritis is sufficiently likely that joint aspiration should be done.

Acute Polyarticular Arthritis

Acute arthritis involving more than one joint in a child usually raises the question of acute rheumatic fever (Chapter 18) or juvenile rheumatoid arthritis (Chapter 10). However, septic arthritis can involve more than one joint, particularly with staphylococcal or gonococcal bacteremia during the newborn period or with intravenous drug use.

Subacute or Chronic Arthritis

Subacute or chronic arthritis can be defined as arthritis with gradual onset and duration of weeks to months, with little or no fever and slow progression. Tenderness, swelling, and limitation of motion may be persistent or recur episodically. The most likely infectious causes are partially treated or subacute septic arthritis. Lyme disease and tuberculosis are possibilities in the patient with an appropriate exposure history. Juvenile rheumatoid arthritis (JRA), aseptic necrosis, and neoplasm should be considered. Occasionally, a congenital coagulation defect will be unrecognized until bleeding into a joint occurs and aspiration reveals a hemarthrosis. A chronic or recurrent monarticular arthritis is often due to JRA and a slit-lamp examination looking for iridocyclitis is indicated. In addition, a therapeutic trial of ibuprofen or other nonsteroidal anti-inflammatory agent is often prescribed.

Acute Tenosynovitis

Acute tenosynovitis is characterized by swelling, tenderness, and pain on motion of the tendon sheaths, especially over the wrist, foot, or ankle. In the sexually active adolescent, gonococcal infection is a common cause.

Acute Arthralgia

Acute arthralgia is characterized by joint aching without objective signs on physical examination. If more than one joint is involved the term "polyarthralgia" is used. The causes of acute polyarthritis should be considered first, because objective findings might be subtle or delayed. However, fever from any cause is often associated with polyarthralgia. Muscle aches (myalgia) are often associated with acute viral infections such as influenza and may be mistaken for polyarthralgia.

Acute Myalgia

Acute polymyalgia, like acute polyarthralgia, is often a nonspecific manifestation of a febrile illness. The term "acute myositis" should be reserved for cases of muscle inflammation proved by biopsy or by an increased serum concentration of muscle enzymes, such as creatinine kinase and aldolase.

■ INFECTIOUS ARTHRITIS

Importance of Septic Arthritis

Septic arthritis is a medical emergency. Early diagnosis and proper treatment can usually prevent permanent disability. The most important characteristic of septic arthritis in children is that subsequent growth is likely to exaggerate any deformity caused by the illness, especially in the hip joint. Diagnostic aspiration should be done as soon as joint swelling or tenderness is recognized, and maximum therapeutic efforts should be made as soon as the diagnosis is confirmed by aspiration of pus. This is particularly true of septic arthritis of the hip, where destruction of the epiphyseal growth plate can result in unequal leg length or fusion of the joint, with severe gait disturbance. Several studies have demonstrated the importance of prompt surgical drainage. A delay of more than 4 days from onset of symptoms to decompression of the hip joint is the most important prognostic risk factor for permanent sequelae.[1–4]

Mechanisms

Septic arthritis in children most commonly occurs via hematogenous seeding of the synovial space. Occasionally, it occurs by local spread of contiguous infection or is secondary to trauma or surgery. The blood supply to the head of the femur and to the humerus is by way of the proximal metaphyseal (retinacular) arteries, which lie within the joint cavity.[5] These vessels can be compressed by increased intra-articular pressure, with resultant ischemia and destruction of the epiphyseal growth plate. Compromised blood supply can also lead to avascular necrosis of the femur or humerus. Therefore, most orthopedic surgeons strongly urge prompt open

drainage of purulent arthritis, especially when these joints are involved.

The action of proteolytic enzymes in pus, even when it is sterile, can destroy joint cartilage, with resultant joint deformity and crippling.[6] Therefore, preservation of joint cartilage is another reason for thorough removal of pus from joint spaces. Often, as much as 100 mL of pus can be removed from a joint during an operation after the joint was thought to have been tapped dry by needle aspiration. This may be explained by loculation of the pus, especially if the onset has been subacute.

Presentation

The most frequent joints involved are those of the lower extremity, and thus the child will usually present with acute onset of limp or refusal to walk. The child with septic arthritis of the hip will occasionally complain only of referred knee pain. If a joint in the upper extremity is involved, the child will usually refuse to move the arm. The joint is typically held in the position of least pain (usually flexion). Most children will have fever, but occasionally it is low-grade. In one study of children less than 2 years old with septic arthritis, 14 (35%) of 40 had a temperature less than 38.3°C.[7] A careful examination will reveal a red, swollen, and tender joint with pain on motion. Detecting infection in joints that are not easily isolated on examination, such as the sacroiliac and sternoclavicular joints, is difficult and requires a high index of suspicion.

■ BACTERIAL CAUSES OF ARTHRITIS

Pyogenic Organisms

Staphylococcus aureus is the most common cause of septic arthritis in all ages, although Group B streptococcus is also a common cause in newborns. Prior to the routine use the of conjugated vaccine in the early 1990s, *Haemophilus influenzae* type B (Hib) was a common cause of septic arthritis in children but has now become rare.[8] *Kingella kingae* has become the most frequent gram-negative organism causing septic arthritis in young children.[9] The common causes of bacterial arthritis and predisposing factors are shown in Table 16-1.

Acute bacterial arthritis is usually monarticular but is often polyarticular in neonates and in adolescents with gonococcal arthritis. Polyarticular pneumococcal arthritis has been described in children with HIV infection.[10] Occasionally, previously

TABLE 16-1. PREDISPOSING FACTORS AND CAUSES OF BACTERIAL ARTHRITIS

BACTERIA	PREDISPOSING FACTORS/COMMENTS
More Common Causes	
Staphylococcus aureus	Any age
Haemophilus influenzae	Now rare in areas with high vaccine coverage
Group A streptococcus	Convalescent from varicella[285]
Group B streptococcus	Newborns
Streptococcus pneumoniae	HIV infection
Borrelia burgdorferi	Residence in Lyme-endemic area, history of deer tick exposure
Salmonella spp.	Hemoglobinopathies, systemic lupus
Neisseria gonorrheae	Newborns, sexually-active adolescents
Kingella kingae	Children <24 months old;[7,9] direct inoculation of joint fluid into blood culture bottle increases yield[102]
Less Common Causes	
Neisseria meningitidis	Complement deficiency;[286] more commonly causes a reactive arthritis[287]
Gram-negative enteric bacilli	Newborns
Mycoplasma spp.	Hypogammaglobulinemia[14]
Ureaplasma urealyticum	Hypogammaglobulinemia[14]
Group G streptococcus	Underlying systemic or joint disease[288]
Pseudomonas aeruginosa	Puncture wound to foot;[161] injection drug use
Streptobacillus moniliformis (rat bite fever)	Rat bite or scratch[289]
Brucella spp.	Goat milk ingestion; >50% of children with brucellosis develop arthritis[290]
Nocardia asteroides	Puncture wound;[93,291] immunocompromise[292]
Fusobacterium necrophorum	Lemierre syndrome[293]
Rickettsia rickettsii (Rocky Mountain spotted fever)	Arthralgia is very common, but arthritis is rare[294]
Coxiella burnetii (Q fever)	Exposure to cattle, sheep, and goats[295]
Polymicrobial	Usually after trauma

healthy children will present with multiple joint involvement in the context of severe staphylococcal sepsis, with or without meeting the criteria for toxic shock syndrome.[11] In addition, acute polyarthritis can occur as a complication of a systemic bacterial infection without infection of the joint. Bacterial endocarditis is often associated with musculoskeletal manifestations, such as arthritis, arthralgia, and myalgia.[12] These patterns are probably best classified with the reactive arthritides.

Recurrent bacterial arthritis is uncommon and should suggest underlying immunodeficiency, such as agammaglobulinemia.[13] In one series of patients

with hypogammaglobulinemia, 8 (38%) of 21 episodes of septic arthritis were attributed to Mycoplasma or Ureaplasma.[14] Patients with chronic lymphedema are also predisposed to recurrent arthritis in the involved limb.[15] Septic arthritis due to *Salmonella* occurs with greater frequency in patients with sickle cell anemia as well as those with systemic lupus erythematosus.[16,17]

Lyme Arthritis

In a child who lives in or has visited an endemic area (primarily the northeastern and mid-Atlantic states and parts of Wisconsin and Minnesota), Lyme disease is a possible cause of arthritis. Characteristically, one or two large joints suddenly become swollen and warm, but there is often minimal pain or erythema.[18] The knee is the most frequently affected joint. There may or may not be a history of a tick bite or an erythema migrans rash. However, by the time arthritis develops (usually several weeks after infection), a specific IgG and IgM antibody response in the serum to *Borrelia burgdorferi* is nearly always present.[19] Synovial fluid leukocyte counts are typically less than 50,000 per mcL but range from 500–100,000 per mcL, usually with a neutrophil predominance.[20] Using PCR, *B. burgdorferi* DNA can be detected in the synovial fluid of patients with Lyme arthritis.[21] In the small percentage of patients who develop chronic arthritis despite antimicrobial therapy, PCR testing is negative.[21] Thus, in addition to causing infectious arthritis, *B. burgdorferi* can apparently cause a form of reactive arthritis in some genetically-predisposed people.[22] Chronic arthritis in children with Lyme disease is uncommon; greater than 95% of children treated with an appropriate course of antibiotics have no long-term symptoms.[23]

It is not uncommon for a parent to request testing for Lyme disease in a child with nonspecific symptoms, such as headache, fatigue, and arthralgia. In the absence of a history of erythema migrans or objective findings (such as arthritis, carditis, meningitis, or neuritis), the likelihood of Lyme disease is remote. In such children the positive predictive value of serologic testing is less than 5%; that is, nearly all positive tests are false-positives.[24] For persons not residing in a Lyme-endemic region, the positive predictive value of serologic tests approaches zero. Testing for Lyme disease in such patients is counterproductive, because a positive test is likely to result in delayed treatment of the correct diagnosis, such as fibromyalgia or chronic fatigue syndrome.[25]

Septic Arthritis in the Neonate and Young Infant

The young infant with septic arthritis may present acutely with lethargy, fever or hypothermia, and poor feeding. However, the presentation is often subtle and subacute, without systemic symptoms.[26] Redness and warmth may be absent and swelling may be difficult to appreciate, especially in the hip. Irritability during diaper changes, lack of movement of an extremity (which may be misdiagnosed as an isolated nerve palsy), or even limb cyanosis may be the only clue to the diagnosis.[27,28] Decreased extremity movement is usually secondary to pain (so-called "pseudoparalysis") but is occasionally the result of true paralysis from nerve impingement, especially when the shoulder is involved.[29] In the case of hip joint infection, the child will prefer to hold the extremity in external rotation, abduction, and flexion to reduce intra-articular pressure. Polyarticular infection and concomitant osteomyelitis are common (as discussed in the section on osteomyelitis).[30] Risk factors include prematurity, indwelling intravascular catheters (especially umbilical arterial lines), and femoral venipuncture.[26,31]

Postoperative Septic Arthritis

In comparison with adults, a history of previous joint surgery in children is very uncommon. However, prosthetic joints are occasionally placed in children or adolescents after limb salvage, resection of bone tumors, after major trauma, or in children with severe disability from rheumatoid arthritis or other conditions.[32,33] Infection in such joints may be subtle; fever and joint swelling occur in a minority of cases.[34] Joint pain, which is nearly always present, may be the only symptom.[34] Constant pain is suggestive of infection, whereas mechanical loosening commonly causes pain only with motion and weight bearing. Nearly any organism, including those normally considered contaminants, can cause prosthetic joint infection. In one study over a 23-year period, prosthetic joint infection occurred in 466 (1.8%) of 26,505 recipients.[35] The most common etiologic agents were *S. aureus* (22%), coagulase-negative staphylococci (19%), streptococci (9%), gram-negative bacilli (8%), anaerobes (6%), and other agents (5%). In addition, 19% of infections were polymicrobial. Independent risk factors for infection included malignancy, postoperative surgical site infection, and a history of previous joint arthroplasty. Removal of the prosthesis is usually required for successful treatment. For some bone cancer patients this would necessitate limb amputation, and thus lifelong antibiotic therapy may be used instead in an attempt to chronically suppress infection.

Septic arthritis after arthroscopic anterior cruciate ligament reconstruction is even less common, occurring in 7 (0.3%) of 2500 patients in one study.[36] As in the case with prosthetic joint infections, the allograft must usually be removed to effect a cure.

Mycobacterial and Fungal Arthritis

Bone or joint involvement occurs in about 5% of cases of extra-pulmonary tuberculosis in children.[37] Presentation may mimic bacterial arthritis[38] or JRA.[39] For any child with arthritis, risk factors for exposure to tuberculosis should be elicited (see Chapter 8) and, if present, a chest x-ray and tuberculin skin test should be performed. Keep in mind, however, that these tests are often negative in the child with extrapulmonary tuberculosis.[40] Joint fluid will typically have fewer than 50,000 leukocytes per mcL with a neutrophilic predominance, but these findings are variable. When suspected, a smear for acid-fast bacilli and mycobacterial culture should be performed on the joint fluid. Occasionally, synovial biopsy is required to make the diagnosis.[40] Joint involvement with nontuberculous mycobacteria is most commonly reported in the setting of HIV infection[41] but has been described in an immunocompetent child.[42]

Candidal arthritis is uncommon, with the notable exception being premature neonates. In one study, *Candida* species were responsible for 17% of episodes of hospital-acquired neonatal septic arthritis, second in frequency only to staphylococci.[43]

Besides prematurity, other risk factors often present in these infants include central venous catheters, prolonged use of antibiotics, hyperalimentation, and recent surgery.[44,45] Septic arthritis is an uncommon manifestation of disseminated candidiasis in patients with chemotherapy-induced neutropenia.[46]

Other fungal infections rarely causing arthritis include histoplasmosis,[47] blastomycosis,[48] cryptococcosis,[49] coccidioidomycosis,[50] sporotrichosis,[51] and aspergillosis,[52] most commonly—but not exclusively—in immunocompromised hosts. Patients with histoplasmosis can also develop a reactive arthritis, sometimes in association with other inflammatory phenomena, such as erythema nodosum.[53]

Viral Arthritis

Several viruses have been associated with arthritis (Table 16-2). In many cases, such as with parvovirus B19,[54] the process resembles a reactive arthritis rather than viral infection of the synovial space. Patients with HIV infection have a higher incidence of several types of arthritis, including septic arthritis and Reiter syndrome.[55] In addition, there appears to be an entity of HIV-associated arthritis, which occurs in up to 8% of infected patients.[56] Like other viral arthritides, it is typically an acute-onset oligoarticular arthritis of relatively brief duration and does not cause permanent joint damage. Both natu-

TABLE 16-2. VIRAL CAUSES OF ARTHRITIS

VIRUS	COMMENTS
Varicella[296]	May occur before, during, or after rash
Parvovirus B19[54]	Knee most commonly affected joint; may or may not have erythema infectiosum rash
HIV[56]	Usually lasts about 2 weeks
Rubella[297]	Also rarely occurs 10–28 days after rubella immunization
Mumps[298]	May be associated with fever and leukocytosis
Hepatitis A, B, C[281–283]	Probably a form of reactive arthritis in all three instances
Cytomegalovirus[299]	Especially in the immunocompromised host
Coxsackievirus B[300]	Associated with fever and oral ulcerations; may have synovial fluid leukocyte count >50,000 per mcL
Herpes simplex virus[301]	Uncommon
Epstein-Barr virus[302]	Uncommon; probably a reactive arthritis
Echovirus[303]	Hypogammaglobulinemia is a risk factor
Adenovirus[304]	A possible cause of recurrent arthritis

ral rubella infection and, much less commonly, vaccination with live-attenuated rubella vaccine are associated with inflammation of the small joints.[57] As with parvovirus B19-associated arthritis, young adult women are more likely to develop rubella-associated arthritis.

Differential Diagnosis of Infectious Arthritis

Many diseases resemble septic arthritis. Some of the more common of these can be brought to mind by recalling the acrostic JOINT STARTS HOT (Table 16-3).

Osteomyelitis

The most important consideration in suspected septic arthritis of the hip is osteomyelitis of the femoral neck or, less commonly, of a pelvic bone (see the section on osteomyelitis). It is also important to remember that osteomyelitis and septic arthritis sometimes occur together.[30]

Joint Effusion Near Osteomyelitis

Sometimes called a "sympathetic effusion," joint fluid near an osteomyelitis closely resembles septic arthritis clinically. However, aspiration of the joint reveals relatively clear fluid, without bacteria present on the Gram stain. Only joint aspiration can distinguish between a purulent and a sympathetic effusion in a joint adjacent to an area of osteomyelitis, although range of motion is usually less limited in a sympathetic effusion. The pus formed in the metaphysis in osteomyelitis may break through into the joint space, especially in joints where the metaphyseal spongiosa lies within the attachments of the joint capsule, as in the hip and shoulder.[58] To avoid the damaging effects of pressure and pus, it is essential to aspirate such joints to recognize a purulent arthritis. When the joint tap is nonpurulent in suspected septic arthritis of the hip, a bone scan should be done to look for femoral neck osteomyelitis.

Transient Synovitis of the Hip

Transient synovitis, also called "toxic synovitis" or "irritable hip," is manifested by unilateral hip pain,

TABLE 16-3. DIFFERENTIAL DIAGNOSIS OF SEPTIC ARTHRITIS: JOINT STARTS HOT

CAUSE	COMMENTS
Juvenile rheumatoid arthritis	Associated features variable, depending on type (pauciarticular, polyarticular, or systemic onset); rash, uveitis, often with very high serum ferritin[305]
Osteomyelitis	Focal pain and point tenderness; may coexist with septic arthritis[58]
Inflammatory systemic diseases	Inflammatory bowel disease,[84] systemic lupus erythematosis,[80] dermatomyositis,[82] juvenile ankylosing spondylitis[81a]
Neoplastic diseases	Leukemia,[89] neuroblastoma,[90] lymphoma,[306] Ewing sarcoma[307]
Transient synovitis	Fever, elevated ESR less common than with septic arthritis, but substantial overlap exists[60]
Soft-tissue infection	Cellulitis, pyomyositis,[308] bursitis[63]
Trauma	Hemarthrosis secondary to abuse or coagulopathy
Acute rheumatic fever	Migratory polyarthritis of large joints, often with dramatic response to aspirin[83]
Reactive arthritis	Many possible causes (see Box 16–1)
Tenosynovitis	Gonococcal infection is a common cause in the sexually-active adolescent[309]
Serum sickness	Polyarthritis, usually with urticarial rash and recent infection or drug exposure[87]
Henoch-Schöenlein purpura	Purpuric rash with normal platelet count, abdominal pain, and hematuria; arthritis is the presenting symptom in 1/4 of patients[86]
Other	Kawasaki disease (arthritis occurs in about 30% of cases),[85,310] Lyme disease (arthritis occurs in about 6% of cases in children)[23,311]
Tuberculosis	History of exposure is key to diagnosis; chest x-ray and tuberculin skin test will sometimes be negative[37]

refusal to walk, or limping, and is a frequent cause of arthritis in children. In fact, it is the most common cause of atraumatic limp in children presenting to the emergency department, accounting for about 40% of such visits in one study.[59] Fever, if present, is usually low-grade. Transient synovitis is much more frequent than septic arthritis of the hip. Nevertheless, the physician must not assume that a child with a swollen, painful hip joint has transient synovitis rather than septic arthritis. The risks of diagnostic joint aspiration performed by a physician who is experienced in this procedure are small compared with the dangers of a destructive septic arthritis. Ultrasound is not helpful in distinguishing transient synovitis from septic arthritis because an effusion is found in both conditions.

Several algorithms have been developed to assist in determining the likelihood of septic arthritis vs. transient synovitis. Kocher et al.[60] reviewed the charts of all children presenting to Children's Hospital in Boston with an irritable hip over an 18-year period. Of 262 children, 82 were diagnosed with confirmed or presumed septic arthritis, 86 were diagnosed with transient synovitis, and 114 were excluded. Lack of synovial fluid studies was the most common reason for exclusion, and, presumably, many of these children had transient synovitis. In multivariate analysis, four variables were found to be independent predictors of septic arthritis: a history of subjective fever, non-weight-bearing, ESR 40 mm/hour or greater, and peripheral WBC greater than 12,000 per mcL. The probability of septic arthritis could be calculated based on the number of these variables present (Table 16-4). Using this algorithm, children with three or four

predictors should usually undergo hip aspiration in the operating room, given the high likelihood that arthrotomy and drainage will be needed. Children with two predictors may be good candidates for aspiration in the outpatient setting. Depending on clinical suspicion, some children with fewer than two predictors will be appropriate candidates for careful observation without aspiration. Other similar algorithms have been developed.[61,62] It is important to remember that the utility of such algorithms may be lower in children less than 18–24 months of age, in whom transient synovitis is less common and in whom the presentation of septic arthritis is often subtle.

The cause of transient synovitis of the hip is unknown. Symptoms usually last only a few days, although it can be recurrent. Legg-Calve-Perthes disease (aseptic necrosis of the femoral capital epiphysis) in its early stage may cause synovitis that is indistinguishable from transient synovitis, so that patients with synovitis should have careful evaluation and follow-up, with referral to an orthopedic surgeon if symptoms persist.

Cellulitis

Cellulitis near a joint may resemble acute arthritis. However, with septic arthritis the erythema is usually symmetrically distributed around the joint, and the borders of redness are diffuse. Motion of the joint is usually exquisitely painful. Cellulitis will typically have more well-demarcated erythema, often with evidence of a local wound, and joint motion causes little discomfort. Despite these generalizations, it is often difficult to tell whether the

TABLE 16-4. PREDICTED PROBABILITY OF SEPTIC ARTHRITIS VS. TRANSIENT SYNOVITIS BASED ON THE PRESENCE OF FOUR VARIABLES[60]

NO. OF PREDICTORS PRESENT*	TRANSIENT SYNOVITIS (N=86)	SEPTIC ARTHRITIS (N=82)	PREDICTED PROBABILITY OF SEPTIC ARTHRITIS
0	19 (22%)	0 (0%)	<0.2%
1	47 (55%)	1 (1%)	3%
2	16 (19%)	12 (15%)	40%
3	4 (5%)	44 (54%)	93%
4	0 (0%)	25 (31%)	99.6%

* The four predictors are (1) a history of subjective fever, (2) non-weight-bearing, (3) ESR ≥40 mm per hour, and (4) peripheral WBC >12,000 per mcL.

joint is involved. Diagnostic aspiration (avoiding the cellulitis, if possible) should usually be done if there is reasonable suspicion of increased fluid in the joint. The risk of introducing bacteria from cellulitis into the joint is small compared with the risk of delay in diagnosing septic arthritis. In certain cases, ultrasound may be performed first and, if there is no joint effusion, arthrocentesis can be avoided. However, the ultrasound must be done in a timely fashion by a radiologist expert in interpreting the results. Sonography is useful for excluding joint effusion in the hip but may be less sensitive in detecting fluid in smaller joints. If no joint fluid is present by clinical or ultrasound examination (and osteomyelitis is not suspected or has been ruled out), blood cultures should be obtained and the patient should be treated with intravenous antibiotics such as oxacillin or cefazolin to cover *S. aureus* and Group A streptococcus. The patient usually responds promptly when cellulitis without underlying septic arthritis is present, as discussed in Chapter 17.

Septic Bursitis

Bacterial infection of a bursa is usually secondary to a local laceration or abrasion of the skin.[63] In children, this condition is most frequently observed in the prepatellar bursa after an abrasion of the knee. Septic prepatellar bursitis can usually be distinguished from septic arthritis of the knee by physical examination, because there is less pain on motion in bursitis. Treatment with drainage and antibiotics is similar to that for a skin abscess.

Reactive Arthritis

Reactive arthritis is defined as a nonpurulent arthritis that occurs simultaneously or subsequent to an infection elsewhere in the body. The larger joints are more commonly affected. Onset is typically acute and fever may be present. The most well recognized associations are with various causes of bacterial enteritis and genital infection (see Box 16-1). There remains considerable debate as to whether such arthritis is caused by occult infection in the joint or by an immune response to infection.[64] It is possible that different mechanisms are operative depending on the pathogen responsible. Nucleic acid of *Chlamydia trachomatis* and, less frequently, *C. pneumoniae* has been found in the synovial tissue of patients with reactive arthritis.[65,66] *Chlamydia*

> **BOX 16-1 ■ Some Causes of Post-Infectious Reactive Arthritis**
>
> **Diarrheal**
> *Salmonella**†[264]
> *Campylobacter**[265]
> *Yersinia**[266]
> *Shigella*[267,268]
> *Clostridium difficile*[269,270]
> *Giardia*[271]
>
> **Meningeal**
> *Neisseria meningitidis*†[272]
> *Haemophilus influenzae* type b†[273]
>
> **Genital**
> *Chlamydia trachomatis**[274]
> *Neisseria gonorrheae*†[275]
> *Ureaplasma urealyticum*[276]
> *Mycoplasma hominis*[277]
>
> **Other**
> *Chlamydia pneumoniae*[278]
> Group A streptococci†[279]
> Group C and G streptococci[280]
> *Mycoplasma pneumoniae*[277]
> Hepatitis A, B, and C[281–283]
> *Propionibacterium acnes*[284]
>
> * more common cause of reactive arthritis
> † also causes purulent arthritis

DNA is present in the synovial tissue of a small percentage of asymptomatic subjects as well.[67]

Some patients are genetically predisposed—there is a higher incidence of the HLA-B27 phenotype in patients with reactive arthritis—but this does not explain all cases. Some infectious agents, such as meningococcus[68] and Group A streptococcus,[69,70] can cause either purulent arthritis or reactive arthritis. The mechanism of arthritis for many viral infections may be immune-related, and these can be considered a form of reactive arthritis. Several vaccines have been anecdotally associated with the development of reactive arthritis.[71–77] "Reiter's syndrome" is the term used for the subset of patients with reactive arthritis who also have nongonococcal urethritis and ocular inflammation.[78]

Arthritis Associated with Systemic Disease

Many systemic inflammatory diseases may have arthritis as part of the clinical presentation. These include collagen vascular diseases such as JRA,[79] systemic lupus erythematosis,[80] mixed connective tissue disease,[81] juvenile ankylosing spondylitis,[81a] and polymyositis and dermatomyositis.[82] Other systemic diseases that may present with arthritis include acute rheumatic fever,[83] inflammatory bowel disease,[84] Kawasaki disease,[85] sarcoidosis,[85a] and Henoch-Schöenlein purpura.[86] Serum sickness is also a consideration, particularly in the child who has received medication in the previous 2 weeks.[87] Approximately 5–10% of children with cystic fibrosis have episodic arthritis that is probably immune-mediated.[88]

Arthritis Associated with Malignancies

Several malignant conditions in childhood may initially manifest joint involvement, especially leukemia and neuroblastoma.[89] Laboratory clues to the presence of malignancy include anemia, elevated erythrocyte sedimentation rate (ESR) in the presence of a normal or decreased platelet count, and elevated serum lactate dehydrogenase (LDH).[90]

Trauma

Trauma with bleeding into the joint may mimic septic arthritis. A history of only mild trauma resulting in significant joint swelling should raise suspicion for child abuse or an underlying coagulation disorder. It should also be kept in mind that a history of recent trauma to the joint is very common in children with septic arthritis, and such a history should not decrease suspicion for this diagnosis.

Penetrating foreign body injury to the joint may result in a presentation identical to septic arthritis.[91,92] Cultures are usually sterile, but such injury can occasionally inoculate bacteria into the joint resulting in a traumatic septic arthritis.[93,94] Clenched fist human bite injuries commonly cause infection of the underlying metacarpal-phalangeal joint.[95] Early surgical exploration is indicated for such injuries, and prophylaxis with amoxicillin-clavulanate is appropriate to cover the commonly implicated organisms (streptococci, *S. aureus*, *Eikenella corrodens*, and anaerobes).

Diagnostic Approach

Ordinary Roentgenograms

Radiologic examination may be useful to indicate the presence of fluid in the hip joint, which is difficult to detect by physical examination (Figs. 16-1

and 16-2), although ultrasound is superior for this purpose. Plain film x-rays are most helpful to detect an unsuspected fracture or chronic bone or joint disease, and thus their use is justified. However, they are not helpful in excluding the diagnosis of septic arthritis.

Ultrasound

Ultrasound can reliably detect fluid in the hip joint,[96] and may be useful in detecting fluid in other joints as well.[97] However, sonography cannot distinguish whether a joint effusion is purulent, sterile, or hemorrhagic.[96]

Radionuclide Scan

Scanning with radioactive technetium (^{99m}Tc) is especially useful to detect septic arthritis in joints that are difficult to examine clinically, such as the sacroiliac area.[98] On bone scan, septic arthritis usually

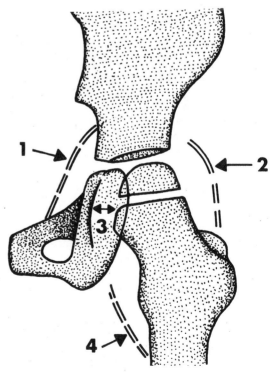

■ **FIGURE 16-1** Septic arthritis of the hip. Two views of the full pelvis should be examined: legs together and frog-leg positions. If pain limits motion, the degree of rotation should be the same on each side for comparative measurements. Diagram showing possible radiologic findings: (1) obturator internus muscle swelling; (2) joint capsule distention; (3) medial joint space widening, indicating lateral displacement of femoral head; (4) iliopsoas muscle swelling.

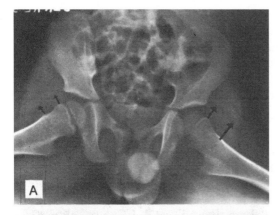

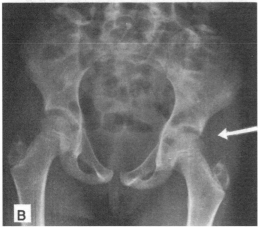

■ **FIGURE 16-2** (**A**) Hip roentgenograms of patient with septic arthritis showing obturator internus swelling and edema in muscle planes (*long arrows*). (**B**) Capsular distention in another patient (*arrow*). (Photo A from Dr. Thomas Carter; B from Dr. Peter Karofsky.)

reveals diffuse, faintly increased tracer uptake on both sides of the joint. In osteomyelitis, the increased tracer uptake is usually unilateral and more intense, but differentiating the two conditions may be difficult.[99] In some cases of septic arthritis of the hip, fluid in the joint under pressure causes impaired perfusion and decreased tracer uptake ("cold-hip" sign).[100]

Computed Tomography (CT) and Magnetic Resonance Imaging (MRI)

These studies are of limited usefulness, because joint fluid and synovial enhancement will be seen on CT or MRI with arthritis of any cause.[99] Their main utility in this setting is in looking for an associated osteomyelitis.

Arthrocentesis

If a joint effusion is suspected because of clinical or imaging findings, an arthrocentesis should be done. Some of the fluid should be put in a tube containing an anticoagulant for use in studies that cannot be done with clotted blood. Such clotting is due to fibrin, which is not present in normal joints. A white cell count and differential should be done, and the joint fluid should be Gram stained, noting the frequency of leukocytes as well as looking for bacteria. Bacterial antigen detection tests are neither approved for use with joint fluid nor helpful in diagnosing or excluding septic arthritis.[101]

The highest yield for bacterial culture is obtained by inoculating several milliliters of joint fluid directly into a standard blood culture bottle for use in an automated detection system.[102] A small amount of fluid can also be inoculated into a lysis-centrifugation tube, but these tubes are not as commonly available, and whether their use increases the yield over that of the standard blood culture bottle is unclear.[103] Either of these methods is superior to directly plating synovial fluid onto solid media, especially for recovery of fastidious organisms such as *Kingella kingae*.[104] The microbiology laboratory should be notified if an unusual organism is suspected because of the patient's exposure history. Stain and culture for fungi and mycobacteria are not necessary for most cases with an acute presentation. These tests should be considered in the immunocompromised host, the patient with a subacute or chronic course, or if an initial joint tap was culture negative and the response to empiric antibacterial therapy has been slow. Keep in mind, however, that the most common reason for a poor response to therapy is inadequate surgical drainage. Examination for crystals, an important part of synovial fluid analysis in adults, is rarely necessary in children.

Interpretation of Synovial Fluid

A presumptive diagnosis of septic arthritis can be made by immediate examination of the joint fluid, which is usually cloudy. Bacteria and a predominance of segmented neutrophils are often seen on the Gram stain. Leukocyte counts greater than 50,000 per mcL are strongly suggestive of bacterial infection, although some patients will have lower counts. Occasionally, patients with other causes of arthritis will have leukocyte counts greater than 50,000 per mcL.[105] Decreased glucose and increased protein concentrations in the joint fluid are supportive but not universal findings and should not be relied upon. Only about 30–60% of synovial fluid cultures will be positive, even in the child who has not received recent antibiotics.[4,106–108] Thus, a negative culture does not rule out the possibility of bacterial arthritis.

Other Studies

Positive blood cultures are found in approximately 40% of children with septic arthritis.[108] Thus, at least one and, preferably, two blood cultures should be obtained. The erythrocyte sedimentation rate (ESR) and C-reactive protein (CRP) are both useful for following response to therapy and should be obtained at baseline.[109] A complete blood count and peripheral smear should also be obtained, remembering that anemia, extreme leukocytosis or leukopenia, and decreased platelet count in a patient with an elevated ESR are clues to possible malignancy. If Lyme disease is suspected, a two-step approach to serologic testing is used. An enzyme immunoassay or indirect immunofluorescent assay is done first. If these screening tests are positive, they require confirmation with a Western blot assay. At least five bands must be present on the Western blot for the test to be considered positive. Caution is indicated, as we have seen children with culture-positive *S. aureus* septic arthritis who also had positive Western blot testing for Lyme disease. This could be secondary to an unrecognized infection with *B. burgdorferi* in the past, current coinfection, or a false-positive test.

Treatment

Surgical Drainage

Drainage of pus from a joint may be done by intermittent aspiration, by open incision with drainage (followed by continuous suction drainage) or by arthroscopy. The risk of severe deformity from septic arthritis in children leads most orthopedic surgeons to argue for open decompression and removal of pus. However, repeated aspiration may be acceptable for the knee, elbow, or ankle, if there is rapid improvement. In the hip and shoulder, open incision and drainage is advisable.

Antibiotic Therapy

If the joint fluid shows more than 10,000 leukocytes per mcL with a predominance of neutrophils,

the working diagnosis should be "purulent arthritis, probably septic." Antibiotic therapy should not be delayed until culture results are available. Rather, immediate intravenous therapy should be given based on the Gram stain. If the Gram stain is negative, then antibiotic therapy should be based on the most frequent organisms recovered. In most settings, empiric therapy using an agent with good activity against *S. aureus*, such as oxacillin or cefazolin, is appropriate. Vancomycin may be used in areas with a high prevalence of community-acquired MRSA. Clindamycin is also an option, depending on local susceptibility profiles.[109a] If *S. pneumoniae, H. influenzae, Salmonella,* or *N. gonorrheae* are suspected, ceftriaxone or cefotaxime is added. For the neonate, oxacillin plus cefotaxime or gentamicin may be used to cover the most likely pathogens (*S. aureus,* Group B streptococcus, and enteric gram-negative rods). For all patients, as soon as definite culture and sensitivity results are obtained, the initial therapy can be changed, if necessary. If the isolate (usually *S. aureus*) is shown to be sensitive to a β-lactam antibiotic, this should be used preferentially because of greater inherent antistaphylococcal activity than vancomycin.

Rarely, slow response to therapy with a β-lactam antibiotic is the result of bacterial tolerance, rendering the antibiotic bacteriostatic instead of bactericidal.[110] More commonly, poor response is secondary to inadequate drainage. Culture-negative septic arthritis is common and should be treated as aggressively as culture-positive cases,[107] with therapy that ensures good coverage against *S. aureus* (the most frequent and serious cause).

Intra-articular antibiotics have not been shown to improve outcome.[111] In addition, their use may exacerbate the inflammatory response of the synovium. A recent prospective, randomized study of septic arthritis in children reported improved outcome among patients receiving a 4-day course of intravenous dexamethasone compared with placebo controls.[111a] However, the incidence of residual joint dysfunction was higher in the control group than is generally seen. These findings require replication in larger studies before the use of carticosteroids in the treatment of septic arthritis becomes routine.

Lyme arthritis is treated effectively with a 4-week course of doxycycline for children older than 8 years and with amoxicillin for those 8 years old or younger.[24] For the few patients with persistent arthritis despite appropriate therapy, a single

14–21-day course with ceftriaxone is sometimes used, although this approach has been shown to be of no benefit in controlled trials.[112] Prolonged use of intravenous antibiotics in patients with a history of possible Lyme disease and persistent nonspecific symptoms is inappropriate. This practice has been associated with severe complications from the use of central catheters, including death.[113]

Route of Therapy

Initial therapy should be by the intravenous route. It has become common practice to switch to high-dose oral therapy after about a week in the child who has an excellent initial response to therapy, with normalization of temperature and decreased pain and swelling of the joint. Other criteria sometimes used include (1) decreasing ESR or CRP, (2) assurance of compliance, (3) identification of the organism, and (4) documentation of adequate serum levels of antibiotics. Serum bactericidal levels have also been advocated. In this test, the infecting organism must be recovered from the blood or joint fluid. The patient's serum is obtained at the expected peak or trough concentration of the oral antibiotic and serially diluted. If the organism is killed at a 1:8 dilution at peak or 1:2 dilution at trough, the oral antibiotic is likely to be effective.[114] For most antibiotics with time-dependent killing (such as the β-lactam antibiotics), trough titers are expected to be more predictive of therapeutic efficacy, and this was found to be true in a study of adults.[115] In practice, serum bactericidal testing is technically difficult, and very few microbiology laboratories offer this service.

For cephalexin (the most commonly used oral agent in this setting), the peak joint fluid concentration is approximately 65% of the peak serum concentration,[116] providing theoretic rationale for this approach. If oral antibiotics are to be used, the dose should generally be two to three times the usual oral dose (e.g., for cephalexin, 100–150 mg/kg/day divided every 6 hours). It is important to realize that no studies of sufficient power have been done to evaluate oral vs. intravenous therapy for septic arthritis, and they are not likely to be done. At least 8% of children with septic arthritis develop significant sequelae.[4] To detect a doubling of this rate to 16% with 80% power, at least 500 children would need to be studied (250 in each group).[117] This is not to imply that oral therapy should never be used. In the patient with good initial response to intravenous therapy and excellent compliance with the oral regimen, it is likely to be as effective as the intravenous route (and with fewer potential complications). However, as with much of medicine, this decision must be made in the absence of data to support or refute it.

Duration of Therapy

The optimal duration of therapy is likewise unknown, but it is certainly influenced by several factors, including the etiologic agent and its antimicrobial susceptibility, the joint involved (and whether there is concomitant osteomyelitis), the initial response to therapy, and the immune status of the host.[118] For example, infections caused by S. aureus, those involving the hip or shoulder, or those occurring in an immunocompromised host (including a neonate) should probably be treated for a minimum of 3–4 weeks, occasionally longer. Infections of joints other than the hip or shoulder caused by susceptible strains of H. influenzae, S. pneumoniae, Group A streptococcus, Kingella, or Neisseria species can often be effectively treated with 2–3 weeks of therapy.

Other Therapy

Adequate pain control is often neglected. Intravenous narcotic analgesics are appropriate initially. Traction is often necessary to relieve the pain of muscle spasms, to decrease intra-articular pressure, and to prevent contractures. The more proximal the joint, the more likely traction is to be of value.

Crutches should be used to avoid weight-bearing after septic arthritis of the hip for several weeks after discharge from the hospital. Children may not understand or obey such instructions, and special supervision is often necessary. The physician should always keep in mind the adverse psychologic effects in children of restraints, immobilization, and parental separation. Special attention to the unexpressed needs and fears of the young inarticulate child is especially important.

Prognosis

Sequelae of septic arthritis have been reported to occur in 8–25% of children and include abnormal growth, poor joint mobility, and unstable articulation.[4,101,119] Risk factors for sequelae include age less than 6 months, infection involving the hip or shoulder, concomitant osteomyelitis, infection with

> **BOX 16-2 ■ Classification of Osteomyelitis**
>
> **Hematogenous**
> Acute
> Subacute
>
> **Nonhematogenous**
> Traumatic
> Postoperative
> Secondary to adjacent infection
>
> **Special Situations**
> Chronic
> Multifocal
> Chronic recurrent multifocal osteomyelitis
> Unusual microorganisms
> Unusual bones
> Culture-negative
> Immunocompromised host

S. aureus, and most importantly, delay in surgical drainage.[4]

■ OSTEOMYELITIS

Osteomyelitis is defined as an infection in a bone. When not further modified, the term osteomyelitis usually means acute hematogenous osteomyelitis in a long bone, as this is the common clinical pattern in children. However, osteomyelitis can also be subacute or chronic. Osteomyelitis can involve a variety of bones and organisms, and special cases can be identified that differ from the classic pattern (Box 16-2).

Common Clinical Patterns

Acute Hematogenous Osteomyelitis

The classic presentation of a child with acute hematogenous osteomyelitis is that of high fever and focal pain with marked redness, swelling, and tenderness, along with an elevated white blood cell count. Unfortunately, this pattern is evident in less than half of cases by the time of presentation, and the soft-tissue changes described previously are usually late findings.[120–124] The most common site of involvement is the region of the knee (distal femur and proximal tibia), and thus most children present with limp or refusal to bear weight. Pain is usually constant. The level of pain may fluctuate, but it does not usually disappear.[124a] Fever, although common, is not universal, and in one recent large series occurred in less than half of children.[123] Con-

sistent across series is a male-to-female ratio of nearly 2:1.[120,121–124] One-third of cases occur in the first 2 years of life and more than half in the first 5 years.[124] The median time to presentation is 3 days.[123] A history of minor trauma to the affected site is common, occurring in about one-third of cases and frequently distracts the physician into suspecting a noninfectious etiology.[120,125]

On physical examination, swelling is present in about half of cases, erythema in about one-third, and warmth in about one-quarter.[122,123] If sought carefully, point tenderness can be elicited in over three-fourths of patients.[123] However, it is sometimes difficult to detect the site of bony involvement in the young child. A toddler who refuses to bear weight may have pain anywhere from the spine to the foot. If the child had previously been walking but will now only crawl, the pain is likely below the knee.

It is important to remember that the white blood cell count is normal in the majority of children with acute hematogenous osteomyelitis.[121–123] The ESR, however, is typically elevated unless the child presents within the first couple days of illness.[124] The ESR typically peaks between 3 to 5 days after onset; in contrast, the peak CRP value is reached on day 2.[126]

The importance of establishing an etiologic diagnosis cannot be overemphasized. Blood cultures are positive in about one-third of cases, although the yield is lower if the child has recently received antibiotics.[123] Culture of bone (either by needle aspirate or from a surgical specimen) has a higher yield, with about 75% being positive.[121–123] *S. aureus* is by far the most common cause.[120–124]

Subacute Hematogenous Osteomyelitis

The term "Brodie abscess" is sometimes used to describe a minimally symptomatic pyogenic abscess of a bone. Fever is almost always absent or low-grade. Symptoms, such as pain, swelling, or limp, cause little functional impairment and are usually present for at least 2 weeks before presentation.[127] The fever and symptoms may also be modified by analgesic agents, particularly nonsteroidal anti-inflammatory drugs, such as ibuprofen, which can profoundly suppress inflammation and pain. In some patients, the infection becomes localized without antibiotic therapy. Radiologic studies are nonspecific, and a bone tumor is often the initial diagnosis.[128,129] The diagnosis is made by histologic examination of a bone biopsy specimen.[127]

This subacute presentation occurs in 10–30% of cases of hematogenous osteomyelitis.[123,128,130] Compared with the acute form, bone cultures are less frequently positive (about 30%) and blood cultures are nearly always negative.[127,129] However, when an etiologic agent is identified it is usually *S. aureus*.[127,129] Treatment should be vigorous, just as for the acute-onset type, although surgical debridement is less often needed.[131] Subacute hematogenous osteomyelitis appears to have become more common in recent years, in part related to the use of antibiotics without recognition of the source of fever.

Primary Chronic Osteomyelitis

Chronic osteomyelitis may be classified as primary or secondary. Intracellular bacteria, fungi, or mycobacteria are the usual causes of primary chronic osteomyelitis, if there has been no preceding antibiotic therapy. Cat scratch disease is occasionally associated with osteolytic bone lesions and should especially be considered in the child with cat exposure and regional adenopathy.[132]

Tuberculosis can be a cause of osteomyelitis, particularly of the vertebra or phalanges.[133] In any case of subacute or chronic osteomyelitis of unknown cause, a tuberculin skin test and chest roentgenogram should be done to look for evidence of tuberculosis. Taking a thorough history of possible exposures is also important, because there is often no evidence of pulmonary involvement to make the clinician suspect tuberculosis.[134] Actinomycosis, blastomycosis, cryptococcosis, coccidioidomycosis, sporotrichosis, brucellosis, and nontuberculous mycobacteria can also cause a chronic granulomatous osteomyelitis.[135–137] *Aspergillus* osteomyelitis should raise suspicion of chronic granulomatous disease (discussed later).[138] Occasionally, *Candida* is a cause in a neonate or other immunocompromised host.[139,140] For each of these causes, biopsy of bone is critical for histologic and microbiologic diagnosis.

Secondary Chronic Osteomyelitis

Secondary chronic osteomyelitis occurs as a complication of previous acute hematogenous or traumatic osteomyelitis. Less than 5% of children with acute hematogenous osteomyelitis typically develop chronic infection, although this number is higher if therapy is partial or incomplete or if a piece of dead bone (sequestrum) has not been removed. *S. aureus* is the most common cause, although cultures are often negative.

A Brodie abscess is often mistaken for a tumor or cyst because of the lack of fever, relief of pain by anti-inflammatory agents, location in the diaphysis, and atypical radiologic appearance.[141] Hence, it is important to get a culture of the operative specimen even when chronic osteomyelitis is not suspected, because frozen sections can be misread. More commonly, chronic osteomyelitis is secondary to previous trauma. Infections are often polymicrobial, with gram-negative organisms and anaerobes predominating.[58] Symptoms include ongoing pain, limitation of activity, and, often, draining fistulous tracts. Eradicating infection is difficult because of poor penetration of antibiotics into avascular, necrotic areas of bone.

Effective treatment of chronic osteomyelitis usually requires wide excision of dead bone and prolonged antimicrobial therapy.[142] Bony defects may require bone grafting, placement of antibiotic beads, and application of a local muscle flap.[143,144] Duration of antibiotic therapy is dictated by clinical and radiographic response but is usually a minimum of 8 weeks and sometimes several months. CT is usually the imaging modality of choice in these patients, because it is useful for demonstrating the development of sequestra, sinus tracts, and cortical destruction.[145,146] The presence of an internal fixation device makes eradication of infection difficult, but occasionally infection can be cured without hardware removal.[147]

Mechanisms and Age Factors

Acute hematogenous osteomyelitis can occur in any bone, but the usual sites are the long bones (femur, tibia, and humerus) near either end (metaphyses), where the blood supply is greatest (Fig. 16-3).[148] As blood slows to pass through the tiny blood vessels that form the metaphyseal loops, bacteria present in the blood begin to replicate. A local inflammatory response within the marrow ensues, increasing pressure within the metaphysis, and allowing pus to perforate through the cortex and lift up the periosteum. The increased local pressure may compromise the vascular supply to the cortex, leading to an area of dead bone (sequestrum). Within 10–14 days, new bone is formed over the area, producing an involucrum.[58] The blood supply

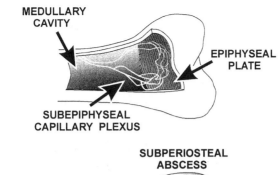

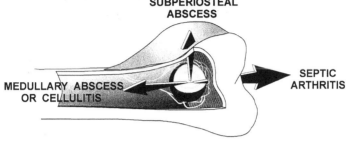

■ **FIGURE 16-3** Acute hematogenous osteomyelitis can occur in any bone, but the usual sites are the long bones (femur, tibia, and humerus) near either end (metaphyses), where the blood supply is greatest.

differs with age and influences the clinical pattern, as described next.

Infantile Form

In children younger than ages 12–18 months, transphyseal vessels are present. They arise in the metaphyseal loops and cross the growth plates into the epiphysis. Thus, infection can spread directly into the epiphyses and from there through epiphyseal vessels into the joint.[118] In addition, the metaphyses of some joints, such as the hip and shoulder, lie within the joint capsule, and the thin infantile periosteum allows rupture of a subperiosteal abscess directly into the joint space. These two mechanisms explain the higher rate of concomitant septic arthritis in young infants with osteomyelitis.[30] In addition, epiphyseal growth centers may be damaged, with shortening of a limb, if a long bone is involved.

Neonatal Form

In the first month of life, osteomyelitis has many of the characteristics of the infantile form, particularly invasion of the joints with the potential for residual deformity. The rate of joint involvement has ranged from 25–75% in various studies.[149–151] Special features of neonatal osteomyelitis include the involvement of the facial bones (especially the maxilla),

involvement of the proximal humerus (presumably secondary to birth trauma), and the frequent infection of multiple bones.[149,151] Whereas multiple foci are involved in only about 5% of cases in older children,[121,122] this occurs in more than one-third of neonatal cases.[149,150] Most cases are the result of hematogenous dissemination, but direct inoculation and extension of infection from surrounding soft tissue can occur.[149] Direct inoculation may occur secondary to intrauterine fetal monitoring electrodes,[152] femoral venipuncture,[153] or heel puncture.[154] Rarely, an infected cephalohematoma can progress to involve the adjacent skull bones.[155]

The onset is typically subtle, with swelling or decreased motion; fever and leukocytosis are often absent.[149,150] In some premature infants, the presence of septicemia is clinically evident, but the involvement of the skeleton is not, emphasizing the importance of a careful daily physical examination. As with neonatal septic arthritis, risk factors include prematurity and umbilical artery catheterization.[26,150] S. aureus accounts for over half of cases, with Group B streptococcus and enteric gram-negative rods the next most frequent cause.[149]

A bone scan may detect clinically unrecognized foci of bony involvement, although the sensitivity of bone scan in neonates (about 85%) is slightly lower than in older children.[99,150] Ultrasound can be used to detect effusions in adjacent joints, which should be drained promptly. Drilling or windowing the bone is usually not necessary in newborns.

Childhood Form

This type occurs in patients about 1 year of age to puberty. By 12–18 months of age the transphyseal vessels are obliterated, and thus infection is usually localized to the metaphysis and does not spread to the epiphysis. Consequently, damage to the growth cartilage is uncommon. In the past, the incidence of concomitant septic arthritis has been about 15%, much lower than the rate in neonates and young infants.[124] However, a recent study of 66 children with osteomyelitis found no difference in the rate of septic arthritis based on age.[156] In that study, 16 (31%) of 52 children older than 18 months had involvement of the adjacent joint, most commonly the knee.

Adult Form

Acute hematogenous osteomyelitis after the age of 16 years is uncommon.[130] However, when it does occur, chronic infection is more likely to result. Osteomyelitis in adults is more often secondary to a local injury or due to vascular insufficiency (e.g., diabetes), when it usually occurs in the feet.[157]

Specific Bones

Long Bones

The patterns described previously for hematogenous osteomyelitis are typical for long bones. The femur or tibia is involved in greater than 50% of cases. In most series, the next most commonly involved bones are the humerus, fibula, radius, and ulna.[120–123] The diagnosis may be more difficult when the area of osteomyelitis is not, as usual, in the metaphysis but rather in the diaphysis (center) or epiphysis (end) of the long bone.[158,159] Osteomyelitis of the femoral neck can also be difficult to diagnose because it may resemble arthritis of the hip, with negative findings in the joint. It can lead to severe hip-joint complications as a result of interruption of the blood supply to the femoral head or penetration into the joint.[160]

Foot

The foot is uncommonly involved in acute hematogenous osteomyelitis, although in one recent series the calcaneus was affected more frequently than the humerus.[123] More typically, osteomyelitis of the foot occurs secondary to a puncture wound, as described later.[161]

Pelvis

Although uncommon, pelvic osteomyelitis is not rare, accounting for 5–10% of cases in most series.[121–124] The ilium, ischium, or pubis may be involved.[162] Pain is a common manifestation, but it may be poorly localized, and an intra-abdominal source may be considered initially. The most common admitting diagnosis is presumed septic arthritis of the hip.[162]

Unfortunately, the sensitivity of bone scan is somewhat lower than for other sites, especially early in the course. In one series, the bone scan was positive in 17 (68%) of 25 children with pelvic osteomyelitis.[162] MRI may have greater sensitivity for diagnosing osteomyelitis of the pelvis.[163] In our experience, several studies (bone scan, CT, and MRI) are sometimes needed to confirm the diagnosis, and imaging should be repeated if pelvic osteomyelitis is still suspected despite negative studies early in the diagnostic evaluation.

Vertebrae

In children, infection of the vertebral body is quite uncommon, accounting for about 2% of cases of osteomyelitis.[121,124] Infection of the intervertebral disk ("diskitis") is more common and is covered in a separate section at the end of this chapter.

Bacteremia results in localization at the anterior part of the vertebral body, at the greatest distance from the nutrient artery (and the spinal cord), and spread can occur anteriorly, lifting up the anterior longitudinal ligament, and through the disk to the adjacent vertebrae.[164]

Children usually have fever and back or neck pain, which may be constant or intermittent. Sometimes symptoms are present for several days or weeks prior to diagnosis.[165] As with pelvic osteomyelitis, bone scan is relatively insensitive, and MRI is the diagnostic study of choice, demonstrating high signal intensity within the vertebral body on T2-weighted images.[99,165,166] It can also demonstrate the presence of disk space involvement as well as soft tissue extension in the form of paravertebral or epidural abscess.[166]

S. aureus is the most common cause, but other organisms, including *Bartonella henselae* (the agent of cat scratch disease), are occasionally implicated.[132,165] In children, usually no predisposing factor is found. Adults will often have one or more predisposing conditions, such as intravenous drug use, diabetes mellitus, or preceding bacteremia. Unusual organisms, especially *Mycobacterium tuberculosis* and *Brucella* species, are also more common in adults.[167]

Fingers

Pyogenic osteomyelitis occurs as a complication in many fingertip abscesses (felons), usually secondary to trauma.[168] Nail biting and atopic dermatitis have also been reported as predisposing conditions.[169,170] Osteomyelitis of a phalanx without an adjacent infection may be due to tuberculosis.[171]

Clavicle

The clavicle is occasionally the site of infection, accounting for about 2% of bone infections.[122,123] The process may present acutely or subacutely and is frequently confused with a fracture or malignancy.[172] Occasionally, a risk factor is found, such as trauma,[173] recent clavicular fracture,[174] or an infected central venous line.[175,176] Subsequent pathologic fracture may occur in the infected bone.[177] The clavicle has also been described as a site of involvement with chronic recurrent multifocal osteomyelitis (discussed later).[178]

Cranium

Cranial osteomyelitis is typically an extension of malignant otitis externa in an immunocompromised host (in which case *Pseudomonas* is the usual cause) or secondary to mastoiditis or sinusitis in an adolescent (in which case *S. pneumoniae, H. influenzae*, and anaerobes are commonly implicated).[179] The patient presents with fever, intense headache, and sometimes facial swelling, often during or after a course of antibiotics for sinus infection. Bony involvement may not be detected by conventional CT, and fine cut CT with bone window settings is usually needed.[180]

Patella

Osteomyelitis of the patella is very rare, and thus, diagnosis is usually delayed. It should be considered in any child with persistent peripatellar pain and swelling as well as any child with suspected cellulitis, prepatellar bursitis, or septic arthritis of the knee that does not respond to standard therapy.[181]

Rib

Osteomyelitis of a rib is also rare and may be caused by bacteria, fungi, or mycobacteria. Chest pain, swelling, and fever are usually present, often for several weeks before diagnosis.[182] Although antimicrobial therapy is also effective, excision of the rib cures the osteomyelitis and provides material to exclude Ewing sarcoma or other tumor.[183]

Possible Infectious Etiologies

Acute or Subacute Osteomyelitis

In acute or subacute hematogenous osteomyelitis, *S. aureus* is the most common organism in children of all ages, accounting for 50–75% of cases.[120–124] In most series, Group A streptococcus is second in frequency.[120,121,124] Among neonates, Group B streptococcus is the second most common cause, followed by gram-negative enteric organisms.[149] *S. pneumoniae* is an occasional cause of osteomyelitis.[184] *Salmonella* should be suspected in the child with sickle cell anemia (discussed later). Whether coagulase-negative staphylococcus can cause hematogenous osteomyelitis is controversial. In most instances, isolation of this organism from bone cultures probably represents contamination from skin flora. However, recovery of the same strain of coagulase-negative staphylococcus from multiple cultures or from both bone and blood may indicate an etiologic role.[124]

In osteomyelitis secondary to a penetrating injury, an operation, or a compound fracture, *S. aureus* is still the most common organism.[185] However, in this instance, coagulase-negative staphylococci can certainly play a role, particularly if foreign material is in place. *Pseudomonas, E. coli, Enterobacter*, and other enteric organisms have also been implicated.[185] Polymicrobial infection is common in this setting. Anaerobic osteomyelitis typically has predisposing factors, such as trauma or chronic skin, sinus, or mastoid infections.[186] Fungi are commonly cultured in the setting of compound fractures that are grossly contaminated with soil, but their significance depends upon demonstration of invasion or repeatedly positive cultures inpatients undergoing serial debridement.

Chronic Osteomyelitis

The common etiologies depend on whether the infection is primary or secondary, as discussed in previous sections.

Infections Resembling Osteomyelitis

Cellulitis

Severe cellulitis of an extremity is often a manifestation of underlying osteomyelitis (Fig. 16-4). Although the two may be difficult to differentiate, with osteomyelitis the swelling is usually more circumferential and the margins of the erythema less distinct. Cellulitis is more likely to occur in the area of a local wound, whereas no wound is typically present in osteomyelitis, because the mechanism is hematogenous seeding. If a bone scan is done, the initial blood flow images will show a generalized increase in radiotracer uptake in the affected soft tissue. Adjacent bone may also demonstrate mild

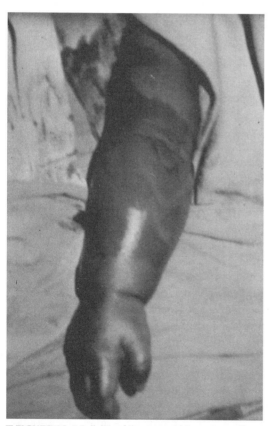

■ FIGURE 16-4 Cellulitis of the arm, which was a manifestation of underlying osteomyelitis of the radius. (Photo from Dr. Dennis Lyne.)

diffuse increased uptake secondary to hyperemia. However, in the case of cellulitis no abnormal uptake in bone is identified on the delayed phase.[187] If cellulitis of an extremity does not show significant improvement within 24 hours of antimicrobial therapy, or if bony tenderness is present, a presumptive diagnosis of osteomyelitis should be made, and bone aspiration or open drainage should be performed.

Soft-Tissue Abscess

A soft-tissue abscess should be drained, and antibiotics should be administered based on Gram stain and culture results. If the infection fails to respond to these measures after 2–3 days, underlying bone infection should be considered, especially in an extremity.

Septic Arthritis

As already mentioned, septic arthritis is a possible complication of osteomyelitis.[156] It is especially a concern in the hip but may also occur in the knee, shoulder, or ankle. The ESR is usually higher and remains elevated longer if a joint becomes involved.[188] The possibility of concomitant septic arthritis can be detected even more quickly by monitoring CRP. In one study of 46 children with osteomyelitis, the CRP returned to normal an average of 6 days after starting therapy in children without septic arthritis compared with 11 days in the children with septic arthritis.[189]

Muscle Abscess (Pyomyositis)

Pyomyositis is more common in tropical countries but also occasionally occurs in temperate climates. Deep muscles of the hip and thigh are the most common sites, and a history of trauma or vigorous exercise can be elicited about 25% of the time.[190,191] Fever, pain, and limp are present in most children, mimicking septic arthritis and pelvic osteomyelitis. Sometimes an intra-abdominal process is suspected.[190] S. aureus is the most common cause, accounting for about 75% of culture-positive cases, followed in frequency by Group A streptococcus.[190,191] Although gallium scan is able to detect muscle abscess with good sensitivity,[192] MRI has become the imaging modality of choice in recent years.[187,190,191] In addition to the increased signal intensity in muscle on T2-weighted images, reactive inflammatory changes are often seen in adjacent bone.[187] This does not usually indicate the presence of bone involvement, although occasionally an associated osteomyelitis can be found if the bone is aspirated.[190]

Management of pyomyositis depends on how early in the process the diagnosis is made. If there is not yet a discrete abscess, but only diffuse inflammation of the muscle (phlegmon), antibiotics alone are likely to be sufficient. If an abscess has formed, either percutaneous or surgical drainage will usually be required for cure. Antistaphylococcal antibiotics are usually given for 3–4 weeks.

Wound Infection

A purulent operative or traumatic wound infection, especially in an extremity, may resemble osteomyelitis. Unfortunately, children who sustain open fractures are susceptible to developing osteomyelitis, and distinguishing bone infection from soft tissue infection can be extremely difficult. As discussed later in the section on traumatic osteomyelitis, if this diagnosis is suspected, bone biopsy is required to identify the organism and confirm the diagnosis.

Congenital Syphilis

In infants in the first few months of life, congenital syphilis may resemble osteomyelitis (see Chapter 19). Metaphyseal abnormalities are present in greater than 90% of infants with symptomatic congenital syphilis and in up to 20% of those with asymptomatic disease.[193] The infant may have fever, decreased spontaneous movement, and swelling of the involved extremity, with radiographic evidence of bony destruction.[194] Syphilis results in an obliterative vasculitis with decreased blood flow to the bone and, as a result, radioactive tracer does not accumulate at the site of syphilic osseus lesions.[195,196] Congenital syphilis should therefore be considered in the young infant with clinically suspected osteomyelitis but a normal bone scan.

Other Congenital Infections

Rubella and cytomegalovirus can produce bone changes resembling osteomyelitis after congenital infection. Typically, radiolucencies are seen in the metaphysis. These are caused by abnormal growth rather than by destruction from infection.

Noninfectious Differential Diagnosis

Bone Infarction

This is covered in the subsequent section on osteomyelitis in children with sickle-cell disease.

Bone Injury

Often, a history of trauma cannot be elicited from a child, so that a subperiosteal hematoma, traumatic periostitis, or occult fracture may be mistaken for acute osteomyelitis.[197] Bone scan in a child with an extremity fracture usually shows subtle uniform increased uptake along the entire length of the bone as compared with much more focal uptake in acute osteomyelitis.[198]

Preceding trauma in an area that develops osteomyelitis is quite common; such a history is present in about one-third of cases. Usually, fever and local erythema are the first clues that the persistently painful area is infected.

Bone Cyst

A bone cyst may resemble a Brodie abscess clinically and radiographically. Most unicameral bone cysts are asymptomatic until diagnosis, which usually follows a pathologic fracture. In contrast, aneurysmal bone cysts are expansile lesions that typically cause pain and swelling. Histologic examination of material obtained at biopsy can distinguish between different types of cysts, infection, and tumors.

Tumor

Some bone tumors, such as Ewing sarcoma, may produce a clinical picture resembling that of subacute or chronic osteomyelitis.[89] Osteoid osteoma, a benign bone tumor, produces gradually increasing pain that is usually relieved by aspirin.[199] Eosinophilic granuloma is a form of Langerhans' cell histiocytosis without extraskeletal involvement. The skull is the most common site, but any bone can be affected, and the presentation may be indistinguishable from a Brodie abscess.[200] Patients with subacute or chronic osteomyelitis can have eosinophils on frozen section, which may be mistaken for an eosinophilic bone cyst and thus not cultured. For all these conditions, definitive diagnosis requires a biopsy with culture.

Acute Leukemia

Fever, bone pain, elevated ESR, and relatively acute onset can occur in acute childhood leukemia. In one series, 22 (21%) of 107 children with acute leukemia presented with orthopedic complaints.[201] The bone scan usually shows localized intense uptake in one or several metaphyses and diaphyses but may instead show "cold" areas.[202–204] The presence of anemia, thrombocytopenia, or liver or spleen enlargement may be clues to the diagnosis and would provide an indication for bone marrow aspiration.

Infantile Cortical Hyperostosis

Also called Caffey's disease, this rare disorder of unknown cause can produce fever, swelling, and periosteal elevation—especially in the mandible—that can be mistaken for acute osteomyelitis.[205]

Garre Sclerosing Osteomyelitis

Also known as "chronic nonsuppurative sclerosing osteomyelitis" or "proliferative periostitis," this condition is characterized by localized swelling of a bone, often the mandible, that may or may not be tender. Fever, leukocytosis, and elevated ESR are not usually present. Dental infection or trauma may be inciting stimuli, but bone cultures are usually negative. Histologically, there are supracortical foci of reactive bone formation with pronounced osteoblastic activity. In the case of mandibular involvement, the patient should be referred to an oral surgeon.[206]

Diagnostic Plan

Acute or subacute hematogenous osteomyelitis is suspected based on the history and physical examination and confirmed by aspiration or biopsy of bone. However, other tests can be helpful in limiting the diagnostic possibilities or in recovering the etiologic agent. The usefulness of imaging studies depends on the child's presentation. In the child with classic acute hematogenous osteomyelitis of a long bone, no imaging studies are usually necessary, and immediate bone aspiration is appropriate. In more complex cases, imaging studies can be useful, as discussed later.

Blood Culture

About a third of patients will have positive blood cultures. Before starting therapy for presumed cellulitis, at least one and preferably two blood cultures should be obtained. If osteomyelitis is suspected, bone aspirate or biopsy should also be performed and material sent for culture.

Laboratory Tests

A complete blood count should be obtained. Anemia may be a clue to malignancy masquerading as a bone infection,[89] although patients with a subacute presentation of osteomyelitis may also have significant anemia of inflammation.[207] The ESR is usually elevated and can be used to follow response to therapy, although it tends to normalize slowly. The CRP rises faster with infection, reaching a peak value by the second day of illness in children with osteomyelitis. It also reaches normal values much more quickly, usually within a week of therapy.[126] Persistent elevation of the CRP may be an indication of an undrained subperiosteal abscess or concurrent septic arthritis.[189,208] CRP levels may rise in response to any tissue injury, making interpretation difficult in the child with traumatic or postoperative osteomyelitis. However, needle aspiration or bone biopsy does not appear to affect the CRP level.[126]

Radiologic Examinations

Plain films should usually be obtained in the child with suspected osteomyelitis. Abnormalities on plain radiographs indicative of acute osteomyelitis include evidence of bone destruction and periosteal new bone formation (Figs. 16-5 and 16-6). However, these changes generally take at least 7–10 days to become apparent,[209] and thus less than one-quarter of patients have plain film findings suggestive of osteomyelitis at the time of presentation.[123] Deep soft-tissue swelling may be seen as early as 48 hours after the onset of symptoms, but this finding is not as specific for osteomyelitis as are the subsequent skeletal changes.[210] As expected, children with subacute hematogenous osteomyelitis much more frequently have radiographic changes at the time of presentation.[127] The classic Brodie abscess appears as a well-defined radiolucent lesion surrounded by a rim of dense sclerosis.[211]

Although radiographs cannot be used to exclude the possibility of acute osteomyelitis at the time of presentation, they remain useful to diagnose diseases that can be confused with osteomyelitis, such as unsuspected fracture and bone tumors. In addition, if the plain film does show findings consistent with osteomyelitis (or if clinical suspicion for osteo-

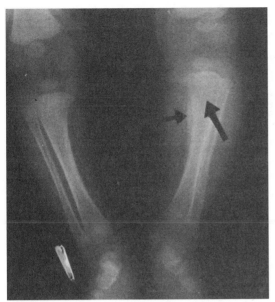

■ **FIGURE 16-5** Elevated periosteum (*short arrow*) in infant with tibial osteomyelitis caused by Group A streptococcus. Soft-tissue swelling and some radiolucency (*long arrow*) can also be seen.

myelitis is high), further imaging is unnecessary and one can proceed directly to bone aspirate or biopsy.

Bone Scans

Skeletal scintigraphy is most helpful when either the diagnosis or the location is in doubt, such as in the case of a toddler with refusal to bear weight but no localizing findings on physical examination. In such instances, bone scan can be very useful in the evaluation of acute osteomyelitis because abnormalities are demonstrated early in the course, usually at the time of initial evaluation (Fig. 16-6). Using proper technique and both early and delayed views, the examination can reliably distinguish skeletal from soft-tissue involvement.[212] Bone scan is less expensive than MRI and rarely requires sedation.[99] In addition, scintigraphy has the benefit of detecting clinically inapparent multifocal infection, which is especially common in the neonate.

Although a focal abnormality on bone scan does not distinguish between infection, trauma, or tumor, clinical and radiographic correlation will usually permit proper interpretation. Atypical patterns must be recognized, such as a "cold" area, which may be seen early and is caused by ischemia from high intramedullary pressure and decreased periosteal blood supply. In one study, 7 (9%) of

81 children with osteomyelitis had this pattern of decreased radionuclide uptake.[213] These children appeared to have a more aggressive bone infection, with higher fever and ESR on admission, as well as longer hospital stay, than children with increased tracer uptake on bone scan.

Although scintigraphy can be very helpful in detecting acute osteomyelitis, it is not perfect; both sensitivity and specificity are about 90–95% in most patients.[99,211] As with any diagnostic test in the practice of medicine, a normal study in a patient thought likely to have the diagnosis should be viewed with caution. In the case of suspected osteomyelitis, if focal erythema and tenderness are present, the bone should be aspirated. If these signs are absent, either the bone scan should be repeated or it should be supplemented with a gallium scan or, preferably, an MRI.[163,214] Note that gallium scan may be more specific than bone scan, but it is usually not more sensitive.[215] If a bone scan is negative, a gallium scan is likely to be negative also. In addition, the gallium scan requires at least 24–36 hours for an adequate study.

MRI, CT, and Ultrasound

As discussed previously, for routine acute hematogenous osteomyelitis in a long bone, these imaging studies are unnecessary. In certain anatomic sites, such as the pelvis and vertebral bodies, clinical findings may be nonspecific and bone scans may be difficult to interpret. For these areas, the sensitivity of MRI is higher.[99,166] MRI also has the advantage of detecting intramedullary and subperiosteal abscesses and thus may indicate whether surgical drainage is necessary. Although MRI is highly sensitive, its specificity is lower, as increased signal in marrow may sometimes be due to fracture, infarction, or nearby soft-tissue infection.[216] In addition, MRI is not useful for differentiating infarction from osteomyelitis in children with sickle-cell disease.[217]

CT is superior to MRI for visualizing cortical destruction, gas in the bone, and bony sequestra,[99] findings that are often indications for surgical debridement. CT is also helpful in detecting associated soft-tissue abscesses and in planning a surgical approach to debridement. In addition, CT is usually cheaper and easier to obtain on short notice. Thus, for practical reasons CT is usually obtained first and, if negative, MRI can be done. For the young child, general anesthesia may be required, and a CT-guided bone aspiration can be done at the same

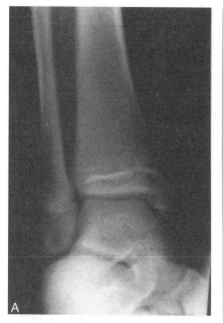

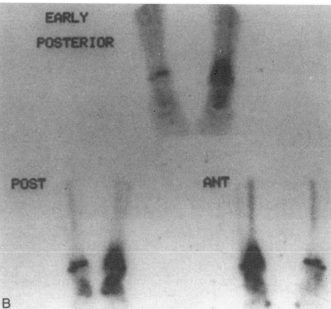

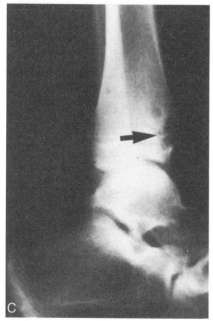

■ **FIGURE 16-6** Acute osteomyelitis of right distal tibia. (**A**) Normal roentgenogram 1 day after onset of fever. (**B**) Abnormal bone scan the same day. (**C**) Destructive bony changes apparent 12 days later. (Photo from Dr. Richard Shore.)

time. CT is also useful to follow response to therapy in cases of chronic osteomyelitis.

Ultrasound may be useful if a subperiosteal abscess is present,[218] but otherwise it is insensitive[219] and generally not used for the diagnosis of acute osteomyelitis.[99]

Bone Aspiration

Pus can often be aspirated from the center of the area of maximum erythema and tenderness. This procedure is relatively easy for superficial bones, such as the tibia, if the pus is just below the periosteum. The needle is inserted just to the outer cortex of the bone, and the subperiosteal space is aspirated. If no pus is encountered, the needle is advanced through the cortex into the medullary cavity, and the marrow is aspirated. Even if no pus is found, the marrow should be cultured, because it is often positive.[215] If an abscess is found, surgical drainage is usually indicated. It is important to note that needle aspiration does not alter the results of subsequent bone scans.[220] Thus, if osteomyelitis is suspected based on the presence of focal erythema and tenderness over the metaphysis, bone aspiration should not await the results of imaging studies.

Treatment

Antibiotics

Early antibiotic therapy is essential to prevent severe anatomic changes.[221] However, a concerted effort to obtain appropriate cultures should be undertaken before starting therapy. Two blood samples should be taken for culture, the bone should be aspirated, if possible, and intravenous antibiotics should be begun.

In the newborn, the initial treatment can be oxacillin and cefotaxime or gentamicin. In other age groups, oxacillin or cefazolin can be used. Vancomycin or, possibly, clindamycin should be considered in areas with high rates of community-acquired MRSA.[109a] Children with sickle-cell disease should receive agents to cover *Salmonella* and *S. aureus*, such as oxacillin plus ceftriaxone. Although no data are available, cefepime as a single agent would also cover these two organisms.

Most semisynthetic penicillins and cephalosporins typically used to treat osteomyelitis penetrate adequately into intramedullary pus and bone,[222] although the concentration may be less than that in joints.[116] In addition, a sequestrum or ischemic area may be poorly penetrated by antibiotics, requiring more prolonged therapy and, usually, surgical debridement. In addition to the β-lactam antibiotics, clindamycin is also effective in the treatment of osteomyelitis in children and can be used when penicillin allergy is present.[223] Clindamycin also has the advantage of excellent bone penetration.

If the osteomyelitis is secondary to a contaminated fracture or follows an operation, an antibiotic effective against *Pseudomonas* and enteric gram-negative bacteria, such as gentamicin, should be added until bone culture results are available. Empiric treatment without obtaining bone cultures in this setting is not advised, because the range of possible organisms is large, and polymicrobial infection is common.[185] If all organisms are later found to be susceptible to a single agent, such as a carbapenem, therapy can then be consolidated.[224] Antibiotics are usually given for 4 to 6 weeks, unless retained hardware is present, in which case a longer duration of therapy is necessary.

Route of Therapy

The decision of whether to use oral antibiotics is similar to the situation with septic arthritis. As with septic arthritis, initial therapy should be by the intravenous route, and an assessment of response to therapy is then made. Most experts believe that if the response to initial therapy is prompt, therapy can be switched to the oral route, particularly if serum bactericidal titers are monitored.[114] Doses used are two to three times the usual recommended oral dose. Approximately 10–15% of children do not absorb oral antibiotics sufficiently to produce a peak serum bactericidal titer of at least 1:8 and require even higher doses or the addition of probenicid to obtain adequate titers.[225] In practice, however, bactericidal titers are often not monitored.[123,226]

Serious complications, such as chronic osteomyelitis, occur in about 3–6% of children with acute osteomyelitis.[120,123,124] The difference between a 3% incidence and a 6% incidence of chronic osteomyelitis is a clinically significant one. To detect such a difference based on route of therapy with 80% power would require a sample size of 1600 children (800 in each group).[117] One recent series reported no complications among 50 children with acute osteomyelitis who were switched to oral antibiotics within 4 days of therapy and completed a mean total duration of therapy of 23 days.[226] Serum bactericidal titers were not measured. With a sample size of 50, the upper limit of the 95% confidence interval can be estimated by dividing 3 by 50, which is 6%.[227] Thus, the true rate of chronic osteomyelitis with this approach could be as high as 6%.

As with septic arthritis, if oral therapy is used it should be understood that there are no data to support or refute its being equivalent to the intravenous route. Clinical experience, though often cited as rationale for oral therapy, is of limited reassurance in this instance, because adverse outcomes are relatively uncommon with either route. If oral therapy is used, the importance of strict adherence to the regimen cannot be overemphasized. Indeed, one of the benefits of measuring serum bactericidal titers is that they are an indirect measure of both adherence and drug absorption. Adherence to prescribed medication use is generally lower than physicians believe, especially once the symptoms have subsided.[228] Many experts prefer to treat osteomyelitis with intravenous antibiotics for the duration of therapy, particularly if the child is less than age 2 years, if there is extensive bony involvement, or if the initial response to therapy is slow. A peripherally inserted central catheter (PICC) is placed, and therapy can usually be given at home. If the catheter tip is located centrally (superior vena cava or right atrium), the complication rate is less than 5%. Complications are generally not serious and include occlusion, phlebitis, leaking, and infection.[229]

Although necessary to treat the infection, prolonged administration of antibiotics (by any route) is frequently associated with side effects, such as diarrhea, neutropenia, elevated liver enzymes, and occasionally, renal insufficiency. In addition to following the patient's response to therapy with weekly ESR and CRP, tests to monitor for these side effects (CBC and serum ALT and creatinine) should be obtained weekly as well.

Development of normocytic anemia is extremely common in children with bone or joint infections. This anemia of inflammation is secondary to sequestration of iron within macrophages.[207] It is not due to iron deficiency, and iron supplementation is of no benefit. The degree of anemia can sometimes be severe, with hemoglobin levels as low as 7 g/dL.[207] However, the temptation to transfuse red blood cells should be resisted unless the child is symptomatic, which is uncommon. Treatment of the infection will result in correction of the anemia.

Duration of Therapy

In general, osteomyelitis is treated for longer than septic arthritis because of decreased penetration of antibiotics into bone. A study published in the 1970s reported a 19% treatment failure rate for cases treated for 3 weeks or less and a 2% treatment failure rate for those treated longer than 3 weeks.[130] Duration must be individualized and is based on the etiologic agent, the clinical response, and the decrease in laboratory measures of inflammation. Although the ESR and CRP can be used to follow the response to therapy, the duration of therapy should not be based on these values alone; early normalization of the values is encouraging but is not an indication for stopping therapy. We generally treat osteomyelitis due to S. aureus or gram-negative enteric bacilli for a minimum of 4–6 weeks. Other agents, such as Group A streptococcus and S. pneumoniae, can sometimes be treated for a shorter duration.

Surgical Drainage

If an abscess is found upon bone aspiration, or if there has been no response after 48 hours of antibiotic therapy, surgical drainage through the cortex should probably be done.[215] However, in infants less than 1 year of age, such drainage is sometimes not necessary, particularly if needle aspiration can be done for identification of the organism. For children of any age, if bone destruction is evident by imaging studies, surgical debridement of necrotic bone is usually necessary.

Irrigation

After open drainage, closed irrigation with an antibiotic solution is sometimes used. There is no evidence that this is necessary. Many orthopedic surgeons prefer to simply close the wound over a penrose drain, which is removed in 2–4 days.[215]

Special Situations

Osteomyelitis with Negative Cultures

Osteomyelitis with negative cultures may occur because of preceding antibiotic therapy, a fastidious organism, low inoculum, or a noninfectious cause. Treatment must be a judgment based on the most likely or most severe situation. Usually, antistaphylococcal therapy is given and the patient's response monitored closely.

Osteomyelitis in Children with Sickle Cell Disease (SCD)

Two groups of children are at particularly increased risk for osteomyelitis and deserve special mention: those with sickle cell disease and those with chronic granulomatous disease.[230] Children with SCD frequently develop bone infarction, but they also have an increased incidence of osteomyelitis.[16] In one series of 113 children, bone infarction was 60 times more common than infection.[231] Osteomyelitis and infarction can both cause swelling, tenderness, warmth, and erythema. They can both be associated with increased inflammatory markers and with fever, although the fever is more often high-grade in those with osteomyelitis.[16] Both processes usually result in an abnormal bone scan. A 24-hour observation period without antibiotic therapy can be of value to see whether the symptoms respond dramatically to hydration and analgesia. If response to therapy for presumed infarction is slow, or if the patient has high fever, elevated WBC count and focal bone pain with erythema, osteomyelitis should be suspected and the bone aspirated.

In most series, *Salmonella* is the most common agent of osteomyelitis in children with SCD,[232] although other gram-negative enteric organisms and *S. aureus* are also commonly implicated, and the relative frequency varies by location.[233] Once the diagnosis is made, management is similar to that for children without SCD. They may require a longer duration of parenteral therapy because of poorer perfusion of bone.[124a]

Pain and swelling of the hands or feet can occur in infants with SCD. This hand-foot dactylitis is usually caused by multiple small bone infarcts but can also be caused by osteomyelitis.[234]

Osteomyelitis in Children with Chronic Granulomatous Disease (CGD)

CGD is a primary immunodeficiency disease in which phagocytic cells are unable to reduce molecular oxygen and thus unable to kill certain bacteria or fungi after ingesting them (see Chapter 23). These children are particularly susceptible to infections with catalase-positive organisms. Of 368 patients with CGD in a national registry, 90 (24%) developed osteomyelitis.[235] The most common organisms responsible were *Serratia* (29%), *Aspergillus* (22%), *Paecilomyces* (8%), *S. aureus* (6%), *Nocardia* (3%), and *Burkholderia*, *Klebsiella*, and *Pseudomonas* (2% each). Infection may occur as a result of direct spread from an adjacent focus (most commonly seen with fungal or mycobacterial infection) or from hematogenous spread (usually with bacterial infection).[236] Vertebrae, ribs, and metatarsals are commonly involved bones.[236] Attempts to isolate the etiologic agent should be made vigorously. Wide operative debridement along with prolonged administration of antimicrobials is necessary to effect a cure.[236] If the child is not already receiving γ-interferon, this should be added as well.[138]

Children with other immunocompromising conditions are also at risk for osteomyelitis. Virtually any organism may be responsible, especially fungi, and unusual sites, such as the jaw, may be involved.[237–239]

Traumatic Osteomyelitis

Traumatic osteomyelitis includes osteomyelitis secondary to animal bites (commonly due to *Pasteurella multocida*),[240] needle puncture of the new-born's heel for blood tests,[154] bone-marrow aspiration,[241] puncture wounds,[242] and fractures. The incidence of infection after internal fixation of closed fractures is less than 2%, whereas the infection rate of open fractures can be higher than 30%, depending on the type of fracture.[147,243,244] The infection rate of open fractures can be decreased by 24 hours of intravenous antibiotic active against *S. aureus*. *Aeromonas* or other unusual bacteria may cause osteomyelitis in water-contaminated trauma.[245]

Children with osteomyelitis secondary to trauma (particularly open fractures) frequently present over several days to weeks with purulent discharge, sometimes accompanied by pain and swelling. Fever and erythema are usually absent, and the WBC count and ESR are often normal.[185] Because of the associated bony trauma, the bone scan is usually positive and does not assist in excluding osteomyelitis. One study found that the combination of bone scan and indium-labeled WBC scan had a sensitivity of 86% and a specificity of 84% for the diagnosis of osteomyelitis.[246] Treating empirically for osteomyelitis is not appropriate because wound cultures, including sinus tract drainage, fail to predict bone culture results 75% of the time.[185] Infection is often polymicrobial, with *S. aureus* and gram-negative enteric organisms predominating. If osteomyelitis is suspected, prompt operative bone culture is the only reliable way of making the diagnosis.

Fever to 102°F (38.8°C) commonly occurs for about 4 days during hospitalization for closed femoral-shaft fractures, presumably due to tissue injury and hematoma formation as the fracture site is healing. Usually, it begins several days after the injury, and should not, by itself, be attributed to infection.[247]

Postoperative Osteomyelitis

Postoperative osteomyelitis can follow open reduction of closed fractures, craniotomies, median sternotomies, and other operations involving bone.[248]

Osteochondritis After Nail Puncture Wounds to the Foot

Osteomyelitis of the foot most commonly occurs after a nail puncture, usually through a tennis shoe.[161] Bone and cartilage are typically both infected (osteochondritis), and associated septic arthritis occurs in about 20% of patients. Infections occurring within the first few days after a puncture wound are usually cellulitis caused by *S. aureus* or Group A streptococcus. Osteochondritis usually occurs 5–10 days after the puncture wound, and *P. aeruginosa* is the responsible organism in 95% of cases.[249] Local pain and erythema are common and may involve the dorsum of the foot. Fever and leukocytosis are typically absent, although the ESR is often modestly elevated.[161] Plain films are most often normal, but bone scans are usually positive (Fig. 16-7).[161]

The primary management is surgical, with thorough debridement of infected bone and cartilage via a dorsal incision. Antibiotics are very unlikely to cure the infection without surgical intervention. The vast majority of patients have complete recovery after a 7–10-day course of antipseudomonal therapy following aggressive surgical debridement.[161] There is no evidence that administration of prophylactic antibiotics (even those with antipseudomonal activity) at the time of a nail puncture wound prevents subsequent osteochondritis. In one retrospective study, patients receiving prophylactic antibiotics had a higher incidence of *Pseudomonas osteochondritis*.[249]

Multifocal Osteomyelitis

As discussed previously, multifocal osteomyelitis is often seen in neonates, occurring in at least one-third of cases.[149] Osteomyelitis occurring postoperatively or in injection drug users is also frequently multifocal. Multiple foci of increased uptake on bone scan can also represent malignancy.

Chronic Recurrent Multifocal Osteomyelitis (CRMO)

This condition is an inflammatory bone disease of unknown etiology, usually occurring in children and characterized by exacerbations and spontaneous remissions. Bone pain is the presenting symptom, and almost all patients have more than one focus over time.[250] Fever occurs in about one-third of episodes, and the ESR is often elevated during exacerbations but not usually as high as in acute hematogenous osteomyelitis. The tibia, femur, clavicles, feet, and vertebral bodies are the sites most commonly affected. Females are affected nearly twice as often as males.[251]

About one-third of children have associated extraosseous conditions, especially palmo-plantar

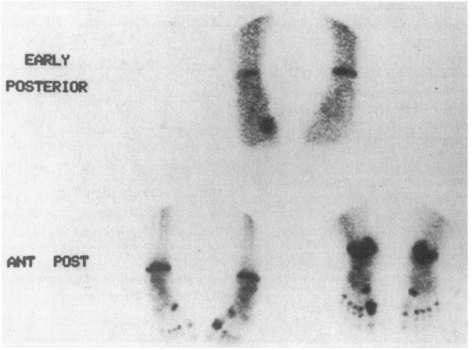

■ **FIGURE 16-7** Bone scan of both feet showing increased uptake at the left first metatarsal-intraphalangeal joint and osteomyelitis on each side of the joint after an 11-year-old boy stepped on a nail that penetrated his tennis shoe. (Photo from Dr. Richard Shore.)

pustulosis. Some children have a constellation of findings described by the acronym SAPHO syndrome (synovitis, acne, pustulosis, hyperostosis, and osteitis).[252,253] Inflammatory bowel disease, psoriasis, pyoderma gangrenosum, and Sweet syndrome have also been described in children with CRMO.[250,254,255] Histologic features include acute and chronic inflammation with occasional areas of necrosis.[250,251] However, cultures are sterile, and there is no response to antimicrobial therapy. Most children respond to nonsteroidal anti-inflammatory agents, and the long-term prognosis is good, although exacerbations may continue to occur for years.

■ DISKITIS

Definitions

Narrowing of the disk space without evidence of herniation of the disk is called diskitis (or discitis). Spondylitis is an obsolete term used primarily for vertebral body osteomyelitis (which was called Pott's disease when it was almost invariably secondary to tuberculosis).

Early publications did not often distinguish between infection of the vertebral body and that of the intervertebral disk space, although the age distribution, pathogenesis, causes, and prognosis differ. The vertebral blood supply undergoes involution from richly anastomotic intraosseus arteries in the young child to end-arteries in the adolescent and adult.[256] The disk itself is avascular at all ages and is probably a bystander in the disease process, which occurs at the disk-vertebral interface. Diskitis is more common in young children (median age, 20 months), and vertebral osteomyelitis is more common in older children and adults.[165] It is hypothesized that a septic embolus in the young child with abundant anastomoses leads to a small infarction and a lower likelihood of vertebral body involvement than seen in adults with vertebral osteomyelitis.[256]

The third to fifth lumbar disks are most frequently involved.[257] Cultures of the disk space are usually negative,[165,258] but they occasionally reveal *S. aureus* or, less commonly, other pathogens.[256,259] Even in culture-positive cases, the outcome does not appear to be affected by antimicrobial therapy. The current belief is that diskitis is probably the result of low-grade bacterial infection with sterilization of the area via host defenses in most cases.

Diagnosis

The onset of diskitis is gradual and subtle, and the spinal column is not often suspected as the site of difficulty. Fever is usually absent or low-grade. Occasionally, an intra-abdominal source is suspected.[165] Children less than 3 years old present with irritability and limp, followed by refusal to walk, sit, or stand. The child's irritability is greater than expected for the systemic findings. Older children usually complain of back pain. As with septic arthritis and osteomyelitis, a history of preceding trauma is common.

One review of 155 cases distinguished three patterns of presenting syndromes: the back pattern, the hip-leg pattern, and the meningeal pattern.[260] The back pattern is by far the most common and presents as described previously. Motion of the pelvis or thighs, percussion of the soles of the feet, or lying prone produces discomfort. Increased lumbar lordosis is often present. The spine is often tender to direct pressure or compression (elicited by pressing on the top of the child's head). Flexing the hips fully with the child supine (to eliminate the normal lordosis) produces pain, as do pelvic tilt maneuvers.

The hip-leg pattern is defined by poorly localized pain in these areas, referred from the lumbar area. Gower sign (using hands to push on the knees to rise to a standing position) has been observed in some children with diskitis who had no muscular weakness.[261] Rarely, diskitis presents a meningeal pattern, with signs of meningeal irritation, hyperreflexia, and back pain. A spinal tumor may be suspected.

The WBC count is usually normal, but the ESR is nearly always modestly elevated.[165] Blood cultures should be obtained but are rarely positive in diskitis; a positive blood culture suggests vertebral osteomyelitis. A history of possible exposure to tuberculosis should be obtained, and tuberculin skin testing and chest roentgenography should be considered.

The first radiographic sign of diskitis is diminished width of the disk space, which takes at least 10 days to become apparent.[211] Because children often present several days after initial onset of symptoms, radiographs are abnormal at presentation in about three-fourths of patients.[165] Scintigraphic changes occur earlier than plain film findings. Bone scans show increased uptake in the disk space and the contiguous ends of the adjoining vertebrae on both the blood pool and delayed bone images.[211] However, this pattern is not specific for diskitis and is seen in vertebral osteomyelitis as well. In the child with symptoms compatible with diskitis and characteristic plain film findings, further imaging is rarely necessary. If the plain films are negative, bone scan or MRI should be considered. If vertebral osteomyelitis is suspected, MRI should be performed, because it is highly sensitive and specific for this diagnosis, demonstrating vertebral body and paravertebral soft-tissue involvement.

In the past, aspiration or biopsy of the affected disk was recommended but is now rarely done in children for whom the diagnosis of diskitis is straightforward. Aspiration can usually be reserved for the child who does not respond to initial therapy.

Differential Diagnosis

The two most important conditions to exclude in the child with suspected diskitis are vertebral osteomyelitis and spinal tumors. If the history includes sudden onset of symptoms, high fever, elevated WBC count, positive blood culture, neurologic impairment, or radiologic evidence of a paraspinous mass or vertebral lesion not adjacent to the disk, MRI is indicated.[256] Sacroiliac septic arthritis may also resemble diskitis clinically. In adolescents, Scheuermann disease (osteochondritis of the vertebral body) is a consideration.[262] Rarely, idiopathic calcification of the intervertebral disk occurs in children.[263]

Possible Etiologies

In some series, 50% or more of patients have positive cultures on disk aspiration or biopsy, but in most series the yield is much lower.[165,256,258] *S. aureus* is the most frequently identified organism. *S. epidermidis*, *S. pneumoniae*, *Moraxella*, *Salmonella*, *Proteus*, *Pseudomonas*, *Corynebacterium*, *Kingella*, and other low-virulence bacteria are occasionally cultured. Involvement of the intervertebral disk can be an early finding in spinal tuberculosis, which has become uncommon in the United States.

Treatment

Most children with diskitis are made more comfortable by immobilization of the spine. This is usually done with a rigid body cast; sometimes, a body brace can be substituted. Immobilization is usually done for 4 weeks, but shorter periods may be sufficient. Failure of immobilization to relieve discomfort suggests another diagnosis and should lead to biopsy or aspiration of the lesion.[256] Nonsteroidal anti-inflammatory agents are usually given. Although patients seem to have a satisfactory outcome even if antimicrobial therapy is withheld, most physicians treat with an antistaphylococcal antibiotic. The most cautious choice is to treat with an intravenous antibiotic for 5–7 days and then switch to an oral agent for another 7–14 days. If response to therapy is slow, vertebral osteomyelitis should be considered, biopsy should be performed, and duration of therapy should be extended. The outcome is generally good. Although narrowed disk spaces may persist, most children have no long-term functional impairment or pain.

■ REFERENCES

1. Bennett OM, Namnyak SS. Acute septic arthritis of the hip joint in infancy and childhood. Clin Orthop 1992; 281:123–32.
2. Lunseth PA, Heiple KG. Prognosis in septic arthritis of the hip in children. Clin Orthop 1979;139:81–5.
3. Morrey BF, Bianco AJ, Rhodes KH. Suppurative arthritis of the hip in children. J Bone Joint Surg Am 1976;58: 388–92.
4. Welkon CJ, Long SS, Fisher MC, et al. Pyogenic arthritis in infants and children: a review of 95 cases. Pediatr Infect Dis 1986;5:669–76.
5. Obletz B. Suppurative arthritis of the hip joint in infants. Clin Orthop 1962;22:27–33.
6. Curtiss PH, Klein L. Destruction of articular cartilage in septic arthritis. II: *In vivo* studies. J Bone Joint Surg Am 1965;47:1595–604.
7. Yagupsky P, Bar-Ziv Y, Howard CB, et al. Epidemiology, etiology, and clinical features of septic arthritis in children younger than 24 months. Arch Pediatr Adolesc Med 1995;149:537–40.
8. Howard AW, Viskontas D, Sabbagh C. Reduction in osteomyelitis and septic arthritis related to *Haemophilus influenzae* type B vaccination. J Pediatr Orthop 1999;19: 705–9.
9. Lundy DW, Kehl DK. Increasing prevalence of *Kingella kingae* in osteoarticular infections in young children. J Pediatr Orthop 1998;18:262–267.
10. Arlievsky N, Li KI, Munoz JL. Septic arthritis with osteomyelitis due to *Streptococcus pneumoniae* in human immunodeficiency virus-infected children. Clin Infect Dis 1998;27:898–9.
11. Paterson MP, Hoffman EB, Roux P. Severe disseminated staphylococcal disease associated with osteitis and septic arthritis. J Bone Joint Surg Br 1990;72:94–7.
12. Churchill MA Jr, Geraci JE, Hunder GG. Musculoskeletal manifestations of bacterial endocarditis. Ann Intern Med 1977;87:754–9.
13. Peters TR, Brumbaugh DE, Lawton AR, et al. Recurrent

pneumococcal arthritis as the presenting manifestation of X-linked agammaglobulinemia. Clin Infect Dis 2000; 31:1287–8.

14. Furr PM, Taylor-Robinson D, Webster AD. Mycoplasmas and ureaplasmas in patients with hypogammaglobulinaemia and their role in arthritis: microbiological observations over twenty years. Ann Rheum Dis 1994;53:183–7.

15. Albornoz MA, Myers AR. Recurrent septic arthritis and Milroy's disease. J Rheumatol 1988;15:1726–8.

16. Chambers JB, Forsythe DA, Bertrand SL, et al. Retrospective review of osteoarticular infections in a pediatric sickle cell age group. J Pediatr Orthop 2000;20:682–5.

17. Chen JY, Luo SF, Wu YJ, et al. *Salmonella* septic arthritis in systemic lupus erythematosus and other systemic diseases. Clin Rheumatol 1998;17:282–7.

18. Szer IS, Taylor E, Steere AC. The long-term course of Lyme arthritis in children. N Engl J Med 1991;325: 159–63.

19. Craft JE, Grodzicki RL, Steere AC. Antibody response in Lyme disease: evaluation of diagnostic tests. J Infect Dis 1984;149:789–95.

20. Steere AC. Diagnosis and treatment of Lyme arthritis. Med Clin North Am 1997;81:179–94.

21. Nocton JJ, Dressler F, Rutledge BJ, et al. Detection of *Borrelia burgdorferi* DNA by polymerase chain reaction in synovial fluid from patients with Lyme arthritis. N Engl J Med 1994;330:229–34.

22. Sigal LH. Lyme arthritis: lessons learned and to be learned. Arthritis Rheum 1999;42:1809–12.

23. Gerber MA, Zemel LS, Shapiro ED. Lyme arthritis in children: clinical epidemiology and long-term outcomes. Pediatrics 1998;102:905–8.

24. Shapiro ED, Gerber MA. Lyme disease. Clin Infect Dis 2000;31:533–42.

25. Sigal LH, Patella SJ. Lyme arthritis as the incorrect diagnosis in pediatric and adolescent fibromyalgia. Pediatrics 1992;90:523–8.

26. Frederiksen B, Christiansen P, Knudsen FU. Acute osteomyelitis and septic arthritis in the neonate, risk factors and outcome. Eur J Pediatr 1993;152:577–80.

27. McLario DJ, Burton LJ, Bruce RW, et al. Pseudoparalysis of the lower extremity in an infant. Pediatr Emerg Care 1998;14:277–9.

28. Mordehai J, Kurzbart E, Cohen E, et al. Cyanotic limb in a newborn: a peculiar presentation of septic hip. Pediatr Emerg Care 1997;13:408–9.

29. Lejman T, Strong M, Michno P. Radial-nerve palsy associated with septic shoulder in neonates. J Pediatr Orthop 1995;15:169–71.

30. Jackson MA, Burry VF, Olson LC. Pyogenic arthritis associated with adjacent osteomyelitis: identification of the sequela-prone child. Pediatr Infect Dis J 1992;11:9–13.

31. Chacha PB. Suppurative arthritis of the hip joint in infancy. A persistent diagnostic problem and possible complication of femoral venipuncture. J Bone Joint Surg Am 1971;53:538–44.

32. Sim FH, Pritchard DJ, Ivins JC, et al. Total joint arthroplasty. Applications in the management of bone tumors. Mayo Clin Proc 1979;54:583–9.

33. Klassen RA, Parlasca RJ, Bianco AJ Jr. Total joint arthroplasty. Applications in children and adolescents. Mayo Clin Proc 1979;54:579–82.

34. Inman RD, Gallegos KV, Brause BD, et al. Clinical and microbial features of prosthetic joint infection. Am J Med 1984;77:47–53.

35. Berbari EF, Hanssen AD, Duffy MC, et al. Risk factors for prosthetic joint infection: case-control study. Clin Infect Dis 1998;27:1247–54.

36. Williams RJ III, Laurencin CT, Warren RF, et al. Septic arthritis after arthroscopic anterior cruciate ligament reconstruction. Diagnosis and management. Am J Sports Med 1997;25:261–7.

37. Maltezou HC, Spyridis P, Kafetzis DA. Extra-pulmonary tuberculosis in children. Arch Dis Child 2000;83:342–6.

38. Zahraa J, Johnson D, Lim-Dunham JE, et al. Unusual features of osteoarticular tuberculosis in children. J Pediatr 1996;129:597–602.

39. Al-Matar MJ, Cabral DA, Petty RE. Isolated tuberculous monoarthritis mimicking oligoarticular juvenile rheumatoid arthritis. J Rheumatol 2001;28:204–6.

40. Jacobs JC, Li SC, Ruzal-Shapiro C, et al. Tuberculous arthritis in children. Diagnosis by needle biopsy of the synovium. Clin Pediatr (Phila) 1994;33:344–8.

41. Friedman AW, Ike RW. *Mycobacterium kansasii* septic arthritis in a patient with acquired immune deficiency syndrome. Arthritis Rheum 1993;36:1631–2.

42. Frosch M, Roth J, Ullrich K, et al. Successful treatment of *Mycobacterium avium* osteomyelitis and arthritis in a non-immunocompromised child. Scand J Infect Dis 2000;32:328–9.

43. Dan M. Neonatal septic arthritis. Isr J Med Sci 1983;19: 967–71.

44. Murphy O, Gray J, Wagget J, et al. *Candida* arthritis complicating long term total parenteral nutrition. Pediatr Infect Dis J 1997;16:329.

45. Swanson H, Hughes PA, Messer SA, et al. *Candida albicans* arthritis one year after successful treatment of fungemia in a healthy infant. J Pediatr 1996;129:688–94.

46. Fainstein V, Gilmore C, Hopfer RL, et al. Septic arthritis due to Candida species on patients with cancer: report of five cases and review of the literature. Rev Infect Dis 1982;4:78–85.

47. Darouiche RO, Cadle RM, Zenon GJ, et al. Articular histoplasmosis. J Rheumatol 1992;19:1991–3.

48. Abril A, Campbell MD, Cotten VR Jr, et al. Polyarticular blastomycotic arthritis. J Rheumatol 1998;25:1019–1.

49. Stead KJ, Klugman KP, Painter ML, et al. Septic arthritis due to *Cryptococcus neoformans*. J Infect 1988;17:139–45.

50. Holt CD, Winston DJ, Kubak B, et al. Coccidioidomycosis in liver transplant patients. Clin Infect Dis 1997;24: 216–21.

51. Schwartz DA. *Sporothrix* tenosynovitis—differential diagnosis of granulomatous inflammatory disease of the joints. J Rheumatol 1989;16:550–3.

52. Gunsilius E, Lass-Florl C, Mur E, et al. *Aspergillus* osteoarthritis in acute lymphoblastic leukemia. Ann Hematol 1999;78:529–30.

53. Rosenthal J, Brandt KD, Wheat LJ, et al. Rheumatologic manifestations of histoplasmosis in the recent Indianapolis epidemic. Arthritis Rheum 1983;26:1065–70.

54. Nocton JJ, Miller LC, Tucker LB, et al. Human parvovirus B19-associated arthritis in children. J Pediatr 1993;122: 186–90.

55. Kaye BR. Rheumatologic manifestations of infection with

human immunodeficiency virus (HIV). Ann Intern Med 1989;111:158–67.

56. Berman A, Cahn P, Perez H, et al. Human immunodeficiency virus infection associated arthritis: clinical characteristics. J Rheumatol 1999;26:1158–62.

57. Tingle AJ, Allen M, Petty RE, et al. Rubella-associated arthritis. I. Comparative study of joint manifestations associated with natural rubella infection and RA 27/3 rubella immunisation. Ann Rheum Dis 1986;45:110–4.

58. Sonnen GM, Henry NK. Pediatric bone and joint infections. Diagnosis and antimicrobial management. Pediatr Clin North Am 1996;43:933–47.

59. Fischer SU, Beattie TF. The limping child: epidemiology, assessment and outcome. J Bone Joint Surg Br 1999;81: 1029–34.

60. Kocher MS, Zurakowski D, Kasser JR. Differentiating between septic arthritis and transient synovitis of the hip in children: an evidence-based clinical prediction algorithm. J Bone Joint Surg Am 1999;81:1662–70.

61. Beach R. Minimally invasive approach to management of irritable hip in children. Lancet 2000;355:1202–3.

62. Eich GF, Superti-Furga A, Umbricht FS, et al. The painful hip: evaluation of criteria for clinical decision-making. Eur J Pediatr 1999;158:923–8.

63. Meyers S, Lonon W, Shannon K. Suppurative bursitis in early childhood. Pediatr Infect Dis 1984;3:156–8.

64. Hughes RA, Keat AC. Reiter's syndrome and reactive arthritis: a current view. Semin Arthritis Rheum 1994;24: 190–210.

65. Schumacher HR Jr, Gerard HC, Arayssi TK, et al. Lower prevalence of *Chlamydia pneumoniae* DNA compared with *Chlamydia trachomatis* DNA in synovial tissue of arthritis patients. Arthritis Rheum 1999;42:1889–93.

66. Branigan PJ, Gerard HC, Hudson AP, et al. Comparison of synovial tissue and synovial fluid as the source of nucleic acids for detection of *Chlamydia trachomatis* by polymerase chain reaction. Arthritis Rheum 1996;39: 1740–46.

67. Schumacher HR Jr, Arayssi T, Crane M, et al. *Chlamydia trachomatis* nucleic acids can be found in the synovium of some asymptomatic subjects. Arthritis Rheum 1999; 42:1281–4.

68. Mader R, Zu'bi A, Schonfeld S. Recurrent sterile arthritis following primary septic meningococcal arthritis. Clin Exp Rheumatol 1994;12:531–3.

69. Feder HM Jr, Lawrence C. Group A streptococcal multifocal septic arthritis: a case report. Clin Pediatr (Phila) 1999;38:481–3.

70. Ahmed S, Ayoub EM, Scornik JC, et al. Poststreptococcal reactive arthritis: clinical characteristics and association with HLA-DR alleles. Arthritis Rheum 1998;41: 1096–102.

71. Adachi JA, D'Alessio FR, Ericsson CD. Reactive arthritis associated with typhoid vaccination in travelers: report of two cases with negative HLA-B27. J Travel Med 2000; 7:35–6.

72. Maillefert JF, Tonolli-Serabian I, Cherasse A, et al. Arthritis following combined vaccine against diphtheria, polyomyelitis, and tetanus toxoid. Clin Exp Rheumatol 2000; 18:255–6.

73. Maillefert JF, Sibilia J, Toussirot E, et al. Rheumatic disorders developed after hepatitis B vaccination. Rheumatology (Oxford) 1999;38:978–3.

74. Ferrazzi V, Jorgensen C, Sany J. Inflammatory joint disease after immunizations. A report of two cases. Rev Rheum Engl Ed 1997;64:227–32.

75. Nussinovitch M, Harel L, Varsano I. Arthritis after mumps and measles vaccination. Arch Dis Child 1995; 72:348–9.

76. Biasi D, Carletto A, Caramaschi P, et al. A case of reactive arthritis after influenza vaccination. Clin Rheumatol 1994;13:645.

77. Slater PE, Ben-Zvi T, Fogel A, et al. Absence of an association between rubella vaccination and arthritis in underimmune postpartum women. Vaccine 1995;13:1529–32.

78. Keat A. Reiter's syndrome and reactive arthritis in perspective. N Engl J Med 1983;309:1606–15.

79. Gallagher KT, Bernstein B. Juvenile rheumatoid arthritis. Curr Opin Rheumatol 1999;11:372–6.

80. Mills JA. Systemic lupus erythematosus. N Engl J Med 1994;330:1871–9.

81. Hoffman RW, Greidinger EL. Mixed connective tissue disease. Curr Opin Rheumatol 2000;12:386–90.

81a. Law LA, Haftel HM, Shoulder, knee, and hip pain as initial symptoms of juvenile ankylosing spondylitis: a case report. J Orthop Sports Phys Ther 1998;27:167–72.

82. Schumacher HR, Schimmer B, Gordon GV, et al. Articular manifestations of polymyositis and dermatomyositis. Am J Med 1979;67:287–92.

83. Stollerman GH. Rheumatic fever. Lancet 1997;349: 935–42.

84. Gravallese EM, Kantrowitz FG. Arthritic manifestations of inflammatory bowel disease. Am J Gastroenterol 1988; 83:703–09.

85. Hicks RV, Melish ME. Kawasaki syndrome. Pediatr Clin North Am 1986;33:1151–75.

85a. Hoffman AL, Milman N, Byg KE. Childhood Sarcoidosis in Denmark 1979-1994: incidence, clinical features, and laboratory results at presentation. Acta Paediatr 2004;93: 30–6.

86. Saulsbury FT. Henoch-Schonlein purpura in children. Report of 100 patients and review of the literature. Medicine (Baltimore) 1999;78:395–409.

87. Kunnamo I, Kallio P, Pelkonen P, et al. Serum-sickness-like disease is a common cause of acute arthritis in children. Acta Paediatr Scand 1986;75:964–9.

88. Wulffraat NM, de Graeff-Meeder ER, Rijkers GT, et al. Prevalence of circulating immune complexes in patients with cystic fibrosis and arthritis. J Pediatr 1994;125: 374–8.

89. Cabral DA, Tucker LB. Malignancies in children who initially present with rheumatic complaints. J Pediatr 1999; 134:53–7.

90. Aston JW Jr. Pediatric update #16. The orthopaedic presentation of neuroblastoma. Orthop Rev 1990;19: 929–32.

91. Reginato AJ, Ferreiro JL, O'Connor CR, et al. Clinical and pathologic studies of twenty-six patients with penetrating foreign body injury to the joints, bursae, and tendon sheaths. Arthritis Rheum 1990;33:1753–62.

92. O'Connor CR, Reginato AJ, DeLong WG Jr. Foreign body reactions simulating acute septic arthritis. J Rheumatol 1988;15:1568–71.

93. Freiberg AA, Herzenberg JE, Sangeorzan JA. Thorn synovitis of the knee joint with *Nocardia* pyarthrosis. Clin Orthop 1993;233–6.

94. De Champs C, Le Seaux S, Dubost JJ, et al. Isolation of *Pantoea agglomerans* in two cases of septic monoarthritis after plant thorn and wood sliver injuries. J Clin Microbiol 2000;38:460–1.

95. Phair IC, Quinton DN. Clenched fist human bite injuries. J Hand Surg [Br] 1989;14:86–7.

96. Miralles M, Gonzalez G, Pulpeiro JR, et al. Sonography of the painful hip in children: 500 consecutive cases. Am J Roentgenol 1989;152:579–82.

97. Lim-Dunham JE, Ben-Ami TE, Yousefzadeh DK. Septic arthritis of the elbow in children: the role of sonography. Pediatr Radiol 1995;25:556–9.

98. Miller JH, Gates GF. Scintigraphy of sacroiliac pyarthrosis in children. JAMA 1977;238:2701–4.

99. Jaramillo D, Treves ST, Kasser JR, et al. Osteomyelitis and septic arthritis in children: appropriate use of imaging to guide treatment. Am J Roentgenol 1995;165:399–403.

100. Uren RF, Howman-Giles R. The "cold hip" sign on bone scan. A retrospective review. Clin Nucl Med 1991;16:553–6.

101. Barton LL, Dunkle LM, Habib FH. Septic arthritis in childhood. A 13-year review. Am J Dis Child 1987;141:898–900.

102. Yagupsky P, Dagan R, Howard CW, et al. High prevalence of *Kingella kingae* in joint fluid from children with septic arthritis revealed by the BACTEC blood culture system. J Clin Microbiol 1992;30:1278–81.

103. Yagupsky P, Press J. Use of the isolator 1.5 microbial tube for culture of synovial fluid from patients with septic arthritis. J Clin Microbiol 1997;35:2410–12.

104. Moylett EH, Rossmann SN, Epps HR, et al. Importance of *Kingella kingae* as a pediatric pathogen in the United States. Pediatr Infect Dis J 2000;19:263–5.

105. Baldassare AR, Chang F, Zuckner J. Markedly raised synovial fluid leucocyte counts not associated with infectious arthritis in children. Ann Rheum Dis 1978;37:404–9.

106. Luhmann JD, Luhmann SJ. Etiology of septic arthritis in children: an update for the 1990s. Pediatr Emerg Care 1999;15:40–2.

107. Lyon RM, Evanich JD. Culture-negative septic arthritis in children. J Pediatr Orthop 1999;19:655–9.

108. Nelson JD, Koontz WC. Septic arthritis in infants and children: a review of 117 cases. Pediatrics 1966;38:966–71.

109. Kallio MJ, Unkila-Kallio L, Aalto K, et al. Serum C-reactive protein, erythrocyte sedimentation rate and white blood cell count in septic arthritis of children. Pediatr Infect Dis J 1997;16:411–3.

109a. Martinez-Aguilar G, Hammerman WA, Mason EO Jr, et al. Clindamycin treatment of invasive infections caused by community-acquired, methicillin-resistant and methicillin-susceptible Staphylococcus aureus in children. Pediatr Infect Dis J 2003;22:593–8.

110. Thometz JG, Lamdan R, Kehl KS, et al. Microbiological tolerance in orthopaedic infections: delayed response of septic arthritis and osteomyelitis of the hip due to infection with tolerant *Staphylococcus aureus*. J Pediatr Orthop 1996;16:518–21.

111. Argen RJ, Wilson CH Jr, Wood P. Suppurative arthritis. Clinical features of 42 cases. Arch Intern Med 1966;117:661–6.

111a. Odio CM, Ramirez T, Arias G, et al. Double blind, randomized, placebo-controlled study of dexamethasone therapy for hematogenous septic arthritis in children. Pediatr Infect Dis J 2003;22:883-8.

112. Klempner MS, Hu LT, Evans J, et al. Two controlled trials of antibiotic treatment in patients with persistent symptoms and a history of Lyme disease. N Engl J Med 2001;345:85–92.

113. Patel R, Grogg KL, Edwards WD, et al. Death from inappropriate therapy for Lyme disease. Clin Infect Dis 2000;31:1107–9.

114. Prober CG, Yeager AS. Use of the serum bactericidal titer to assess the adequacy of oral antibiotic therapy in the treatment of acute hematogenous osteomyelitis. J Pediatr 1979;95:131–5.

115. Weinstein MP, Stratton CW, Hawley HB, et al. Multicenter collaborative evaluation of a standardized serum bactericidal test as a predictor of therapeutic efficacy in acute and chronic osteomyelitis. Am J Med 1987;83:218–22.

116. Nelson JD, Howard JB, Shelton S. Oral antibiotic therapy for skeletal infections of children. I. Antibiotic concentrations in suppurative synovial fluid. J Pediatr 1978;92:131–4.

117. Dupont WD, Plummer WD Jr. Power and sample size calculations. A review and computer program. Control Clin Trials 1990;11:116–28.

118. Prober CG. Current antibiotic therapy of community-acquired bacterial infections in hospitalized children: bone and joint infections. Pediatr Infect Dis J 1992;11:156–9.

119. Howard JB, Highgenboten CL, Nelson JD. Residual effects of septic arthritis in infancy and childhood. JAMA 1976;236:932–5.

120. Vaughan PA, Newman NM, Rosman MA. Acute hematogenous osteomyelitis in children. J Pediatr Orthop 1987;7:652–5.

121. Scott RJ, Christofersen MR, Robertson WW, et al. Acute osteomyelitis in children: a review of 116 cases. J Pediatr Orthop 1990;10:649–52.

122. Faden H, Grossi M. Acute osteomyelitis in children. Reassessment of etiologic agents and their clinical characteristics. Am J Dis Child 1991;145:65–9.

123. Karwowska A, Davies HD, Jadavji T. Epidemiology and outcome of osteomyelitis in the era of sequential intravenous-oral therapy. Pediatr Infect Dis J 1998;17:1021–1026.

124. Nelson JD. Acute osteomyelitis in children. Infect Dis Clin North Am 1990;4:513–522.

124a. Darville T, Jacobs RF. Management of acute hematogenous osteomyelitis in children. Pediatr Infect Dis J 2004;23:255–7.

125. Guler N, Ones U, Yazicioglu M, et al. Community-acquired severe staphylococcal septicemia in children: the relationship with blunt trauma. Acta Paediatr Jpn 1998;40:441–5.

126. Unkila-Kallio L, Kallio MJ, Eskola J, et al. Serum C-reactive protein, erythrocyte sedimentation rate, and white blood cell count in acute hematogenous osteomyelitis of children. Pediatrics 1994;93:59–62.

127. Rasool MN. Primary subacute haematogenous osteomyelitis in children. J Bone Joint Surg Br 2001;83:93–8.

128. Roberts JM, Drummond DS, Breed AL, et al. Subacute hematogenous osteomyelitis in children: a retrospective study. J Pediatr Orthop 1982;2:249–54.

129. Cottias P, Tomeno B, Anract P, et al. Subacute osteomyelitis presenting as a bone tumour. A review of 21 cases. Int Orthop 1997;21:243–8.

130. Dich VQ, Nelson JD, Haltalin KC. Osteomyelitis in infants and children. A review of 163 cases. Am J Dis Child 1975;129:1273–8.

131. Ross ER, Cole WG. Treatment of subacute osteomyelitis in childhood. J Bone Joint Surg Br 1985;67:443–8.

132. Hulzebos CV, Koetse HA, Kimpen JL, et al. Vertebral osteomyelitis associated with cat-scratch disease. Clin Infect Dis 1999;28:1310–2.

133. Vohra R, Kang HS, Dogra S, et al. Tuberculous osteomyelitis. J Bone Joint Surg Br 1997;79:562–6.

134. Wang MN, Chen WM, Lee KS, et al. Tuberculous osteomyelitis in young children. J Pediatr Orthop 1999;19:151–5.

135. Friduss ME, Maceri DR. Cervicofacial actinomycosis in children. Henry Ford Hosp Med J 1990;38:28–32.

136. Weigl JA, Haas WH. Postoperative *Mycobacterium avium* osteomyelitis confirmed by polymerase chain reaction. Eur J Pediatr 2000;159:64–9.

137. Blais RE, Cesani F, Ali S, et al. Blastomycotic osteomyelitis of the pelvis: a case report. Am Surg 1997;63:414–6.

138. Pasic S, Abinun M, Pistignjat B, et al. *Aspergillus* osteomyelitis in chronic granulomatous disease: treatment with recombinant gamma-interferon and itraconazole. Pediatr Infect Dis J 1996;15:833–4.

139. Jonnalagadda S, Veerabagu MP, Rakela J, et al. *Candida albicans* osteomyelitis in a liver transplant recipient: a case report and review of the literature. Transplantation 1996;62:1182–4.

140. Oleinik EM, Della-Latta P, Rinaldi MG, et al. *Candida lusitaniae* osteomyelitis in a premature infant. Am J Perinatol 1993;10:313–5.

141. Miller WB Jr, Murphy WA, Gilula LA. Brodie abscess: reappraisal. Radiology 1979;132:15–23.

142. Simpson AH, Deakin M, Latham JM. Chronic osteomyelitis. The effect of the extent of surgical resection on infection-free survival. J Bone Joint Surg Br 2001;83:403–7.

143. Fitzgerald RH Jr, Ruttle PE, Arnold PG, et al. Local muscle flaps in the treatment of chronic osteomyelitis. J Bone Joint Surg Am 1985;67:175–85.

144. Patzakis MJ, Mazur K, Wilkins J, et al. Septopal beads and autogenous bone grafting for bone defects in patients with chronic osteomyelitis. Clin Orthop 1993;295:112–8.

145. Wing VW, Jeffrey RB Jr, Federle MP, et al. Chronic osteomyelitis examined by CT. Radiology 1985;154:171–4.

146. Seltzer SE. Value of computed tomography in planning medical and surgical treatment of chronic osteomyelitis. J Comput Assist Tomogr 1984;8:482–7.

147. Zimmerli W, Widmer AF, Blatter M, et al. Role of rifampin for treatment of orthopedic implant-related staphylococcal infections: a randomized controlled trial. Foreign-Body Infection (FBI) Study Group. JAMA 1998;279:1537–41.

148. Trueta J. The three types of acute hematogenous osteomyelitis: a clinical and vascular study. J Bone Joint Surg Br 1959;41:671–80.

149. Asmar BI. Osteomyelitis in the neonate. Infect Dis Clin North Am 1992;6:117–32.

150. Wong M, Isaacs D, Howman-Giles R, et al. Clinical and diagnostic features of osteomyelitis occurring in the first three months of life. Pediatr Infect Dis J 1995;14:1047–53.

151. Fox L, Sprunt K. Neonatal osteomyelitis. Pediatrics 1978;62:535–42.

152. McGregor JA, McFarren T. Neonatal cranial osteomyelitis: a complication of fetal monitoring. Obstet Gynecol 1989;73:490–2.

153. Nelson DL, Hable KA, Matsen JM. *Proteus mirabilis* osteomyelitis in two neonates following needle puncture. Successful treatment with ampicillin. Am J Dis Child 1973;125:109–10.

154. Lilien LD, Harris VJ, Ramamurthy RS, et al. Neonatal osteomyelitis of the calcaneus: complication of heel puncture. J Pediatr 1976;88:478–80.

155. Lee PY. Infected cephalhaematoma and neonatal osteomyelitis. J Infect 1990;21:191–3.

156. Perlman MH, Patzakis MJ, Kumar PJ, et al. The incidence of joint involvement with adjacent osteomyelitis in pediatric patients. J Pediatr Orthop 2000;20:40–3.

157. Lew DP, Waldvogel FA. Osteomyelitis. N Engl J Med 1997;336:999–1007.

158. Tountas AA, Kwok JM. Acute hematogenous diaphyseal osteomyelitis in childhood. Can Med Assoc J 1985;132:1287–8.

159. Rosenbaum DM, Blumhagen JD. Acute epiphyseal osteomyelitis in children. Radiology 1985;156:89–92.

160. Kemp HB, Lloyd-Roberts GC. Avascular necrosis of the capital epiphysis following osteomyelitis of the proximal femoral metaphysis. J Bone Joint Surg Br 1974;56(B):688–97.

161. Jacobs RF, McCarthy RE, Elser JM. *Pseudomonas* osteochondritis complicating puncture wounds of the foot in children: a 10-year evaluation. J Infect Dis 1989;160:657–61.

162. Mustafa MM, Saez-Llorens X, McCracken GH Jr, et al. Acute hematogenous pelvic osteomyelitis in infants and children. Pediatr Infect Dis J 1990;9:416–21.

163. Mazur JM, Ross G, Cummings J, et al. Usefulness of magnetic resonance imaging for the diagnosis of acute musculoskeletal infections in children. J Pediatr Orthop 1995;15:144–7.

164. Messer HD, Litvinoff J. Pyogenic cervical osteomyelitis. Chondro-osteomyelitis of the cervical spine frequently associated with parenteral drug use. Arch Neurol 1976;33:571–6.

165. Fernandez M, Carrol CL, Baker CJ. Discitis and vertebral osteomyelitis in children: an 18-year review. Pediatrics 2000;105:1299–304.

166. Mahboubi S, Morris MC. Imaging of spinal infections in children. Radiol Clin North Am 2001;39:215–22.

167. Colmenero JD, Jimenez-Mejias ME, Sanchez-Lora FJ, et al. Pyogenic, tuberculous, and brucellar vertebral osteomyelitis: a descriptive and comparative study of 219 cases. Ann Rheum Dis 1997;56:709–15.

168. Morse TS, Pryles CV. Infections of the bone and joints in children. N Engl J Med 1960;262:846–52.

169. Waldman BA, Frieden IJ. Osteomyelitis caused by nail biting. Pediatr Dermatol 1990;7:189–90.

170. Boiko S, Kaufman RA, Lucky AW. Osteomyelitis of the distal phalanges in three children with severe atopic dermatitis. Arch Dermatol 1988;124:418–23.

171. Corbella X, Carratala J, Rufi G, et al. Unusual manifestations of miliary tuberculosis: cutaneous lesions, phalanx osteomyelitis, and paradoxical expansion of tenosynovitis. Clin Infect Dis 1993;16:179–80.

172. Morrey BF, Bianco AJ Jr. Hematogenous osteomyelitis of the clavicle in children. Clin Orthop 1977;125:24–8.

173. Morrey BF, Bianco AJ, Rhodes KH. Hematogenous osteomyelitis at uncommon sites in children. Mayo Clin Proc 1978;53:707–13.

174. Valerio PG, Harmsen P. Osteomyelitis as a complication of perinatal fracture of the clavicle. Eur J Pediatr 1995; 154:497–8.

175. Judich A, Haik J, Rosin D, et al. Osteomyelitis of the clavicle after subclavian vein catheterization. J Parenter Enteral Nutr 1998;22:245–6.

176. Kravitz AB. Osteomyelitis of the clavicle secondary to infected Hickman catheter. J Parenter Enteral Nutr 1989; 13:426–7.

177. Lowden CM, Walsh SJ. Acute staphylococcal osteomyelitis of the clavicle. J Pediatr Orthop 1997;17:467–9.

178. Jurik AG, Moller BN. Chronic sclerosing osteomyelitis of the clavicle. A manifestation of chronic recurrent multifocal osteomyelitis. Arch Orthop Trauma Surg 1987;106: 144–51.

179. Chandler JR, Grobman L, Quencer R, et al. Osteomyelitis of the base of the skull. Laryngoscope 1986;96:245–51.

180. Saxton VJ, Boldt DW, Shield LK. Sinusitis and intracranial sepsis: the CT imaging and clinical presentation. Pediatr Radiol 1995;25(suppl 1):S212–7.

181. Roy DR. Osteomyelitis of the patella. Clin Orthop 2001: 30–4.

182. Bishara J, Gartman-Israel D, Weinberger M, et al. Osteomyelitis of the ribs in the antibiotic era. Scand J Infect Dis 2000;32:223–7.

183. Seashore JH, Touloukian RJ, Pickett LK. Acute hematogenous osteomyelitis of the rib. Primary surgical treatment in two cases. Clin Pediatr (Phila) 1973;12:379–80.

184. Bradley JS, Kaplan SL, Tan TQ, et al. Pediatric pneumococcal bone and joint infections. The Pediatric Multicenter Pneumococcal Surveillance Study Group (PMPSSG). Pediatrics 1998;102:1376–82.

185. Dubey L, Krasinski K, Hernanz-Schulman M. Osteomyelitis secondary to trauma or infected contiguous soft tissue. Pediatr Infect Dis J 1988;7:26–34.

186. Brook I. Anaerobic osteomyelitis in children. Pediatr Infect Dis 1986;5:550–6.

187. Struk DW, Munk PL, Lee MJ, et al. Imaging of soft tissue infections. Radiol Clin North Am 2001;39:277–303.

188. Morrey BF, Peterson HA. Hematogenous pyogenic osteomyelitis in children. Orthop Clin North Am 1975;6: 935–51.

189. Unkila-Kallio L, Kallio MJ, Peltola H. The usefulness of C-reactive protein levels in the identification of concurrent septic arthritis in children who have acute hematogenous osteomyelitis. A comparison with the usefulness of the erythrocyte sedimentation rate and the white blood-cell count. J Bone Joint Surg Am 1994;76:848–53.

190. Spiegel DA, Meyer JS, Dormans JP, et al. Pyomyositis in children and adolescents: report of 12 cases and review of the literature. J Pediatr Orthop 1999;19:143–50.

191. Gubbay AJ, Isaacs D. Pyomyositis in children. Pediatr Infect Dis J 2000;19:1009–12.

192. Hirano T, Srinivasan G, Janakiraman N, et al. Gallium 67 citrate scintigraphy in pyomyositis. J Pediatr 1980;97: 596–8.

193. Brion LP, Manuli M, Rai B, et al. Long-bone radiographic abnormalities as a sign of active congenital syphilis in asymptomatic newborns. Pediatrics 1991;88:1037–40.

194. Rasool MN, Govender S. The skeletal manifestations of congenital syphilis. A review of 197 cases. J Bone Joint Surg Br 1989;71:752–5.

195. Lim HK, Smith WL, Sato Y, et al. Congenital syphilis mimicking child abuse. Pediatr Radiol 1995;25:560–1.

196. Torchinsky MY, Shulman H, Landau D. Radiological case of the month. Congenital syphilis presenting as osteomyelitis with normal radioisotope bone scan. Arch Pediatr Adolesc Med 2001;155:613–4.

197. Friedman MS. Traumatic periostitis in infants and children. JAMA 1958;166:1840–5.

198. Park HM, Kernek CB, Robb JA. Early scintigraphic findings of occult femoral and tibial fractures in infants. Clin Nucl Med 1988;13:271–5.

199. Abril JC, Castillo F, Casas J, et al. Brodie's abscess of the hip simulating osteoid osteoma. Orthopedics 2000;23: 285–7.

200. Yoshikawa M, Sugawara Y, Kikuchi T, et al. Two cases of pediatric bone disease (eosinophilic granuloma and Brodie's abscess) showing similar scintigraphic and radiographic findings. Clin Nucl Med 2000;25:986–90.

201. Rogalsky RJ, Black GB, Reed MH. Orthopaedic manifestations of leukemia in children. J Bone Joint Surg Am 1986; 68:494–501.

202. Caudle RJ, Crawford AH, Gelfand MJ, et al. Childhood acute lymphoblastic leukemia presenting as "cold" lesions on bone scan: a report of two cases. J Pediatr Orthop 1987;7:93–5.

203. Clausen N, Gotze H, Pedersen A, et al. Skeletal scintigraphy and radiography at onset of acute lymphocytic leukemia in children. Med Pediatr Oncol 1983;11:291–6.

204. Bernard EJ, Nicholls WD, Howman-Giles RB, et al. Patterns of abnormality on bone scans in acute childhood leukemia. J Nucl Med 1998;39:1983–6.

205. Greer LW, Friedman AC, Madewell JE. Periosteal reaction of the femur in an infant with fever. JAMA 1981;245: 1765–6.

206. Eversole LR, Leider AS, Corwin JO, et al. Proliferative periostitis of Garre: its differentiation from other neoperiostoses. J Oral Surg 1979;37:725–31.

207. Abshire TC. The anemia of inflammation. A common cause of childhood anemia. Pediatr Clin North Am 1996; 43:623–37.

208. Roine I, Faingezicht I, Arguedas A, et al. Serial serum C-reactive protein to monitor recovery from acute hematogenous osteomyelitis in children. Pediatr Infect Dis J 1995; 14:40–4.

209. Waldvogel FA, Medoff G, Swartz MN. Osteomyelitis: a review of clinical features, therapeutic considerations and unusual aspects. N Engl J Med 1970;282:198–206.

210. Capitanio MA, Kirkpatrick JA. Early roentgen observa-

tions in acute osteomyelitis. Am J Roentgenol 1970;108: 488–96.

211. Mandell GA. Imaging in the diagnosis of musculoskeletal infections in children. Curr Probl Pediatr 1996;26: 218–37.

212. Howie DW, Savage JP, Wilson TG, et al. The technetium phosphate bone scan in the diagnosis of osteomyelitis in childhood. J Bone Joint Surg Am 1983;65:431–7.

213. Pennington WT, Mott MP, Thometz JG, et al. Photopenic bone scan osteomyelitis: a clinical perspective. J Pediatr Orthop 1999;19:695–8.

214. Handmaker H, Giammona ST. Improved early diagnosis of acute inflammatory skeletal-articular diseases in children: a two-radiopharmaceutical approach. Pediatrics 1984;73:661–9.

215. Green NE, Edwards K. Bone and joint infections in children. Orthop Clin North Am 1987;18:555–76.

216. Erdman WA, Tamburro F, Jayson HT, et al. Osteomyelitis: characteristics and pitfalls of diagnosis with MR imaging. Radiology 1991;180:533–9.

217. Frush DP, Heyneman LE, Ware RE, et al. MR features of soft-tissue abnormalities due to acute marrow infarction in five children with sickle cell disease. Am J Roentgenol 1999;173:989–93.

218. Kaiser S, Rosenborg M. Early detection of subperiosteal abscesses by ultrasonography. A means for further successful treatment in pediatric osteomyelitis. Pediatr Radiol 1994;24:336–9.

219. Larcos G, Antico VF, Cormick W, et al. How useful is ultrasonography in suspected acute osteomyelitis? J Ultrasound Med 1994;13:707–9.

220. Canale ST, Harkness RM, Thomas PA, et al. Does aspiration of bones and joints affect results of later bone scanning? J Pediatr Orthop 1985;5:23–6.

221. Aronoff SC, Scoles PV. Treatment of childhood skeletal infections. Pediatr Clin North Am 1983;30:271–80.

222. Tetzlaff TR, Howard JB, McCracken GH, et al. Antibiotic concentrations in pus and bone of children with osteomyelitis. J Pediatr 1978;92:135–40.

223. Kaplan SL, Mason EO Jr, Feigin RD. Clindamycin versus nafcillin or methicillin in the treatment of Staphylococcus aureus osteomyelitis in children. South Med J 1982;75: 138–42.

224. Freij BJ, Kusmiesz H, Shelton S, et al. Imipenem and cilastatin in acute osteomyelitis and suppurative arthritis. Therapy in infants and children. Am J Dis Child 1987; 141:335–42.

225. Nelson JD. Oral antibiotic therapy for serious infections in hospitalized patients. J Pediatr 1978;92:175–6.

226. Peltola H, Unkila-Kallio L, Kallio MJ. Simplified treatment of acute staphylococcal osteomyelitis of childhood. The Finnish Study Group. Pediatrics 1997;99:846–50.

227. Hanley JA, Lippman-Hand A. If nothing goes wrong, is everything all right? Interpreting zero numerators. JAMA 1983;249:1743–5.

228. Matsui DM. Drug compliance in pediatrics. Clinical and research issues. Pediatr Clin North Am 1997;44:1–14.

229. Racadio JM, Doellman DA, Johnson ND, et al. Pediatric peripherally inserted central catheters: complication rates related to catheter tip location. Pediatrics 2001;107:E28.

230. Wald ER. Risk factors for osteomyelitis. Am J Med 1985; 78:206–12.

231. Dalton GP, Drummond DS, Davidson RS, et al. Bone infarction versus infection in sickle cell disease in children. J Pediatr Orthop 1996;16:540–4.

232. Burnett MW, Bass JW, Cook BA. Etiology of osteomyelitis complicating sickle cell disease. Pediatrics 1998;101: 296–7.

233. Aken'Ova YA, Bakare RA, Okunade MA, et al. Bacterial causes of acute osteomyelitis in sickle cell anaemia: changing infection profile. West Afr J Med 1995;14: 255–8.

234. Bennett OM. Salmonella osteomyelitis and the hand-foot syndrome in sickle cell disease. J Pediatr Orthop 1992; 12:534–8.

235. Winkelstein JA, Marino MC, Johnston RB Jr, et al. Chronic granulomatous disease. Report on a national registry of 368 patients. Medicine (Baltimore) 2000;79: 155–69.

236. Sponseller PD, Malech HL, McCarthy EF Jr, et al. Skeletal involvement in children who have chronic granulomatous disease. J Bone Joint Surg Am 1991;73:37–51.

237. Williams RL, Fukui MB, Meltzer CC, et al. Fungal spinal osteomyelitis in the immunocompromised patient: MR findings in three cases. Am J Neuroradiol 1999;20: 381–5.

238. Hovi L, Saarinen UM, Donner U, et al. Opportunistic osteomyelitis in the jaws of children on immunosuppressive chemotherapy. J Pediatr Hematol Oncol 1996;18: 90–4.

239. Berman S, Jensen J. Cytomegalovirus-induced osteomyelitis in a patient with the acquired immunodeficiency syndrome. South Med J 1990;83:1231–2.

240. Szalay GC, Sommerstein A. Inoculation osteomyelitis secondary to animal bites. The clinical course differs from acute hematogenous osteomyelitis. Clin Pediatr (Phila) 1972;11:687–9.

241. Shah M, Watanakunakorn C. Staphylococcus aureus sternal osteomyelitis complicating bone marrow aspiration. South Med J 1978;71:348–9.

242. Chang MJ, Barton LL. Mycobacterium fortuitum osteomyelitis of the calcaneus secondary to a puncture wound. J Pediatr 1974;85:517–9.

243. Buckley SL, Smith GR, Sponseller PD, et al. Severe (type III) open fractures of the tibia in children. J Pediatr Orthop 1996;16:627–34.

244. Hutchins CM, Sponseller PD, Sturm P, et al. Open femur fractures in children: treatment, complications, and results. J Pediatr Orthop 2000;20:183–8.

245. Karam GH, Ackley AM, Dismukes WE. Posttraumatic Aeromonas hydrophila osteomyelitis. Arch Intern Med 1983;143:2073–4.

246. Nepola JV, Seabold JE, Marsh JL, et al. Diagnosis of infection in ununited fractures. Combined imaging with indium-111-labeled leukocytes and technetium-99m methylene diphosphonate. J Bone Joint Surg Am 1993; 75:1816–22.

247. Barlow B, Niemirska M, Gandhi R, et al. Response to injury in children with closed femur fractures. J Trauma 1987;27:429–30.

248. Edwards MS, Baker CJ. Median sternotomy wound infections in children. Pediatr Infect Dis 1983;2:105–9.

249. Fitzgerald RH Jr, Cowan JD. Puncture wounds of the foot. Orthop Clin North Am 1975;6:965–72.

250. Schultz C, Holterhus PM, Seidel A, et al. Chronic recurrent multifocal osteomyelitis in children. Pediatr Infect Dis J 1999;18:1008–13.

251. King SM, Laxer RM, Manson D, et al. Chronic recurrent multifocal osteomyelitis: a noninfectious inflammatory process. Pediatr Infect Dis J 1987;6:907–11.

252. Beretta-Piccoli BC, Sauvain MJ, Gal I, et al. Synovitis, acne, pustulosis, hyperostosis, osteitis (SAPHO) syndrome in childhood: a report of ten cases and review of the literature. Eur J Pediatr 2000;159:594–601.

253. Letts M, Davidson D, Birdi N, et al. The SAPHO syndrome in children: a rare cause of hyperostosis and osteitis. J Pediatr Orthop 1999;19:297–300.

254. Bousvaros A, Marcon M, Treem W, et al. Chronic recurrent multifocal osteomyelitis associated with chronic inflammatory bowel disease in children. Dig Dis Sci 1999; 44:2500–7.

255. Omidi CJ, Siegfried EC. Chronic recurrent multifocal osteomyelitis preceding pyoderma gangrenosum and occult ulcerative colitis in a pediatric patient. Pediatr Dermatol 1998;15:435–8.

256. Cushing AH. Diskitis in children. Clin Infect Dis 1993; 17:1–6.

257. Hensey OJ, Coad N, Carty HM, et al. Juvenile discitis. Arch Dis Child 1983;58:983–7.

258. Brown R, Hussain M, McHugh K, et al. Discitis in young children. J Bone Joint Surg Br 2001;83:106–11.

259. Amir J, Shockelford PG. *Kingella kingae* intervertebral disk infection. J Clin Microbiol 1991;29:1083–6.

260. Rocco HD, Eyring EJ. Intervertebral disk infections in children. Am J Dis Child 1972;123:448–51.

261. Amir N, Hurvitz H, Korn-Lubetzki I, et al. Gowers' sign in discitis in childhood. Clin Pediatr (Phila) 1986;25: 459–61.

262. Wenger DR, Bobechko WP, Gilday DL. The spectrum of intervertebral disc-space infection in children. J Bone Joint Surg Am 1978;60:100–8.

263. Smith RA, Vohman MD, Dimon JH III, et al. Calcified cervical intervertebral discs in children. Report of three cases. J Neurosurg 1977;46:233–8.

264. Carroll WL, Balistreri WF, Brilli R, et al. Spectrum of *Salmonella*-associated arthritis. Pediatrics 1981;68: 717–20.

265. Bremell T, Bjelle A, Svedhem A. Rheumatic symptoms following an outbreak of *Campylobacter* enteritis: a five year follow up. Ann Rheum Dis 1991;50:934–8.

266. Taccetti G, Trapani S, Ermini M, et al. Reactive arthritis triggered by *Yersinia enterocolitica:* a review of 18 pediatric cases. Clin Exp Rheumatol 1994;12:681–4.

267. Lauhio A, Lahdevirta J, Janes R, et al. Reactive arthritis associated with *Shigella sonnei* infection. Arthritis Rheum 1988;31:1190–3.

268. Sieper J, Braun J, Wu P, et al. The possible role of *Shigella* in sporadic enteric reactive arthritis. Br J Rheumatol 1993;32:582–5.

269. Mermel LA, Osborn TG. *Clostridium difficile* associated reactive arthritis in an HLA-B27 positive female: report and literature review. J Rheumatol 1989;16:133–5.

270. Cron RQ, Gordon PV. Reactive arthritis to *Clostridium difficile* in a child. West J Med 1997;166:419–21.

271. Letts M, Davidson D, Lalonde F. Synovitis secondary to giardiasis in children. Am J Orthop 1998;27:451–4.

272. Edwards MS, Baker CJ. Complications and sequelae of meningococcal infections in children. J Pediatr 1981;99: 540-5.

273. DiLiberti JH, Tarlow S. Bone and joint complications of *Hemophilus influenzae* meningitis. Clin Pediatr (Phila) 1983;22:7–10.

274. Inman RD, Whittum-Hudson JA, Schumacher HR, et al. *Chlamydia* and associated arthritis. Curr Opin Rheumatol 2000;12:254–62.

275. Kerr JM, LeBlanc W, Heagarty MC. Genitourinary gonorrhea presenting as mild arthritis. Clin Pediatr (Phila) 1991;30:388–9.

276. Vittecoq O, Schaeverbeke T, Favre S, et al. Molecular diagnosis of *Ureaplasma urealyticum* in an immunocompetent patient with destructive reactive polyarthritis. Arthritis Rheum 1997;40:2084–9.

277. Poggio TV, Orlando N, Galanternik L, et al. Microbiology of acute arthropathies among children in Argentina: *Mycoplasma pneumoniae* and *hominis* and *Ureaplasma urealyticum.* Pediatr Infect Dis J 1998;17:304–8.

278. Hannu T, Puolakkainen M, Leirisalo-Repo M. Chlamydia pneumoniae as a triggering infection in reactive arthritis. Rheumatology (Oxford) 1999;38:411–4.

279. Bont L, Brus F, Dijkman-Neerincx RH, et al. The clinical spectrum of post-streptococcal syndromes with arthritis in children. Clin Exp Rheumatol 1998;16:750–2.

280. Jansen TL, Janssen M, de Jong AJ. Reactive arthritis associated with group C and group G beta-hemolytic streptococci. J Rheumatol 1998;25:1126–30.

281. Schiff ER. Atypical clinical manifestations of hepatitis A. Vaccine 1992;10:S18–20.

282. Segool RA, Lejtenyi C, Taussig LM. Articular and cutaneous prodromal manifestations of viral hepatitis. J Pediatr 1975;87:709–12.

283. Buskila D. Hepatitis C-associated arthritis. Curr Opin Rheumatol 2000;12:295–9.

284. Delyle LG, Vittecoq O, Bourdel A, et al. Chronic destructive oligoarthritis associated with *Propionibacterium acnes* in a female patient with acne vulgaris: septic-reactive arthritis? Arthritis Rheum 2000;43:2843–7.

285. Mills WJ, Mosca VS, Nizet V. Orthopaedic manifestations of invasive group A streptococcal infections complicating primary varicella. J Pediatr Orthop 1996;16:522–8.

286. Rottem M, Miron D, Shiloah E, et al. Properdin deficiency: rare presentation with meningococcal bone and joint infections. Pediatr Infect Dis J 1998;17:356–8.

287. Dillon M, Nourse C, Dowling F, et al. Primary meningococcal arthritis. Pediatr Infect Dis J 1997;16:331–2.

288. Konrad D, Zbinden R, Kuster H, et al. Group G streptococcus sacroilitis with sepsis in a 15-y-old adolescent. Scand J Infect Dis 1999;31:100–2.

289. Hockman DE, Pence CD, Whittler RR, et al. Septic arthritis of the hip secondary to rat bite fever: a case report. Clin Orthop 2000:173–6.

290. Zaks N, Sukenik S, Alkan M, et al. Musculoskeletal manifestations of brucellosis: a study of 90 cases in Israel. Semin Arthritis Rheum 1995;25:97–102.

291. Dinulos JG, Darmstadt GL, Wilson CB, et al. *Nocardia asteroides* septic arthritis in a healthy child. Pediatr Infect Dis J 1999;18:308–10.

292. Ray TD, Nimityongskul P, Ramsey KM. Disseminated *No-*

cardia asteroides infection presenting as septic arthritis in a patient with AIDS. Clin Infect Dis 1994;18:256–7.

293. Stahlman GC, DeBoer DK, Green NE. *Fusobacterium* osteomyelitis and pyarthrosis: a classic case of Lemierre's syndrome. J Pediatr Orthop 1996;16:529–32.

294. Sundy JS, Allen NB, Sexton DJ. Rocky Mountain spotted fever presenting with acute monarticular arthritis. Arthritis Rheum 1996;39:175–6.

295. Cottalorda J, Jouve JL, Bollini G, et al. Osteoarticular infection due to *Coxiella burnetii* in children. J Pediatr Orthop B 1995;4:219-21.

296. Quintero-Del-Rio AI, Fink CW. Varicella arthritis in childhood. Pediatr Infect Dis J 1997;16:241–3.

297. Grahame R, Armstrong R, Simmons NA, et al. Isolation of rubella virus from synovial fluid in five cases of seronegative arthritis. Lancet 1981;2:649–51.

298. Harel L, Amir J, Reish O, et al. Mumps arthritis in children. Pediatr Infect Dis J 1990;9:928–9.

299. Burns LJ, Gingrich RD. Cytomegalovirus infection presenting as polyarticular arthritis following autologous BMT. Bone Marrow Transplant 1993;11:77–9.

300. David JJ, Dietz FR, Jones MM. Coxsackie-B monarthritis with hepatitis. A case report. J Bone Joint Surg Am 1993; 75:1685–6.

301. Remafedi G, Muldoon RL. Acute monarticular arthritis caused by herpes simplex virus type I. Pediatrics 1983; 72:882–3.

302. Berger RG, Raab-Traub N. Acute monoarthritis from infectious mononucleosis. Am J Med 1999;107:177–8.

303. Ackerson BK, Raghunathan R, Keller MA, et al. Echovirus 11 arthritis in a patient with X-linked agammaglobulinemia. Pediatr Infect Dis J 1987;6:485–8.

304. Ford DK, Stein HB, Schulzer M, et al. Lymphocytes from the site of disease suggest adenovirus is one cause of persistent or recurrent inflammatory arthritis. J Rheumatol 1993;20:310–3.

305. Fujikawa S, Okuni M. Clinical analysis of 570 cases with juvenile rheumatoid arthritis: results of a nationwide retrospective survey in Japan. Acta Paediatr Jpn 1997;39: 245–9.

306. Falcini F, Bardare M, Cimaz R, et al. Arthritis as a presenting feature of non-Hodgkin's lymphoma. Arch Dis Child 1998;78:367–70.

307. Pouchot J, Barge J, Marchand A, et al. Ewing's sarcoma of the ilium mimicking an infectious sacroiliitis. J Rheumatol 1992;19:1318–20.

308. Chen WS, Wan YL. Iliacus pyomyositis mimicking septic arthritis of the hip joint. Arch Orthop Trauma Surg 1996; 115:233–5.

309. Schaefer RA, Enzenauer RJ, Pruitt A, et al. Acute gonococcal flexor tenosynovitis in an adolescent male with pharyngitis. A case report and literature review. Clin Orthop 1992:212–5.

310. Calvo Rey C, Borque Andres C, del Castillo Martin F, et al. [Kawasaki disease; complications and clinical course. Apropos of 38 cases]. An Esp Pediatr 1993;39: 423–7.

311. Gerber MA, Shapiro ED, Burke GS, et al. Lyme disease in children in southeastern Connecticut. Pediatric Lyme Disease Study Group. N Engl J Med 1996;335:1270–4.

CHAPTER 17

Skin and Soft-Tissue Syndromes

Skin infections should be distinguished from exanthems, which are rashes associated with a generalized febrile disease and are discussed in Chapter 11. A primary skin infection is one in which the principal and original manifestation of the infection is in the skin. Examples of such infections that are discussed below include cellulitis, gangrene, impetigo, pustules, boils, abscesses, scalded skin syndrome, tinea, and skin ulcers. A secondary skin infection is one occurring because of a change in the skin's protective mechanism. Examples include acne, burns, diaper dermatitis, and wounds, either surgical or traumatic. Some skin infections only involve the epidermis or dermis, whereas others may also involve the underlying subcutaneous fat and fascia, in which case the broader term, soft-tissue infection, is used. Infection of muscle (pyomyositis) is addressed in Chapter 16. Animal and human bites are discussed in Chapter 21.

■ NORMAL SKIN FLORA

Normally, bacteria of the skin can be found on the surface, in the hair follicles, or beneath the superficial cells of the stratum corneum.[1] Skin flora can be divided into two groups: resident and transient. The resident flora exist in relatively stable numbers and consist primarily of *Staphylococcus epidermidis*, micrococci, and aerobic and anaerobic diphtheroids, such as *Propionibacterium* species.[2] Transient flora are introduced from the environment and usually only reside on the skin temporarily. The most important of the transient flora are *Staphylococcus aureus* and group A β-hemolytic streptococcus. *S. aureus* is found so frequently (approx. 30%) in the nose, axilla, groin, perineum, and the newborn umbilicus that it is sometimes regarded as normal flora of these areas.[3–5] Children with underlying skin disease such as atopic dermatitis have much higher rates of colonization with *S. aureus* (approx. 90%).[6] Hospitalized persons, especially those in intensive care units, often become colonized with a wide variety of organisms.[7] Exposure to antibiotics, even as an outpatient, changes the composition of skin flora, primarily increasing colonization with *Candida*.[8]

Most superficial skin infections occurring in outpatients are caused by either *S. aureus* or group A streptococci, although occasionally other organisms are implicated.[2] Among hospitalized patients, a greater array of organisms is seen. Among 1562 bacterial isolates recovered from hospitalized patients with skin and soft tissue infections in the United States and Canada, the most common pathogens were *S. aureus* (43%), *Pseudomonas aeruginosa* (11%), *Enterococcus* spp. (8%), *Escherichia coli* (7%), *Enterobacter* spp. (5%), and β-hemolytic streptococci (5%).[9]

■ CELLULITIS

Cellulitis is defined as a localized inflammation of the skin, recognized by an area of redness and warmth. Fever may be present, and underlying subcutaneous tissue is often involved. Note that this broad definition includes noninfectious diseases that may mimic bacterial cellulitis. Lymphangitis, which may accompany cellulitis, is a thin line of redness typically extending from an infected wound along the route of the lymphatic drainage. If the erythema and warmth are more generalized, the diagnosis of scarlet fever or scalded skin syndrome should be considered.

Cellulitis is a diagnosis that can often be subclassified according to its location, which gives a clue to the etiology, as described later. Cellulitis can also be described by adjectives that imply more severe disease than "simple" cellulitis, which is manifested only by redness, warmth, and swelling of the soft tissues.

Necrotizing Cellulitis

In the past, a distinction was made between necrotizing cellulitis and necrotizing fasciitis.[10] In necrotizing cellulitis the skin is involved early with hemorrhage and necrosis. In necrotizing fasciitis, the skin and subcutaneous tissues are lifted up by dissection of infection along fascial planes, and the skin is pale and shiny. However, the distinction between these two conditions is not always easy, and the precise label is of little importance. Early recognition and urgent operative intervention is critical for both conditions (see section on necrotizing soft-tissue infections).

Crepitant Cellulitis

As discussed in the section on necrotizing soft-tissue infections, crepitance of a cellulitic area should be presumed to be early gangrene.

Location

The location of the cellulitis is very important, and the descriptive diagnosis should always state the location, because there may be a serious infection underneath the cellulitis. The center point of the cellulitis may give a clue to the underlying disease (Table 17-1). Important possible underlying diseases include osteomyelitis, septic arthritis, peritonitis, sinusitis, neck space infections, or deep wound infections, all of which are discussed in other chapters.

Cellulitis of an Extremity

Cellulitis of an arm or leg is often associated with local injury and a minor wound. Lymphangitic streaking, local tenderness, erythema, fever, malaise, and tender regional adenopathy are common.[2] A poorly defined border of erythema could simply be due to cellulitis deep in the subcutaneous tissue or could signal an underlying osteomyelitis, especially if there is tenderness over the metaphysis (see Chapter 16). Blood cultures are usually negative in simple cellulitis of an extremity, and aspirate cultures are positive in about one-quarter of cases.[11,12] Many experts recommend aspirating the leading edge as opposed to the center of the lesion, although a study comparing the two techniques found no difference in the yield.[13] Swab cultures of pus give higher yields, but visible pus is not frequently present.

S. aureus is the most common cause, followed by group A streptococcus. In the majority of cases, mild cellulitis of an extremity in a normal child can be treated with an oral antibiotic (e.g., cephalexin)

TABLE 17-1. POSSIBLE CAUSES OF CELLULITIS IN VARIOUS LOCATIONS

LOCATION	CONSIDER
Eye and periorbital	Ethmoid sinusitis
Abdomen	Peritonitis
Arm or leg	Osteomyelitis or pyomyositis
Joint	Septic arthritis
Around a wound	Wound infection
Over an enlarged lymph node	Adenitis or abscess
Perianal or perineal	Group A streptococci
Cheek	Dental abscess, maxillary sinusitis, *Haemophilus influenzae* buccal cellulitis
Both tibias	Erythema nodosum
Sacrum	Pilonidal cyst infection
Scalp	Kerion (inflammatory tinea capitis)
Behind ear	Mastoiditis
Junction of ear and scalp	Infected atopic dermatitis
Entire ear	Malignant otitis externa or auricular perichrondritis
Scrotum	Fournier syndrome, epididymitis
Around neck	Neck space infections

that covers these two organisms. For immunocompromised children (including neonates) and children with manifestations of a severe infection (such as high fever or toxicity), blood cultures should be obtained, and parenteral therapy (e.g., oxacillin or cefazolin) should be started.

Sacral Cellulitis

Infection of a pilonidal cyst is the usual cause of midline sacral cellulitis. It occurs predominantly in males and usually manifests clinically near the end of the second decade of life. Pilonidal cysts are asymptomatic until they become infected. The primary therapy of an infected pilonidal cyst is surgical, either excision or incision and curettage.[14] The cyst abscess usually contains mixed anaerobic and aerobic flora, so ampicillin-sulbactam or clindamycin with gentamicin is reasonable perioperative coverage, although healing time is similar whether or not antibiotics are given.[15,16]

Perianal Cellulitis

This is a relatively common problem in young children, and group A streptococcus is the usual cause. Children usually present with a sharply demarcated area of perianal erythema, pruritis, painful defecation and, occasionally, blood-streaked stools.[17] Vaginal involvement may occur in girls. A swab for culture of group A streptococcus should be performed (rapid tests are neither approved nor appropriate for diagnosis of this condition). Treatment is with oral penicillin or amoxicillin.

External Ear

Cellulitis of the ear may be a manifestation of malignant otitis externa (discussed in Chapter 5). More commonly, infection of the pinna is secondary to ear piercing. Infection of the earlobe, which has its own blood supply, is usually a minor problem and responds to removal of the embedded earring and oral antistaphylococcal antibiotics. In contrast, infection of the upper ear cartilage, termed auricular perichondritis, is more difficult to treat (Fig. 17-1).[18] P. aeruginosa is the most common cause.[19] The ear cartilage does not have its own blood supply, so antibiotics alone are usually ineffective. Early referral to a plastic surgeon for debridement of infected cartilage is appropriate.

Infectious Etiologies

Group A Streptococcus

Group A streptococcus (GAS) and S. aureus are the two most common causes of cellulitis. Streotococcal cellulitis is infrequently associated with fluctuance; the infection may progress rapidly. Perineal streptococcal carriage in surgical personnel has been associated with outbreaks of postoperative wound infections.[20] Erysipelas is a form of cellulitis that is almost always due to GAS and involves the more superficial layers of the skin. In erysipelas, the area of inflammation is raised above the surrounding skin, and there is a distinct demarcation between involved and normal skin.[21]

Staphylococcus aureus

S. aureus is currently the most commonly implicated organism in cellulitis following a surgical procedure[22] and is also a common cause after nonsurgical wounds. Cellulitis caused by S. aureus is generally more indolent, and fluctulance is more likely to develop. Facial cellulitis in a newborn infant can be a manifestation of staphylococcal osteomyelitis.[23]

Haemophilus influenzae and Streptococcus pneumoniae

Prior to the introduction of the conjugate vaccine, H. influenzae type b (Hib) was a common cause of cellulitis of the periorbital area and of the cheek (buccal cellulitis) in infants under 2 years of age.[24,25] Cellulitis due to Hib results from bacteremic spread and is classically associated with a violacious hue, although occasionally S. pneumoniae can cause a similar pattern.[26,27]

Groups B, C, and G Streptococci

Group B streptococcal (GBS) infection in the newborn or young infant can occasionally present as focal cellulitis, sometimes with an associated adenitis.[28] As with cellulitis caused by Hib and S. pneumoniae, cellulitis in this setting is the result of bacteremic spread. Lumbar puncture is indicated to rule out concomitant GBS meningitis, which may be clinically inapparent.[29,30] Other streptococcal groups (e.g., C and G) may occasionally be associated with cellulitis, especially in the extremities of patients with poor venous or lymphatic drainage.[31]

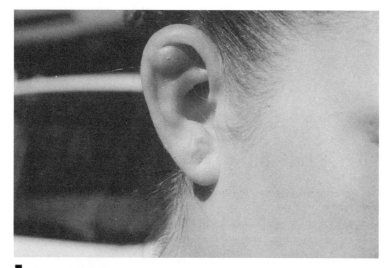

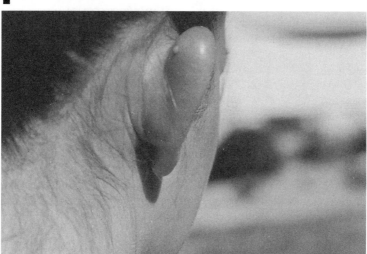

■ **FIGURE 17-1** 13-year-old girl with auricular perichondritis caused by *Pseudomonas aeruginosa* infection of an upper ear piercing. Despite treatment with oral ciprofloxacin, she required surgical excision of the infected cartilage.

Erysipelothrix rhusiopathiae

This gram-positive rod is associated with three distinct syndromes, the most common of which is a mild cutaneous infection known as erysipeloid. The diffuse cutaneous form and the septicemic form are much less common.[32] Erysipeloid manifests as a sharply demarcated red to purple patch at the site of inoculation, usually the finger or hand. Rare in the United States, the infection is usually acquired occupationally by exposure to contaminated animals, birds, fish, or their products. Penicillin is the drug of choice.

Vibrio Species

Vibrios (especially *V. vulnificus*, *V. alginolyticus*, and *V. damsela*) are uncommon causes of cellulitis. Patients usually have a history of sustaining a wound while having direct contact with seawater or while cleaning shellfish. Patients typically have fever and bullous cellulitis with intense pain at the wound site. Secondary fasciitis or septicemia may ensue, with a mortality rate of 25%.[33] Studies in a mouse model as well as in vitro synergy studies suggest that the optimal antibiotic treatment should include both tetracycline and cefotaxime.[34,35]

Other Organisms

Several other causes (e.g., cutaneous anthrax, sporotrichosis, and *Nocardia*) may resemble cellulitis initially but usually progress to form ulcerative lesions. They are discussed later in the chapter in the section on skin ulcers.

Laboratory Approach

The white blood cell (WBC) count and differential suggest infection in most patients with an infectious cellulitis, although in mild cases sometimes the WBC count is normal. Blood should usually be obtained for culture before starting therapy, especially for the more severe cases, because once therapy is begun the yield of subsequent cultures falls dramatically. Needle aspiration of an area of cellulitis for Gram stain and culture may be helpful,[36] especially if there is a bleb or underlying abscess, elevated periosteum, or joint effusion.

Treatment

The treatment of cellulitis depends on the cause. For most cases of cellulitis, empiric therapy should be directed against Group A streptococcus and *S. aureus*. For mild cases, a 7–10-day course of an oral antibiotic, such as cephalexin or dicloxacillin is reasonable. A follow-up appointment in 24–48 hours should be made to ensure that the patient is responding to therapy. Cases of cellulitis accompanied by high fever, toxicity, extensive lymphangitis, or rapid progression require hospitalization and intravenous antibiotics. Reasonable choices include oxacillin, cefazolin, or clindamycin. Once the child has improved clinically, a 10-day course can be completed with an oral agent. If the location of the cellulitis suggests a possible underlying cause, the initial antibiotic therapy should be directed at that cause (see Table 17-1). Adjunctive therapy, such as warm compresses and elevation of the affected extremity have not been subjected to rigorous study but probably provide symptomatic relief.

Immunosuppressed Children

Agents that rarely produce cellulitis in normal individuals can cause cellulitis in immunosuppressed children. This is explained, in part, by unusual host susceptibility and, in part, by the frequent prior use of antibiotics in these patients, which selects for altered flora. A vigorous attempt to determine the causative organism should be made. *P. aeruginosa* and enteric gram-negative organisms are often implicated, and empiric therapy should cover these organisms as well as staphylococci and streptococci. Initial therapy should be given intravenously. Examples of empiric therapy include cefepime or an antistaphylococcal penicillin and an aminoglycoside. Fungi, especially *Cryptococcus*, as well as mycobacteria, are occasionally implicated.

Mucor and other zygomycetes are primitive fungi that can produce a necrotizing cellulitis resembling necrotizing fasciitis, especially in the newborn period, under adhesive dressings or bandages.[37]

Noninfectious Cellulitis

Eosinophilic Cellulitis

This self-limited condition usually presents with sudden onset of single or multiple erythematous swellings affecting the extremities or trunk. Histologically, there are diffuse dermal infiltrates of eosinophils, but peripheral eosinophilia is variably present.[38] The condition may be familial, and it has been reported in newborns.[39] Lesions usually respond to corticosteroids. The term "Wells syndrome" is usually reserved for recurrent cases of eosinophilic cellulitis.

Scleredema

This rare entity is sometimes referred to as "scleredema adultorum" (although it is probably more common in children) or as "scleredema of Buschke." It is characterized by dermal deposits of mucopolysaccharides, which cause nonpitting induration of the skin, sometimes with erythema. The induration often has a cape-like distribution spreading from the neck and shoulders to the back and trunk. It may occur as a postinfectious phenomenon[40,41] or, in adults, as a complication of long-standing diabetes mellitus.[42] The disease usually resolves spontaneously over a period of weeks to months.

Erythema Nodosum

Erythema nodosum is often initially mistaken for cellulitis of the legs. The hallmark is tender, bright-red subcutaneous nodules over the tibias, although other areas are occasionally affected. New nodules are round and poorly demarcated, with diameters from 1–10 cm; over days they become purple and bruise-like (Fig. 17-2). A prodromal period of low-grade fever, arthralgia, and leg pain is common. The erythrocyte sedimentation rate (ESR) is typically elevated, but other laboratory results are usually normal.

Erythema nodosum should be considered a clue that another disease may be present (see Box 17-1). More common in females, it is caused by inflammation in the septae between subcutaneous fat lobules (septal panniculitis) and occurs as an immunologic response to various stimuli.[43] In children, infectious triggers are the most common, especially recent group A streptococcal pharyngitis.[44,45]

In the past, tuberculosis was the infection most commonly associated with erythema nodosum. The lesions can antedate skin test conversion.[46] Rarely, the skin test itself, as well as BCG vaccine, is associated with erythema nodosum. Nontuberculous mycobacterial infection may also be associated with

> **BOX 17-1 ■ Conditions Associated with Erythema Nodosum**
>
> ***Infectious***
> Group A streptococcus
> Tuberculosis and nontuberculous mycobacteria
> Systemic fungal infections (histoplasmosis, coccidioidomycosis, blastomycosis)
> Epstein-Barr virus
> Toxoplasmosis
> Leptospirosis
> Enteric infections (yersiniosis, salmonellosis, campylobacteriosis)
> Psittacosis
>
> ***Noninfectious***
> Sarcoidosis
> Inflammatory bowel disease
> Malignancy (leukemia, lymphoma)
> Drug reactions (sulfas, others)
> Idiopathic

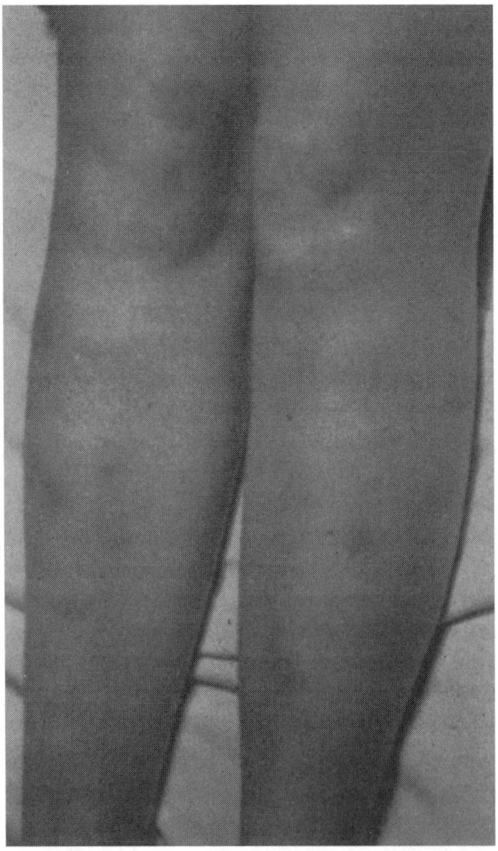

■ **FIGURE 17-2** Erythema nodosum, with red tender nodules. This is sometimes mistaken for cellulitis. (Photo from Dr. Gordon Tuffli.)

erythema nodosum.[47] In addition, the nodules caused by infection with *Mycobacterium marinum* infection in patients with exposure to fish tanks or swimming pools may sometimes resemble erythema nodosum.[48]

Other common triggers for erythema nodosum include Epstein-Barr virus (EBV) infection and systemic fungal disease, such as histoplasmosis and coccidioidomycosis.[45,49] Some of the more common noninfectious conditions that are associated with erythema nodosum include sarcoidosis, inflammatory bowel disease, Hodgkin's disease, and use of certain drugs (especially sulfonamides and oral contraceptive agents).[43] Other causes of panniculitis, as well as vasculitides, such as polyarteritis nodosa, may sometimes mimic erythema nodosum.[43,50]

A careful history of possible exposures should be elicited and a thorough physical examination performed. Unless the underlying condition is obvious, a complete blood count, chest roentgenograph, ESR, and a tuberculin skin test should be done. In selected cases, other tests, such as throat culture, antistreptococcal antibodies, EBV titers, and fungal serologies may be indicated.

In children, between one-quarter and one-third of cases of erythema nodosum are idiopathic.[44,45] The lesions most often resolve within a few weeks. Usually, only analgesics are necessary for treatment, although severe cases respond to systemic corticosteroids. Before steroids are prescribed, it is important to exclude an underlying infection that may be worsened by their use.

■ NECROTIZING SOFT-TISSUE INFECTIONS

Classification of necrotizing soft-tissue infections may be based on the anatomic structure involved, the infecting organisms, and the clinical manifestations. Because of considerable overlap in these parameters, the nomenclature is confusing. For example, what was once commonly referred to as streptococcal gangrene is now usually called necrotizing fasciitis. However, organisms other than Group A streptococcus may cause necrotizing fasciitis. Some authors define *gangrenous* infections as those with onset within 24–48 hours after trauma or surgery and *necrotizing* infections as those with more delayed onset.[51]

Any classification of necrotizing soft-tissue infections should emphasize that awaiting bacterial classification of the etiology can lead to unnecessary delay and worsened outcome. In one series, operations performed more than 24 hours after recognition of infection resulted in a 70% mortality rate compared with a 36% rate if the time was less than 24 hours.[52] An experienced surgeon should be consulted as soon as possible after the recognition of any necrotizing skin infection.

Necrotizing Fasciitis

Guiliano's classification of necrotizing fasciitis into two types seems to have withstood the test of time.[53] Type I is caused by mixed anaerobic and gram-negative aerobic bacilli and usually occurs as a postoperative complication. Type II is caused by Group A streptococcus and most commonly occurs after penetrating injuries, trauma, or during convalescence with varicella. The presentation and initial management of both types are similar.

The affected area is erythematous, warm, shiny, and swollen, with or without bullae, and often with indistinct margins. The appearance is often described as peau d'orange (orange peel) in character. The presence of fever, severe pain out of proportion to the local findings, and systemic toxicity should suggest the possibility of necrotizing fasciitis. Associated laboratory findings include leukocytosis, thrombocytopenia, hyponatremia, hypocalcemia, azotemia, and increased serum creatine phosphoki-

nase.[54–56] Of patients with streptococcal toxic shock syndrome, about half will have concomitant necrotizing fasciitis.[21]

In children, systemic toxicity and marked tissue edema may be the only initial clues to the presence of necrotizing fasciitis; fever and leukocytosis are not uniformly present.[57] Most infections are either due to Group A streptococcus or are polymicrobial.[57,58] In newborns, necrotizing fasciitis can be a complication of omphalitis. Initial periumbilical erythema and swelling can progress rapidly to involve the entire abdominal wall and may progress to involve the flank and chest.[59]

Fournier Gangrene

Necrotizing fasciitis of the perineal, genital, or perianal regions is referred to as Fournier gangrene.[60] This condition is very uncommon in children, with approximately fifty reported cases in the literature.[61] In adults, gram-negative bacilli and anaerobes predominate, whereas in children, staphylococcal and streptococcal species are more common. The presentation may be subacute, and the child may not appear systemically ill initially. Management is as for other forms of necrotizing fasciitis.

Clostridial Myonecrosis (Gas Gangrene)

Although historically referred to as "gas gangrene," clostridial myonecrosis indicates the causal agent and the tissue involved and thus is the preferred term.[54] Three major groups are recognized: posttraumatic, postoperative, and spontaneous (which is rare). Clostridial myonecrosis is characterized by crepitation, the crackling feeling consequent to palpation of bubbles of gas under the skin. Crepitant cellulitis should be presumed to be early gas gangrene. The triad of severe pain, tachycardia out to proportion to fever, and crepitus strongly suggests the diagnosis.[54] *Clostridium perfringens* is the usual species recovered in these cases. The course of tissue destruction is usually rapid and severe, with pain, shiny pallor, edema, vesiculation, and crepitus progressing to hemorrhagic darkening and softening of the tissues. Gas may be seen in the subcutaneous tissues on roentgenography. Gram stain of wound discharge or tissue reveals gram-positive rods, usually without neutrophilic infiltration.

Non-Clostridial Gas Gangrene

Aerogenic coliform infections, such as with *E. coli*, *Enterobacter*, or *Aeromonas*, may produce gas in the tissues but are usually less necrotizing and destructive than clostridial infection.[62] Gas introduced by trauma into the tissues may be mistaken for gas gangrene.[63]

Necrotizing Cellulitis (Wet Gangrene)

This type is characterized by swollen, boggy tissues, with erythema and blister formation along with tissue destruction. It resembles cellulitis early in its course.

Dry Gangrene

This type is usually secondary to interruption of the blood supply, most often affecting an extremity. The area initially appears dusky, then dark purple, and finally black. If there is no blood vessel disease and an infection is suspected, the diagnosis may be purpura fulminans. The most common cause is meningococcemia,[64] which is discussed in Chapters 10 and 11. Neonates with an inherited deficiency of protein C or protein S may present with purpura fulminans.[65,66]

Meleney's Synergistic Gangrene

This is caused by co-infection with *S. aureus* and a microaerophilic streptococcus.[67] It is usually a post-surgical complication, especially of the abdomen or chest. It manifests as a slowly expanding ulceration of the superficial fascia. The wound is typically tender and purple.

Compartment Syndromes

Ischemic extremities can result from a compartment syndrome (the compression of a muscle mass within a fascial compartment) as a result of traumatic swelling or vascular occlusion. The syndrome can occur in any age group, including newborns, in whom it can be a consequence of septicemia.[68]

Diagnosis and Management of Necrotizing Soft-Tissue Infections

Fluid from vesicles or exudate may reveal gram-positive rods (clostridia), gram-positive cocci in pairs and chains (streptococci), or a mixture of organisms in polymicrobial infection. However, caution is indicated, as the Gram stain frequently suggests a single organism when subsequent cultures reveal multiple pathogens.[57] In patients with wounds exposed to salt water, *Vibrio* infection should be considered (see previous section, Cellulitis). Necrotic tissue should be cultured for anaerobes and aerobes. Blood cultures may be positive in up to 50% of cases.[59] Imaging studies can sometimes be useful if the diagnosis is in doubt, but negative studies cannot exclude the possibility of necrotizing infection. In clostridial myonecrosis, plain films often show soft-tissue gas dissecting into the muscle. Gas in the tissues is an inconsistent finding in other forms of necrotizing fasciitis. CT may show asymmetric thickening of deep fascia, and MRI may demonstrate abnormal high signal intensity along deep fascial planes on T2-weighted images.[69] However, necrotizing fasciitis is a clinical diagnosis, and surgical intervention should not be delayed awaiting imaging studies.

Because most patients with necrotizing fasciitis are in shock, fluid and electrolyte replacement is necessary. Prompt and aggressive surgical debridement of all necrotic tissue is critical. In a series of 20 children with necrotizing fasciitis, all 15 survivors underwent surgical debridement within 3 hours of admission.[57] Multiple repeat operations may be required in the first few days.

Initial antibiotic coverage should be broad and include coverage for streptococci, gram-negative bacilli, and anaerobes, even if the initial Gram stain indicates a single organism. The combination of ampicillin, gentamicin, and clindamycin is reasonable empiric therapy. If operative cultures grow only GAS, penicillin plus clindamycin is appropriate. In deep tissue infections with large inocula, streptococcal replication may be slow and penicillin-binding protein expression may be inadequate for a cell-wall active agent, such as penicillin, to kill optimally.[70] The addition of a protein synthesis inhibitor, such as clindamycin, may speed killing and decrease toxin production. Penicillin plus clindamycin is also appropriate antibiotic therapy for clostridial myonecrosis.[54]

The role of nonsteroidal anti-inflammatory drugs (NSAIDS) in the pathogenesis of necrotizing fasciitis is controversial. Some studies have found an association between recent NSAID use and the development of necrotizing fasciitis,[71] whereas others have not.[72] It is possible that these agents delay the diagnosis of necrotizing fasciitis by masking the symptoms. Given the ready availability of an alternate antipyretic agent, it is probably wise to avoid NSAIDS in children with varicella.[73] It is also reasonable to avoid their use in a child with severe cellulitis in whom the possibility of early necrotizing fasciitis is being considered.

The use of intravenous immune globulin (IVIG)

in the treatment of severe, invasive GAS infections has been reported anecdotally[74] but not subjected to clinical trials. In a mouse model of group A streptococcal necrotizing fasciitis, the addition of immune globulin did not result in increased bacterial clearance.[75] However, given the high mortality rate of necrotizing fasciitis and the biologically plausible consideration that IVIG could neutralize the effect of streptococcal superantigens, its use may be justified.

The use of hyperbaric oxygen in the treatment of necrotizing fasciitis is likewise controversial. A retrospective study reported a case-fatality rate of 23% among patients receiving hyperbaric oxygen and 66% among those not receiving that therapy.[76] Given that the overall case-fatality rate of necrotizing fasciitis in most series is approximately 25%, it is unlikely that the benefit of hyperbaric oxygen is as dramatic as this study would suggest. Its use should not delay surgical intervention.

■ TRAUMATIC WOUND INFECTIONS

Traumatic wounds encompass a spectrum from clean lacerations to contaminated compound fractures. This section deals with the prophylaxis and treatment of infections associated with simple lacerations, severe contaminated wounds, penetrating abdominal injuries, and open (compound) fractures. Animal and human bite infections are discussed in Chapter 21.

General Management

Established surgical principles, irrigation, and debridement are the most important factors in the management of traumatic wounds. Antibiotics do not prevent infection in the absence of thorough wound decontamination.[77] Saline is the safest and most effective irrigant.[78] All devitalized tissue should be carefully debrided. Wounds at low risk for infection can be closed as late as 12–24 hours after the injury, whereas high-risk wounds (contaminated wounds, those in locations with poor blood supply, and those in immunocompromised patients) should be closed within 6 hours.[77]

A history of tetanus vaccination should be obtained from all persons with traumatic wounds. A guide to the use of tetanus toxoid and tetanus immune globulin is given in Table 17-2.

Follow-up cultures should be done every 2–3 days if drainage is present, to detect the emergence of resistant organisms. Ordinarily, such organisms are present in small numbers and proliferate when the susceptible organisms are inhibited.

Simple Lacerations

The routine use of prophylactic antibiotics in simple, nonbite wound lacerations is not recommended. A meta-analysis of seven randomized, controlled trials demonstrated no difference in the rate of wound infection among those receiving antibiotics as compared with placebo recipients.[79]

Simple lacerations uncommonly become infected. If signs and symptoms of infection are apparent but no discharge is present to culture, antibiotic therapy directed against *S. aureus* and group A streptococcus is reasonable, e.g., cephalexin. For infected wounds associated with freshwater exposure, *Pseudomonas* and *Aeromonas* are possibilities,

TABLE 17-2. INDICATIONS FOR PROPHYLAXIS WITH TETANUS TOXOID AND TETANUS IMMUNE GLOBULIN (TIG) AFTER WOUNDS

NO. OF PREVIOUS DOSES	CLEAN, MINOR WOUNDS		OTHER WOUNDS*	
	TETANUS TOXOID	TIG	TETANUS TOXOID	TIG
<3 or unknown ≥3	Yes	No	Yes	Yes
≥3 (Last dose <5 yr ago)	No	No	No	No
≥3 (Last dose 5–10 yr ago)	No	No	Yes	No
≥3 (Last dose >10 yr ago)	Yes	No	Yes	No

* Such as wounds contaminated with dirt, feces, and saliva; puncture wounds; avulsions; and wounds resulting from missiles, crushing, burns, and frostbite.

(Modified from Centers for Disease Control and Prevention. Diphtheria, tetanus, and pertussis: recommendations for vaccine use and other preventative measures. Recommendations of the Immunization Practices Advisory Committee (ACIP). MMWR Recomm Rep 1991:40:1–28.)

and the use of a fluoroquinolone should be entertained.[80] If the infection does not respond promptly to therapy, the incision may need to be reopened and the wound irrigated and debrided.

Severe Contaminated Wounds

No data exist on the effectiveness of prophylactic antibiotics in this setting, although most experts recommend their use. Using antibiotics in patients with grossly contaminated wounds is probably more appropriately considered empiric therapy than prophylaxis. The appropriate duration of therapy is likewise unknown but is usually about 5–7 days.

In established infection of severe wounds, the responsible organism varies depending on whether or not the patient has received prophylactic antibiotics. Unfortunately, not all reports give those details. In a study in the Vietnam war, severe extremity wounds were cultured on the first, third, and fifth day in a field hospital.[81] *Bacillus* species and *S. epidermidis* were the most common organisms recovered initially, but *Enterobacter, E. coli, Serratia, Klebsiella*, and *Acinetobacter* were also common. *Proteus* and *Pseudomonas* were rarely found at first but were commonly recovered from cultures on the fifth day, after antibiotics had been given. A reasonable regimen for empiric therapy in the setting of severe contaminated wounds would be ampicillin-sulbactam or clindamycin plus either gentamicin or ceftazidime.

Open Fractures

Gas gangrene has been reported as an important complication in open forearm fractures of children when antibiotics have not been given.[82] Patients with open fractures should receive empiric antimicrobial therapy. Despite the use of antibiotics, the rates of infection are approximately 10–15%.[83]

It is likely that local factors play a greater role in the risk of infection than antibiotics. In a study of 240 consecutive open fractures of the arm or leg, the most significant risk factors for infection were fracture grade, internal or external fixation, and fracture of the lower leg.[84] Timing and duration of antimicrobial therapy did not affect the risk of infection. In a randomized trial, a 24-hour course of antistaphylococcal therapy was as effective as a 5-day regimen.[83] A first generation cephalosporin (e.g., cefazolin) can be used for open fractures. Cefazolin does not have activity against *Clostridia*, however. For heavily contaminated open fractures, coverage against anaerobes and gram-negative organisms should be considered, such as with ampicillin-sulbactam or the combination of clindamycin and gentamicin.

The necessity of antimicrobial prophylaxis in closed fractures is less clear. However, a randomized placebo-controlled trial in 2195 adults with closed extremity fractures found that a single preoperative dose of a cephalosporin reduced the rate of superficial and deep wound infection from 8% down to 4%.[85]

Penetrating Abdominal Wounds

The use of prophylactic antimicrobials for abdominal injury is predicated on the assumption that hollow visceral injury with resultant bacterial contamination of the intraperitoneal cavity has occurred.[86] However, at the time of surgery, definitive evidence of intra-abdominal contamination may be lacking. The use of prophylactic antibiotics in this setting has been demonstrated to be superior to placebo in a randomized controlled trial.[87] Injury to the colon carries the highest risk of infection.[88] Administration of antibiotics *before* surgery is associated with a lower incidence of postoperative wound infection and intra-abdominal abscess than initial administration of antibiotics in the intraoperative or postoperative period.[89] Antibiotic regimens should cover gut anaerobes, such as *Bacteroides fragilis* as well as enteric gram-negative rods, such as *E. coli*. Timing of antibiotic administration (preoperative vs. later) is more important than duration.[90] Two studies have demonstrated no difference in infection rates in patients receiving antibiotics for 12–24 hours as compared to 5 days, regardless of degree of injury.[91,92]

Overall, the incidence of peritonitis and intra-abdominal abscess following abdominal trauma is less than 5%.[93] However, the risk increases to greater than 25% in patients with colonic injury, especially if there is concomitant injury to the spleen.[94] Bedside ultrasound is sometimes used because of convenience, but computed tomography (CT) is more sensitive in detecting intra-abdominal abcesses.[95] Open surgical drainage or, more commonly, CT-guided percutanous drainage of abscesses is usually necessary. The principles of antibiotic therapy in this situation are similar to those for ruptured appendix with peritonitis, as discussed in Chapter 12. Several options exist, including single-drug regimens (e.g., ampicillin-sulbactam or meropenem) and multiple-drug regimens (e.g., ampicillin, gentamicin, and metronidazole or clindamycin). The initial regimen can then be modified, if necessary, based on results of Gram stain and culture. Duration of therapy is usually 7–14 days.

■ BURN INFECTIONS

Despite remarkable advances in burn care over the past 2 decades, infection remains an important cause of morbidity and mortality in these patients. The increased susceptibility of the burned child to infection relates to impairment in both local and systemic immune response, the loss of the skin barrier, and the frequent need for invasive devices (such as central venous lines, urinary catheters, and endotracheal tubes), which further breach host defenses.

Approximately one-third of infections in burned children involve the burn wound, one-third are secondary to catheter-related bacteremia, and one-third involve other sites (most notably pneumonia and urinary tract infection).[96] Depth, type, and extent of the burn are the greatest factors influencing the risk of infection. Age of the child and location of the burn appear to be less important factors.

Among 70 consecutive children cared for in a burn unit, 18 (38%) of 47 of children with full thickness burns developed an infection compared with only 1 (4%) of 23 children with partial thickness burns.[96] All nine children who sustained both flame and inhalation injury developed infection as compared with 2 (14%) of 14 children with flame burns that were not accompanied by inhalation injury and eight (19%) of 43 children with scald burns. All 6 children with greater than 30% of the total body surface area burned developed infection; in contrast, infection occurred in 10 (16%) of 64 children with less extensive burns.

Possible Etiologies

Gram-positive organisms (especially *S. aureus* and *S. epidermidis*) are the most common cause of infections in burn patients. *P. aeruginosa*, once the most common cause of infection in this setting, remains the most prominent of the gram-negative pathogens. However, any organism can cause infection in the burn patient. Patients with a history of treatment with systemic antibiotics are at increased risk

for late infections with *Candida* spp., as well as *Aspergillus* spp. or other filamentous fungi.[96,97] Both primary infection and reactivation of herpes viruses may occur, including herpes simplex virus (HSV), varicella-zoster virus (VZV), and cytomegalovirus. Vesicular lesions should raise suspicion of HSV or VZV infection. CMV infection typically presents several weeks after the burn as persistent fever and lymphocytosis.[98]

Diagnostic Approach

All burn wounds become colonized with bacteria, and distinguishing colonization from infection is critical. The peak incidence of burn wound infection (sometimes referred to as "burn wound sepsis") is from 6–10 days post burn, but infection can occur at any point during the patient's course.[99] Local signs of burn wound infection include purulence; gray, green, black, or hemorrhagic discoloration; erythema or edema at the wound margin; unexpected eschar separation; conversion of partial thickness to full thickness necrosis; and nonadherence of grafts.[96,97] Although the above findings may provide clues to the presence of infection, burn wound biopsy with quantitative cultures demonstrating greater than 10^5 organisms per gram of tissue in conjunction with histologic evidence of tissue invasion by bacteria is considered the gold standard.[97] Systemic signs of infection (tachycardia, fever or hypothermia, leukocytosis or leukopenia, and hypotension) are often present in patients with burn wound infection but may also be present in the severely burned patient in the absence of infection. Blood cultures in burn wound infection are positive in approximately half of cases.

Diagnosis of catheter-associated bacteremia, urinary tract infection, and ventilator-associated pneumonia is similar to that in children without burns. Persistent bacteremia or a new murmur should suggest the possibility of endocarditis.[100] Infection with toxin-producing staphylococci or streptococci can lead to toxic shock syndrome.[101] Other possible infections include meningitis, suppurative chondritis of ear burns, suppurative thrombophlebitis, osteomyelitis, septic arthritis, and sinusitis consequent to long-term nasotracheal intubation. Multisystem organ failure is the most common cause of death in burn patients and may occur in association with overwhelming infection. However, it can also occur in the clinically uninfected burn patient who has a history of multiple previous infections during the hospital course. It is postulated that uncontrolled systemic inflammation persists despite control of infection, leading to multiple organ failure.[102]

Treatment

Burn Wound Infection

The penetration of various systemic antibiotics into the burn eschar has not been well-studied, and thus these agents cannot be relied upon as the sole treatment modality.[103] Prompt surgical removal of the infected tissue is necessary, as is the use of topical antimicrobial agents. Topical agents are discussed further in the next section.

The choice of systemic antibiotic is best made from the results of burn wound biopsy culture or blood culture. The empiric use of antibiotics pending culture results should be based on the most commonly cultured invasive pathogens in the burn unit, as well as the results of surveillance burn wound cultures. As soon as culture results are available, therapy should be adjusted to the narrowest spectrum agent with efficacy against the organism. The pharmacokinetics of antibiotics are altered in burn patients, and serum levels should be monitored if assays are available. The duration of therapy should be tailored to the clinical response and the results of repeat cultures.

Other Infections

Treatment of catheter-associated bloodstream or urinary tract infections may require removal of the foreign device. As with therapy for burn wound infection, prolonged courses of systemic antibiotics are discouraged because of the high likelihood of selecting for resistant organisms and of predisposing to infection with opportunistic pathogens, such as fungi.

Prevention

Burn Wound Infection

In general, the initial treatment of a burn wound includes removing all necrotic tissue, ruptured blisters, and debris. Most experts recommend early tangential excision, which involves surgical debridement of graduated amounts of necrotic tissue until viable tissue is reached.[104] Early closure of the burn wound with grafting protects against infection. The role of routine surveillance wound cultures is de-

bated. If they are used, it is important that physicians understand that a positive culture is not an indication for administering systemic antibiotics; it is simply a guide for future empiric therapy when it is necessary.

Topical antimicrobial agents play a key role in burn wound management. Several agents are available, each with advantages and disadvantages to their use. Silver sulfadiazine (Silvadene) is probably the most commonly used agent. It has the advantage of broad spectrum of activity, especially against gram-negative organisms but also against gram-positives and anaerobes, as well as fungi and some viruses (e.g., HSV). It is also effective in reducing pain. Disadvantages include allergic reactions in 5–10% of patients and reversible neutropenia in a smaller percentage.

Mafenide acetate (Sulfamylon) also has a relatively broad spectrum of coverage. It has especially good activity against *P. aeruginosa*. Its main advantage is that it penetrates burn eschar, enabling it to be used for treatment of deeply infected wounds. It is also the agent of choice for serious burns to the ear to help prevent chondritis.[104] Its main disadvantage is the tendency to produce metabolic acidosis, which is especially troublesome in the patient with inhalation injury and subsequent respiratory acidosis. Its application is painful to intact nerve endings. Also, prolonged use may allow overgrowth of *Candida* spp.

Other topical agents with narrower spectra that may be used in certain circumstances, sometimes in combination with other agents, include silver nitrate, nitrofurantoin, mupirocin, and nystatin. Acticoat, a silver-coated dressing material, has shown promise in a small trial comparing its use to that of silver nitrate.[105]

Dressing changes are typically performed once or twice daily. The incidence of bacteremia during burn wound manipulation varies depending on the extent of the burn. In one recent study the overall rate was 13%.[106] The prophylactic use of systemic antibiotics is generally discouraged, primarily because of the risks of selecting for resistant bacteria and causing fungal overgrowth, but also because of a lack of demonstrated efficacy.[107]

After being debrided and cleaned, many small, partial thickness burns can be treated as an outpatient, as long as follow-up can be assured. The caretaker can be instructed in the application of a topical agent (usually silver sulfadiazine) with twice-daily dressing changes.

Other Measures

The value of isolation measures in the prevention of colonization and infection of burns is difficult to assess. One study using historic controls demonstrated a decrease of gram-negative bacteremia from 31% in patients cared for in an open ward to 12% among patients in single-patient rooms.[108] Other factors that changed during the 10-year study period could account for some of this effect. Techniques such as single room, sterile linens, gowning, masking, and gloving are generally used. Strict attention to handwashing should be observed. Laminar airflow units are used in some hospitals but do not prevent infection with the patient's own organisms.

Prevention of urinary tract infection can be accomplished by early removal of the urinary catheter. The further the insertion site of a central venous catheter from the burn wound the lower the likelihood of catheter-associated bacteremia.[109] Measures that have not been demonstrated to prevent infection in patients with burns include selective decontamination of the digestive tract[110] and the use of IVIG.[111]

◼ PUSTULES AND SKIN ABSCESSES

Definitions

Purulent localized bacterial skin infections have a variety of names, depending on the size, severity, and the area of the skin or skin organ infected. A *pustule* is a small (1–5 mm in diameter) raised lesion with a yellow fluid exudate (containing necrotic tissue and leukocytes). An *abscess* is a large (1 cm or greater) spherical collection of pus, usually walled off by a capsule. Abscesses may occur in any body organ. When they occur in the skin, they are termed *furuncles*. The lay term for a furuncle is a *boil*. A *carbuncle* is a larger lesion formed by the coalescence of furuncles; carbuncles usually have multiple openings to the skin.

Special Locations

Special names are used for infections of various areas of the skin or skin organs. A *paronychia* is an infection around the fingernail or toenail. A *hordeolum* (or *sty*) is an infection of a gland of the eyelid and is discussed in Chapter 5. *Folliculitis* is a pustular infection of the hair follicles. An abscess of the subcutaneous fat pad of the fingertip is called a *felon* or *whitlow*. The latter has come to be used more commonly to describe herpetic lesions. A superficial blistering lesion over the a finger's distal fat pad with thin pus has been called "blistering distal dactylitis" and is classically caused by group A streptococcal infection,[112] although cases attributed to *S. aureus* and group B streptococcus, have been described.[113,114]

Periporitis is a synonym for multiple small sweat-gland abscesses, usually occurring in infancy. These dome-shaped pustules are not hot or tender and usually do not "point" or drain spontaneously.[115] *Hidradenitis suppurativa* presents as infection with acute inflammation of the apocrine sweat glands of adolescents or adults and occurs particularly in the axilla, perianal region, perineum, or buttocks. In at least some cases, a predisposition to this condition is inherited as an autosomal dominant disorder.[116] A careful history of the occurrence of boils or abscesses in relatives of the patient may be helpful in establishing the diagnosis (and in differentiating this condition from recurrent furunculosis). It may become chronic with persistent pain, sinus tract and fistula formation, purulent discharge, and dermal scarring. Treatment of patients with severe disease can be difficult and may require complex surgical intervention.[117] The prognosis in patients with the familial form is almost always poor. Frequent and sometimes lifelong recurrences are common.

A *pyogenic granuloma* is a painless pink or red pea-sized nodule that develops after a minor injury, especially on the hands or face. It is not an infection but a proliferation of vascular tissue.

Erythema toxicum occurs in the first week of life and is characterized by papules and pustules. Smear of the pustules reveals eosinophils, but not bacteria, as described in Chapter 11.

Mastitis is a cellulitis or abscess of the breast, usually occurring in nursing mothers. *S. aureus* is the most common cause. Usually, it need not interfere with nursing the infant. In women with HIV infection, mastitis is a risk factor for postpartum transmission of infection to the nursing infant.[118]

Infectious mastitis can be distinguished from two other conditions, milk stasis, and noninfectious inflammation of the breast, by quantifying the number of leukocytes and bacteria per mL of milk. In both milk stasis and noninfectious inflammation, bacterial counts are less than 10^3, but leukocyte counts are less than 10^6 in the former condition and greater than 10^6 in the latter. In infectious mastitis, leukocyte counts are greater than 10^6 and bacterial counts are greater than 10^3.[119,120] Infectious mastitis is treated with systemic antibiotics and emptying the breast. Surgical drainage is done if a breast abscess develops.

Breast abscess or mastitis occasionally occurs in the newborn or young infant.[121–123] Systemic symptoms may be minimal. *S. aureus* is the most common cause, but occasionally group B streptococcus or gram-negative organisms are cultured. Most cases respond to systemic antibiotics.

Recurrent Furunculosis

Some patients, typically during adolescence, develop the frustrating problem of recurrent furuncles. *S. aureus* is the usual cause. Moist areas, such as the axilla and groin, are the most common areas affected. The abscess begins as a very tender, raised nodule with stretched, shiny skin and an indurated base.[124] The boils usually enlarge, soften, and then rupture, yielding a purulent discharge. Fever is variable. Treatment consists of incision and drainage and warm compresses. Oral antibiotics are sometimes necessary, if there are large or multiple lesions. Prevention is discussed later.

A history of recurrent boils in a young child should prompt testing for immune deficiency, especially neutrophil function disorders. Job-Buckley syndrome (hyper-IgE syndrome) may present with recurrent furunculosis, eczema, and coarse facial features. There is almost always a history of recurrent sinopulmonary infections.

Previously healthy teenagers with new onset of recurrent boils rarely have detectable immune disorders. However, they are often chronic carriers of *S. aureus* in the nose, groin, axilla, or rectum. Occasionally, there is an exposure history, such as the use of steam baths.[125]

Possible Infectious Etiologies

Most pustules and skin abscesses are caused by bacterial infections (Box 17-2). *S. aureus* is the most common cause, although many skin abscesses contain mixed anaerobic and aerobic bacteria.[126] *P. aeruginosa* causes folliculitis in persons exposed to contaminated hot tubs or spas.[127] The pustules are most prominent in areas covered by the swimming suit, because the warmer environment allows the bacteria to proliferate. The disease is self-limited in immunocompetent hosts and requires no therapy.

Perirectal abscesses can occur in children without any underlying disease. The most common causes are *S. aureus*, *Bacteroides*, and enteric bacteria. In one review of twenty-nine cases, one-quarter of children had an underlying illness.[128] Perirectal abscess in a child should always bring to mind the possibility of chronic granulomatous disease (CGD). In a series of 368 children with CGD, 51 (14%) developed a perirectal abscess.[129] Subcutaneous abscesses on other parts of the body are also common in children with CGD. They may also be a clue to other neutrophil disorders, such as leukocyte adhesion deficiency or hyper IgE syndrome (see Chapter 23).[130–132]

Cutaneous gonococcal infection of the finger can appear as grouped pustules, mimicking herpetic whitlow. Patients with disseminated gonorrhea may also develop skin pustules as well as oligoarthritis; this clinical pattern has been termed the "gonococcal dermatitis-arthritis syndrome."[133]

Group A streptococcus is an occasional cause of skin abscesses,[134] but *S. pneumoniae* and *H. influenzae* are rarely implicated.[135,136] Other rare causes of skin abscesses include *Streptococcus milleri*,[137] *Listeria monocytogenes*,[138] *Mycoplasma*,[139] *Nocardia*,[140,141] *Salmonella*,[142] *Yersinia*,[143] *Legionella*,[144] and various mycobacterial species.[145–147] Most of these rare causes occur predominantly in immunocompromised hosts or in patients with a specific risk factor (such as injection drug use).

Fungal causes, such as *Candida*[148] and *Coccidioides*,[149] are likewise rare. *Rhizopus* species have caused pustular and ulcerative skin lesions in orthopedic patients from contact with contaminated elastic bandages.[150] A travel history should be obtained as occasionally myiasis (botfly infestation) may mimic furunculosis in the patient with a recent visit to the tropics.[151]

Noninfectious Etiologies

Acropustulosis of Infancy

As described in Chapter 11, this condition consists of pruritic pustules on the distal extremities of in-

---

BOX 17-2 ■ Some Possible Causes of Pustules

Bacteria, particularly *S. aureus*
Erythema toxicum (in newborns)
Herpes simplex (especially fingertips)
Pustules secondary to bacteremia
Scabies
Acropustulosis of infancy

fants. It is often mistaken for impetigo or scabies.[152,153]

Acute Febrile Neutrophilic Dermatosis

Also called Sweet syndrome after the author who originally described it,[154] this condition is characterized microscopically by infiltration with neutrophils and clinically by waxy papules that progress to form violaceous papular or pustular nodules that may resemble intracutaneous abscesses. Fever and leukocytosis are common. Although sometimes idiopathic, many cases are associated with underlying disorders, including malignancies, infections, and autoimmune diseases.[155–157]

Eosinophilic Pustular Folliculitis (Ofuji Disease)

Most reports of this condition have been in young Japanese adult males, but children can get the disease, and there are several reports in infants. The disorder presents as recurrent crops of pruritic papules and pustules, primarily affecting the scalp and variably extending to the face, limbs, and trunk.[158] Systemic symptoms are absent, but there is usually leukocytosis and peripheral eosinophilia. It may occur in neonates, in which case it must be distinguished from erythema toxicum, transient neonatal pustular melanosis, infantile acropustulosis, and Langerhans' cell histiocytosis.[159] Histologically, there is a dense dermal infiltrate with perifollicular and perivascular eosinophilia.[160] Most cases are idiopathic, but the condition may occur in association with HIV infection[161] or hematologic malignancy.[162] One report describes a case of carbamazepine-induced eosinophilic pustular folliculitis, and another describes an association with skin test hypersensitivity to the house dust mite *Dermatophagoides pteronyssinus* in three children.[163] Various treatments have been reported as successful, including topical and systemic corticosteroids, indomethacin, interferon-α, and dapsone. It should be emphasized that the condition is self-limited, and thus therapies with the lowest incidence of side effects should be considered.

Diagnostic Approach and Treatment

Gram stain and culture of pustular skin lesions is a simple and useful diagnostic procedure. It is especially important to do this procedure in newborn infants, including those with mastitis.

Aspiration or incision and drainage of boils should be done when the surface of the lesion has a necrotic center. If they are few or small, this may be all that is needed. However, most clinicians use an antistaphylococcal antibiotic in addition (such as cephalexin), and this is certainly reasonable, especially if there is cellulitis surrounding the boil. In neonates, blood cultures should be obtained and intravenous antibiotics started.

Differentiation of bacterial felon from herpetic whitlow is important, because immediate drainage is indicated for the former and contradicted for the latter. Grouped vesicles on a red base are typical of herpetic lesions. In a series of 26 children with herpetic whitlow, 15 (65%) were initially misdiagnosed as a bacterial felon.[164] Incision of herpetic whitlow is unnecessary because the condition is self-limited. In adults, incision has been reported to be a risk factor for secondary bacterial infection, but firm data are lacking. A single case of HSV encephalitis has been reported after incision of whitlow in a child.[164] This seems likely to have been coincidental.

The early presentation of bacterial felon may be subtle and can be detected by increased opacity of the fingertip upon transillumination in a dark room.[165] If the felon has been caused by progression of a deep paronychia, in addition to incising the abscess, the nail should be removed.

Treatment of recurrent furunculosis is challenging. Cultures of the nose, groin, axilla, and rectum are often done to determine whether the patient is a *S. aureus* carrier. After treatment of the boils, several regimens have been used in an attempt to eradicate carriage and prevent further recurrences. If the isolate is susceptible to rifampin, this agent may be used in addition to another antistaphylococcal agent (such as cephalexin or clindamycin) for 10–14 days.[166] We also prescribe a 5-day course of topical mupirocin (Bactroban) to the nares and ask that the child bathe with an antistaphylococcal soap once daily for 5 days and then weekly for 6 months; chlorhexidine (Hibiclens) or hexachlorophene (Phisohex) may be used. In general, staphylococcal carriers carry staphylococci; thus, even if carriage is eradicated, the patient is usually recolonized within 6 months.[167] Therefore, in order to effect a long-term solution to this problem, some experts recommend repeating the mupirocin treatment every 6 months. Sometimes the source of the child's recurrent infection is an asymptomatic family member, in which case all members of the household can be treated with mupirocin and chlorhexidine. Multiple other regimens have been reported to have anecdotal success in preventing recurrences, including supplemental iron,[168] pentoxifyllin,[169] vitamin C,[170] and cycling antibiotics 1 of every 4 weeks for 6 months.[171]

■ STAPHYLOCOCCAL SCALDED SKIN SYNDROME

Staphylococcal scalded skin syndrome (SSSS) is best defined as the acute onset of generalized erythema with tenderness and exfoliation of the superficial epidermis. These features of redness, tenderness, blister formation, and skin sloughing resemble the features of a scald burn. A positive Nikolsky sign is often present,[172] elicited by pressing laterally against intact skin and sliding the epidermal layer off like the skin of an overripe peach. The disease is most common in children less than 5 years old. In one study of 15 children with generalized SSSS, the median age was 12 months, with a range of 23 days to 6 years.[173]

SSSS is caused by strains of *S. aureus* (usually phage group II) that produce one of two exfoliative toxins, ETA or ETB. Approximately 5% of all *S. aureus* produce exfoliative toxins,[174] which are variously referred to in the literature as "epidermolytic toxins," "epidermolysins," and "exfoliatins." In the generalized form, toxin is produced at a distant site and absorbed into the bloodstream. The source may be a focal infection (such as pneumonia or conjunctivitis), but most often it is a site of colonization only (such as the nares). Antitoxin antibody is protective and is found in nearly 90% of adults and full-term newborns (reflecting passive acquisition of maternal antibody), but in only 30% of children between 3 months and 2 years old.[175]

Spectrum of Illness

Newborn SSSS (Ritter's Disease)

In this age group, SSSS can be extensive (Fig. 17-3), and newborns are at high risk for complications due to loss of the protective epidermis, such as hypothermia, dehydration, and secondary infection.[174] Initially, the infant may not appear very ill, but staphylococcal disease in newborns should be regarded as potentially serious. Outbreaks in neonatal nurseries have been reported.[176] Rigorous infection control measures, such as isolation of cases, treatment of colonized staff, and strict attention to handwashing, are indicated.[177]

Childhood SSSS

After the newborn period, SSSS is usually less severe. Skin creases in the groin, axilla, and neck are often involved. Even if the area of skin involvement is extensive, children usually do not appear toxic, and with proper treatment the case-fatality rate is less than 4%.[178]

Adult SSSS

In adults, SSSS usually occurs in the setting of immunocompromise or renal failure,[179] in the latter case presumably due to inability to excrete the toxin. In contrast to children, the blood culture is frequently positive, and the mortality rate is greater than 50%.[179] Occasionally, children with the above risk factors may develop "adult type" SSSS, as has been reported in an anephric child.[180]

Bullous Impetigo

Bullous impetigo may occur in any age group and is best thought of as a localized form of SSSS (Fig. 17-4). Commonly occurring on the extremities, there are one to several isolated flaccid bullae that easily rupture, releasing clear fluid. In contrast to nonbullous impetigo, which is characterized by a honey-crusted lesion and may be caused by either *S. aureus* or group A streptococcus, bullous impetigo is nearly always caused by exfoliative toxin-producing strains of *S. aureus*.[173] The blisters in bullous impetigo are culture positive, in contrast to generalized SSSS in which the *S. aureus* is present at a distal site and toxin spreads hematogenously to the epidermis.

Differential Diagnosis

Staphylococcal Scarlet Fever

Once thought to be the mild end of the SSSS spectrum, staphylococcal scarlet fever is now understood to be a separate entity. This was demonstrated by a study of 60 *S. aureus* isolates from children with generalized SSSS (n = 15), bullous impetigo (n = 28), or staphylococcal scarlet fever (n = 17).[173] All strains isolated from children with generalized SSSS or bullous impetigo produced ETA and/or ETB. However, only 1 of 17 isolates from children with staphylococcal scarlet fever produced exfoliative toxin. The remaining 16 isolates produced a toxic shock syndrome toxin (TSST-1) and/or an enterotoxin. Thus, staphylococcal scarlet fever is

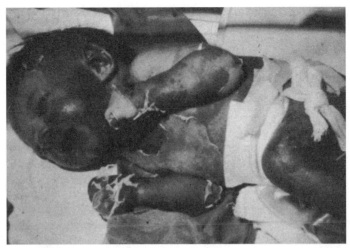

■ **FIGURE 17-3** Scalded-skin syndrome produced by staphylococcal epidermolytic toxin. (From: Melish Me, Glasgow LA. The staphylococcal scalded-skin syndrome. N Engl J Med 1970;282:114–9.)

probably better understood as a mild form of toxic shock syndrome. It is characterized by an erythematous rash that resolves by fine peeling or flaking with minimal exfoliation. There is no strawberry tongue and no circumoral pallor, which occur in the streptococcal form of scarlet fever (discussed in Chapter 11).

Toxic Epidermal Necrolysis (TEN)

In 1956, Lyell[181,182] introduced the term "toxic epidermal necrolysis" to describe patients with exten-

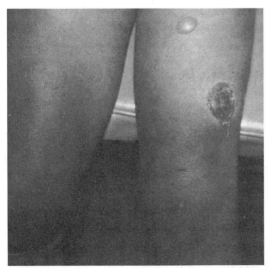

■ **FIGURE 17-4** Bullous impetigo showing an unruptured bulla and an older, crusted lesion. (Photo from Dr. Norman Fost.)

sive loss of epidermis due to necrosis that leaves the skin surface looking scalded. Once regarded as the same condition, it is now clear that SSSS and TEN are distinct conditions, with different causes, clinical presentation, and course. TEN is usually drug-induced and is best considered the severe end of the spectrum of Stevens-Johnson syndrome (SJS). As with SJS, TEN begins with small blisters on dusky purpuric macules accompanied by mucosal lesions in 90% of cases.[182] Unlike SJS, patients with TEN slough large sheets of necrotic epidermis with a total detachment greater than 30% of body surface area. The exposed skin is wrinkled and with varying degrees of erythema, which represents full-thickness necrosis of the epidermis.

In contrast, the peeling due to SSSS is more superficial and leaves an area of uniform erythema and no necrosis. TEN and SSSS are easily distinguished on skin biopsy. In SSSS, the separation is midepidermal, at the level of the zona granulosa, whereas the separation in TEN occurs at the dermal-epidermal junction.[183] For a rapid differentiation of the two conditions, a frozen section of peeled skin can be analyzed.[184,185] TEN is a multisystem disease, with fever, leukopenia, and lesions of the respiratory and gastrointestinal tracts being common findings. The case-fatality rate is approximately 25%.[186]

Epidermolysis Bullosa

This is the term for a clinically and genetically heterogeneous group of blistering skin disorders that are inherited in an autosomal-dominant or autosomal recessive fashion.[187,188] There is also a rare acquired form characterized by IgG anti-basement membrane autoantibodies to collagen VII.[189] Epidermolysis bullosa may be distinguished from SSSS by the frequently positive family history, the absence of systemic manifestations of infection, and the occurrence of bullae after minimal trauma.

Toxic Shock Syndromes (TSS)

As discussed in Chapter 11, staphylococcal TSS is caused by strains of *S. aureus* elaborating TSST-1 and/or enterotoxin, whereas streptococcal TSS is caused by strains of GAS elaborating streptococcal pyrogenic exotoxins (SPE) A and/or C.[190] TSS is characterized by fever, hypotension, generalized erythematous rash, and multiple organ involvement. The desquamation occurs 1–2 weeks after the rash, which is considerably later than that in SSSS.

Kawasaki Disease

As discussed in Chapter 11, desquamation of the fingertips, palms, and soles usually occurs 1 to 2 weeks after the erythema and swelling of the hands and feet.

Other Conditions

Several other conditions may mimic SSSS and can usually be distinguished on the basis of history. Sunburn, chemical burns, and scald burns, including those occurring from a nonaccidental injury, must be a consideration.[183] Infants with zinc deficiency may present with a bullous eruption resembling SSSS.[191] In recipients of allogenic stem cell transplants, graft versus host disease often causes a generalized erythroderma. In the neonate, bullous ichthyosis presents with generalized erythema and superficial blisters that are frequently mistaken for SSSS.[192]

Diagnostic Approach

The diagnosis of SSSS is usually made by the characteristic presentation in a young child of well-demarcated superficial bullae with fragile roofs that easily rupture leaving a weepy, uniformly red base.[183] Blood cultures should be performed, although they are rarely positive in children with SSSS. Cultures of bullous lesions as well as any foci of infection (such as purulent conjunctivitis) are

also often performed. However, the organism is not often present in the bullae, and a positive culture could simply be the result of colonization. Testing *S. aureus* isolates for the production of exfoliative toxin is done in research laboratories but is helpful only in confirming the diagnosis in retrospect. As mentioned previously, SSSS can be reliably distinguished from TEN by histologic examination of skin biopsy or even peeled skin.

Treatment

In neonates with any form of SSSS, intravenous antibiotics are indicated. They are also indicated in older children with generalized SSSS. A penicillinase-resistant penicillin, such as oxacillin, or a first-generation cephalosporin, such as cefazolin, may be used. Early, localized presentations of SSSS outside the neonatal period may be treated with an oral antibiotic, such as cephalexin. In many cases, new exfoliating lesions appear for 24–36 hours after starting treatment; if new lesions continue to appear after this time, hospital admission for intravenous antibiotics is indicated.[183] In vitro studies show that clindamycin can significantly inhibit toxin production by *S. aureus*, and many experts add this agent for severe cases, although data in humans are lacking. In areas where community-acquired MRSA infections are common, an additional advantage to the use of clindamycin is that most of these strains remain susceptible.[193] Although controversial in the management of TEN, corticosteroids are clearly contraindicated in the patient with SSSS, so differentiation of these two entities is critical. For patients with severe forms of either of these diseases, management in a burn center may be appropriate.

■ IMPETIGO

Impetigo typically begins as a red macule or papule that rapidly becomes pustular. Pain and fever are absent. The pustule then ruptures, revealing an oozing, sticky, honey-like exudate crusted over a shallow ulcerated base. This is the classic honey-crusted lesion of impetigo. Papular and bullous forms (see previous section) occur less commonly. Characteristically, the patient has a number of lesions, apparently spread by the fingers. Often another family member or other contact acquires similar lesions.

Possible Etiologies

S. aureus is responsible for nearly all cases of bullous impetigo and for about 75% of cases of nonbullous impetigo. Most of the remaining cases are caused by either group A streptococcus alone or by polymicrobial infection.[194] Primary nonbacterial processes, such as varicella or eczema, can become secondarily impetiginized, resulting in diagnostic confusion.

Treatment

Topical mupirocin has excellent activity against the agents of impetigo, and for localized lesions it is the drug of choice. Other topical agents (such as bacitracin and neomycin/polymyxin) have little effect.[195,196] For widespread lesions, those near the mouth, and those with associated cellulitis, a systemic antibiotic, such as cephalexin, should be used.[196,197] Although penicillin continues to have excellent activity against GAS, nearly all *S. aureus* isolates are now resistant. Approximately one-quarter of *S. aureus* are resistant to the macrolides as well, although they may be used for the patient who is allergic to cephalexin. Recalcitrant cases may sometimes be cured by the addition of rifampin.[198] Often, failure to respond promptly to therapy is due to the presence of other diseases that resemble impetigo, especially HSV infection, scabies, or a kerion (pustular tinea of the scalp).

Complications

Local complications, such as cellulitis or lymphangitis, are uncommon. Post-streptococcal glomerulonephritis (PSGN) can occur about 3 weeks after a case of impetigo caused by nephritogenic strains of *S. pyogenes*.[199] Fortunately, this complication has become uncommon, probably because of decreasing circulation of nephritogenic M-types.[200] Patients present with edema, hematuria, and hypertension. Complement levels (especially C3) are decreased, and patients will usually have elevation of anti-streptococcal antibodies (particularly anti-DNAse B). Antimicrobial treatment of the impetigo has no bearing on the likelihood of developing PSGN. Acute rheumatic fever does not occur as a complication of streptococcal skin infections.[201]

■ SKIN ULCERS

Ulcers of the skin are usually circular or oval crater-shaped erosions. The ulcers may be superficial, involving only the epidermis, or deep, extending into the dermis or even muscle. Many skin ulcers are secondary to pressure (bedsores) or to poor venous drainage (stasis ulcers). This section deals with infectious causes of skin ulcers (Box 17-3). Genital ulcers are discussed in Chapter 15.

Decubitus Ulcers

Decubitus (pressure) ulcers uncommonly become infected in children. Infections in decubitus ulcers are often polymicrobial, with *S. aureus*, gram-negative enteric organisms, and anaerobes most frequently isolated. Debridement and antibiotic therapy based on susceptibility tests are indicated. Application of simple granulated sugar, which prevents bacterial growth by an osmotic effect, has also been advocated but is not widely practiced.[202] In hospitalized adults, bacteremia secondary to pressure ulcers is associated with a high mortality rate.[203] In one study, the bacteria most commonly isolated were *Proteus mirabilis*, *S. aureus*, *E. coli*, and *Bacteroides* species.[203] Ampicillin-sulbactam or clindamycin and gentamicin are reasonable choices for empiric therapy. For infected pressure ulcers that are refractory to therapy, the possibility of underlying osteomyelitis should be considered. The specificity of bone scan in this setting is low; MRI may be the best imaging modality. Antibiotic therapy is directed at the bacteria obtained by bone biopsy.[204]

Specific Syndromes

Ulcerograndular Syndrome

When there is an enlarged lymph node that receives lymphatic drainage from an infected skin ulcer, the condition is called ulceroglandular or ulceronodular syndrome. Most commonly, the ulcer is on the hand or foot, and the lymph node is in the axilla or inguinal region. In addition to *S. aureus* and group A streptococcus, additional agents should be

---

BOX 17-3 ■ Some Infectious Causes of Skin Ulcers

Secondary bacterial invasion
Herpes simplex virus
Syphilis (chancre)
Tularemia
Blastomycosis, sporotrichosis, histoplasmosis
Nontuberculous mycobacteria
Leishmaniasis
Amebiasis

considered in the patient with an appropriate exposure history. These less common causes of ulcerograndular syndrome include cat-scratch disease, tularemia, plague, and atypical mycobacteria.

Ulceroglandular tularemia is the most common presentation of infection with *Francisella tularensis*. The ulcer occurs at the site of entry, which is usually on the finger or hand if the patient has contracted the infection by handling a contaminated rabbit. However, it is more commonly transmitted by infected ticks. There is usually marked regional adenopathy, which is generally quite painful. Systemic symptoms such as fever and malaise are prominent and many precede the ulceroglandular stage. Intramuscular streptomycin is the traditional therapy, but gentamicin is equally effective and can be given intravenously.[205]

Yersinia pestis, the agent of plague, sometimes produces an ulceroglandular illness. A few plague cases occur annually in the southwestern United States, where fleas from the wild rodent reservoir are the usual vectors. In addition, approximately 20% of cases in the United States are acquired through contact with mammals, including domestic cats.[206] Bubonic plague, the most common form, presents with sudden onset of fever, chills, and weakness, and the development of an acutely swollen tender lymph node (or bubo). Occasionally, skin ulcerations occur at the site of a flea bite.[207] *Yersinia enterocolitica*, which ordinarily causes diarrhea, has also been reported to produce a plague-like ulceroglandular illness.[208]

Lymphocutaneous Syndrome

Lymphocutaneous syndrome is characterized by a primary skin lesion (which may or may not ulcerate), regional adenopathy, and satellite nodules along the lymphatics. The most common cause of this syndrome is sporotrichosis,[209] but multiple other agents have been implicated as well, including bacteria, such as *Nocardia*, and mycobacteria, especially *M. marinum*.[210]

Infectious Causes of Ulcerative Skin Lesions

Bacteria

Beta-hemolytic streptococci are frequent secondary invaders of superficial ulcers that fail to heal promptly. Other bacteria, such as *S. aureus* and enteric bacteria, can produce chronic ulcers after subcutaneous injection, such as during use of nonsterile needles for injections of illicit drugs. Syphilis may produce ulcers near the breasts or mouth that resemble the chancres of the genital area. *Nocardia brasiliensis* can cause primary skin and soft tissue infection, often with a lymphocutaneous syndrome resembling sporotrichosis. The exposure history is also similar to that of sporotrichosis cases, and often includes rose thorn punctures or wood splinter injuries.[211] Incision and drainage of lesions and affected lymph nodes is indicated, and diagnosis is made by culture of drainage. The treatment of choice is trimethoprim-sulfamethoxazole, generally for about 2 months in a patient with a normal immune system.

B. anthracis may cause inhalational, gastrointestinal, or cutaneous syndromes, depending on the route of exposure. Cutaneous anthrax typically presents as a painless and pruritic vesicle with erythema and edema, which evolves into a black eschar.[212,213] Without therapy, secondary septicemia may ensue, with a mortality rate of about 20%.[214] Previously, anthrax was rare and seen almost exclusively in those with exposure to contaminated goat products. However, it is now being used as an agent of bioterrorism and disseminated through the mail, resulting in both inhalational and cutaneous disease.[215]

Mycobacteria

Tuberculosis of the skin can produce a chronic ulcer. Characteristically, this occurs where a lymph node has suppurated and broken down, often in the neck. Several of the nontuberculous mycobacteria cause skin ulcers. "Fish-tank granuloma" is caused by infection with *M. marinum* in persons who sustain minor trauma in water contaminated with the mycobacterium. The diagnosis is frequently delayed, often because the exposure has been forgotten. In a review of 40 cases with known incubation periods, the median incubation period was 21 days, but the longest was 9 months.[216] Patients with ulcerating nodules should be questioned about possible exposures to fresh or salt water in the recent and remote past. In the study mentioned above, 193 infections had known exposures; 49% were aquarium-related, 27% were related to fish or shellfish injuries, and 9% were related to injuries associated with saltwater. Successful treatment has been reported with several regimens, including clarithromycin, doxycycline, trimethoprim-sulfamethoxasole, and rifampin plus ethambutol.[217] At least 3 months of therapy is necessary.

Caused by infection with *Mycobacterium ulcerans*, Buruli ulcer disease most commonly affects children living in areas of tropical rain forest, especially West Africa.[218] After contact with contaminated water or soil, the child develops a painless nodule or plaque—typically on an extremity—which eventually ulcerates, and then becomes necrotic. Healing results in scarring and disabling contractures. Early excision of the preulcerative lesion is curative. Antimycobacterial therapy is of little benefit.

Mycobacterium haemophilum infection usually occurs in immunocompromised hosts.[219] Lesions begin as tender papules or nodules that then suppurate and begin to ulcerate. Bone, joint, and lung involvement may occur as well. Prolonged combination therapy is required. Other mycobacteria (such as *M. fortuitum* and *M. chelonae*) may occasionally cause ulcerating skin lesions, particularly in immunocompromised patients.[220]

Fungi

As mentioned previously, sporotrichosis is the classic cause of the lymphocutaneous syndrome. *Sporothrix schenckii* grows best in sphagnum moss, decaying vegetation, soil, or hay, and most cases occur after direct inoculation into skin, such as from a thorn injury.[221] Zoonotic transmission, especially from armadillos and cats, has also been described.[222] The lesion begins as a papule or nodule, which then ulcerates and may drain serosanguinous fluid. Pain is mild, and systemic symptoms are typically absent.[221] Progression of infection is characterized by lymphangitic streaking and nodular lesions that appear along the lymphatic distribution proximal to the initial lesion.[221] Definitive diagnosis is by culture, and the treatment of choice is a 3- to 6-month course of itraconazole.

Cutaneous blastomycosis usually occurs in patients with concomitant pulmonary involvement, but primary cutaneous blastomycosis has been reported to occur after inoculation injuries or dog bites.[223] It usually begins as a papule or nodule that clears in the center, leaving a verrucous or ulcerated scar. Lymphadenopathy is usually absent. The disease occurs primarily in the Mississippi and Ohio valley areas. Diagnosis usually requires biopsy and special fungal staining. Mild cases may be self-limited, but most experts would treat immunocompe-

tent hosts with a 6-month course of itraconazole. Immuncompromised patients should usually receive initial treatment with amphotericin B followed by a prolonged course of itraconazole.

Like blastomycosis, cutaneous coccidioidomycosis is usually the result of disseminated disease but can occur after direct inoculation. Coccidioidomycosis is endemic in the desert southwest United States and parts of Central and South America. The primary cutaneous syndrome begins as a mildly painful, deeply indurated, dusky lesion, followed shortly by ulceroglandular disease and, in many cases, nodular lymphangitis (lymphocutaneous syndrome).[210] It is important to distinguish primary cutaneous disease from skin lesions associated with disseminated disease, because the former may be self-limiting, whereas the latter requires prolonged antifungal therapy, often with amphotericin B initially, followed by itraconazole or fluconazole.

Cutaneous involvement with other endemic fungi (such as histoplasmosis and cryptococcosis) is uncommon but is sometimes seen in the immunocompromised host.

Cutaneous forms of aspergillosis have also been reported in severely immunocompromised patients. In these cases, the physician's principal task is distinguishing cutaneous infection from disseminated infection with cutaneous manifestations.[224]

Viruses

Cutaneous infections with HSV are often easily diagnosed clinically by the characteristic painful grouped vesicles on a red base. However, the vesicles may coalesce and ulcerate, especially in an immunocompromised host, making their distinction from other causes difficult. The diagnosis can be made by sending a scraping of the lesion for HSV identification; viral culture, direct fluorescent antibody testing, and polymerase chain reaction are used in different laboratories. Treatment is with acyclovir or valacyclovir.

A case of severe skin ulceration due to cytomegalovirus has been reported in an immunocompromised patient.[225]

Parasites

Cutaneous amebiasis is a rare complication of amebic liver disease.[226] Patients with acanthamoeba encephalitis may develop granulomatous skin lesions.[227]

Transmitted by the bite of the sandfly, cutaneous

leishmaniasis is a common cause of ulcerated skin lesions in certain parts of the world (Latin America, the Middle East, Asia, and Africa), and it should be considered in travelers returning from these areas. It typically begins as a papule and then becomes a nodule with a central crust that drops off to expose a painless ulcer. The lesions become chronic and many have a raised border with satellite lesions.[228] Two excellent reviews discuss this and other ulcerating skin lesions to consider in the returned traveler.[228,229]

Noninfectious Causes of Ulcerative Skin Lesions

Pyoderma Gangrenosum

The lesions of pyoderma gangrenosum begin as tender papules or pustules that develop into painful ulcers with ragged, overhanging, dusky purple edges and surrounding induration and erythema.[230] The name is a misnomer because the lesions are the result of neither infection nor gangrene. The lower extremities are the predominant location in 75% of cases.[230] Approximately half of cases are associated with an underlying disease, such as ulcerative colitis, Crohn's disease, rheumatoid arthritis, and malignancy. Histologically, there may be a neutrophilic infiltrate resembling Sweet syndrome or chronic inflammation with ulceration. The pathogenesis is unknown. Corticosteroids and other immunosuppressive agents are the mainstays of therapy.[231]

Necrotic Arachnidism

The bites of a number of spiders indigenous to the United States can produce necrotic lesions. The most common of these is the brown recluse (*Loxosceles reclusa*). The brown recluse resides in the midwest, south-central, and southeastern United States,[232] where *Chiracanthium* species are also found. In the northwest United States, the brown recluse has been blamed for necrotic wounds despite the fact that this spider is not found there. Necrotic wounds there are likely caused by the "northwestern brown spider" (*Tegenaria agrestis*).[232,233]

Most spiders do not bite unless they are trapped or otherwise provoked. A common scenario involves being bit when putting on shoes or clothing that were lying on the floor during the night. Alternatively, the spider may crawl into the popliteal or

antecubital fossa and then be trapped when the child flexes the joint. The bite of the northwestern brown spider is entirely painless; that of the recluse produces a mild, transient, burning sensation; and that of members of the species *Chiracanthium* is said to be very painful. All are followed by increasing pain and erythema several hours later. Systemic symptoms may occur with any necrotic spider bite, and include fever, chills, headache, nausea, and arthralgia. Over the next few days, blistering occurs, accompanied by the "red, white, and blue" sign: erythema, ischemia, and necrosis.[234] An eschar forms in the center and then sloughs off, leaving an ulcer, which may take months to heal. Skin grafting procedures are occasionally required. Although no controlled trials in humans have been done, some experts recommend therapy with dapsone.

Other Conditions

Behçet disease is rare in children. It is characterized by recurrent mouth and genital ulcers, as well as uveitis and skin lesions. Other than in the genital region, the skin lesions do not ulcerate. They are usually either erythema nodosum or papulopustular lesions resembling acne.[235] In children, sarcoidosis usually presents with arthritis, uveitis, and a follicular skin rash. Ulcerative skin lesions have occasionally been reported in adults.[236] Chronic ulceration can also be secondary to Langerhans' cell histiocytosis or other malignancies.[237] Lesions should be biopsied, and some tissue should be saved for special stains for microorganisms and cultures.

■ SUPERFICIAL FUNGAL INFECTIONS

"Tinea" (Latin for "worm") is the general term for any superficial fungal infection of the skin. The location of the infection is described in a second term, such as "tinea pedis" (athlete's foot), "tinea cruris" (jock itch), "tinea capitis" (ringworm of the scalp) (Fig. 17-5), and "tinea corporis" (ringworm of the body). Most superficial fungal infections are caused by dermatophytes (fungi of the *Trichophyton*, *Microsporum*, or *Epidermophyton* genera), but occasionally *Candida* is the cause. *Malassezia furfur* is a lipophilic yeast that is the cause of tinea versicolor. In addition, some microorganisms mentioned in this section cause tinea-like skin disease but are not fungi. Tinea is occasionally acquired from animals or the soil, but the vast majority of infections are transmitted person to person. A hypersensitivity re-

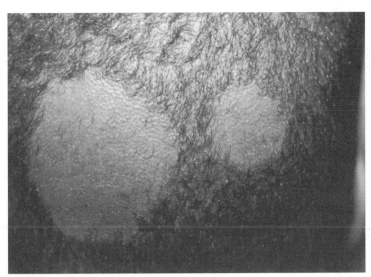

■ **FIGURE 17-5** Tinea capitis.

action to fungal antigens may develop, called a dermatophytid or "id" reaction.[238] This often presents as a rash with red, scaly plaques on the face, neck, trunk, and proximal extremities.

Locations and Etiologies

Tinea Capitis

This common infection in childhood was once primarily caused by *Microsporum audouini*, but *Trichophyton tonsurans* is now the predominant cause.[239] Tinea capitis often results in breakage of hairs close to the scalp, resulting in a "black-dot" appearance (Fig. 17-5). Occasionally, an exuberant inflammatory response leads to a boggy, pustular lesion called a "kerion," which may be mistaken for a bacterial infection. Occipital or retroauricular adenopathy is common.

Tinea Corporis

This form is also very common in childhood. *T. rubrum* is the most common cause, but many cases are now caused by *T. tonsurans*. It presents as a round, scaly patch with a prominent, enlarging border and relatively clear central portion.[240] Pruritus is variable. There may be multiple lesions.

Tinea Cruris

Usually caused by *T. rubrum* or *E. floccosum*, tinea cruris typically occurs in males and is uncommon prior to adolescence. The lesion often extends over the adjacent upper inner thigh.[240] If *Candida* infection is the cause, the border is irregular with satellite lesions and, frequently, scrotal involvement.

Tinea Pedis

Caused predominantly by *T. rubrum*, this presents as erythema, scaling, and maceration in the web spaces, often with intense itching. It may be confused with erythrasma, caused by *Corynebacterium minutissimum*, which produces coral red fluorescence under a Wood's light.

Tinea Versicolor

This condition is common in adolescents and presents as multiple pink scaly lesions of the upper trunk, neck, and shoulders. The lesions usually appear hyperpigmented in light-skinned persons and hypopigmented in dark-skinned persons. It is caused by infection with *M. furfur*.

Tinea Unguium (Onychomycosis)

Fungal infection of the nail plate may be caused by dermatophytes or other fungi (*Candida* or *Aspergillus*). It presents as discoloration, ridging, thickening, and fragility of the nail, with little or no inflammation.[238]

Diagnostic Approach

Ultraviolet Light

The most common causes of tinea capitis and tinea corporis do not fluoresce under a Wood's lamp (long wave ultraviolet light), and this procedure should not be relied upon for diagnosis. It is useful for certain conditions, however. Tinea versicolor fluoresces yellow-green under a Wood's lamp, and erythrasma fluoresces a coral red color. *Microsporum* species, which cause about 10% of tinea capitis, fluoresce bluish green.[241]

Smear

This is usually not necessary for initial diagnosis if the presentation is typical. However, for atypical or refractory cases, it is a simple test that can be performed in the office. The active border is scraped onto a glass slide and 10–20% potassium hydroxide is added. It is then left to digest for 30 minutes or heated gently and then examined under a microscope for evidence of spores or fungal hyphae.[238] The sensitivity is reported as approaching 90% for tinea corporis but only 50% for tinea capitis.[241]

Culture for Fungus

This can be done but is seldom needed. Most species can be identified by colony characteristics. *C. albicans* may be recovered in 1–2 days, but *Microsporum* or *Trichophyton* species usually take 1 or 2 weeks.

Treatment

For tinea corporis, tinea cruris, and most cases of tinea pedis, topical therapy is sufficient. Multiple preparations are available both by prescription and over the counter.[242] The azoles (e.g., clotrimazole, econazole, and miconazole) and the newer allylamines (e.g., terbinafine, naftifine, and butenafine) are probably equivalent in efficacy. Cure rates with tolnaftate are slightly lower; they are considerably lower with undecylenic acid.[242] Nystatin has activity against *Candida* but not the dermatophytes. Topical preparations containing the combination of an antifungal agent and a corticosteroid have no rational basis for their use. Treatment is usually twice daily for 2–4 weeks.

Tinea capitis, tinea unguium, and severe cases of tinea pedis require systemic therapy for cure. Griseofulvin is safe, inexpensive, and effective but has several limitations. Because it is fungistatic, it must be given for a prolonged period of time, often about 6–12 weeks (and at least 2 weeks after complete clearing of the lesion). The liquid preparation must be taken with fatty food or drink to enhance absorption. Nausea is a common side effect. The dose is 20 mg/kg/day of the microsize (liquid) preparation or 10 mg/kg/day of the ultramicrosized tablets. Routine monitoring of liver enzymes is generally unnecessary.[238]

A recent randomized trial compared 6 weeks of griseofulvin to 3 weeks of terbinafine, itraconazole, or fluconazole in 200 children with tinea capitis (50 children in each group). The cure rates at 12 weeks were 92% for griseofulvin, 94% for terbinafine, 86% for itraconazole, and 84% for fluconazole ($P = 0.33$).[243] All four drugs were well tolerated. The newer agents may provide additional options, although none are yet FDA-approved for this use in children. Fluconazole, itraconazole, and terbinafine are all dosed at 3–5 mg/kg daily for tinea capitis, but only the first two are available in a liquid preparation.

For tinea capitis, in addition to oral antifungal agents, sporicidal shampoo, such as selenium sulfide, may be used two to three times per week for the first 2 weeks of therapy to reduce transmission. For patients with a severe localized inflammatory response (kerion), 1–2 mg/kg/day of prednisolone for 7–10 days may be added as well. Dermatophytid reactions are treated with a similar course of corticosteroids.

Both topical and oral agents are used in the treatment of tinea versicolor. Twice daily application of selenium sulfide shampoo or lotion is often used, as is terbinafine, econzole, or ketoconazole applied topically for 2–4 weeks. Recurrences are common and may be less frequent if a short course of oral therapy with itraconazole is used.[240]

■ INFECTED DIAPER DERMATITIS

Diaper rashes, which are very common, are usually erythematous, but some have vesicular or pustular components. Most diaper rashes are presumably noninfectious and due to irritation. Prompt changing of soiled diapers and use of a barrier paste, such as zinc oxide, are often all that is needed to clear up the diaper rash. Removing the diaper and exposing the diaper area to air as long as possible is also effective.[244]

Possible Etiologies

Candida albicans is the most frequent secondary infection in the diaper area. It usually starts in the perianal area and then spreads to involve the perineum and sometimes the upper thighs.[245] The rash is usually well-defined and beefy red, with occasional satellite lesions, which are papules separated from the confluent rash. In a placebo-controlled trial, no additional benefit was found to adding oral nystatin to local therapy with nystatin cream.[246] However, about half the babies required 3 weeks of therapy, instead of the originally planned 10 days.

Occasionally, the reason for refractory diaper dermatitis is dermatophyte infection (e.g., *Trichophyton rubrum*).[247] Typically the lesions are more circinate or serpiginous. Nystatin does not have activity against the dermatophytes, so empiric therapy with clotrimazole or a similar agent is appropriate if these agents are suspected.

Secondary bacterial infection can sometimes occur in denuded skin in the diaper area. Beta-hemolytic streptococcus and *S. aureus* are the most common causes, and an oral agent (e.g., cephalexin) may be necessary. Herpes simplex occasionally infects denuded skin in the diaper area. Vesicular diaper rashes should be cultured for HSV.

Noninfectious etiologies of dermatitis in the diaper area include seborrhea, atopic dermatitis, and contact dermatitis from detergents. Uncommon causes include epidermolysis bullosa, Leiner disease (intractable seborrhea-like dermatitis with diarrhea, failure to thrive, and immune dysfunction), acrodermatitis enteropathica (zinc deficiency), and Langerhans' cell histiocytosis.

■ ACNE

Acne is generally regarded as beginning with obstruction of the pilosebaceous structures (hair follicle and sebaceous glands) with secondary inflammation and infection in more severe forms. Mild, non-inflammatory acne consists of open comedones (blackheads) and closed comedones (whiteheads). Inflammatory acne may be papular, pustular, cystic, nodular, or a combination, and is often infected.[248] The peak incidence is ages 14–16 years in girls and 16–19 years in boys.

Propionibacterium acnes is a microaerophilic diphtheroid that plays a role in acne, both by liberating lipases and secreting chemotactic factors that attract neutrophils and other inflammatory mediators.[248] Medications (such as steroids) can predispose to acne.

Treatment

Local Therapy

Topical therapies are often all that is necessary for mild to moderate acne. Benzoyl peroxide is the only remedy of any value that is available over the counter.[249] It is active against both inflammatory and noninflammatory acne, and is available in multiple forms and strengths. The gel is the most effective form. Topical retinoids are an extremely effective class of medications for the treatment of acne. The creams are less irritating than the gels. For patients who do not respond to the combination of topical benzoyl peroxide and topical retinoids, a topical antibiotic, such as erythromycin or clindamycin, may be added.

Systemic Therapy

Patients with severe inflammatory lesions, those with involvement of large areas of the trunk, and those who fail a 6- to 12-week course of topical therapy usually require systemic therapy for control of the acne. Oral antibiotics such as doxycycline and minocycline are the mainstay of oral therapy. Patients should be reminded of the high incidence of photosensitivity with doxycycline and the importance of protective sunscreen. Patients with severe nodulocystic acne may require therapy with oral isotretinoin. It is very effective but has several side effects. Importantly, it is highly teratogenic and should generally not be given to females of childbearing potential. Because of the potential severe complications of using this drug, it should probably be prescribed only by dermatologists.[249]

■ INFECTED ECZEMA

Eczema (atopic dermatitis) is a chronic, relapsing, pruritic, inflammatory skin disease that usually develops in early childhood.[250] There is often a personal or family history of atopy, as well as elevated IgE. These children are typically colonized with *S. aureus*. One placebo-controlled trial showed improvement in skin lesions with the use of mupirocin, suggesting that *S. aureus* may play a pathogenic role in eczema.[251]

In children with atopic dermatitis, herpes simplex can produce either localized infections with vesicles and ulcers or a severe disseminated eruption termed eczema herpeticum (Fig. 17-6). If it is suspected to be severe eczema only, it may be treated with ever increasing potencies of topical steroids, with disastrous results. If a child has severe eczema, skin lesions should be cultured for HSV and the empiric use of intravenous acyclovir should be considered while awaiting culture results.[252] In older children with milder disease, oral acyclovir

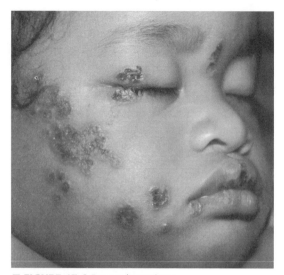

■ **FIGURE 17-6** Eczema herpeticum.

has been effective.[253] Superinfection with scabies can also occur in children with eczema.[254] As in the case of HSV superinfection, it can be made worse by the use of topical steroids.

■ **REFERENCES**

1. Montes LF, Wilborn WH. Anatomical location of normal skin flora. Arch Dermatol 1970;101:145–59.
2. Magee JS, Schutze GE. Bacterial infections of the skin. Semin Pediatr Infect Dis 1997;8:215–9.
3. Dancer SJ, Noble WC. Nasal, axillary, and perineal carriage of Staphylococcus aureus among women: identification of strains producing epidermolytic toxin. J Clin Pathol 1991; 44:681–4.
4. Shopsin B, Mathema B, Martinez J, et al. Prevalence of methicillin-resistant and methicillin-susceptible Staphylococcus aureus in the community. J Infect Dis 2000;182: 359–62.
5. Stark V, Harrisson SP. Staphylococcus aureus colonization of the newborn in a Darlington hospital. J Hosp Infect 1992;21:205–11.
6. Hoeger PH, Lenz W, Boutonnier A, et al. Staphylococcal skin colonization in children with atopic dermatitis: prevalence, persistence, and transmission of toxigenic and nontoxigenic strains. J Infect Dis 1992;165:1064–8.
7. Larson EL, Cronquist AB, Whittier S, et al. Differences in skin flora between inpatients and chronically ill outpatients. Heart Lung 2000;29:298–305.
8. Brook I. The effects of amoxicillin therapy on skin flora in infants. Pediatr Dermatol 2000;17:360–3.
9. Doern GV, Jones RN, Pfaller MA, et al. Bacterial pathogens isolated from patients with skin and soft tissue infections: frequency of occurrence and antimicrobial susceptibility patterns from the SENTRY Antimicrobial Surveillance Program (United States and Canada, 1997). SENTRY Study Group (North America). Diagn Microbiol Infect Dis 1999; 34:65–72.
10. Baxter CR. Surgical management of soft tissue infections. Surg Clin North Am 1972;52:1483–99.
11. Brook I, Frazier EH. Clinical features and aerobic and anaerobic microbiological characteristics of cellulitis. Arch Surg 1995;130:786–92.
12. Hook EW III, Hooton TM, Horton CA, et al. Microbiologic evaluation of cutaneous cellulitis in adults. Arch Intern Med 1986;146:295–7.
13. Newell PM, Norden CW. Value of needle aspiration in bacteriologic diagnosis of cellulitis in adults. J Clin Microbiol 1988;26:401–4.
14. da Silva JH. Pilonidal cyst: cause and treatment. Dis Colon Rectum 2000;43:1146–56.
15. Sondenaa K, Nesvik I, Andersen E, et al. Bacteriology and complications of chronic pilonidal sinus treated with excision and primary suture. Int J Colorectal Dis 1995;10: 161–6.
16. Kronborg O, Christensen K, Zimmermann-Nielsen C. Chronic pilonidal disease: a randomized trial with a complete 3-year follow-up. Br J Surg 1985;72:303–4.
17. Kokx NP, Comstock JA, Facklam RR. Streptococcal perianal disease in children. Pediatrics 1987;80:659–63.
18. Bassiouny A. Perichondritis of the auricle. Laryngoscope 1981;91:422–31.
19. Cumberworth VL, Hogarth TB. Hazards of ear-piercing procedures which traverse cartilage: a report of Pseudomonas perichondritis and review of other complications. Br J Clin Pract 1990;44:512–3.
20. Berkelman RL, Martin D, Graham DR, et al. Streptococcal wound infections caused by a vaginal carrier. JAMA 1982; 247:2680–2.
21. Bisno AL, Stevens DL. Streptococcal infections of skin and soft tissues. N Engl J Med 1996;334:240–5.
22. National Nosocomial Infections Surveillance (NNIS) report, data summary from October 1986-April 1996, issued May 1996. A report from the National Nosocomial Infections Surveillance (NNIS) System. Am J Infect Control 1996;24:380–8.
23. Cavanaugh F. Osteomyelitis of the superior maxilla in infants: a report of 24 personally treated cases. Br Med J 1962;5171:468–72.
24. Ginsburg CM. Buccal cellulitis. Pediatr Infect Dis 1983;2: 381–2.
25. Fisher RG, Benjamin DK Jr. Facial cellulitis in childhood: a changing spectrum. South Med J 2002;95:672–4.
26. Thirumoorthi MC, Asmar BI, Dajani AS. Violaceous discoloration in pneumococcal cellulitis. Pediatrics 1978;62: 492–3.
27. Givner LB, Mason EO Jr, Barson WJ, et al. Pneumococcal facial cellulitis in children. Pediatrics 2000;106:E61.
28. Hauger SB. Facial cellulitis: an early indicator of group B streptococcal bacteremia. Pediatrics 1981;67:376–7.
29. Albanyan EA, Baker CJ. Is lumbar puncture necessary to exclude meningitis in neonates and young infants: lessons from the group B streptococcus cellulitis-adenitis syndrome. Pediatrics 1998;102:985–6.
30. Rathore MH. Group B streptococcal cellulitis and adenitis concurrent with meningitis. Clin Pediatr (Phila) 1989;28: 411.
31. Baddour LM, Bisno AL. Non-group A beta-hemolytic streptococcal cellulitis. Association with venous and lymphatic compromise. Am J Med 1985;79:155–9.

32. Brooke CJ, Riley TV. *Erysipelothrix rhusiopathiae*: bacteriology, epidemiology and clinical manifestations of an occupational pathogen. J Med Microbiol 1999;48:789–99.

33. Klontz KC, Lieb S, Schreiber M, et al. Syndromes of *Vibrio vulnificus* infections. Clinical and epidemiologic features in Florida cases, 1981-1987. Ann Intern Med 1988;109:318–23.

34. Chuang YC, Liu JW, Ko WC, et al. In vitro synergism between cefotaxime and minocycline against *Vibrio vulnificus*. Antimicrob Agents Chemother 1997;41:2214–7.

35. Chuang YC, Ko WC, Wang ST, et al. Minocycline and cefotaxime in the treatment of experimental murine *Vibrio vulnificus* infection. Antimicrob Agents Chemother 1998;42:1319–22.

36. Fleisher G, Ludwig S, Campos J. Cellulitis: bacterial etiology, clinical features, and laboratory findings. J Pediatr 1980;97:591–3.

37. White CB, Barcia PJ, Bass JW. Neonatal zygomycotic necrotizing cellulitis. Pediatrics 1986;78:100–2.

38. Ferreli C, Pinna AL, Atzori L, et al. Eosinophilic cellulitis (Well's syndrome): a new case description. J Eur Acad Dermatol Venereol 1999;13:41–5.

39. Kuwahara RT, Randall MB, Eisner MG. Eosinophilic cellulitis in a newborn. Pediatr Dermatol 2001;18:89–90.

40. Cron RQ, Swetter SM. Scleredema revisited. A poststreptococcal complication. Clin Pediatr (Phila) 1994;33:606–10.

41. Parmar RC, Bavdekar SB, Bansal S, et al. Scleredema adultorum. J Postgrad Med 2000;46:91–3.

42. Vereecken P, Lutz R, De Dobbeleer G, et al. Nonpitting induration of the back. Scleredema adultorum of Buschke type III. Arch Dermatol 1997;133:649–52.

43. Fox MD, Schwartz RA. Erythema nodosum. Am Fam Physician 1992;46:818–22.

44. Kakourou T, Drosatou P, Psychou F, et al. Erythema nodosum in children: a prospective study. J Am Acad Dermatol 2001;44:17–21.

45. Garty BZ, Poznanski O. Erythema nodosum in Israeli children. Isr Med Assoc J 2000;2:145–6.

46. Weinstein L. Erythema nodosum. Dis Mon 1969:1–30.

47. Garty B. Swimming pool granuloma associated with erythema nodosum. Cutis 1991;47:314–6.

48. King AJ, Fairley JA, Rasmussen JE. Disseminated cutaneous *Mycobacterium marinum* infection. Arch Dermatol 1983;119:268–70.

49. Ozols, II, Wheat LJ. Erythema nodosum in an epidemic of histoplasmosis in Indianapolis. Arch Dermatol 1981;117:709–12.

50. Mocan H, Mocan MC, Peru H, et al. Cutaneous polyarteritis nodosa in a child and a review of the literature. Acta Paediatr 1998;87:351–3.

51. Nichols RL, Florman S. Clinical presentations of soft-tissue infections and surgical site infections. Clin Infect Dis 2001;33(suppl 2):S84–93.

52. Freischlag JA, Ajalat G, Busuttil RW. Treatment of necrotizing soft tissue infections. The need for a new approach. Am J Surg 1985;149:751–5.

53. Giuliano A, Lewis F Jr, Hadley K, et al. Bacteriology of necrotizing fasciitis. Am J Surg 1977;134:52–7.

54. Chapnick EK, Abter EI. Necrotizing soft-tissue infections. Infect Dis Clin North Am 1996;10:835–55.

55. Wilson GJ, Talkington DF, Gruber W, et al. Group A streptococcal necrotizing fasciitis following varicella in children: case reports and review. Clin Infect Dis 1995;20:1333–8.

56. Wall DB, de Virgilio C, Black S, et al. Objective criteria may assist in distinguishing necrotizing fasciitis from nonnecrotizing soft tissue infection. Am J Surg 2000;179:17–21.

57. Moss RL, Musemeche CA, Kosloske AM. Necrotizing fasciitis in children: prompt recognition and aggressive therapy improve survival. J Pediatr Surg 1996;31:1142–6.

58. Brook I. Microbiology of necrotizing fasciitis associated with omphalitis in the newborn infant. J Perinatol 1998;18:28–30.

59. Hsieh WS, Yang PH, Chao HC, et al. Neonatal necrotizing fasciitis: a report of three cases and review of the literature. Pediatrics 1999;103:e53.

60. Smith GL, Bunker CB, Dinneen MD. Fournier's gangrene. Br J Urol 1998;81:347–55.

61. Adams JR Jr, Mata JA, Venable DD, et al. Fournier's gangrene in children. Urology 1990;35:439–41.

62. Bessman AN, Wagner W. Nonclostridial gas gangrene. Report of 48 cases and review of the literature. JAMA 1975;233:958–63.

63. Filler RM, Griscom NT, Pappas A. Post-traumatic crepitation falsely suggesting gas gangrene. N Engl J Med 1968;278:758–61.

64. Darmstadt GL. Acute infectious purpura fulminans: pathogenesis and medical management. Pediatr Dermatol 1998;15:169–183.

65. Marlar RA, Neumann A. Neonatal purpura fulminans due to homozygous protein C or protein S deficiencies. Semin Thromb Hemost 1990;16:299–309.

66. Paret G, Barzilai A, Barzilay Z. Purpura fulminans skin lesions in a newborn with complete protein C deficiency. J Pediatr 1998;132:558.

67. Daly JW, Lukowski MJ, Monif GR. The spontaneous occurrence of progressive synergistic bacterial gangrene on the abdominal wall. Am J Obstet Gynecol 1978;131:624–7.

68. Christiansen SD, Desai NS, Pulito AR, et al. Ischemic extremities due to compartment syndromes in a septic neonate. J Pediatr Surg 1983;18:641–3.

69. Struk DW, Munk PL, Lee MJ, et al. Imaging of soft tissue infections. Radiol Clin North Am 2001;39:277–303.

70. Stevens DL, Yan S, Bryant AE. Penicillin-binding protein expression at different growth stages determines penicillin efficacy in vitro and in vivo: an explanation for the inoculum effect. J Infect Dis 1993;167:1401–5.

71. Zerr DM, Alexander ER, Duchin JS, et al. A case-control study of necrotizing fasciitis during primary varicella. Pediatrics 1999;103:783–90.

72. Lesko SM, O'Brien KL, Schwartz B, et al. Invasive group A streptococcal infection and nonsteroidal antiinflammatory drug use among children with primary varicella. Pediatrics 2001;107:1108–15.

73. American Academy of Pediatrics. Committee on Infectious Diseases. Severe invasive group A streptococcal infections: a subject review. Pediatrics 1998;101:136–40.

74. Lamothe F, D'Amico P, Ghosn P, et al. Clinical usefulness of intravenous human immunoglobulins in invasive group A Streptococcal infections: case report and review. Clin Infect Dis 1995;21:1469–70.

75. Patel R, Rouse MS, Florez MV, et al. Lack of benefit of intravenous immune globulin in a murine model of group

A streptococcal necrotizing fasciitis. J Infect Dis 2000;181: 230–4.

76. Riseman JA, Zamboni WA, Curtis A, et al. Hyperbaric oxygen therapy for necrotizing fasciitis reduces mortality and the need for debridements. Surgery 1990;108:847–50.

77. Singer AJ, Hollander JE, Quinn JV. Evaluation and management of traumatic lacerations. N Engl J Med 1997;337: 1142–8.

78. Dire DJ, Welsh AP. A comparison of wound irrigation solutions used in the emergency department. Ann Emerg Med 1990;19:704–8.

79. Cummings P, Del Beccaro MA. Antibiotics to prevent infection of simple wounds: a meta-analysis of randomized studies. Am J Emerg Med 1995;13:396–400.

80. Gold WL, Salit IE. *Aeromonas hydrophila* infections of skin and soft tissue: report of 11 cases and review. Clin Infect Dis 1993;16:69–74.

81. Tong MJ. Septic complications of war wounds. JAMA 1972;219:1044–7.

82. Fee NF, Dobranski A, Bisla RS. Gas gangrene complicating open forearm fractures. Report of five cases. J Bone Joint Surg Am 1977;59:135–8.

83. Dellinger EP, Caplan ES, Weaver LD, et al. Duration of preventive antibiotic administration for open extremity fractures. Arch Surg 1988;123:333–9.

84. Dellinger EP, Miller SD, Wertz MJ, et al. Risk of infection after open fracture of the arm or leg. Arch Surg 1988;123: 1320–7.

85. Boxma H, Broekhuizen T, Patka P, et al. Randomised controlled trial of single-dose antibiotic prophylaxis in surgical treatment of closed fractures: the Dutch Trauma Trial. Lancet 1996;347:1133–7.

86. Malangoni MA, Jacobs DG. Antibiotic prophylaxis for injured patients. Infect Dis Clin North Am 1992;6:627–42.

87. Rowlands BJ, Clark RG, Richards DG. Single-dose intraoperative antibiotic prophylaxis in emergency abdominal surgery. Arch Surg 1982;117:195–9.

88. Nichols RL, Smith JW, Klein DB, et al. Risk of infection after penetrating abdominal trauma. N Engl J Med 1984; 311:1065–70.

89. Fullen WD, Hunt J, Altemeier WA. Prophylactic antibiotics in penetrating wounds of the abdomen. J Trauma 1972; 12:282–9.

90. Dellinger EP. Antibiotic prophylaxis in trauma: penetrating abdominal injuries and open fractures. Rev Infect Dis 1991;13(suppl 10):S847–57.

91. Dellinger EP, Wertz MJ, Lennard ES, et al. Efficacy of short-course antibiotic prophylaxis after penetrating intestinal injury. A prospective randomized trial. Arch Surg 1986; 121:23–30.

92. Fabian TC, Croce MA, Payne LW, et al. Duration of antibiotic therapy for penetrating abdominal trauma: a prospective trial. Surgery 1992;112:788–94; discussion 94–5.

93. Gibson DM, Feliciano DV, Mattox KL, et al. Intraabdominal abscess after penetrating abdominal trauma. Am J Surg 1981;142:699–703.

94. Dawes LG, Aprahamian C, Condon RE, et al. The risk of infection after colon injury. Surgery 1986;100:796–803.

95. Gerzof SG, Oates ME. Imaging techniques for infections in the surgical patient. Surg Clin North Am 1988;68:147–65.

96. Rodgers GL, Mortensen J, Fisher MC, et al. Predictors of infectious complications after burn injuries in children. Pediatr Infect Dis J 2000;19:990–5.

97. Pruitt BA Jr, McManus AT, Kim SH, et al. Burn wound infections: current status. World J Surg 1998;22:135–45.

98. Deepe GS Jr, MacMillan BG, Linnemann CC Jr. Unexplained fever in burn patients due to cytomegalovirus infection. JAMA 1982;248:2299–301.

99. Bang RL, Gang RK, Sanyal SC, et al. Burn septicaemia: an analysis of 79 patients. Burns 1998;24:354–61.

100. Cartotto RC, Macdonald DB, Wasan SM. Acute bacterial endocarditis following burns: case report and review. Burns 1998;24:369–73.

101. Childs C, Edwards-Jones V, Heathcote DM, et al. Patterns of *Staphylococcus aureus* colonization, toxin production, immunity and illness in burned children. Burns 1994;20: 514–21.

102. Sheridan RL, Ryan CM, Yin LM, et al. Death in the burn unit: sterile multiple organ failure. Burns 1998;24: 307–11.

103. Dacso CC, Luterman A, Curreri PW. Systemic antibiotic treatment in burned patients. Surg Clin North Am 1987; 67:57–68.

104. Kao CC, Garner WL. Acute burns. Plast Reconstr Surg 2000;105:2482–92.

105. Tredget EE, Shankowsky HA, Groeneveld A, et al. A matched-pair, randomized study evaluating the efficacy and safety of Acticoat silver-coated dressing for the treatment of burn wounds. J Burn Care Rehabil 1998;19: 531–7.

106. Mozingo DW, McManus AT, Kim SH, et al. Incidence of bacteremia after burn wound manipulation in the early postburn period. J Trauma 1997;42:1006–10.

107. Rodgers GL, Fisher MC, Lo A, et al. Study of antibiotic prophylaxis during burn wound debridement in children. J Burn Care Rehabil 1997;18:342–6.

108. McManus AT, Mason AD Jr, McManus WF, et al. A decade of reduced gram-negative infections and mortality associated with improved isolation of burned patients. Arch Surg 1994;129:1306–9.

109. Franceschi D, Gerding RL, Phillips G, et al. Risk factors associated with intravascular catheter infections in burned patients: a prospective, randomized study. J Trauma 1989; 29:811–6.

110. Barret JP, Jeschke MG, Herndon DN. Selective decontamination of the digestive tract in severely burned pediatric patients. Burns 2001;27:439–45.

111. Waymack JP, Jenkins ME, Alexander JW, et al. A prospective trial of prophylactic intravenous immune globulin for the prevention of infections in severely burned patients. Burns 1989;15:71–6.

112. Hays GC, Mullard JE. Blistering distal dactylitis: a clinically recognizable streptococcal infection. Pediatrics 1975;56: 129–31.

113. Norcross MC Jr, Mitchell DF. Blistering distal dactylitis caused by Staphylococcus aureus. Cutis 1993;51:353–4.

114. Benson PM, Solivan G. Group B streptococcal blistering distal dactylitis in an adult diabetic. J Am Acad Dermatol 1987;17:310–1.

115. Maibach HI, Kligman AM. Multiple sweat gland abscesses. JAMA 1960;174:140–2.

116. Von Der Werth JM, Williams HC, Raeburn JA. The clinical

genetics of hidradenitis suppurativa revisited. Br J Dermatol 2000;142:947–53.

117. Parks RW, Parks TG. Pathogenesis, clinical features and management of hidradenitis suppurativa. Ann R Coll Surg Engl 1997;79:83–9.

118. John GC, Nduati RW, Mbori-Ngacha DA, et al. Correlates of mother-to-child human immunodeficiency virus type 1 (HIV-1) transmission: association with maternal plasma HIV-1 RNA load, genital HIV-1 DNA shedding, and breast infections. J Infect Dis 2001;183:206–12.

119. Scott-Conner CE, Schorr SJ. The diagnosis and management of breast problems during pregnancy and lactation. Am J Surg 1995;170:401–5.

120. Thomsen AC, Espersen T, Maigaard S. Course and treatment of milk stasis, noninfectious inflammation of the breast, and infectious mastitis in nursing women. Am J Obstet Gynecol 1984;149:492–5.

121. Walsh M, McIntosh K. Neonatal mastitis. Clin Pediatr 1986;25:395–9.

122. Nelson JD. Letter: Bilateral breast abscess due to group B streptococcus. Am J Dis Child 1976;130:567.

123. Rudoy RC, Nelson JD. Breast abscess during the neonatal period. A review. Am J Dis Child 1975;129:1031–4.

124. Jain A, Daum RA. Staphylococcal infections in children: part 1. Pediatr Rev 1999;20:183–91.

125. Baggett HC, Hennessy TW, Rudolph K. Community-onset methicillin-resistant *Staphylococcus aureus* associated with antibiotic use and the cytotoxin Panton-Valentine leukocidin during a furunculosis outbreak in rural Alaska. J Infect Dis 2004;189:1565–73.

126. Brook I, Finegold SM. Aerobic and anaerobic bacteriology of cutaneous abscesses in children. Pediatrics 1981;67: 891–5.

127. Gregory DW, Schaffner W. *Pseudomonas* infections associated with hot tubs and other environments. Infect Dis Clin North Am 1987;1:635–48.

128. Krieger RW, Chusid MJ. Perirectal abscess in childhood. A review of 29 cases. Am J Dis Child 1979;133:411–2.

129. Winkelstein JA, Marino MC, Johnston RB Jr, et al. Chronic granulomatous disease. Report on a national registry of 368 patients. Medicine (Baltimore) 2000;79:155–69.

130. Buckley RH. The hyper-IgE syndrome. Clin Rev Allergy Immunol 2001;20:139–54.

131. Paller AS, Nanda V, Spates C, et al. Leukocyte adhesion deficiency: recurrent childhood skin infections. J Am Acad Dermatol 1994;31:316–9.

132. Lakshman R, Finn A. Neutrophil disorders and their management. J Clin Pathol 2001;54:7–19.

133. English JC, Monk JS. Gonococcal dermatitis-arthritis syndrome. Am Fam Physician 1986;34:77–9.

134. Kontiainen S, Rinne E. Bacteria isolated from skin and soft tissue lesions. Eur J Clin Microbiol 1987;6:420–2.

135. Liston TE. Pneumococcal subcutaneous abscess in immunocompetent children. Am J Dis Child 1982;136:947–8.

136. Medina FA. Unusual case of *Haemophilus influenzae* type b: *Haemophilus influenzae* type b meningitis cellulitis and subcutaneous abscess. Pediatr Emerg Care 1987;3:28–9.

137. Muller F, von Graevenitz A, Ferber T. *Streptococcus milleri* subcutaneous abscesses in drug addicts. Infection 1987; 15:201.

138. Owen CR, Meis A, Jackson JW, et al. A case of primary cutaneous listeriosis. N Engl J Med 1960;262:1024–1025.

139. Sacker I, Walker M, Brunell PA. Abscess in newborn infants caused by *Mycoplasma*. Pediatrics 1970;46:303–4.

140. Clark NM, Braun DK, Pasternak A, et al. Primary cutaneous *Nocardia otitidiscaviarum* infection: case report and review. Clin Infect Dis 1995;20:1266–70.

141. Freites V, Sumoza A, Bisotti R, et al. Subcutaneous *Nocardia asteroides* abscess in a bone marrow transplant recipient. Bone Marrow Transplant 1995;15:135–6.

142. Nice CS, Panigrahi H. Cutaneous abscesses caused by *Salmonella enteritidis*: an unusual presentation of salmonellosis. J Infect 1993;27:204–5.

143. Krogstad P, Mendelman PM, Miller VL, et al. Clinical and microbiologic characteristics of cutaneous infection with *Yersinia enterocolitica*. J Infect Dis 1992;165:740–3.

144. Ampel NM, Ruben FL, Norden CW. Cutaneous abscess caused by *Legionella micdadei* in an immunosuppressed patient. Ann Intern Med 1985;102:630–2.

145. Hendrick SJ, Jorizzo JL, Newton RC. Giant *Mycobacterium fortuitum* abscess associated with systemic lupus erythematosus. Arch Dermatol 1986;122:695–7.

146. Stellbrink HJ, Koperski K, Albrecht H, et al. *Mycobacterium kansasii* infection limited to skin and lymph node in a patient with AIDS. Clin Exp Dermatol 1990;15:457–8.

147. Wallace RJ Jr, Brown BA, Onyi GO. Skin, soft tissue, and bone infections due to *Mycobacterium chelonae*: importance of prior corticosteroid therapy, frequency of disseminated infections, and resistance to oral antimicrobials other than clarithromycin. J Infect Dis 1992;166:405–12.

148. Feldman WE, Hedaya E, O'Brien M. Skin abscess caused by *Candida albicans*: unusual presentation of *C. albicans* disease. J Clin Microbiol 1980;12:44–5.

149. Feigin RD, Shackelford PG, Lins RD, et al. Subcutaneous abscess due to *Coccidioides immitis*. Am J Dis Child 1972; 124:734–5.

150. Dennis JE, Rhodes KH, Cooney DR, et al. Nosocomial *Rhizopus* infection (zygomycosis) in children. J Pediatr 1980; 96:824–8.

151. Gewirtzman A, Rabinovitz H. Botfly infestation (myiasis) masquerading as furunculosis. Cutis 1999;63:71–72.

152. Dorton DW, Kaufmann M. Palmoplantar pustules in an infant. Acropustulosis of infancy. Arch Dermatol 1996; 132:1365–1366, 1368–9.

153. Kahn G, Rywlin AM. Acropustulosis of infancy. Arch Dermatol 1979;115:831–3.

154. Sweet RD. An acute febrile neutrophilic dermatosis. Br J Dermatol 1964;74:349–56.

155. Collins P, Rogers S, Keenan P, et al. Acute febrile neutrophilic dermatosis in childhood (Sweet's syndrome). Br J Dermatol 1991;124:203–6.

156. Kibbi AG, Zaynoun ST, Kurban AK, et al. Acute febrile neutrophilic dermatosis (Sweet's syndrome): case report and review of the literature. Pediatr Dermatol 1985;3: 40–4.

157. Hensley CD, Caughman SW. Neutrophilic dermatoses associated with hematologic disorders. Clin Dermatol 2000; 18:355–67.

158. Darmstadt GL, Tunnessen WW Jr, Swerer RJ. Eosinophilic pustular folliculitis. Pediatrics 1992;89:1095–8.

159. Buckley DA, Munn SE, Higgins EM. Neonatal eosinophilic pustular folliculitis. Clin Exp Dermatol 2001;26:251–5.

160. Patrone P, Bragadin G, Stinco G, et al. Ofuji's disease: diagnostic and therapeutic problems. A report of three cases. Int J Dermatol 2001;40:512–5.

161. Ramdial PK, Morar N, Dlova NC, et al. HIV-associated eosinophilic folliculitis in an infant. Am J Dermatopathol 1999;21:241–6.

162. Jang KA, Chung ST, Choi JH, et al. Eosinophilic pustular folliculitis (Ofuji's disease) in myelodysplastic syndrome. J Dermatol 1998;25:742–6.

163. Boone M, Dangoisse C, Andre J, et al. Eosinophilic pustular folliculitis in three atopic children with hypersensitivity to *Dermatophagoides pteronyssinus*. Dermatology 1995;190: 164–8.

164. Szinmai G, Schaad UB, Heininger U. Multiple herpetic whitlow lesions in a 4-year-old girl: case report and review of the literature. Eur J Pediatr 2001;160:528–33.

165. Samuel EP. Transillumination of whitlows of terminal phalanx. Lancet 1950;258:763.

166. Hoss DM, Feder HM Jr. Addition of rifampin to conventional therapy for recurrent furunculosis. Arch Dermatol 1995;131:647–8.

167. Peacock SJ, de Silva I, Lowy FD. What determines nasal carriage of *Staphylococcus aureus*? Trends Microbiol 2001; 9:605–10.

168. Weijmer MC, Neering H, Welten C. Preliminary report: furunculosis and hypoferraemia. Lancet 1990;336:464–6.

169. Wahba-Yahav AV. Intractable chronic furunculosis: prevention of recurrences with pentoxifylline. Acta Derm Venereol 1992;72:461–2.

170. Levy R, Shriker O, Porath A, et al. Vitamin C for the treatment of recurrent furunculosis in patients with impaired neutrophil functions. J Infect Dis 1996;173:1502–5.

171. Sweetman L, Ellis-Pegler RB. Treatment of recurrent staphylococcal furunculosis. Med J Aust 1992;156:292.

172. Moss C, Gupta E. The Nikolsky sign in staphylococcal scalded skin syndrome. Arch Dis Child 1998;79:290.

173. Lina G, Gillet Y, Vandenesch F, et al. Toxin involvement in staphylococcal scalded skin syndrome. Clin Infect Dis 1997;25:1369–73.

174. Ladhani S. Recent developments in staphylococcal scalded skin syndrome. Clin Microbiol Infect 2001;7:301–7.

175. Melish ME, Chen FS, Sprouse S, et al. Epidermolytic toxin in staphylococcal infection: toxin levels and host response. Zentralbl Bakteriol 1981;10(suppl):287–98.

176. Dancer SJ, Simmons NA, Poston SM, et al. Outbreak of staphylococcal scalded skin syndrome among neonates. J Infect 1988;16:87–103.

177. Saiman L, Jakob K, Holmes KW, et al. Molecular epidemiology of staphylococcal scalded skin syndrome in premature infants. Pediatr Infect Dis J 1998;17:329–34.

178. Farrell AM. Staphylococcal scalded-skin syndrome. Lancet 1999;354:880–1.

179. Cribier B, Piemont Y, Grosshans E. Staphylococcal scalded skin syndrome in adults. A clinical review illustrated with a new case. J Am Acad Dermatol 1994;30:319–24.

180. Borchers SL, Gomez EC, Isseroff RR. Generalized staphylococcal scalded skin syndrome in an anephric boy undergoing hemodialysis. Arch Dermatol 1984;120:912–8.

181. Lyell A. Toxic epidermal necrolysis: an eruption resembling scalding of the skin. Br J Dermatol 1956;68:355–61.

182. Roujeau JC, Stern RS. Severe adverse cutaneous reactions to drugs. N Engl J Med 1994;331:1272–85.

183. Ladhani S, Joannou CL. Difficulties in diagnosis and management of the staphylococcal scalded skin syndrome. Pediatr Infect Dis J 2000;19:819–21.

184. Feder HM Jr, Hoss DM, Dimond RL. Toxic epidermal necrolysis. N Engl J Med 1996;334:922.

185. Amon RB, Dimond RL. Toxic epidermal necrolysis. Rapid differentiation between staphylococcal- and drug-induced disease. Arch Dermatol 1975;111:1433–7.

186. Revuz J, Penso D, Roujeau JC, et al. Toxic epidermal necrolysis. Clinical findings and prognosis factors in 87 patients. Arch Dermatol 1987;123:1160–5.

187. Eady RA. Epidermolysis bullosa: scientific advances and therapeutic challenges. J Dermatol 2001;28:638–40.

188. Uitto J, Pulkkinen L, McLean WH. Epidermolysis bullosa: a spectrum of clinical phenotypes explained by molecular heterogeneity. Mol Med Today 1997;3:457–65.

189. Hallel-Halevy D, Nadelman C, Chen M, et al. Epidermolysis bullosa acquisita: update and review. Clin Dermatol 2001;19:712–8.

190. McCormick JK, Yarwood JM, Schlievert PM. Toxic shock syndrome and bacterial superantigens: an update. Annu Rev Microbiol 2001;55:77–104.

191. Palma PA, Conley SB, Crandell SS, et al. Zinc deficiency following surgery in zinc-supplemented infants. Pediatrics 1982;69:801–3.

192. Hoeger PH, Harper JI. Neonatal erythroderma: differential diagnosis and management of the "red baby." Arch Dis Child 1998;79:186–91.

193. Hussain FM, Boyle-Vavra S, Bethel CD, et al. Current trends in community-acquired methicillin-resistant *Staphylococcus aureus* at a tertiary care pediatric facility. Pediatr Infect Dis J 2000;19:1163–6.

194. Brook I, Frazier EH, Yeager JK. Microbiology of nonbullous impetigo. Pediatr Dermatol 1997;14:192–5.

195. Wilkinson RD, Carey WD. Topical mupirocin versus topical neosporin in the treatment of cutaneous infections. Int J Dermatol 1988;27:514–5.

196. Bass JW, Chan DS, Creamer KM, et al. Comparison of oral cephalexin, topical mupirocin and topical bacitracin for treatment of impetigo. Pediatr Infect Dis J 1997;16: 708–10.

197. Demidovich CW, Wittler RR, Ruff ME, et al. Impetigo. Current etiology and comparison of penicillin, erythromycin, and cephalexin therapies. Am J Dis Child 1990;144: 1313–5.

198. Feder HM Jr, Pond KE. Addition of rifampin to cephalexin therapy for recalcitrant staphylococcal skin infections—an observation. Clin Pediatr 1996;35:205–8.

199. Nordstrand A, Norgren M, Holm SE. Pathogenic mechanism of acute post-streptococcal glomerulonephritis. Scand J Infect Dis 1999;31:523–37.

200. Schwartz B, Facklam RR, Breiman RF. Changing epidemiology of group A streptococcal infection in the USA. Lancet 1990;336:1167–71.

201. Dillon HC Jr. Post-streptococcal glomerulonephritis following pyoderma. Rev Infect Dis 1979;1:935–45.

202. Topham J. Sugar for wounds. J Tissue Viability 2000;10: 86–9.

203. Bryan CS, Dew CE, Reynolds KL. Bacteremia associated with decubitus ulcers. Arch Intern Med 1983;143:2093–5.

204. Sugarman B, Hawes S, Musher DM, et al. Osteomyelitis beneath pressure sores. Arch Intern Med 1983;143:683–8.

205. Cross JT Jr, Schutze GE, Jacobs RF. Treatment of tularemia with gentamicin in pediatric patients. Pediatr Infect Dis J 1995;14:151–2.

206. Gage KL, Dennis DT, Orloski KA, et al. Cases of cat-associated human plague in the Western US, 1977-1998. Clin Infect Dis 2000;30:893–900.

207. Inglesby TV, Dennis DT, Henderson DA, et al. Plague as a biological weapon: medical and public health management. Working Group on Civilian Biodefense. JAMA 2000; 283:2281–90.

208. Alvin R, Middleton DB. Plaguelike presentation of *Yersinia enterocolitica* disease. J Pediatr 1986;109:79–80.

209. Orr ER, Riley HD Jr. Sporotrichosis in childhood: report of ten cases. J Pediatr 1971;78:951–7.

210. Smego RA Jr, Castiglia M, Asperilla MO. Lymphocutaneous syndrome. A review of non-sporothrix causes. Medicine (Baltimore) 1999;78:38–63.

211. Smego RA Jr, Gallis HA. The clinical spectrum of *Nocardia brasiliensis* infection in the United States. Rev Infect Dis 1984;6:164–80.

212. Dixon TC, Meselson M, Guillemin J, et al. Anthrax. N Engl J Med 1999;341:815–26.

213. Freedman A, Afonja O, Chang MW, et al. Cutaneous anthrax associated with microangiopathic hemolytic anemia and coagulopathy in a 7-month-old infant. JAMA 2002; 287:869–74.

214. Inglesby TV, Henderson DA, Bartlett JG, et al. Anthrax as a biological weapon: medical and public health management. Working Group on Civilian Biodefense. JAMA 1999; 281:1735–45.

215. Centers for Disease Control and Prevention. Update: Investigation of bioterrorism-related anthrax and interim guidelines for exposure management and antimicrobial therapy, October 2001. MMWR 2001;50:909–19.

216. Jernigan JA, Farr BM. Incubation period and sources of exposure for cutaneous *Mycobacterium marinum* infection: case report and review of the literature. Clin Infect Dis 2000;31:439–43.

217. Anonymous. Diagnosis and treatment of disease caused by nontuberculous mycobacteria. Am J Respir Crit Care Med 1997;156:S1–25.

218. van der Werf TS, van der Graaf WT, Tappero JW, et al. Mycobacterium ulcerans infection. Lancet 1999;354: 1013–8.

219. Shah MK, Sebti A, Kiehn TE, et al. Mycobacterium haemophilum in immunocompromised patients. Clin Infect Dis 2001;33:330–7.

220. Okano A, Shimazaki C, Ochiai N, et al. Subcutaneous infection with *Mycobacterium fortuitum* after allogeneic bone marrow transplantation. Bone Marrow Transplant 2001; 28:709–11.

221. Kauffman CA. Sporotrichosis. Clin Infect Dis 1999;29: 231–6.

222. Reed KD, Moore FM, Geiger GE, et al. Zoonotic transmission of sporotrichosis: case report and review. Clin Infect Dis 1993;16:384–7.

223. Larson DM, Eckman MR, Alber RL, et al. Primary cutaneous (inoculation) blastomycosis: an occupational hazard to pathologists. Am J Clin Pathol 1983;79:253–5.

224. Isaac M. Cutaneous aspergillosis. Dermatol Clin 1996;14: 137–40.

225. Colsky AS, Jegasothy SM, Leonardi C, et al. Diagnosis and treatment of a case of cutaneous cytomegalovirus infection with a dramatic clinical presentation. J Am Acad Dermatol 1998;38:349–51.

226. Rimsza ME, Berg RA. Cutaneous amebiasis. Pediatrics 1983;71:595–8.

227. Gullett J, Mills J, Hadley K, et al. Disseminated granulomatous acanthamoeba infection presenting as an unusual skin lesion. Am J Med 1979;67:891–6.

228. Wilson ME. Skin problems in the traveler. Infect Dis Clin North Am 1998;12:471–88.

229. Kain KC. Skin lesions in returned travelers. Med Clin North Am 1999;83:1077–102.

230. Bennett ML, Jackson JM, Jorizzo JL, et al. Pyoderma gangrenosum. A comparison of typical and atypical forms with an emphasis on time to remission. Case review of 86 patients from 2 institutions. Medicine 2000;79:37–46.

231. Chow RK, Ho VC. Treatment of pyoderma gangrenosum. J Am Acad Dermatol 1996;34:1047–60.

232. Forks TP. Brown recluse spider bites. J Am Board Fam Pract 2000;13:415–23.

233. Fisher RG, Kelly P, Krober MS, et al. Necrotic arachnidism. West J Med 1994;160:570–2.

234. Masters EJ. Images in clinical medicine. Loxoscelism. N Engl J Med 1998;339:379.

235. Kontogiannis V, Powell RJ. Behcet's disease. Postgrad Med J 2000;76:629–37.

236. Albertini JG, Tyler W, Miller OF III. Ulcerative sarcoidosis. Case report and review of the literature. Arch Dermatol 1997;133:215–9.

237. Modi D, Schulz EJ. Skin ulceration as sole manifestation of Langerhans-cell histiocytosis. Clin Exp Dermatol 1991; 16:212–5.

238. Stein DH. Tineas—superficial dermatophyte infections. Pediatr Rev 1998;19:368–72.

239. Elewski BE. Tinea capitis: a current perspective. J Am Acad Dermatol 2000;42:1–20.

240. Zuber TJ, Baddam K. Superficial fungal infection of the skin. Where and how it appears help determine therapy. Postgrad Med 2001;109:117–20, 123–6, 131–2.

241. Berg D, Erickson P. Fungal skin infections in children. New developments and treatments. Postgrad Med 2001; 110:83–4, 87–8, 93–4.

242. Topical butenafine for tinea pedis. Med Lett Drugs Ther 1997;39:63–4.

243. Gupta AK, Adam P, Dlova N, et al. Therapeutic options for the treatment of tinea capitis caused by *Trichophyton* species: griseofulvin versus the new oral antifungal agents, terbinafine, itraconazole, and fluconazole. Pediatr Dermatol 2001;18:433–8.

244. Wolf R, Wolf D, Tuzun B, et al. Diaper dermatitis. Clin Dermatol 2000;18:657–60.

245. Hoppe JE. Treatment of oropharyngeal candidiasis and candidal diaper dermatitis in neonates and infants: review and reappraisal. Pediatr Infect Dis J 1997;16:885–94.

246. Munz D, Powell KR, Pai CH. Treatment of candidal diaper dermatitis: a double-blind placebo-controlled comparison of topical nystatin with topical plus oral nystatin. J Pediatr 1982;101:1022–5.

247. Cavanaugh RM Jr, Greeson JD. *Trichophyton rubrum*. Infection of the diaper area. Arch Dermatol 1982;118: 446.

248. Mancini AJ. Acne vulgaris: a treatment update. Contemp Pediatr 2000;17:122–33.

249. Hurwitz S. Acne treatment for the 90s. Contemp Pediatr 1995;12:19–32.

250. Turvey SE. Atopic diseases of childhood. Curr Opin Pediatr 2001;13:487–95.

251. Lever R, Hadley K, Downey D, et al. Staphylococcal colonization in atopic dermatitis and the effect of topical mupirocin therapy. Br J Dermatol 1988;119:189–98.

252. Jawitz JC, Hines HC, Moshell AN. Treatment of eczema herpeticum with systemic acyclovir. Arch Dermatol 1985; 121:274–5.

253. Woolfson H. Oral acyclovir in eczema herpeticum. Br Med J (Clin Res Ed) 1984;288:531–2.

254. Camassa F, Fania M, Ditano G, et al. Neonatal scabies. Cutis 1995;56:210–2.

255. Centers for Disease Control and Prevention. Diphtheria, tetanus, and pertussis: recommendations for vaccine use and other preventive measures. Recommendations of the Immunization Practices Advisory committee (ACIP). Morb Mortal Wkly Rep 1991;40:1–28.

CHAPTER 18

Cardiovascular Syndromes

Inflammatory processes involving the heart are usually classified as pericarditis, myocarditis, or endocarditis, including valvulitis. When all three of these processes are present, the inflammation is called "pancarditis." Infections of the heart or blood vessels are uncommon in children, in whom they are usually secondary to underlying anatomic defects.

Inflammatory diseases involving the blood vessels can be classified as arteritis or phlebitis. These diseases, too, are rare in children except as a complication of indwelling catheters, as discussed in Chapter 10.

■ ACUTE MYOCARDITIS

The clinical findings of acute myocarditis may differ considerably depending upon the age of the patient. In infants, it is often found in association with a severe systemic illness resembling sepsis. Enteroviruses, in particular, may cause infants to suffer a severe and rather acute myocarditis in addition to signs of systemic inflammatory response syndrome. This condition, often called "enteroviral sepsis," is a serious illness with a high mortality rate. In older children and adolescents, myocarditis is usually best defined by the following findings: presumed acute onset, usually over a week or so; congestive heart failure, conduction abnormalities, or arrhythmias; fever or history of recent fever; and no alternate explanation for the cardiac findings, such as congenital heart disease. Often, the time of onset is difficult to determine in retrospect, so that subacute and chronic myocarditis are diagnosed based on the course rather than the history. The usual clinical findings include gallop rhythm, enlarged heart, and other signs of congestive heart failure (CHF). Distant or soft heart sounds are unusual unless there is severe CHF or pericarditis. Possible electrocardiographic (ECG) abnormalities include low voltage, prolonged conduction time, depressed ST segments and inverted T waves, widened QRS complex, and multifocal extrasystoles.[1–5] In older adolescents and adults, the presentation of myocarditis may mimic acute myocardial infarction.[6] In one large prospective study of over 672,000 military recruits, 98 (92%) of 107 subjects who developed myocarditis had signs and symptoms suggestive of myocardial infarction.[7] In ten (9%) patients, myocarditis caused dilated cardiomyopathy or sudden death.

Classification

There are three general types of myocarditis:

1. Primary. Here, myocarditis is the chief clinical problem.
2. Complicating. Examples of this type include myocarditis complicating severe influenza, meningococcemia, or diphtheria.
3. Incidental. This type may occur as an autopsy finding without apparent clinical manifestation[8] or as a minor ECG abnormality in another disease, such as measles, without any significant clinical manifestation.[2]

Causes of Primary Myocarditis

Primary Viral Myocarditis

The enteroviruses, especially coxsackievirus B are the most common causes of primary viral myocarditis.[1] The simultaneous occurrence in the community of aseptic meningitis, pleurodynia, or fever without localizing signs supports coxsackievirus B as the cause. Studies utilizing PCR have also shown enteroviruses in heart biopsy samples of patients suffering from myocarditis.

Coxsackievirus A may be an important, but often unproved, cause of primary myocarditis. Unlike coxsackieviruses B, coxsackieviruses A are not readily grown in tissue culture. They do, however, produce skeletal necrosis in mice. Therefore, in the past, mouse inoculation was used to prove a suspected diagnosis of coxsackieviruses A infection. Most laboratories no longer have this capability.

This group of viruses should be suspected when there is herpangina in the community (see Chapter 2).

Molecular techniques have shown that adenoviruses may be one of the most common causes of myocarditis in childhood. In one study utilizing PCR of myocardial tissue to establish the etiologic diagnosis, adenovirus was even more common than Coxsackie B virus,[12] although this has not been the case in other studies.[13]

Other viruses that have been established as a cause of myocarditis by recovery from the myocardial tissue include poliovirus, influenza, mumps virus, and echovirus. During the 1998–1999 influenza epidemic, a single hospital reported nine cases of myocarditis that developed 4–7 days into a course of typical influenza.[14] Echoviruses can be considered less-virulent enterovirus relatives of the coxsackieviruses A and B. A 5-month-old with serologically confirmed roseola who developed a rapidly fatal case of acute myocarditis suggests that HHV-6 can cause myocarditis.[15]

Acute Rheumatic Fever

This has been the most common cause of clinically apparent myocarditis in childhood and is discussed in detail in the following section. The myocarditis in this disease is often associated with a prolonged PR interval on the ECG and with findings of valvulitis, most frequently manifested by the murmurs of mitral or aortic insufficiency.

Other Infectious Causes

Many other microorganisms or parasites that have the capacity to invade skeletal muscle may also involve cardiac muscle. These include trichinosis, toxoplasmosis, and visceral larval migrans.[16] *Mycoplasma pneumoniae* infection and Lyme disease can also produce myocarditis.[17,18] *Chlamydia trachomatis* is a rare but treatable cause of myocarditis. Several cases have occurred during acute bacterial enteritis due to *Shigella sonnei*[19] and *Campylobacter jejuni*.[20]

Hypersensitivity Vasculitis

Drug hypersensitivity has been reported as a rare cause of myocarditis in adults.[21] 5-fluorouracil has been implicated as a cause of myocarditis in those with malignancies.[22]

Idiopathic Primary Myocarditis

In many cases an etiologic diagnosis cannot be established. Perhaps many or most of these cases are caused by a virus, but laboratory evidence does not usually confirm a concurrent infection with a virus known to be capable of producing myocarditis.

Myocarditis Complicating Other Diseases

Myocarditis Complicating Common Childhood Infections

The ECG changes of myocarditis are no more common in children with acute respiratory infections than in a normal control group.[23] However, mild myocarditis can complicate measles and mumps.[2,24] Rarely, cases associated with varicella[25] or with Epstein-Barr virus infection have been reported.[26] In these latter cases, direct proof of causation is lacking. Cytomegalovirus has been known to cause myocarditis in immune-suppressed patients after organ transplantation.[27]

Myocarditis Secondary to Severe Bacterial Infection

In severe bacterial infections, particularly sepsis and meningitis, myocarditis may occur. It is rarely the primary cause of death except in diphtheria, however. In fatal cases of meningococcemia, histologic evidence of myocarditis is frequently found. In non-fatal cases of septicemia with *Staphylococcus aureus*, clinical evidence of myocarditis may be present. Staphylococcal toxic shock syndrome is occasionally complicated by myocarditis.

Myocarditis Complicating Vasculitis

Juvenile rheumatoid arthritis of systemic onset can include myocarditis (Chapter 10). Dermatomyositis, systemic lupus erythematosus, and scleroderma are rarely complicated by myocarditis. The early stages of Kawasaki disease (Chapter 11) are associated with myocarditis in greater than 50% of cases.[28]

Human Immunodeficiency Virus Infection (HIV)

Patients with HIV infection often develop myocarditis or cardiomyopathy. It may be caused by the viruses implicated above or may be related to the underlying disease process. In one autopsy study, histologic evidence of myocarditis was found in 11 (34%) of 32 patients with HIV infection, and borderline myocarditis was seen in another 13 (41%). Adenovirus and CMV were the principal pathogens. No myocarditis was found in 32 age-matched controls (patients with structural heart disease).[29] The onset may be insidious, and patients may be asymptomatic or marginally symptomatic for long periods of time. The situation may be further complicated by lymphocytic interstitial pneumonitis, which provides the clinician with another suspect for the gradual loss of cardiovascular vigor. Alternatively, patients with HIV may rapidly develop myocarditis and profound loss of function, especially in late stages of HIV disease or in cases where the myocarditis is due to the mitochondrial toxicity of nucleoside analogue antiretroviral agents (see Chapter 20).

Diagnostic Approach

Perhaps the most difficult task is establishing the diagnosis of myocarditis, because signs and symptoms can be nonspecific. In relatively sick children with fever, vomiting, and even mild shock, myocarditis should be on the clinician's "pessimist list" (see Chapter 1), and a chest x-ray and an ECG should be ordered.

If carried out early in the disease process, cultures (or PCR testing) of the nasopharynx and/or rectum may yield coxsackievirus or adenovirus. Acute and convalescent antibody titers to coxsackieviruses A and B, adenovirus, and EBV may be obtained. Serologic studies should also include antistreptococcal antibody titer measurement, as described in the following section on acute rheumatic fever (ARF). If respiratory symptoms are prominent, and influenza virus is known to be circulating, rapid testing for influenza virus should also be done.[30] Because metabolic disturbances may cause similar symptoms, blood glucose and serum calcium levels should be sent. If the patient is highly febrile, blood cultures are reasonable. Complete blood count, erythrocyte sedimentation rate, C-reactive protein, troponin T, LDH, and CPK round out the nonspecific studies. Studies to evaluate heart size and function include the ECG, chest roentgenogram, and echocardiogram. Magnetic resonance imaging (MRI) offers a good picture of acute myocarditis because it can clearly image all parts of the heart, including the apex of the right ventricle.[31] Some investigators have used contrast media-enhanced MRI to follow the progress of the disease from focal to diffuse inflammatory changes over the first 2 weeks of illness.[32] Endomyocardial biopsy may be helpful in some cases, but its yield in patients who have only dysrhythmias is very low.[33]

Complications

Arrhythmia or complete heart block can occur in acute myocarditis.[34,35] Acute CHF with acute pulmonary edema can occur.

In children, chronic myocardial failure (cardiomyopathy) sometimes occurs without preceding fever or other evidence of an acute infection.[34] Cardiomyopathies are usually idiopathic but are occasionally related to infiltrative diseases, toxins, primary muscle or neurologic diseases, nutritional deficiencies, or hypersensitivity reactions. A previous attack of subclinical viral myocarditis has been postulated as a cause of idiopathic cardiomyopathy. In some cases, biopsy of heart muscle will yield the offending virus by PCR testing. In animal models, chronic myocarditis has been linked to ongoing virus replication, but in humans the situation is not entirely clear. Chronic myocarditis is a serious disease with a high mortality rate.[34]

Treatment

Bed Rest

The emphasis on bed rest, which is recommended for 2 weeks or so, depending on the clinical course, is based in part on the evidence obtained from the experimental model of coxsackievirus B myocarditis in mice, in which exercise worsens disease.[36] There is also some evidence in humans that strenuous exercise, in particular, may lead to worsened outcome.[37]

Digitalization

Digoxin is often helpful, especially in those with signs and symptoms of congestive heart failure, but it should be administered with caution because the inflamed myocardium is exceedingly sensitive to this drug.

Immunosuppressive Agents

Treatment of acute myocarditis with steroids, azathioprine, or other immunosuppressive agents is controversial. In a mouse model of experimental myocarditis, steroids given during the acute phase of the illness worsened the degree of inflammation and reduced survival.[38] Small, retrospective or uncontrolled studies in humans, on the other hand, have suggested some benefit. In one prospective trial 84 patients with dilated cardiomyopathy and increased HLA expression were randomized to receive immunosuppressive therapy or placebo. Short-term improvement was noted, but by 2 years there were no significant differences in the primary end points of death, cardiac transplant, or hospital readmission.[39]

Intravenous Immunoglobulin (IVIG)

Isolated case reports of patients with severe myocarditis who survived after receiving high-dose IVIG in addition to conventional supportive measures have been published.[40] The authors of one prospective study gave IVIG in conventional 2 g/kg dosages to twenty-one consecutive children with signs and symptoms of acute myocarditis. No contemporaneous controls were used, but left ventricular function and survival in treated subjects was compared with that of historic controls.[41] In this analysis, the group given IVIG was more likely to achieve normal left ventricular function by 1 year after diagnosis ($P = 0.03$). There was a trend toward improved survival. No adverse events of IVIG administration were noted.

Consultation

A cardiologist should be consulted about children with myocarditis because of the complications outlined above. Inotropic agents, diuretics, vasodilators, antiarrhythmia drugs, and regulation of intravascular volume all need careful consideration, usually in an intensive care setting.

Prognosis

Myocarditis has a 1-year case-fatality rate of 15–20%.[42] A small but significant percentage of survivors will require cardiac transplantation at a later stage. McCarthy and colleagues have demonstrated that patients who present with fulminant myocarditis have a better long-term prognosis than those who are less severely ill at the time of presentation.[42] Of 15 patients with fulminant myocarditis, 14 (93%) were alive without having received a transplant 11 years after presentation as compared to only 59 (45%) of 132 patients with nonfulminant myocarditis. Thus, an aggressive approach, including the use of mechanical circulatory assistance, is warranted in patients with severe fulminant myocarditis.

■ ACUTE RHEUMATIC FEVER

Acute rheumatic fever (ARF) is an acute, active disease that should be distinguished from rheumatic heart disease (RHD), which is a permanent valvular deformity usually manifested by a heart murmur. In most cases, the diagnosis of ARF is suspected when a patient has carditis, polyarthritis, or both in temporal proximity to an episode of pharyngitis. Occasionally, chorea is a late sole manifestation of the disease. However, the definition of ARF is complex and is based on a combination of findings called the "Jones criteria," described later.

In the past, ARF was overdiagnosed, and at present, accurate diagnosis is essential because of the possibility of long-term consequences and the need for antibiotic prophylaxis. Consultation with a cardiologist who will use modern technologic aids is strongly advised.[43]

Frequency

Once the leading cause of death among children in the United States, the frequency of ARF has been decreasing since the 1940s, when sulfonamide prophylaxis was shown to prevent recurrences in patients with previous rheumatic fever, and penicillin therapy of streptococcal pharyngitis was shown to prevent first attacks.

After 30 years of a steadily decreasing frequency of ARF, in the 1980s there was a resurgence, for reasons that are not entirely clear. Within a period of 5 years, the tone of article titles changed from describing "a vanishing disease" to "the comeback of a disappearing disease."[44-48] Rheumatic heart disease is a frequent cause of death in developing countries, and the decrease in the United States had been attributed to "higher standards of living."[48] The outbreaks in the 1980s and 1990s often occurred in middle-class children, a category of children not usually thought to be at high risk for the disease.[44]

The resurgence of ARF was localized to several areas and has not been sustained. One theory to explain the fluctuating incidence in the United States points to virulence factors or cofactors that are not yet adequately defined.[46-48] Certain M-types of GAS are more rheumatogenic than others, and the M-types that circulate in the United States change over time.[49]

In addition, there are probably other factors that determine susceptibility to ARF that are yet to be described. For example, the Aboriginal population of Australia has rates of ARF and RHD that are among the highest in the world. However, Group A streptococcus (GAS) throat colonization is uncommon, and symptomatic Streptococcal pharyngitis is rare.[50]

Many other studies show a higher attack rate for urban racial minorities, suggesting either a genetic factor or factors related to accessibility of medical care and treatment of the preceding streptococcal illness.[51–54]

Etiology

ARF is a late nonsuppurative sequela of Group A β-hemolytic streptococcal pharyngitis (Chapter 2), often called the preceding or antecedent illness. The pharyngitis is not recognized as an illness by the patient or by the parents in 10–33% of cases, although 50–60% of this subset of patients do remember having had a sore throat.[55–57] This illness is followed by a latent period ranging from 1 to 5 weeks (average 19 days) before the symptoms of ARF appear.[58]

About 0.5–2% of children with nonepidemic, untreated exudative pharyngitis and a culture positive for group A streptococci develop ARF.[59] The frequency is even less, if the patient group taken as the denominator includes those with less severe or less precisely diagnosed streptococcal infections. This variation in frequency of ARF according to the denominator is an important concept and is clearly demonstrated in the one controlled study done in children[59] (Table 18-1). The suggestion is that the development of ARF is likely to follow only infection with rheumatogenic strains of S. pyogenes.[60] The types of GAS that usually cause skin infection (impetigo), for example, may precede glomerulonephritis but do not cause ARF. The relatively avirulent phenotypes that are frequently carried in the throats of schoolchildren, also, are not associated with ARF.[61] The incidence of ARF following GAS pharyngitis that is treated with appropriate antibiotics is exceedingly low (<0.05%).[62]

It is probably a combination of pathogen and host factors that allow this small percentage of patients to develop ARF. Rheumatogenic strains of GAS are rich in M protein and thickly encapsulated with hyaluronic acid.[63] No specific host factors that predispose to the development of ARF have been clearly identified; however, in some studies HLA-DR7 was found with greater frequency in patients with ARF than in controls.[64] In developing countries, malnutrition and failure to thrive have been associated with the development of ARF.[65]

Both the arthritis and the carditis are thought to be autoimmune. The arthritis is mediated by antigen-antibody complexes, but the carditis is caused by cytotoxic T lymphocytes.[66] There may be antigens in GAS that are closely related to heart antigens, which causes the host to produce heart-di-

TABLE 18-1. THE FREQUENCY OF ACUTE RHEUMATIC FEVER FOLLOWING UNTREATED STREPTOCOCCAL PHARYNGITIS*

FINDINGS IN UNTREATED CHILDREN WITH PHARYNGITIS	DENOMINATOR (NUMBER WITH FINDING)	NUMERATOR (NUMBER DEVELOPING RHEUMATIC FEVER)	PER CENT
Beta-hemolytic streptococci	608	2	0.3
Group A streptococci	519	2	0.4
Typable Group A streptococci	273	2	0.9
Exudate and Group A streptococci	186	2	1.1
Exudate and ASO titer rise	95	2	2.1
Exudate and positive culture for 21 days	81	2	2.5

* The percent of children who develop acute rheumatic fever depends on the denominator used to define the accuracy, severity, and persistence of the streptococcal pharyngitis. (Modified from Siegel AC, Johnson EE, Stellerman GH, et al. Controlled studies of streptococcal pharyngitis in a pediatric population. I. Factors related to the attack rate of rheumatic fever. N Engl J Med 1961; 265:559.)

rected immune responses. The current medical practice is to treat all episodes of streptococcal pharyngitis in order to prevent ARF (Chapter 2).

Age Factors

First attacks of rheumatic fever usually occur in children over 5 years of age and in young adults, presumably because previous streptococcal infections are necessary to sensitize the patient. First attacks of ARF rarely occur in patients less than 3 years of age.[67]

Jones Criteria

As modified in 1992,[68] the Jones criteria are applicable only to the initial attack of ARF. Although designed as an epidemiologic tool, the Jones criteria are now often used as a guide in diagnosis. The criteria require either two major manifestations or one major and two minor manifestations plus, in either case, evidence of a preceding streptococcal infection (Box 18-1).[69] The diagnosis should always state the major manifestations present (e.g., ARF with carditis and polyarthritis).[69]

Major Manifestations

The usual major manifestations are polyarthritis (not polyarthralgia) and carditis (defined by mur-

murs, pericarditis, cardiomegaly, or CHF). The three murmurs that suggest rheumatic carditis are described in the Jones Criteria:[69]

1. Apical systolic murmur. This long, blowing, high-pitched murmur is best heard at the apex and has variable loudness. It is transmitted toward the axilla and suggests *mitral regurgitation*.
2. Apical mid-diastolic (Carey-Coombs) murmur. This is best heard with the bell of the stethoscope with the patient lying on the left side with the breath held in expiration. This murmur is a result of rapid ventricular filling, as in left *ventricular dilatation* and may occur in conditions other than acute carditis.
3. Basal diastolic murmur. This high-pitched blowing murmur is best heard with the diaphragm of the stethoscope at the right upper or the left midsternal border with the patient sitting and leaning forward with the breath held after deep expiration. It suggests *aortic regurgitation*.

Many patients who do not have physical examination evidence of carditis have been shown to have mitral insufficiency and/or aortic insufficiency by Doppler echocardiography.[70] The importance of this so-called silent carditis, and whether echocardiographic evidence of carditis should be counted as fulfilling the diagnostic criteria for ARF, are topics of some debate.[66,70] Most of these clinically silent valvular abnormalities are transient but a small percentage may persist.[70,71]

The arthritis of ARF is a characteristic migratory polyarthritis. It typically involves the large joints (knees, ankles, wrists, and elbows) and is manifested by swelling, warmth, and exquisite tenderness. Joint inflammation usually lasts for only a few days and then another joint becomes affected. The arthritis is so responsive to aspirin and other NSAIDS that a trial of these agents is sometimes used as a "diagnostic test." The arthritis of ARF is not deforming, and unlike the cardiac manifestations, there are no long-term sequelae of joint involvement. This led to the description of ARF as a disease that "licks the joints but bites the heart."[72]

The other major manifestations are much less common and consist of chorea,[73] subcutaneous nodules, and erythema marginatum. The nodules are better seen than felt. They may occur with other diseases, and it has been recommended by some observers that they be dropped from the list of major manifestations of ARF.[74] Erythema marginatum is an evanescent, usually rapidly migratory,

---

BOX 18-1 ■ Jones Criteria (Modified) for the Diagnosis of ARF

Two major OR
One major and two minor manifestations
PLUS Preceding Group A streptococcal infection
    (recent scarlet fever, throat culture positive for
    Group A streptococci, high or rising
    antistreptococcal antibody titer [ASO or anti-
    DNAse B])

Major Manifestations
Polyarthritis
Carditis
Chorea
Erythema marginatum
Subcutaneous nodules

Minor Manifestations
Arthralgia
Prolonged PR interval
Fever
Elevated erythrocyte sedimentation rate or
    C-reactive protein

nonpruritic pink rash with serpiginous raised borders. The rash resembles smoke rings, expanding and leaving a clearing center. Adequate pictures of this rash are rare, and it is seldom seen now.[75] In the largest of the 1980s outbreaks (107 confirmed cases), no erythema marginatum was seen.[76] Sydenham's chorea (St. Vitus' dance) is more common than subcutaneous nodules or erythema marginatum, occurring in 15–20% of patients. It has a longer latent period than arthritis or carditis, with symptoms starting several months after an episode of GAS pharyngitis. Importantly, it may occur as the sole manifestation of the disease ("pure chorea"). In one study of 22 children with pure chorea, however, 14 (63%) were demonstrated to have valvulitis by echocardiography, the long-term consequences of which are unclear.[77] Chorea is manifested by erratic jerky movements of the extremities and facial grimacing, as well as emotional lability. Physical findings suggestive of chorea include spooning (hyperextension of the fingers and wrists when the arms are held in extension) and tongue fasciculations.

Minor Manifestations

The minor manifestations are arthralgia (not counted as a minor manifestation if polyarthritis is used as a major), fever in excess of 100.4°F (38.0°C) rectally, abnormal acute-phase reactants (erythrocyte sedimentation rate or C-reactive protein), and conduction changes detected by ECG, primarily prolonged PR interval (not counted as a minor manifestation if carditis is used as a major). Rarely, ARF presents as Stokes-Adams attacks, complete heart block,[78] or torsade de pointes.[79]

Differential Diagnosis

The differential diagnosis of ARF includes a number of other diagnoses or syndromes, which are discussed in the sections on myocarditis and pericarditis, rheumatoid arthritis, septic arthritis, gonococcal arthritis, reactive arthritis (Chapter 16), and infective endocarditis. Common errors include making the diagnosis of ARF when a single joint is involved, when an innocent murmur is present, when a nonspecific rash (especially an urticarial or an erythema multiforme rash) is erroneously called erythema marginatum, and when other causes of chorea are overlooked.[80]

Acute rheumatic fever can produce a tenosynovitis resembling that of disseminated gonococcemia, and the two diseases may be very difficult to distinguish.[81]

Misdiagnosis of ARF is not unusual, and in one series, only 68 of 100 children originally thought to have ARF had illnesses clearly meeting the modified Jones criteria.[82] Of the 32 with illnesses not meeting these criteria, 14 had a different diagnosis (such as congenital heart disease, rheumatoid arthritis, and undiagnosed fever), 9 had suspected ARF without heart disease, and 9 had evidence of RHD (mitral or aortic valvular disease) without a history of ARF.[82] The difficulties of "delabeling" patients with an uncertain diagnosis make it essential that all patients with suspected ARF receive diagnostic evaluations that are as thorough as possible at the time of the initial episode. If the diagnosis of ARF is made, the reasoning behind the diagnosis should be carefully documented in the medical record.

The flip side of the coin is that ARF can sometimes be a difficult diagnosis to establish. The arthritis may be short-lived[83] or even monoarticular.[84] The carditis may be silent. Physicians who see patients in areas where ARF is uncommon may not have ever seen a case. Therefore, the thought that a particular set of symptoms may represent ARF may never enter the mind. When one case occurs, the physician should be on the lookout for others, because it tends to come in groups as a rheumatogenic strain is passed around the community.

Post-Streptococcal Reactive Arthritis (PSRA)

This entity has now been well-described and can be distinguished from the arthritis of ARF on the basis of several characteristics.[85]

The latent period from the onset of GAS pharyngitis to onset of arthritis is shorter in PSRA than in ARF and is usually less than 2 weeks. In contrast to the arthritis of ARF, PSRA is nonmigratory and affects small joints as well as large ones. The arthritis of ARF usually lasts only a few weeks and is very responsive to salicylates. PSRA has a more protracted course and responds poorly to aspirin and other NSAIDs. A small subset of children (about 6%) who seemingly have PSRA will develop carditis over time, primarily manifested by subtle mitral valve disease.[86,87] Finally, patients with PSRA do not meet the modified Jones Criteria for the diagnosis of ARF. Criteria for the diagnosis of PSRA have recently been proposed and include the distinguishing features discussed previously.[88]

A survey of rheumatologists and infectious disease specialists in Canada showed that there is no consensus on the utility or the duration of prophylactic therapy for PSRA.[89] The American Heart Association recommends that patients with PSRA receive penicillin prophylaxis for 1 year. If, at that time, there is no evidence of carditis, prophylaxis is discontinued.[90] This seems to be a reasonable approach and one that we have adopted, although others have argued for longer prophylaxis in these patients.[91] Longer prophylaxis (i.e., as for ARF) should probably be prescribed for patients with post-streptococcal arthritis whose symptoms are more typical of ARF than PRSA (e.g., large joints, migratory, responsive to aspirin).

Chorea

Sydenham's chorea (the chorea of ARF) can be mimicked by chorea induced by oral contraceptives, that following infectious mononucleosis,[92,93] that associated with systemic lupus erythematosis,[94] or paroxysmal choreoathetosis, which is usually familial.[95] Chorea may also be a complication of surgery for congenital heart disease.[96]

Sydenham's chorea may leave some residual deficits.[97] The chorea may recur after streptococcal infections that are too mild and transient to be readily detectable or possibly after stimuli other than streptococcal infection.[98]

Treatment

Bed Rest

As soon as the diagnosis is made, bed rest is advisable for a minimum of 2–3 weeks until it is certain no carditis is present. If carditis is present, bed rest for 1 to 3 months may be advisable. When the heart rate and sedimentation rate are normal and the arthritis is over, gradual resumption of normal activities can begin. Every patient in whom this diagnosis is considered should be thoroughly evaluated, ideally by a cardiologist, in terms of the Jones criteria, before being put on bed rest.

Salicylates and Other Nonsteroidal Anti-Inflammatory Agents

Patients with arthritis or carditis in the absence of cardiomegaly are generally treated with anti-inflammatory agents. Aspirin at a starting dose of 100 mg/kg per day for 1 week up to 10 g per day and then 60 mg/kg per day for 3–4 weeks has been used.

In the past, salicylate levels of 15–25 mg/dL were sought and levels followed. Most experts now believe that obtaining levels is unnecessary unless signs of salicylate toxicity occur or the therapy is not producing the desired result.

Because of the small risk of Reye syndrome in patients on aspirin therapy, alternate anti-inflammatory therapy has been evaluated. A small, noncomparative group of patients had rapid resolution of fever and arthritis on naproxen sodium.[99]

For patients with frank cardiomyopathy or signs of congestive heart failure, corticosteroids are generally used in place of aspirin (see later).

Whenever applicable, vaccination against influenza and varicella should be considered for patients who may require long-term aspirin therapy.

Treatment of Congestive Heart Failure

Treatment usually includes digitalization and diuretics.[100,101] Some older children and adults with severe valve damage may require valve replacement. Serious arrhythmias, such as ventricular tachycardia, are rare.[55,102]

Corticosteroids

The value of steroids for treatment of acute rheumatic carditis is controversial.[103] Most authorities agree that steroids are not necessary if there are no significant murmurs and that these agents probably *should* be used in very ill patients with severe carditis manifested by congestive failure or pericarditis. In patients with significant murmurs but without congestive failure, the superiority of steroid therapy to aspirin therapy is not proved. If steroids are used, the recommended dose is 2 mg/kg per day of prednisone, up to 60 mg/day, until clinical improvement (about 2–4 weeks), followed by a gradual taper in the dose (reduce by 5 mg every 2–3 days). Salicylates are begun at the time the prednisone taper is started and continued for 6–12 weeks.[80] No adequately randomized and controlled trials have demonstrated the utility of corticosteroids in the treatment of ARF.

Intravenous Immunoglobulin (IVIG)

Because of potent immunomodulatory effects, it has been thought by some physicians that IVIG might be beneficial in severe cases of ARF. Very small case series in which IVIG was thought to have been beneficial have appeared.[104] However, a randomized, prospective, double-blinded trial in 59 patients with ARF showed no detectable benefit from the administration of large, repeated dosages of IVIG.[105]

Prognosis

A rebound (transient worsening) occurs in about one-third of children within 4 weeks of stopping steroid or salicylate therapy and presumably represents the original suppressed disease.[106] Recurrences tend to have the same manifestations as the original attack.[107] Death caused directly by ARF is now rare in the United States.

Prevention

Prevention of the First Attack

Reviews of the histories of patients with a first attack of ARF indicate that the majority had a sore throat or fever or both.[56,57] The details of the diagnosis and treatment of Group A streptococcal infections are discussed in the sections on pharyngitis in Chapter 2.

Prevention of Recurrences

Once a patient has had an episode of rheumatic fever, prophylaxis against β-hemolytic streptococcal infections is imperative.[108] ARF is much more common in someone who has had a previous episode. In addition, if the original episode manifested carditis, the heart is likely to be involved in recurrent cases as well. Secondary prophylaxis is achieved with oral penicillin V, 250 mg twice a day, or intramuscular benzathine penicillin (1.2 million units) every 3–4 weeks. The intramuscular route is advisable if the patient is unreliable about taking oral medication. A systematic review of six studies concluded that monthly intramuscular benzathine penicillin is more effective ARF than oral penicillin.[109] In addition, injections every 3 weeks appear to be more effective than montly injections.[109] The American Heart Association recommends lifelong prophylaxis (or at least well into adulthood) for patients with cardiac involvement. Patients with ARF without carditis are given prophylaxis for 5 years or until age 21 years, whichever is longer.[90]

Erythromycin or clindamycin is an adequate substitute for oral penicillin if there is significant penicillin allergy,[110] as is a sulfonamide, such as sulfadiazine or sulfisoxazole.

■ PERICARDITIS

Pericarditis is defined by a pericardial friction rub, a pericardial effusion, or diagnostic ECG findings. Pericarditis can be acute or chronic, idiopathic or with a specific etiology, and with or without clinical valvulitis or myocarditis.

Clinical Diagnosis

The most common symptoms of acute pericarditis are fever, chest or abdominal pain, tachypnea, and tachycardia. Acute chest pain is sometimes absent in children. Occasionally, abdominal pain may be severe. Acute pericarditis can be diagnosed clinically when a friction rub or pericardial effusion is present.

Friction Rub

The rub is precordial and synchronous with the heartbeat and is usually associated with central chest pain.[111] A variety of rubs or clicks may be heard.[112] Rubs can sometimes be heard more clearly when the patient is kneeling or leaning forward. In childhood pericarditis, a friction rub is by no means common; only 7 (23%) of 30 patients in one series had discernable friction rubs at the time of initial evaluation.[113] A rub may be less likely in cases where the effusion is large.

Pericardial Effusion

An effusion is usually first suspected when the heart sounds are distant. The patient may also have an expiratory grunt or rapid, splinted breathing.[112] The chest roentgenogram typically shows a widened heart shadow, which could also be caused by acute cardiac failure. If the lung fields are relatively clear, without pulmonary congestion, the large heart shadow is usually secondary to a pericardial effusion rather than to a dilated heart in failure. If the effusion develops rapidly, patients may have symptoms of pericarditis even when the effusion is small and the chest x-ray picture appears normal.

A pericardial effusion can best be confirmed by echocardiogram. An effusion can also be diagnosed by observing the findings of cardiac tamponade, as described later.

Other Studies

Electrocardiogram (ECG) Changes

Typical ECG changes of acute pericarditis include decreased voltage if effusion is present, ST-segment

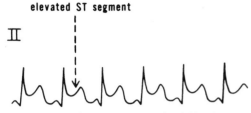

■ FIGURE 18-1 Electrocardiogram of a child with purulent pericarditis caused by *S. aureus*. Note the elevated ST segments. Heart sounds were very distant, and an emergency pericardiocentesis was required. The child had respiratory distress but did not appear toxic.

elevation, and T-wave inversion or splitting (Fig. 18-1).

Echocardiogram

An M-mode echocardiogram is very accurate and sensitive for detecting a pericardial effusion.[111,114] It is also helpful for demonstrating pericardial tamponade.[111,114]

Early Complications

Cardiac Tamponade

The principal physiologic disturbance that may occur in pericarditis is cardiac tamponade. It is much more likely to occur in purulent pericarditis than in other types, and rapid accumulation of fluid is more likely to produce tamponade than is gradual accumulation. Signs include hypotension, dyspnea, orthopnea, tachycardia, and distention of the neck veins.[111] Paradoxical pulse is one of the chief diagnostic findings, in which the radial pulse becomes weaker or disappears during inspiration. Jugular venous pressure also, paradoxically, increases during inspiration (Kussmaul sign). When the blood pressure is taken, the force of the pulse varies greatly with the phase of breathing. The systolic pressure is decreased in inspiration, and the pulse pressure is narrowed. The difference between the systolic pressures at the end of expiration and inspiration is the magnitude of the paradoxical pulse. Values greater than 10 mm Hg during quiet breathing suggest cardiac tamponade.

Congestive Heart Failure

Systemic venous congestion is the usual presenting manifestation of chronic pericarditis but may also be the first indication of acute pericarditis.

Chronic Pericarditis

This is extremely rare in children but can follow acute bacterial pericarditis. It is much more subtle and may be manifested only by chronic CHF. Chronic or recurrent pericarditis has been shown, in adults, to occasionally be due to enterovirus infection.[115] As in acute pericarditis, the findings of effusion, tamponade, a rub, or low voltage on ECG are practically diagnostic.

Emergency Treatment

Cardiac tamponade should be treated by pericardiocentesis. This is best done with the patient in the upright position. A needle should be inserted just to the left of the xiphoid notch and directed toward the right shoulder. Occasionally, a patient suspected of having pericarditis may instead have acute dilatation of the heart secondary to severe CHF. Therefore, an ECG and echocardiogram should be done, if possible, to confirm pericardial effusion before attempting the procedure. Pericardiocentesis can be lifesaving. However, it can also be dangerous if performed by inexperienced physicians. If the patient is stable, echocardiogram-guided drainage of pericardial fluid is best accomplished in the controlled environment of the operating suite. Digoxin is usually said to be contraindicated because it slows the heart rate and interferes with diastolic filling, both of which are useful compensatory mechanisms in cardiac tamponade. Vigorous diuretic therapy should not be used.

■ PERICARDITIS SYNDROMES

A number of patterns of pericarditis can be distinguished clinically, of which the purulent type is the most common in children.

Purulent Pericarditis

An effusion may be suspected for the reasons described earlier and can be confirmed by echocardiogram. Pericardiocentesis should be done in patients with an effusion if there is a suspicion of purulent pericarditis,[116–118] and any fluid obtained should be Gram stained and cultured for bacteria.

Purulent pericarditis is most common in infants or preschool children. Typically, it accompanies sepsis or localized infection elsewhere in the body. The most commonly associated condition is pneumonia, often with pleural effusion, but purulent pericarditis may also accompany septic arthritis or osteomyelitis. It occasional occurs without accompanying infection. *S. aureus* is the most common cause, accounting for 24 (80%) of 30 patients in one series.[113] In times when access to antimicrobial treatment was limited, *S. pneumoniae* was a fairly common cause, accompanied by pneumonia in 105 (93%) of 113 cases. Pericarditis in this setting is thought to be a consequence of delayed treatment of the primary pneumonia.[119] *H. influenzae* type b was seen occasionally as a comorbidity of pneumonia or meningitis, but the conjugated Hib vaccine has made this etiologic diagnosis rare. Nontypeable *H influenzae* may cause pericarditis in immunocompromised hosts,[120] but no reports in persons of normal immunity have appeared. Acute meningococcemia with or without meningitis is a rare cause of purulent pericarditis in children.[121,122] Rarely, septic arthritis and pericarditis may be the presenting features of acute meningococcemia or of disseminated gonococcemia.[123]

Treatment of purulent pericarditis should include surgical drainage of pus with partial pericardectomy to prevent recurrences or constrictive pericarditis.[121,122,124,125] Antibiotics used should be based first on the Gram stain and then on culture and susceptibility results. Empiric therapy usually includes a penicillinase-resistant penicillin (nafcillin or oxacillin) along with a third-generation cephalosporin. When an etiologic diagnosis is made and susceptibilities are available, antibiotic therapy can be tailored. Intravenous antibiotics are usually continued for 3–4 weeks.

Acute Nonpurulent Pericarditis

This syndrome has been called acute painful pericarditis and acute benign pericarditis. The term "benign" should not be used because myocardial infarction, purulent pericarditis, rheumatic fever, and other serious causes of pericarditis must be excluded. Acute nonpurulent pericarditis is characterized by the sudden onset of precordial pain that is often mistaken for the pain of an acute myocardial infarction in adults but is usually aggravated by inspiration and certain positions. Friction rub and ECG changes typical of pericarditis may be found. An effusion may be present, but tamponade is rare. The patient is usually neither as febrile nor as ill-appearing as patients with acute purulent pericarditis. Laboratory diagnostic procedures should include viral cultures and serology, as described in

the section on myocarditis, because coxsackievirus B infections are the main cause of this syndrome.[126] Some laboratories have PCR testing available for enteroviruses. Serum transaminase concentrations may be elevated.

If serious causes of pericarditis are excluded, treatment is usually only rest and reassurance, provided aspiration is not necessary to treat or prevent tamponade. Many cases of acute benign pericarditis must be classified as idiopathic in spite of viral studies.[127]

Viral pericarditis with effusion can be caused by coxsackievirus B[126] and influenza virus.[128] Adenovirus and coxsackievirus A have also been recovered from pericardial fluid during pericarditis.[129] *Mycoplasma pneumoniae* infection and infectious mononucleosis have been associated with pericarditis.[130,131] In one case, in situ hybridization performed on pericardial tissue was positive for Epstein-Barr virus in a patient with pericarditis.[132]

Acute rheumatic fever may cause pericarditis, as discussed in the previous section. In most situations, the appearance of a pericardial friction rub occurs in association with valvulitis.

Tuberculous Pericarditis

In the United States, pericarditis due to *Mycobacterium tuberculosis* is rare. When it does occur, it is more likely to be subacute or chronic, rather than acute. Sometimes pericarditis accompanies miliary tuberculosis. Most patients with tuberculous effusions have enlarged hilar lymph nodes.[133] Effusions may be bloody. Acid-fast staining (AFB) of aspirated pericardial fluid is unlikely to be positive. Adenine deaminase (ADA) levels are very high in the pericardial fluid of patients with tuberculous pericarditis. In one study, a level of 75 IU/L was 100% sensitive and 94% specific for the diagnosis.[134] Pericardial effusions associated with neoplastic diseases may also have an elevated ADA level. With the exception of the patient with miliary disease, almost all patients have a positive PPD, because the effusion represents a florid immune response to *M. tuberculosis*. Diagnosis is usually confirmed with a biopsy of the pericardium. Appropriate drainage procedures and antituberculous chemotherapy must be provided.

Fungal Pericarditis

In areas of endemicity, histoplasmosis is a common cause of pericarditis. Histoplasmal pericarditis arises late in the course of an outbreak and late in the course of an individual patient's disease process.[135] Unlike patients with disseminated histoplasmosis, who are usually immunocompromised, patients with pericardial involvement are generally immunocompetent adolescents or adults. The pericardial fluid tends to be bloody. Stains and cultures of aspirated fluid are almost always negative, and the condition responds to anti-inflammatory therapy, so it is thought to be a post-infectious complication of primary histoplasmosis.

Coccidioidomycosis and blastomycosis may also cause a similar clinical syndrome, but do so with much lower frequency.

Other Causes

Another cause of pericarditis with effusion is juvenile rheumatoid arthritis with systemic onset. In this disease, pericardial effusion, or even cardiac tamponade, is recognized after a febrile illness of 1–4 weeks' duration. Systemic lupus erythematosus and amebiasis are rare causes of pericarditis. A familial syndrome of recurrent pericarditis associated with arthritis and camptodactyly (flexion contractures of the fingers) has been described.[136]

Purulent pericarditis can occur after cardiac operations, but postpericardiotomy syndrome (PPS) is a more likely diagnosis. PPS is common, occuring after 15–20% of cardiac operations.[137,138] This syndrome is characterized by fever a few days to 2 weeks after a heart operation.[137,138] There is usually chest pain, which is often precordial but sometimes pleuritic. Pericardial friction rub or pericardial effusion and ECG findings of pericarditis are usually present. Pleural effusion can occur.[138] Typically, the disease has a self-limited course of 1–4 weeks. Bacterial endocarditis should be excluded by stopping antibiotics and obtaining blood cultures. This syndrome may represent a hypersensitivity reaction to blood in the pericardial sac and resembles the findings in posttraumatic or post-myocardial infarction pericarditis. After other causes have been excluded, aspirin or nonsteroidal anti-inflammatory drugs are the agents of choice for PPS.[138]

■ INFECTIVE ENDOCARDITIS

Infective endocarditis is a general term used to describe infection of the heart valves or endocardium. Usually, the infection is bacterial and occurs on an abnormal valve or a congenital defect, possibly one repaired with a patch or sutures, and, especially, on prosthetic valves or conduits. Older adults often have heart valves with some fibrotic changes, so infective endocarditis is much more common in adults than in children. The term "infective endocarditis" should be used instead of "bacterial endocarditis" until the etiology is known because nonbacterial agents, such as yeast, may be the infecting organisms. The term should be considered to include infection of the aorta, because a patent ductus arteriosus or a coarctation of the aorta may become infected, just as may the heart valves or endocardial surfaces.

Clinical Patterns

Fever and Heart Disease

This can be a useful problem-oriented descriptive diagnosis to help the physician remember the importance of excluding infective endocarditis. Children with rheumatic or congenital heart disease may have fever from the same causes as any other patient, as well as fever related to their heart disease (e.g., a recurrence of ARF). However, the principal diagnostic concern in a patient with heart disease and fever is to exclude infective endocarditis.

The initial approach to a child with heart disease and fever is the same as that to any child with fever, with one exception: if there is doubt about the cause of the fever, the child with heart disease should have at least two blood samples obtained for culture before starting antibiotic therapy. In most cases, the patient will not have endocarditis. However, if a positive blood culture is found, the patient should be hospitalized for further evaluation.

Fever after Cardiac Surgery

This is a general, problem-oriented diagnosis that can be regarded as a special case of fever and heart disease. Although the most common causes are catheter-associated bacteremia and ventilator-associated pneumonia, the most important cause to be excluded is infective endocarditis. The post pericardiotomy syndrome is another cause and can be defined as fever and pericardial rub or effusion persisting longer than 1 week after cardiac surgery.[139,140]

Fever after cardiac surgery can also be caused by infection with cytomegalovirus (see postperfusion syndrome) transmitted by blood transfusions containing fresh leukocytes at the time of the operation.[141,142] The fever typically occurs for a period of 3–7 weeks after the operation and is associated with atypical lymphocytosis, often with splenomegaly. The presence of serum antibodies to cytomegalovirus preoperatively does not rule out this cause.[142,143]

Subacute Bacterial Endocarditis (SBE)

Until the etiology is confirmed, this is more appropriately called "subacute infective endocarditis." The disease can be defined as a slowly progressive infection of the endocardium or heart valve. A presumptive diagnosis of SBE should be made when the triad of changing heart murmur, fever, and embolic phenomena is noted. However, a minority of children with IE will have all three of these factors at the time of presentation. Therapy should usually not be begun until three to five blood samples are obtained for culture over a period of a few hours. If the patient does not appear very sick, and embolic phenomena are not seen, the blood cultures may be spaced over 24 hours. The diagnosis is confirmed in the laboratory by positive blood cultures, usually with a low-virulence organism, such as the viridans group of streptococci or other normal flora of the respiratory tract.

Acute Bacterial Endocarditis

In acute bacterial endocarditis, the patient usually appears septic and acutely ill. The pathogen is usually one of well-defined virulence for areas outside the heart, such as *S. aureus,* and the course is rapidly progressive. Therapy is urgent; it should not be delayed for spaced cultures or to get culture results. The clinical distinction between subacute and acute bacterial endocarditis is important, because progressive valvular damage by a virulent organism may be lessened by immediate antibiotic therapy.

Endocarditis in Normal Hearts

The usual predisposing condition for this disease is intravenous inoculation of high doses of bacteria, as from contaminated intravenous catheters, which is more frequent in children, or from contaminated needles and illegal drugs, which is more common in adults.

Neonatal Endocarditis

Bacteremia can cause endocarditis in newborn infants with normal hearts, especially if there is an indwelling central venous catheter, in which case coagulase-negative staphylococcus is a possible cause.[144,145]

Predisposing Conditions

Congenital Heart Disease

In adults, infective endocarditis occurs most frequently in patients with degenerative cardiac lesions, such as a calcified mitral annulus. In children, congenital heart disease is now the usual underlying problem[143] and infective endocarditis is becoming more frequent in children because survival with congenital heart disease has increased. Rheumatic heart disease as a predisposing factor in children is now rare (Table 18-2).[146–158]

The location of the endocarditis depends on the hemodynamics of the particular defect. The congenital heart lesions most frequently associated with infective endocarditis are tetralogy of Fallot, small ventricular septal defect, aortic stenosis, and bicuspid aortic valve. Infective endocarditis complicating patent ductus arteriosus is unusual. Prosthetic valves, patches, and conduits can also become a focus of endocarditis in children, and this problem is discussed in the section on cardiac operations.

Mitral Valve Prolapse

Mitral valve prolapse is a disorder that can occur in adolescents. A flail mitral valve leaflet, detectable by echocardiography, can produce mitral regurgitation and be a focus of endocarditis.[159]

Precipitating Event

In endocarditis occurring in patients with heart disease, a transient bacteremia may have been produced by a precipitating event, such as dental extraction, urinary tract instrumentation, or minor operations (i.e., incision and drainage of a boil, nasal packing for nosebleeds). In patients with known heart disease, antibiotic prophylaxis may be given just before procedures known to be associated with bacteremia, as described in the later section on prevention of endocarditis. In a retrospective study in adults, the "incubation period" between the potential precipitating event and the onset of symptoms was usually about 1 week, and almost always (84%) less than 2 weeks.[160] About half of the cases do not have a recognized precipitating event. Transient bacteremia following chewing food or brushing teeth is nearly as common as with minor dental procedures.[161]

Cardiac Operations

Usually done with antibiotic prophylaxis, these operations may be followed by endocarditis from unu-

TABLE 18-2. CONDITIONS PREDISPOSING TO ENDOCARDITIS ESTIMATED FROM EIGHT PEDIATRIC SERIES

PREDISPOSING CONDITION	PERCENTAGE OF CASES
Septal defects (VSD, AV canal)	20–25
Cyanotic complex (Tetralogy of Fallot, truncus arteriosus, transposition of the great vessels)	20–25
Aortic defects (stenosis, insufficiency, subaortic coarctation, PDA)	10–15
Mitral or pulmonary group (stenosis, insufficiency, prolapse)	5–10
Other complex*	5–10
Rheumatic heart disease	1–5
Central venous catheter-associated	10–15
No predisposing condition	5–10

* More than one defect was present in the other categories listed by the predominant defect.
VSD, ventricular septal defect; AV, arteriovenous; PDA, patent ductus arteriosus.

sual pathogens, such as gram-negative bacteria. *Candida albicans* or *S. epidermidis* may colonize artificial valves, which may have to be removed.[162,163] Occasionally, children with prosthetic material (patches, grafts) will be able to be cured by antibiotics alone.[146]

Staphylococcus aureus Septicemia

The frequency of unrecognized endocarditis complicating *S. aureus* bacteremia in children is much lower than in adults but must always be considered. In one study, transthoracic echocardiography demonstrated endocardial involvement in 4 (11%) of 36 children with *S. aureus* bacteremia.[164]

Drug Addiction

Intravenous abuse of drugs is the prototype situation for *S. aureus* acute endocarditis, most commonly involving the tricuspid valve. With right-sided endocarditis, a murmur may not be present, and pulmonary findings may dominate the clinical picture.

Intravenous Catheters

As discussed in Chapter 10, intravascular devices are increasingly a source of sepsis, septic phlebitis, and, rarely, endocarditis in normal valves in a situation somewhat analogous to the exposure of the drug user. Intravascular devices were the usual pre-

disposing factor in a series of infective endocarditis in children without underlying heart disease (see Table 18-2).

Clinical Diagnosis

The three classic findings of infective endocarditis are fever, heart murmur, and embolic phenomena. Fever is present in almost all cases and can be used to date the probable onset of the disease. However, in SBE the fever is often low-grade, and associated symptoms, such as malaise and fatigue, are nonspecific. Embolic phenomonena are the exception, rather than the rule, in patients with SBE. Thus, for patients with structural heart lesions that are known to predispose to infective endocarditis, a high index of suspicion for this diagnosis should be maintained at all times. In most patients with infective endocarditis, the murmur cannot be recognized early as a "changing murmur." A changing murmur implies structural change and is heard more frequently in acute endocarditis, where it implies valvular destruction with resulting insufficiency. In patients with a surgical shunt, SBE may cause disappearance of a murmur, and the shunt murmur is heard again with a cure. However, in most such patients, no change in murmur is appreciated.

For early clinical diagnosis, it is critical to consider infective endocarditis whenever fever occurs in a situation known to be associated with the disease or whenever embolic phenomena are observed.

Microscopic hematuria, petechiae, and splenomegaly are the most common embolic phenomena. The usual emboli in SBE appear as small (1–2 mm) circular flat spots. At first, these spots are faint pink but within a few hours become dark red, then purple. These spots need to be distinguished in size and appearance from freckles or common brown nevi ("moles"). They are usually distinctive in their round character, early pink appearance, and the transition from pink to darker red. Such emboli may be sterile if the patient is receiving antibiotics. The release of such emboli during antibiotic therapy does not necessarily indicate a failure of antibiotics, because it may indicate release of sterile emboli from vegetations.

If embolic phenomena are noted only below the waist, infection of a coarctation of the aorta or a patent ductus arteriosus should be suspected. Roth's spots are embolic lesions in the retina seen by funduscopic examination. Brain emboli may be manifested as convulsions, hemiplegia, or meningitis. Spleen emboli may be the cause of splenomegaly, which is usually related to the duration of the disease. Pulmonary emboli may be manifested as septic pulmonary infarcts, especially associated with right-sided endocarditis, particularly with involvement of the tricuspid valve or a ventricular septal defect.

Diagnostic Approach

Blood Cultures

Blood cultures are necessary to confirm the diagnosis. A single culture positive for *S. epidermidis* may reflect a skin contaminant. However, an α-hemolytic streptococcus or an enterococcus is rarely a contaminant, and, in the appropriate clinical setting, a single culture positive for either is strong evidence for SBE. There is no particular time to obtain the culture in relation to the fever because the bacteremia in SBE is continuous.[151] Although the bacteremia is continuous, it is not uncommon for only some of the cultures obtained to be positive. This may be because of the fastidious nature of some of the common causes of SBE, such as viridans streptococci. Three to five samples should be taken in the first 24 hours. While these results are pending, antibiotic therapy may be started if sufficient clinical evidence of bacterial endocarditis is noted. However, if the patient is stable and suspicion is

relatively low, therapy can be withheld until cultures return positive. In our experience the most common mistake is for clinicians, faced with a clinically stable patient, to start antibiotic therapy too soon and with an insufficient number of preantibiotic blood cultures, thus masking the diagnosis. Anaerobic cultures are rarely helpful, as most reviews indicate that anaerobes, with the occasional exception of some streptococci, are rarely recovered in this disease. The laboratory should be notified that endocarditis is suspected, so that the blood cultures can be held for an extended incubation.

Nonspecific Tests

Leukocytosis is often not present in SBE, so that a normal total white blood cell count with a shift to the left is perfectly consistent with the diagnosis. The erythrocyte sedimentation rate is usually elevated in SBE. Serum complement may be low and is associated with focal or diffuse glomerulonephritis, and antigammaglobulin factors such as rheumatoid factor may appear, reflecting antigen–antibody reactions.

Circulating Immune Complexes

The complexes of IgG, complement, and bacterial antigen that form frequently in infective endocarditis can be detected by several methods, including the Raji cell radioimmunoassay. Circulating immune complexes are also found in sepsis and some other conditions, but generally at lower levels. Levels greater than 100 mcg/mL are highly suggestive of endocarditis.[165] This test, although seldom used in pediatrics, may correlate with the course and severity of the disease and may prove useful in establishing the diagnosis of culture-negative endocarditis or in distinguishing endocarditis from bacteremia without endocarditis.[153]

Echocardiogram

Echocardiograms may detect valvular vegetations, myocardial abscesses, or other complications.[154,155] However, as with any diagnostic modality, echocardiography is most useful when the pretest probability of disease is high.[166–168] The sensitivity of transthoracic echocardiography for detection of vegetations in children with infective endocarditis ranges from 25–50%.[156,158] It is lowest in those with complex congenital heart disease.[158]

■ ENDOCARDITIS WITH NEGATIVE BLOOD CULTURES

Endocarditis is a difficult diagnosis to make without positive blood cultures.[151,153] However, reviews of patients with negative cultures indicate that the disease can be diagnosed in retrospect on the basis of the response to antibiotic therapy, the presence of embolic phenomena, a change in the murmur, elevated rheumatoid factor, vegetations seen on an echocardiogram, or decreased serum complement.[153]

One explanation for negative blood cultures is that the patient may have congenital heart disease with a left-to-right shunt, so that the bacteria released from vegetations go to the lungs. In such cases, an echocardiogram can be very helpful to detect vegetations or signs of right-sided endocarditis. Pulmonary infarction should be seen by roentgenogram or noted clinically. However, it should be recognized that blood from systemic veins contains bacteria that have passed through systemic capillaries, and there is no reason to assume that the pulmonary capillaries are any more effective than the systemic capillaries in removing bacteria. In fact, blood cultures are usually positive in right-sided SBE, although somewhat less frequently than in left-sided SBE.

Another explanation for negative blood cultures is the low concentration of bacteria in the blood, usually fewer than 100 organisms per mL. Sometimes, the patient has had recent antibiotics, and it then may take many days for the culture to become positive.[170] There may be embolization of sterile vegetation particles after the infection has been cured.

A third explanation is that endocarditis can be caused by microorganisms that are difficult to culture with conventional techniques. These organisms, described in the following section, include fastidious streptococci with special growth requirements, anaerobic bacteria, L forms of bacteria, *Mycoplasma hominis*, *Brucella*, and unusual bacteria or nonbacterial organisms, such as those of Q fever or psittacosis, fungi, and some viruses.[171,172] There can also be noninfectious thrombotic endocarditis.[171–173]

Causes of Infective Endocarditis

The approximate frequencies of various microorganisms as causes of endocarditis in children are summarized in Table 18-3.

TABLE 18-3. APPROXIMATE FREQUENCIES OF BACTERIOLOGIC CAUSES OF ENDOCARDITIS IN CHILDREN*

Viridans group streptococci	39%
Staphylococcus aureus	31%
Coagulase-negative staphylococci	6%
Streptococcus pneumoniae	3%
Enterococci	3%
HACEK organisms	3%
Culture negative	6%
Other organisms (gram-negatives, fungi, etc.)	9%

* Pooled data from three separate reports containing a total of 336 cases[156,179,189]

Common Bacteria

Approximately three-quarters of the infecting organisms in pediatric endocarditis are the viridans group of streptococci or *S. aureus* (Table 18-3). Enterococci, so common in adults, are less common causes of endocarditis in children[152] but have become more frequent in recent years.[156]

Fastidious Streptococci

Some streptococci require active forms of vitamin B6 and so cannot be recovered unless these factors are added to culture media. Other bacteria may provide growth requirements for fastidious streptococci, so the streptococcal colonies appear near other colonies streaked in a line by the microbiology technologist (so-called "satellite phenomenon"). Nutritionally deficient or satelliting streptococci formerly were a common cause of SBE with negative blood cultures but are now recovered by most laboratories.[174]

Other Bacteria

Pneumococcal endocarditis is rare but typically severe. In children, unlike adults, it tends to occur without pneumonia or meningitis.[175] The so-called HACEK group (*Haemophilus aphrophilus, Actinobacillus actinomycetemcomitans, Cardiobacterium hominis, Eikenella corrodens,* and *Kingella kingae*) are mouth flora associated with endocarditis. They are more common in adult patients than in children. Gram-negative enteric bacteria, such as *P. aerugi-*

nosa or *E. coli,* are an occasional cause of SBE, especially after cardiac surgery.

Occasionally, recovery of an unusual organism or suspected contaminant may delay diagnosis unless the physician is alert. Uncommon gram-negative rods, such as *Acinetobacter* or *Haemophilus*-like species, may be difficult for some laboratories to isolate and identify. The physician should also recognize that coagulase-negative staphylococci can cause SBE, especially if a valve prosthesis has been inserted. Premature neonates with indwelling catheters are also subject to endocarditis from coagulase-negative staphylococci.

Fungal Endocarditis

Fungi sometimes cause endocarditis, particularly following cardiac operations.[176,177] Patches, sutures, homografts, and prosthetic valves often become foci of infection following cardiac surgery.

Viral Endocarditis

There is experimental evidence that coxsackieviruses B can produce mural and valvular endocarditis in mice. This type of endocarditis in no way resembles SBE but rather is a valvulitis resembling that of RHD.

Rickettsial Endocarditis

Coxiella burneti, the agent of Q fever, is a rare cause of endocarditis. Patients will have negative blood cultures but respond to proper antibiotic therapy.

Duke Criteria for Diagnosis of Infective Endocarditis

Because the diagnosis of infective endocarditis can be difficult, several sets of diagnostic criteria have been proposed. Currently, the most commonly used are the modified Duke criteria, which are analogous to the Jones criteria for ARF in that they include both major and minor criteria. Designed for diagnosis of endocarditis in adults, they have been validated for use in children as well.[178,179]

Table 18-4 lists the two major and five minor criteria in the Duke classification, and Table 18-5 details how the criteria are used to classify cases of endocarditis as definite, probable, or rejected.

Complications

A number of complications can occur, including myocardial infarction, rupture of the spleen, and heart block. The most serious is probably embolization to a vital area, such as the brain. Embolic glomerulonephritis can also occur. Congestive heart failure may occur because of destruction of a heart valve. This is especially dangerous in acute endocarditis, in which aortic insufficiency may occur. Emergency replacement of the aortic valve with a prosthesis may be lifesaving.

Mycotic Aneurysm

"Mycotic" is derived from the Greek word for "fungus" *(mykis).* However, mycotic aneurysms, which are weaknesses in an arterial wall, are usually caused by bacteria such as staphylococci or *Salmonella.* A mycotic aneurysm is more likely to occur in acute bacterial endocarditis than in SBE and is a life-threatening emergency if it should rupture in a vital area. When the embolized bacteria go to a coronary artery, an abscess of the myocardium can ensue.

Indications for Surgery

In adults, the generally accepted indications for surgical intervention (usually valve replacement) during active endocarditis are as follows: (1) refractory CHF; (2) more than one serious embolic episode; (3) uncontrolled infection; (4) physiologically significant valve dysfunction as demonstrated by echocardiography; (5) ineffective antimicrobial therapy (as in fungal endocarditis); (6) resection of mycotic aneurysms; (7) most cases of prosthetic valve endocarditis caused by certain pathogens (e.g., *S. aureus,* enteric gram-negative bacilli); and (8) local suppurative complications, including perivalvular or myocardial abscesses.[180,181]

In a series of children undergoing operative intervention for endocarditis, the most common indications for surgery were persistent infection, embolic phenomena, and increasing CHF. *S. aureus* and viridans streptococci were the most common etiologic agents.[182]

Treatment

The most critical factor in successful treatment probably is early administration of antibiotic therapy with maximum safe doses to minimize vegetation growth and valve destruction. Treatment of endocarditis requires prolonged intravenous therapy with at least one bactericidal antibiotic. There is no role for oral therapy. The vegetations of endocardi-

TABLE 18-4. MAJOR AND MINOR CRITERIA USED IN THE MODIFIED DUKE CRITERIA FOR DIAGNOSIS OF INFECTIVE ENDOCARDITIS (IE)

MAJOR CRITERIA	MINOR CRITERIA
1. Positive blood culture(s)	1. Predisposing heart condition or IV drug use
• Typical microorganism from ≥2 blood cultures (viridans streptococci, *S. bovis,* HACEK group, *S. aureus*), or	2. Fever ≥38 °C
• Enterococci, in the absence of a primary focus, or	3. Vascular phenomena
• Persistently positive blood culture with an organism consistent with IE from blood cultures drawn >12 h apart, or	• Major arterial emboli • Septic pulmonary infarcts • Mycotic aneurysm • Intracranial hemorrhage • Conjunctival hemorrhages
• All 3 or a majority of 4 or more separate blood cultures, with the first and last drawn at least 1 h apart, or	• Janeway lesions
• Positive serology for Q fever	4. Immunologic phenomena • Osler's nodes • Roth spots
2. Evidence of endocardial involvement by echocardiogram	• Glomerulonephritis • Rheumatoid factor
• Vegetation	
• Abscess	5. Microbiologic evidence
• New partial dehiscence of prosthetic valve	• Positive blood culture but not meeting major criterion
• New valvular regurgitation	• Serologic evidence of active infection with an organism consistent with IE

Adapted from Milazzo AS Jr, and Li JS. Bacterial endocarditis in infants and children, Pediatr Infect Dis J 2001;20:799–801.

TABLE 18-5. INTERPRETATION OF DUKE CRITERIA TO CLASSIFY CASES OF INFECTIVE ENDOCARDITIS (IE)

DEFINITE IE	POSSIBLE IE	REJECTED
Pathologic criteria	• At least 1 major criterion and 1 minor criterion, or	• Alternative diagnosis made, or
• Microorganisms (by culture or histology in a vegetation or intracardiac abscess)	• 3 minor criteria	• Resolution of manifestations with antibiotic therapy for ≤4 days, or
• Histology (vegetation or intracardiac abscess showing active IE)		• No pathologic evidence of IE at surgery or autopsy, with antibiotic therapy for ≤4 days
Clinical criteria (see Table 18-4)		
• 2 major criteria, or		
• 1 major and 3 minor, or		
• 5 minor		

Adapted from Milazzo AS Jr, Li JS. Bacterial endocarditis in infants and children. Pediatr Infect Dis J 2001;20:799–801.

tis are well protected from the host immune response, as illustrated by the 100% mortality of infective endocarditis in the preantibiotic era. The selection of an antibiotic to treat bacterial endocarditis can be based on the preliminary use of likely antibiotic susceptibilities but as soon as possible should be based on the special studies (described later) made on the organism recovered in blood cultures. In the absence of any positive bacterial culture or while awaiting culture results, the recommended drugs for a pediatric patient are either nafcillin and gentamicin or penicillin, nafcillin, and gentamicin, with vancomycin substituted for the β-lactams if prostheses or deep central venous lines are present.[151] In suspected acute endocarditis, vanomycin, nafcillin, and gentamicin should be used until susceptibility results are available because of the possibility of MRSA or a gram-negative organism.

In one series of 75 episodes of pediatric infective endocarditis, the mean duration of fever after initiation of appropriate therapy was 4.3 days. Over one-third experienced secondary fever.[156]

Guidelines have been published for antibiotic treatment of adults with infective endocarditis due to common pathogens.[183] In the absence of similar guidelines for children, the adult guidelines are generally followed with doses adjusted appropriately.[184]

For penicillin-sensitive viridans streptococci (MIC ≤0.1 mcg/mL), aqueous crystalline penicillin G, 200,000 units/kg per day (up to 18 million units per day total dose) is recommended. It may be given by continuous infusion or divided every 4 hours. An alternative is ceftriaxone 100 mg/kg daily up to 2 g daily. Treatment of native valve infection is usually for 4 weeks. Prosthetic valve infections are treated for 6 weeks with the addition of gentamicin (1 mg/kg every 8 hours) for the first 2 weeks of therapy. Similarly, for patients with endocarditis due to viridans streptococci with penicillin MIC greater than 0.1 mcg/ml or due to nutritionally variant streptococci, 4 weeks of penicillin G is given, with gentamicin given concomitantly for the first 2 weeks. Alternatively, 4 weeks of vancomycin may be used.

Enterococcal endocarditis is especially difficult to treat. Treatment with two bactericidal agents is required. Depending on susceptibility testing, penicillin G, ampicillin (300 mg/kg/day), or vancomycin (40 mg/kg/day) along with gentamicin is given for 4–6 weeks. Vancomycin trough levels should be maintained between 5 and 10 mcg/mL. The levels of gentamicin required for synergy are lower than those required to treat gram-negative infections. The goal is a peak of 3 ug/mL and trough less than 1 ug/mL.

Treatment of native-valve *S. aureus* endocarditis is with a penicillinase-resistant antibiotic such as nafcillin (200 mg/kg/day divided every 4–6 hours with a maximum of 12 g/day) for 6 weeks. Gentamicin is often given for the first 3–5 days of therapy. For methicillin-resistant *S. aureus* (MRSA), vancomycin is given for 6 weeks.

Prosthetic-valve endocarditis due to *S. aureus* requires 6 weeks or greater of therapy. Agents used are those discussed previously for native-valve *S. aureus* endocarditis. In addition, rifampin is given for the entire treatment course and gentamicin is given for the first 2 weeks of therapy. If a prosthetic valve is infected with methicillin-resistant *S. aureus*, treatment is the same, except that vancomycin is substituted for nafcillin. Valve replacement is often required with *S. aureus* disease, regardless of its susceptibility.

Endocarditis caused by the slow-growing fastidious gram-negative organisms of the HACEK group is generally treated with ceftriaxone. The duration is 4 weeks for native-valve IE and 6 weeks for prosthetic-valve IE. Culture negative IE is generally treated with nafcillin and gentamicin for 6 weeks.

Patients who have any foreign material in their heart or great vessels are treated with the guidelines used for prosthetic valve endocarditis. This is true regardless of whether the material is a homograft or artificial material and regardless of whether the area of suspected IE involves the foreign material or not.

Many experts recommend a repeat set of blood cultures one week after completion of antibiotic therapy.

Special Susceptibility Studies

Infective endocarditis is the most important indication for special antibiotic susceptibility studies.[151] Routine studies using the paper disc method should not be considered adequate if special studies are available in a reference laboratory.

Minimal Bactericidal Concentration (MBC)

This term defines the concentration necessary to kill (not merely inhibit) the patient's organism, using a standard inoculum. The MBC is more important

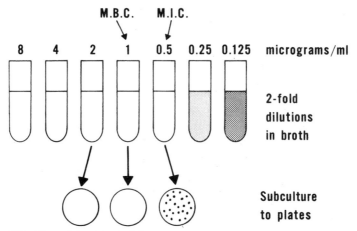

■ **FIGURE 18-2** Minimal inhibitory concentration (MIC) and minimal bactericidal concentration (MBC) for a patient's staphylococcus tested against nafcillin. The MIC is the lowest concentration with no turbidity from bacterial growth (0.5 μg/mL). The MBC is the lowest concentration with no turbidity from bacterial growth on subculture (1 μg/mL).

than the MIC (minimal inhibitory concentration) because inhibition of the organism is insufficient to eradicate it from the fibrin matrix. Usually, the MIC is defined by lack of turbidity in the incubated broth-organism mixture, whereas the MBC is defined by lack of growth on subculture of the previously incubated broth-organism mixture (Fig. 18-2). The MBC is used in infective endocarditis to determine whether the patient's organism can be killed by attainable serum concentrations of a particular antibiotic and detects tolerance of the organ-

ism (inhibition but not killing), especially for streptococci.

Serum Bactericidal Titer

This test defines the ability of the patient's antibiotic-containing serum to kill the organism isolated (Fig. 18-3). The serum specimens should be obtained at the time of the anticipated peak and trough concentrations after administration of an antibiotic. Usually, a peak bactericidal titer of 1:32

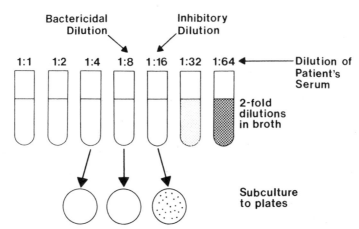

■ **FIGURE 18-3** Measurement of patient's serum antibacterial inhibitory and killing titer (Schlicter test) (See Fig. 18-2).

TABLE 18-6. CARDIAC CONDITIONS ASSOCIATED WITH ENDOCARDITIS[186]

ENDOCARDITIS PROPHYLAXIS RECOMMENDED

High-Risk Category

- Prosthetic cardiac valves, including bioprosthetic and homograft valves
- Previous bacterial endocarditis
- Complex cyanotic CHD (e.g., single ventricle, TGA, TOF)
- Surgically constructed systemic-pulmonary shunts or conduits

Moderate-Risk Category

- Most other congenital cardiac malformations (other than those listed)
- Acquired valvular dysfunction (e.g., RHD)
- Hypertrophic cardiomyopathy
- MVP with valvular regurgitation and/or thickened leaflets

ENDOCARDITIS PROPHYLAXIS NOT RECOMMENDED

Negligible-Risk Category (no greater risk than the general population)

- Isolated secundum ASD
- Surgical repair of ASD, VSD, or PDA (without residua beyond 6 months)
- Previous CABG surgery
- MVP without valvar regurgitation
- Innocent heart murmurs
- Previous Kawasaki disease without valvular dysfunction
- Previous rheumatic fever without valvular dysfunction
- Cardiac pacemakers and implanted defibrillators

CHD, congenital heart disease; TGA, transposition of the great arteries; TOF, tetralogy of Fallot; RHD, rheumatic heart disease; MVP, mitral valve prolapse; ASD, atrial septal defect; VSD, ventricular septal defect; PDA, patent ductus arteriosus; CABG, coronary artery bypass graft.

TABLE 18-7. PROCEDURES FOR WHICH IE PROPHYLAXIS IS RECOMMENDED[186]

DENTAL PROCEDURES

- Dental extractions
- Periodontal procedures including surgery, scaling and root planing, probing, and recall maintenance
- Dental implant placement and reimplantation of avulsed teeth
- Endodontic (root canal) instrumentation or surgery only beyond the apex
- Subgingival placement of antibiotic fibers or strips
- Initial placement of orthodontic bands but not brackets
- Intraligamentary local anesthetic injections
- Prophylactic cleaning of teeth or implants where bleeding is anticipated

RESPIRATORY TRACT PROCEDURES

- Tonsillectomy and/or adenoidectomy
- Surgical operations that involve respiratory mucosa
- Rigid bronchoscopy

GASTROINTESTINAL TRACT PROCEDURES*

- Sclerotherapy for esophageal varices
- Esophageal stricture dilation
- Endoscopic retrograde cholangiography with biliary obstruction
- Biliary tract surgery
- Surgical operations that involve intestinal mucosa

GENITOURINARY TRACT PROCEDURES

- Prostatic surgery
- Cystoscopy
- Urethral dilation

* Prophylaxis is recommended for high-risk patients; optional for moderate-risk patients.

TABLE 18-8. PROPHYLACTIC REGIMENS AGAINST IE FOR DENTAL, ORAL, RESPIRATORY TRACT, OR ESOPHAGEAL PROCEDURES IN CHILDREN[186]

SITUATION	AGENT	REGIMEN
Standard general prophylaxis	Amoxicillin	50 mg/kg (max 2 g) orally*
Unable to take oral medications	Ampicillin	50 mg/kg (max 2 g) IV† or IM†
Allergic to penicillin	Clindamycin or	20 mg/kg (max 600 mg) orally*
	Cephalexin‡ or	50 mg/kg (max 2 g) orally*
	Azithromycin	15 mg/kg (max 500 mg) orally*
Allergic to penicillin and unable to take oral medications	Clindamycin or	20 mg/kg (max 600 mg) IV†
	Cefazolin‡	25 mg/kg (max 1 g) IV† or IM†

* Oral doses are given 1 hour before the procedure.
† IV or IM doses are given so that the infusion/injection is completed 30 min before the procedure.
‡ Cephalosporins should not be used in patients with immediate-type hypersensitivity reaction (urticaria, angioedema, or anaphylaxis) to penicillins.

and a trough titer of 1:8 is associated with successful therapy.[148,150,151] However, serum bactericidal testing has not been standardized, and many clinical laboratories do not perform it.

Prophylaxis

Updated recommendations by the American Heart Association (AHA) for prevention of endocarditis in patients with underlying heart defects were pub-lished in 1997.[186] The recommendations stress that most cases of endocarditis are not attributable to an invasive procedure.[187] In fact, in a study of 273 patients with infective endocarditis, recent dental treatment was no more common among cases than among controls.[188]

In addition, it is important to remember that no randomized controlled trials have been done to establish that antibiotic prophylaxis provides pro-tection against development of endocarditis during

TABLE 18-9. PROPHYLACTIC REGIMENS AGAINST IE FOR GENITOURINARY AND GASTROINTESTINAL (EXCLUDING ESOPHAGEAL) PROCEDURES IN CHILDREN[186]

SITUATION	AGENTS	REGIMEN
High-risk patients	Ampicillin plus gentamicin	Ampicillin 50 mg/kg IV† or IM† (max 2 g) plus gentamicin‡ 1.5 mg/kg (max 120 mg) IV† or IM†; 6 h later, ampicillin 25 mg/kg IV or IM or amoxicillin 25 mg/kg orally
High-risk patients allergic to penicillin	Vancomycin plus gentamicin	Vancomycin‡ 20 mg/kg (max 1 g) IV† over 1–2 h plus gentamicin‡ 1.5 mg/kg (max 120 mg) IV or IM†
Moderate-risk patients	Amoxicillin or ampicillin	Amoxicillin 50 mg/kg (max 2 g) orally* or ampicillin 50 mg/kg (max 2 g) IV or IM†
Moderate risk patients allergic to penicillin	Vancomycin	Vancomycin‡ 20 mg/kg (max 1 g) IV† over 1–2 h

* Initial oral doses are given 1 hour before the procedure.
† Initial IV or IM doses are given so that the infusion/injection is completed 30 min before the procedure.
‡ No second dose of vancomycin or gentamicin is recommended.

bacteremia-inducing procedures. Nevertheless, the use of antibiotic prophylaxis is such a commonly accepted practice that it may be wise to follow the AHA guidelines, if only for medicolegal purposes.

Whether a patient is a candidate for endocarditis prophylaxis depends on his or her underlying heart defect (current guidelines divide patients into three categories—high-risk, moderate-risk, and negligible-risk) and on what procedure he or she is about to undergo. Tables 18-6 through 18-9 summarize the current AHA recommendations.

■ REFERENCES

1. Levine HD. Viral myocarditis: a critique of the literature from clinical electrocardiographic, and pathologic standpoints. Am J Med Sci 1979;277:132–44.
2. Ross LJ. Electrocardiographic findings in measles. Am J Dis Child 1952;83:282–90.
3. Rodriguez-Torres R, Lin JS, Berkovich S. A sensitive electrocardiographic sign in myocarditis associated with viral infection. Pediatrics 1969;43:846–51.
4. Feldman AM, McNamara D. Myocarditis. N Engl J Med 2000;343:1388–98.
5. Abelmann WH. Virus and the heart. Circulation 1971;44:950–6.
6. Silverman AJ, Kapadia N, Borin AJ. Acute myocarditis presenting as acute myocardial infarction. J Am Osteopath Assoc 1995;95:278–80.
7. Karjalainen J, Heikkila J. Incidence of three presentations of acute myocarditis in young men in military service. A 20-year experience. Eur Heart J 1999;20:1120–5.
8. DeSa DJ. Isolated myocarditis in the first year. Arch Dis Child 1985;60:484–5.
9. Kaplan MH, Klein SW, McPhee J, et al. Group B Coxsackievirus infections in infants younger than three months of age: a serious childhood illness. Rev Infect Dis 1983;5:1019–32.
10. Burch GE, Sun SC, Chu KC, et al. Interstitial and Coxsackie B myocarditis in infants and children. JAMA 1968;203:18.
11. Sainani GS, Krompotic E, Slodki SJ. Adult heart disease due to the Coxsackie virus B infection. Medicine 1968;47:133–47.
12. Martin AB, Webber S, Fricker FJ, et al. Acute myocarditis. Rapid diagnosis by PCR in children. Circulation 1994;90:330-9.
13. Grumbach IM, Heim A, Pring-Akerblom P, et al. Adenoviruses and enteroviruses as pathogens in myocarditis and dilated cardiomyopathy. Acta Cardiol 1999;54:83–8.
14. Onitsuka H, Imamura T, Miyamoto N, et al. Clinical manifestations of influenza A myocarditis during the influenza epidemic of winter 1998–1999. J Cardiol 2001;37:315–23.
15. Yoshikawa T, Ihira M, Suzuki K, et al. Fatal acute myocarditis in an infant with human herpesvirus 6 infection. J Clin Pathol 2001;54:792–5.
16. Cunningham T. Pancarditis in acute toxoplasmosis. Am J Clin Pathol 1982;78:403–5.
17. Chen SC, Tsai CC, Nouri S. Carditis associated with Myco-

plasma pneumoniae infection. Am J Dis Child 1986;140:471–2.
18. Jacobs JC, Rosen JM, Szer IS. Lyme myocarditis diagnosed by gallium scan. J Pediatr 1984;105:950–2.
19. Rubenstein JS, Noah ZL, Zales VR, et al. Acute myocarditis associated with Shigella sonnei gastroenteritis. J Pediatr 1993;122:82–4.
20. Cox ID, Fluck DS, Joy MD. Campylobacter myocarditis; loose bowels and a baggy heart. Eur J Heart Fail 2001;3:105–7.
21. Taliercio CP, Olney BA, Lie JT. Myocarditis related to drug hypersensitivity. Mayo Clin Proc 1985;60:463–8.
22. Sasson Z, Morgan CD, Wang B, et al. 5-fluorouracil related toxic myocarditis: case reports and pathological confirmation. Can J Cardiol 1994;10:861–4.
23. Scott LP III, Gutelius MF, Parrott RH. Children with acute respiratory infections: an electrocardiographic study. Am J Dis Child 1970;119:111–3.
24. Batra AS, Lewis AB. Acute myocarditis. Curr Opin Pediatr 2001;13:234–9.
25. Moore CM, Henry J, Benzing G III, et al. Varicella myocarditis. Am J Dis Child 1969;118:899–902.
26. Fraisse A, Paut O, Zandotti C, et al. Epstein-Barr virus. An unusual cause of acute myocarditis in children. Arch Pediatr 2000;7:752–5.
27. Stack WA, Mulcahy HE, Fenelon L, et al. Cytomegalovirus myocarditis following liver transplantation. Postgrad Med J 1994;70:658–60.
28. Hiraishi S, Yashiro K, Oguchi K, et al. Clinical course of cardiovascular involvement in the mucocutaneous lymph node syndrome. Relation between clinical signs of carditis and development of coronary arterial aneurysm. Am J Cardiol 1981;47:323–30.
29. Bowles NE, Kearney DL, Ni J, et al. The detection of viral genomes by polymerase chain reaction in the myocardium of pediatric patients with advanced HIV disease. J Am Coll Cardiol 1999;34:857–65.
30. Onitsuka H, Imamura T, Miyamoto N, et al. Clinical manifestation of influenza A myorcaditis during the influenza epidemic of winter 1998-1999. J Cardiol 2001;37:315–23.
31. Di Cesare E. MRI of the cardiomyopathies. Eur J Radiol 2001;38:179–84.
32. Friedrich MG, Strohm O, Schulz-Menger J, et al. Contrast media-enhanced magnetic resonance imaging visualizes myocardial changes in the course of viral myocarditis. Circulation 1998;12:1802–9.
33. Webber SA, Boycle GJ, Jaffe R, et al. Role of right ventricular endomyocardial biopsy in infants and children with suspected or possible myocarditis. Br Heart J 1994;72:360–3.
34. Greenwood RD, Nadas AS, Fyler DC. The clinical course of primary myocardial disease in children. Am Heart J 1976;12:549–60.
35. Mahoney LT, Marvin WJ Jr, Atkins DL, et al. Pacemaker management for acute onset of heart block in children. J Pediatr 1985;107:207–11.
36. Reyes MP, Ho KL, Smith F, et al. A mouse model of dilatedtype cardiomyopathy due to Coxsackie virus B3. J Infect Dis 1981;144:232–6.
37. Friman G, Larsson E, Rolf C. Interaction between infection and exercise with special reference to myocarditis and the

increased frequency of sudden deaths among young Swedish orienteers 1979–1992. Scand J Infect Dis Suppl 1997;104:41–9.

38. Tomioka N, Kishimoto C, Matsumori A, et al. Effects of prednisolong on acute viral myocarditis in mice. J Am Coll Cardiol 1986;7:868–72.

39. Wojnicz R, Nowalany-Kozielska E, Wojciechowska C, et al. Randomized, placebo-controlled study for immunosuppressive treatment of inflammatory dilated cardiomyopathy: two-year follow-up results. Circulation 2001;104:39–45.

40. Briassoulis G, Papadopoulos G, Zavras N, et al. Cardiac troponin I in fulminant adenovirus myocarditis treated with a 24-hour infusion of high-dose intravenous immunoglobulin. Pediatr Cardiol 2000;21:391–4.

41. Drucker NA, Colan SD, Lewis AB, et al. Gamma-globulin treatment of acute myocarditis in the pediatric population. Circulation 1994;89:252–7.

42. McCarthy RE 3rd, Boehmer JP, Hruban RH, et al. Long-term outcome of fulminant myocarditis as compared with acute (nonfulminant) myocarditis. N Engl J Med 2000;342:690–5.

43. Vardi P, Markiewicz W, Weiss Y, et al. Clinical echocardiographic correlations in acute rheumatic fever. Pediatrics 1983;71:830–4.

44. Veasy LG, Wiedemeier SE, Orsmond GS, et al. Resurgence of acute rheumatic fever in the Intermountain area of the United States. N Engl J Med 1987;316:421–7.

45. Hosier DM, Craenen JM, Teske DW, et al. Resurgence of acute rheumatic fever. Am J Dis Child 1987;141:730–3.

46. Ferried P. Acute rheumatic fever: the comeback of a disappearing disease [editorial]. Am J Dis Child 1987;141:725–7.

47. Congeni B, Rizzo C, Congeni J, et al. Outbreak of acute rheumatic fever in northeast Ohio. J Pediatr 1987;111:176–9.

48. Kaplan EL, Hill HR. Return of rheumatic fever: consequences, implications, and needs [editorial]. J Pediatr 1987;111:244–6.

49. Schwartz B, Facklam RR, Breiman RF. Changing epidemiology of group A streptococcal infection in the USA. Lancet 1990;336:1167–71.

50. McDonald M, Curie BJ, Carapetis JR. Acute rheumatic fever: a chink in the chain that links the heart to the throat? Lancet Infect Dis 2004;4:240–5.

51. Odic, A. The incidence of acute rheumatic fever in a suburban area of Los Angeles. West J Med 1986;144:179–84.

52. Chun LT, Reddy DV, Yamamoto LG. Rheumatic fever in children and adolescents in Hawaii. Pediatrics 1987;79:549–52.

53. Tolaymat A, Goudarzi T, Soler GP, et al. Acute rheumatic fever in North Florida. South Med J 1984;77:819–23.

54. Markowitz M. The decline of rheumatic fever: role of medical intervention. J Pediatr 1985;106:545–50.

55. Zagala JG, Feinstein AR. The preceding illness of acute rheumatic fever. JAMA 1962;179:863–6.

56. Grossman BJ, Stamler J. Potential preventability of first attacks of acute rheumatic fever in children. JAMA 1963;183:985–8.

57. Czoniczer G, Lees M, Massell BF. Streptococcal infection: the need for improved recognition and treatment for the prevention of rheumatic fever. N Engl J Med 1961;265:951–2.

58. Rammelkamp CH, Stolzer BL. The latent period before the onset of acute rheumatic fever. Yale J Biol Med 1961;34:386–98.

59. Siegel AC, Johnson EE, Stollerman GH. Controlled studies of streptococcal pharyngitis in a pediatric population I: factors related to the attack rate of rheumatic fever. N Engl J Med 1961;265:559–66.

60. Stollerman GH. Rheumatic fever. Lancet 1997;349:935–42.

61. Stollerman GH, Siegel AC, Johnson EE. Variable epidemiology of streptococcal disease and the changing pattern of rheumatic fever. Mod Concepts Cardiovasc Dis 1965;34:45–8.

62. Adam D, Scholz H, Helmerking M. Short-course antibiotic treatment of 4782 culture-proven cases of group A streptococcal tonsillopharyngitis and incidence of poststreptococcal sequelae. J Infect Dis 2000;182:509–16.

63. Bisno AL. The Concept of Rheumatogenic and Non-rheumatogenic Group A Streptococci. In: Read SE, Zabriski JB, eds. Streptococcal Diseases and the Immune Response. New York: Academic Press, 1980:789–803.

64. Visentainer JE, Pereira FC, Dalalio MM, et al. Association of HLA-DR7 with rheumatic fever in the Brazilian population. J Rheumatol 2000;27:1518–20.

65. Zaman MM, Yoshiike N, Chowdhury AH, et al. Nutritional factors associated with rheumatic fever. J Trop Pediatr 1998;44:142–7.

66. Stollerman GH. Rheumatic fever in the 21st century. Clin Infect Dis 2001;33:806–14.

67. Rosenthal A, Czoniczer G, Massell BF. Rheumatic fever under 3 years of age: a report of 10 cases. Pediatrics 1968;41:612–9.

68. Guidelines for the diagnosis of rheumatic fever. Jones Criteria, 1992 update. Special Writing Group of the Committee on Rheumatic Fever, Endocarditis, and Kawasaki Disease of the Council on Cardiovascular Disease in the Young of the American Heart Association. JAMA 1992;268:2069–73.

69. Shulman ST, Kaplan EL, Bisno AL, et al. Jones criteria (revised) for guidance in the diagnosis of rheumatic fever. Circulation 1984;69:204A–8A.

70. Figueroa FE, Fernandez MS, Valdes P, et al. Prospective comparison of clinical and echocardiographic diagnosis of rheumatic carditis: long-term follow-up of patients with subclinical disease. Heart 2001;85:407–10.

71. Ozkutlu S, Ayabakan C, Saraclar M. Can subclinical valvitis detected by echocardiography be accepted as evidence of carditis in the diagnosis of acute rheumatic fever? Cardiol Young 2001;11:255–60.

72. Hoey J. The disease that "bites the heart and licks the joints." CMAJ 1998;158:1335–6.

73. Aron AM, Freeman JM, Carter S. The natural history of Syndenham's chorea. Am J Med 1965;38:83–95.

74. Dagan B, Herman J, Kaufman B, et al. Pseudorheumatoid subcutaneous nodules and the poststreptococcal state. Arch Intern Med 1983;143:2316–7.

75. Bywaters EGL. Skin Manifestations of Rheumatic Disease. In: Fitzpatrick TB, ed. Dermatology in General Medicine. New York: McGrawHill, 1971:1534–45.

76. Centers for Disease Control and Prevention. Acute rheumatic fever—Utah. MMWR 1987;36:108–10.

77. Elevli M, Celebi A, Tombul T, et al. Cardiac involvement in Sydenham's chorea: clinical and echocardiographic findings. Acta Paediatr 1999;88:1074–7.

78. Lenox CC, Zuberbuhler JR, Park SC, et al. Arrhythmias and strokes—Adams attacks in acute rheumatic fever. Pediatrics 1978;61:599–603.

79. Liberman L, Hordof AJ, Alfayyadh M, et al. Tosade de pointes in a child with acute rheumatic fever. J Pediatr 2001;138:280–2.

80. Kaplan EL. Acute rheumatic fever. Pediatr Clin North Am 1978;25:817–29.

81. Cherian S, Tabatabai MR, Cummings NA. Rheumatic fever and gonococcal pharyngitis in an adult. South Med J 1979; 72:319–22.

82. Blackman NS, Kuskin L. Should prophylactic therapy be given to patients with an uncertain history of rheumatic fever? Clin Pediatr 1972;11:15–9.

83. Williamson L, Bowness P, Mowat A, et al. Lesson of the week: difficulties in diagnosing acute rheumatic fever—arthritis may be short lived and carditis silent. Br Med J 2000;320:362–5.

84. Carapetis JR, Currie BJ. Rheumatic fever in a high-incidence population: the importance of monoarthritis and low-grade fever. Arch Dis Child 2001;85:223–7.

85. Shulman ST, Ayoub EM. Poststreptococcal reactive arthritis. Curr Opin Rheumatol 2002;14:562–5.

86. Ahmed S, Ayoub EM, Scornik JC, et al. Poststreptococcal reactive arthritis: clinical characteristics and association with HLA-DR alleles. Arthritis Rheum 1998;41:1096–102.

87. Lehman TJ, Edelheit BS. Clinical trials for post-streptococcal reactive arthritis. Curr Rheumatol Rep 2001;3:363–4.

88. Ayoub EM, Ahmed S. Update on complications of group A streptococcal infections. Curr Probl Pediatr 1997;27: 90–101.

89. Birdi N, Hosking M, Clulow MK, et al. Acute rheumatic fever and poststreptococcal reactive arthritis: diagnostic and treatment practices of pediatric subspecialists in Canada. J Rheumatol 2001;28:1681–8.

90. Dajani A, Taubert K, Ferrieri P, et al. Treatment of acute streptococcal pharyngitis and prevention of rheumatic fever: a statement for health professionals. Committee on Rheumatic Fever, Endocarditis, and Kawasaki Disease of the Council on Cardiovascular Disease in the Young, the American Heart Association. Pediatrics 1995;96:758–64.

91. De Cunto CL, Giannini EH, Fink CW, et al. Prognosis of children with poststreptococcal reactive arthritis. Pediatr Infect Dis J 1988;7:683–6.

92. Friedland R, Yahr MD. Meningoencephalopathy secondary to infectious mononucleosis: unusual presentation with stupor and chorea. Arch Neurol 1977;34:186–8.

93. Leavell R, Ray CG, Ferry PC, et al. Unusual neurologic presentations with Epstein–Barr virus infection. Arch Neurol 1986;43:186–7.

94. Herd JK, Medhi M, Uzendoski DM, et al. Chorea associated with systemic lupus erythematosus: report of two cases and review of the literature. Pediatrics 1978;61:308–15.

95. Kinast M, Erenberg G, Rothner AD. Paroxysmal choreoathetosis: report of five cases and review of the literature. Pediatrics 1980;65:74–7.

96. Wong PC, Barlow CF, Hickey PR, et al. Factors associated with choreoathetosis after cardiopulmonary bypass in children with congenital heart disease. Circulation 1992;86(5 suppl):II 118–26.

97. Bird MT, Palkes H, Prensky AL. A follow-up study of Sydenham's chorea. Neurology 1976;26:601–6.

98. Berrios X, Quesney F, Morales A, et al. Are all recurrences of "pure" Syndenham chorea true recurrences of acute rheumatic fever? J Pediatr 1985;107:867–72.

99. Uziel Y, Hashkes PJ, Kassem E, et al. The use of naproxen in the treatment of children with rheumatic fever. J Pediatr 2000;137:269–71.

100. Spagnuolo M, Feinstein AR. Congestive heart failure and rheumatic activity in young patients with rheumatic heart disease. Pediatrics 1964;33:653–60.

101. Feinstein AR, Arevalo AC. Manifestations and treatment of congestive heart failure in young patients with rheumatic heart disease. Pediatrics 1964;33:661–71.

102. Freed MS, Sacks P, Ellman MH. Ventricular tachycardia in acute rheumatic fever. Arch Intern Med 1985;145: 1904–5.

103. Editorial. Treatment of rheumatic fever. N Engl J Med 1965;272:101–2.

104. Diab KA, Timani MA, Bitar FF. Treatment of rheumatic carditis with intravenous gammaglobulin: is there a beneficial effect? Cardiol Young 2001;11:565–7.

105. Voss LM, Wilson NJ, Neutze JM, et al. Intravenous immunoglobulin in acute rheumatic fever: a randomized controlled trial. Circulation 2001;23:401–6.

106. Holt KS. "Rebound" in acute rheumatic fever. Am J Dis Child 1965;31:444–51.

107. Feinstein AR, Spagnuolo M. Mimetic features of rheumatic fever recurrences. N Engl J Med 1960;262:533–40.

108. Committee on Prevention of Rheumatic Fever, American Heart Association: Prevention of rheumatic fever. Circulation 1984;70:1118A–22A.

109. Manyemba J, Mayosi BM. Intramuscular penicillin in secondary prevention of rheumatic fever: a systematic reveiw. S Afr Med J 2003;93:212–8.

110. Massell BF. Prophylaxis of streptococcal infections and rheumatic fever: a comparison of orally administered clindamycin and penicillin. JAMA 1979;241:1589–94.

111. Spodick DH. Acute pericardial disease. Heart Lung 1985; 14:599–604.

112. Spodick DH. Acoustic phenomena in pericardial disease. Am Heart J 1971;81:114–24.

113. Jayashree M, Singhi SC, Singh RS, et al. Purulent pericarditis: clinical profile and outcome following surgical drainage and intensive care in children in Chandigarh. Ann Trop Pediatr 1999;19:377–81.

114. Jacobs WR, Talano JV, Loeb HS. Echocardiographic interpretation of pericardial effusion. Arch Intern Med 1978; 138:622–5.

115. Muir P, Nicholson F, Tilzey AJ, et al. Chronic relapsing pericarditis and dilated cardiomyopathy: serological evidence of persistent enterovirus infection. Lancet 1989;1: 804–7.

116. Garvin PJ, Danis RK, Lewis JE Jr, et al. Purulent pericarditis in children. Surgery 1978;84:471–5.

117. Feldman WE. Bacterial etiology and mortality of purulent pericarditis in pediatric patients. Am J Dis Child 1979; 133:641–4.

118. Stroobant J, Leanage R, Deanfield J, et al. Acute infective pericarditis in infancy. Arch Dis Child 1982;57:73–4.

119. Kauffman CA, Watanakunakorn C, Phair JP. Purulent pneumococcal pericarditis: a continuing problem in the antibiotic era. Am J Med 1973;54:743–50.

120. Ligtenberg JJ, van der Werf TS, Zijlstra JG, et al. Non-surgical treatment of purulent pericarditis, due to non-encapsulated *mophilus influenzae*, in an immunocompromised patient. Neth J Med 1999;55:151–4.

121. Blaser NU, Reingold AL, Alsever RN, et al. Primary meningococcal pericarditis: a disease of adults associated with serogroup C *Neisseria meningitidis*. Rev Infect Dis 1984;6:625–32.

122. Herman RA, Rubin HA. Meningococcal pericarditis without meningitis presenting as tamponade. N Engl J Med 1974;290:143–4.

123. Watring WG, Vaughn DL. Gonococcemia in pregnancy. Obstet Gynecol 1976;48:428–30.

124. Fyfe DA, Hagler DJ, Puga FJ, et al. Clinical and therapeutic aspects of *Haemophilus influenzae* in pediatric patients. Mayo Clin Proc 1984;59:415–22.

125. Ricketts RR, Ilbawi MN, Idriss FS. Management of *Haemophilus influenzae* pericarditis. J Pediatr Surg 1982;17:285–9.

126. Gillett RL. Acute benign pericarditis and the Coxsackie virus. N Engl J Med 1959;261:838–43.

127. Christian HA. Nearly ten decades of interest in idiopathic pericarditis. Am Heart J 1951;42:645–51.

128. Hildebrandt HM, Maassat HF, Willis PW. Influenza virus pericarditis. Am J Dis Child 1962;104:579–82.

129. Van Reken D, Hernandez A, Feigin RD. Infectious pericarditis in children. J Pediatr 1974;85:165–9.

130. Sands MG, Satz JE, Turner WE Jr, et al. Pericarditis and perimyocarditis associated with active *Mycoplasma pneumoniae* infection. Ann Intern Med 1977;86:544–8.

131. Shapiro SC, Dimich I, Steier M. Pericarditis as the only manifestation of infectious mononucleosis. Am J Dis Child 1973;126:662–3.

132. Satoh T, Kojima M, Ohshima K. Demonstration of the Epstein-Barr genome by the polymerase chain reaction and in situ hybridization in a patient with viral pericarditis. Br Heart J 1993;69:563–4.

133. Orbtals DW, Avioli LV. Tuberculous pericarditis. Arch Intern Med 1979;139:231–4.

134. Aggeli C, Pitsavos C, Brili S, et al. Relevance of adenosine deaminase and lysozyme measurements in the diagnosis of tuberculous pericarditis. Cardiology 2000;94:81–5.

135. Wheat LJ, Stein L, Corya BC, et al. Pericarditis as a manifestation of histoplasmosis during two large urban outbreaks. Medicine (Baltimore) 1983;62:110–9.

136. Martinez-Lavin M, Buendia A, Delgado E, et al. A familial syndrome of pericarditis, arthritis, and camptodactyly. N Engl J Med 1983;309:224–5.

137. Clapp SK, Garson A Jr, Gutgesell HP, et al. Postoperative pericardial effusion and its relation to postpericardiotomy syndrome. Pediatrics 1980;66:585–8.

138. Horneffer PJ, Miller RH, Pearson TA, et al. The effective treatment of postpericardiotomy syndrome after cardiac operations: a randomized placebo-controlled trial. J Thorac Cardiovasc Surg 1990;100:292–6.

139. Strauss AW, SantaMaria M, Goldring D. Chronic pericarditis in children. Am J Dis Child 1975;129:822–6.

140. Rooney JJ, Crocco JA, Lyons HA. Tuberculous pericarditis. Ann Intern Med 1970;72:73–78.

141. Lang DJ, Hanshaw JB. Cytomegalovirus infection and the postperfusion syndrome: recognition of primary infections in four patients. N Engl J Med 1969;280:1145–9.

142. Foster KM, Jack I. A prospective study of the role of cytomegalovirus in posttransfusion mononucleosis. N Engl J Med 1969;280:1312–6.

143. Adler SP, Baggett J, McVoy M. Transfusion-acquired cytomegalovirus infections in seropositive cardiac surgery patients. Lancet 1985;2:743–5.

144. Oelberg DG, Fisher DJ, Gross DM, et al. Endocarditis in high-risk neonates. Pediatrics 1983;71:392–7.

145. Noel GJ, O'Loughlin JE, Edelson PJ. Neonatal *Staphylococcus epidermidis* right-sided endocarditis: description of five catheterized infants. Pediatrics 1988;82:234–9.

146. Stanton BF, Baltimore RS, Clemens JD. Changing spectrum of infective endocarditis in children: analysis of 26 cases, 1970–1979. Am J Dis Child 1984;138:720–5.

147. Johnson CM, Rhodes KH. Pediatric endocarditis. Mayo Clin Proc 1982;57:86–94.

148. Moy RJD, George RH, DeGiovanni JV, et al. Improving survival in bacterial endocarditis. Arch Dis Child 1986;61:394–9.

149. Mendelsohn G, Hutchens GM. Infective endocarditis during the first decade of life: an autopsy review of 33 cases. Am J Dis Child 1979;133:619–22.

150. Shulman ST. Infective endocarditis: 1986. Pediatr Infect Dis 1986;5:691–4.

151. Cleary TG, Kohl S. Antiinfective therapy of infectious endocarditis. Pediatr Clin North Am 1983;30:349–64.

152. Teixeira OHP, Carpenter B, Flad P. Enterococcal endocarditis in early infancy. Can Med Assoc J 1982;127:612–3.

153. Waterspiel JN, Kaplan SL. Incidence and clinical characteristics of "culture negative" infective endocarditis in a pediatric population. Pediatr Infect Dis 1986;5:328–32.

154. Kavey RE W, Frank DM, Byrum CJ, et al. Two-dimensional echocardiographic assessment of infective endocarditis in children. Am J Dis Child 1983;137:851–6.

155. Bricker JT, Larson LA, Huhta JC, et al. Echocardiographic evaluation of infective carditis in children. Clin Pediatr 1985;24:312–7.

156. Martin JM, Neches WH, Wald ER. Infective endocarditis: 35 years of experience at a children's hospital. Clin Infect Dis 1997;24:669–75.

157. Morris CD, Reller MD, Menashe VD. Thirty-year incidence of infective endocarditis after surgery for congenital heart defect. JAMA 1998;279:599–603.

158. Saiman L, Prince A, Gersony WM. Pediatric infective endocarditis in the modern era. J Pediatr 1993;122:847–53.

159. Jennings RB Jr, Johnson DH, Chrenka BA, et al. Bacterial endocarditis with flail mitral valve leaflet. J Pediatr 1981;98:426–9.

160. Starkebaum M, Durak D, Beeson P. The "incubation period" of subacute bacterial endocarditis. Yale J Biol Med 1977;50:49–58.

161. Hall G, Heimdahl A, Nord CE. Bacteremia after oral surgery and antibiotic prophylaxis for endocarditis. Clin Infect Dis 1999;29:1–8.

162. Walsh TJ, Hutchins GM. Postoperative *Candida* infections of the heart in children: clinicopathologic study of a con-

tinuing problem of diagnosis and therapy. J Pediatr Surg 1980;15:325–31.

163. Wilson WR, Danielson GK, Giuliani ER, et al. Prosthetic valve endocarditis. Mayo Clin Proc 1982;57:155–61.

164. Friedland IR, du Plessis J, Cilliers A. Cardiac complications in children with *Staphylococcus aureus* bacteremia. J Pediatr 1995;127:746–8.

165. Williams RC, Kunkel HG. Rheumatoid factors and their disappearance following therapy in patients with SBE. Arthritis Rheum 1962;5:126.

166. Milazzo AS Jr, Li JS. Bacterial endocarditis in infants and children. Pediatr Infect Dis J 2001;20:799–801.

167. Sable CA, Rome JJ, Martin GR, et al. Indications for echocardiography in the diagnosis of infective endocarditis in children. Am J Cardiol 1995;75(12):801–4.

168. Lindner JR, Case RA, Dent JM, et al. Diagnostic value of echocardiography in suspected endocarditis. An evaluation based on the pretest probability of disease. Circulation 1996;93:730–36.

169. VanScoy RE. Culture negative endocarditis. Mayo Clin Proc 1982;57:149–54.

170. Pazin GJ, Saul S, Thompson ME. Blood culture positivity: suppression by outpatient antibiotic therapy in patients with bacterial endocarditis. Arch Intern Med 1982;142:263–8.

171. Pesanti EL. Infective endocarditis with negative blood cultures: an analysis of 52 cases. Am J Med 1979;66:43–50.

172. Cannady PB, Sanford JP. Negative blood cultures in infective endocarditis: a review. South Med J 1976;69:1420–4.

173. Biller J, Challa VR, Toole JF, et al. Nonbacterial thrombotic endocarditis. Arch Neurol 1982;39:95–8.

174. Feder HM Jr, Olsen N, McLaughlin JC, et al. Bacterial endocarditis caused by vitamin B6–dependent viridans group Streptococcus. Pediatrics 1980;66:309–12.

175. Tolaymat A, Rhatigan RM, Levin S. Pneumococcal endocarditis in infants. South Med J 1979;72:448–51.

176. Walsh TJ, Hutchins GM. Postoperative *Candida* infections of the heart in children: clinicopathologic study of a continuing problem of diagnosis and therapy. J Pediatr Surg 1980;15:325–31.

177. Barst RJ, Prince AS, Neu HC. *Aspergillus* endocarditis in children: case report and review of the literature. Pediatrics 1981;68:73–8.

178. Del Pont JM, De Cicco LT, Vartalitis C, et al. Infective endocarditis in children: clinical analysis and evaluation of two diagnostic criteria. Pediatr Infect Dis J 1995;14:1079–86.

179. Stockheim JA, Chadwick EG, Kessler S, et al. Are the Duke criteria superior to the Beth Israel criteria for the diagnosis of infective endocarditis in children? Clin Infect Dis 1998;27:1451–6.

180. Citak M, Rees A, Mavroudis C. Surgical management of infective endocarditis in children. Ann Thorac Surg 1992;54:755-60.

181. Ferrieri P, Gewitz MH, Gerber MA, et al. Unique features of infective endocarditis in childhood. Pediatrics 2002;109:931–43.

182. Tolan RW Jr, Kleiman MB, Frank M, et al. Operative intervention in active endocarditis in children: report of a series of cases and review Clin Infect Dis 1992;14:852–62.

183. Wilson WR, Karchmer AW, Dajani AS, et al. Antibiotic treatment of adults with infective endocarditis due to streptococci, enterococci, staphylococci, and HACEK microorganisms. American Heart Association. JAMA 1995;274:1706–13.

184. Brook MM. Pediatric bacterial endocarditis. Treatment and prophylaxis. Pediatr Clin North Am 1999;46:275–87.

185. Shulman ST, Amren DP, Bisno AL, et al. Prevention of bacterial endocarditis. Am J Dis Child 1985;139:232–6.

186. Dajani AS, Taubert KA, Wilson W, et al. Prevention of bacterial endocarditis. Recommendations by the American Heart Association. JAMA 1997;277:1794–801.

187. Roberts GJ. Dentists are innocent! "Everyday" bacteremia is the real culprit: a review and assessment of the evidence that dental surgical procedures are a principal cause of bacterial endocarditis in children. Pediatr Cardiol 1999;20:317–25.

188. Strom BL, Abrutyn E, Berlin JA, et al. Dental and cardiac risk factors for infective endocarditis. A population-based, case-control study. Ann Intern Med 1998;129:761–9.

189. Johnson DH, Rosenthal A, Nadas AS. A forty-year review of bacterial endocarditis in infancy and childhood. Circulation 1975;51:581–8.

CHAPTER 19

Perinatal Syndromes

This chapter is divided into the following sections:

1. Prenatal infections (alphabetized by disease)
2. Exposures during pregnancy
3. Chronic congenital infection ("TORCH syndrome")
4. Neonatal sepsis and meningitis
5. Miscellaneous neonatal infections (alphabetized by organ system)
6. Use of antimicrobial agents in pregnancy and lactation

The field of neonatal infectious diseases has expanded and is thoroughly covered in large reference books such as that edited by Drs. Remington and Klein,[1] to which the reader is referred for more detailed discussion of the topics presented in this chapter.

Some neonatal infections are covered elsewhere in this book. For example, neonatal hepatitis is discussed in Chapter 13, neonatal osteomyelitis is covered in Chapter 16, and prevention of respiratory syncytial virus (RSV) in premature infants is covered in Chapter 7.

■ PRENATAL INFECTIONS

Prenatal infection means any infection that occurs before birth and involves either the pregnant woman or the fetus, although maternal infections usually do not damage the fetus.[2] Congenital infections are infections of the fetus acquired in utero and are usually manifest at the time of birth. Neonatal infections are acquired during delivery or shortly after birth; they may be evident at birth but are usually manifest later (within the first 4 weeks of life). "Natal infections" or "intrapartum infections" are expressions sometimes used to describe infections acquired during delivery; these terms constitute a subset of neonatal infections.

Possible Outcomes

Infection of the pregnant woman can lead to six possible results in the fetus. More than one of these results may be present.

1. *Death.* Abortion, stillbirth, or neonatal death can be produced by infection in the pregnant woman.
2. *Low birth weight.* Low-birth-weight infants may be a result of maternal infection because of either intrauterine growth retardation or premature onset of labor and delivery.
3. *Teratogenic malformations.* Rubella virus is the infectious agent most clearly documented as capable of producing teratologic malformation, such as pulmonic stenosis. Reports that other maternal infections can cause such anomalies in infants should be examined carefully. Intrauterine infection of a particular fetus can be confirmed by recovery of the agent, by demonstration of an antibody titer rise, or by detecting agent-specific IgM (immunoglobulin M) antibodies in the newborn infant. However, prospective studies of women with carefully diagnosed infections must be compared with findings in matched controls to determine whether the malformation is statistically associated with infection by that particular agent. Some infections produce damage without teratogenic anomalies, as described in item 5.
4. *Active congenital infection.* This infection occurs before birth with an infectious agent still present after birth. Often, the infant clearly has an illness at the time of birth. The congenital infection can be defined as chronic if the onset is at least a month before birth or if active disease continues after birth. Because the time of onset of infection in the fetus usually cannot be determined, the diagnosis of chronic active congenital infection is usually suspected on the basis of findings suggesting earlier infection, particularly low birth weight for gestational age or congenital malformation. The phrase "chronic active congenital infection" is useful to describe an active disease process, as in "active tuberculosis" or "chronic active hepatitis." Expanded congenital rubella syndrome (CRS) and congenital cytomegalovi-

rus (CMV) infection are examples of chronic active congenital infections.

5. *Organ damage.* Some fetal infections produce damage to an organ, such as the brain or eye, without teratogenesis. This outcome is common in congenital toxoplasmosis.
6. No disease or damage. CMV and rubella virus are examples of viruses that can infect the fetus without any apparent damage.

Multiple Causal Factors

Fetal teratogenesis has multiple possible causes including genetics, exposure to drugs, and environmental exposures. The causes of most birth defects are unknown. Infection is a very uncommon cause of birth defects, and with the exception of a small number of infectious agents, infection of the fetus is not associated with teratogenesis. Several other prenatal infections can be associated with poor fetal outcomes, and are discussed in the following text.

Specific Infections

The risks of prenatal infection are discussed in the following short sections in alphabetical order, with unusual and miscellaneous infections discussed at the end. Perinatal AIDS is discussed in Chapter 20.

Appendicitis

Large studies have demonstrated that the incidence of acute appendicitis during pregnancy is approximately 1:1400, which is lower than that of the general population of the same age.[3] The most common presenting symptom is right lower quadrant abdominal pain. White blood cell (WBC) count and temperature do not differentiate patients with histologically proven appendicitis from those with pseudoappendicitis.[4] Rarely, the symptoms may be misinterpreted as preterm labor.[5] Outcome after appendectomy, whether open or laparoscopic, is usually quite good.[4,6] Fetal loss is rare in patients who present past the first trimester.[7] For those who present after 24 weeks' gestational age, premature labor is a frequent complication; fortunately, preterm delivery is uncommon.[4]

Babesiosis

Babesiosis is a condition not unlike malaria, in which the pathogen, *Babesia microti*, infects red blood cells. Successful treatment of a pregnant woman, with no adverse consequences for the fetus, has been described.[8] Infantile babesiosis, without proof of intrauterine infection, was first reported in 1986.[9] A more recent case describes a 5-week-old baby whose mother was bitten by a tick 7 weeks prior to delivery; the baby was pale, lethargic, and mildly icteric. The platelet count was 87,000/μl and the serum bilirubin was 9.7 mg/dL. More than 4% of the baby's red blood cells demonstrated ring forms, and the illness resolved with quinine, clindamycin, and azithromycin. Both mother and baby mounted a serologic response to *B. microti*.[10]

Bacterial Vaginosis

As discussed in Chapter 15, bacterial vaginosis during pregnancy is associated with premature rupture of membranes, preterm delivery, and low birth weight.

Bartonella henselae

No known human cases of congenital bartonellosis exist. In an experimental feline model, bacteremic cats had difficulty conceiving; none of the offspring suffered ill effects of the maternal infection.[11]

Brucellosis

Brucella abortus is a well-known cause of fetal demise in farm animals. Because it had not been carefully studied, humans were thought to be protected from such effects by an unknown mechanism. However, in a report from Saudi Arabia of 92 pregnant women with brucellosis, 40 (43%) underwent spontaneous abortions during the first and second trimesters.[12] There was a 2% incidence of intrauterine death in the third trimester. Antepartum antimicrobial treatment of the infection was protective against spontaneous abortion (relative risk 0.14, p <0.0001).

Candidiasis

About 20–25% of pregnant women have vaginal candidiasis, but intrauterine candidiasis is rare.[13] Babies who are infected while in the womb may develop congenital cutaneous candidiasis. The name is somewhat inappropriate, because babies born prematurely with this condition often have positive blood, urine, and/or cerebrospinal fluid cultures.[14] In full-term babies who are otherwise healthy, disease is almost always restricted to the skin, and the prognosis is excellent, with or without topical antifungal therapy.[14] In its most common presentation, the baby is born with a rash or develops it within the first few days of life. The rash is usually widespread, including the palms and soles, and consists of discreet macules, papules, or pustules. Over a few days, it evolves toward a more pustular or vesicular appearance, and sometimes to bullous lesions. Involvement is worst on the back and extensor surfaces of the extremities. The diaper area is usually less involved than the back and trunk. Lesions should be unroofed for microscopic examination and culture.

Extremely low-birth-weight infants more commonly have a flat red rash that resembles a burn, or extensive areas of denudation. This rash heralds a higher likelihood of systemic infection and mortality.[14]

Chickenpox

See varicella and zoster.

Chlamydia

Cervical *Chlamydia trachomatis* is transmitted to about half the babies who pass through the infected birth canal.[15,16] Of these, between 10–20% develop pneumonia, and between 20–45% develop conjunctivitis.[16] These infections are discussed in detail in Chapters 5 and 8. Risk factors for *C. trachomatis* infection include age less than 24 years at the time of pregnancy, unmarried status, and unemployment.[17]

There is evidence that cervical *C. trachomatis* infection is a risk factor for premature birth and, perhaps, low birth weight.[18] Study of a cohort of 264 babies with perinatal problems resulting in neonatal intensive care unit (NICU) admission and 274 control babies without significant perinatal complications revealed that 15% of the former versus 6% of the latter had an IgM (immunoglobulin M) response to *C. trachomatis*.[18] Average gestational age at delivery was 32 weeks for those seropositive for chlamydia, and 34 weeks for those who were seronegative. A much larger, prospective study compared outcomes in 1,110 *C. trachomatis*–positive but untreated women with 1,323 who were treated during pregnancy; treatment decreased the risk of premature rupture of membranes (odds ratio 0.56). There was also a trend toward increased perinatal survival in babies whose mothers were treated.[19]

There is no evidence that *C. trachomatis* infection is associated with respiratory distress syndrome or chronic lung disease.[20]

Coxsackievirus

See enteroviruses.

Cytomegalovirus

Congenital infection with this virus is represented by the C in the "TORCH" acrostic, discussed later. Primary infections and those occurring in the first trimester are most likely to lead to adverse perinatal outcomes.[21,22] If the maternal infection represents a reactivation rather than a primary infection, a poor fetal outcome is unlikely.[23]

Diarrhea

If a pregnant woman has an apparently infectious diarrhea, she should be placed in enteric isolation, and cultures should be done. Salmonellosis probably represents the greatest risk through colonization during delivery, with a risk of neonatal meningitis developing later. Other bacterial pathogens, such as *Campylobacter* or *Shigella*, should be treated and the mother and baby isolated.

Echovirus

See enteroviruses.

Enteroviruses

Enteroviruses rarely cause intrauterine infection that results in severe disease or death of the fetus. Echovirus 71 was found in the midbrain and liver of a stillborn baby who, by the use of ultrasound, was found to have hepatosplenomegaly, liver calcifications, and ascites at 25 weeks of gestation.[24] One neonate was born with a disseminated papulovesicular, nodular, ulcerated and partially necrotic rash, and developed pneumonia, carditis, and hepatitis in the days after birth. This disease was attributed to late prenatal acquisition of coxsackievirus B3 after the virus was cultured from throat and rectal swabs of both the mother and the baby, and serologic results suggested intrauterine transmission.[25] Infection early in gestation may result in an increased number of spontaneous abortions.[26,27] Coxsackievirus infection can be suspected clinically in the pregnant woman because of pleurodynia or ulcerative pharyngitis, and has been proposed as a cause of congenital heart disease and digestive and urogenital anomalies.[28] Increased frequency of fetal death or prematurity also appear to follow maternal coxsackievirus infections.[28] There may be an association with rare central nervous system defects after early pregnancy infections.[29] Disseminated coxsackievirus disease can also occur in the early weeks of life, possibly by intrauterine or postpartum transmission.

Epidemiologic and case-control studies suggest that intrauterine infection with enteroviruses may predispose to the development of insulin-dependent diabetes mellitus (IDDM); however, this is controversial. In one study of 55 mothers whose children developed IDDM and 55 matched controls who delivered at the same hospital and in the same month, IgM antibodies to coxsackievirus B3 were found more frequently in the case population, with an odds ratio of 2.57 (95% CI, 1.02-7.31).[30] A second study of 96 pregnant mothers and matched controls revealed similar findings. These authors found the association was stronger when IDDM developed at or before age 3 years.[31] There is a potential physiologic basis for this association (based on molecular mimicry), and postnatal acquisition of enteroviral infections has also been postulated as a potential risk factor for IDDM.[32] However, a prospective study that examined coxsackievirus infections at delivery in 16 mothers whose children later developed islet-cell autoantibodies and in 110 HLA (histocompatibility locus antigen)-matched control mothers found no association between maternal coxsackievirus infection and IDDM in their offspring.[33] Research in this area is ongoing.

Epstein-Barr virus

More than half of all women of childbearing age are seropositive for Epstein-Barr virus (EBV) and asymptomatic reactivation is common. However, in one study of 67 mother-infant pairs, only 2 of the babies were polymerase chain reaction (PCR) positive for EBV in peripheral blood lymphocytes.[34] The literature contains one case of suspected intrauterine EBV infection in which the baby was born with hypotonia, petechiae, anemia, elevated liver enzymes, and thrombocytopenia. Other intrauterine infections were systematically excluded. The mother was shown to have suffered a primary EBV infection during the pregnancy.[35]

Ehrlichiosis

Experience with this infection during pregnancy is limited. Two pregnant women diagnosed with ehr-

lichiosis during pregnancy and successfully treated with rifampin have been reported. Neither of the fetuses suffered any illness.[36] One reported case was strongly suggestive of intrauterine transmission, in which the mother developed fever and malaise the day after delivery and the baby was admitted at age 9 days with a fever, poor eating, and lethargy. A buffy coat smear showed 23% of the neonate's granulocytes had morulae, and a PCR was positive. Both the mother and the baby mounted a serologic response to the pathogen.[37]

Erythema Infectiosum

See parvovirus B19.

Gonorrhea

Intrauterine infection with fetal death can occur via aspirated contaminated amniotic fluid.[38] Early diagnosis and effective treatment of gonococcal salpingitis or disseminated gonococcemia during pregnancy is likely to spare the fetus from adverse effects. In one case, a 7-day-old baby whose mother had tested negative for *Neisseria gonorrhoeae* during pregnancy presented with septic arthritis of the right hip with gram-negative diplococci. The mother's sexual partner had been seen in the emergency department 10 days prior to the baby's delivery sick with fever, malaise, and dysuria, and his urethral culture grew *N. gonorrheae*.[39]

One study of 256 pregnant women in South Africa suggests that in areas of high prevalence, untreated gonorrhea is an independent risk factor for premature delivery and low birth weight.[40]

Group B Streptococci

This is the most important cause of sepsis in newborns, and is discussed in detail in the section on neonatal sepsis.

Hansen Disease (Leprosy)

Very little is known about pregnancy risk in patients with Hansen disease. Pregnancy causes a relative decrease in cellular immunity, which can lead to development of primary lesions or cause reactivation of previously treated disease.[41] It is thought that the principal risk to the fetus is the antimicrobial agents used to treat the disease.

Human Herpesvirus 6 and 7 (HHV-6, HHV-7)

Both of these herpes group viruses are ubiquitous, and infection usually occurs within the first two years of life. Seroprevalence in pregnant women approaches 100% for HHV-6 and is almost as high for HHV-7. In one study of 569 women, 345 of whom were pregnant, the seroprevalence of HHV-6 was 100%; genital shedding was found in 7 (2.4%) of 297 pregnant women tested versus 8 (3.7%) of 214 nonpregnant women.[42] Another study demonstrated that reactivation of latent HHV-6 occurred in more than 40% of those studied at some time during pregnancy, but HHV-6 was found in only 1% of cord blood samples.[43] A study of 106 pregnant women found HHV-6 reactivating during the first trimester in 28 (25%); outcomes of these pregnancies did not differ from those of women who did not have active replication.[44] Taken together, these data suggest that neither HHV-6 nor HHV-7 cause fetal harm.

Human Herpesvirus 8 (HHV-8)

This virus, the cause of Kaposi's sarcoma in patients with HIV infection, can be transmitted transplacentally. Blood from 2 (2.2%) of 89 babies born to mothers seropositive for HHV-8 had HHV-8 DNA detectable within their peripheral blood mononuclear cells.[45] No known adverse pregnancy outcome or disease in newborns has been associated with HHV-8.

Hepatitis A, B, C, and E Viruses

Management of these infections during pregnancy and issues of maternal-fetal transmission are discussed in Chapter 13.

Herpes Simplex Virus

The incidence of herpes simplex virus (HSV) infection in newborns in the United States is approximately 1 in 1,500–3,200.[46,47]

Pregnant women with genital herpes can transmit the virus to the fetus by three different pathways. Transmission to the baby as it passes through the vaginal canal (intrapartum) is by far the most common. Infection can also be transmitted via the amniotic fluid (ascending route; usually when membranes have been ruptured, but in rare cases despite membranes thought to be intact) or via the blood (transplacentally; rare). Although rare, transplacental (intrauterine) HSV infection is associated with severe manifestations present at birth, including skin lesions and scars, chorioretinitis, micro-

cephaly, hydrocephalus, and microphthalmia. Surviving infants have severe neurologic sequelae.[48]

Pregnant women who develop disseminated HSV infection should be treated with intravenous acyclovir. Intravenous acyclovir also crosses the placenta. Data on outcomes from more than 1,100 prospectively followed acyclovir-exposed pregnancies (more than 700 involving first-trimester exposure) have been compiled. The findings do not show an increase in the number of birth defects identified among the prospective reports when compared with those expected in the general population. However, this sample size is insufficient to detect small increases in risk to the fetus.[49]

The most important consideration is that of neonatal infection acquired via intrapartum transmission. Intrapartum transmission is most common with primary infection because of the higher viral titers present in vaginal secretions and because of the lack of placentally transferred type-specific HSV antibodies in the newborn. In the absence of Cesarean birth, the infection rate of babies delivered vaginally through a primarily infected birth canal is 30–50%; the rate in cases of recurrent disease is less than 5%. A large prospective trial of women with asymptomatic shedding at the time of delivery disclosed a 33% infection rate among babies born to mothers with asymptomatic shedding and serologic evidence of primary infection, and a 3% rate among a similar group of babies whose mothers had asymptomatic recurrent disease.[50]

Prevention of neonatal herpes infection is a complicated process, mainly because cervical shedding of the virus can occur in either primary or recurrent disease, and often occurs in the absence of either physical signs or symptoms of maternal infection. In the past, attempts were made to predict HSV shedding using weekly cervical cultures as a guide; unfortunately, if cervical cultures are obtained more than 48 hours apart, only 20% of the culture pairs are concordant; thus, it is virtually impossible to predict viral shedding at the time of delivery by the use of cervical cultures.[51] The presence of maternal antibodies against HSV at the time of pregnancy augurs a low risk of neonatal herpes infection, probably because transmission of the virus is most common from primary infection, and the presence of antibodies suggests past infection. However, it is important to note that although primary maternal infection confers the highest risk to the fetus, nearly half of all neonatal HSV infections are the result of recurrent disease in the mother. This is because recurrent infections are so much more common than primary infections. Decision analysis suggests that screening for the presence of type-specific antibodies is not a practical method for preventing neonatal herpes infection.[52] The most commonly used mechanism for prevention of disease is visual inspection at the time of labor, with cesarean delivery of babies whose mothers have clinically apparent lesions. In a recent study, cesarean delivery reduced the HSV transmission rate among women from whom HSV was isolated during labor from 7.7% to 1.2%.[47]

Unfortunately, this practice will not prevent all cases of transmission because of the possibility of asymptomatic shedding. A prospective study of 143 women with known risk factors for acquisition of HSV infection revealed that of 123 who were asymptomatic at the time of delivery, only 3 (2.4%) were found to be shedding the virus. In addition, 2 of 5 women who had prodromal symptoms (itching or burning) in the absence of overt herpetic lesions had positive cervical cultures.[53] Therefore, the absolute magnitude of the problem (asymptomatic shedding) is not overwhelming; however, children born to women without a history of genital herpes who are asymptomatic at the time of delivery are overrepresented in the patient population of neonates with herpes infections, mainly because steps are taken to avert the infection in babies whose mothers have clinically obvious disease.

Prophylactic oral acyclovir treatment of women with recurrent genital herpes lesions decreases the percent who are shedding the virus or have active disease at the time of labor; and this, in turn, decreases the number of cesarean deliveries.[54] However, because viral shedding may still occur, neonatal infection is still possible.[54a] In addition, this intervention would be expected to have minimal effect on the number of babies infected with HSV, however, because the risk of infection with recurrent disease is about ten-fold lower than the risk with primary infection. There are currently insufficient data to justify the routine use of suppressive therapy in pregnant women who have had genital herpes.[54a]

Pregnant women who deliver herpes simplex–infected babies tend to be young and nulliparous, without a significantly increased frequency of nonherpetic venereal disease. They often deliver between 30 and 37 weeks' gestation. Acute neonatal herpes is discussed in the next section.

Infectious Mononucleosis

See Epstein-Barr virus.

Influenza

Transplacental transmission of influenza virus at term in a febrile woman has been reported, without adverse effects on mother or baby.[55] A prospective study showed that such transmission is certainly uncommon; of 138 babies born to women with serologically proven influenza virus infection, none had cord blood IgM antibodies, and IgG seroreversion occurred within the first 6–12 months of life in all, suggesting passive transfer of maternal antibody and no in utero infections.[56] There has been much speculation in the literature about the possibility that influenza virus infection during pregnancy sets the stage for later development of schizophrenia in the offspring of those pregnancies.[57] All carefully designed trials testing this hypothesis have been unable to find an association.[58–61]

Pregnant women are certainly at higher risk of morbidity and hospitalization from influenza, especially during the third trimester, at which time they are approximately 5 times more likely to be hospitalized for respiratory illness than are postpartum women.[62] These data are the impetus for the recommendation that women who will be beyond the first trimester of pregnancy during influenza season receive the influenza vaccine.[63]

Leishmaniasis (Kala Azar)

Visceral leishmaniasis is transmitted by the bite of the sandfly. Transmission through other means (such as blood transfusion and organ transplants) has been documented. Vertical transmission occurs, but is rare. Parasites have been found in the placenta of a 5-month fetus.[64] In other cases, the time between transmission and presentation with overt disease ranged from weeks to 16 months; in utero spread was suspected for epidemiologic reasons.[65] Presentation is with fever, hepatosplenomegaly, and diffuse lymphadenopathy. Diagnosis is usually established by bone marrow biopsy, liver biopsy, or both.

Leptospirosis

Rare in the United States, leptospirosis during pregnancy can be devastating to the fetus. A review of 16 cases revealed that 8 pregnancies ended in abortion and 4 babies were born with active disease.[66]

Spontaneous abortion is reportedly more common when infection occurs early in the course of pregnancy.

Listeriosis

Listeria monocytogenes is a fastidious, intracellular gram-positive rod that contaminates foodstuffs, especially processed meats and soft cheeses. Contact with this bacterium is apparently common; about 10% of all refrigerated food is contaminated.[67] An intact cellular immune system prevents infection and disease.

Unfortunately, pregnant women have a predilection for development of disease due to pregnancy-induced diminishment of cellular immunity. The risk appears to be higher for women with multiple gestations than for those with singleton pregnancies. In Los Angeles women with multiple gestations accounted for 4% of all cases of listeriosis, although they made up only 1% of the population. Infection was even more common in triplet pregnancies, in which the relative risk was estimated to be 38.[68] Rates are also higher in mothers with HIV infection and AIDS.[69]

The infection in mothers usually presents as an indolent, "flu-like" illness, with fever, myalgias, arthralgias, and headache. Premature labor is also a common sign. In one series of 21 untreated patients, there were 5 perinatal deaths and one fetal loss at 18 weeks.[70] In general, about a fifth of perinatal infections result in neonatal death or stillbirth. Prompt treatment during pregnancy considerably improves outcomes.

Babies may be born with diffuse microabscesses and granulomas and die in the first day of life from listeriosis; this presentation is known as granulomatosis infantiseptica. Usually, though, listerial infection in the newborn period resembles that of group B streptococci, with early-onset and late-onset forms. Gram staining of the meconium may provide an early clue to the diagnosis while cultures are incubating. Treatment is with ampicillin. Gentamicin is given for synergy until sterilization is documented.

General recommendations for preventing listeriosis are similar to those for other foodborne illnesses (Chapter 12), and include avoidance of unpasteurized milk and cheeses. Persons at high risk for complications from listeriosis (i.e., pregnant women and immunocompromised persons) should adhere to these additional precautions: (a) avoid soft cheeses (i.e., feta, Brie, Camembert, blue-veined, and Mexican-style cheese); (b) cook leftover foods or ready-to-eat foods (e.g., hot dogs) until steaming hot; and (c) consider avoiding deli meats.[71]

Lyme Disease

Lyme disease during pregnancy is evidently a rare occurrence. A serologic survey of 1,416 mothers and their 1,434 babies found a prevalence (in the mothers) of only 0.85%.[72] Only 1 of the 12 women with elevated titers to *Borrelia burgdorferi* had active disease. There is some evidence that the spirochete is transmissible to the fetus; however, proof of adverse outcome as a result of such transmission is lacking. When 60 placentas from women with serologic evidence of Lyme disease were silver stained, 3 (5%) of 60 stained positive for spirochetes, and in two of these cases PCR was positive for *B. burgdorferi*.[73] The babies were healthy. There is a case report in the literature of a 37-year-old pregnant woman who was bitten by a tick, developed an erythema migrans rash, was treated with penicillin for 7 days, and seroconverted to *B. burgdorferi*, whose baby died of unclear reasons 23 hours after birth.[74] Postmortem examination demonstrated rare spirochetes in brain and liver without any accompanying inflammation. The child died of respiratory causes, and no spirochetes were found in the lung.

Lymphocytic Choriomeningitis Virus (LCMV)

This arenavirus, carried and spread by asymptomatic rodents, causes a congenital infection syndrome marked by chorioretinitis, microcephaly or macrocephaly, and periventricular calcifications.[75] Long-term neurologic deficits, including cerebral palsy, mental retardation, and visual problems, are the rule in affected babies. At birth, the syndrome resembles that caused by CMV, toxoplasmosis, or rubella virus. The unique features of LCMV disease are principally that hepatosplenomegaly and hearing deficits are uncommon.[75]

If infection occurs early in pregnancy, fetal loss may occur.[76] Occasionally, nonimmune hydrops fetalis has been reported.

A history of known or suspected rodent exposure is present in about half of cases. Diagnosis is established by serologic evaluation. An immunofluorescence-based test is commercially available and reasonably sensitive. Complement fixation–based antibody testing is not sufficiently reliable and should not be used.

Malaria

Although traditionally regarded as an infection without much risk to the fetus, parasitized red blood cells tend to get sequestered in the placenta, causing decreased blood flow to the fetus,[77] which may be the pathophysiologic mechanism behind the four-fold increase in low birth weight babies and the two-fold increased risk of stillbirth that has been documented in mothers with malaria.[78] In areas of malaria endemicity, low birth weight increases infant mortality by 300%. Mathematical modeling suggests that malaria may, in fact, indirectly account for up to 6% of infant deaths in those areas.[79]

In endemic areas, congenital malaria has been thought to occur in less than 1% of newborns.[80] However, two different prospective studies in sub-Saharan Africa found congenital malaria in 7% of newborns.[81,82] Cases are occasionally reported in the United States.[83]

Congenital malaria should be considered in any infant less than 4 months of age whose mother has a suspect travel history and who presents with fever, anemia, and splenomegaly.[83a] Jaundice and respiratory distress are also common findings in neonates with congenital malaria.[84]

Appropriate antimalarial prophylaxis of the mother protects against maternal and fetal malaria, low birth weight, and perinatal death.[82]

Measles

Fortunately, most women of childbearing age are not susceptible to measles because of vaccine receipt. In one study of 26 pregnant women with measles, fetal mortality was 8%; the risk of fetal loss was higher if measles virus infection occurred early in pregnancy.[85] Another study compared the outcomes of pregnancy in 40 women who contracted measles during gestation with 120 controls without evidence of measles virus infection. Mothers with measles were more likely to be hospitalized with pneumonia and fever; and perinatal morbidity was higher, with premature delivery, neonatal hospital admission, and neonatal length of stay significantly increased in the group that contracted measles.[86] Prematurity may result from premature onset of labor.[87] Congenital malformations were not documented in a small prospective study.[88]

Measles vaccine is contraindicated during pregnancy. However, pregnancy is listed as a situation where prevention with immune globulin is indicated for susceptible household contacts of measles patients (Table 21-9).[89]

Immune globulin has also been recommended for the newborn exposed just prior to birth.[90]

Meningococcus

Perinatal infection with *Neisseria meningitidis* appears to be extremely rare. In one case, a 25-year-old mother presented at 38 weeks' gestation with sepsis, meningitis, petechiae, and purpura; her baby had Apgar scores of zero and one at 1 and 5 minutes, had a purpuric rash, and ultimately succumbed at age 72 hours. Although the neonate's cultures were sterile, the mother's blood and cerebrospinal fluid cultures were both positive for *N. meningitidis*. She had received antibiotics for 18 hours prior to delivery, which probably accounts for his negative cultures.[91]

Mumps Virus

In the first trimester, mumps virus infection is associated with significantly increased fetal death rates.[92] Maternal mumps virus infection is not statistically associated with prematurity.[87] Congenital malformations have been ascribed to maternal mumps, but the evidence is not conclusive. Hydrocephalus secondary to aqueductal stenosis can be produced in experimental fetal infections in rodents and has been observed after acquired infection in children but may be coincidental. It has not yet been observed in a statistical study of human pregnancies.[93] In a small prospective study of 19 pregnant women with mumps infection, there was no increased frequency of congenital anomalies.[94] In a larger study of 117 newborns, the frequency of congenital anomalies was the same as in a control group.[88]

Case reports describe babies who were born severely ill and required mechanical ventilation following maternal mumps infection late in pregnancy.[95,96] Mumps IgM was present in both babies; mumps virus RNA was found in cord blood by PCR in one, and postmortem examination revealed intra-alveolar multinucleated giant cells in the other. Neonatal thrombocytopenia and splenomegaly have been reported following perinatal mumps infection.[97]

Whether intrauterine mumps infection is a cause

of endocardial fibroelastosis has been a subject of debate. The incidence of both of these entities has decreased dramatically in recent years.[98] In a study of myocardial tissue from 29 children with autopsy-proven endocardial fibroelastosis, 21 (72%) of samples were positive for mumps viral RNA by PCR as compared with none of 65 control samples.[99]

Mycoplasmas

Low birth weight is statistically associated with pre-natal cervical *Mycoplasma hominis* colonization.[100] A very small percentage of extremely low-birth-weight premature neonates have respiratory tract colonization with *M. hominis*; this has not been conclusively linked to any particular clinical syndrome.

Papillomaviruses

Human papillomaviruses (HPV) cause genital warts and some are precursors for cervical cancer (Chapter 15). The idea that pregnancy increased the prevalence of cervical infections with these viruses has been around for years; some investigators even found that the prevalence increased with increasing gestational age.[101] However, the largest study of its type to date found that the prevalence of HPV did not differ between 752 pregnant and 504 nonpregnant women.[102]

The principal disease associated with perinatal acquisition of HPV infection is laryngeal papillomatosis, an intractable cause of stridor. Intact membranes and cesarean delivery are not absolutely protective against perinatal transmission; in fact, 23[103]–33%[104] of babies whose mothers have genital warts and who are born by cesarean delivery are PCR positive for HPV at birth. One study of 37 babies showed that the risk of being PCR positive for HPV increased with a longer duration of ruptured membranes. These investigators also showed, however, that all 11 of the "infected" babies cleared the virus, some as early as 5 weeks after delivery.[105] They suggest that babies are "contaminated" rather than infected. Given the disparity between the large numbers of women that are PCR positive for these viruses during pregnancy (one-fourth to one-half of all women) and the small number of children with laryngeal papillomatosis, the concept of "contamination" (or, more palatably, transient colonization) may well be correct.

Parasites

Onchocerciasis appears to be a cause of spontaneous abortion. Gross rates of pregnancy loss in endemic areas are decreased when women of child-bearing age receive ivermectin treatment every six months.[106] Infection later in pregnancy can cause congenital disease. The syndrome principally consists of an intensely pruritic body rash, with or without intermittent fever. The diagnosis is established by skin snip.[107,108]

Various helminthic infections are common during pregnancy in developing countries.[109] Hookworm infestation is associated with low iron stores and anemia.[110,111] In one case a spontaneous abortion was attributed to infestation with *Ascaris lumbricoides*.[112]

Parvovirus B19

Much has been made about parvovirus B19 infection in pregnancy because of the sometimes dramatic outcomes associated with this condition. The most commonly associated problem is nonimmune hydrops fetalis (NIHF). It is estimated that parvovirus infection is responsible for 15–27% of all cases of NIHF.[113,114] Parvovirus infects red blood cell precursors, thus arresting their maturation. In the fetus, this can lead to severe anemia.[114a] The anemia, coupled (in some cases) with myocarditis, causes cardiac failure, which leads to the anasarca characteristic of NIHF. In most cases, the primary infection in the mother is asymptomatic, and the problem is discovered by routine ultrasound. In addition to NIHF, parvovirus infection during the first and second trimesters can lead to fetal loss; one study found parvovirus B19 in the placentas of 7 (15%) of 47 cases of intrauterine fetal death after 22 weeks' gestation versus zero of 53 placentas from full-term deliveries. The virus was also found in 2 (5%) of 37 products of spontaneous abortion versus none of 29 elective abortions.[115] Parvovirus B19 is not a common cause of premature labor and premature delivery.[116]

Although the consequences can certainly be dire, there are several facts that mitigate against hysteria when it comes to parvovirus B19 in pregnancy. First, one-half to two-thirds of women of childbearing age have serologic evidence of past infection.[117,118] Second, the incidence of seroconversion (thus, primary infection) during pregnancy is approximately 1.5%[119] The exact incidence of NIHF or fetal death among fetuses of mothers who undergo primary infection has not been clearly defined; however, in one prospective study, the fetuses of only 3 (8%) of 38 mothers who underwent seroconversion developed NIHF.[120] Outcomes were good in all babies. Mathematically, this works out to a risk of about 2.5 cases per 10,000 pregnancies. Seroconversion rates can be considerably higher (up to 15%) during outbreak situations, however.[118] Women with occupational exposure to children (e.g., pediatric nursing and child care work) are at increased risk of acquiring infection, but this risk is lower than the presence of other children in the home.[118,119]

Counseling of pregnant women who become *exposed* during pregnancy can be simplified into the following: about 50% of women are susceptible, approximately 30% of exposed susceptible hosts become infected, approximately 25% of exposed fetuses become infected, and approximately 10% of infected fetuses die. Thus, the risk of fetal death in a woman with known exposure to parvovirus B19 is approximately $0.5 \times 0.3 \times 0.25 \times 0.1 = 0.4\%$. If the woman is seropositive, the risk approximates zero; if she is seronegative, the risk is about 0.8%.

Outcomes for fetuses with NIHF is improved by intrauterine transfusion.[121]

Q Fever

The agent of Q fever, *Coxiella burnetii*, is an abortifacient in animals, both in the wild and in experimental situations.[122] In one review of more than a thousand cases of Q fever, 15 were diagnosed during pregnancy; only 5 babies were delivered, and only 2 of these were of normal birth weight.[123] Chronic infection with *C. burnetii* can be reactivated during subsequent pregnancies.[124]

Rocky Mountain Spotted Fever

There have been no documented cases of maternal-fetal transmission of *Rickettsia rickettsiae*, the agent of Rocky Mountain spotted fever (RMSF). Treatment of infected pregnant women is tricky, because the drug of choice, doxycycline, is contraindicated during pregnancy.[125] However, because of the severe consequences of inadequately treated RMSF, the use of doxycycline in this case is probably justified.

Rubella Virus

A very high fetal death rate occurs in pregnancies complicated by first-trimester rubella virus infections.[126] Transmission of the virus across the placenta reaches its maximum during the first trimester (more than 80%), goes down to less than 25% by the end of the second trimester, and then rises again during the third trimester (more than 60%).[127,128]

About 20% of maternal rubella infections occurring in the first trimester result in spontaneous abortion. Among live births, congenital defects occur in more than 80% of children infected during the first trimester, and in about one-third of children infected between 13 and 16 weeks' gestation. Virtually no defects attributable to rubella are found in those infected after 16 weeks.[127]

The time from maternal rash to infection of the embryo is 20–30 days.[128] The pathophysiology behind the teratogenic effects of rubella virus infection in embryos is not completely understood; the virus spreads through the vascular system and causes widespread vessel damage.[129] A direct cytopathic effect through necrosis and apoptosis may disrupt organogenesis.[130]

Postnatally acquired rubella ("German measles") is generally a mild disease. Immunization against rubella is principally aimed at preventing congenital rubella syndrome (CRS). In the United States, rubella immunization is done in childhood, during adolescent birth-control counseling, for the mother by the primary care physician when her child is immunized, and as a requirement for college entry, military service, or hospital employment. Despite widespread use of the vaccine, a small percentage of women of childbearing age remain susceptible to rubella virus infection.[131] In addition, only about half the world's population resides in areas where rubella vaccination is routinely given.[132] As a consequence, CRS continues unabated in those areas. In Russia, for example, CRS accounts for 15% of all birth defects.[133] Immigrants who come to the United States from countries not practicing rubella vaccination represent opportunities for possible outbreaks.[134-136]

Prematurity and intrauterine growth retardation occur. Active congenital infections and many congenital malformations can be produced and are discussed in the section on chronic congenital infections (TORCH syndrome). Patent ductus arteriosus, pulmonic stenosis, cataracts, glaucoma, and deafness deserve emphasis.

All women should know their immune status for rubella before risking pregnancy. The importance of knowing this status is, however, not sufficiently appreciated. There is a small but measurable risk of transmitting the attenuated vaccine virus to the fetus.[137] Therefore, patients who may be pregnant should not be given the vaccine, and vaccine recipients should avoid becoming pregnant within 28 days of being vaccinated.[138]

Syphilis

The outcome of maternal infection with *Treponema pallidum*, the causative agent of syphilis, depends on the timing and stage of the disease. A woman may (i) become pregnant while in the primary or secondary stages of the disease, or (ii) become infected during pregnancy. In the former situation, the longer a woman has had syphilis prior to conception, the less likely the fetus will be infected; chances of infection are highest when the fetus is conceived during primary or secondary stages.[139] In the latter situation, morbidity and mortality are increased when the pregnant mother is infected during the first or second trimester.[139] Infection of the fetus often results in stillbirth. Alternatively, the baby may be born with congenital syphilis, which may be asymptomatic, or carry the signs and symptoms outlined in the section on chronic congenital infections. Signs of syphilis in the mother may be subtle or absent. In one study, 121 (78%) of 155 pregnant women with syphilis were asymptomatic.[140] Therefore, prevention of congenital syphilis must depend on serologic testing and adequate treatment of pregnant women. The risk of congenital syphilis is highest in those with less frequent prenatal visits.[141] Unfortunately, outbreak investigation has shown that even when prenatal appointments are kept, many physicians do not offer appropriate screening tests.[142] Of all 451 cases of congenital syphilis reported in the US in 2002, a total of 333 (74%) occurred because the mother had no documented treatment or received inadequate treatment of syphilis.[142a]

Because routine serologic testing of women early in pregnancy will not detect syphilis acquired later in pregnancy, a serologic test for syphilis should be repeated later in high-risk pregnancies.

Antibiotic therapy should be given to the pregnant woman with a serologic diagnosis of syphilis. A total of three shots of benzathine penicillin, given one week apart, is recommended and appears to have been effective over the years.[143] Women who are allergic to penicillin should undergo desensitization and treatment with penicillin. Alternative antibiotics or alternate schedules of penicillin are not acceptable. Babies born to mothers with incomplete or improper treatment should be considered infected. Fetal infection has been observed in a few instances despite appropriate treatment with benzathine penicillin.[143] The optimal penicillin treatment regimen has not really been scientifically established; a recent Cochrane database review revealed no clinical studies that randomized subjects into treatment groups.[144]

Toxoplasmosis

Infection with toxoplasmosis during pregnancy is usually asymptomatic, and only a rise in titer of paired sera early and later in pregnancy is a reliable method of diagnosis. Physicians who order such titers must be able to rely on the accuracy of those tests, offer further testing such as amniotic fluid PCR,[145] and discuss risks and prognosis with the prospective parents. In general, infection of the fetus is most likely to occur when the mother seroconverts later in pregnancy, but the severity of the congenital illness is greater when infection occurs early.[146] The transmission rate is about 6% for mothers infected in the first 13 weeks of pregnancy, but up to 72% for those infected at 36 weeks. The risk of infection and the frequency of severe consequences counterbalance, so that women who seroconvert between 24 and 30 weeks' gestation have the highest chances of having a symptomatic congenitally infected child.[146] However, it should be remembered that even babies with asymptomatic congenital infection usually go on to have adverse outcomes, especially chorioretinal lesions and learning disabilities.

If infection of the mother is confirmed during pregnancy, treatment can be offered, although the scientific basis for the efficacy of this treatment is shaky. One group attempted to do a systematic review of published studies about the utility of maternal treatment; of 2,591 published studies, none was rigorous enough to meet inclusion criteria, so the review had to be scrapped.[147] In countries with a high number of toxoplasmosis infections in pregnant women (such as France), most practitioners do treat the maternal infection. Small, nonrandomized studies suggest that the rate of transmission is *not* affected by maternal treatment, but the severity of the illness may be lessened.[148]

Pregnant women should avoid unnecessary exposure to possible sources of toxoplasmosis, such as cat feces or undercooked meat. (Fig. 19-1). In

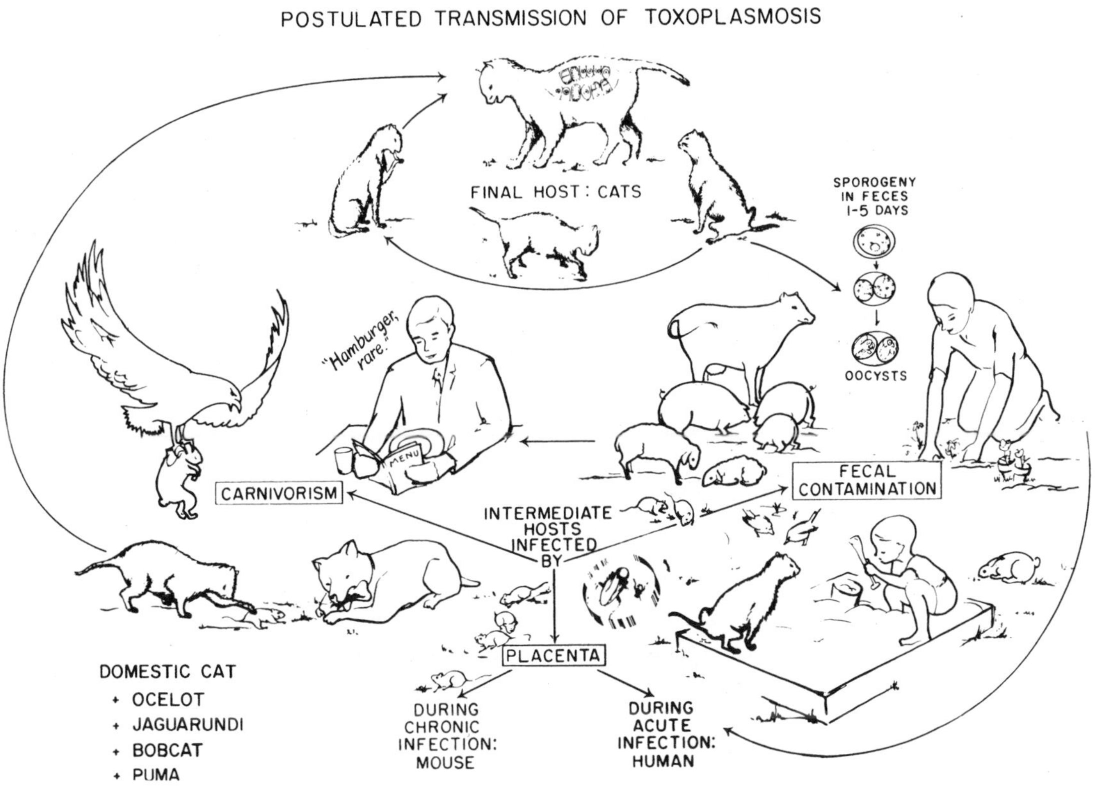

POSTULATED TRANSMISSION OF TOXOPLASMOSIS

■ FIGURE 19-1 Possible sources of infections with *Toxoplasma gondii*. (From Frenkel JK. Toxoplasmosis. In: Marcial-Rojas RA. *Pathology of Protozoal and Helminthic Diseases.* Baltimore: Williams & Wilkins, 1971.)

the United States, physicians have done a good job of alerting pregnant mothers to the dangers of cat litter; however, the dangers of undercooked meat have not been adequately trumpeted. Overseas, where consumption of raw or undercooked meats is more common, this has become the principal risk factor for the acquisition of toxoplasmosis during pregnancy.[149]

Tuberculosis

Tuberculosis during pregnancy is important to diagnose, because as many as two-thirds of pregnant women with pulmonary tuberculosis are asymptomatic[150–152] and newborns are at very high risk of disseminated tuberculosis if exposed to an active case.[153,154] Congenital tuberculosis is very uncommon and is discussed later in this chapter.

All of the first-line drugs (isoniazid, rifampin, ethambutol, and pyrazinamide) have an excellent safety record in pregnancy and have not been associated with congenital malformations.[155] Streptomycin is strongly associated with hearing and bal-

ance problems in children exposed in utero, and its use is contraindicated during pregnancy.[155]

Pregnant women with latent tuberculosis infection who have recent acquisition of infection, and those with HIV infection, may have rapid progression to active disease and should be treated promptly with isoniazid for 9 months.[156] Although no harmful effects of isoniazid to the fetus have been observed, some experts delay therapy of latent infection until after the delivery in the absence of HIV infection, immunosuppression, or recent tuberculosis infection. Pregnant and nursing women on isoniazid should receive pyridoxine (vitamin B6) 25 mg daily.[156]

Pregnancy is associated with progressive suppression of tuberculin sensitivity (and other lymphocyte functions), which is maximal between 36 weeks' gestation and delivery.[157]

Ureaplasmas

Colonization of the cervix with *Ureaplasma urealyticum* probably occurs in about half of pregnant women.[158] Ascending intrauterine infection is a major cause of premature labor; ureaplasmas are some of the most common of the organisms thought to be associated with early induction of labor.[159] Antibiotic treatment aimed at *U. urealyticum* in laboring mothers does not, however, alter the rate of preterm birth.[159]

There has been controversy surrounding the possible role of *U. urealyticum* in the pathogenesis of chronic lung disease ("bronchopulmonary dysplasia") in premature neonates. The hypothesis is that ascending infection from the cervix causes an increase in inflammatory mediators in the intrauterine environment, and colonizes the infant's respiratory tract with the organism.[160] After birth, ongoing inflammation due to the presence of *Ureaplasma* in the trachea and lung causes arrest of normal lung development and initiates fibrosis, both of which contribute to the development of chronic lung disease (CLD). In vitro studies demonstrate that *U. urealyticum* causes neonatal macrophages to overproduce proinflammatory cytokines.[161] Some clinical studies demonstrate an increased incidence of CLD in colonized versus uncolonized babies,[162–164] while others do not.[165–168] Finally, a histopathologic study showed more interstitial fibrosis in the lungs of babies colonized by *Ureaplasma*.[169]

Prospective, placebo-controlled trials of erythromycin treatment show no benefit.[168] Taken together, these data suggest that a link between *Ureaplasma* colonization and CLD, if it exists at all, is tenuous and of a small magnitude.

Ureaplasmas have rarely been isolated from cerebrospinal fluid specimens, sometimes in concert with pleocytosis and sometimes without. Cases of spontaneous resolution have been described.[170] In the largest study to date, *U. urealyticum* was isolated from the spinal fluid of only 2 (0.2%) of 920 infants.[168] One very low-birth-weight infant developed osteomyelitis of the right femur and had a blood culture positive for *U. urealyticum*.[171]

Urinary Infections

Preterm delivery is statistically more common in women with bacteriuria, and the mortality rate of infants is significantly higher if the infection occurs within 15 days of delivery.[172]

Varicella

Varicella tends to be particularly severe in pregnant women, in whom life-threatening pneumonitis may occur. Maternal varicella between 8 and 20 weeks of gestation results approximately in a 1–2% incidence of congenital varicella syndrome.[173] In one study of 1,373 women with varicella during pregnancy, the risk of congenital varicella syndrome was 2% if infection occurred between 13 and 20 weeks' gestation and 0.4% before 13 weeks' gestation.[174]

The syndrome consists of limb hypoplasia, cicatricial (scar-like) rash, microcephaly, chorioretinitis or other ophthalmic defects (optic atrophy, microphthalmia, cataracts, or keratoconjunctivitis), and sometimes intracranial calcifications. Incomplete forms may exist; one report describes finding antivaricella-zoster virus (VZC) antibodies in the cerebrospinal fluid of 4 babies who presented with seizures and mild hypotonia.[175] Congenital varicella syndrome is rare for two reasons: (a) most women of childbearing age, with or without a clinical history of varicella, are immune to the disease,[176] and (b) most cases of proven varicella during pregnancy do not lead to the syndrome.[177] In the first trimester, maternal chickenpox is associated with slightly increased fetal death rates.[92]

Fatal neonatal infections can occur, especially in infants born to mothers who developed a chickenpox rash 5 or fewer days before delivery or within 2 days after delivery.[178] The probable reason for the severity of primary varicella in these babies is that the mother passes the virus to the baby transplacentally before she has had time to mount an antibody response, thus leaving the baby infected and unprotected. Varicella-zoster immune globulin (VZIG) is recommended for the baby after birth (Table 21-9).[179] Acyclovir may provide some additional protection; in one small prospective study, 2 of 4 babies given VZIG alone versus none of ten given both VZIG and acyclovir developed symptoms of varicella.[180] Most experts withhold acyclovir unless the baby develops signs or symptoms of disease.[181]

Infants who develop zoster in the first few years of life without a history of preceding chickenpox[182] probably had primary varicella in the womb. Most of these babies will not have any of the findings of congenital varicella syndrome, although unrecognized chorioretinitis should be sought.

About 90% of women of childbearing age who have a negative or unknown history of chickenpox have serologic evidence of past infection;[176] those who are seronegative and wish to be protected can be offered varicella vaccine. Because the vaccine is a live attenuated virus, it should not be given to women who are already pregnant. There is a theoretical risk of congenital varicella syndrome or fetal loss if it is inadvertently administered to pregnant women, but there have not been any reported cases.[183]

VZIG should be administered to susceptible women exposed to active varicella during pregnancy (Table 21-9). If the mother's immune status is uncertain, VZIG can be withheld pending serologic results. Most will be immune. However, the consequences of varicella to both the mother and fetus can be severe; therefore, VZIG should not be withheld if serologic results cannot be returned in a timely fashion.

West Nile Virus

A single case of intrauterine transmission of West Nile virus (WNV) infection has been reported in which both the mother and infant had WNV-specific IgM in both the serum and spinal fluid.[184] The newborn had bilateral chorioretinitis and severe cerebral abnormalities, but whether these were the result of WNV infection is not known. A case of transmission via breast milk has also been reported.[185] In this case, the mother acquired the infection via a blood transfusion postpartum, ruling out transplacental acquisition. The baby developed a serum IgM response but remained asymptomatic.

Zoster (Shingles)

Herpes zoster in pregnancy does not appear to result in congenital malformations or an unfavorable prognosis. In a prospective study of 366 pregnant women with zoster, none of the infants had clinical evidence of intrauterine infection.[174]

Miscellaneous Prenatal Infections

Infections during pregnancy that are diagnosed and treated promptly with a specific effective therapy usually do not result in an adverse fetal outcome, especially in the second half of pregnancy. In addition to those previously listed alphabetically, reported infections appropriately treated that had no adverse fetal effects include bacterial endocarditis, botulism, *Clostridium perfringens*, cryptococcosis,[186] disseminated blastomycosis, disseminated histoplasmosis, *Haemophilus influenzae* meningitis, pertussis, pneumococcal pneumonia, psittacosis, and many other infections uncommon in the United States.[187]

Maternal infections for which there is no specific therapy may have an adverse outcome for the fetus, with spontaneous abortion early in pregnancy or stillbirth or postnatal death if the infection occurs shortly before delivery. Infection with dengue virus late in gestation may result in transmission of infection to the fetus, with coagulopathy and multiorgan dysfunction in the newborn.[188]

One disease with a specific treatment that nevertheless has a poor prognosis for the fetus infected near term is relapsing fever (caused by various species of *Borreliae* and usually transmitted by ticks or lice).[189]

■ EXPOSURES DURING PREGNANCY

Exposure to Rubella-Like Illness

The most urgent clinical situation in prevention of congenital rubella syndrome is the management of a pregnant woman with suspected exposure to rubella. This situation is also avoidable by serologic testing before pregnancy. The problem has three parts.

1. Is the pregnant woman susceptible to rubella? This can be determined by testing her serum for rubella antibody. A history of clinical rubella is of no value because it is unreliable.
2. Does the exposing individual really have rubella? Laboratory documentation of rubella in the exposing individual is best done by determination of rubella IgM antibodies. Even if the pregnant woman is not susceptible to rubella, it may be of value to determine whether the exposing individual really has rubella, because this is of importance to other women at risk in the community.
3. If the pregnant woman is susceptible and really exposed to rubella, has she become infected? A follow-up serum specimen should be obtained in 3 and 6 weeks to determine if seroconversion has occurred. If rubella IgG remains negative, infection has not occurred.

If rubella infection has occurred prior to 16 weeks' gestation, the risk for severe fetal malformation is very high. A realistic portrayal of the likely outcome should be explained. Some parents are philosophically opposed to elective abortion and may decide to continue the pregnancy. In this case, intramuscular administration of immune globulin 0.55 mL/kg should be given as soon after exposure as possible (before determining if the woman has been infected). This has been shown to decrease clinically apparent infection in an exposed susceptible person from 87% to 18%.[190]

High Rubella Titers

It is not unusual for a pregnant woman to have a high rubella titer (1:256 or higher) at her first prenatal visit. This does not necessarily indicate recent infection and again illustrates the importance of knowing the woman's rubella titer before pregnancy. Unfortunately, testing a high-titer serum for the presence of specific rubella IgM may not be helpful, because the IgM antibody can indicate infection any time in the preceding 10–12 months.[191]

Rubella Immunization During Pregnancy

The live rubella virus vaccine can infect the fetus but rarely causes rubella-related defects.[192] Nevertheless, the rubella vaccine is labeled as contraindicated in pregnancy, although if given, it "should not be a reason to consider interruption of pregnancy" (because of possible congenital rubella defects).[192]

Exposure to Other Viral Illnesses

Most women of childbearing age have been immunized against measles and mumps and had chickenpox as children, although the infection may have been subclinical. If the woman has not previously had measles vaccine or illness, prevention by immune globulin is probably indicated, using 0.25 mL/kg (maximum 15 mL), if the woman is exposed.[89] Mumps hyperimmune globulin is generally not available and is not recommended for the exposed pregnant woman. VZIG for the prevention of chickenpox is available for the newborn infant, and for the pregnant susceptible woman, as previously described.

Exposure to paravirus is discussed in a previous section.

Pre-exposure Immunity Testing

As with rubella, measles and chickenpox immunity testing is feasible, but it is not publicized or used. Women whose occupations make them especially likely to be exposed (teachers, health care professionals) would benefit from a readily available screen on one specimen of blood for rubella, measles, and chickenpox. Detection of unsuspected immunity before exposure would eliminate the need for immunoglobulin prophylaxis in the pregnant woman who is later exposed to measles or chickenpox.

■ CHRONIC CONGENITAL INFECTION SYNDROMES

Chronic congenital infection syndrome is a more comprehensive preliminary diagnosis than "TORCH syndrome" for a newborn infant who has one or more abnormalities that can result from an intrauterine infection. The term "TORCH" was originally coined as a mnemonic to emphasize that herpes simplex could produce effects similar to those already recognized as attributable to other agents. The word is an acronym for toxoplasma, other (especially syphilis), rubella, cytomegalovirus, and herpes.[193–195] A new acronym, CHEAP TORCHES, has been proposed.[196] This acronym broadens the differential diagnosis for congenital infections, reminding the clinician of other possible causes. It also solves one of the problems with the TORCH acronym; that is, it specifically mentions syphilis. The acronym is explained in Box 19-1.

A chronic congenital infection can be defined as an infection that has apparently been present for more than a month with manifestations still present at birth. Some chronic congenital infections are active; that is, associated with evidence of an active inflammatory response, as well as with recovery of

---

BOX 19-1 ■ Cheap Torches Acronym

This is a memory device to recall some important causes of congenital and neonatal infections. It is not meant to imply that the entities on the list are similar in clinical presentation.

C Chickenpox
H Hepatitis B, C, E
E Enteroviruses
A AIDS (HIV)
P Parvovirus B19

T Toxoplasmosis
O Other (GBS, *Listeria*, *Candida*, tuberculosis, LCMV
R Rubella
C Cytomegalovirus
H Herpes simplex virus
E Everything else sexually transmitted (gonorrhea, *Chlamydia*, *Ureaplasma*, papillomavirus)
S Syphilis

GBS, Group B streptococcus; LCMV, lymphocytic choriomeningitis virus; AIDS, acquired immunodeficiency syndrome; HIV, human immunodeficiency virus.

the infectious agent from the infant. Other chronic congenital infections are probably inactive or "burned out," with only the congenital anomaly or damaged organ remaining as evidence of past infection.

Clinical Diagnosis

Chronic congenital infection should be considered when any of the 3 following general findings is present.

1. *Intrauterine growth retardation.* Intrauterine growth retardation is defined as a low birth weight for the period of gestation (small for gestational age), as estimated by dates and by physical examination. It can occur with congenital infections but usually has other causes.[197]
2. *Congenital defects indicating teratogenesis or damaged organs.* The defects most frequently associated with congenital infections are heart disease (especially patent ductus arteriosus and pulmonic stenosis), central nervous system abnormalities (especially microcephaly, hydrocephalus, intracranial calcifications, and psychomotor retardation), eye abnormalities (especially cataracts, glaucoma, and chorioretinitis), and deafness.
3. *Signs suggesting chronic active infection.* Several clinical patterns should suggest the possibility of an active congenital infection. Jaundice with hepatosplenomegaly suggests infection involving the liver. Thrombocytopenic purpura suggests infection involving the bone marrow. Other signs include a petechial, pustular, or bullous rash; pleocytosis of the cerebrospinal fluid; lytic bone lesions; pneumonitis; myocarditis; rhinitis; vomiting; or diarrhea.

Many combinations of the above findings have been observed in chronic congenital infections, and the presence of one should stimulate a search for other signs of congenital infection. Occasionally, however, a single malformation or a transient sign of active infection is observed.

Asymptomatic infection with no detectable abnormalities can occur with all of these congenital infections. Some of the abnormalities most frequently associated with specific congenital infections are described in the following text. The patterns of involvement of various organ systems, the laboratory approach, and the spectrum of disease produced by these agents have been well reviewed.[193–195,197]

Causes of Chronic Congenital Infections

Rubella Virus

Congenital rubella infection can be classified into several major patterns.

1. Classical congenital rubella syndrome was originally described before the virus could be cultured in the laboratory. The major features are congenital heart disease (particularly patent ductus arteriosus and pulmonic stenosis) and eye defects (particularly cataracts, glaucoma, and microphthalmia). Microcephaly and deafness may also be present.
2. Expanded congenital rubella syndrome was defined during the severe epidemic in the United States in 1964, when a number of other manifestations were clearly recognized for the first time. These included intrauterine growth retardation, jaundice with hepatosplenomegaly, thrombocytopenic purpura, encephalitis, and myocarditis in various combinations. The term "blueberry muffin" baby was coined to describe the yellow baby with purple spots because of jaundice and purpura or dermal erythropoiesis. Other possible manifestations are a large anterior fontanel, transient longitudinal bone radiolucencies, failure to grow well, unusual dermatoglyphics, and dental enamel defects. Retinitis manifested by excessive pigmentation or depigmentation is neither progressive nor associated with decreased vision.
3. Late-onset rubella syndrome is a form in which there are minimal symptoms at birth but acute severe multisystem disease develops after 3–6 months, with interstitial pneumonia, skin rash, diarrhea, hypogammaglobulinemia, and circulating immune complexes.[198] Aseptic meningitis, hepatosplenomegaly, thrombocytopenia, and *Pneumocystis* pneumonia may also occur.

    Diabetes mellitus has been observed later in childhood in follow-up studies of some infants with congenital rubella infection. Hypotonia or convulsions or a chronic progressive panencephalitis can also occur in later childhood.[199]
4. Isolated defects can occur, particularly language retardation,[200] strabismus, deafness, and neonatal hepatitis.[201]

Congenital Rubella Syndrome (Revised Classification)

In 1980, new definitions were proposed for the classification of congenital rubella syndrome (CRS) cases because of the difficulty in some situations.[202] The Centers for Disease Control and Prevention recommended a revised classification with criteria to define confirmed, probable, possible infection without defects, and absent CRS.

The current CDC classification can be found here: http://www.cdc.gov/nip/publications/pink/rubella.pdf

Toxoplasmosis

The "classic triad" of chorioretinitis, intracranial calcifications, and hydrocephalus is uncommon. Several clinical patterns of toxoplasmosis can be defined.[203]

1. Asymptomatic infection is the most common pattern. Most babies with congenital toxoplasmosis do not have any obvious symptomatology and are discharged from the nursery as well babies. In one study that looked at using a routine IgM-capture assay for toxoplasmosis in all newborns, 100 (0.02%) of 635,000 had a positive screening test. Additional serologic testing (IgM and IgG) of the infant and mother confirmed congenital toxoplasmosis in 52 (52%) of the newborns with a positive screening test. Of those 52 children identified through screening, 50 (96%) had been judged to be normal newborns. However, after the test results became known, and more thorough neurologic and ophthalmologic examinations were performed, 19 (40%) of 48 infants evaluated were found to have subtle abnormalities.[204] Children who are asymptomatic at birth have more favorable outcomes than those with symptomatic disease; however, they are less likely to be treated, and treatment has been shown to improve outcomes dramatically.[205] The child with asymptomatic congenital toxoplasmosis who receives no therapy is most likely to come to medical attention because of visual changes associated with chorioretinitis, which may develop years later.

2. Jaundice with hepatosplenomegaly may occur without evidence of blood group incompatibility. Fever, rash, lymphadenopathy, pneumonitis, vomiting, or diarrhea may also be present. This acute pattern has been called the gene-

ralized form of congenital toxoplasmosis. The patient may also have some neurologic manifestations.

3. Neurologic manifestations occur in various combinations and may include hydrocephalus or microcephaly, cerebral calcifications, chorioretinitis, and convulsions. These abnormalities often are not recognized until the child is several months of age but occasionally are noted in infants with the jaundice pattern. Calcifications tend to be widely spread, rather than periventricular as they are in CMV infection. The majority of these lesions resolve with long-term antitoxoplasma therapy.[206]

4. Isolated defects, particularly mental retardation, deafness, or microphthalmia, may occur.

Repeated spontaneous abortions resulting from toxoplasmosis have been described. Repeated congenital disease in newborn infants of the same woman is rare. Very rarely, congenital toxoplasmosis is seen in babies born to mothers who were immune prior to conception,[207] or who contracted the infection just prior to conception.[208]

Cytomegalovirus

Between 0.5–2% of all newborns are infected with CMV in utero. A recent study evaluated maternal serostatus to CMV during the previous pregnancy as a risk for delivering a newborn with congenital CMV. Of 604 babies born to initially seronegative mothers, congenital CMV infection occurred in 18 (3%). In contrast, of 2,857 babies born to immune mothers, congenital CMV infection occurred in 29 (1%).[209]

About 95% of infants with congenital CMV infection are asymptomatic at birth. It should be noted that it is not unusual for CMV shedding to continue for months to years. If the urine is not tested (by culture or PCR) for CMV before 3–4 weeks after birth, any later positive results may represent an acquired CMV infection, which occurs in about 10–30% of infants in the first year of life. Seropositivity may be even higher in breastfed babies; a prospective study showed that 11 (65%) of 17 babies breastfed by mothers who were seropositive for CMV developed antibodies to CMV prior to their first birthday versus 24 (28%) of 87 bottle-fed babies (P = 0.005).[210]

Several patterns of congenital infection can be defined.

1. Jaundice with marked hepatosplenomegaly may

be due to CMV infection. Transient hepatosplenomegaly may also occur. Portal hypertension is an uncommon late complication of neonatal CMV hepatitis. The kidney is usually involved in severe cases, and cytomegalic inclusions can usually be seen in renal tubule cells excreted into the urine (Fig. 19-2). CMV can readily be grown in cell culture of urine.

2. Thrombocytopenic purpura often occurs with the jaundice pattern. Transient petechiae may also be attributed to CMV infection.

3. Neurologic abnormalities resembling those of toxoplasmosis can occur in various combinations or as isolated defects, including microcephaly, chorioretinitis, cerebral calcifications, spastic diplegia, and psychomotor retardation. Cerebral calcifications, when found, are usually periventricular in distribution. A single such neurologic abnormality may be the only abnormality. The presence of any abnormality on computed tomography (CT) scans of the head during the newborn period is highly predictive of adverse outcome. A prospective study of 56 babies with symptomatic congenital CMV showed that 90% of children with abnormal CT scans had at least one sequela, whereas only 29% of those with normal CT scans had identifiable sequelae.[211] Sequelae included mental retardation, seen in 59% of those with abnormal scans, and hearing impairment. In a study of 180 children with symptomatic congenital CMV infection, evidence of disseminated infection (petechiae and intrauterine growth retardation) was most predictive of subsequent hearing loss. The presence of microcephaly and other neurologic abnormalities was not predictive of hearing loss.[212]

4. Persistent interstitial pneumonia can result from infection acquired before or during birth or in the newborn period (from blood transfusions containing the virus). Fortunately, transmission via blood transfusion has become rare. Acquired neonatal CMV pneumonia is often associated with hepatosplenomegaly and atypical lymphocytosis. Chronic interstitial pneumonia is also discussed in Chapters 8 and 22.

5. Asymptomatic infection, with excretion of the virus at birth, is the most common pattern of congenital CMV infection. Detailed studies about the prognosis of this form of congenital CMV have been performed. Approximately 15% of asymptomatic CMV-shedding babies develop sensorineural hearing loss.[213,214] Unfortunately, universal newborn hearing screening is of very limited benefit, because only about 5% of them have abnormal screens at the time of hospital discharge.[214] In addition, the severity of the hearing loss tends to be progressive over time, even in those whose hearing is found to be abnormal at the time of the initial screening examination.[213]

Some controversy exists about whether developmental delay, mental retardation, or other neurologic outcomes are more frequent in patients who were asymptomatically shedding CMV at the time of birth. One study evaluated the development and intelligence quotient of 204 children with asymptomatic CMV infection and used 177 uninfected siblings as controls; no significant difference in neurodevelopmental status could be found.[215]

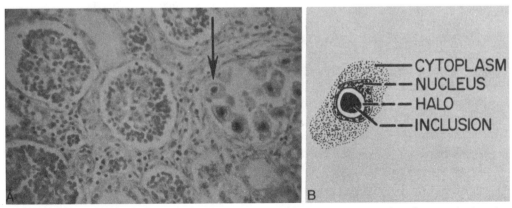

■ **FIGURE 19-2** Cytomegalovirus inclusions. (**A**) In renal tubular cells. (**B**) Diagram of a cell as seen in the urine. (Photo from Dr. Enid Gilbert).

Syphilis

In the case of syphilis, several clinical patterns can be observed in the newborn period.[216,217]

1. Asymptomatic infection is the most common pattern of congenital syphilis. Even infection that is clinically silent at first can be devastating; therefore, identifying and treating these babies is of utmost importance. The prevention of congenital syphilis depends on testing and treatment of infected mothers. The mother's test results should always be transcribed onto the newborn's record. A negative screening test early in pregnancy does not eliminate the possibility of syphilis, as women can become infected during gestation.[218]
2. Symptomatic disease is usually manifested by a rash. Typically, the rash is vesicular or bullous, sharply demarcated, and involves the face, diaper area, palms, and soles. An erythema multiforme rash may also be seen.
3. Chronic rhinitis ("the snuffles") and fissures of the lips can be a manifestation of syphilis in the newborn period. Babies sent home from the nursery may present within the first days to weeks of life with rhinitis, with or without rash. The rhinitis of syphilis is often blood-tinged.
4. Jaundice with hepatosplenomegaly may occur. The serum bilirubin is mostly the direct (conjugated) form.
5. Monocytosis may be present; an absolute monocyte count higher than 1,500/mcL occurs.[219] Hemolytic anemia can occur.
6. Lytic bone lesions, with periosteal reaction or metaphyseal destruction, may be observed on long-bone x-rays, which are usually taken because the infant fails to use an arm or leg, or as part of a workup for congenital syphilis.
7. Nephrotic syndrome may be the principal manifestation of congenital syphilis during the newborn period.
8. Neurosyphilis in an infected infant is usually discovered by Venereal Disease Research Laboratory (VDRL) testing of the CSF, rather than by clinical observation of an abnormality referable to the central nervous system.

Herpes Simplex Virus

Neonatal infections with herpes simplex virus (HSV) have traditionally been divided into three classifications. As seen from the following descriptions, there may be overlap among the three categories.

1. *Disseminated disease.* This is the most devastating form of neonatal HSV infection. Babies with disseminated HSV tend to present with symptoms suggestive of sepsis.[220] Acute hepatic failure may be the presenting syndrome.[221] Bleeding secondary to poor production of coagulation factors may dominate the clinical picture. The mortality rate of disseminated HSV infection in the neonate is high (57–80%). The course may be rapidly fulminant or more indolent, with the initial presentation one of persistent neonatal fever without other symptoms. However, even in those with an indolent presentation, eventually overwhelming infection will occur if treatment is not instituted. For infants in the first 6 weeks of life who present with fever and whose workup for bacterial infection (blood culture, CSF culture, urine culture) is negative, the possibility of HSV infection should be considered. Clues include elevated aminotransferase levels and depressed platelet count. In such patients, HSV PCR should be sent on the spinal fluid, cultures of HSV from mouth and any skin lesions, and empiric acyclovir considered. The drug can be discontinued when testing for HSV is negative or another diagnosis is made.
2. *Central nervous system (CNS) disease.* The principal manifestation of CNS disease is encephalitis. Involvement may be relatively minor, or it may be devastating. Patients may have gaze preferences, seizures, partial or complete paraplegia, and disorders of sensory processing. The mortality of CNS disease is about 15%, but long-term morbidity is high (40–80% have residual neurologic deficits).[222] All neonates with suspected bacterial meningitis but a negative Gram stain should have an HSV PCR sent from the CSF and acyclovir started empirically. As with disseminated disease, about half of neonates with CNS disease do not have any skin lesions at the time of presentation (and some patients never develop skin lesions).
3. *Skin, eye, and mucous membrane disease (SEM).* Some infants have HSV infection that appears to be limited to the skin, eyes, mucous membranes, or some combination of these 3 sites. Outcome for these patients is considerably better than that of children with either disseminated or CNS disease. Untreated, the infection

usually progresses to CNS or disseminated disease. Differentiation of SEM disease from the other two categories can be difficult, because skin lesions may also be associated with CNS or disseminated disease. The delineation of disease as "SEM" may be somewhat artificial, as some patients develop learning disabilities in the long term. Infants with apparent SEM disease must undergo a lumbar puncture to exclude the possibility of CNS involvement. Some children experience frequent recurrences of their skin disease; these can be suppressed with long-term oral acyclovir therapy.[223] Patients who undergo more than 3 recurrences have been shown to be at higher risk of long-term cognitive defects than those with fewer than 3.[223]

Laboratory Approach

After clinical examination for cataracts, retinopathy, murmurs, hepatosplenomegaly, and other signs

mentioned earlier, there is a reasonable set of laboratory studies to be considered when a congenital infection is suspected (Box 19-2). Nonspecific studies might include ultrasonography for intracranial calcifications, long-bone roentgenograms for bone destruction, chest roentgenogram, electrocardiogram (ECG) for heart lesions, CSF examination, and more common studies such as a platelet count. Although total IgM has traditionally been measured in children with possible congenital infections, this test is neither a sensitive nor specific indicator of infection.[224]

Herpes Simplex Virus

Babies with skin, eye, or mucous membrane lesions consistent with HSV should have viral cultures and direct fluorescent antibody stains (DFA) of the lesional material sent. DFA is a relatively sensitive and rapid test that may give the clinician results within a couple of hours. Visible lesions that are

---

BOX 19-2 ■ Laboratory Approach to Congenital and Neonatal Infections

Nonspecific studies
Complete blood count with differential and platelets, liver enzymes, bilirubin, and blood culture
CSF cell count, glucose, and protein

Specific smears[a]
Darkfield examination of lesions for spirochetes

Specific serologies
RPR (or VDRL), with confirmatory syphilis tests if RPR is positive
Toxoplasmosis, rubella[a], parvovirus[a], HIV[a], and lymphocytic choriomeningitis virus[a]

Specific CSF studies[a]
VDRL, HSV PCR, Toxoplasma IgM (and PCR), and enterovirus PCR

Urine tests
CMV culture and/or PCR
Culture for rubella virus[a]

Surface cultures[a]
DFA and culture (or PCR) for HSV from skin lesions, eyes, nasopharynx or oropharynx, and rectum
Nasopharyngeal and conjunctival swabs for rubella culture
Nasopharyngeal and rectal swabs for enterovirus (culture or PCR)

Amniotic fluid (if available)
Toxoplasma PCR[a]

Other studies
Head CT, hearing test, retinal examination

Abbreviations: Ig, immunoglobulin; CSF, cerebrospinal fluid; RPR, rapid plasma reagin; VDRL, venereal disease research laboratory test; HIV, human immunodeficiency virus; HSV, herpes simplex virus; PCR, polymerase chain reaction; DFA, direct fluorescent antibody; CT, computed tomography.
[a] Test for specific entity if it is clinically suspected (see Table 19–1).

caused by HSV are teeming with virus; therefore, viral cultures of these lesions usually turn positive within 36–48 hours. Cerebrospinal fluid is generally sent for HSV PCR to rule out involvement of the central nervous system. Results may be available within a day or two, or, if shipped out and run in batches, they may take longer. Hospitals should contract with a laboratory that runs these tests on a daily basis to minimize delay. In disseminated disease, liver function studies are usually elevated. Pneumonitis may or may not be present. Serum may also be sent for HSV PCR. Babies with neonatal HSV are viremic more frequently than was previously believed.[225]

Toxoplasmosis

Toxoplasmosis is usually diagnosed by serologic methods. Direct identification of the pathogen is less readily available because it involves injecting tissues or fluids from the baby into the peritoneal cavity of a mouse, and requires 6 weeks of incubation time. Tissue culture methods are more rapid, but less sensitive. Because maternal IgM does not cross the placenta, identification of toxoplasma-specific IgM in the infant's serum provides evidence of congenital infection. Unfortunately, this testing is not always positive. Specialized testing, including Western blotting to identify bands of IgG that exist in baby's serum but not in maternal samples,[226] and IgG avidity assays, has been shown to have validity. Placental examination, culture, and PCR testing may also be helpful. Unfortunately, no test is 100% sensitive. In one study, even the combination of placental examination, cord blood IgM and IgA testing, and Western blot for differential IgG assay failed to identify 2 (10%) of 20 children who eventually were proven to be infected.[227] The criterion standard in this study was presence of antibody in the infant's blood beyond 1 year of age.

Syphilis

Any baby born to a mother with a measurable RPR (rapid plasma reagin) titer should be screened for active congenital infection, even if the baby is asymptomatic and has a normal physical examination. Most cases of congenital syphilis result from nontreatment, inadequate treatment, or undocumented treatment of maternal syphilis.[228] The physician should obtain a history of the mother's RPR titer, precisely what therapy the mother received, the timing of therapy, and a posttreatment RPR

titer. If the mother received appropriate benzathine penicillin therapy (2.4 million units IM once; some experts recommend 2 doses a week apart), had therapy completed more than 30 days prior to delivery, and had a posttreatment RPR that was at least four-fold less than the pretreatment titer, the baby should receive a careful examination monthly until the RPR reverts to negative. In all other circumstances, the baby should get a full physical examination, complete blood count, metabolic profile (to include liver function studies); CSF VDRL, cell count, glucose, and protein; and long-bone films in addition to an RPR. Some have argued that long-bone films add little to the diagnostic workup and should be abandoned.[229] However, a large epidemiologic study showed that death from congenital syphilis was more likely when x-rays and/or CSF evaluations were omitted.[228]

Many TORCH test kits are commercially available but should be avoided. Instead, use the techniques of laboratories that participate in proficiency testing.[230] Results of TORCH titer kits have a poor diagnostic record for prenatal screening and for evaluation of young infants.[231]

In general, it is preferable to develop a differential diagnosis of the likely possibilities and then test for each of them instead of reflexively ordering "TORCH titers" (Table 19-1). Some tests are only helpful if negative. For example, if the baby's serum IgG to CMV or rubella is negative, those entities can be ruled out. However, if they are positive, it could be from passive transfer and does not necessarily indicate infection in the baby. Unfortunately, IgM assays for many of the agents of congenital infection (CMV, rubella, and HSV) are not reliable.

Treatment

Syphilis

Elaborate criteria for withholding treatment have been proposed on the basis of the infant's serial RPR results. However, treatment should usually be given if there is a reasonable possibility of congenital syphilis. This includes any cases where the mother's adequate and appropriate treatment, and a response thereto, cannot be clearly documented. Starting one's life with 10 days of intravenous penicillin is infinitely preferable to starting it with undiagnosed and untreated congenital syphilis. No treatment is necessary if the infant's RPR result is negative and the mother is known to have received adequate treatment.

TABLE 19-1. DIFFERENTIATING FEATURES OF SOME CAUSES OF CONGENITAL AND NEONATAL INFECTIONS

CLINICAL FEATURE	ETIOLOGIC AGENT							
	CMV[a]	ENTEROVIRUS	HIV[a]	HSV	LCMV	PARVOVIRUS	RUBELLA[a]	SYPHILIS[a]
General								
Fetal loss	+	−	+	−	+	++	++	++
IUGR	++	−	+	+	−	−	++	++
Prematurity	++	−	+	+	−	++	++	++
Failure to thrive	+	−	++	−	−	−	+	+
Hematologic								
Anemia	+	−	+	+	+	++	+	+
Thrombocytopenia	++	+	+	++	−	++	+	+
Fetal hydrops	+	−	−	+	+	++	−	+
CNS								
Hydrocephaly	+	−	−	+	++	−	−	−
Microcephaly or macrocephaly	++	−	−	+	++	−	+	−
Intracranial calcification[b]	++	−	+	+	++	−	−	−
Retinopathy	++	−	−	+	++	−	+	+
Cataracts	−	−	−	−	−	−	++	−
Deafness	++	−	−	+	−	−	++	+
Gastrointestinal								
Jaundice	++	+	−	+	−	−	++	+
Hepatosplenomegaly	++	+	++	+	−	+	++	++
Elevated ALT	++	++	−	++	−	−	++	++
Cardiac								
Congenital defects	−	−	−	−	−	−	++	−
Myocarditis	−	++	−	+	+	+	−	−
Other organs								
Lymphadenopathy	−	−	++	−	−	−	++	++
Skin rash	+[c]	+[d]	+[e]	++[f]	−	+[c]	++[c]	++[c,g]
Conjunctivitis	−	+	−	++	−	−	−	−
Bony lesions	−	−	−	−	−	−	++	++

Abbreviations: CMV, cytomegalovirus; HIV, human immunodeficiency virus; HSV, herpes simplex virus; LCMV, lymphocytic choriomeningitis virus; IUGR, intrauterine growth retardation; CNS, central nervous system; ALT, alanine aminotransferase.
Key: −, rare or not reported; +, occasionally seen; ++, common finding.
[a] May be asymptomatic in the neonatal period but cause progressive abnormalities later in life.
[b] CMV and LCMV, periventricular; HIV, basal ganglia calcification; HSV, rare reports of diffuse intracerebral calcification secondary to in utero HSV transmission; toxoplasmosis, diffuse intracerebral calcification.
[c] Petechial or purpuric rash.
[d] Erythematous maculopapular rash.
[e] Eczema; also prone to candidal rash and thrush.
[f] Vesicular rash.
[g] Copper-colored maculopapular rash involving palms and soles.

Antibiotic therapy of the newborn infant with proven or suspected congenital syphilis should consist of aqueous penicillin, 50,000 U/kg intravenously (IV) twice a day over a 10-day period, since neurosyphilis is difficult to exclude (Table 15-1).[232] Procaine penicillin 50,000 U/kg per dose given IM once a day may be substituted. Procaine penicillin has a small risk of producing a sterile abscess. Failure of procaine penicillin therapy to eradicate severe infection has been reported.[233] Some advocate the use of a single IM dose of 50,000 U/kg of benzathine penicillin for babies at low risk for congenital syphilis (for example, those whose mother's treatment response was not documented, and who have normal screening evaluations). This treatment option is based on a study that demonstrated good outcomes for a cohort of babies treated in this fashion.[234] The number of babies in the study was not sufficient to convince us that IM benzathine penicillin is a reliable option. It is conceptually and practically more rational to dichotomize infants into those who require treatment and those who do not. Those who need treatment should be given a full course of IV penicillin.

Toxoplasmosis

Treatment for congenitally infected infants, whether symptomatic or asymptomatic, is advocated. The combination of pyrimethamine and sulfadiazine is synergistic. Folinic acid (leucovorin) must be administered with pyrimethamine or severe anemia may develop. Dosages are as follows: pyrimethamine, 2 mg/kg per day for 2 days, then 1 mg/kg per day for 2–6 months, then 1 mg/kg per day MWF (Monday, Wednesday, Friday) out to 1 year; sulfadiazine, 100 mg/kg per day for 2–6 months, then MWF to 1 year; leukovorin, 5 mg to 10 mg 3 times a week. Because of the long half-life of pyrimethamine, leukovorin should be continued for 1 week after therapy is stopped. Some experts recommend adding prednisone, 1 mg/kg per day divided every 12 hours if the CSF protein is greater than 1 g/dL, or if the patient has active chorioretinitis that threatens vision.

Outcomes are better with prolonged treatment. The exact optimal duration has not been determined. Studies clearly show that outcome is better with 12 months of therapy than with one month.[205] A retrospective study of 78 children with congenital toxoplasmosis treated for 12 months versus 24 months suggested that outcome was slightly better in babies treated for 24 months.[235] Immunologic rebounds, mostly asymptomatic, occurred in 90% of cases regardless of treatment duration. Results of properly treated congenital toxoplasmosis are encouraging: CNS lesions generally resolve or stabilize, and intellectual functioning, although generally lower than siblings, seems to be stable over time.[205]

Cytomegalovirus

Ganciclovir inhibits the replication of CMV in vitro and in vivo, and is effective against CMV infection in immunocompromised hosts. However, its role in the treatment of congenital CMV infection remains uncertain. Recently, the results of a randomized, controlled trial of ganciclovir in neonates with symptomatic CMV were published.[236] Infants younger than 1 month of age, more than 32 weeks gestation, and weighing more than 1200 g at birth were eligible for participation. Patients were randomized to receive ganciclovir (6 mg/kg/dose given intravenously every 12 hours for 6 weeks) or no treatment. Hearing, as measured by brain stem evoked response (BSER) at 6 and 12 months, was the primary outcome measured. Twenty-one (84%) of 25 ganciclovir recipients had improved hearing or maintained normal hearing between baseline and 6 months versus 10 (59%) of 17 control patients ($P = 0.06$). By one year, 21% of ganciclovir recipients had worsening of their hearing from baseline as compared with 68% of controls ($P < 0.01$).

Although these results are encouraging, there are several caveats. The intervention is not benign. Nearly two-thirds of ganciclovir recipients developed drug-induced neutropenia. In addition, treatment requires the placement of a central venous catheter. If treatment with ganciclovir is considered, these issues should be discussed openly with the family. Pharmacokinetic studies of oral valganciclovir infants are ongoing. The availability of an oral drug for this population may allow more infants to be treated.

Herpes Simplex Virus

The treatment of HSV infection in neonates, particularly the treatment for CNS disease, is evolving. Vidarabine, the original treatment of choice, has been replaced by acyclovir. The dose of IV acyclovir has been doubled, from 30 mg/kg per day to 60 mg/kg per day divided t.i.d. for term infants with normal renal function. The duration of therapy has lengthened; current standard of care includes 21 days of IV acyclovir for CNS or disseminated disease and 14 days for SEM disease. Most experts recommend a follow-up lumbar puncture (LP), with repeat PCR at the end of the 3 weeks of therapy, with prolongation of the IV course if the PCR remains positive. We generally retest the CSF weekly until the HSV PCR is negative. Quantitation of virus in CSF is now possible; the exact clinical correlate of these numbers is not clearly defined.

Case reports suggest that endogenous reactivation of HSV inside the CNS may also occur,[237] analogous to the recurrences seen in SEM disease. When skin lesions do not accompany the CNS disease, reactivation may be difficult to detect. Some patients begin to lose developmental milestones previously attained. This can be accompanied by elevated cell counts and protein levels in the CSF.[238] Symptomatic reactivation, producing recurrences of HSV encephalitis, have also been reported.[239] In one case, reactivation CNS disease accompanied by recurrent skin lesions was managed with long-term oral acyclovir, with an excellent outcome.[240] Oral acyclovir is poorly absorbed; doses of between 1,000 and 2,500 mg/m^2/dose are required to attain serum levels of greater than 2 μg/mL.[241] Much smaller doses have been successfully employed to suppress recurrences of SEM disease.[223] It is likely that the recommended treatment for HSV encephalitis will continue to evolve. As durations of therapy have increased, outcomes have improved. Supportive care measures have improved during this period as well. A randomized trial of suppressive therapy is ongoing.

■ NEONATAL SEPSIS AND MENINGITIS

The diagnosis of septicemia of the newborn is one of the most difficult in the field of pediatric infectious diseases, primarily because diagnostic studies are not helpful soon enough and the possible consequences of delayed therapy are severe morbidity or death. The risk is even greater in premature infants, who may already have numerous other physiological handicaps.

Definitions

As discussed in Chapter 10, "sepsis" is usually the presumptive diagnosis when there is clinical suspicion of infection and evidence of a systemic response (tachycardia, tachypnea, hyperthermia, hypothermia).[242] Suspected sepsis becomes confirmed sepsis when the blood culture proves positive.

Sources

Most newborns with confirmed early-onset sepsis do not have any apparent source of infection. However, in the first days of life, aspiration of contaminated amniotic fluid is probably the source of the bacteremia, as it usually is for group B streptococcal sepsis and meningitis. In premature infants requiring ventilation or surgical procedures, the risk of colonization or infection can persist for weeks, as they stay in an intensive care unit and are exposed to various necessary invasive procedures.

Time of Onset

Early-onset Sepsis

This is defined as the occurrence of septicemia in the first 7 days after birth. In this form, the infection of the infant usually began in utero. In the worst form of early-onset septicemia, the infant is born macerated with a generalized disseminated bacterial infection. In less severe forms, there may be no external evidence of generalized infection except for fetal distress before birth and respiratory distress, apnea, or limpness after birth. The mortality rate is generally higher in early-onset than in late-onset sepsis, especially in fulminant cases. In such patients, it is advisable to obtain cultures of blood, urine, and spinal fluid (if the patient is sufficiently stable), and to begin antibiotic therapy immediately.

Late-onset Sepsis

Late-onset sepsis is defined as septicemia occurring after day 7 of life. The baby typically is normal at birth. The clinical manifestations of sepsis then develop. The identity of the infecting pathogen is a more important predictor of the prognosis of neonatal sepsis than is the timing of the infection, although early-onset Group B streptococcal and *Listeria* infections have a worse prognosis than do the late-onset forms.

In late-onset sepsis, the full-term baby does well in the first week of life and is discharged from the hospital gaining weight and having no difficulty. However, the appearance of fever, subnormal temperature, tachypnea or apnea, jaundice, vomiting, or failure to eat well any time in the first month of life should be considered a possible indication of septicemia of the late-onset type (Box 19-3). In such cases, the baby should be hospitalized and cultures obtained of blood, spinal fluid, urine, and any area that appears to be a source of infection. A diagnosis of presumptive sepsis should be made and antibiotic therapy started without awaiting the results of cultures.

In the premature infant in the intensive care nursery, the bacteria are likely to be those related to procedures such as ventilation and intravascular catheters, and the signs of illness are subtler than in the term infant (Box 19-3).

Predisposing Factors

Predisposing factors can be divided into maternal, neonatal, and treatment related (Box 19-4).[243] Prolonged rupture of membranes and amnionitis may exert their major influence by predisposing to prematurity, the most significant of the many factors in neonatal sepsis.

Neonatal Factors

The newborn has greater susceptibility to infections than older infants for several reasons, but princi-

---

BOX 19-3 ■ Signs Suggesting Neonatal Sepsis

Early Onset
Fetal distress before delivery
Meconium staining of amniotic fluid
Respiratory distress
*Persistent tachycardia
*Hypothermia or hyperthermia
*Apneic and bradycardic spells
Meconium aspiration
*Hypotension

Late Onset in Full-term Infants
*Jaundice
*Poor sucking, poor feeding, vomiting, poor
   weight gain
*Lethargy, decreased muscle tone, seizures
*Abdominal distention, diarrhea
*Skin mottling or cold skin
*Fever

Late Onset in Premature Infant in Intensive Care
*Same as for above infants
Increasing ventilator oxygen requirement
Decreased perfusion detected by pulse and blood
   pressure

---

pally because of the immaturity of almost all measurable functions of immunity.[251] In addition, labor often results in relative hypoxemia and acidosis in the infant. Developmental abnormalities can contribute to the risk of infection.

Maternal Factors

Management of premature rupture of the membranes involves the risks of delivery of a premature infant, balanced with the risks of maternal or fetal ascending infection.[244] Adverse fetal outcome is related to the premature delivery as much as to the infection.[245] Amniocentesis may provide information on fetal lung maturity, provide cultures useful in the treatment of amnionitis, and allow continuation of pregnancy; however, these steps do not always improve the fetal outcome.[246] Group B streptococcus (GBS) is the most common cause of neonatal sepsis; the bacterium is carried in the genital tract and/or rectum of 15% – 30% of all women of childbearing age. Not much is known about why some women are carriers and others are not. One study suggests that the rate of GBS carriage is higher in women who smoke.[247] In this analysis, age, weight, race, income level, marital status, number of prenatal visits, parity, and history of drug use were found not to be associated with the carriage of GBS.[247] The purported association between cigarette smoking and GBS carriage has not been previously reported, nor has the study yet been replicated.

Repeated or prolonged courses of antenatal steroids are not associated with antenatal maternal fever, chorioamnionitis, or neonatal sepsis.[248] Maternal epidural receipt causes more patients to have prolonged rupture of membranes, induces fetal tachycardia, and leads to low-grade temperature elevations in the laboring mother, ultimately causing a higher percentage of their babies to undergo sepsis evaluations (20% versus 9%); however, the incidence of sepsis in their offspring is not increased.[249]

Treatment-related Factors

As listed in Box 19-4, the process of resuscitation and treatment of neonatal problems adds to the risk of infection, especially when monitoring or treatment devices are needed.

Prevention

Prevention of neonatal sepsis has focused primarily on reducing the risk of GBS. In the past, two differ-

BOX 19-4 ■ Predisposing Factors in Neonatal Sepsis

Neonatal
Prematurity
Congenital anomalies
Skin or umbilical cord infection
Necrotizing enterocolitis
Asphyxia

Maternal
Amnionitis
Bleeding
Prolonged labor
Difficult delivery
Fetal distress
Premature rupture of membranes
Prolonged (> 12 hours) rupture of membranes
Urinary tract infection
Lack of prenatal care
Coitus in prepartum week[251]

Treatment Related
Intravascular catheters
Respiratory intubation
Scalp electrodes
Hand contamination of health care workers
Contaminated equipment
Parenteral nutrition

ent approaches to this clinical problem were advocated. One approach had all pregnant women undergo screening cultures of the rectum and vagina at 35–37 weeks' gestation, and all women who screened positive were given intrapartum antibiotic prophylaxis (IAP). The other approach was risk-based. This approach was based on the fact that mothers who are GBS carriers are much more likely to transmit infection when certain risk factors are present, namely prolonged (> 18 hours) or premature (prior to 37 weeks) rupture of membranes, or maternal fever (greater than 38.0°C). Both strategies lead to IAP of approximately the same percentage of mothers, as the GBS carriage rate is around 20%, and approximately 20% of laboring mothers develop the risk factors mentioned.[252] Studies that compared the protective efficacy of the two strategies head-to-head have clearly demonstrated the superiority of the culture-based screening approach.[253] Therefore, the risk-based approach is no longer endorsed.[254] A large study involving more than 52,000 births estimated that the screen and treat approach decreased GBS sepsis by 68%.[255]

All pregnant women should undergo rectovaginal (not just vaginal) culture at 35–37 weeks' gestation. The culture should be incubated in selective broth medium, rather than on plain agar plates. Mothers whose cultures are positive for GBS should be given IAP, preferably using penicillin, starting at least 4 hours prior to delivery if possible. A history of penicillin allergy should be carefully investigated; many patients who claim to be allergic to penicillin lack a convincing history and can be safely given penicillin. Those judged to be at high risk for anaphylaxis can be given clindamycin. Those deemed to be penicillin allergic but at low risk for anaphylaxis should be given cefazolin. Antibiotic prophylaxis is not necessary for nonlaboring women undergoing planned cesarean delivery over intact membranes.

For women who do not undergo GBS screening (either because of delivery prior to scheduled screening or because screening was inadvertently omitted), IAP should be administered if any of the following apply: (a) delivery before 37 weeks, (b) rupture of membranes longer than 18 hours, or (c) intrapartum temperature greater than 38°C.

Women with GBS bacteriuria during their current pregnancy or who previously gave birth to an infant with GBS disease should also receive IAP.

Management of the baby born to a woman who received IAP is shown in Box 19-5.

Concerns about GBS Prevention Protocols

Some have been concerned that focusing prevention efforts on GBS might lead to a compensatory increase in sepsis attributable to other pathogens. Most studies of this issue show that the incidence of non-GBS sepsis remained the same,[256,257] or even decreased slightly[258] after GBS-prevention methods were introduced.

Others expressed concern that widespread use of IAP might lead to increased antibiotic resistance in GBS isolates or in other bacteria that cause neonatal sepsis. No change in antibiotic susceptibilities of GBS isolates has been noted. Ampicillin resistance among *E. coli* isolates has been increasing in recent years; it is not clear how much of this trend can be blamed on IAP protocols. However, in one study, the amount of ampicillin resistance in clinical isolates from babies with sepsis correlated positively with the number of doses of ampicillin the mother received prenatally.[259] This issue is potentially important and needs further study; in one report, am-

---

BOX 19-5 ■ Approach to the Baby Whose Mother Received Intrapartum Antibiotic Prophylaxis (IAP)

1. Ascertain the rationale behind the IAP. Suspected chorioamnionitis? Workup and treat for sepsis.
2. Assess the baby. Ill appearing? Workup and treat for sepsis. Well appearing but less than 35 weeks' EGA[a]? Limited evaluation and observation for at least 48 hours.
3. Ascertain duration of IAP. Less than 4 hours? Limited evaluation and observation.
4. Babies >35 weeks' EGA whose mothers received IAP for >4 hours as prophylaxis because of GBS carrier state and who are well-appearing at initial evaluation can be observed for at least 48 hours. Evaluation and therapy are not required, provided that the baby maintains a well state.

[a] EGA, estimated gestational age.

---

picillin resistance was associated with increased mortality.[255] It should be remembered, however, that because GBS is a much more common cause of early-onset neonatal sepsis than are the gram-negative rods, the overall impact of GBS-prevention protocols has been decreased perinatal mortality. In addition, the vast majority of *E. coli* isolates remain sensitive to gentamicin and cefotaxime, one of which should be used along with ampicillin for empiric treatment in the newborn with suspected sepsis.

Clinical Diagnosis

The diagnosis of presumptive neonatal sepsis is based on a history of predisposing factors, physical findings, and laboratory results other than blood cultures. The diagnosis of "suspected sepsis" needs to be made as early as possible, and treatment needs to begin without waiting for the results of a blood culture to confirm sepsis. If the blood culture is negative at 48 hours, the decision to continue antibiotics depends on clinical suspicion of sepsis. If the clinical suspicion is low, antibiotics may be stopped. The problem-oriented diagnosis is then "evaluation for possible sepsis." If the baby is clinically improved, but based on the baby's initial presentation the suspicion of sepsis is high, antibiotics are sometimes continued even with negative cultures. The problem-oriented diagnosis is then "culture-negative sepsis." If the baby's clinical condition is not improving, in addition to continuing antibiotics (or adding new ones) a vigorous search for a focus should be undertaken (e.g., repeat lumbar puncture (LP) to include HSV PCR, and/or imaging studies).

Signs suggesting sepsis are listed in Box 19-3. One study indicated that persistent tachycardia exceeding 160 beats/minute in infants less than 72 hours old is a useful sign of early-onset sepsis.[260] A prospective study in a neonatal intensive care unit found that otherwise well-appearing babies had decreased baseline heart-rate variability and short-lived decelerations starting about 24 hours prior to abrupt sepsis or sepsis-like events.[261]

Laboratory Approach

Cultures

Blood, spinal fluid, urine, and any apparently infected lesion should usually be cultured. Small newborns with severe respiratory distress need not be routinely subjected to LP. However, a single negative blood culture does not reliably exclude meningitis. An LP should usually be performed once the infant is stable (and especially if the blood culture is positive). A study of 43 infants with bacterial meningitis in the first 3 days of life found that the diagnosis would have been delayed or missed in 16 (37%) had selective criteria for LP been used.[262]

Urine cultures have a low yield of additional information in the first few days of life and may usually be omitted. They should not be omitted in the child with late-onset disease. If a urine culture is obtained, the specimen should be obtained by catheter or bladder puncture for maximum accuracy. Microscopic examination of the cerebrospinal fluid, or occasionally the urine, may provide immediate information about the likely infecting organism. Microscopic examination of a gastric aspirate shortly after birth may indicate amniotic fluid inflammation (leukocytosis) and may show bacteria, but rarely adds new information, except to indicate unsuspected amnionitis.

Automated blood-culture systems have made recovery of organisms more rapid and more reliable.[263] In newborns with suspected sepsis, 77%,

89%, and 94% of blood cultures that are eventually going to turn positive have done so by 24, 36, and 48 hours of incubation, respectively.[264] It should be remembered that even a negative blood culture does not eliminate the possibility of serious nonbacteremic bacterial infections. Indeed, in one study, 18% of 100 autopsied infants who died of a serious bacterial infection did not have a positive blood culture, indicating that "blood cultures may be negative in newborns dying with significant foci of bacterial infection."[265] Furthermore, abnormalities of the white blood cell count, differential, and platelet counts were not invariably specific for bacterial infection[265] (see following text).

Nonspecific Laboratory Tests

Hematologic Parameters

In the late 1970s, Manroe and colleagues studied hematologic values in both well and sick babies in an attempt to establish norms.[266] Many nurseries have used the immature to total neutrophil count ("I/T ratio") as a screening tool for sepsis. A more recent survey of neutrophil and band counts in healthy term newborns suggests that variability is greater than previously suspected; the mean I/T ratio was 0.16, but the 10th to 90th percentile range was from 0.05 to 0.27.[267] The same investigators also found that there was a wide interreader variability in the interpretation of cells as being either "neutrophils" or "bands."[268] This would obviously change the value of the I/T ratio, calling its utility into question. In addition, others have found that the absolute neutrophil count and I/T ratios evolve; therefore, the test is better when it is repeated.[269] In a large clinical trial, a normal initial I/T ratio, even when followed by a normal immature to mature (I/M) ratio and coupled with a platelet count greater than 150,000 per mcL, had a negative predictive value of only 94% for the absence of sepsis.[270] In another study, an I/T ratio cut-off of 0.2 had a sensitivity of 78% and specificity of 73% in predicting sepsis.[271]

In one study, 18 of 18 premature neonates with late-onset coagulase-negative staphylococcal septicemia had elevated mean platelet volumes, which returned to normal values with correction of sepsis.[272]

C-reactive Protein (CRP)

Compared with other measures of inflammation, most investigators feel that the CRP is the "best test."[273] Even so, a value of greater than 1 mg/dL has a sensitivity of only 85% and a specificity of only 62% for sepsis.[273] Other investigators found that the initial CRP did not reliably discriminate infected from noninfected neonates, but that a repeat CRP 24–48 hours later that was less than 1 mg/dL had a negative predictive value of 99%.

Interleukin-6 (IL-6) and Interleukin-8 (IL-8) Levels

IL-6 levels are elevated in both maternal serum[274] and in cord blood[275] of babies who develop early-onset sepsis. In late-onset sepsis, IL-6 levels go up 1–2 days prior to the onset of sepsis or sepsis-like episodes.[276] One group of investigators found, however, that IL-6 levels were highly elevated in the cord blood of *all* sick babies, not just in those with infectious diseases.[277] Another group found that IL-6 levels were helpful in the diagnosis of sepsis or serious bacterial infections in premature neonates but not in term babies.[278]

Unlike IL-6, elevated IL-8 levels are specific for infectious illness,[277] but the sensitivity of IL-8 levels for sepsis are not as good as those of IL-6, no matter what cutoff value is established.[275] In Germany, a nursery used IL-8 levels of greater than 53 pg/dL and/or a CRP of greater than 1 mg/dL as a screening tool for late-onset sepsis in their premature neonate population; this yielded a 94% sensitivity and decreased antibiotic use by 73%.[279]

Although helpful adjuncts, normal nonspecific laboratory tests never rule out the possibility of neonatal sepsis. The three broad categories to evaluate—risk factors for sepsis, postnatal clinical signs, and laboratory tests—must each be considered. Concern with any *one* of these three factors is sufficient reason to initiate a sepsis evaluation and begin empiric antibiotic therapy in a newborn.

Bacterial Causes

Group B streptococci and *E. coli* remain the most frequent causes of neonatal sepsis and meningitis in the first month of life.[280] Other enteric gram-negative bacteria (especially *Klebsiella*), *Listeria*,[281] *Staphylococcus aureus*, and viridans streptococci,[282] are other possible causes.

Infants with long stays in intensive care units, repeated episodes of suspected sepsis, and many courses of antibiotics can have sepsis with *Staphylococcus epidermidis* (usually from intravascular catheters),[283] *Candida albicans* or *Candida parapsilosis* (especially very low-birth-weight infants),[284] and bacteria that have become colonizing flora in such patients (*Pseudomonas aeruginosa*, *Stenotrophomonas maltophilia*, *Enterobacter cloacae*, *Citrobacter freundii*, *Acinetobacter* spp., and anaerobes). Unsuspected serious infection is common at postmortem examination in infants from this setting.[285] *Mycoplasma*, *Ureaplasma*, and *Lactobacillus* species (from the mother's cervix) are very rare causes of sepsis.[286–288]

Many other bacterial species have been reported as rare causes of neonatal sepsis and meningitis, including meningococci, pneumococci, *Campylobacter*, and a host of maternal genital normal flora (Chapter 15).[286–288] Since the development of better anaerobic techniques, *Bacteroides*, *Clostridium*, *Peptococcus*, *Peptostreptococcus*, and *Veillonella* species have been recovered in neonatal sepsis.[289,290]

Atypical mycobacteria are a rare cause of sepsis in the newborn.[291] The nursery environment might be a source. Standard blood culture or acid-fast stain of an abscess may be useful for detection.

Meningitis

Neonatal septicemia is associated with meningitis about 30% of the time.[280] The same principles of early diagnosis and therapy apply to meningitis as to septicemia, except that the drugs selected should penetrate the spinal fluid well. Meningitis in the newborn and young infant is discussed in Chapter 9.

Diseases Resembling Sepsis

While treating a newborn for "suspected sepsis," the clinician should consider the long list of conditions resembling sepsis, so they can be looked for and treated if found (Box 19-6).

Antibiotic Treatment

The most important feature in treatment of neonatal sepsis is that antibiotic therapy not be delayed while awaiting results of cultures. When neonatal sepsis is suspected, specimens should be taken and treatment begun immediately. As a rule, any infant who is thought to be sick enough to require a sepsis evaluation should be regarded as sick enough to be treated with antibiotics for sepsis.

The initial antibiotics, before culture results are available, should be chosen in view of the probability of various causative organisms. Many bacteria

---

BOX 19-6 ■ Some Diseases Resembling Neonatal Bacterial Sepsis

Other Infections
Disseminated viral infections: herpesvirus, enterovirus
Viral meningitis
Chronic active congenital infection
Fungal sepsis
Pneumonia, diarrhea, urinary tract infection, peritonitis

Respiratory Diseases
Respiratory distress syndrome, transient tachypnea
Pneumothorax, hemorrhage, meconium aspiration

Neurologic Diseases
Intracranial hemorrhage, seizures, malformations

Cardiovascular Diseases
Patent ductus arteriosus, hypoplastic left heart syndrome

Hematologic Diseases
ABO incompatibility, polycythemia, anemia

Metabolic Diseases
Urea cycle disorders, other congenital enzymatic defects
Accidental poisoning

Gastrointestinal Diseases
Necrotizing enterocolitis
Congenital malformations

---

can be causes of neonatal sepsis, as discussed in the preceding section, which explains the variety of regimens recommended for use before culture results are available. The best reference on antibiotic selection and dosages, especially for newborns and premature infants, is Nelson's *Pocketbook of Pediatric Antimicrobial Therapy*, which is revised every other year. Regimens may vary somewhat depending on local susceptibility patterns. In most locations, the best empiric regimen for suspected neonatal sepsis remains ampicillin and gentamicin. If meningitis is suspected based on CSF findings, cefotaxime should be added to the above regimen. Therapy can then be adjusted based on culture and sensitivity results.

If *S. aureus* is suspected, nafcillin or oxacillin may be substituted for ampicillin. Empiric vancomycin is not necessary, even for babies with intravascular catheters, as coagulase-negative staphylococcal infection is rarely fulminant.[292] For infants who have been long-term intensive care patients, ceftazidime is appropriate as it has activity against most strains of *Pseudomonas,* which carries the highest case-fatality rate of any bacterial cause of late-onset sepsis in these patients.[292] Risk factors for candidemia include prematurity, intravascular catheters, hyperalimentation, prolonged intensive care unit (ICU) stays (particularly if endotracheal intubation is prolonged), and, most importantly, frequent or prolonged antibacterial therapy.[293,294]

Mucocutaneous candidiasis is also a predictor of subsequent invasive candidal infection. In one prospective study of infants less than 1,500 g, 9 (32%) of 28 infants with mucocutaneous candidiasis developed invasive disease compared with 7 (2%) of 330 infants without mucocutaneous candidiasis.[295]

In patients with the above risk factors who fail to respond to initial empiric therapy, evidence for invasive fungal disease (renal ultrasound, retinal examination) should be done and consideration should be given to adding amphotericin B or fluconazole.

Nonantibiotic Treatment

Fresh whole-blood exchange transfusions, leukocyte transfusions, fresh adult human plasma, and intravenous immune globulin have been used to treat neonatal sepsis. None of these interventions have been clearly shown to be of benefit.

Prevention

Antibiotic prophylaxis should not be given on the basis of prematurity alone. Antibiotics should be administered to premature neonates who have other risk factors or signs of sepsis, such as hypoglycemia, prolonged premature rupture of membranes, respiratory distress, maternal fever, and the like. This practice results in most premature babies receiving antibiotics for 48–72 hours while blood cultures are incubating.

A recent study suggests that prophylactic fluconazole, given intravenously for the first 6 weeks of life to very low-birth-weight infants, reduced both colonization and infection with fungal pathogens.[296] A concern about the development of fluconazole resistance has kept most nurseries from adopting this practice.

■ MISCELLANEOUS NEONATAL INFECTIONS

This section discusses some selected focal infections, by organ system. Newborn infections of other anatomic areas are covered in their appropriate chapters.

Bone and Joint Infections

Septic arthritis and osteomyelitis in neonates are discussed in Chapter 16.

Ear Infections

Absent or limited mobility of the tympanic membranes is frequently found by pneumatic otoscopy in the first 72 hours of life.[297] In the normal newborn of this age, the tympanic membrane may appear pink or red without crying.

Young infants in an intensive care nursery who had tympanocentesis because of a clinical diagnosis of acute otitis media had a higher frequency of enteric bacteria in their middle ear compared with outpatients, who are more likely to have respiratory flora, such as *Streptococcus pneumoniae* and *Haemophilus influenzae*.[298]

Gastrointestinal Infections

Necrotizing Enterocolitis (NEC)

Newborns with NEC initially present with abdominal distention and retention of feedings. They may then progress rapidly to a picture resembling sepsis. About one-quarter of patients develop bloody stools. NEC is most common in the first 2 weeks of life but onset may be delayed in very low-birth-weight babies. Evidence of pneumatosis intestinalis on abdominal plain films is highly specific for NEC but has a sensitivity of less than 75%. CT may be more sensitive. Portal vein gas is a sign of severe disease; pneumoperitoneum indicates a perforation.

Despite the fact that NEC has been a recognized complication of extreme prematurity for decades, the pathogenesis of this clinical entity remains mysterious. The principal risk factors are prematurity, enteral feeding, and bacterial colonization.[299] Hypoxia or ischemia/reperfusion injury may also be involved,[300] although in animal models the full-term gut is much more susceptible to this type of insult.[301] Infection may be a contributory or precipitating cause, because outbreaks occur.[302] Experimentally, endotoxin in stool filtrates from *E. coli, K. pneumoniae, Enterobacter* spp, and *Clostridium* spp correlates with risk of NEC.[303] In one small outbreak, blood cultures from 3 of 6 patients were positive for a new species of *Clostridium*, dubbed *C. neonatale*.[304] Perhaps the strongest link to infection is a study of contamination of enteral feeding tubes. During the course of this study, 7 babies developed NEC; all of them had been fed formula found to be contaminated with more than 100,000 cfu/mL of gram-negative rods.[305] Four of the seven required surgery, and surgical cultures recovered the same bacteria found in their feeding tubes.[305]

Breast milk feeding appears to offer significant protection.[306] Supplementing tube feeds with lactobacilli is fruitless,[307] as are oral immunoglobulins.[308] Oral antibiotic prophylaxis decreases the incidence of NEC somewhat, but at the cost of producing antibiotic-resistant organisms.[309] Premature babies are generally arginine deficient, and low plasma arginine levels have been postulated as a possible risk factor. A large, blinded, placebo-controlled trial of L-arginine supplementation demonstrated a decrease incidence of NEC from 27% to 7%.[310] Unfortunately, the incidence in the control group was very high, and stage 1 NEC (which can be a rather subjective diagnosis) was used as one endpoint.[310]

Treatment is with bowel rest, nasogastric suction, and antibiotics (such as ampicillin, gentamicin, and metronidazole). Although many cases can be managed nonoperatively, consultation with a pediatric surgeon is strongly recommended. Surgical intervention is indicated for patients with evidence of perforation or in cases that progressively worsen despite optimal medical management.[311]

The mortality rate associated with laparotomy for perforated necrotizing enterocolitis is significantly higher among neonates with a body weight of less than 1,000 g. For this reason, bedside placement of peritoneal drains is used initially in place of laparotomy for the management of perforation in the smallest newborns. Approximately one-third of neonates treated with the placement of drains die from the disease, one-third require subsequent laparotomy and bowel resection for necrotizing enterocolitis-related obstruction or undrained abscess, and one-third do not require further surgery.[312]

Neonatal Appendicitis

Appendicitis is rare in the newborn infant and is likely to be discovered only if the patient is operated on for necrotizing enterocolitis.[313] Mucormycosis is a rare cause of appendicitis or bowel perforation in premature or young infants.[314]

Diarrhea

Common diarrheal pathogens can be transmitted to the newborn, including *Salmonella, Shigella, Campylobacter, Yersinia*, rotavirus, and others. The infections may be mistaken for necrotizing enterocolitis.[315,316]

Pulmonary Infections

Afebrile Interstitial Pneumonitis

A variety of aspirated maternal cervical flora can be recovered from infants with pneumonia in the first weeks of life, especially in those born prematurely. These organisms include CMV, *Chlamydia trachomatis, C. albicans*, mycoplasmas, ureaplasmas, trichomonas, herpes simplex, *Pneumocystis jiroveci* (formerly *carinii*) and *Bacteroides* species.[317–325] Some of these isolates may be coincidental in a particular infant, but etiologic associations are well documented for many of these pathogens in neonates from 2–12 weeks of age [317] *Bacteroides* spp, *Candida* spp, and *Trichomonas vaginalis* lack a proven association.

In one series of CMV infections with diffuse interstitial pneumonia, the infants were noted to have a gray pallor, enlarged liver and spleen, atypical lymphocytosis, deteriorating respiratory function, and a septic appearance.[318] Most of the babies apparently acquired the disease after birth, perhaps from blood transfusions.

Outbreaks of acquired interstitial pneumonia can occur in nurseries and are usually attributed to respiratory syncytial virus or parainfluenza viruses. Mumps can produce severe pneumonia in the newborn in the absence of transplacental antibodies.

Erythromycin is the treatment of choice for chlamydial pneumonia, which is the most likely treatable infectious cause of afebrile interstitial pneumonia. Metronidazole has been effective when *Trichomonas* has been documented.[322]

Fulminant Pneumonia

Herpes simplex virus can cause rapidly fatal pneumonia without skin lesions and may respond to acyclovir.[325] Adenoviruses and *Pneumocystis jiroreci* can also cause relentlessly progressive pneumonia.[326,327]

Newborn Exposed to Tuberculosis (TB)

Newborns exposed to patients with active pulmonary TB are at high risk of becoming infected. Cases should be reported promptly to public health authorities, as a contact investigation to detect additional cases is critical. If the active case is the mother, the infant should be evaluated for the possibility of congenital tuberculosis (see following text). The baby should generally receive isoniazid even if there is no evidence of disease and despite a negative skin test and normal chest x-ray. Ideally, the infant is separated from the adult with active TB until noncontagiousness is ensured. However, when the active case is the mother, this is usually not practical. The infant's isoniazid may be discontinued at 4–6 months if the condition is asymptomatic and a repeat chest x-ray and tuberculin skin test are negative.

If a household contact of a newborn is found to have latent TB infection (LTBI) only (not active disease), a contact investigation is again critical to make sure there are no cases of active disease to which the infant may have been exposed. Separation is not necessary, and the baby does not need isoniazid (unless the contact investigation is delayed). The baby may continue to breast-feed. If the mother is taking isoniazid, both mother and nursing baby should receive pyridoxine (vitamin B6).[328] For the baby, this can be in the form of a standard liquid multivitamin.

Congenital Tuberculosis

Although uncommon, congenital tuberculosis is becoming increasingly recognized. About half of cases are a result of hematogenous spread via the placenta and about half are due to aspiration of infected amniotic fluid.[329]

The presenting symptoms are nonspecific. The most common signs are hepatosplenomegaly, respiratory distress, and fever. Chorioretinitis may be present, mimicking other causes of congenital infection, such as CMV and toxoplasmosis. Occasionally, infants may present with a fulminant picture of septic shock and disseminated intravascular coagulation.[330]

The median age at onset is 24 days (range, 1–84 days). In one review, 24 (75%) of 32 mothers were completely asymptomatic prior to delivery.[331] This underscores the importance of performing a tuberculin skin test on all pregnant women with epidemiologic risk factors for tuberculosis (such as being foreign-born).

Making the diagnosis promptly is critical to patient survival. If suspected, tuberculin skin testing should be performed (though it is usually negative in infants); any induration is suggestive of TB. Gastric aspirates, endotracheal aspirates (if the child is intubated), and spinal fluid should be sent for acid-fast bacteria stain and mycobacterial culture. If still available, the placenta should be examined for histological evidence of TB. The mother should undergo an evaluation to exclude pulmonary and extrapulmonary tuberculosis. If suspicion for congenital tuberculosis is high, four-drug therapy is initiated (usually isoniazid, rifampin, pyrazinamide, and streptomycin) and continued for 2 months. If isolates are susceptible to isoniazid and rifampin, these agents are continued to complete a 12-month course. Unlike most young children with tuberculosis, infants with congenital tuberculosis may be contagious and should be cared for using airborne precautions.[332]

Pulmonary Candidiasis

In the full-term infant with candidal pneumonia, the infant usually has thrush, and the mother is found to have vaginal candidiasis. Typically, the infant has cyanosis, rales, and a pulmonary infiltrate. In premature infants, pulmonary candidiasis occurs in association with disseminated candidiasis.[333] It is difficult to be certain of the antemortem diagnosis in term infants, because secretions obtained from the trachea by bronchoscopy or direct laryngoscopy may be contaminated by *Candida* from the oropharynx.

Lung Abscess

A report of 6 cases of neonatal lung abscess indicated the causes were group B streptococci, *E. coli*, and *Klebsiella pneumoniae*.[334] Two patients had previously unrecognized congenital cystic malformations. In four patients, partial lung resection was required.

Noninfectious Pulmonary Diseases

Many abnormal chest roentgenograms reflect congenital anatomic abnormalities, aspiration, and

---

BOX 19-7 ■ Noninfectious Neonatal
Pulmonary Diseases

Bronchopulmonary dysplasia
Transient tachypnea of the newborn (aspirated
   amniotic fluid)
Respiratory distress syndrome (immature
   surfactant system)
Aspiration pneumonia
Meconium aspiration
Pulmonary hemorrhage
Postextubation lobar opacification
Congenital lung abnormalities
Pneumatoceles, lung cysts, interstitial air
Pulmonary alveolar proteinosis
Necrotizing tracheobronchitis

---

complications of ventilator therapy, such as necrotizing tracheobronchitis (Box 19-7).[335]

Skin Infections

Pyogenic Infections

Scalp abscesses may occur at the site of intrauterine electrodes and can be caused by maternal cervical flora.[336,337] Neonatal mastitis is usually caused by *S. aureus*, but can be caused by any bacteria, including group B streptococci and gram-negative organisms.[338]

Umbilical cord infection (omphalitis) is usually secondary to *S. aureus* or streptococci.[339] Moist or "smelly" cords need to be distinguished from true omphalitis, which will have associated erythema, swelling, or drainage. The most serious complication of omphalitis is necrotizing fasciitis (Chapter 17), which occurs in 13–26% of cases.[340,341]

Prevention of omphalitis is by good cord care, which usually consists of triple dye application in the nursery and once or twice daily alcohol until the cord separates.[342]

Noninfectious rashes are often a concern in newborns because they can be mistaken for infections, as described in the following text.

Transient Neonatal Pustular Melanosis

This skin disorder occurs more frequently in black infants and can resemble erythema toxicum. However, the lesions contain segmented neutrophils rather than the eosinophils of erythema toxicum.[343,344]

Acropustulosis of Infancy

Beginning in the first few months of life, small vesicles rapidly progress to pustules.[344,345] The disease can be mistaken for HSV infection.

Incontinentia Pigmenti

This hereditary disease is worth mentioning only because the linear vesicles can be mistaken for herpes infection.[346] The vesicular lesions later become pigmented macules.

Linear IgA Bullous Dermatosis

This immunobullous disease may also present in the newborn period and can mimic the vesicles of HSV infection.[347]

Maternal Mastitis

Although mastitis in the nursing mother is a logical source of staphylococcal infection to the baby, such infection rarely occurs.[348] Emptying the breast (including by breast feeding) and antistaphylococcal antibiotics traditionally clear the maternal infection.[349] Breast abscess occurs in about 10% of patients with mastitis. Management is similar, except that the abscess should be drained and breastfeeding should be limited to the unaffected side until the infection is cleared.[349]

■ USE OF ANTIMICROBIAL AGENTS IN PREGNANCY AND LACTATION

Although using antibiotics only when there is a clear-cut indication is good advice in caring for any patient, it is particularly salient when approaching the treatment of a pregnant or lactating woman. Because it is ethically unfeasible to perform prospective, controlled trials of antibiotics in these circumstances, no currently available antibiotic has been deemed completely safe. However, the Food and Drug Administration has placed drugs in risk categories for use in pregnancy, and the American Academy of Pediatrics has developed similar risk categories for nursing infants.[350]

Breastfeeding has many advantages, including prevention of infections in infants, and thus it should be encouraged. Most antibiotics are compatible with nursing, and breastfeeding can usually be continued safely. Similarly, in a pregnant woman with an infection, treatment necessity often outweighs potential risks for fetal anomalies. For exam-

TABLE 19-2. SELECTED ANTIMICROBIAL AGENTS AND THEIR RISK CATEGORIES IN PREGNANCY AND LACTATION

ANTIMICROBIAL AGENTS	FDA PREGNANCY RISK CATEGORY*	BREASTFEEDING
Antibacterial agents		
Aminoglycosides	D	Compatible
Azithromycin	B	Compatible
Cephalosporins	B	Compatible
Clindamycin	B	Compatible
Clarithromycin	C	Unknown
Chloramphenicol	C	Unknown but may be of concern
Dapsone	C	Compatible
Erythromycin	B	Compatible (concentrated in human milk)
Fluoroquinolones	C	Compatible
Imipenem	C	Unknown
Isoniazid	C	Compatible–place mother and infant on vitamin B6 (pyridoxine)
Meropenem	B	Unknown
Metronidazole	B	Unknown but may be of concern
Nitrofurantoin	B	Compatible
Penicillins	B	Compatible
Pyrazinamide	C	Unknown
Rifampin	C	Compatible
Sulfonamides	C	Compatible (caution in infant with jaundice or prematurity)
Tetracyclines	D	Compatible
Vancomycin	C	Unknown
Antifungal agents		
Amphotericin B	B	Unknown
Fluconazole	C	Compatible
Itraconazole	C	Unknown
Terbinafine	B	Contraindicated
Antiparasitic agents		
Albendazole	C	Unknown
Atovaquone/proguanil	C	Unknown
Chloroquine	C+	Compatible
Furazolidone	C	Unknown (contraindicated <1 mo old due to hemolytic anemia)
Ivermectin	C	Compatible
Mebendazole	C	Compatible
Mefloquine	C†	Unknown
Paromomycin	C	Compatible
Praziquantel	B	Unknown
Quinidine	C	Compatible

TABLE 19-2. (continued)

Quinine	X	Compatible
Antiviral agents		
Acyclovir	B	Compatible (concentrated in human milk)
Ganciclovir	C	Unknown
Oseltamivir	C	Unknown
Ribavirin	X	Unknown
Valacyclovir	B	Unknown

* FDA pregnancy categories: A, studies in pregnant women, no risk to fetus; B, no risk in animal studies but human studies inadequate *or* toxicity in animal studies but no risk in human studies; C, animal studies show toxicity, human studies are inadequate but benefit may exceed risk; D, evidence of human risk, but benefits may outweigh risks; X, fetal abnormalities in humans, risk outweighs benefits.

⁺ In general, for pregnant women traveling to areas with malaria, the risks to the mother and fetus from acquiring malaria outweigh the risks of adverse effects of antimalarial medication.

ple, the antituberculous drugs should not be withheld from pregnant patients with active tuberculosis.

Table 19-2 lists some commonly used antimicrobial agents and their risk categories for both pregnancy and lactation. Reference texts may be consulted for a more comprehensive discussion.[351]

■ REFERENCES

1. Remington JS, Klein JO. Infectious diseases of the fetus and newborn infant, 5th ed. Philadelphia, PA: WB Saunders, 2001.
2. Waterson AP. Virus infections (other than rubella) during pregnancy. Br Med J 1979;2:564–6.
3. Andersson RE, Lambe M. Incidence of appendicitis during pregnancy. Int J Epidemiol 2001;30:1281–5.
4. Mourad J, Elliott JP, Erickson L, Lisboa L. Appendicitis in pregnancy: new information that contradicts long-held clinical beliefs. Am J Obstet Gynecol 2000;182:1027–9.
5. Auguste T, Murphy B, Oyelese Y. Appendicitis in pregnancy masquerading as recurrent preterm labor. Int J Gynaecol Obstet 2002;76:181–2.
6. Lyass S, Pikarsky A, Eisenberg VH, et al. Is laparoscopic appendectomy safe in pregnant women? Surg Endosc 2001;15:377–9.
7. Andersen B, Nielsen TF. Appendicitis in pregnancy: diagnosis, management and complications. Acta Obstet Gynecol Scand 1999;78:758–62.
8. Raucher HS, Jaffin H, Glass JL. Babesiosis in pregnancy. Obstet Gyneco 1984;63:S7–S9.
9. Scimeca PG, Weinblatt ME, Schonfeld G, et al. Babesiosis in two infants from eastern Long Island, New York. Am J Dis Child 1986;140:971.
10. New DL, Quinn JB, Qureshi MZ, et al. Vertically transmitted babesiosis. J Pediatr 1997;131:163–4.
11. Guptill L, Slater LN, Wu CC, et al. Evidence of reproductive failure and lack of perinatal transmission of *Bartonella henselae* in experimentally infected cats. Vet Immunol Immunopathol 1998;23:177–89.
12. Khan MY, Mah MW, Memish ZA. Brucellosis in pregnant women. Clin Infect Dis 2001;32:1172–7.
13. Maudsley RF, Brix GA, Hinton NA, et al. Placental inflammation and infection. A prospective bacteriologic and histologic study. Am J Osbstet Gynecol 1966;95:648–59.
14. Darmstadt GL, Dinulos JG, Miller Z. Congenital cutaneous candidiasis: clinical presentation, pathogenesis, and management guidelines. Pediatrics 2000;105:438–44.
15. Gencay M, Koskiniemi M, Fellman V, et al. *Chlamydia trachomatis* infection in mothers with preterm delivery and in their newborn infants. APMIS 2001;109:636–40.
16. Wu S, Shen L, Liu G. Study on vertical transmission of *Chlamydia trachomatis* using PCR and DNA sequencing. Chin Med J 1000;112:396–9.
17. Nyari T, Woodward M, Meszaros G, et al. *Chlamydia trachomatis* infection and the risk of perinatal mortality in Hungary. J Perinat Med 2001;29:55–9.
18. Gencay M, Koskiniemi M, Saikku P, et al. *Chlamydia trachomatis* seropositivity during pregnancy is associated with perinatal complications. Clin Infect Dis 1995;21:424–6.
19. Ryan GM Jr, Abdella TN, McNeeley SG, et al. *Chlamydia trachomatis* in pregnancy and effect of treatment on outcome. Am J Obstet Gynecol 1990;162:34–9.
20. Garland SM, Bowman ED. Role of *Ureaplasma urealyticum and chlamydia trachomatis* in lung disease in low birth weight infants. Pathology 1996;28:266–9.
21. Stagno S, Pass RF, Cloud G, et al. Primary cytomegalovirus infection in pregnancy: incidence, transmission to fetus, and clinical outcome. JAMA 1986;256:1904–8.
22. Stagno S, Whitley RJ. Herpesvirus infections of pregnancy Part I: Cytomegalovirus and Epstein-Barr virus infections. N Engl J Med 1985;313:1270–4.
23. Nankervis GA, Kumar ML, Cox FE, et al. A prospective study of maternal cytomegalovirus infection and its effect on the fetus. Am J Obstet Gynecol 1984;149:435–40.
24. Chow KC, Lee CC, Lin TY, et al. Congenital enterovirus 71 infection: a case study with virology and immunohistochemistry. Clin Infect Dis 2000;31:509–12.
25. Sauerbrei A, Gluck B, Jung K, et al. Congenital skin le-

sions caused by intrauterine infection with coxsackievirus B3. Infection 2000;28:326–8.

26. Axelsson C, Bondestam K, Frisk G, et al. Coxsackie B virus infections in women with miscarriage. J Med Virol 1993;39:282–5.

27. Frisk G, Diderholm H. Increased frequency of Coxsackie B virus IgM in women with spontaneous abortion. J Infect 1992;24:141–5.

28. Brown GC, Karunas RS. Relationship of congenital anomalies and maternal infection with selected enteroviruses. Am J Epidemiol 1972;95:207–17.

29. Gauntt CJ, Gudvangen RJ, Brans YW, et al. Coxsackievirus group B antibodies in the ventricular fluid of infants with severe anatomic defects in the central nervous system. Pediatrics 1985;76:64–8.

30. Dahlquist G, Frisk G, Ivarson SA, et al. Indications that maternal coxsackie B virus infection during pregnancy is a risk factor for childhood-onset IDDM. Diabetologia 1995;38:1371–3.

31. Hyoty H, Hiltunen M, Knip M, et al. a prospective study of the role of coxsackie B and other enterovirus infections in the pathogenesis of IDDM. Childhood Diabetes in Finland (DiMe) Study Group. Diabetes 1995;44:652–7.

32. Oldstone MBA. Molecular mimicry and autoimmune disease. Cell 1987;50:819–20.

33. Fuchtenbusch M, Irnstetter A, Jager G, et al. No evidence for an association of coxsackie virus infection during pregnancy and early childhood development of islet auto-antibodies in offspring of mothers or fathers with type 1 diabetes. J Autoimmun 2001;17:333–40.

34. Meyohas MC, Marechal V, Desire N, et al. Study of mother-to-child Epstein-Barr virus transmission by means of nested PCRs. J Virol 1996;70:6816–9.

35. Schusgter V, Janssen W, Seidenspinner S, et al. Congenital Epstein-Barr virus infection. Monatsscgr Kinderheilkd 1993;141:401–4.

36. Buitrago MI, Ijdo JW, Rinaudo P, et al. Human granulocytic ehrlichiosis during pregnancy treated successfully with rifampin. Clin Infect Dis 1998;27:213–5.

37. Horowitz HW, Kochevsky E, Haber S, et al. Perinatal transmission of the agent of human granulocytic ehrlichiosis. New Engl J Med 1998;339:375–8.

38. Oppenheimer EH, Winn KJ. Fetal gonorrhea with deep tissue infection occurring in utero. Pediatrics 1982;69:74–6.

39. Babl FE, Ram S, Barnett ED, et al. Neonatal gonococcal arthritis after negative prenatal screening and despite conjunctival prophylaxis. Pediatr Infect Dis J 2000;19:346–9.

40. Donders GG, Desmyter J, De Wet DH, et al. The association of gonorrhoea and syphilis with premature birth and low birthweight. Ginotourin Med 1993;69:98–101.

41. Lyde CB. Pregnancy in patients with Hansen disease. Arch Dermatol 1997;133:623–7.

42. Baillargeon J, Piper J, Leach CT. Epidemiology of human herpesvirus 6 (HHV-6) infection in pregnant and non-pregnant women. J Clin Virol 2000;16:149–57.

43. Dahl H, Fjaertoft G, Norsted T, et al. Reactivation of human herpesvirus 6 during pregnancy. J Infect Dis 1999;180:2035–8.

44. Maeda T, Okuno T, Hayashi K, et al. Outcomes of infants whose mothers are positive for human herpesvirus-6

DNA within the genital tract in early gestation. Acta Pediatr Jpn 1997;39:653–7.

45. Mantina H, Kankasa C, Klaskala W, et al. Vertical transmission of Kaposi's sarcoma-associated herpesvirus. Int J Cancer 2001;94:749–52.

46. Jacobs RF. Neonatal herpes simplex virus infections. Semin Perinatol 1998;22:64–71.

47. Brown ZA, Wald A, Morrow RA, et al. Effect of serologic status and cesarean delivery on transmission rates of herpes simplex virus from mother to infant. JAMA 2003;289:203–9.

48. Hutto C, Arvin A, Jacobs R, et al. Intrauterine herpes simplex virus infections. J Pediatr 1987;110:97–101.

49. Physicians Desk Reference 2003, 1707.

50. Brown ZA, Benedetti J, Ashley R, et al. Neonatal herpes simplex virus infection in relation to asymptomatic maternal infection at the time of labor. N Engl J Med 1991;325:965–6.

51. Garland SM, Lee TN, Sacks S. Do antepartum herpes simplex virus cultures predict intrapartum shedding for pregnant women with recurrent disease? Infect Dis Obstet Gynecol 1999;7:230–6.

52. Rouse DJ, Stringer JS. An appraisal of screening for maternal type-specific herpes simplex virus antibodies to prevent neonatal herpes. Am J Obstet Gynecol 2000;183:400–6.

53. Catalano PM, Merritt AO, Mead PB. Incidence of genital herpes simplex virus at the time of delivery in women with known risk factors. Am J Obstet Gynecol 1991;164:1303–6.

54. Braig S, Luton D, Sibony O, et al. Acyclovir prophylaxis in late pregnancy prevents recurrent genital herpes and viral shedding. Eur J Obstet Gynecol Reprod Biol 2001;96:55–8.

54a. Kimberlin DW, Rouse DJ. Genital herpes. N Engl J Med 2004;350:1970–7.

55. McGregor JA, Burns JC, Levin MJ et al. Transplacental passage of influenza A/Bangkok (H_3N_2) mimicking amniotic fluid infection syndrome. Am J Obstet Gynecol 1984;149:856–9.

56. Irving WL, James DK, Stephenson T, et al. Influenza virus infection in the second and third trimesters of pregnancy: a clinical and seroepidemiologic study. BJOG 2000;107:1292–9.

57. Brown AS, Susser ES. In utero infection and adult schizophrenia. Ment Retard Dev Disabil Res Rev 2002;8:51–7.

58. Mino Y, Oshima I, Tsuda T, et al. No relationship between schizophrenic birth and influenza epidemics on Japan. J Psychiatr Res 2000;34:133–8.

59. Selten JP, Brown AS, Moons KG, et al. Prenatal exposure to the 1957 influenza pandemic and non-affective psychosis in The Netherlands. Schizophr Res 1999;17:85–91.

60. Grech A, Takei N, Murray RM. Maternal exposure to influenza and paranoid schizophrenia. Schizophr Res 1997;29:121–5.

61. Morgan V, Castle D, Page A, et al. Influenza epidemics and incidence of schizophrenia, affective disorders and mental retardation in Western Australia: no evidence of major effect. Schizophr Res 1997;25:25–39.

62. Neuzil KM, Reed GW, Mitchel EF, et al. Impact of influ-

enza on acute cardiopulmonary hospitalizations in pregnant women. Am J Epidemiol 1998;148:1094–102.

63. Bridges CB, Fukuda K, Uyeki TM, et al. Prevention and control of influenza. Recommendations of the Advisory Committee on Immunization Practices (ACIP). MMWR Recomm Rep 2002;51:1–31.

64. Eltoum IA, Zijlstra EE, Ali MS, et al. Congenital kala-azar and leishmaniasis in the placenta. Am J Trop Med Hyg 1992;46:57–62.

65. Meinecke CK, Schottelius J, Oskam L, et al. Congenital transmission of visceral leishmaniasis (kala azar) from an asymptomatic mother to her child. Pediatrics 1999;104: e65.

66. Shaked Y, Shpilberg O, Samra D, et al. Leptospirosis in pregnancy and its effect on the fetus: case report and review. Clin Infect Dis 1993;17:241–3.

67. Pinner RW, Schuchat A, Swaminathan B, et al. Role of foods in sporadic listeriosis II. Microbiologic and epidemiologic investigation. JAMA 1992;267:2046–50.

68. Mascola L, Ewert DP, Eller A. Listeriosis: a previously unreported medical complication in women with multiple gestations. Am J Obstet Gynecol 1994;45:284–5.

69. Smith KJ, Skelton HG 3rd, Angritt P, et al. Cutaneous lesions of listeriosis in a newborn. J Cutan Pathol 1991; 18:474–6.

70. Craig S, Permezel M, Doyle L, et al. Perinatal infection with Listeria monocytogenes. Aust N Z J Obstet Gynaecol 1996;36:286–90.

71. Centers for Disease Control and Prevention. Multistate outbreak of listeriosis—United States, 1998. MMWR Morb Mortal Wkly Rep 1999;47:1085–6.

72. Nadal D, Hunziker UA, Bucher HU, et al. Infants born to mothers with antibodies against Borrelia burgdoreri at delivery. Eur J Pediatr 1989;148:426–7.

73. Figueroa R, Bracero LA, Aguero-Rosenfeld M, et al. Confirmation of Borrelia burgdorferi spirochetes by polymerase chain reaction in placentas of women with reactive serology for Lyme antibodies. Gynecol Obstet Invest 1996;41:240–3.

74. Weber K, Bratzke HJ, Neubert U, et al. Borrelia burgdorferi in a newborn despite oral penicillin for Lyme borreliosis during pregnancy. Pediatr Infect Dis J 1988;7:286–9.

75. Barton LL, Mets MB. Congenital lymphocytic choriomeningitis virus infection: decade of rediscovery. Clin Infect Dis 2001;33:370–4.

76. Enders G, Varho-Gobel M, Lohler J, et al. Congenital lymphocytic choriomeningitis virus infection: an underdiagnosed disease. Pediatr Infect Dis J 1999;18:652–5.

77. Dorman EK, Shulman CE, Kingdom J, et al. Impaired uteroplacental blood flow in pregnancies complicated by falciparum malaria. Ultrasound Obstet Gynecol 2002;19: 165–70

78. Okoko BJ, Ota MO, Yamuah LK, et al. Influence of placental malaria infection on foetale outcome in the Gambia: twenty years after Ian McGregor. J Health Popul Nutr 2002;20:4–11.

79. Guyatt HL, Snow RW. Malaria in pregnancy as an indirect cause of infant mortality in sub-Saharan Africa. Trans R Soc Trop Med Hyg 2001;95:569–76.

80. Edwards B. Congenital malaria. [Letter] N Engl J Med 1997;336(1):71; author reply 72.

81. Fischer PR. Congenital malaria: an African survey. Clin Pediatr 1997;36:411–3.

82. Nyirjesy P, Kavasya T, Axelrod P, Fischer PR. Malaria during pregnancy: neonatal morbidity and mortality and the efficacy of chloroquine chemoprophylaxis. Clin Infect Dis 1993;16(1):127–32.

83. Centers for Disease Control and Prevention. Congenital malaria as a result of Plasmodium malariae—North Carolina, 2000. MMWR—Morb Mortal Wkly Rep March 1, 2002;51(08):164–5.

83a. Fisher PR. Malaria and newborns. J Trop Pediatr 2003; 49:132–4.

84. Hulbert TV. Congenital malaria in the United States: report of a case and review. [Review] Clin Infect Dis 1992; 14:922–6.

85. Noia G, Masini L, De Santis M, et al. Fetal infection from rubeola virus or cytomegalovirus: correlation among maternal serological profiles, invasive diagnostic procedures, and long-term follow-up. J Matern Fetal Med 1998;7: 36–42.

86. Ali ME, Albar HM. Measles in pregnancy: maternal morbidity and perinatal outcome. Int J Gynaecol Obstet 1997; 59:109–13.

87. Siegel M, Fuerst HT. Low birth weight and maternal virus diseases: a prospective study of rubella, measles, mumps, chickenpox and hepatitis. JAMA 1966;197:680-4.

88. Siegel M. Congenital malformations following chickenpox, measles, mumps, and hepatitis: results of a cohort study. JAMA 1973;226:1521–4.

89. Centers for Disease Control and Prevention. Leads from the MMWR—Morb Mortal Wkly Rep Measles prevention. JAMA 1987;258:890–5.

90. Gazala E, Karplus M, Liberman JR, et al. The effect of maternal measles on the fetus. Pediatr Infect Dis J 1985; 4:203–4.

91. Bhutta ZA, Khan IA, Agha Z. Fatal intrauterine meningococcal infection. Pediatr Infect Dis J 1991;10:868–9.

92. Siegel M, Fuerst HT, Peress NS. Comparative fetal mortality in maternal virus diseases: a prospective study on rubella, measles, mumps, chickenpox, and hepatitis. N Engl J Med 1966;274:768–71.

93. Bray PF. Mumps—a cause of hydrocephalus. Pediatrics 1972;42:446–9.

94. Korones SB, Todaro J, Roane JA, et al. Maternal virus infection after the first trimester of pregnancy and status of offspring to 4 years of age in a predominantly Negro population. J Pediatr 1970;77:245–51.

95. Takahashi Y, Teranishi A, Yamada Y, et al. A case of congenital mumps infection complicated with persistent pulmonary hypertension. Am J Perinatol 1998;15:409–12.

96. Groenendaal F, Rothbarth PH, van den Anker JN, et al. Congenital mumps pneumonia: a rare cause of neonatal respiratory distress. Acta Paediatr Scand 1990;79: 1252–4.

97. Lacour M, Maherzi M, Vienny H, et al. Thrombocytopenia in a case of neonatal mumps infection: evidence for further clinical presentations. Eur J Pediatr 1993;152: 739–41.

98. van Loon FP, Holmes SJ, Sirotkin BI, et al. Mumps surveillance: United States 1988-1995. MMWR CDC Surveill Summ 1995;44:1–14.

99. Ni J, Bowles NE, Kim YH, et al. Viral infection of the

myocardium in endocardial fibroelastosis. Molecular evidence for the role of mumps virus as an etiologic agent. Circulation 1997;95:133–9.

100. Berman SM, Harrison HR, Boyce WT, et al. Low birth weight, prematurity, and postpartum endometritis: association with prenatal cervical *Mycoplasma hominis* and *Chlamydia trachomatis* infections. JAMA 1987;257:1189–94.

101. Armbruster-Moraes E, Ioshimoto LM, Leao E, et al. Prevalence of "high risk" human papillomavirus in the lower genital tract of Brazilian gravidas. Int J Gynaecol Obstet 2000;69:223–37.

102. Tenti P, Zappatore R, Migliora P, et al. Latent human papillomavirus infection in pregnant women at term: a case-control study. J Infect Dis 1997;176:277–80.

103. Xu S, Liu L, Lu S, et al. Clinical observation on vertical transmission of human papillomavirus. Chin Med Sci J 1998;13:29–31.

104. Wang X, Zhu Q, Rao H. Maternal-fetal transmission of human papillomavirus. Chin Med J 1998;111:726–7.

105. Tenti P, Zappatori R, Migliora P, et al. Perinatal transmission of human papillomavirus from gravidas with latent infections. Obstet Gynecol 1999;93:475–9.

106. Guderian RH, Lovato R, Anselmi M, et al. Onchocerciasis and reproductive health in Ecuador. Trans R Soc Trop Med Hyg. 1997;91:315-7.

107. Anosike JC, Onwiliri CO. A probable case of vertical transmission of *Onchocerca volvulus* microfilariae. J Helminthol 1993;67:83–4.

108. Ufomadu GO, Sato Y, Takahashi H. Possible transplacental transmission of *Onchocerca volvulus*. Trop Geogr Med 1990;42:69–71.

109. Egwunyenga AO, Ajayi JA, Nmorsi OP, et al. Plasmodium/intestinal helminth co-infections among pregnant Nigerian women. Mem Inst Oswaldo Cruz 2001;96:1055–9.

110. Dreyfuss ML, Stoltzfus RJ, Shrestha JB, et al. Hookworms, malaria, and vitamin A deficiency contribute to anemia and iron deficiency among pregnant women in the plains of Nepal. J Nutr 2000;130:2527–36.

111. Nurdia DS, Sumarni S, Suyoko K, et al. Impact of intestinal helminth infection on anemia and iron status during pregnancy: a community based study in Indonesia. Southeast Asian J Trop Med Public Health 2001;32:14–22.

112. Deveci S, Tanyuksel M, Deveci G, et al. Spontaneous missed abortion caused by Ascaris lumbricoides. Cent Eur J Public Health 2001;9:188–9.

113. Yaegashi N, Niinuma T, Chisaka H, et al. The incidence of, and factors leading to, parvovirus B19-related hydrops fetalis following maternal infection; report of 10 cases and meta-analysis. J Infect 1998;37:28–35.

114. Von Kaisenberg CS, Jonat W. Fetal parvovirus B19 infection. Ultrasound Obstet Gynecol 2001;18:280–8.

114a. Young NS, Brown KE. Parvovirus B19. N Engl J Med 2004;350:580–92.

115. Tolfvenstam T, Papadogiannakis N, Norbeck O, et al. Frequency of human parvovirus B19 infection in intrauterine fetal death. Lancet 2001;357:1494–7.

116. Koga M, Matsuoka T, Katayama K, et al. Human parvovirus B19 in cord blood of premature infants. Am J Perinatol 2001;18:237–40.

117. Karunajeewa H, Siebert D, Hammond R, et al. Seroprevalence of varicella zoster virus, parvovirus B19 and *Toxoplasma gondii* in a Melbourne obstetric population: implications for management. Aust N Z J Obstet Gynaecol 2001;41:23–8.

118. Jensen IP, Thorsen P, Jeune B, et al. An epidemic of parvovirus B19 in a population of 3,596 pregnant women: a study of sociodemographic and medical risk factors. BJOG 2000;107:637–43.

119. Valeur-Jensen AK, Pedersen CB, Westergaard T, et al. Risk factors for parvovirus B19 infection in pregnancy. JAMA 1999;281:1099–105.

120. Odibo AO, Campbell WA, Feldman D, et al. Resolution of human parvovirus B19-induced nonimmune hydrops after intrauterine transfusion. J Ultrasound Med 1998;17:547–50.

121. Rodis JF, Borgida AF, Wilson M, et al. Management of parvovirus infection in pregnancy and outcomes of hydrops: a survey of members of the Society of Perinatal Obstetricians. Am J Obstet Gynecol 1998;179:985–8.

122. Stein A, Lepidi H, Mege JL, et al. Repeated pregnancies in BALB/c mice infected with *Coxiella burnetii* cause disseminated infection, resulting in stillbirth and endocarditis. J Infect Dis 2000;181:188–94.

123. Raoult D, Tissot-Dupont H, Foucault C, et al. Q fever 1985-1998. Clinical and epidemiologic features of 1,383 infections. Medicine (Baltimore) 2000;79:109–23.

124. Stein A, Raoult D. Q fever during pregnancy: a public health problem in southern France. Clin Infect Dis 1998;27:592–6.

125. Stallings SP. Rocky Mountain spotted fever and pregnancy: a case report and review of the literature. Obstet Gynecol Surv 2001;56:37–42.

126. Koskimies O, Lapinleimu K, Saxén L. Infections and other maternal factors as risk indicators for congenital malformations: a case-control study with paired serum samples. Pediatrics 1978;61:832–7.

127. Miller E, Cradock-Watson JE, Pollock TM. Consequences of confirmed maternal rubella at successive stages of pregnancy. Lancet 1982;2:781–4.

128. Katow S. Rubella virus genome diagnosis during pregnancy and mechanism of congenital rubella. Intervirology 1998;41:163–9.

129. Webster WS. Teratogen update: congenital rubella. Teratology 1998;58:13–23.

130. Lee JY, Bowden DS. Rubella virus replication and links to teratogenicity. Clin Microbiol Rev 2000;13:571–87.

131. McElhaney RD Jr, Ringer M, DeHart DJ, et al. Rubella immunity in a cohort of pregnant women. Infect Control Hosp Epidemiol 1999;20:64–6.

132. Plotkin S. Rubella eradication. Vaccine 2001;19:3311–9.

133. Semerikov VV, Lavrentyeva IN, Popov VF, et al. Rubella in the Russian Federation: epidemiologic features and control measures to prevent the congenital rubella syndrome. Epidemiol Infect 2000;125:359–6.

134. Centers for Disease Control and Prevention. Control and prevention of rubella: evaluation and management of suspected outbreaks, rubella in pregnant women, and surveillance for congenital rubella syndrome. MMWR Recomm Rep 2001;50:1–23.

135. Rangel MC, Sales RM, Valeriano EN. Rubella outbreaks

among Hispanics in North Carolina: lessons learned from a field investigation. Ethn Dis 1999;9:230–6.

136. Danovaro-Holliday MC, LeBaron CW, Allensworth C, et al. A large rubella outbreak with spread from the workplace to the community. JAMA 2000;284:2733–9.

137. Hofmann J, Kortung M, Pustowoit B, et al. Persistent fetal rubella vaccine virus infection following inadvertant vaccination during early pregnancy. J Med Virol 2000; 61:155–8.

138. Anonymous. Revised ACIP recommendation for avoiding pregnancy after receiving a rubella-containing vaccine. MMWR Morb Mortal Wkly Rep 2001;50:1117.

139. Wicher V, Wicher K. Pathogenesis of maternal-fetal syphilis revisited. Clin Infect Dis 2001;33:354–63.

140. Mavrov GI, Goubenko TV. Clinical and epidemiologic features of syphilis in pregnant women: the course and outcome of pregnancy. Gynecol Obstet Invest 2001;52: 114–8.

141. Warner L, Rochat RW, Fichtner RR, et al. Missed opportunities for congenital syphilis prevention in an urban southeastern hospital. Sex Transm Dis 2001;28:92–8.

142. Southwick KL, Guidry HM, Weldon MM, et al. An epidemic of congenital syphilis in Jefferson County, Texas, 1994-1995: inadequate prenatal syphilis testing after an outbreak in adults. Am J Public Health 1999;89:557–60.

142a. Centers for Disease Control and Prevention. Congenital syphilis—United States, 2002. MMWR 2004;53:716–9.

143. Jones JE Jr, Harris RE: Diagnostic evaluation of syphilis during pregnancy. Obstet Gynecol 1979;54:611–4.

144. Walker GJ. Antibiotics for syphilis diagnosed during pregnancy. Cochrane Database Syst Rev 2001;3: CD001143.

145. Hohlfeld P, Daffos F, Costa JM, et al. Prenatal diagnosis of congenital toxoplasmosis with a polymerase chain reaction text on amniotic fluid. N Engl J Med 1994;331: 695–9.

146. Dunn D, Wallon M, Peyron F, et al. Mother-to-child transmission of toxoplasmosis: risk estimates for clinical counselling. Lancet 1999;353:1829–33.

147. Peyron F, Walllon M, Liou C, et al. Treatments for toxoplasmosis in pregnancy. Cochrane Database Syst Rev 2000;CD001684.

148. Foulon W, Villena I, Stay-Pedersen B, et al. Treatment of toxoplasmosis during pregnancy: a multicenter study of impact on fetal transmission and children's sequelae at age 1 year. Am J Obstet Gynecol 1999;180:410–5.

149. Cook AJ, Gilbert RE, Buffolano W, et al. Sources of toxoplasma infection in pregnant women: European multicentre case-control study. European Research Network on Congenital Toxoplasmosis. Br Med J 2000;321: 142–7.

150. Carter EJ, Mates S. Tuberculosis during pregnancy. The Rhode Island experience, 1987 to 1991. Chest 1994;106: 1466–70.

151. Schaefer G, Zervoudakis IA, Fuchs FF, et al. Pregnancy and pulmonary tuberculosis. Obstet Gynecol 1975;46: 706–15.

152. Wilson EA, Thelin TJ, Dilts PV Jr. Tuberculosis complicated by pregnancy. Am J Obstet Gynecol 1973;115: 526–9.

153. Comstock GW, Livesay VT, Woolpert SF. The prognosis

154. Mehta JB, Bentley S. Prevention of tuberculosis in children: missed opportunities. Am J Prev Med 1992;8: 283–6.

155. Bothamley G. Drug treatment for tuberculosis during pregnancy: safety considerations. Drug Safety 2001;24: 553–65.

156. Targeted tuberculin testing and treatment of latent tuberculosis infection. Am J Respir Crit Care Med 2000; 161: S221–47.

157. Covelli HD, Wilson RT. Immunologic and medical considerations in tuberculin-sensitized pregnant patients. Am J Obstet Gynecol 1978;132:256–9.

158. Chua KB, Ngeow YF, Ng KB, et al. Ureaplasma urealyticum and Mycoplasma hominis isolation from cervical secretions of pregnant women and nasopharyngeal secretions of their babies at delivery. Singapore Med J 1998; 39:300–2.

159. Goncalves LF, Chaiworapongsa T, Romero R. Intrauterine infection and prematurity. Ment Retard Dev Disabil Res Rev 2002;8:3–13.

160. Lyon A. Chronic lung disease of prematurity. The role of intra-uterine infection. Eur J Pediatr 2000;159:798–802.

161. Li YH, Brauner A, Jonsson B, et al. Ureaplasma urealyticum-induced production of proinflammatory cytokines by macrophages. Pediatr Res 2000;48:114–9.

162. Hannaford K, Todd DA, Jeffery H, et al. Role of *Ureaplasma urealyticum* in lung disease of prematurity. Arch Dis Child Fetal Neonatal Ed 1999;81:F162–7.

163. Abele-Horn M, Genzel-Boroviczeny O, Uhlig T, et al. *Ureaplasma urealyticum* colonization and bronchopulmonary dysplasia: a comparative prospective multicentre study. Eur J Pediatr 1998;157:1004–11.

164. Pacifico L, Panero A, Roggini M, et al. *Ureaplasma urealyticum* and pulmonary outcome in a neonatal intensive care population. Pediatr Infect Dis J 1997;16:579–86.

165. Heggie AD, Bar-Shain D, Boxerbaum B, et al. Identification and quantification of ureaplasmas colonizing the respiratory tract and assessment of their role in the development of chronic lung disease in preterm infants. Pediatr Infect Dis J 2001;20:854–9.

166. Ollikainen J, Korppi M, Heiskanene-Kosma T, et al. Chronic lung disease of the newborn is not associated with *Ureaplasma urealyticum*. Pediatr Pulmonol 2001;32: 303–7.

167. Da Silva O, Gregson D, Hammerberg O. Role of *Ureaplasma urealyticum* and *Chlamydia trachomatis* in development of bronchopulmonary dysplasia in very low birth weight infants. Pediatr Infect Dis J 1997;16:579–86.

168. Heggie AD, Jacobs MR, Butler VT, et al. Frequency and significance of isolation of *Ureaplasma urealyticum* and *Mycoplasma hominis* from cerebrospinal fluid and tracheal aspirate specimens from low birth weight infants. J Pediatr 1994;124:956–61.

169. Viscardi RM, Manimtim WM, Sun CC, et al. Lung pathology in premature infants with *Ureaplasma urealyticum*. Pediatr Dev Pathol 2002;5:141–50.

170. Neal TJ, Roe MF, Shaw NJ. Spontaneously resolving *Ureaplasma urealyticum* meningitis. Eur J Pediatr 1994;153: 342–3.

171. Gjuric G, Prislin-Muskic M, Nikolic E, et al. *Ureaplasma*

urealyticum osteomyelitis in a very low birth weight infant. J Perinat Med 1994;22:79–81.

172. Naeye RL. Causes of the excessive rates of perinatal mortality and prematurity in pregnancies complicated by maternal urinary-tract infections. N Engl J Med 1979;300:819–23.

173. Bruder E, Ersch J, Hebisch G, et al. Fetal varicella syndrome: disruption of neural development and persistent inflammation of non-neural tissues. Virchows Arch 2000;437:440–4.

174. Enders G, Miller E, Cradock-Watson J, et al. Consequences of varicella and herpes zoster in pregnancy: prospective study of 1739 cases. Lancet 1994;343:1548–51.

175. Mustonen K, Mustakangas P, Valanne L, et al. Congenital varicella-zoster virus infection after maternal subclinical infection: clinical and neuropathologic findings. J Perinatol 2001;21:141–6.

176. Linder N, Ferber A, Kopilov U, et al. Reported exposure to chickenpox: a predictor of positive anti-varicella-zoster antibodies in parturient women. Fetal Diagn Ther 2001;16:423–6.

177. Harger JH, Ernest JM, Thurnau GR, et al. Frequency of congenital varicella syndrome in a prospective cohort of 347 pregnant women. Obstet Gynecol 2002;100:260–5.

178. Meyers JD. Congenital varicella in term infants: risk reconsidered. J Infect Dis 1974;129:215–7.

179. American Academy of Pediatrics. varicella-zoster infections. In: Pickering LK, ed. 2003 Red Book: Report of the Committee on Infectious Diseases. Elk Grove Village, IL: American Academy of Pediatrics, 2003:672–86.

180. Huang YC, Lin TY, Lin YJ, et al. Prophylaxis of intravenous immunoglobulin and acyclovir in perinatal varicella. Eur J Pediatr 2000;160:91–4.

181. Bakshi SS, Miller TC, Kaplan M, et al. Failure of varicella-zoster immunoglobulin in modification of severe congenital varicella. Pediatr Infect Dis 1986;5:699–702.

182. Brunnell PA, Kotchmar JR. Zoster in infancy: Failure to maintain virus latency following intrauterine infection. J Pediatr 1981;98:71–3.

183. Shields KE, Galil K, Seward J, et al. Varicella vaccine exposure during pregnancy: data from the first 5 years of the pregnancy registry. Obstet Gynecol 2001;98:14–9.

184. Centers for Disease Control and Prevention. Intrauterine West Nile virus infection—New York, 2002. MMWR—Morb Mortal Wkly Rep 2002;51:1135–6.

185. Centers for Disease Control and Prevention. Possible West Nile virus transmission to an infant through breast-feeding—Michigan, 2002. MMWR—Morb Mortal Wkly Rep 2002;51:877–8.

186. Catanzaro A. Pulmonary mycoses in pregnant women. Chest 1984;86(suppl):145–95.

187. Brabin BJ. Epidemiology of infection in pregnancy. Rev Infect Dis 1985;7:579–603.

188. Chye JK, Lim CT, Ng KB, Lim JM, George R, Lam SK. Vertical transmission of dengue. Clin Infect Dis 1997;25:1374–7.

189. Jongen VH, van Roosmalen J, Tiems J, et al. Tick-borne relapsing fever and pregnancy outcome in rural Tanzania. A Obstet Gynecol Scan 1997;76:834–8.

190. American Academy of Pediatrics. In: Pickering LK, ed. 2003 Red Book: Report of the Committee on Infectious Diseases. Elk Grove Village, IL: American Academy of Pediatrics, 2003:536–41.

191. Pattison JR, Dane DS, Mace JE. Persistence of specific IgM after natural infection with rubella virus. Lancet 1975;1:185–7.

192. Centers for Disease Control and Prevention. Leads from the MMWR: Rubella vaccination during pregnancy-United States, 1971-1986. JAMA 1987;258:753–7.

193. Plotkin SA, Starr SE, eds. Symposium on perinatal infections. Clin Perinatal 1981;8:395–654.

194. Alford CA, Pass RF: Epidemiology of chronic congenital infections of man. Clin Perinatol 1981;8:397–414.

195. Stagno S. Diagnosis of viral infections in the newborn infant. Clin Perinatol 1981;8:579–89.

196. Ford-Jones EL, Kellner JD. "Cheap Torches": an acronym for congenital and perinatal infections. Pediatr Infect Dis J 1995;14:638–9.

197. Primhak RA, Simpson RM. Screening small for gestational age babies for congenital infection. Clin Pediatr 1982;21:417–20.

198. Tardieu M, Grospierre B, Durandy A, et al. Circulating immune complexes containing rubella antigens in late-onset rubella syndrome. J Pediatr 1980;97:370–3.

199. Weil ML, Itabashi HH, Cremer NE, et al. Chronic progressive panencephalitis due to rubella virus simulating subacute sclerosing panencephalitis. N Engl J Med 1975;292:994–8.

200. Chess S, Fernandez P, Korn S. Behavioral consequences of congenital rubella. J Pediatr 1979;93:699–703.

201. Stern H, Williams BM. Isolation of rubella virus in a case of neonatal giant-cell hepatitis. Lancet 1966;1:293–5.

202. Centers for Disease Control and Prevention: Leads from the MMWR. Rubella and congenital rubella-United States, 1984-1986. JAMA 1987;258:2491.

203. Stagno S. Congenital toxoplasmosis. Am J Dis Child 1980;134:635–7.

204. Guerina NG, Hsu HW, Meissner HC, et al. Neonatal serologic screening and early treatment for congenital *Toxoplasma gondii* infection. The New England Regional Toxoplasma Working Group. N Engl J Med 1994;330:1858–63.

205. Roizen N, Swisher CN, Stein MA, et al. Neurologic and developmental outcome in treated congenital toxoplasmosis. Pediatrics 1995;95:11–20.

206. Patel DV, Holfels EM, Vogel NP, et al. Resolution of intracranial calcifications in infants with treated congenital toxoplasmosis. Radiology 1996;199:433–40.

207. Gavinet MF, Robert F, Firtion G, et al. Congenital toxoplasmosis due to maternal reinfection during pregnancy. J Clin Microbiol 1997;35:1276–7.

208. Vogel N, Kirisits M, Michael E, et al. Congenital toxoplasmosis transmitted from an immunologically competent mother infection before conception. Clin Infect Dis 1996;23:1055–60.

209. Fowler KB, Stagno S, Pass RF. Maternal immunity and prevention of congenital cytomegalovirus infection. JAMA 2003;289:1008–11.

210. Minamishima I, Ueda K, Minematsu T, et al. Role of breast milk in acquisition of cytomegalovirus infection. Microbiol Immunol 1994;38:549–52.

211. Boppana SB, Fowler KB, Vaid Y, et al. Neuroradiographic findings in the newborn period and long-term outcome

in children with symptomatic congenital cytomegalovirus infection. Pediatrics 1997;99:409–14.

212. Rivera LB, Boppana SB, Fowler KB, et al. Predictors of hearing loss in children with symptomatic congenital cytomegalovirus infection. Pediatrics 2002;110:762–7.

213. Williamson WD, Demmler GJ, Percy AK, et al. Progressive hearing loss in infants with asymptomatic congenital cytomegalovirus infection. Pediatics 1992;90:862–6.

214. Fowler KB, Dahle AJ, Boppana SB, et al. Newborn hearing screening: will children with hearing loss caused by congenital cytomegalovirus infection be missed? Pediatrics 1999;135:60–4.

215. Kashden J, Frison S, Fowler K, et al. Intellectual assessment of children with asymptomatic congenital cytomegalovirus infection. J Dev Behav Pediatr 1998;19:254–9.

216. Pickering LK. Diagnosis and therapy of patients with congenital and primary syphilis. Pediatr Infect Dis J 1985; 4:602–5.

217. Mascola L, Pelosi R, Blount JH, et al. Congenital syphilis revisited. Am J Dis Child 1985;139:575–80.

218. Richardson MP, Palfreeman A, Nielsen PB, et al. Congenital syphilis following negative antenatal screening. Commun Dis Public Health 2002;5:72–3.

219. Karayalycin G, Chanijou A, Young KY, et al. Monocytosis in congenital syphilis. Am J Dis Child 1977;131:782–3.

220. Jones CL. Herpes simplex virus infection in the neonate: clinical presentation and management. Neonatal Netw 1996;15:11–15.

221. Greenes DS, Rowitch D, Thorne GM, et al. Neonatal herpes simplex virus infection presenting as fulminant liver failure. Pediatr Infect Dis J 1995;14:242–4.

222. Malm G, Forsgren M, el Azazi M, et al. A follow-up study of children with neonatal herpes simplex virus infections with particular regard to late nervous disturbances. Acta Paediatr Scand 1991;80:226–34.

223. Kimberlin D, Powell D, Gruber W, et al. Administration of oral acyclovir suppressive therapy after neonatal herpes simplex virus disease limited to the skin, eyes and mouth: Results of a phase 1/2 trial. Pediatr Infect Dis J 1996;15: 247–54.

224. Mahon BE, Yamada EG, Newman TB. Problems with serum IgM as a screening test for congenital infection. Clin Pediatr 1994;33:142–6.

225. Diamond C, Mohan K, Hobson A, et al. Viremia in neonatal herpes simplex virus infections. Pediatr Infect Dis J 1999;18:487–9.

226. Gross U, Luder CG, Hendgen V, et al. Comparative immunoglobulin G antibody profiles between mother and child (CGMC test) for early diagnosis of congenital toxoplasmosis. J Clin Microbiol 2000;38:3619–22.

227. Robert-Gangneux F, Gavinet MF, Ancelle T, et al. Value of prenatal diagnosis and early postnatal diagnosis of congenital toxoplasmosis: retrospective study of 110 cases. J Clin Microbiol 1999;37:2893–8.

228. Gust DA, Levine WC, St Louis ME, et al. Mortality associated with congenital syphilis in the United States, 1992-1998. Pediatrics 2002;109:E79–E89.

229. Moyer VA, Schneider V, Yetman R, et al. Contribution of long-bone radiographs to the management of congenital syphilis in the newborn infant. Arch Pediatr Adolesc Med 1998;152:353–7.

230. Sever JL. TORCH tests and what they mean. Am J Obstet Gynecol 1985;152:495–8.

231. Leland D, French MLV; Kleiman MB, et al. The use of TORCH titers. Pediatrics 1983;72:41–3.

232. Speer ME, Mason EO, Scharnberg JT. Cerebrospinal fluid concentrations of aqueous procaine penicillin G in the neonate. Pediatrics 1981;67:387–8.

233. Hardy JB, Hardy PH, Oppenheimer EH, et al. Failure of penicillin in a newborn with congenital syphilis. JAMA 1970;212:1345–9.

234. Paryani SG, Vaughn AJ, Crosby M, et al. Treatment of asymptomatic congenital syphilis: benzathine versus procaine penicillin G therapy. J Pediatr 1994;125:471–5.

235. Villena I, Aubert D, Leroux B, et al. Pyrimethamine-sulfadoxine treatment of congenital toxoplasmosis: follow-up of 78 cases between 1980-1997. Reims Toxoplasmosis Group. Scand J Infect Dis 1998;30:295–300.

236. Kimberlin DW, Chin-Yu L, Sanchez PJ, et al. Effect of ganciclovir therapy on hearing in symptomatic congenital virus disease involving the central nervous system: a randomized, controlled trial. J Pediatr 2003;143:16–25.

237. Ito Y, Kimura H, Yabuta Y, et al. Exacerbation of herpes simplex encephalitis after successful treatment with acyclovir. Clin Infect Dis 2000;30:185–7.

238. Gutman LT, Wilfert CM, Eppes S. Herpes simplex virus encephalitis in children: analysis of cerebrospinal fluid and progressive neurodevelopmental deterioration. J Infect Dis 1986;154:415–21.

239. VanLandingham KE, Marsteller HB, Ross GW, et al. Relapse of herpes simplex encephalitis after conventional acyclovir therapy. JAMA 1988;259:1051–3.

240. Bergstrom T, Trolifors B. Recurrent herpes simplex virus type 2 encephalitis in a preterm neonate. Favorable outcome after prolonged acyclovir treatment. Acta Paediatr Scand 1991;80:878–81.

241. Rudd C, Rivadeneira ED, Gutman LT. Dosing considerations for oral acyclovir following neonatal herpes disease. Acta Paediatr 1994;83:1237–43.

242. Jafari HS, McCracken GH Jr. Sepsis and septic shock: a review for clinicians. Pediatr Infect Dis J 1992;11: 739–48.

243. Marks MI, Welch DF. Diagnosis of bacterial infections of the newborn infant. Clin Perinatal 1981;8:537–58.

244. Garite TJ. Premature rupture of the membranes: the enigma of the obstetrician. Am J Obstet Gynecol 1985; 151:1001–5.

245. Ferguson MG, Rhodes PG, Morrison JC, et al. Clinical amniotic infection and its effect on the neonate. Am J Obstet Gynecol 1985;151:1058–61.

246. Feinstein SJ, Vintzileos AM, Lodeiro JG, et al. Amniocentesis with premature rupture of membranes. Obstet Gynecol 1986;68:147–52.

247. Terry RR, Kelly FW, Gauzer C, et al. Risk factors for maternal colonization with group B beta-hemolytic streptococci. J Am Osteopath Assoc 1999;99:571–3.

248. Thorp JA, Jones AM, Hunt C, et al. The effect of multidose antenatal betamethasone on maternal and infant outcomes. Am J Obstet Gynecol 2001;184:196–202.

249. Goetzl L, Cohen A, Frigoletto F Jr, et al. Maternal epidural use and neonatal sepsis evaluation in afebrile mothers. Pediatrics 2001;108:1099–102.

250. Naeye RL, Ross. S. Coitus and chorioamnionitis: a prospective study. Early Hum Dev 1982;6:91–7.

251. Wilson CB. Immunologic basis for increased susceptibility of the neonate to infection. J Pediatr 1986;108:1–12.

252. Towers CV, Rumney PJ, Minkiewicz SF, et al. Incidence of intrapartum maternal risk factors for identifying neonates at risk for early-onset group B streptococcal sepsis: a prospective study. Am J Obstet Gynecol 1999;181: 1197–202.

253. Gilson GJ, Christensen F, Romero H, et al. Prevention of group B streptococcus early-onset neonatal sepsis: comparison of the Centers for Disease Control and Prevention screening-based protocol to a risk-based protocol in infants at greater than 37 weeks' gestation. J Perinatol 2000; 20:491–5.

254. Schrag S, Gorwitz R, Fultz-Butts K, et al. Prevention of perinatal Group B streptococcal disease. Revised guidelines from the CDC. MMWR – Morb Mortal Wkly Rep 2002;51 (RR11):1–22.

255. Schuchat A, Zywicki SS, Dinsmoor MJ, et al. Risk factors and opportunities for prevention of early-onset neonatal sepsis: a multicenter case-control study. Pediatrics 2000; 105:21–6.

256. Baltimore RS, Huie SM, Meek JI, et al. Early-onset neonatal sepsis in the era of group B streptococcal prevention. Pediatrics 2001;108:1094–8.

257. Reisner DP, Haas MJ, Zingheim RW, et al. Performance of a group B streptococcal prophylaxis protocol combining high-risk treatment and low-risk screening. Am J Obstet Gynecol 2000;182:1335–43.

258. Chen KT, Tuomala RE, Cohen AP, et al. No increase in rates of early-onset neonatal sepsis by non-group B streptococcus or ampicillin-resistant organisms. Am J Obstet Gynecol 2001;185:854–8.

259. Terrone DA, Rinehart BK, Einstein MH, et al. Neonatal sepsis and death caused by resistant *Escherichia coli*: possible consequences of extended maternal ampicillin administration. Am J Obstet Gynecol 1999;180:1345–8.

260. Graves GR, Rhodes PG. Tachycardia as a sign of early onset neonatal sepsis. Pediatr Infect Dis J 1984;3:404–6.

261. Griffin MP, Moorman JR. Toward the early diagnosis of neonatal sepsis and sepsis-like illness using novel heart rate analysis. Pediatrics 2001;107:97–104.

262. Wiswell TE, Baumgart S, Gannon CM, et al. No lumbar puncture in the evaluation for early neonatal sepsis: will meningitis be missed? Pediatrics 1995;95:803–6.

263. Lee CS, Tang RB, Chung RL, et al. Evaluation of different blood culture media in neonatal sepsis. J Microbiol Immunol Infect 2000;33:165–8.

264. Garcia-Prats JA, Cooper TR, Schneider VF, et al. Rapid detection of microorganisms in blood cultures of newborn infants utilizing an automated blood culture system. Pediatrics 2000;105:523–7.

265. Squire E, Favara B, Todd J. Diagnosis of neonatal bacterial infection: hematologic and pathologic findings in fatal and nonfatal cases. Pediatrics 1979;64:60–4.

266. Manroe BL, Weinberg AG, Rosenfeld CR, et al. The neonatal blood count in health and disease. I. Reference values for neutrophilic cells. J Pediatr 1979;95:89–98.

267. Schelonka RL, Yoder BA, desJardins SE, et al. Peripheral leukocyte count and leukocyte indexes in healthy newborn term infants. J Pediatr 1994;125:603–6.

268. Schelohka RL, Yoder BA, Hall RB, et al. Differentiation of segmented and band neutrophils during the early newborn period. J Pediatr 1995;127:298–300.

269. Greenberg DN, Yoder BA. Changes in the differential white blood cell count in screening for group B streptococcal sepsis. Pediatr Infect Dis J 1990;9:886–9.

270. Ghosh S, Mittal M, Jaganathan G. Early diagnosis of neonatal sepsis using a hematological scoring system. Indian J Med Sci 2001;55:495–500.

271. Berger C, Uehlinger J, Ghelfi D, et al. Comparison of C-reactive protein and white blood cell count with differential in neonates at risk for septicemia. Eur J Pediatr 1995; 154:138–44.

272. O'Connor TA, Ringer KM, Gaddis ML. Mean platelet volumes during coagulase-negative staphylococcal sepsis in neonates. Am J Clin Pathol 1993;99:69–71.

273. Dollner H, Vatten L, Austgulen R. Early diagnostic markers for neonatal sepsis: Comparing c-reactive protein, interleukin-6, soluble tumor necrosis factor receptors and soluble adhesion molecules. J Clin Epidemiol 2001;54: 1251–7.

274. Lewis DF, Barrilleaux PS, Wang Y, et al. Detection of interleukin-6 in maternal plasma predicts neonatal and infectious complications in preterm premature rupture of membranes. Am J Perinatol 2001;18:387–91.

275. Krueger M, Nauck MS, Sang S, et al. Cord blood levels of interleukin-6 and interleukin-8 for the immediate diagnosis of early-onset infection in premature infants. Biol Neonate 2001;80:118–23.

276. Kuster H, Weiss M, Willeitner AE, et al. Interleukin-1 receptor antagonist and interleukin-6 for early diagnosis of neonatal sepsis 2 days before clinical manifestation. Lancet 1998;352:1271–7.

277. Santana C, Guindeo MC, Gonazalez G, et al. Cord blood levels of cytokines as predictors of early neonatal sepsis. Acta Paediatr 2001;90:1176–81.

278. Dollner H, Vatten L, Linnebo I, et al. Inflammatory mediators in umbilical plasma from neonates who develop early-onset sepsis. Biol Neonate 2001;80:41–7.

279. Franz AR, Steinbach G, Kron M, et al. Reduction of unnecessary antibiotic therapy in newborn infants using interleukin-8 and C-reactive protein as markers of bacterial infections. Pediatrics 1999;104:447–53.

280. Bradley JS. Neonatal infections. Pediatr Infect Dis 1985; 4:315–20.

281. Evans JR, Allen AC, Stinson DA, et al. Perinatal listeriosis: report of an outbreak. Pediatr Infect Dis 1985;4:237–41.

282. Spigelblatt L, Saintonge J, Chicoine R, et al. Changing pattern of neonatal streptococcal septicemia. Pediatr Infect Dis 1985;4:56–8.

283. Baumgart S, Hall SE, Campos JM, et al. Sepsis with coagulase-negative staphylococci in critically ill newborns. Am J Dis Child 1983;137:461–3.

284. Faix RG. Systemic *Candida* infections in infants in intensive care nurseries: high incidence of central nervous system involvement. J Pediatr 1984;105:616–22.

285. Pierce JR, Merenstein GB, Stocker JT. Immediate postmortem cultures in an intensive care nursery. Pediatr Infect Dis 1984;3:510–3.

286. Litknukul S, Kusmiez H, Nelson JD, et al. Role of genital mycoplasmas in young infants with suspected sepsis. J Pediatr 1986;109:971–4.

287. Cox SM, Phillips LE, Mercer LJ, et al. Lactobacillemia of amniotic fluid origin. Obstet Gynecol 1986;68:134–5.

288. Garland SM, Murton LJ. Neonatal meningitis caused by *Ureaplasma urealyticum*. Pediatric Infect Dis J 1987;6: 868–70.

289. Chow AW, Leake RD, Yamauchi T, et al. The significance of anaerobes in neonatal bacteremia: analysis of 23 cases and review of the literature. Pediatrics 1974;54:736–45.

290. Bogdan JC, Rapkin RH. *Clostridia* infection in the newborn. Pediatrics 1976;58:120–2.

291. Speert DP, Munson D, Mitchell C, et al. *Mycobacterium chelonei* septicemia in a premature infant. J Pediatr 1980; 96:681–3.

292. Karlowicz MG, Buescher ES, Surka AE. Fulminant late-onset sepsis in a neonatal intensive care unit, 1988-1997, and the impact of avoiding empiric vancomycin therapy. Pediatrics 2000;106:1387–90.

293. Baley JE, Kliegman RM, Fanaroff AA. Disseminated fungal infections in very low-birth-weight infants: clinical manifestations and epidemiology. Pediatrics 1984;73:144–2.

294. Weese-Mayer DE, Fondriest DW, Brouillette RT, et al. Risk factors associated with candidemia in the neonatal intensive care unit: a case-control study. Pediatr Infect Dis J 1987;6:190–6.

295. Faix RG, Kovarik SM, Shaw TR, et al. Mucocutaneous and invasive candidiasis among very low birth weight (<1,500 grams) infants in intensive care nurseries: a prospective study. Pediatrics 1989;83:101–7.

296. Kaufman D, Boyle R, Hazen KC, et al. Fluconazole prophylaxis against fungal colonization and infection in preterm infants. N Engl J Med 2001;345(23):1660–6.

297. Cavanaugh RM Jr. Pneumatic otoscopy in healthy fullterm infants. Pediatrics 1987;79:520–3.

298. Berman SA, Balkany TJ, Simmons MA. Otitis media in infants less than 12 weeks of age: differing bacteriology among in-patients and out-patients. J Pediatr 1978;93: 453–4.

299. Claud EC, Walker WA. Hypothesis: inappropriate colonization of the premature intestine can cause necrotizing enterocolitis. FASEB J 2001;15:1398–403.

300. Ewer AK. Role of platelet activating factor in the pathophysiology of necrotizing enterocolitis. Acta Paediatr Suppl 2002;91:2–5.

301. Chan KL, Hui CW, Chan KW, et al. Revisiting ischemia and reperfusion injury as a possible cause of necrotizing enterocolitis: role of nitric oxide and superoxide dismutase. J Pediatr Surg 2002;37:828–34.

302. Rotbart HA, Levin MJ. How contagious is necrotizing enterocolitis? Pediatr Infect Dis 1983;2:406–13.

303. Duffy LC, Zielezny MA, Carrion V, et al. Bacterial toxins and enteral feeding of premature infants at risk for necrotizing enterocolitis. Adv Exp Med Biol 2001;501:519–27.

304. Alfa MJ, Robson D, Davi M, Bernard K, et al. An outbreak of necrotizing enterocolitis associated with a novel clostridium species in a neonatal intensive care unit. Clin Infect Dis 2002;35:S101–5.

305. Mehall JR, Kite CA, Saltzman DA, et al. Prospective study of the incidence and complications of bacterial contamination of enteral feeding in neonates. J Pediatr Surg 2002; 37:1177–82.

306. Schanler RJ. The use of human milk for premature infants. Pediatr Clin North Am 2001;48:207–19.

307. Dani C, Biadaioli R, Bertini G, et al. Probiotics feeding in prevention of urinary tract infection, bacterial sepsis and necrotizing enterocolitis in preterm infants. A prospective, double-blind study. Biol Neonate 2002;82: 103–8.

308. Foster J, Cole M. Oral immunoglobulin for preventing necrotizing enterocolitis in preterm and low birth-weight neonates. Cochrane Database Syst Rev 2001;(3): CD001816.

309. Bury RG, Tudehope D. Enteral antibiotics for preventing necrotizing enterocolitis in low birthweight or preterm infants. Cochrane Database Syst Rev 2001;(1): CD000405.

310. Amin HJ, Zamora SA, McMillan DD, et al. Arginine supplementation prevents necrotizing enterocolitis in the premature infant. J Pediatr 2002;140:425–31.

311. Caplan MS. Jilling T. New concepts in necrotizing enterocolitis. Curr Opin in Pediatr 2001;111–5.

312. Adzick NS, Nance ML. Pediatric surgery. First of two parts. N Engl J Med 2000;342(22):1651–7.

313. Kwong MS, Dinner M. Neonatal appendicitis masquerading as necrotizing enterocolitis. J Pediatr 1980;96:917–8.

314. Michalak DM, Cooney PR, Rhodes KH, et al. Gastrointestinal mucormycosis in infants and children: a cause of gangrenous intestinal cellulitis and perforation. J Pediatr Surg 1980;15:320–4.

315. Starke JR, Baker CJ. Neonatal shigellosis with bowel perforation. Pediatr Infect Dis 1985;4:405–7.

316. Youngs ER, Roberts C, Davidson DC. *Campylobacter* enteritis and bloody stools in the neonate. Arch Dis Child 1985;60:480–1.

317. Brasfield DM, Stagno S, Whitley, RJ, et al. Infant pneumonitis associated with cytomegalovirus, *Chlamydia*, *Pneumocystis*, and *Ureaplasma*: follow-up. Pediatrics 1987;79: 76–83.

318. Ballard RA, Drew L, Hugnagle KG, et al. Acquired cytomegalovirus infection in preterm infants. Am J Dis Child 1979;133:482–5.

319. Attenburrow AA, Barker CM. Chlamydial pneumonia in the low birthweight neonate. Arch Dis Child 1985;60: 1169–72.

320. Sagy M, Barzilay Z, Yahar J, et al. Severe neonatal chlamydial pneumonitis. Am J Dis Child 1980;134:89–91.

321. Taylor-Robinson D, Furr PM, Liberman MM. The occurrence of genital mycoplasmas in babies with and without respiratory disease. Acta Paediat Scand 1984;73:383–6.

322. Hiemstra I, VanBel F, Berger HM. Can *Trichomonas vaginalis* cause pneumonia in newborn babies? Lancet 1984; 2:355–6.

323. Brook I, Martin WJ, Finegold SM. Neonatal pneumonia caused by members of the *Bacteroides fragilis* group. Clin Pediatr 1980;19:541–4.

324. Anderson RD. Herpes simplex virus infection of the neonatal respiratory tract. Am J Dis Child 1987;141:274–6.

325. Mascola L, Cable DC, Walsh P, et al. Neonatal herpes simplex virus death manifested as rapidly progressive pneumonia. Clin Pediatr 1984;23:400–3.

326. Bhat AM, Meny RG, Aranas EA, et al. Fatal adenovirus (type 7) respiratory disease in neonates. Clin Pediatr 1984;23:409–411.

327. Stagno S, Pifer LL, Hughes WT, et al. *Pneumocystis carinii*

pneumonitis in young immunocompetent infants. Pediatrics 1980;66:56–62.

328. Blumberg HM, Burman WJ, Chaisson RE, et al. American Thoracic Society/Centers for Disease Control and Prevention/Infectious Diseases Society of America: treatment of tuberculosis. Am J Respir Crit Care Med 2003;167:603–62.

329. Cantwell MF, Shehab ZM, Costello AM, et al. Brief report: congenital tuberculosis. N Engl J Med 1994;330:1051–4.

330. Mazade MA, Evans EM, Starke JR, et al. Congenital tuberculosis presenting as sepsis syndrome: case report and review of the literature. Pediatr Infect Dis J 2001;20:439–42.

331. Abughali N, Van der Kuyp F, Annable W, Kumar ML. Congenital tuberculosis. Pediatr Infect Dis J 1994;13:738–41.

332. Lee LH, LeVea CM, Graman PS. Congenital tuberculosis in a neonatal intensive care unit: case report, epidemiological investigation, and management of exposures. Clin Infect Dis 1998; 27:474–7.

333. Kassner EG, Kaufmann SL, Yoon JJ, et al. Pulmonary candidiasis in infants: clinical, radiologic, and pathologic features. AJR 1981;137:707–16.

334. Siegel JD, McCracken GH. Neonatal lung abscess. Am J Dis Child 1979;133:947–9.

335. Boros SJ, Mammel MC, Lewallen PK, et al. Necrotizing tracheobronchitis: a complication of high-frequency ventilation. J Pediatr 1986;109:95–100.

336. Glaser JB, Engelberg M, Hammerschlag M. Scalp abscess associated with *Mycoplasma hominis* infection complicating intrapartum monitoring. Pediatr Infect Dis 1983;2:468–70.

337. Wagener MM, Rycheck RR, Yee RB, et al. Septic dermatitis of the neonatal scalp and maternal endomyometritis with intrapartum internal fetal monitoring. Pediatrics 1984;74:81–5.

338. Walsh M, McIntosh K. Neonatal mastitis. Clin Pediatr 1986;25:395–9.

339. Cushing AH. Omphalitis: a review. Pediatr Infect Dis 1985;4:282–5.

340. Ameh EA, Nmadu PT. Major complications of omphalitis in neonates and infants. Pediatr Surg Int 2002;18:413–6.

341. Samuel M, Freeman V, Vaishnav A, et al. Necrotizing fasciitis: a serious complication of omphalitis in neonates. J Pediatr Surg 1994;29:1414–6.

342. Janssen PA, Selwood BL, Dobson SR, et al. To dye or not to dye: a randomized, clinical trial of a triple dye/alcohol regime versus dry cord care. Pediatrics 2003;111:15–20.

343. Ramamurthy RS, Reveri M, Esterly NG, et al. Transient neonatal pustular melanosis. J Pediatr 1976;88:831–5.

344. Caputo RV. Recent advances in pediatric dermatology. Pediat Clin North Am 1983;30:735–7.

345. Kahn G, Rywlin AM. Acropustulosis of infancy. Arch Dermatol 1979;115:831–3.

346. Batson WJ, Reiner CB. Coxsackievirus B-2 infection in a neonate with incontinentia pigmenti. Pediatrics 1986;77:897–900.

347. Hruza LL, Mallory SB, Fitzgibbons J, et al. Linear IgA bullous dermatosis in a neonate. Pediatr Dermatol 1993;10:171–6.

348. Katzman DK, Wald ER. Staphylococcal scalded skin syndrome in a breast-fed infant. Pediatr Infect Dis 1987;6:295–6.

349. Thomsen AC, Espersen T, Maigaard S. Course and treatment of milk stasis, noninfectious inflammation of the breast, and infectious mastitis in nursing women. Am J Obstet Gynecol 1984;149:492–5.

350. American Academy of Pediatrics Committee on Drugs. Transfer of drugs and other chemicals into human milk. Pediatrics 2001;108:776–89.

351. Briggs GG, Freeman RK, Yaffe SJ. Drugs in Pregnancy and Lactation, 6th ed. Philadelphia: Williams & Wilkins, 2001.

CHAPTER 20

HIV Infection and AIDS

■ INTRODUCTION

This chapter will discuss several aspects of HIV infection and AIDS, including maternal-infant transmission, diagnostic tests, treatments, and prognosis. Detailed information about management of these children is beyond the scope of this book. Care of the HIV-infected baby, child, or adolescent is complex and rapidly evolving. It is hoped that the clinician can learn enough from this chapter to feel comfortable about the basics. Once HIV infection has been definitively diagnosed, care of these children should be done in concert with a physician who has specific training in pediatric infectious diseases and experience caring for children with HIV infection.

■ MODES OF TRANSMISSION

Maternal-Fetal (Vertical Acquisition)

Vertical transmission remains the most common way that pediatric patients become infected with HIV. It may occur during gestation, during the intrapartum period, or in the immediate postpartum period. In the absence of any steps to prevent transmission, 20–40% of babies born to HIV-positive mothers will become infected.[1-3] It is thought that most babies who become infected do so in the peripartum period. Earlier infection does occur, as HIV has been found by in situ PCR (polymerase chain reaction) in the tissues of aborted fetuses during the second trimester.[4] Transmission to babies after they have been born usually occurs through breastfeeding. This remains a problem in the developing world, where breast milk may be the only form of nutrition available, but it has been virtually eliminated in the United States, where clean water for formula is readily available.

The single most important factor in determining the risk of transmission is the viral load in maternal plasma. In one study of 552 maternal-infant pairs, none of 57 babies whose mother's viral load was less than 1,000 copies/mL became infected, but 26 (41%) of 64 babies whose maternal viral loads were greater than 100,000 copies/mL became infected.[2] The plasma viral load has been shown to correlate with the amount of HIV in both cervical mucus and in vaginal secretions,[5] which is a plausible explanation for the phenomenon. Transmission of HIV is also augmented by concomitant maternal syphilis.[6]

In the early 1990s, Pediatric AIDS Clinical Trials Group (PACTG) Protocol 076 demonstrated the effective prevention of maternal-infant transmission. This double-blind, prospective, placebo-controlled trial showed that the administration of zidovudine (ZDV or sometimes called azidothymidine [AZT]) to pregnant mothers during the last trimester of pregnancy, coupled with intravenous AZT in the immediate peripartum period and six weeks of oral AZT therapy for their neonates decreased maternal-infant transmission from 28% to 8%.[3] Maternal-infant transmission decreased greatly after this standard was adopted. Of course, the success of this form of prophylaxis depends upon knowing which mothers are HIV infected. This, in turn, relies upon prenatal counseling and universal HIV testing of pregnant women. When testing is offered to pregnant women, the majority accepts it. In one exemplary early program, counseling and testing increased from 21% to 95% of pregnancies, and the perinatal HIV transmission rate in North Carolina was documented to decrease from 31% to 3.1% statewide.[7] Testing pregnant women for HIV infection should be routine, similar to testing for syphilis or rubella immunity.

At any plasma viral load, adherence to the 076 AZT protocol decreases transmission rates. Factors that decrease the chances that a mother-infant pair will receive all three components of the protocol include older maternal age, CD4 counts greater than 500/μL, and cocaine or heroin use.[8] Because following all three parts of the 076 protocol is cumbersome and expensive, it has been difficult to implement in developing countries. Trials in which the maternal portion, the neonatal portion, or both were truncated suggest that a longer maternal component is more important than a longer neonatal component.[9] In these trials, the intrapartum intravenous AZT was replaced with frequent oral AZT. In another attempt at simplification, mothers and their infants were each given a single dose of nevirapine.[10] This regimen decreased transmission significantly only in mothers not already receiving standard antiretroviral therapy.[11] In one open-label trial, the combination of AZT and lamivudine (3TC) was also shown to be effective in preventing transmission. However, a common 3TC resistance mutation was demonstrated in 52 (39%) of 132 neonates, and adverse events, including severe anemia and thrombocytopenia, were common. Two children who were subsequently proven to be uninfected with HIV died before the age of 12 months from mitochondrial toxicities thought to be related to the combination therapy.[12]

Ultimately, antiretroviral therapies that best treat the mother's disease probably result in the best possible outcomes for both mother and baby.[13] The standard of care for pregnant women with HIV infection now includes use of multiple-drug therapy, at least one of which should be AZT. Fears that there would be long-term adverse outcomes in HIV-uninfected babies whose mothers received AZT during pregnancy have been largely assuaged. One study showed a slightly increased risk of first febrile seizure in these children,[14] but another study that followed, for a mean of 4.2 years, HIV-uninfected children whose mothers were enrolled in protocol 076 showed no significant difference in growth, cognition, or development in those whose mothers received AZT compared with those whose mothers received placebo.[15]

Other factors shown to be independently associated with increased risk of maternal-infant transmission include maternal obesity and procedures that cause the baby to contact maternal blood or cervical secretions.[16] In light of this finding, it is not surprising that elective cesarean delivery prior to rupture of membranes decreases transmission by about half.[17] However, the efficacy of cesarean delivery in the era of highly active antiretroviral therapy (HAART) has not been evaluated. Enthusiasm for elective cesarean birth has been waning, due, in part, to the fact that transmission rates are already less than 2% in many populations, and that cesarean delivery is not without risk, especially because wound healing may be poor in patients with advanced HIV disease.

Postnatal transmission via breast milk occurs in about 15% of babies who are exclusively breastfed.[18] Thus, HIV-positive mothers should not breastfeed their babies unless there is no possible alternative source of nutrition.

Sexual and Parenteral Transmission (Horizontal Transmission)

Horizontal transmission of HIV is usually from either sexual contact or through intravenous drug use. In recent years, there has been an increase in the number of teenagers being infected, usually through unprotected sex. It has been estimated that at least half of all new HIV infections in the United States occur among people below the age of 25, and that the majority of these young people are infected through sexual activity.[19] The message of so-called safe sex (more appropriately termed "safer sex") has been preached to a large number of people at risk. Unfortunately, adherence to this idea has been declining as improved therapies for HIV have become widely used.[20] Some of this laxity is due to the perception that persons on HAART are unlikely to transmit the infection. Remarkably, surveys reveal that the relaxed attitude toward HIV transmission is largely attributable to the perception that HIV infection is now a manageable disease. In one survey of 80 women, whereas only 5% of respondents believed that safer sex was no longer important, 15% said that they no longer insist on condom use, and 40% agreed that "AIDS is now a less serious threat."[21] Many teenagers, in particular, engage in high-risk behavior even though they understand the risk factors for HIV infection. This may be caused by the tendency of teenagers to feel a sense of immortality.

Injection drug use is a risk for acquisition of infection not only through needle sharing, but also because people who use injection drugs engage in riskier sexual behavior.[22] Even alcohol use has been identified as a risk factor.[23]

■ PRESENTING FEATURES OF HIV INFECTION

Most perinatally-infected babies are born to known HIV-positive mothers. Testing pregnant women for HIV during prenatal care identifies the risk to the fetus early, and mothers are given antiretroviral therapy. Babies born to these mothers are followed very closely and serially tested for the presence of the virus. Management of these babies is outlined in Box 20-1. With the exception of babies infected in utero, who may be born prematurely and develop severe signs and symptoms early in life, most babies with known exposure who prove to be infected are not symptomatic at the time of their diagnosis. There is a tendency for HIV-infected babies to be born slightly prematurely, and to be small for gestational age.[24] Other early signs, if present, include generalized lymphadenopathy, eczema,* hepatosplenomegaly, recalcitrant thrush, chronic diarrhea, failure to thrive, spasticity/hypertonicity, or recurrent bacterial infections. Dramatic presentation in the first months of life with life-threatening *Pneumocystis jiroveci* (formerly *carinii*) pneumonia is now uncommon.

Sometimes babies are born to mothers whose HIV status is unknown, either because they received no prenatal care or because they refused or were not offered HIV testing during pregnancy. Others test negative early but become infected with HIV during the course of the pregnancy. Rapid oral tests for HIV infection have been developed and may become important in the management of these high-risk mothers and their babies.

The natural course of HIV infection in vertically infected infants varies greatly. Most develop very high viral loads early in life, which may spontaneously drop within the first few months, but may plateau at a steady state that is still quite high (usually greater than 100,000/mL). Failure to thrive is a frequent problem. Linear growth is decreased within the first 6 months of life in HIV-infected infants, and the severity of the problem correlates with the magnitude of the viral load.[25,26] Neurodevelopmental delays are also common.[25,26] Decreased growth patterns are sustained through at least age five years. In a study that compared 95 infected children with 439 uninfected controls, poor growth was associated with history of pneumonia (relative risk [RR] 9), maternal cocaine use (RR 3), low CD4 cell counts (RR 2), and receipt of

---

BOX 20-1 ■ Management of the Known HIV-exposed Baby

In the hospital:
Thorough physical examination
Careful maternal history (maternal viral load, CD4 cell count, antiretroviral therapy, receipt of intrapartum IV AZT, other blood borne or sexually transmitted diseases)
Begin oral AZT, 2 mg/kg per dose,[a] every 6 hours; first dose within 4–6 hours of birth
HIV DNA PCR at time of hospital discharge (never use cord blood)
Ensure that mother seeks a general pediatrician to assume primary care

After discharge:
Follow-up visits with both a general pediatrician and an infectious diseases specialist
Thorough physical examinations, with special emphasis on growth, presence or absence of lymphadenopathy and hepatosplenomegaly, skin condition, and neurologic exam
Recalculate AZT dose, as rapid growth may lead to inadequate dosing
Repeat DNA PCRs, preferably at ages 2–4 weeks and more than 4 months (some experts recommend one RNA PCR at some point during the first 4 months, as limited data suggest it may be slightly more sensitive)
Stop AZT at 6 weeks of age
At 6 weeks, babies whose growth, development, and physical examinations are entirely normal and who have two negative PCR tests have a posttest probability of HIV infection that approaches 1/10,000. Therefore, trimethoprim-sulfamethoxazole prophylaxis is probably not necessary
Any baby who does not fulfill *all* of the above criteria should be started on trimethoprim sulfamethoxazole until the post-4 month PCR is obtained and proved to be negative
When the baby is at least 4-months-old, has had at least 3 negative PCR tests, and is clinically well, he or she can be discharged from the Infectious Diseases clinic with a "clean bill of health." Documenting seroreversion is not necessary

[a]Anecdotally, 3 mg/kg taken orally every 8 hours is functionally equivalent to 2 mg/kg every 6 hours, easier on family. For term babies requiring IV AZT because they cannot take by mouth for any reason, the dosage is 1.5 mg/kg IV every 6 hours. For premature babies (less than 34 weeks) able to take medicines orally, the experimental dosage is 1.5 mg/kg every 12 hours for 2 weeks, then 2 mg/kg every 8 hours thereafter until they are the size of a normal newborn baby.
Source: Modified from: Benjamin DK Jr, Miller WC, Fiscus SA, et al. Rational testing of the HIV-exposed infant. *Pediatrics* 2001;108:e3, with permission.

antiretroviral therapy by age 3 months (RR 3). After adjusting for pneumonia and antiretroviral therapy, the child's viral load remained associated with failure to thrive.[27]

Classification

The Centers for Disease Control and Prevention (CDC) classification scheme for infants and children with HIV infection has changed several times. The scheme currently in use is quite straightforward. Patients are classified based on symptoms designated by letters—N, for no symptoms; A, for mild symptoms; B, for moderate symptoms; and C, for severe symptoms—and immune suppression designated by numbers: 1, for no suppression; 2, for moderate suppression; and 3, for severe

suppression. The type of clinical conditions and degree of immune suppression that qualify a patient for the various designations is shown in Box 20-2.

■ TREATMENT OPTIONS

Antiretroviral Therapy

An introduction to the various classes of antiretroviral agents, their uses, and their side effects and limitations follows. The actual clinical approach to using these agents is discussed briefly thereafter.

Nucleoside Analogue Reverse Transcriptase Inhibitors (NRTIs)

The first class of effective antiretrovirals was the nucleoside analogues. These agents work by block-

---

BOX 20-2 ■ CDC Classification Scheme for Patients with HIV Infection

Letter Designations

N. No symptoms, or only one of the symptoms from A, below.

A. Mild symptoms. Two of more of the following, without any symptoms from B or C, below. Lymphadenopathy, hepatosplenomegaly, dermatitis, parotitis, recurrent or persistent upper respiratory tract infections, sinusitis, or otitis media

B. Moderate symptoms. Anemia, neutropenia, or thrombocytopenia; invasive bacterial infection (sepsis, pneumonia, meningitis); persistent thrush at age greater than 6 months; cardiomyopathy; recurrent or chronic diarrhea; herpes group virus infections (CMV prior to age 1 month; recurrent HSV stomatitis; HSV bronchitis, pneumonitis, or esophagitis before age 1 month; two episodes or two-dermatomal herpes zoster [shingles]; complicated chickenpox; LIP; leiomyosarcoma; nephropathy; nocardiosis; toxoplasmosis before 1 month of age; fever for greater than 1 month.

C. Severe symptoms. Multiple or recurrent invasive bacterial infections; esophageal or pulmonary candidiasis; disseminated fungal infections (coccidioidomycosis, histoplasmosis, or extrapulmonary cryptococcosis); severe herpes group virus infections (persistent mucocutaneous ulcer; bronchitis, pneumonitis, or esophagitis in child greater than 1 month of age; CMV disease anywhere but liver, spleen, or lymph nodes, onset after 1 month of age; Kaposi sarcoma); diarrhea for greater than one month caused by protozoans (cryptosporidiosis, isosporiasis); PCP; PML(progressive multifocal leukoencephalopathy); severe mycobacterial infection (extrapulmonary TB, disseminated nontuberculous mycobacterial infection); recurrent *Salmonella* sepsis; toxoplasmosis of the brain after age 1 month; oncologic problem (primary brain lymphoma, Burkitt lymphoma, large-cell lymphoma); encephalopathy; wasting syndrome.

Number designations

IMMUNE CATEGORY	<12 MONTHS		1–5 YEARS		≥6 YEARS	
	NO./MM³	(%)	NO./MM³	(%)	NO./MM³	(%)
Category 1: No suppression	≥1500	≥25%	≥1000	≥25%	≥500	≥25%
Category 2: Moderate suppression	750–1499	15–24%	500–999	15–24%	200–499	15–24%
Category 3: Severe suppression	<750	<15%	<500	<15%	200	<15%

Abbreviations: CMV, cytomegalovirus; HSV, herpes simplex virus; LIP, lymphoid interstitial pneumonitis (see text); PCP, *Pneumocystis jiroveci* pneumonia (see text); PML, progressive multifocal leukoencephalopathy (rare in children); TB, tuberculosis.

ing the action of reverse transcriptase. Reverse transcriptase is an enzyme that the virus uses to change its genomic RNA into DNA. Once DNA is formed, it is integrated into the host cell genome. When reverse transcription is inhibited, RNases (ribonucleases) in the cytoplasm are able to destroy the viral RNA.

AZT is the prototype nucleoside analogue drug. Many others have been developed (see Box 20-3). The virus is able to develop resistance to these agents very rapidly; thus, they should never be used alone for treatment. The combination of AZT and 3TC has been used extensively because resistance to AZT tends to confer susceptibility to 3TC, and vice versa.[28] Because they are analogues of the same nucleoside (thymidine), AZT and d4T (stavudine) compete with each other and should never be used together.

In a typical regimen, a pair of nucleoside analogues is coupled with a non-nucleoside reverse transcriptase inhibitor or with a protease inhibitor. These types of combination or "cocktail" therapies

---

BOX 20-3 ■ Antiretroviral Agents

Nucleoside reverse transcriptase inhibitors
AZT (azidothymidine, ZDV, zidovudine, Retrovir)
3TC (lamivudine, Epivir)
d4T (stavudine, Zerit)
ddI (didanosine, Videx)
ddC (zalcitabine, dideoxycytidine, Hivid)
abacavir (Ziagen)
emtricitabine (Emtriva)
tenofovir (Viread, technically a nucleoTIDE RT
   inhibitor)

Non-nucleoside reverse transcriptase inhibitors
Nevirapine (Viramune)
Efavirenz (Sustiva)
Delavirdine (Rescriptor)

Protease Inhibitors
Nelfinavir (Viracept)
Saquinavir (Fortovase, Invirase)
Ritonavir (Norvir)
Indinavir (Crixivan)
Amprenavir (Agenerase)
Lopinavir/ritonavir (Kaletra)
Fosamprenavir (Levitra)
Atazanavir (Reyataz)

Fusion Inhibitors
T-20 (enfuvirtide, Fuzeon)

---

have been called highly active antiretroviral therapy (HAART).

Non-nucleoside Reverse Transcriptase Inhibitors (NNRTIs)

These drugs also inhibit reverse transcriptase, but do it by a different mechanism. Non-nucleoside agents are much more potent than nucleosides. The combination of two nucleoside agents and a non-nucleoside has been shown to be just as effective as two nucleosides and a protease inhibitor.[29,30] Nevirapine, a non-nucleoside agent, is given twice a day. It has been associated with severe and even fatal hepatotoxicity. Rarely, nevirapine has been associated with untoward events in pregnant women, particularly in those with CD4 cell counts greater than $250/\mu L$.

Efavirenz is the other commonly used non-nucleoside agent. Its principal toxicity involves the central nervous system (CNS). Patients taking efavirenz may experience dysphoria and complain of feeling "spaced out," and dreams have been reported to be vivid and sometimes frightening. This side effect is much more common in adults than in children and tends to subside with continued therapy. There are concerns of teratogenicity based upon animal studies. Therefore, efavirenz should never be used in pregnant patients or in adolescents in whom the possibility of becoming pregnant cannot be eliminated.

Protease Inhibitors (PIs)

During replication, HIV produces a polyprotein (a long chain of amino acids that includes multiple protein molecules linked together). This polyprotein is not functional and must be broken up into its constituent proteins by a viral enzyme called protease. Protease inhibitors act by preventing this enzyme from cleaving the polyprotein into usable protein molecules. These drugs are highly effective when used in combination with other antiretrovirals. If used alone or with only one other drug, resistance develops rapidly.

Of all the protease inhibitors currently available (Box 20-3), nelfinavir is the one that has the longest track record in the treatment of childhood HIV infection, mainly because it was the first to be available in liquid form. Ritonavir, difficult to tolerate as the only PI, is now being used in combination with other PIs because it boosts levels by its strong inhibition of cytochrome P450 in the liver.

Side effects of protease inhibitors are numerous. Perhaps most troublesome are hypertriglyceridemia, hypercholesterolemia, and lipodystrophy (discussed follows).

New Classes of Antiretroviral Agents

Although other targets have been identified, such as integrase, development of agents to suppress targets other than reverse transcriptase and protease has been difficult. Enfuvirtide (T-20, Fuzeon) is a new drug whose function is to inhibit fusion of the viral envelope with cell membranes. It has recently been FDA-approved for use in adults and children aged 6 years and older. Inhibition of fusion inhibits cell-to-cell spread of the virus as well as slowing the penetration phase of viral replication. In highly antiretroviral-experienced patients, the addition of enfurvitide versus placebo to an optimized background regimen improves viral control, and concomitant increases in CD4 cell counts are also seen.[31] As with other classes of antiretrovirals, resistance develops very quickly if they are used alone. T-20, the prototype of the class, must be administered by subcutaneous injection twice a day, which can be a major impediment for some patients. Injection site reactions (including subcutaneous nodules, itching, redness, swelling, and rarely cellulitis) were seen in 98% of participants in one clinical trial, although the majority of these were manageable and not dose limiting.[31]

Highly Active Antiretroviral Therapy (HAART)

Optimally, antiretroviral therapies are given in combination. The principal reason for this is that resistance emerges very quickly when they are used alone. Beyond this simple concept, the clinical work of initiating, monitoring, maintaining, and changing antiretroviral therapies is vastly complicated and generally not the subject of much consensus; thus, a thorough discussion is beyond the scope of this book.

Increasingly, physicians are realizing that antiretroviral therapy is probably best when individualized. Much of the success of any regimen is dependent on the patient's adherence to it. A study in adults demonstrated a striking difference in rates of virologic failure (defined as more than 400 viral copies/mL a median of 6 months later) between those with 95% adherence or more (22% had virologic failure) and those with 80–94.9% adherence

(61% had virologic failure).[32] Eighty percent of those who took less than 80% of the prescribed doses experienced virologic failure.[32] This problem is compounded somewhat in pediatrics, because adherence is often the job of someone other than the patient, usually the primary caregiver. Primary caregivers may also be HIV infected, and are sometimes ill or even suffer from dementia associated with HIV infection. They may not be well organized and may not be able to remember each dose. In addition, young children (particularly from about age 18 months to 4 years) may refuse to take their medications. In these children, consideration should be given to the placement of a gastrostomy tube for medication administration.[33]

The physician caring for children with HIV infection is faced with many difficult decisions. HIV infection should be conceptualized as a "decades-long" disease, and the approach to therapy tempered by that concept. In other words, sometimes one most forego the "optimal" short-term regimen in favor of one the patient is more likely to adhere to and tolerate. In pediatric HIV, especially, it is distressingly easy to "burn" regimens and entire classes of antiretroviral drugs, leaving the patient with extremely limited options for future treatment. The complexities involved in deciding exactly when and how to switch ARV treatment regimens are beyond the scope of this chapter. These decisions need to be made by (or in concert with) a physician with appropriate training and clinical experience. Even if adherence is perfect, antiretroviral therapies often cause side effects and complications that can become dose limiting and affect the patient's quality of life. Some of these complications are discussed in the following text. General ideas about appropriate antiretroviral regimens are shown in Box 20-4.

Complications of Antiretroviral Therapy

Lipodystrophy

As more experience with HAART is gained, more long-term side effects of therapy are discovered. One of the more troubling of these is called lipodystrophy, the essence of which is fat redistribution. There are many different forms of the condition: some patients have peripheral fat wasting, some have truncal fat accumulation, some have dyslipidemia and hypercholesterolemia, and some have insulin resistance. In most cases, patients have a combination of two or more of these problems.

BOX 20-4 ■ Combination Antiretroviral Therapies

2 NRTIs[a] plus 1 PI[b]
2 NRTIs plus 1 NNRTI
3 NRTIs (AZT/3TC/abacavir)[c]
1 or 2 NRTIs plus 1 NNRTI plus 1 PI[b]

Abbreviations: NRTI, nucleoside reverse transcriptase inhibitor; NNRTI, non-nucleoside reverse transcriptase inhibitor; PI, protease inhibitor.
[a] The following NRTI combinations are not recommended: AZT plus d4T or 3TC plus FTC (competitive inhibition), ddI plus d4T (too much toxicity), tenofovir plus either ddI or abacavir, ?{AQ4} ddI plus abacavir.
[b] PIs (saquinavir, indinavir, and amprenavir but *not* nelfinavir) can be boosted with low-dose ritonavir.
[c] Recently shown to be less effective than PI-containing or NNRTI-containing regimens.

Lipodystrophy occurs with distressing frequency. Large surveys and prospective studies have documented that up to 41% of patients on HAART regimens experience increased abdominal girth,[34] 32% have decreased facial fat, and 57% have hypercholesterolemia.[35] In one small study of children with HIV infection, even the 28 children without clinically apparent lipodystrophy had increased central fat and peripheral lipoatrophy documented by dual-energy x-ray absorptiometry ("dexa") scanning.[36] Risk factors for the development of lipodystrophy include advanced disease,[37] duration of HIV positivity,[34] use of stavudine (d4T) for longer than a year,[37] and use of indinavir or ritonavir.[34]

Long thought to principally be a complication of protease inhibitor therapy, it has now been clearly established that nucleoside reverse transcriptase inhibitors (especially stavudine and didanosine) can also lead to lipodystrophy. One hypothesis is that a combination of these NRTIs and the protease inhibitors leads to the full syndrome of lipodystrophy, with the NRTI affecting the mitochondrial function of the adipocytes and the protease inhibitor causing insulin resistance and impaired adipocyte maturation.[38]

Patients with lipodystrophy say that their quality of life is impaired; self-esteem issues are the primary determinant of this problem.[37] Adherence to therapy may also suffer, as patients often stop taking the medications in an effort to treat the syndrome.[39] Unfortunately, lipodystrophy is not that easily reversed. An exercise program combined with a moderate-fat, low-glycemic-index, high-fiber diet, however, has been shown to improve several aspects of lipodystrophy.[40] Interestingly, even though many patients with lipodystrophy syndrome have elevated levels of triglycerides and cholesterol, lipodystrophy in patients with HIV does not present as large a risk factor for atherosclerotic coronary vascular disease as similar cholesterol and triglyceride levels would in the HIV-uninfected patient.[41]

Mitochondrial Toxicity

The principal toxicity of the nucleoside analogue drugs occurs in the mitochondria, and is a direct extension of the pharmacologic activity of these agents. Mitochondria contain reverse transcriptases (principally polymerase gamma and telomerase), and these are inhibited to varying degrees by reverse transcriptase inhibitors. Any drug of this class can produce mitochondrial toxicity, but ddC (dideoxycytidine), ddI (didanosine), and d4T are more likely to do so than are 3TC and AZT. Abacavir is the least mitochondria-toxic of all the NRTIs. When suppression of mitochondrial polymerases occurs, tissues with high metabolic needs are the most likely to be affected. Clinically, the syndrome usually presents with vague symptoms, such as gastrointestinal upset, dyspnea, and fatigue. Occasionally, it manifests as severe myalgias and/or myocarditis. Laboratory studies show mildly elevated aminotransferase levels and elevated lactate. Obesity, female gender, and preexisting liver disease are risk factors for the development of symptomatic mitochondrial toxicity states. Micronutrient deficiencies may increase the risk of developing the syndrome. Symptoms of mitochondrial toxicity syndrome usually resolve when the offending nucleoside is discontinued.[42]

Immune Reconstitution Inflammatory Syndrome (IRIS)

Soon after the advent of HAART, it became clear that some patients were developing worsening symptoms of illness as their immune systems were recovering function. The symptoms are based upon the newfound ability of the immune system to mount an inflammatory response to a variety of antigens. This phenomenon has been seen with a number of infectious agents, but is most frequently described with *Mycobacterium avium* complex (MAC) infection.[43] When symptoms of MAC develop in patients on HAART, they usually do so within a month of effective antiretroviral therapy.[43] Disease tends to be more localized, and may include caseating granulomas.[44] In one study, 12 (36%) of 33 adult patients co-infected with *Mycobacterium tuberculosis* and HIV developed "paradoxical worsening" of symptoms when HAART was begun.[45] Subclinical CMV (cytomegalovirus) infection of the eye may turn into severe, sometimes sight-threatening inflammation, termed "immune recovery uveitis."[46] Most cases of IRIS have been described in adults, but the phenomenon also occurs in children.

Evaluation of the Pediatric HIV-infected Patient with Fever

The workup of any HIV-infected child who presents with fever begins with an assessment of the child's immune status. Causes of fever in children with category 1 disease (i.e., CD4 count 25% or greater) do not differ significantly from those seen in non-HIV-infected children. They are likely to have common community-acquired infections, as would any child with fever. The exception would be that HIV-infected children have a much higher incidence of pneumococcal infection than their uninfected peers (see text that follows). Children in category 2 (i.e., CD4 cell count 15–24%) are still more likely to acquire common diseases than opportunistic infections. Patients with low absolute lymphocyte counts, those in the lower end of CDC class 2, may have relatively compromised immunity, which might predispose to a broader array of infections. In all children with HIV and fever, if an obvious local source cannot be found, or if the source is pneumonia, a set of blood cultures should be obtained prior to administration of any antibiotic agent. Selected antibiotics should have good activity against *Streptococcus pneumoniae*, the most common pathogen. As with infections in other immunocompromised patients, the intravenous route may be necessary initially and duration of therapy may need to be longer than in the healthy host.

For patients with category 3 immune suppression (CD4 less than 15%), infection with a wide variety of pathogens is possible (including concomitant infection with more than one pathogen). As immunity is severely suppressed, signs and symptoms of disease may be mild. Evaluation needs to be thorough, and, when febrile, these patients often require admission to the hospital. It is prudent to involve an infectious-diseases trained pediatrician from the outset. Workup is more extensive than expected by the severity of symptoms; for example, intermittent or persistent headache with low-grade fever in this type of patient might be an indication for a computed tomography (CT) scan and a lumbar puncture. Blood cultures, including special cultures for *Mycobacterium avium* complex (see following text), should be obtained. If any localizing signs or symptoms are found, investigation can begin by focusing on those areas. Many of the problems children with HIV and AIDS may encounter are discussed in the remainder of this chapter.

◼ COMMON PROBLEMS IN PATIENTS WITH HIV INFECTION

Central Nervous System (CNS) Problems

Encephalopathy

HIV enters the CNS of babies early during the course of infection.[47] In some patients, this gives rise to HIV encephalopathy, a condition that usually manifests as peripheral spasticity, followed or accompanied by developmental delay or loss of developmental milestones and cognitive decline, with or without microcephaly.[48] The course may be progressive or it may plateau and become static. It may resemble, and may be difficult to differentiate from, cerebral palsy. The severity of HIV encephalopathy is related to the cerebrospinal fluid (CSF) viral load.[49] CSF viral load does not necessarily correlate with plasma viral load, is not readily measurable, and is seldom used clinically.

Clinical changes consistent with HIV encephalopathy are usually accompanied by neuroradiographic changes, including cerebral atrophy, white matter lesions, and basal ganglia calcifications. Of these, atrophy is most closely related to the clinical findings of HIV encephalopathy.[50] In general, baseline CD4 cell count, viral load, and clinical examination correlate with the severity of atrophy on head CT scanning.[50,51] Serial routine neuroimaging, therefore, is usually redundant. In one study of 58 children with HIV infection, treatment was not altered by follow-up CT scanning in any patient.[52] A thorough neurologic and developmental evaluation is probably the most sensitive indicator of cortical dysfunction associated with HIV encephalopathy.

Much of the literature on HIV encephalopathy concerns this condition in the pre-HAART era. Treatment of HIV infection with HAART probably has had some effect on both the incidence and severity of HIV encephalopathy. The case of an 8-year-old boy with rather severe encephalopathy who recovered much of his brain function after effective treatment of his HIV infection has been published.[47] Anecdotally, the percentage of our HIV-infected patients who suffer from moderate to severe neurodevelopmental problems has decreased over the past several years.

Cryptococcal Meningitis

Cryptococcal meningitis is a disease that occurs only in patients with advanced immunosuppression. It is more common in adults with AIDS than it is in children. Of 1,478 pediatric AIDS cases reported to one registry from 1985–1994, 20 (1.4%) were diagnosed with cryptococcosis.[53] In the largest pediatric series published to date, 19 (63%) of 30 cases occurred in children between the ages of 6 and 12 years. The median CD4 cell count within three months of cryptococcal meningitis was 54/μL, and more than half of these children had a prior AIDS-defining illness.[53]

The diagnosis should be suspected in any patient with advanced AIDS who has headache and fever, even if both of these symptoms are subtle. Cryptococcal meningitis can have a very indolent course. Altered mental status, focal neurologic signs, or seizures are uncommon, and indicate a poor prognosis.[54] The inflammatory response to cryptococci in the CSF is generally not impressive. Therefore, normal CSF white blood cell counts, glucose, and protein levels should not deter the clinician from pursuing the diagnosis with India ink staining, serum and CSF cryptococcal antigen testing, and culture.

Amphotericin B, with or without flucytosine, is the treatment of choice. Mortality is higher in patients in whom clearance of the pathogen from the CSF is delayed.[55] Critical elevation of intracranial pressure may ensue, which sometimes necessitates ventriculoperitoneal shunting.[56] Serial cryptococcal antigen testing of the CSF may be used to monitor response to treatment; antigen levels decrease with proper therapy. The exact duration of therapy for cryptococcal meningitis has not been established; most experts recommend 0.7–1.0 mg/kg per day of amphotericin B for 14 days, followed by 8 weeks of daily oral fluconazole or itraconazole, followed by suppressive therapy with daily fluconazole at half the treatment dose. Suppressive therapy is usually maintained for life. Although prophylaxis against other opportunistic infections can usually be safely discontinued after the patient experiences immune reconstitution (usually defined as CD4 cell count greater than 200/μL for greater than 6 months), data regarding this strategy in cryptococcal meningitis are limited and, as yet, unconvincing.[57] Signs and symptoms of cryptococcal meningitis are often worsened by immune recovery (see section on Immune Reconstitution Inflammatory Syndrome [IRIS]).

Cerebral Toxoplasmosis

Cerebral toxoplasmosis generally represents reactivation of latent toxoplasmosis disease. It is more common in adults than in children. All HIV-positive children outside the infant age group should be tested for antibodies against *Toxoplasma gondii*. If immunoglobulin IgG is measurable, past infection has occurred, meaning the patient will be at risk for disease when immune suppression ensues. Cerebral toxoplasmosis is usually seen in patients with advanced HIV disease.

The incidence of toxoplasmosis has decreased in the HAART era,[58] but not as convincingly as other opportunistic diseases, including *Pneumocystis jiroveci* pneumonia (PCP) and cryptococcal meningitis.[59] Fortunately, TMP-SMX (trimethoprim-sulfamethoxazole), given for PCP prophylaxis, is also an effective prophylaxis against cerebral toxoplasmosis.

The diagnosis is considered when a patient with advanced HIV disease has fever and headache, sometimes accompanied by altered level of consciousness or focal seizures. Differentiating toxoplasmal encephalitis from other conditions of the CNS, especially lymphoma, can be difficult. Single photon emission-computed tomography (SPECT) scanning is not always reliable.[60] Most experts advise treating presumptively for toxoplasmosis in HIV-positive patients who have both positive serology and multiple cerebral lesions by CT scan.[61] Treatment is with pyrimethamine, sulfadiazine, and folinic acid for 3–6 weeks. Follow-up imaging is done in 2 weeks to assess the efficacy of treatment.

Tissue diagnosis should be obtained in patients without AIDS, those with solitary lesions, or those with multiple lesions that are nonresponsive to a trial of therapy.[61] Newer diagnostic modalities, including blood and spinal fluid PCR testing, are promising.[62]

In the past, suppressive antibiotics were recommended for life. In a newer study, suppressive therapy was interrupted in 75 patients with a history of proven toxoplasmosis. These patients had undergone immune reconstitution secondary to HAART therapy. In more than 119 person-years of follow-up, only one relapse of toxoplasmosis occurred.[57] Prevention of toxoplasmosis is discussed in the prevention section.

Hematologic Abnormalities

Anemia

Anemia is the most common hematologic abnormality in patients with HIV infection. By the second month of life, hemoglobin levels are lower in infected than in HIV-exposed but uninfected babies, and the levels diverge throughout the first year of life.[63] The incidence of anemia increases with advancing disease.[64] There are many possible causes of anemia in HIV. Most cases are attributable to anemia of chronic disease,[65] but nutrient deficiencies, autoimmune hemolysis, medication side effects, and persistent parvovirus B19 infection have all been described.[66] AZT is particularly likely to cause broad myelosuppression.[67]

HIV-infected patients with mild-to-moderate anemia are usually symptomatic, although clinicians often overlook the symptoms.[64] The most common symptoms are fatigue and exercise intolerance. Fatigue may be severe enough to adversely affect quality of life.[64] Most important, anemia has been shown to be an independent risk factor for disease progression and death.[68] Resolution of anemia measurably increases quality of life[69] and prolongs survival.[68]

For patients with anemia of chronic disease, successful antiretroviral therapy often resolves the anemia.[70] If an obvious underlying cause can be found, directed therapy is appropriate. Occasionally, medication changes become necessary.[71] If anemia persists despite HAART, weekly treatment with erythropoietin-alfa is often effective.[72] Counterintuitively, the biggest changes in quality of life occur at the higher end of the anemia scale; e.g., raising the hemoglobin level from 11 to 12 produces a more noticeable effect on health than raising it from 8 to 9.[64] In adults, a hemoglobin of 12 for men and 11 for women has been suggested as a reasonable target.[72] Therapies other than erythropoietin have been associated with adverse outcomes; iron causes increased viral replication[73] and transfusions reduce the function of lymphocytes, natural killer cells, and monocytes.[68] Iron should only be administered when iron deficiency is proved by laboratory studies and then only in concert with HAART. Transfusions should be reserved for patients with severe anemia who require emergent correction.[68]

Thrombocytopenia

Defined as a platelet count less than 100,000/mcL, thrombocytopenia is common in HIV-infected persons, occurring in about 11% of patients.[74] Thrombocytopenia can occur through multiple pathways, including shortened survival time and decreased delivery of viable platelets to the peripheral circulation from the bone marrow.[75] In one small study comparing 6 patients with HIV and thrombocytopenia with 98 normal controls, the patients with HIV-mediated thrombocytopenia were found to have about two-thirds the platelet lifespan and about twice the splenic sequestration of the control patients.[75]

Megakaryocyte precursors have been shown to have both CD4[76] and the HIV coreceptor (and chemokine receptor) CXCR4[77] on their surfaces, which could make them potential targets of active HIV replication. In vitro, these precursor cells have been productively infected with HIV.[78]

Children with HIV-associated thrombocytopenia present similarly to children with immune thrombocytopenic purpura (ITP). They may have easy bruising and petechiae, or the low platelet count may be incidentally discovered. Asymptomatic thrombocytopenia with a platelet count greater than 20,000/mcL can usually be safely monitored. Most experts recommend treatment if the platelet count goes below 20,000/mcL or if the condition becomes symptomatic.[79] In most patients, effective antiretroviral therapy produces a sustained increase in platelet counts,[80] but in some the condition persists despite good viral load suppression.[81] When a rapid increase in platelet count is required, low-dose intravenous immune globulin (IVIG) (40 mg/kg per week for 5 weeks) has been successful in most patients, although in one study a sustained response was seen in only a third.[82] Alternatively,

30 μg/kg of anti-RhoD (rhogam) can be given on days 1, 3, and 4, followed by a maintenance dose of 6 μg/kg weekly out to a total of 8 weeks.[83] Although the response to anti-RhoD immunoglobulin therapy is somewhat slower than that to IVIG, about 70–80% of patients respond, and the response seems to be more durable.[83,84] For refractory cases, splenectomy or partial splenectomy[85] may be curative. In response to splenectomy, patients with HIV-related thrombocytopenia recover platelet numbers much more reliably than patients with non-HIV related ITP.[86]

Neutropenia

At some point, neutropenia (defined as an absolute neutrophil count (ANC) less than 1,000/μL) develops in 20–34% of adults with HIV infection.[87] It is also quite common in children. The cause is likely to be multifactorial: (i) HIV may directly infect some precursor cells in the bone marrow, (ii) secondary infection of the bone marrow, such as by *Mycobacterium avium* complex, may occur, (iii) it may be the result of myelosuppressive therapies such as AZT, ganciclovir, or TMP-SMX, (iv) nutritional deficiencies may contribute, (v) neutrophils in patients infected with HIV tend to have an increased rate of programmed cell death, and (vi) cytokine dysregulation is common.[88] Neutropenia in patients with HIV infection does lead to both increased episodes of bacterial infection and increased hospitalizations, but in general it is much better tolerated than in cancer patients.[89]

Severe neutropenia (ANC less than 250) or moderate neutropenia (ANC 251 to 500) that is associated with infectious episodes may be treated with subcutaneous administration of recombinant granulocyte colony-stimulating factor (G-CSF, filgrastim). G-CSF causes not only an increase in neutrophil count but a boost in function as well.[90] In one study, concomitant G-CSF treatment allowed more than 80% of AIDS patients to continue to receive needed but myelosuppressive therapies.[91]

Dermatologic Problems

Atopic and seborrheic dermatitis

Both of these conditions are common in children with HIV infection and AIDS. Sometimes, "bad skin" is the presenting feature of HIV infection in babies. However, seborrheic dermatitis is also common in non-HIV-infected infants, so this finding is nonspecific.

Detailed studies about skin problems in children with HIV infection have not been reported. A prospective study that followed 151 adult HIV patients for 4 months documented dermatologic conditions in 138 (91%).[92] Atopic dermatitis and seborrhea are managed in HIV patients the same way they are managed in patients without HIV. For severe cases, consultation with a dermatologist may be helpful.

Molluscum contagiosum

Children with HIV sometimes develop extensive and refractory molluscum contagiosum. The lesions may be especially numerous on the face, which can cause considerable social problems. Occasionally, the eyelids will be heavily involved, usually in patients with advanced HIV disease. In one series of 11 patients with eyelid molluscum, 10 (91%) of the patients were in CDC stage C3, with a mean CD4 count of 72/μL.[93] In most cases, gaining control over the HIV disease with HAART therapy leads to spontaneous resolution of even the most difficult-to-treat lesions.[94] Topical imiquimod (an immunomodulator)[95] and 1% cidofovir (an antiviral agent)[96] have also been successfully employed in the treatment of refractory molluscum contagiosum.

Zoster (Shingles)

Zoster and recurrent zoster are occasional problems in the HIV-infected population. Zoster is more likely to develop when the patient gets primary varicella when he is already severely immune suppressed.[97] Unlike PCP and MAC, zoster can occur at any stage of HIV infection.[98]

Zoster in patients with HIV infection should be treated promptly with intravenous acyclovir.[97] HIV patients are more likely than non-HIV patients to develop disseminated (multidermatomal) zoster, which is generally considered more contagious than the single dermatomal form. Prolonged,[99] severe, or atypical manifestations have been described, but in our experience are the exception, rather than the rule. Zoster and primary varicella combined accounted for only 44 (2.7%) of 746 hospitalizations of HIV-infected children at one institution (Fisher RG, unpublished data).

The incidence of zoster should decrease with the use of the live attenuated varicella vaccine, which should be given to patients early, when the immune system is still intact (see prevention section).

Pulmonary Problems

Pneumonia

The incidence and severity of bacterial lower respiratory tract infection increases with the degree of immunosupression.[100] In adults with HIV infection, bacterial pneumonia is predictive of decreased survival.[100] In a group of perinatally infected children in Thailand, 16 (52%) of 31 ultimately died of pneumonia, making it the leading cause of death.[101]

The most common pathogen is *Streptococcus pneumoniae*. The radiographic appearance of pneumococcal pneumonia in adults with HIV does not differ from that of patients without HIV.[102] However, viral pneumonia in HIV-infected patients is more likely to produce consolidation, which can sometimes cloud the clinical picture.[103]

A subset of pediatric patients with HIV infection tends to get recurrent pneumonia, generally attributable to the pneumococcus. It is not clear what predisposes this group of patients to this problem. In vitro the alveolar macrophages of patients with HIV infection have defects in neither opsonization nor phagocytosis of *S. pneumoniae*.[104] Issues regarding prevention of pneumococcal infection are discussed in the prevention section.

Patients with advanced AIDS are at risk for pneumonia with opportunistic agents, such as *Rhodococcus equi*, *Pseudomonas aeruginosa*, and *Pneumocystis jiroveci* (formerly *carinii* [see following text]), among others. In severe pneumonia in advanced HIV disease, obtaining a diagnosis by bronchoscopy or lung biopsy is of paramount importance.

Pneumocystis jiroveci (Pneumocystis carinii) Pneumonia (PCP)

Exposure to this ubiquitous protozoan is common, but an intact immune system protects against disease. Patients with relatively advanced HIV disease (usually a CD4 percentage less than 15%) are at risk of acquiring symptomatic PCP. Babies in the first year of life are at higher risk, probably because of additional immunologic shortcomings that accompany being an infant. Although CD4 counts accurately predict risk of PCP in older children and adults, there is no CD4 cell count that is absolutely protective against PCP in infants under the age of 12 months.[105–107] Therefore, PCP has always been the most common AIDS-defining illness in the pediatric population.[107] It has been estimated that without prophylaxis, 7–20% of HIV-infected infants ac-

quire PCP.[108,109] The incidence of PCP peaks between 3 and 8 months of age; as a consequence, in one study, PCP accounted for 60% of AIDS-defining illnesses in the first year of life, but only 19% thereafter.[110] In adults, the incidence of PCP has declined in the HAART era.[111] In pediatrics, the incidence has declined even more dramatically, mostly because of the advent of prenatal screening of pregnant women and the institution of protocol 076 therapy.

Clinically, the disease usually presents acutely with fever, cough, dyspnea, and tachypnea. It may progress rapidly to respiratory failure. In one series of 9 cases in infants, all nine required mechanical ventilation and 4 succumbed to the infection.[112] Chest x-ray generally shows a diffuse reticulonodular pattern, but atypical findings are possible. Most patients are hypoxemic, even if they are not hypercapnic. Hypoxemia may antedate radiographic findings. An elevated lactate dehydrogenase (LDH) is highly suggestive of the diagnosis. Definitive diagnosis requires demonstration of the organism, usually from bronchoalveolar lavage or lung biopsy material. Induced sputum can be diagnostic in older children and adolescents. As *Pneumocystis jiroveci* does not grow in culture, special stains such as methenamine silver, Giemsa, or toluidine blue are used. Experimental PCR studies, including real-time PCR,[113] seem to be effective and rapid substitutes for staining, but may not be readily available.

For treatment of acute PCP, TMP-SMX is so far superior to other regimens that desensitization followed by TMP-SMX is the preferred approach for patients intolerant of TMP-SMX. Atovaquone works better if the suspension, rather than the pills, is given, even for patients who are able to take pills.[114] Prevention of PCP is discussed in the prevention section.

Lymphocytic Interstitial Pneumonitis (Pulmonary Lymphoid Hyperplasia)

Lymphocytic interstitial pneumonitis (LIP) is a chronic lung disease of uncertain pathogenesis that affects 20–40% of children with HIV infection. It is the only AIDS-defining condition that does not also connote CDC class 3 status. It remains the second most common AIDS-defining illness in children with HIV infection, accounting for about 20% of cases.

LIP presents as chronic pulmonary problems including cough and tachypnea. Radiographically there is diffuse interstitial inflammation, usually without enlarged hilar lymph nodes. This latter feature and the patients' otherwise good health help to separate LIP from pulmonary tuberculosis. Patients with LIP often have recurrent or chronic swelling of the parotids or other salivary glands. Generalized lymphadenopathy and hepatosplenomegaly are also frequently associated. As the disease progresses, clubbing of the digits may develop. The disease tends to wax and wane, producing periods of hypoxemia in severe cases. Wheezing or rales that clear with cough may be heard. Patients with LIP may also develop secondary bacterial pneumonia, which is generally accompanied by fever, toxicity, or other systemic signs.

LIP has been etiologically linked to Epstein-Barr virus (EBV), but not all children with LIP show serologic evidence of EBV infection.[115] Histologically there is a mononuclear infiltrate composed of plasma cells, immunoblasts, and CD8 + T lymphocytes. Molecular study of these CD8 + T cells shows that they arise from oligoclonal expansion, similar to what is seen in some mucosa-associated lymphoid tissue (MALT) lymphomas.[116] Both peripheral blood[117] and bronchoalveolar lavage fluid may also have elevated numbers of CD8 cells.

The prognosis is variable. Children with LIP are admitted to the hospital more than twice as often as are those without.[118] Most of these excess admissions are due to bacterial pneumonia. S. pneumoniae is the most frequent pathogen.[118] On the other hand, an early paper about prognosis for children with HIV showed that those with LIP tended to be "long-term nonprogressors." In that observational study, all 8 patients who were given the diagnosis of LIP survived beyond their fifth birthday.[119] Anecdotal evidence also buttresses the supposition that, generally, children with LIP tend to have a slower progression of HIV disease. As for the LIP, in some patients it slowly progresses, in others it stabilizes, and in some cases it regresses completely.

Treatment is supportive. Mild exacerbations may respond to nebulized bronchodilators. Oxygen must be given when patients are hypoxemic. Many patients respond well to oral corticosteroids. Prednisone is usually given at a dose of 1–2 mg/kg per day for 1–2 weeks followed by a slow taper.

Gastrointestinal Tract Problems

Conditions of the Oral Mucosa

The incidence of oral problems in children with HIV infection is much higher than that of the general population. A point prevalence study found some type of oral lesion in 30 (38%) of 80 HIV-infected children, the most common of which was candidiasis.[120] The prevalence of oral problems increased with disease progression.[120] In a 3-month longitudinal study, 30 (79%) of 38 children were found to have some type of oral lesion.[121] Thrush is the most common problem in all series, but other conditions include linear gingival erythema, median rhomboid glossitis,[122] xerostomia,[123] recurrent and refractory aphthous ulcerations, herpetic gingivostomatitis, labial molluscum contagiosum,[124] and oral hairy leukoplakia.[123] In an adult study, the institution of HAART decreased the overall incidence of oral problems.[125] In children, the CD4 count has been shown to inversely correlate with the presence of oral lesions.[121] Therefore, effective treatment of HIV infection might be expected to produce a similar benefit.

Oral candidiasis in children with advanced HIV disease may not have the classic appearance associated with thrush. The tongue may appear to be coated, or it may be erythematous, without white patches.[126] Local treatment may have a high failure rate. Systemic fluconazole therapy (6 mg/kg by mouth on day 1 followed by 6–13 days of 3 mg/kg; adult dose 200 mg on day 1, then 100 mg per day thereafter) is usually effective in eradicating disease.

Aphthous ulcerations may be widespread, extremely painful, and difficult to treat. Anecdotally, some cases respond to short courses of oral prednisone.[127] As a last resort in children with florid aphthous ulceration, most of whom are unable to maintain hydration and nutrition because of pain, thalidomide has been used, with varying success.[128] Because of thalidomide's teratogenicity, extreme caution must be taken with its use in women of childbearing potential. Fortunately, recalcitrant aphthous ulceration seems less common in the HAART era.

Conditions of the Esophagus

Odynophagia and dysphagia are the usual presenting symptoms of esophageal candidiasis, the most common esophageal problem of HIV-infected patients. Risk factors for the development of esophageal candidiasis are a low CD4 cell count and recent antibiotic therapy.[129] Ulcerative disease of the esophagus may also develop, and is usually due to CMV infection. Patients with candidiasis generally have milder symptoms and are more likely to have concomitant thrush than patients with CMV esophagitis.[130] Idiopathic ulcerative disease and HSV infection of the esophagus are much less common.[131]

Endoscopy is required to definitively diagnose esophageal disease in patients with HIV. However, a presumptive diagnosis of candidiasis and a trial of fluconazole prior to endoscopy is a cost-effective approach.[130] In a randomized, prospective trial, 56 (82%) of 68 patients had complete symptomatic relief with empiric fluconazole, usually within a week.[130] Of the 66 patients randomized to endoscopy, 42 (64%) were found to have candidal esophagitis, and 10 (15%) had ulcerative disease.

Esophageal candidiasis usually responds to systemic antifungal therapy. Fluconazole is most commonly used. Refractory cases may require intravenous amphotericin B. Newer antifungal agents such as caspofungin are promising.[132]

Chronic or Recurrent Diarrhea

Patients with HIV infection have a higher incidence of diarrhea than the general population. In early disease, long-term diarrhea is likely to be due to a side effect of antiretroviral medications. Protease inhibitors, especially nelfinavir, cause increased intestinal motility. This can usually be controlled with loperamide.

Patients with advanced HIV disease often have chronic diarrhea. Elucidating the cause can be very difficult. The lower the CD4 cell count the more likely that the diarrhea is caused by an opportunistic infection, especially protozoa.[133] Parasites are also more likely when the diarrhea has persisted for more than 28 days.[133] The most important of these pathogens is *Cryptosporidium parvum*. It is estimated that 10–15% of adults with AIDS develop cryptosporidiosis at some point during their disease.[134] Duration of survival after the diagnosis of cryptosporidiosis is about a third that of matched controls.[134] Antiretroviral therapy is protective against disease (odds ratio 0.072; p = 0.0001).[134]

Microsporidiosis is another important cause of chronic diarrhea. The disease is nonseasonal, and the overall prevalence is decreasing.[135] In most series, it was the second most common identified cause of chronic diarrhea in advanced AIDS. Microsporidiosis is usually caused by *Enterocytozoon bieneusi*[136] and is a marker for advanced AIDS.[137] Other causes such as *Cyclospora cayetanensis* and

Isospora belli are discussed in more detail in Chapter 12.

In patients with advanced HIV disease and chronic diarrhea, repeated stool studies should be sent, followed by endoscopy or colonoscopy, and finally by sigmoidoscopy with biopsy.[138] CMV colitis can also cause chronic diarrhea, even to the point of wasting.[139] Even with full evaluation, the cause of chronic diarrhea remains cryptic in about 40% of patients.[140] Bacterial enteritis is a concern in patients with more acute disease characterized by fever, cramping, and diarrhea, with or without vomiting. Descriptions and principles of therapy for the common bacterial pathogens are outlined in chapter 12. Antibiotics are not indicated for treatment of *Salmonella* gastroenteritis in immunocompetent children but should be used in children with HIV infection to prevent development of extra-intestinal disease. Prevention of chronic diarrhea is discussed in the prevention section.

Uncommon Gastrointestinal Conditions

Pneumatosis intestinalis, a radiologic finding associated with necrotizing enterocolitis in premature infants, was reported in 3 school-aged children with AIDS who presented with fever and severe abdominal pain.[141] Treatment with bowel rest and intravenous antibiotics resulted in clinical and radiographic cure in all cases. No cause was found in any patient, despite extensive laboratory evaluation and even exploratory laparotomy in one case.[141] Intussusception, usually a condition of infancy, has been reported in young adults with HIV infection. It is associated with tumors or, less frequently, gastrointestinal infections.[142]

Miscellaneous or Systemic Problems

Malignancy

Children with HIV infection are at a higher risk of malignancy. A large study of an Italian registry database (7,178 child-years) estimated the risk of cancer in children with HIV infection to be 4.2 cases per 1,000 child-years.[143] As in adults, the most common malignancy is B-cell driven lymphoma.[144] Kaposi's sarcoma, etiologically linked to HHV-8 infection and common in homosexual males with AIDS, is rare in children.

Rarely, malignancy or hemophagocytic syndrome associated with an underlying malignancy is the presenting feature of HIV infection in a vertically infected child.[145,146] EBV-driven tumors, including sarcomas and myosarcomas, are unusual tumors seen in children with AIDS. Sometimes these tumors are intracranial. CNS lymphomas in adults with HIV infection also tend to be EBV driven.[147] Reports of HIV-infected children with refractory cases of "sinusitis" that turned out to be invasive lymphomas serve as reminders that differential diagnoses should remain broad in children with AIDS, even if they appear to have common conditions.[148,149]

Mycobacterium Avium-intracellulare Complex (MAC) Infection

Disseminated infection with organisms of the *Mycobacterium avium-intracellulare* complex occurs only in patients with advanced HIV disease. It is usually said that patients with CD4 cell counts less than $100/\mu L$ are at risk. Young children are probably at risk at a slightly higher number, but most cases in adolescents and adults generally occur in patients with CD4 cell counts less than $50/\mu L$. In a "time of death" study of 58 children who died of AIDS, MAC was the most common infectious isolate, found in 26% of cases.[150] Fortunately, the incidence of disseminated MAC infection has decreased from a baseline of 3.7 to 0.9 cases/100 person-years in the HAART era.[151]

The symptoms of MAC infection are nonspecific, and usually include fever, night sweats, weight loss, and abdominal pain. There may be hematologic abnormalities due to infiltration of the bone marrow. An x-ray study of 16 pediatric patients with MAC infection revealed that 15 (94%) had lymphadenopathy of the retroperitoneal or mesenteric nodes, or both. Two-thirds had hepatosplenomegaly.[152] The diagnosis is established by culturing the organism from blood or bone marrow. Sometimes liver biopsy specimens will provide the diagnosis by acid-fast staining.[153]

Treatment regimens should always include a macrolide unless the organism is known to be macrolide resistant. Although there is some controversy regarding optimal therapy, it appears as though the combination of clarithromycin plus ethambutol *and* rifabutin improves survival compared with clarithromycin plus either ethambutol *or* rifabutin.[154] Because treatment controls but does not eradicate the infection, it is continued for life. In the early days of the epidemic, a diagnosis of MAC infection spelled a very poor prognosis; survival was seldom

longer than 12 months after the diagnosis was made. It is still a poor prognostic factor, but the outlook is no longer universally bleak.

Invasive and Recurrent Pneumococcal Infection

HIV-infected patients have a rate of invasive pneumococcal disease that is approximately 40 times that of the general population.[155] In one study the rate of invasive pneumococcal disease in pediatric HIV patients was 5.5 cases/100 child-years.[156] Risk factors for pneumococcal infection in adult patients are African-American race, CD4 count less than $200/\mu L$, history of any type of pneumonia, and serum albumin of less than 3.0 mg/dL.[157]

In pediatric HIV infection, it has been anecdotally noted that certain children tend to have recurrent pneumococcal infection.[156] These children are not otherwise distinguishable, except perhaps by the presence of LIP and/or parotid swelling, from other HIV-infected children. They do not tend to be "rapid progressors" nor are they always the patients with the most advanced HIV disease. The nasopharyngeal carriage rate of pneumococci does not differ between HIV-infected and HIV-uninfected children.[158] Also, despite the increased frequency, the severity of invasive pneumococcal disease in HIV infection is identical to or perhaps even less than that seen in HIV seronegative patients.[159] Sometimes in HIV-infected children, pneumococci will be recovered from infections expected to be staphylococcal, such as bacterial parotitis,[160] soft tissue abscesses,[161] and osteomyelitis. Prevention of pneumococcal infections is discussed in the prevention section.

■ PREVENTION OF INFECTION IN THE CHILD WITH HIV

Conditions and Methods

Recurrent pneumonia and pneumococcal infection

Pneumococcal vaccination has been recommended for patients with HIV, but it is not entirely clear how well this recommendation is being implemented, nor is it clear how well it works.[162] Multiple studies have reached conflicting conclusions about the response of HIV-infected patients to pneumococcal polysaccharide vaccine. Some say that the percentage of patients who mount a response is lower than the general population, but when a response occurs, its magnitude is similar to controls.[163] Others say that the overall response is lacking.[164] Another study provides some measure of reconciliation by finding that responses to some pneumococcal serotypes is comparable to controls, but that others are impaired; specifically, responses to serotype 18C, 19F, and 23F are poor.[165] This also fits well with epidemiologic data in adults with HIV, which universally show that invasive infection in these groups is likely to be due to the "pediatric serotypes," especially types 6, 14, 19, and 23.[166]

Pneumococcal conjugate vaccine (PCV-7) will likely be more effective than the polysaccharide vaccine (PPV-23), because it is more immunogenic. In a randomized trial of 67 adults, those receiving PCV-7 had higher specific antibody concentrations and higher opsonophagocytic titers than those receiving placebo or PPV-23.[167] In another study, there was enhanced antibody response to PPV-23 among HIV-infected adults who had first been primed with pneumococcal conjugate vaccine.[168] However, antibody response was generally poor in all patients with CD4 counts less than 200/μL, regardless of vaccine regimen. See Tables 22-2 and 22-3 for recommendations regarding the use of pneumococcal vaccines in immunocompromised patients, including those with HIV infection.

The protective efficacy of pneumococcal polysaccharide vaccination is fair. In two different studies, receipt of the pneumococcal vaccine was found to cut the risk of invasive pneumococcal infection by half[169] to about three-quarters.[157] In vaccine responders, antibody titers wane with time. Some experts recommend revaccination every 2–4 years, although there are no data to support this approach.[165] Unfortunately, vaccine nonresponders often will not respond to revaccination, even if the amount of antigen is doubled.[163] Newly HIV-infected children should receive the entire conjugated pneumococcal vaccine scheduled injections, just as their noninfected counterparts. For those too old for the primary vaccine schedule, there may be benefit in giving a two-dose schedule. Conjugated pneumococcal vaccination (7-valent) can be followed by polysaccharide vaccine (23-valent) to broaden the spectrum of serotypes for which protection is attempted. At present there are no data concerning the immunogenicity or protective efficacy of this type of regimen in children with HIV infection.

Pneumocystis jiroveci pneumonia (PCP)

Prevention of PCP is quite easily accomplished in pediatric HIV patients. Patients with CD4 cell counts that place them at risk for PCP should be given trimethoprim-sulfamethoxazole (TMP-SMX). Traditionally, the recommended dosage has been 150 mg/m^2 of the trimethoprim component in two divided doses on three consecutive days a week, but it is likely that smaller dosages are also effective.[156] If adherence to the prophylactic regimen is likely to be enhanced, the drug can be given daily. In a retrospective study, 4 mg/kg of the trimethoprim component ($\frac{1}{2}$ mL/kg of TMP-SMX liquid suspension) daily was a sufficient dose.[156] Based on the pathophysiology of *Pneumocystis jiroveci* infection, this same dosage given on three consecutive days per week should also be efficacious, but data are lacking. For older children weighing more 40 kg, 160 mg of the trimethoprim component (one double-strength tablet) can be given once daily on three consecutive days per week. TMP-SMX is the preferred agent not only because it prevents PCP more effectively than the other regimens, but because patients on TMP-SMX also get some protection from toxoplasmosis, salmonellosis, *Haemophilus influenzae* infection, and *Staphylococcus aureus* infection.[170] Alternative regimens for PCP prophylaxis include dapsone and monthly aerosolized pentamidine. However, these regimens are only about 30–50% as effective as TMP-SMX in preventing PCP.[171] In addition, aerosolized pentamidine requires compliance with the therapy, which cannot be ensured in children less than about 6 years old. Thus, in patients with sulfa allergy, consideration for desensitization should be given. Once desensitized, patients need to receive TMP-SMX daily in order to avoid resensitization from intermittent dosing. In adults, atovaquone is as effective as dapsone or aerosolized pentamidine, but it is much more expensive.[172,173] The use of intermittently administered parenteral pentamidine has not been well studied; its use is not recommended.[174]

Intolerance of TMP-SMX is less common in pediatric HIV patients than in adults. In our experience, only 17% had adverse events and only 6% had to discontinue the drug because of side effects.[156] In adult patients who had TMP-SMX discontinued, rechallenge by dose escalation was successful in 75%.[175] When a patient undergoes a rebound in CD4 cell count to greater than 15% or greater than 200/μL and sustains the increase for 3 months or longer, PCP prophylaxis can safely be discontinued. In one study, no PCP was diagnosed in 758 person-years of follow-up.[176] The maximum risk of breakthrough PCP was calculated to be 0.85 cases per 100 person-years for primary cases, and 4.5 cases per 100 person-years for secondary cases.[176]

Enteric infections

Most cases of chronic diarrhea in HIV-infected patients are caused by bacterial or parasitic infections. These infections can be acquired in several ways: consumption of contaminated drinking water or recreational water, transmission from human or animal feces, consumption of raw oysters or inadequately washed produce, or consumption of food contaminated by an infected food handler. Following several common-sense practices can, therefore, decrease the individual patient's risk. HIV-infected patients should avoid contact with animal or human feces, and should practice careful hand washing after such contact occurs. Contact might come from diapering a baby, cleaning up after a dog on a walk, or even from gardening. Young pets, in particular, pose an increased risk. HIV-infected patients should not adopt animals less than 12 months of age unless a veterinarian has screened the animals for fecal pathogens. HIV-infected patients should never adopt stray animals.

Sexual practices that bring the person into contact with feces, such as oral-anal contact, should also be avoided.

It is not safe to drink water directly from lakes, rivers, or streams. In general, patients may drink water from municipal wells, since these are usually tested twice daily for contamination. Patients with private wells should consider drinking either bottled water or installing and maintaining a filter with a pore size of less than 0.6 microns. Swimming in water that is free from visible or known contamination (whether natural bodies of water or chlorinated pools) is acceptable. However, water in recreational facilities (such as water parks, swimming pools, and even water fountains) should not be ingested. In outbreak situations, local authorities may ask residents to boil municipal water for one minute prior to consumption. HIV-infected patients should follow these recommendations. Ice and "fountain drink" sodas or soft drinks are made from tap water. Soft drinks that are canned or bottled at the factory are safe. It is thought that most bottled water is free from contamination, but HIV-infected people should be made aware that regulations regarding bottled water are lax. Distilled water is an always safe, if bland, alternative.

Raw oysters may contain a variety of pathogens and should not be eaten. Raw or undercooked meat, shellfish, or eggs should not be consumed. Patients should remember that raw or marginally cooked eggs are sometimes in certain sauces, mayonnaise, or other salad dressings; cookie, brownie, or cake dough; egg nog; and some Asian foods such as sukiyaki, domburi, and the like. Unpasteurized milk, cheeses, or fruit juices should be avoided, as well as bean or alfalfa sprouts. Deli-style meats, hot dogs, pâtés and soft cheeses are potential vehicles of listeriosis.

Mycobacterium avium intercellular complex (MAC) infection

Disseminated MAC infection is easily preventable with once-weekly azithromycin prophylaxis. Unfortunately, surveys suggest that only about 40% of patients who should get MAC prophylaxis actually receive it. Rates of appropriate prophylaxis are lowest in patients who receive care at practices without many HIV-infected patients.[177] The appropriate CD4 count at which to institute MAC prophylaxis depends on the patient's age as follows: 6 years or older, less than 50 cells/mcL; 2–6 years, less than 75 cells/mcL; 1–2 years, less than 500 cells/mcL; and younger than 12 months, less than 750 cells/mcL.[174] Prophylaxis is best accomplished with azithromycin given in a dose of 20 mg/kg (maximum 1,200 mg) once weekly.

Toxoplasmosis

As mentioned previously, all HIV-positive patients should be checked for antibodies against *Toxoplasma gondii*, as most disease is caused by reactivation of past infection. Those who initially test seronegative should be retested when immune suppression to the level of a CD4 count of less than 100 ensues. Seroconverters and those whose initial antibody tests were positive should be given chemoprophylaxis. The most effective agent is TMP-SMX, which most of these patients will already be receiving for PCP prophylaxis. Those who cannot tolerate TMP-SMX can be given dapsone-pyrimethamine or atovaquone. Adult studies confirm the safety of discontinuing prophylaxis if HAART therapy induces immune reconstitution (CD4 count greater than 200 for 3–6 months).[57] Data regarding this strategy in children are absent, but most experts believe that children also derive a similar benefit from immune reconstitution.

Toxoplasmosis is usually acquired from consumption of raw or undercooked meat, or from contact with animal feces or soil that has been contaminated with animal feces. Patients with HIV infection should avoid eating undercooked meats, especially lamb, beef, or pork. Meats should be thoroughly cooked. A meat thermometer is helpful, as the disappearance of any pink in the cooked meat (i.e., "well done") does not always correlate with the actual meat temperature (175° F is generally safe). Fruits and vegetables should be washed thoroughly before they are eaten. Patients should wash their hands after contact with raw meat or soil. Cat litter boxes should be emptied daily, preferably by someone other than the person infected with HIV. If the HIV-infected patient must empty the litter box, careful hand washing immediately thereafter is strongly encouraged.

Primary Varicella and Zoster

Live-attenuated varicella vaccine can be given to mildly symptomatic or asymptomatic HIV-infected infants who fall into CDC category 1 (i.e., no immune suppression, Box 20-2).[178] It is recommended that a second dose of vaccine be given 3 months or more after the first one.[174] The safety and immunogenicity of the vaccine in other circumstances have not been adequately determined. Early immunization (12–15 months) of healthy HIV-infected toddlers should also decrease the rate of zoster.

HIV-infected patients should avoid exposure to anyone known to have varicella or zoster. Other members of the household who have no history of chickenpox and who are found to be seronegative should be vaccinated in order to decrease the likelihood of exposure. For cases where there is known exposure, the HIV-infected person should receive varicella zoster immune globulin (VZIG) as soon as possible. VZIG must be given within the first 96 hours after exposure. The dose is one vial (125 units) of VZIG per 10 kg of body weight, given intramuscularly (maximum dose 625 units [5 vials]).

Zoonoses

HIV-infected persons should avoid exotic pets, especially reptiles, turtles, and rodents. Cats and dogs should not be adopted before they are 12 months old or if they have diarrheal illness. Scratches from cats should be avoided, either by removal of the claws or by avoidance of rough play. Cats should not be allowed to lick any area of nonintact skin. Cat-associated wounds should be promptly and thoroughly cleansed. Patients with advanced HIV disease should avoid petting zoos and contact with farm animals.

Vaccines

Children with HIV infection should be given all currently recommended vaccines and on the same schedule as HIV-negative children, with the exception of live attenuated vaccines (measles-mumps-rubella [MMR], intranasal influenza vaccine, and varicella vaccine). MMR should be given to children in CDC classes 1 and 2, but withheld for those with severe immunosuppression (category 3). The second dose can be given 1 month after the first dose, rather than waiting until school entry. Varivax can be given to children classified as either N1 or A1 (no suppression, mild or no symptoms). At present there are no data regarding administration of live-attenuated influenza vaccine to children with HIV. As an acceptable alternative exists, the live-attenuated vaccine should not be given until further data become available. Inactivated influenza vaccine should be given yearly to patients with HIV infection and their household contacts.

Passive Antibody

Intravenous immune globulin is not routinely administered to children with HIV infection. However, its use should be considered in patients with documented hypogammaglobulinemia. Some clinicians also give IVIG to patients with recurrent serious bacterial infections despite prophylaxis with TMP-SMX, although its benefit in this setting is unproven.[174] Respiratory syncytial virus infection is more severe in children with HIV infection,[179] but the use of prophylactic respiratory syncytial virus antibodies in this population is not routine.

■ REFERENCES

1. Wiktor SZ, Ekpni E, Karon JM, et al. Short-course oral zidovudine for prevention of mother-to-child transmission of HIV-1 in Abidjan, Cote d'Ivorie: A randomized trial. Lancet 1999;353:781–5.
2. Garcia PM, Kalish LA, Pitt J, et al. Maternal levels of plasma human immunodeficiency virus type 1 RNA and the risk of

perinatal transmission. Women and Infants Transmission Study Group. N Engl J Med 1999;341:441–3.

3. Connor EM, Sperling RS, Gelber R, et al. Reduction of maternal-infant transmission of human immunodeficiency virus type 1 with zidovudine treatment. Pediatric AIDS Clinical Trials Group Protocol 076 Study Group. N Engl J Med 1994;331:1173–80.

4. Soeiro R, Rubinstein A, Rashbaum WK, et al. Maternofetal transmission of AIDS: frequency of human immunodeficiency virus type 1 nucleic acid sequences in human fetal DNA. J Infect Dis 1992;166:699–703.

5. Hart CE, Lennox JL, Pratt-Palmore M, et al. Correlation of human immunodeficiency virus type 1 RNA levels in blood and the female genital tract. J Infect Dis 1999;179:871–82.

6. Lee MJ, Hallmark RJ, Frenkel LM, et al. Maternal syphilis and vertical perinatal transmission of human immunodeficiency virus type-1 infection. Int J Gynaecol Obstet 1998;63:247–52.

7. Fiscus SA, Adimora AA, Schoenbach VJ, et al. Trends in human immunodeficiency virus (HIV) counseling, testing, and antiretroviral treatment of HIV-infected women and perinatal transmission in North Carolina. J Infect Dis 1999;180:99–105.

8. Orloff SL, Bulterys M, Vink P, et al. Maternal characteristics associated with antenatal, intrapartum, and neonatal zidovudine use in four U.S. cities, 1994-1998. J Acquir Immune Defic Syndr 2001;28:65–72.

9. Lallemant M, Jourdain G, Le Coeur S, et al. A trial of shortened zidovudine regimens to prevent mother-to-child transmission of human immunodeficiency virus type 1. Perinatal HIV prevention trial (Thailand) investigators. N Engl J Med 2000;343:982–91.

10. Guay LA, Musoke P, Fleming T, et al. Intrapartum and neonatal single-dose nevirapine compared with zidovudine for prevention of mother-to-child transmission of HIV-1 in Kampala, Uganda: HIVNET 012 randomised trial. Lancet 1999;354:795–802.

11. Dorenbaum A, Cunningham CK, Gelber RD, et al. Two-dose intrapartum/newborn nevirapine and standard antiretroviral therapy to reduce perinatal HIV transmission: a randomized trial. JAMA 2002;288:189–98.

12. Mandelbrot L, Landreau-Mascaro A, Rekacewicz C, et al. Lamivudine-zidovudine combination for prevention of maternal-infant transmission of HIV-1. JAMA 2001;285:2083–93.

13. Mofensen LM, Lambert JS, Stiehm ER, et al. Risk factors for perinatal transmission of human immunodeficiency virus type 1 in women treated with zidovudine. Pediatric AIDS clinical trials group study 185 team. N Engl J Med 1999;341:385–93.

14. Landreau-Mascaro A, Barret B, Mayaux MJ, et al. Risk of early febrile seizure with perinatal exposure to nucleoside analogues. Lancet 2002;359:583–4.

15. Culnane M, Fowler M, Lee SS, et al. Lack of long-term effects of in utero exposure to zidovudine among uninfected children born to HIV-infected women. Pediatric AIDS clinical trials group protocol 219/076 teams. JAMA 1999;281:151–7.

16. Shapiro DE, Sperling RS, Mandelbrot L, et al. Risk factors for perinatal human immunodeficiency virus transmission in patients receiving zidovudine prophylaxis. Pediatric AIDS clinical trials group protocol 076 study group. Obstet Gynecol 1999;94:897–908.

17. Brockelhurst P. Interventions for reducing the risk of mother-to-child transmission of HIV infection (*Cochrane Review*). Cochrane Database Syst Rev. 2002;1:CD000102.

18. Bertolli J, St Louis ME, Simonds RJ, et al. Estimating the timing of mother-to-child transmission of human immunodeficiency virus in a breast-feeding population in Kinshasa, Zaire. J Infect Dis 1996;174:722–6.

19. Rosenberg PS, Biggar RJ, Goedert JJ. Declining age at HIV infection in the United States [letter]. New Engl J Med 1994;330:789–90.

20. Wilson TE, Minkoff H. Brief report: condom use consistency associated with beliefs regarding HIV disease tranmission among women receiving HIV antiretroviral therapy. J Acquir Immune Defic Syndr 2001;27:289–91.

21. Catz SL, Meredith KL, Mundy LM. Women's HIV transmission risk perceptions and behaviors in the era of potent antiretroviral therapies. AIDS Educ Prev 2001;13:239–51.

22. Boyer CB, Tschann JM, Shafer MA. Predictors of risk for sexually transmitted diseases in ninth grade urban high school students. J Adolesc Res 1999;14:448–65.

23. Seage GR 3rd, Holte S, Gross M, et al. Case-crossover study of partner and situational factors for unprotected sex. J Acquir Immune Defic Syndr 2002;31:432–9.

24. Ellis J, Williams H, Graves W, Lindsay MK. Human immunodeficiency virus infection is a risk factor for adverse perinatal outcome. Am J Obstet Gynecol 2002;186:903–6.

25. Pollack H, Kuchuk A, Cowan L, et al. Neurodevelopment, growth, and viral load in HIV-infected infants. Brain Behav Immun 1996;10:298–312.

26. Pollack H, Glasberg H, Lee E, et al. Impaired early growth in infants perinatally infected with human immunodeficiency virus: correlation with viral load. J Pediatr 1997;130:915–22.

27. Miller TL, Easley KA, Zhang W, et al. Maternal and infant factors associated with failure to thrive in children with vertically transmitted human immunodeficiency virus-1 infection: the prospective, P2C2 human immunodeficiency virus multicenter study. Pediatrics 2001;108:1287–96.

28. Miller V, Stark T, Loeliger AE, et al. The impact of the M184V substitution in HIV-1 reverse transcriptase on treatment response. HIV Med 2002;3:135–45.

29. Podzamczer D, Ferrer E, Consiglio E, et al. A randomized clinical trial comparing nelfinavir or nevirapine associated to zidovudine/lamivudine in HIV-infected naïve patients. Antivir Ther 2002;7:81–90.

30. van Leeuwen R, Katlama C, Murphy RL, et al. A randomized trial to study first-line combination therapy with or without a protease inhibitor in HIV-1-infected patients. AIDS 2003;17:987–99.

31. Lazzarin A, Clotet B, Cooper D, et al. Efficacy of enfurvitide in patients infected with drug-resistant HIV-1 in Europe and Australia. N Engl J Med 2003;348:2186–95.

32. Paterson DL, Swindells S, Mohr J, et al. Adherence to protease inhibitor therapy and outcomes in patients with HIV infection. Ann Intern Med 2000;133:21–30.

33. Shingadia D, Viani RM, Yogev R, et al. Gastrostomy tube insertion for improvement of adherence to highly active antiretroviral therapy in pediatric patients with human immunodeficiency virus. Pediatrics 2000;105:e80.

34. Dreezen C, Schrooten W, De Mey I, et al. Self-reported signs of lipodystrophy by persons living with HIV infection. Int J STD AIDS 2002;13:393–8.

35. Saves M, Raffi F, Capeau J, et al. Factors related to lipodystrophy and metabolic alterations in patients with human immunodeficiency virus infection receiving highly active antiretroviral therapy. Clin Infect Dis 2002;34:1396–405.

36. Brambilla P, Bricalli D, Sala N, et al. Highly active antiretroviral-treated HIV-infected children show fat distribution changes even in absence of lipodystrophy. AIDS 2001;15:2441–4.

37. Mauss S, Corzillius M, Wolf E, et al. Risk factors for the HIV-associated lipodystrophy syndrome in a closed cohort of patients after 3 years of antiretroviral treatment. HIV Med 2002;3:49–55.

37a. Taylor P, Worrell C, Steinberg SM, et al. Natural history of lipid abnormalities and fat redistribution among human immunodeficiency virus-infected children receiving long-term, protease inhibitor-containing, highly active antiretroviral therapy regimens. Pediatrics 2004;114:235–42.

38. Nolan D, John M, Mallal S. Antiretroviral therapy and the lipodystrophy syndrome, part 2: concepts in aetiopathogenesis. Antivir Ther 2001;6:145–60.

39. Duran S, Saves M, Spire B, et al. Failure to maintain long-term adherence to highly active antiretroviral therapy: the role of lipodystrophy. AIDS 2001;15:2441–4.

40. Roubenoff R, Schmitz H, Bairos L, et al. Reduction of abdominal obesity in lipodystrophy associated with human immunodeficiency virus infection by means of diet and exercise: case report and proof of principle. Clin Infect Dis 2002;34:390–3.

41. Mercie P, Thiebaut R, Lavignolle V, et al. Evaluation of cardiovascular risk factors in HIV-1 infected patients using carotid intima-media thickness measurement. Ann Med 2002;34:55–63.

42. Dalakas MC, Illa I, Pezeshkpour GH, et al. Mitochondrial myopathy caused by long-term zidovudine therapy. New Engl J Med 1990;322:1098–105.

42a. White AJ. Mitochondrial toxicity and HIV therapy. Sex Transm Infect 2001;77:158–73.

43. Shelburne SA, Hamill RJ, Rodriguez-Barradas MC, et al. Immune reconstitution inflammatory syndrome. Emergence of a unique syndrome during highly active antiretroviral therapy. Medicine 2002;81:213–27.

44. Cabie A, Abel S, Brebion A, Desbois N, et al. Mycobacterial lymphadenitis after initiation of highly active antiretroviral therapy. Eur J Clin Microbiol Infect Dis 1998;17:812–3.

45. Narita M, Ashkin D, Hollender ES, et al. Paradoxical worsening of tuberculosis following antiretroviral therapy in patients with AIDS. Am J Respir Crit Care Med 1998;158:157–61.

46. Holland GN. Immune recovery uveitis. Ocular Immunol Inflamm 1999;7:215–21.

47. Tepper VJ, Farley JJ, Rothman MI, et al. Neurodevelopmental/neuroradiologic recovery of a child with combination antiretroviral therapy using the HIV-specific protease inhibitor ritonavir. Pediatrics 1998;101:e7.

48. Roy S, Geoffroy G, Lapointe N, et al. Neurological findings in HIV-infected children: A review of 49 cases. Can J Neurol Sci 1992;19:453–7.

49. Brouwers P, Civitelo L, DeCarli C, et al. Cerebrospinal fluid viral load is related to cortical atrophy and not to intracerebral calcifications in children with symptomatic HIV disease. J Neurovirol 2000;6:390–7.

50. Pearson DA, McGrath NM, Nozyee M, et al. Predicting HIV disease progression in children using measures of neuropsychological and neurological functioning. Pediatric AIDS clinical trials 152 study team. Pediatrics 2000;106:e76.

51. Brouwers P, Tudor-Williams G, DeCarli C, et al. Relation between stage of disease and neurobehavioral measures in children with symptomatic HIV disease. AIDS 1995;9:713–20.

52. King SM, Edwards V, Blaser S, et al. Evaluation of the role of routine serial cranial computed tomography in the management of children with human immunodeficiency virus infection. Pediatr AIDS HIV infect 1997;8:15–22.

53. Abadi J, Nachman S, Kressel AB, et al. Cryptococcosis in children with AIDS. Clin Infect Dis 1999;28:309–13.

54. Gumbo T, Kadzirange G, Mielke J, et al. *Cryptococcus neoformans* meningoencephalitis in African children with acquired immunodeficiency syndrome. Pediatr Infect Dis J 2002;21:54–6.

55. Pitisuttithum P, Tansuphasawadikul S, Simpson AJ, et al. A prospective study of AIDS-associated cryptococcal meningitis in Thailand treated with high-dose amphotericin B. J Infect 2001;43:226–33.

56. Liliang PC, Liang CL, Chang WN, et al. Use of ventriculoperitoneal shunts to treat uncontrollable intracranial hypertension in patients who have cryptococcal meningitis without hydrocephalus. Clin Infect Dis 2002;34:e64–8.

57. Kirk O, Reiss P, Uberti-Foppa C, et al. Safe interruption of maintenance therapy against previous infection with four common HIV-associated opportunistic pathogens during potent antiretroviral therapy. Ann Intern Med 2002;137:239–50.

58. Abgrall S, Rabaud C, Coastagliola D. Incidence and risk factors for toxoplasmic encephalitis in human immunodeficiency virus-infected patients before and during the highly active antiretroviral therapy era. Clin Infect Dis 2001;15:1747–55.

59. Ives NJ, Gazzard BG, Easterbrook PJ. The changing pattern of AIDS-defining illnesses with the introduction of highly active antiretroviral therapy (HAART) in a London clinic. J Infect 2001;42:134–9.

60. Licho R, Litofsky NS, Senitko M, et al. Inaccuracy of Tl-201 brain SPECT in distinguishing cerebral infections from lymphoma in patients with AIDS. Clin Nucl Med 2002;27:81–6.

61. Nath A, Sinai AP. Cerebral toxoplasmosis. Curr Treat Options Neurol 2003;5:3–12.

62. Joseph P, Calderon MM, Gilman RH, et al. Optimization and evaluation of a PCR assay for detecting toxoplasmic encephalitis in patients with AIDS. J Clin Microbiol 2002;40:4499–503.

63. Galli L, de Martino M, Rossi ME, et al. Hemochrome parameters during the first two years of life in children with perinatal HIV-1 infection. Pediatr AIDS HIV Infect 1995;6:340–5.

64. Volberding P. The impact of anemia on quality of life in human immunodeficiency virus-infected patients. J Infect Dis 2002;185(Suppl 2):S2110–4.

65. Salome MA, Grotto HZ. Human immunodeficiency virus-related anemia of chronic disease: relationship to hemato-

logic, immune, and iron metabolism parameters, and lack of association with serum interferon-gamma levels. AIDS Patient Care STDs 2002;16:361–5.

66. Koduri PR. Parvovirus B19-related anemia in HIV-infected patients. AIDS Patient Care STDs 2000;14:7–11.

67. Moyle G. Anemia in persons with HIV infection: Prognostic marker and contributor to morbidity. AIDS Rev 2002; 4:13–20.

68. Sullivan P. Associations of anemia, treatments for anemia, and survival in patients with human immunodeficiency virus infection. J Infect Dis 2002;185(Suppl 2):S138–42.

69. Abrams DI, Steinhart C, Frascino R. Epietin alfa therapy for anemia in HIV-infected patients: impact on quality of life. Int J STD AIDS 2000;11:659–65.

70. Moore RD, Forney D. Anemia in HIV-infected patients receiving highly active antiretroviral therapy. J Acquir Immune Defic Syndr 2002;29:54–7.

71. Majluf-Cruz A, Luna-Castanos G, Trevino-Perez S, et al. Lamivudine-induced pure red cell aplasia. Am J Hematol 2000;65:189–91.

72. Volberding P. Consensus statement: anemia in HIV infection—current trends, treatment options, and practice strategies. Anemia in HIV Working Group. Clin Ther 2000;22:1004–20.

73. Afacan YE, Hasan MS, Omene JA. Iron deficiency anemia and HIV infection: immunologic and virologic response. Natl Med Assoc 2002;94:73–7.

74. Glatt AE, Anand A. Thrombocytopenia in patients infected with human immunodeficiency virus: treatment update. Clin Infect Dis 1995;21:415–23.

75. Cole JL, Marzec UM, Gunthel CJ, et al. Ineffective platelet production in thrombocytopenic human immunodeficiency virus-infected patients. Blood 1998;91:3239–46.

76. Riviere C, Subra F, Cohen-Solal K, et al. Phenotypic and functional evidence for the expression of CXCR4 receptor during megakaryocytopoiesis. Blood 1999;93:1511–23.

77. Kowalska MA, Ratajczak J, Hoxie J, et al. Megakaryocyte precursors, megakaryocytes and platelets express the HIV co-receptor CXCR4 on their surface: determination of response to stromal-derived factor-1 by megakaryocytes and platelets. Br J Haematol 1999;104:220–9.

78. Chelucci C, Federico M, Guerriero R, et al. Productive human immunodeficiency virus-1 infection of purified megakaryocytic progenitors/precursors and maturing megakaryocytes. Blood 1998;91:1225–34.

79. Glatt AE, Anand A. Thrombocytopenia in patients infected with human immunodeficiency virus: treatment update. Clin Infect Dis 1995;21:415–23.

80. Carbonara S, Fiorentino G, Serio G, et al. Response of severe HIV-associated thrombocytopenia to highly active antiretroviral therapy including protease inhibitors. J Infect 2001;42:251–6.

81. Ndagijimana JM, Kroll H, Niehues T. Severe HIV-associated thrombocytopenia despite effective highly active antiretroviral therapy in a vertically infected child. AIDS 2002; 16:802–3.

82. Majluf-Cruz A, Luna-Castanos G, Huitron S, et al. Usefulness of a low-dose intravenous immunoglobulin regimen for the treatment of thrombocytopenia associated with AIDS. Am J Hematol 1998;59:127–32.

83. Izzi I, Del Borgno C, Marasca G. Treatment of human immunodeficiency virus-related thrombocytopenia with in-travenous anti-rhesus D immunoglobulin [letter]. Clin Infect Dis 1997;25:171.

84. Smith N. Intravenous anti-D immunoglobulin in the management of immune thrombocytopenic purpura. Curr Opin Hematol 1996;3:498–503.

85. Monpoux F, Kurzenne JY, Sirvent N, et al. Partial splenectomy in a child with human immunodeficiency virus-related immune thrombocytopenia. J Pediatr Hematol Oncol 1999;21:441–3.

86. Lord RV, Coleman MJ, Milliken ST. Splenectomy for HIV-related immune thrombocytopenia: comparison with results of splenectomy for non-HIV immune thrombocytopenic purpura. Arch Surg 1998;133:205–10.

87. Murphy MF, Metcalfe P, Waters AH, et al. Incidence and mechanism of neutropenia and thrombocytopenia in patients with human immunodeficiency virus infection. Br J Haematol 1987;66:337–40.

88. Kuritzkes DR. Neutropenia, neutrophil dysfunction, and bacterial infection in patients with human immunodeficiency virus disease: the role of granulocyte colony-stimulating factor. Clin Infect Dis 2000;30:256–60.

89. Moore DAJ, Benepal T, Portsmouth S, et al. Etiology and natural history of neutropenia in human immunodeficiency virus disease: a prospective study. Clin Infect Dis 2001;32:469–76.

90. Allen RC, Stevens PR, Price TH, et al. In vivo effects of recombinant human granulocyte colony-stimulating factor on neutrophil oxidative functions in normal human volunteers. J Infect Dis 1997;175:1184–92.

91. Hermans P, Rozenbaum W, Jou A, et al. Filgrastim to treat neutropenia and support myelosuppressive medication dosing in HIV infection. AIDS 1996;10:1627–33.

92. Uthayakumar S, Nadwani R, Drinkwaater T, et al. The prevalence of skin disease in HIV infection and its relationship to the degree of immunosuppression. Br J Dermatol 1997;137:595–8.

93. Perez-Blazquez E, Villafruela I, Madero S. Eyelid molluscum contagiosum in patients with human immunodeficiency virus infection. Orbit 1999;18:75–81.

94. Cattelan AM, Sasset L, Corti L, et al. A complete remission of recalcitrant molluscum contagiosum in an AIDS patient following highly active antiretroviral therapy (HAART) [letter]. J Infect 1999;38:58–60.

95. Strauss RM, Doyle EL, Mohsen AH, et al. Successful treatment of molluscum contagiosum with topical imiquimod in a severely immunocompromised HIV-positive patient. Int J STD AIDS 2001;12:264–6.

96. Calista D. Topical cidofovir for severe cutaneous human papillomavirus and molluscum contagiosum infections in patients with HIV/AIDS. A pilot study. J Eur Adac Dermatol Venereol 2000;14:484–8.

97. Gershon AA. Prevention and treatment of VZV infections in patients with HIV. Herpes 2001;8:32–6.

98. Dankner WM, Lindsey JC, Levin MJ. Correlates of opportunistic infections in children infected with the human immunodeficiency virus managed before highly active antiretroviral therapy. Pediatr Infect Dis J 2001;20:40–8.

99. Matsuo K, Honda M, Shiraki K, et al. Prolonged herpes zoster in a patient infected with the human immunodeficiency virus. J Dermatol 2001;28:728–33.

100. Mayaud C, Parrot A, Cadranel J. Pyogenic bacterial lower respiratory tract infection in human immunodeficiency

virus-infected patients. Eur Respir J Suppl 2002;36: S28–39.

101. Chearskul S, Chotpitayasunondh T, Simonds RJ, et al. Survival, disease manifestations, and early predictors of disease progression among children with perinatal human immunodeficiency virus infection in Thailand. Pediatrics 2002;110:e25.

102. French N, Williams G, Williamson V, et al. The radiographic appearance of pneumococcal pneumonia in adults in unaltered by HIV-1 infection in hospitalized Kenyans. AIDS 2002;16:2095–6.

103. Madhi SA, Cumin E, Klugman KP. Defining the potential impact of conjugate bacterial polysaccharide-protein vaccines in reducing the burden of pneumonia in human immunodeficiency virus type 1-infected and -uninfected children. Pediatr Infect Dis J 2002;21:393–9.

104. Gordon SB, Molyneux ME, Boeree MJ, et al. Opsonic phagocytosis of *Streptococcus pneumoniae* by alveolar macrophages is not impaired in human immunodeficiency virus-infected Malawian adults. J Infect Dis 2001;15: 1345–9.

105. Simonds RJ, Lindegren ML, Thomas P, et al. Prophylaxis against *Pneumocystis carinii* pneumonia among children with perinatally acquired HIV infection in the United States. N Engl J Med 1995;332:786-90.

106. Israele V, Wittek A, Courville T, et al. *Pneumocystis carinii* pneumonia (PCP) in infants with CD4 counts greater than 2000 cells/mm3 [Abstract]. VIII International Conference on AIDS, Amsterdam, July 1992.

107. Anonymous. 1995 revised guidelines for prophylaxis against *Pneumocystis carinii* pneumonia for children infected with or perinatally exposed to human immunodeficiency virus. National Pediatric and Family HIV Resource Center and National Center for Infectious Diseases, Centers for Disease Control and Prevention. MMWR Recomm Rep 1995;44:1–11.

108. Scott GB, Hutto C, McKuch RW, et al. Survival in children with perinatally acquired human immunodeficiency virus type 1 infection. N Engl J Med 1989;321:1791–6.

109. Zar HJ, Dechaboon A, Hanslo D, et al. *Pneumocystis carinii* pneumonia in South African children infected with human immunodeficiency virus. Pediatr Infect Dis J 2000;19: 603–7.

110. Simonds RJ, Oxtoby MJ, Caldwell MB, et al. *Pneumocystis carinii* pneumonia among US children with perinatally acquired HIV infection. JAMA 1993;270:470–3.

111. San-Andres FJ, Rubio R, Castilla J, et al. Incidence of acquired immunodeficiency syndrome-associated opportunistic diseases and the effect of treatment on a cohort of 1115 patients infected with human immunodeficiency virus, 1989-1997. Clin Infect Dis 2003;36:1177–85.

112. Sheikh S, Bakshi SS, Pahwa SG. Outcome and survival in HIV-infected infants with *Pneumocystis carinii* pneumonia and respiratory failure. Pediatr AIDS HIV Infect 1996;7: 155–63.

113. Palladino S, Kay I, Fonte R, et al. Use of real-time PCR and the LightCycler system for the rapid detection of *Pneumocystis carinii* in respiratory specimens. Diagn Microbiol Infect Dis 2001;39:233–6.

114. Rosenberg DM, McCarthy W, Slavinsky J, et al. Atovaquone suspension for treatment of *Pneumocystis carinii*

pneumonia in HIV-infected patients. AIDS 2001;26: 211–4.

115. Fishback N, Koss M. Update on lymphoid interstitial pneumonitis. Curr Opin Pulm Med 1996;5:429–33.

116. Kurosu K, Yumoto N, Rom WN, et al. Oligoclonal T cell expansions in pulmonary lymphoproliferative disorders: Demonstration of the frequent occurrence of oligoclonal T cells in human immunodeficiency virus-related lymphoid interstitial pneumonia. Am J Respir Crit Care Med 2002; 165:254–9.

117. Simmank K, Meyers T, Galpin J, et al. Clinical features and T-cell subsets in HIV-infected children with and without lymphocytis interstitial pneumonitis. Ann Trop Paediatr 2001;21:195–201.

118. Sharland M, Gibb DM, Holland F. Respiratory morbidity from lymphocytic interstitial pneumonitis (LIP) in vertically acquired HIV infection. Arch Dis Child 1997;76: 334–6.

119. Kline MW, Paul ME, Bohannon B, et al. Characteristics of children surviving to 5 years of age or older with vertically acquired HIV infection. Pediatr AIDS HIV Infect 1995;6: 350–3.

120. Santos LC, Castro GF, de Souza IP, et al. Oral manifestations related to immunosuppression degree in HIV-positive children. Braz Dent J 2001;12:135–8.

121. Flanagan MA, Barasch A, Koenigsberg et al. Prevalence of oral soft tissue lesions in HIV-infected minority children treated with highly active antiretroviral therapies. Pediatr Dent 2000;22:287–91.

122. Barasch A, Safford MM, Catalanotto FA, et al. Oral soft tissue manifestations in HIV-positive vs HIV-negative children from an inner city population: A two-year observational study. Pediatr Dent 2000;22:215–20.

123. Kozinetz CA, Carter AB, Simon C, et al. Oral manifestations of pediatric vertical HIV transmission. AIDS Patient Care STDs 2000;14:89–94.

124. Flaitz C, Wullbrandt B, Sexton J, et al. Prevalence of orodental findings in HIV-infected Romanian children. Pediatr Dent 2001;23:44–50.

125. Patton LL, McKaig R, Strauss R, et al. Changing prevalence of oral manifestations of human immunodeficiency virus in the era of protease inhibitor therapy. Oral Surg Oral Med Oral Pathol Oral Radiol Endod 2000;89:299–304.

126. Nicolatou O, Theodoridou M, Mostrou G, et al. Oral lesions in children with perinatally acquired human immunodeficiency virus infection. J Oral Pathol Med 1999;28: 49–53.

127. de Asis ML, Bernstein LJ, Schliozberg J. Treatment of resistant oral aphthous ulcers in children with acquired immunodeficiency syndrome. J Pediatr 1995;127:663–5.

128. DeVincenzo JP, Burchet SK. Prolonged thalidomide therapy for human immunodeficiency virus-associated recurrent severe esophageal and oral aphthous ulcers. Pediatr Infect Dis J 1996;15:465–7.

129. Abgrall S, Charreau I, Joly V, et al. Risk factors for esophageal candidiasis in a large cohort of HIV-infected patients treated with nucleoside analogues. Eur J Clin Microbiol Infect Dis 2001;20:346–9.

130. Wilcox CM, Alexander LN, Clark WS, Thompson SE 3rd. Fluconazole compared with endoscopy for human immunodeficiency virus-infected patients with esophageal symptoms. Gastroenterology 1996;110:1803–9.

131. Wilcox CM. Esophageal disease in the acquired immunodeficiency syndrome: etiology, diagnosis, and management. Am J Med 1992;92:412–21.

132. Villanueva A, Arathoon EG, Gotuzzo E, et al. A randomized double-blind study of caspofungin versus amphotericin for the treatment of candidal esophagitis. Clin Infect Dis 2001; 33:1529–35.

133. Navin TR, Weber R, Vugia DJ. Declining CD4+ T-lymphocyte counts are associated with increased risk of enteric parasitosis and chronic diarrhea: results of a 3-year longitudinal study. J Acquir Immune Def Syndr Hum Retrovirol 1999;20:154–9.

134. Manabe YC, Clark DP, Moore RD, et al. Cryptosporidiosis in patients with AIDS: correlates of disease and survival. Clin Infect Dis 1998;27:536–42.

135. Conteas CN, Berlin OG, Lariviere MJ, et al. Examination of the prevalence and seasonal variation of intestinal microsporidiosis in the stools of persons with chronic diarrhea and human immunodeficiency virus infection. Am J Trop Med Hyg 1998;58:559–61.

136. Sobottka I, Schwartz DA, Schottelius J, et al. Prevalence and clinical significance of intestinal microsporidiosis in human immunodeficiency virus-infected patients with and without diarrhea in Germany: a prospective coprodiagnostic study. Clin Infect Dis 1998;26:475–80.

137. Brasil P, de Lima DB, de Paiva DD, et al. Clinical and diagnostic aspects of intestinal microsporidiosis in HIV-infected patients with chronic diarrhea in Rio de Janeiro, Brazil. Rev Inst Med Trop Sao Paulo 2000;42:299–304.

138. Monkemuller KE, Wilcox CM. Investigation of diarrhea in AIDS. Can J Gastroenterol 2000;14:933-40.

139. Togawa M, Shiomi M, Okawa K, et al. Encephalopathy and cytomegalovirus colitis in an AIDS child. Acta Paediatr Jpn 1998;40:515–22.

140. Beaugerie L, Carbonnel F, Carrat F, èt al. Factors of weight loss in patients with HIV and chronic diarrhea. J Acquir Immune Defic Syndr Hum Retrovirol 1998;19:34–9.

141. Cunnion KM. Pneumatosis intestinalis in pediatric acquired immunodeficiency syndrome. Pediatr Infect Dis J 1998;17:355–6.

142. Wood BJ, Kumar PN, Cooper C, et al. AIDS-associated intussusception in young adults. J Clin Gastroenterol 1995;21:158–62.

143. Caselli D, Klersy C, de Martino M, et al. Human immunodeficiency virus-related cancer in children: incidence and treatment outcome—report of the Italian Register. J Clin Oncol 2000;18:3854–61.

144. Veneris MR, Tuel L, Seibel NL. Pediatric HIV infection and chronic myelogenous leukemia. Pediatr AIDS HIV Infect 1995;6:292-4.

145. Lee WS, Chan TL, Koh MT, et al. Acquired immunodeficiency syndrome presenting as childhood non-Hodgkin's lymphoma. Singapore Med J 2001;42:530–3.

146. Preciado MV, De Matteo E, Fallo A, et al. EBV-associated Hodgkin's disease in an HIV-infected child presenting with a hemophagocytic syndrome. Leuk Lymphoma 2001;42: 231–4.

147. Antinori A, De Rossi G, Ammassari A, et al. Value of combined approach with thallium-201 single-photon emission computed tomography and Epstein-Barr virus DNA polymerase chain reaction in CSF for the diagnosis of AIDS-related primary CNS lymphoma. J Clin Oncol 1999;17: 554–60.

148. Robinson MR, Salit RB, Bryant-Greenwood PK, et al. Burkitt's/Burkitt's-like lymphoma presenting as bacterial sinusitis in two HIV-infected children. AIDS Patient Care STDS 2001;15:453–8.

149. Campos JM, Simonetti JP, Santos EN, Pone MV, et al. Lymphoma presenting as a tumor of the maxillary sinuses in an HIV-infected child. Pediatr AIDS HIV Infect 1995;6: 18–20.

150. Johann-Liang R, Cervia JS, Noel GJ. Characteristics of human immunodeficiency virus-infected children at the time of death: an experience in the 1990s. Pediatr Infect Dis J 1997;16:1145–50.

151. Tumbarello M, Tacconelli E, de Donati KG, et al. Changes in incidence and risk factors of Mycobacterium avium complex infections in patients with AIDS in the era of new antiretroviral therapies. Eur J Clin Microbiol Infect Dis 2001;20:498–501.

152. Pursner M, Haller JO, Berdon WE. Imaging features of Mycobacterium avium-intracellulare complex (MAC) in children with AIDS. Pediatr Radiol 2000;30:426–9.

153. Poles MA, Dieterich DT, Schwarz ED, et al. Liver biopsy findings in 501 patients infected with human immunodeficiency virus (HIV). J Acquir Immune Defic Syndr Hum Retrovirol 1996;11:170–7.

154. Benson CA, Williams PL, Currier JS, et al. A prospective, randomized trial examining the efficacy and safety of clarithromycin in combination with ethambutol, rifabutin, or both for the treatment of disseminated Mycobacterium avium complex disease in persons with acquired immunodeficiency syndrome. Clin Infect Dis 2003;37:1234–43.

155. Nuorti JP, Butler JC, Gelling L, et al. Epidemiologic relation between HIV and invasive pneumococcal disease in San Francisco County, California. Ann Intern Med 2000;132: 182–90.

156. Fisher RG, Nageswaran S, Valentine ME, et al. Successful prophylaxis against Pneumocystis carinii pneumonia in HIV-infected children using smaller than recommended dosages of trimethoprim-sulfamethoxazole. AIDS Patient Care STDs 2001;15:263–9.

157. Gebo KA, Moore RD, Keruly JC, et al. Risk factor for pneumococcal disease in human immunodeficiency virus-infected patients. J Infect Dis 1996;173:857–62.

158. Polack FP, Flayhart DC, Zahurak ML, et al. Colonization by Streptococcus pneumoniae in human immunodeficiency virus-infected children. Pediatr Infect Dis J 2000; 19:608–12.

159. Lichenstein R, King JC Jr, Farley JJ, et al. Bacteremia in febrile human immunodeficiency virus-infected children presenting to ambulatory care settings. Pediatr Infect Dis J 1998;17:381–5.

160. Hanekom WA, Chadwick EG, Yogev R. Pneumococcal parotitis in a human immunodeficiency virus-infected child. Pediatr Infect Dis J 1995;14:1113–4.

161. Dobroszycki J, Abadi J, Lambert G, et al. Testicular abscess due to Streptococcus pneumoniae in an infant with human immunodeficiency virus infection. Clin Infect Dis 1997;24:84–5.

162. Pierce AB, Hoy JF. Is the recommendation for pneumococcal vaccination of HIV patients evidence based? J Clin Virol 2001;22:255–61.

163. Rodriguez-Barradas MC, Groover JE, Lacke CE, et al. IgG antibody to pneumococcal capsular polysaccharide in human immunodeficiency virus-infected subjects: persistence of antibody in responders, revaccination in nonresponders, and relationship of immunoglobulin allotype to response. J Infect Dis 173:1347–53.

164. Chang Q, Abadi J, Alpert P, Pirofski L. A pneumococcal capsular polysaccharide vaccine induces a repertoire shift with increased VH3 expression in peripheral B cells from human immunodeficiency virus (HIV)-uninfected but not from HIV-infected persons. J Infect Dis 2000;181: 1313–21.

165. Kroon FP, van Dissel JT, Ravensbergen E, et al. Antibodies against pneumococcal polysaccharides after vaccination in HIV-infected individuals: 5-year follow-up of antibody concentrations. Vaccine 1999;14:524–30.

166. Feldman C, Glatthaar M, Morar R, et al. Bacteremic pneumococcal pneumonia in HIV-seropositive and HIV-seronegative adults. Chest 1999;116:107–14.

167. Feikin DR, Elie CM, Goetz MB, et al. Randomized trial of the quantitative and functional antibody responses to a 7-valent pneumococcal conjugate vaccine and/or 23-valent polysaccharide vaccine among HIV-infected adults. Vaccine 2001;20:545–53.

168. Kroon FP, van Dissel JT, Ravensbergen E, et al. Enhanced antibody response to pneumococcal polysaccharide vaccine after prior immunization with conjugate pneumococcal vaccine in HIV-infected adults. Vaccine 2000;19: 886–94.

169. Dworkin MS, Ward JW, Hanson DL, et al. Adult and Adolescent Spectrum of HIV Disease Project. Pneumococcal disease among human immunodeficiency virus-infected persons: incidence, risk factors, and impact of vaccination. Clin Infect Dis 2001;32:794–800.

170. Dworkin MS, Williamson J, Jones JL, et al. Prophylaxis with trimethoprim-sulfamethoxazole for human immunodeficiency virus-infected patients: impact on risk for infectious diseases. Clin Infect Dis 2001;33:393–8.

171. Nachman SA, Mueller BU, Mirochnick M, et al. High failure rate of dapsone and pentamidine as *Pneumocystis carinii* pneumonia prophylaxis in human immunodeficiency virus-infected children. Pediatr Infect Dis J 1994; 13:1004-6.

172. Chan C, Montaner J, Lefebvre EA, et al. Atovaquone suspension compared with aerosolized pentamidine for prevention of *Pneumocystis carinii* pneumonia in human immunodeficiency virus-infected subjects intolerant of trimethoprim or sulfonamides. J Infect Dis 1999;180: 369–76.

173. El-Sadr WM, Murphy RL, Yurik TM, et al. Atovaquone compared with dapsone for the prevention of *Pneumocystis carinii* pneumonia in patients with HIV infection who cannot tolerate trimethoprim, sulfonamides, or both. Community Program for Clinical Research on AIDS and the AIDS Clinical Trials Group. N Engl J Med 1998;339:1889–95.

174. Kaplan JE, Masur H, Holmes KK. Guidelines for preventing opportunistic infections among HIV-infected persons—2002. Recommendations of the U.S. Public Health Service and the Infectious Diseases Society of America. MMWR Recomm Rep 2002;51:1–52.

175. Leoung GS, Stanford JF, Giordano MF, et al. Trimethoprim-sulfamethoxazole (TMP-SMX) dose escalation versus direct rechallenge for *Pneumocystis carinii* pneumonia prophylaxis in human immunodeficiency virus-infected patients with previous adverse reaction to TMP-SMX. J Infect Dis 2001;184:992–7.

176. Lopez Bernaldo De Quiros JC, Miro JM, Pena JM, et al. A randomized trial of the discontinuation of primary and secondary prophylaxis against *Pneumocystis carinii* pneumonia after highly active antiretroviral therapy in patients with HIV infection. N Engl J Med 2001;18:159–67.

177. Asch SM, Gifford AL, Bozzette SA, et al. Underuse of primary Mycobacterium avium complex and *Pneumocystis carinii* prophylaxis in the United States. J Acquir Immune Defic Syndr 2001;28:340–4.

178. American Academy of Pediatrics. Varicella vaccine update. Pediatrics 2000;105:136–41.

179. Madhi SA, Venter M, Madhi A, Petersen MK, et al. Differing manifestations of respiratory syncytial virus-associated severe lower respiratory tract infections in human immunodeficiency virus type 1-infected and uninfected children. Pediatr Infect Dis J 2001;20:164–70.

CHAPTER 21

Exposure Problems

In the patient who presents with symptoms consistent with an infectious process, an exposure history is one of the most important pieces of information to elicit. Many infectious diseases are first suspected on the basis of the exposure history. This involves asking if the patient or parent knows of any similar illnesses in the patient's family, school, job, or community. However, it also involves specific questions about the patient's personal history, such as hobbies, pets, travel, day care attendance, patient or parent occupation, sexual exposures, and self-medication or drug exposures. Exposure to persons with a chronic unexplained cough might be a clue to tuberculosis or pertussis. Unusual diet (such as ingestion of unpasteurized milk) or the use of well water may indicate an enteric pathogen as the cause of illness. A history of tick or mosquito bites is usually present in vector-borne illnesses. A previous history of blood transfusions provides for the possibility of several transfusion-associated infections.

This chapter provides a general approach to exposures so that a differential diagnosis can be generated once the history of present illness and the exposure history are known. Details of the clinical manifestations caused by particular organisms can be found in earlier chapters. The chapter ends with a discussion of a very common problem: head lice infestation.

■ OCCUPATIONAL AND ENVIRONMENTAL EXPOSURES

Possible exposures of this type, and the associated microorganisms and syndromes to be expected, are listed in Table 21-1.

■ BLOOD TRANSFUSION

With current testing procedures, the blood supply is much safer now than in previous decades.[1] However, the exposure may have occurred in the remote past (such as a red cell transfusion given for anemia of prematurity), in which case it may not be recalled by the patient unless the question is specifically asked. Table 21-2 lists infections associated with transfusion of blood products, specifically packed red blood cells and platelets. In the 1990s, certain immune globulin products were implicated in transmission of hepatitis C virus infection.[2] All immune globulin products are currently treated by a cold ethanol fractionation procedure, which is highly effective in inactivating known infectious agents.[3]

■ ANIMAL EXPOSURES

Children have a higher rate of exposure to animals because of their exploratory behavior. Several excellent reviews of animal-associated infections are available.[4–6] The diseases associated with specific animals and the syndromes produced are shown in Table 21-3. Rabies is a frequent concern in animal bites. The approach to prophylaxis for rabies is outlined in Table 21-4.

Dog and Cat Bite Infections

Frequency and Clinical Patterns

Animal bites represent 1% of all emergency department visits, the majority involving children. Between 70–90% of these visits are caused by dog bites; boys aged 5–9 years have the highest incidence.[7] Severe dog bites in children occur most frequently in those younger than 5 years and involve the head and neck. Large dogs that are familiar to the child are usually involved.[8] Cats account for only 3–15% of animal bites,[5] but because they result in puncture wounds, cat bites are much more likely to become infected (more than 50% as compared with 15–20% for dog bites).

Dog bites tend to be crushing injuries rather than clean, sharp lacerations. In children, three-quarters of dog bites occur on the face, neck, or head,[7] and facial scarring is not uncommon. Bites to the head may be complicated by occult skull fracture and subsequent brain abscess.[9]

TABLE 21-1. OCCUPATIONAL AND ENVIRONMENTAL EXPOSURES AND ASSOCIATED MICROORGANISMS[a]

EXPOSURE	MICROORGANISMS (PARTIAL LIST)
Soil, dirt, dust	Histoplasmosis,[49] coccidioidomycosis,[50,51] blastomycosis
Residence near rivers or associated waterways	Blastomycosis[52]
Bird and bat guano (caves, chicken coops, bird roosts, abandoned buildings)	Histoplasmosis;[53] cryptococcosis (esp. pigeon droppings)[54]
Thorny bushes, sphagnum moss	Sporotrichosis (skin ulcers)[55]
Hot tubs, whirlpools	*Pseudomonas* (rashes);[56] amebic keratitis,[57] *Legionella*,[58] *Mycobacterium avium* pneumonitis[59]
Swimming pools, wavepools	*Pseudomonas* (rashes);[56–60] enteroviruses (fever, vomiting);[61] adenovirus (fever, pharyngitis, conjunctivitis);[62] *E. coli* O157:H7,[63] *Shigella*,[64] *Cryptosporidium*,[65] *Giardia*;[66] (diarrhea); *Aeromonas* (bacteremia),[67] molluscum contagiosum;[68] tinea pedis[69]
Fish tanks	*Mycobacterium marinum* (skin ulcers)[70]
Freshwater lake or river	*Schistosoma* larvae (swimmer's itch),[71] schistosomiasis (travelers),[72] leptospirosis,[73] *Edwardsiella* (diarrhea),[74] *Aeromonas* (wound infection),[75] *Naegleria* (encephalitis)[76]
Sea water and brackish water	*Vibrio vulnificus* and *V. damsela* (cellulitis or sepsis), *V. parahaemolyticus* (diarrhea), *Edwardsiella* (diarrhea),[74] *Erysipelothrix*, *Streptococcus iniae*[77]
Creeks, swimming holes	Leptospirosis[78]
Moldy hay; water in air conditioners or humidifiers	Thermophilic actinomycetes (and other agents of hypersensitivity pneumonitis)[79]
New construction	*Legionella*, Histoplasmosis[80]
Insects	See Table 21–6.
Blood transfusion	See Table 21–2.
Contaminated needle injury	Hepatitis B, hepatitis C, HIV[35]
Injection drug use	Same as needle injury; in addition, *S. aureus* (acute endocarditis),[81] *Pseudomonas* (osteomyelitis),[82] wound botulism[83]

[a] See Table 21–7 for geographic distributions.

Infected bite wounds are characterized by swelling, erythema, and warmth at the site of injury.[6] Purulent drainage, abscess formation, fever, regional adenitis, and leukocytosis are variable findings.[10] The interval between the injury and evidence of infection is particularly short in cases of *Pasteurella* infection, often within 6–12 hours.

In asplenic children or those with other immunocompromising conditions, even a seemingly insignificant dog or cat bite may result in *Capnocytophaga canimorsus* infection, a cause of fulminant septicemia in these patients.[11] Rarely, this organism causes sepsis in previously healthy persons with a recent dog or cat bite.[12] *Pasteurella* can also cause bacteremia in immunocompromised hosts, with a mortality of 30% in one small series.[13]

Infecting Bacteria

In the largest prospective study to date, *Pasteurella* species were the most frequently isolated bacteria from both dog (50%) and cat (75%) bites.[10] Most infections are polymicrobial and involve both aerobes and anaerobes. In one study, in which 107

TABLE 21-2. TRANSFUSION-TRANSMITTED INFECTIONS

CATEGORY	ORGANISM	COMMENTS
Bacteria	*Yersinia enterocolitica*	Organism grows well at cooler temperatures at which red blood cells (RBCs) are stored (4°C)[84]
	Pseudomonas fluorescens	Grows well at 4°C; high mortality rate[85]
	Staphylococci, others	Risk is ~ 1 in 500,000 units for PRBCs and ~ 1 in 12,000 units for platelets[86]
Parasites	Malaria	93 cases reported in the United States from 1963–1999[87]
	Babesiosis	Risk is very low, even in endemic areas[88]
	Trypanosomiasis	In endemic areas (parts of Latin America) transfusion is a major source of transmission[89]
Rickettsia	Rocky Mountain spotted fever	Rare[90]
Spirochetes	Syphilis	Rare in the United States[91]
Viruses	Hepatitis A	Risk ~ 1 in 1 million units[86]
	Hepatitis B	Risk ~ 1 in 60,000 units[92]
	Hepatitis C	Risk ~ 1 in 100,000 units[92]
	HIV	Risk ~ 1 in 500,000 units[92]
	HTLV I and II	Risk ~ 1 in 600,000 units[92]
	Cytomegalovirus	Prevented by using CMV-negative or leukocyte filtered blood products for immunocompromised patients (including neonates)
	Epstein-Barr virus	Probably prevented by using leukocyte filtered blood products
	Parvovirus B19	Risk ~ 1 in 10,000 units[86]

HIV, human immunodeficiency virus; HTLV, human T-cell lymphotropic virus

infected dog or cat bite wounds were cultured at a reference laboratory, the median number of bacterial isolates per culture was five.[10] After *Pasteurella*, the most common aerobes are streptococci, staphylococci, diphtheroids, and *Neisseria* species. Gram-negative enteric rods are an occasional cause. The most common anaerobic bacteria implicated include *Fusobacterium*, *Bacteroides*, *Porphyromonas*, *Prevotella*, *Propionibacterium*, and *Peptostreptococcus* species.[10]

Initial Management

Tetanus immunity should be assessed (see Table 17-2), and the risk of rabies should be considered (Table 21-4). Pain control should not be neglected. Wounds should be explored to determine their depth and to see if any underlying structures (such as bone, joint, or tendon) are involved. Thorough irrigation and debridement reduce the rate of infection.[14] Hand wounds have a high rate of infection and should generally not be sutured. Recent, noninfected wounds on other parts of the body can usually be sutured.

The use of prophylactic antibiotics is generally advocated for certain bites thought to be at high risk for infection. Examples include severe bite wounds with crush injury; puncture wounds that cannot be adequately irrigated; bites to the face, hand, foot, or genital region; and wounds in immunocompromised persons.[15] A recent systematic review of eight randomized, controlled trials found that overall, prophylactic antibiotics did not appear to reduce the rate of infection after bites by dogs or cats, and that wound type (laceration versus puncture) did not appear to influence effectiveness. However, the infection rate for hand bites was significantly reduced by the use of antibiotics (2% versus 28%, odds ratio 0.10, 95% confidence interval 0.01–0.86).[16] In none of the above studies was amoxicillin-clavulanate used as a prophylactic agent.

TABLE 21-3. ANIMAL EXPOSURES VIA BITES, SCRATCHES, MEAT INGESTION, OR CONTACT WITH ANIMAL PARASITE

ANIMAL	MICROORGANISM AND SYNDROMES (PARTIAL LIST)
Dogs	Leptospirosis (hepatitis), dog tapeworm, dog heartworm (chronic pneumonia), *Bordetella bronchiseptica* (cough), *Brucella canis* (fever), *Malassezia pachydermatis* (central line infections in neonatal intensive care units [ICUs]—acquired indirectly from health care workers' dogs)[93]
Cats	Cat-scratch disease (cervical adenitis), toxoplasmosis (mono-like illness), Q fever (pneumonia), plague (pneumonia), tularemia (multiple forms of disease)
Dogs and cats	Ringworm (most cases are not animal associated), scabies, cutaneous larva migrans, visceral larva migrans, rabies, salmonellosis, campylobacteriosis, cryptosporidiosis, giardiasis
Dog or cat bites	*Pasteurella, streptococci,* staphylococci, anaerobes, rabies, others[10]
Horses	Salmonellosis, Group C streptococcal pneumonia or pharyngitis, *Rhodococcus equi* (subacute pneumonia in immune-compromised hosts), *Actinobacillus*
Swine	Brucellosis, *Salmonella choleraesuis*
Cattle or unpasteurized milk or cheese	Brucellosis (fever), actinomycosis (cervical adenitis), nocardiosis, leptospirosis, bovine tuberculosis (cervical adenitis), beef tapeworm, *E. coli* O157:H7, campylobacteriosis, *Listeria* (meningitis)
Chickens	Salmonellosis, campylobacteriosis
Sheep, goats	Orf (pustular dermatitis), brucellosis, Q fever (pneumonia), anthrax
Rats, mice, guinea pigs, hamsters	Lymphocytic choriomeningitis virus (aseptic meningitis or fever), campylobacteriosis, rat bite fever (rash, headache, polyarthralgia), hantavirus pulmonary syndrome[94]
Pet fish	*Mycobacterium marinum* (skin ulcer), edwardsiellosis (diarrhea, wound infection)
Reptiles (turtles, snakes, lizards, iguanas)	Salmonellosis, campylobacteriosis, *Aeromonas*
Parakeets, pigeons, other birds, bird feces	Psittacosis (atypical pneumonia), hypersensitivity pneumonitis (pulmonary infiltrates with eosinophilia), histoplasmosis, cryptococcosis
Skunks, foxes, bats, coyotes	Rabies
Rabbits, muskrats, deer, beaver, squirrels	Tularemia, leptospirosis, Q fever, giardiasis, typhus
Monkeys, chimpanzees	Simian B-virus (meningoencephalitis: usually fatal unless treated with acyclovir),[95] melioidosis, tuberculosis, amebiasis, hepatitis A virus
Ferrets	Influenza, salmonellosis, campylobacteriosis[5]
Raccoons	Rabies, visceral larva migrans, raccoon roundworm encephalitis[96]
Any wild or zoo animal bite	*Pasteurella* species[97]

TABLE 21-4. RABIES PROPHYLAXIS

POSTEXPOSURE PROPHYLAXIS GUIDE[a,b]		
ANIMAL	DISPOSITION OF ANIMAL	TREATMENT OF VICTIM
Dog, cat, or ferret	Healthy, available for 10 days of observation	Prophylaxis only if animal develops signs of rabies[c]
	Rabid or suspected rabid	Immediate immunization and RIG
	Unknown (escaped)	Consult public health officials
Skunk, raccoon, fox, coyote, bobcat, other carnivores; bats[d]	Regard as rabid unless proved negative by laboratory testing[e]	Immediate immunization and RIG
Livestock, small rodents, large rodents (woodchucks and beavers), rabbits, other mammals	Consider individually and consult public health officials. Bites of squirrels, hamsters, guinea pigs, gerbils, chipmunk, rats, mice, other rodents, rabbits, and hares almost never require rabies prophylaxis. Large rodents (especially nutria) more likely to carry rabies than small rodents, but risk is still low	
POSTEXPOSURE IMMUNIZATION		
Persons not previously immunized	**RIG:** 20 IU/kg, full dose infiltrated into the wound if possible, (any remaining volume is given IM at a site distant from vaccine)—given on day 0 only; **Vaccine:** HDVC, RVA, or PCEC 1 mL IM (deltoid), on days 0, 3, 7, 14, and 28	
Persons previously immunized[f]	**RIG:** Not given **Vaccine:** HDCV, RVA, or PCEC 1 mL, IM (deltoid), on days 0 and 3	
PRE-EXPOSURE IMMUNIZATION[g]		
Primary	Intramuscular	HDCV, PCEC, or RVA; 1 mL (deltoid), one each on days 0, 7, and 21 or 28
	Intradermal	HDCV; 0.1 mL, one each on days 0, 7, and 21 or 28
Booster[h]	Intramuscular	HDCV, PCEC, or RVA; 1 mL (deltoid), day 0 only
	Intradermal	HDCV; 0.1 mL, day 0 only

Abbreviations: RIG, rabies immune globulin; HDCV, human diploid cell vaccine; PCEC, purified chick embryo cell vaccine; RVA, rabies vaccine adsorbed; IM, intramuscular.

[a] All bites and wounds should be thoroughly cleaned with soap and water and povidone-iodine solution. If rabies prophylaxis is indicated, both rabies immune globulin (RIG) and vaccine should be given as soon as possible, regardless of the time elapsed since the bite. Local reactions to vaccines are common and do not contraindicate continued treatment.

[b] Two types of possible exposures from a rabid animal must be considered—bite and non-bite exposures. If no exposure has occurred (i.e., neither bite exposure nor nonbite exposure), prophylaxis is not necessary. Any penetration of the skin by teeth constitutes a bite exposure and represents a potential risk of rabies transmission. The contamination of open wounds, abrasions, or mucous membranes with saliva from a rabid animal constitutes a nonbite exposure and requires prophylaxis. In addition, two cases of rabies have been attributed to airborne exposures in caves containing countless numbers of bats.

[c] During the 10-day observation period, begin postexposure prophylaxis at the first sign of rabies in a dog, cat, or ferret that has bitten someone. If the animal exhibits clinical signs of rabies, it should be euthanatized immediately and tested.

[d] Bat bites may inflict minor injury and go undetected. Postexposure prophylaxis should be considered when direct contact between a human and bat has occurred, unless the exposed person can be certain that a bite, scratch, or mucous membrane exposure did not occur.

[e] The animal should be euthanatized and tested as soon as possible. Holding for observation is not recommended. Discontinue vaccine if immunofluorescence test results of the animal are negative.

[f] Any person with a history of preexposure vaccination with HDCV, RVA, or PCEC; prior postexposure prophylaxis with HDCV, RVA, or PCEC; or previous vaccination with any other type of rabies vaccine and a documented history of antibody response to the prior vaccination.

[g] Consider preexposure prophylaxis for children traveling to developing areas where dog rabies is enzootic, especially for prolonged stays (>3 months) or if visiting remote areas (> 24 hours from a reliable source of rabies vaccine). All dog bites or scratches in such areas should be taken seriously and postexposure prophylaxis sought, even in persons are already immunized.
[h] Acceptable antibody titer is 1:5. For persons at frequent risk of rabies exposure, test serology every 2 years and boost if titer falls below 1:5.
Source: Adapted from Centers for Disease Control and Prevention. Human rabies prevention—United States, 1999. Recommendations of the Advisory Committee on Immunization Practices (ACIP). MMWR Recomm Rep 1999;48:1–21.

Despite the lack of data, amoxicillin-clavulanate is a reasonable choice if prophylaxis is deemed to be indicated, because of its activity against the broad range of organisms causing wound infections. For the penicillin-allergic child, trimethoprim-sulfamethoxazole plus clindamycin is reasonable.

Prevention

Young children should be closely supervised when around any dog. Dog owners should be educated to be responsible for preventing bites, and both dog owners and parents should be counseled about preventing dog bites.[17]

Human Bite Infections

Frequency

Human bites are the third most common among bite wounds seen in emergency departments, trailing only the bites of dogs and cats. Although human bites have a reputation for being more frequently and more severely infected, data suggest that bites inflicted anywhere other than the hand carry a similar prognosis as bites of other mammals.[18] If properly irrigated, human bite wounds in areas other than the hand become infected in about 10% of cases.[19]

In a study of 322 human bites in children, areas affected included the upper extremities in 42%, face and neck in 33%, and the trunk in 22%.[20] None of the 242 abrasions became infected compared with 16 (38%) of 42 puncture wounds and 13 (37%) of 35 lacerations. Vigorous debridement and irrigation with saline are critical. Most experts recommend avoidance of primary closure if there is a puncture wound or if the injury is greater than 8–12 hours old, except in the case of facial wounds.

Hand Bites

Human bite wounds of the hand come in two varieties: i) occlusal, wherein the patient is actually bitten, and ii) clenched-fist, in which the injury is sustained by striking the teeth of another person with the fist. Both forms of injury carry a high risk of deep tissue infection such as septic arthritis and osteomyelitis.[21] Human bite injuries of the hand should never be dismissed as minor, and prompt surgical debridement is critical.[22] Factors associated with progression to osteomyelitis include delay in surgical debridement beyond 24 hours and failure to appreciate the severity of the injury at the initial patient visit.[23] The importance of prophylactic antibiotics for human hand bites has been confirmed by a randomized trial of 48 patients.[24] Infection occurred in 7 (47%) of 15 placebo recipients; in contrast, there were no infections among the 33 patients who received antibiotics.

Infecting Bacteria

Human bites or wounds inflicted by clenched fists are often associated with crushed tissue and anaerobic conditions. Infected human bite wounds usually harbor bacteria that are part of the normal mouth and/or skin flora. Aerobic cultures of such wounds typically yield alpha-hemolytic or beta-hemolytic streptococci, *Staphylococcus aureus*, *Haemophilus* species, or *Eikenella corrodens*. The latter organism has a propensity to cause severe infections that are difficult to treat. Anaerobic cultures often grow *Bacteroides*, *Fusobacterium*, *Peptococcus*, *Peptostreptococcus*, and *Veillonella* species.[25,26] Most infections are polymicrobial; one study demonstrated an average of five isolates per specimen.[25] Multiple surgical procedures may be required for cure.[23]

Prophylactic Antibiotics

Patients with simple abrasions do not require prophylactic antibiotics. Children with lacerations or puncture wounds from a human bite should probably receive prophylactic antibiotics. A 3-day course is usually sufficient, unless there are visible signs of infection at the time of presentation, in which case a 10-day course is appropriate. Some practitioners also use the longer course of antibiotics in immunocompromised hosts or if bone, joint, or tendon penetration has occurred. An antibiotic regimen with both aerobic and anaerobic coverage is necessary, both for prophylaxis and for empiric treatment of wound infections, even if no anaerobes grow in culture. Amoxicillin-clavulanate is an appropriate choice for prophylaxis. It can also be used for empiric therapy unless an intravenous antibiotic is desired, in which case ampicillin-sulbactam can be used. For the penicillin-allergic child, clindamycin plus trimethoprim-sulfamethoxazole can be used.[27]

Transmission of Viral Infection

If there is a break in the skin, the risk for transmission of human immunodeficiency virus (HIV) and hepatitis B virus (HBV) infection should be considered. Transmission of HIV infection by a human bite is extremely rare; it has only been well-documented in bites among adults that include the exchange of blood.[28,29] This is expected, since replication-competent HIV is absent from the saliva of most HIV-infected patients.[30] For severe human bites, testing the perpetrator's serum for HIV antibodies is reasonable, especially if there is blood in the saliva. If positive, serial testing and postexposure prophylaxis for the victim is appropriate as detailed in the following section on needlestick injuries.

Transmission of HBV infection via human bite is well-documented in the literature.[31] The need for administering HBV vaccine and hepatitis B immune globulin depends on whether the perpetrator is hepatitis B surface antigen positive and on the vaccination history of the victim (see Table 13-4). Although transmission of hepatitis C virus by human bite has been documented,[32] no postexposure prophylaxis exists, and testing is generally not advised.

■ ADDITIONAL EXPOSURE MECHANISMS

Needlestick Exposures

With needlestick and other occupational exposures involving blood, the main concerns are the transmission of hepatitis B virus (HBV), hepatitis C virus (HCV), and the human immunodeficiency virus (HIV). The likelihood of transmission of these agents varies depending on the titer of virus in the source case's blood, the type and gauge of the needle used, the depth of penetration, and glove use.[33] A rough estimate of the comparative risks is approximated by the "rule of threes": HBV is transmitted in approximately 30% of exposures, HCV in 3%, and HIV in 0.3%.[34] The risk of HBV transmission may be as high as 40% if the source case is HBeAg positive and as low as 2% if HBeAg negative.[33]

In the case of a needlestick injury, serologic testing of the source case (HBsAg, antibody to HCV, and antibody to HIV) should be performed. If the source case is HBsAg positive, management depends on whether the exposed person has been vaccinated with HBV vaccine and, if so, whether they are known to have developed an adequate antibody response to vaccination. If lack of immunity is documented, postexposure prophylaxis with hepatitis B immune globulin and HBV vaccine is given as detailed in Table 13-4.

If the source case is HCV antibody positive, the exposed person should undergo baseline testing for HCV antibody and ALT (alanine aminotransferase) with repeat testing in 4–6 months. No postexposure prophylaxis is recommended.[35]

If the source case is known or suspected to be HIV-infected, the exposed person should be evaluated immediately and baseline HIV serology should be obtained. Whether postexposure prophylaxis is indicated and, if so, what regimen should be used, depends on several factors, as outlined in the Centers for Disease Control and Prevention (CDC) recommendations given in Table 21-5. The only postexposure regimen that has been studied is zidovudine (AZT) monotherapy, which has been shown to decrease transmission by 80%.[36] However, suppression of viral replication is better when more than one effective drug is used, and there is a considerable amount of zidovudine resistance in community isolates of HIV. Therefore, most HIV exposures warrant a two-drug regimen using two nucleoside analogues (e.g., zidovudine and lamivudine). For high-risk injuries, the addition of a protease inhibitor (e.g., nelfinavir) is recommended. Patients with needlestick exposures to HIV should have follow-up HIV-antibody testing at 6 weeks, 12 weeks, and 6 months postexposure.

Injuries from needles found in the community are not uncommon, but transmission of infection is rare. A single case of HBV infection transmitted in this fashion has been reported.[37] Transmission of HCV and HIV from needles found in the community has not been reported. With this type of exposure, the HBV vaccination status of the patient

TABLE 21-5. RECOMMENDED HIV POSTEXPOSURE PROPHYLAXIS FOR PERCUTANEOUS INJURIES[35]

EXPOSURE TYPE	INFECTION STATUS OF SOURCE				
	HIV-POSITIVE CLASS 1[a]	HIV-POSITIVE CLASS 2[a]	SOURCE OF UNKNOWN HIV STATUS[b]	UNKNOWN SOURCE[c]	HIV-NEGATIVE
Less severe[d]	2-drug regimen	3-drug regimen	Generally, no PEP warranted; consider 2-drug PEP[e] for source with HIV risk factors[f]	Generally, no PEP warranted; consider 2-drug PEP[e] in settings where exposure to HIV-infected persons likely	No PEP warranted
More severe[g]	3-drug regimen	3-drug regimen	Generally, no PEP warranted; consider 2-drug PEP[e] for source with HIV risk factors[f]	Generally, no PEP warranted; consider 2-drug PEP[e] in settings where exposure to HIV-infected persons likely	No PEP warranted

Abbreviations: PEP, postexposure prophylaxis.
[a] HIV-Positive, Class 1: asymptomatic HIV infection or known low viral load (e.g., ,1,500 RNA copies/mL). HIV-Positive, Class 2: symptomatic HIV infection, AIDS, acute seroconversion, or known high viral load.
[b] For example, deceased source person with no samples available for HIV testing.
[c] For example, a needle from a sharps container.
[d] Less severe examples: solid needle or superficial injury.
[e] "Consider PEP" indicates that PEP is optional and should be based on an individualized decision between the exposed person and the treating clinician.
[f] If PEP is offered and taken and the source is later determined to be HIV-negative, PEP should be discontinued.
[g] More severe examples: large-bore hollow needle, deep puncture, visible blood on device, or needle used in patient's artery or vein.

should be reviewed, and vaccine and HBIG (hepatitis B immunoglobulin) should be administered if the child has not received the complete series. Postexposure prophylaxis for HIV is generally not necessary, but may be considered in some circumstances. Testing the needle or syringe is neither useful nor safe.

Insect Exposures

Many infectious diseases are transmitted by insect vectors (Table 21-6). The animal reservoir usually determines the geographic area where the disease is most frequent.

Geographic Exposures

Geographic exposure is a broad concept that implies that the patient has been in a place offering exposure to a disease that might not ordinarily be suspected in the region where the patient is now. Therefore, it is important to take a history about the travel of every patient suspected of having an infectious disease. There are several geographic areas within North America that have an unusually high incidence of infection with particular microorganisms and some of these are listed in Table 21-7.

The limitation of a disease to a particular geographic area is usually related to the habitat of an animal reservoir or vector but may be related to the climate needed for a soil fungus. The geographic distribution of various tropical diseases is beyond the scope of this book but may be found in many excellent tropical medicine texts and at the CDC's Web site: www.cdc.gov. Malaria and tuberculosis are two serious but treatable diseases that are very common in much of the developing world and should always be considered as possibilities in the ill returning traveler.

Immigrants, Refugees, and Internationally Adopted Children

An excellent overview of the health problems common in these three groups of children is available.[38]

TABLE 21-6. SOME DISEASES TRANSMITTED BY INSECTS

INSECT	DISEASE	CHAPTER/SECTION OF BOOK
Ticks	Rocky Mountain spotted fever	Rashes/Petechial
	Lyme disease	Rashes; Arthritis
	Lyme-like illness[98]	Rashes
	Ehrlichiosis (granulocytic and monocytic)	Fever
	Babesiosis	Fever
	Colorado tick fever	Fever
	Tularemia	Fever, Pneumonia, Skin/Ulcers
	Relapsing fever	Fever
	Tick paralysis	Neurologic/Paralysis
Mosquitoes	La Crosse (California) encephalitis	Neurologic/Encephalitis
	Eastern equine encephalitis	
	Western equine encephalitis	
	St. Louis encephalitis	
	West Nile encephalitis	
	Malaria	
	Dengue fever	
	Yellow fever	
Fleas	Plague	Skin ulcers, lymphadenopathy
Lice	Epidemic typhus	
	Murine typhus	Rashes
Mites	Rickettsialpox	Rashes
Flies	Tularemia (deerfly)	Fever; Pneumonia; Lymphadenopathy

Table 21-8 lists suggested components and screening tests in the initial evaluation of such children.

Exposures to Sick Persons

Prophylaxis for exposures to chickenpox, *H. influenzae*, meningococcus, and measles is given in Table 21-9.

Other Exposures

Foodborne disease is discussed in Chapter 12. Sexual exposures are discussed in Chapter 15. Management of a child exposed to active tuberculosis is discussed in Chapter 8. Management of exposure to rubella is discussed in Chapter 19, to pertussis in Chapter 7, and to mumps in Chapter 4. Hepatitis exposures are discussed in Chapter 13, and exposure to HIV is discussed in Chapter 20.

Head Lice (*Pediculosis capitis*)

Infestation with head lice is very common, with a prevalence of 1–3%; in some elementary schools the rate of infestation is as high as 25%.[39] Lice are harmless, but unfortunately the hysteria that often results from them is not. Infestation is usually asymptomatic; itching generally increases when patients are told they have head lice. People of all socioeconomic levels are affected. Transmission is primarily by head-to-head contact. Most experts believe that sharing of combs, brushes, and hats is capable of transmitting lice, although this has not been proved. Lice do not jump or fly, and pets are not involved in transmission.[39]

Diagnosis

Lice should be visualized to confirm the diagnosis. Nits (egg cases) may persist for several weeks to

TABLE 21-7. SELECTED GEOGRAPHIC EXPOSURES WITHIN NORTH AMERICA

LOCATION	DISEASE (CHAPTER)
Southwestern U.S. (especially CA and AZ) and Mexico	Coccidioidomycosis (Pneumonia)
Southwest: northern NM, northern AZ, and southern CO	Plague (Skin syndromes); Hantavirus (Pneumonia)
Mexico	Cysticercosis (Neurologic syndromes) Tuberculosis (Pneumonia) Typhoid fever, Malaria (Fever) Leishmaniasis (Skin syndromes)
West: CA, southern OR, and far western NV	Plague (Skin syndromes)
Western half of U.S.	Western equine encephalitis (Neurologic syndromes)
Western mountain states	Colorado tick fever (Fever)
Upper midwest and mid-Atlantic states (especially rural WV)	La Crosse encephalitis (Neurologic syndromes)
Upper midwestern United States	Human granulocytic ehrlichiosis (Fever)
East Coast and Gulf Coast	West Nile encephalitis, Eastern Equine encephalitis (Neurologic syndromes); *Vibrio vulnificus* (Skin syndromes)
Gulf Coast (FL, TX), Ohio and Mississippi Valley	St. Louis encephalitis (Neurologic syndromes)
Nantucket, Martha's Vineyard, Shelter Island, and parts of Long Island	Babesiosis (Fever)
South-central, southeastern and midwestern United States (especially, Ohio and Mississippi river valleys)	Blastomycosis; Histoplasmosis (Pneumonia)
South-central and southeastern United States	Rocky Mountain spotted fever (especially NC); human monocytic ehrlichiosis (especially OK); Lyme-like illness (Southern Tick Associated Rash Illness) (Fever); Cat scratch disease, non-tuberculous lymphadenitis (Adenopathy)
South-central and western U.S.	Tularemia (adenopathy)
Northeastern and mid-Atlantic seaboard, upper north-central U.S., a few counties in northern California	Lyme disease (Fever)
Puerto Rico	Dengue (Fever)
Hawaii	Leptospirosis (Fever, Hepatitis)
Maritime Canada and Maine	Q fever from parturient cats

months after effective treatment, so the presence of nits does not necessarily indicate current infestation. Eggs containing nonviable louse remnants or even random debris such as dandruff, fibers, scabs, or epidermal matter are often misidentified as signs of head louse infestation, even by physicians.[40] The use of a fine-toothed louse comb greatly facilitates detection. In one study of 280 school children, lice were found in only 6% of children by direct visualization and in 25% with the use of a louse comb.[41]

Treatment

Several effective topical agents are available. Permethrin 1% (Nix) is available over-the-counter, kills unhatched nits as well as lice, and is safe. Retreatment is recommended in 7–10 days. Pyrethrins (e.g., A-200, Pronto, R&C, Rid, Triple X) are also safe, effective, and available over-the-counter; however, they kill only lice and not unhatched nits. As with permethrin, retreatment in 7–10 days is

TABLE 21-8. SUGGESTED INITIAL EVALUATION AND SCREENING TESTS FOR IMMIGRANTS, REFUGEES, AND INTERNATIONALLY ADOPTED CHILDREN

COMPONENT	COMMENTS
Complete history and physical examination	Review existing medical records; ascertain details of the previous living situation
Update immunization status	Immunity to vaccine-preventable diseases is often inadequate;[99] consider resuming primary series or measuring titers
Tuberculin skin test	Risk of tuberculosis is ~ 100 times that of children born in the United States[38]
Stool examination for ova and parasites	Positive in ~ 15% of children[100]
Hepatitis B serology (HBsAg, anti-HBs, and anti-HBc)	Especially common in children from Asia
Serologic test for syphilis	If positive, evaluate for extent of disease and treat with full course of penicillin, even if a history of treatment in country of origin
HIV serology	Confirm positive test result with Western blot and PCR
Complete blood count	Anemia is common (may be due to iron deficiency, thalassemia trait, lead poisoning, hemoglobinopathies, malnutrition, chronic disease, or a combination of the above factors)
Nutritional assessment	Rickets and iodine deficiency especially common in children from China and Russia[38]
Vision, hearing, and dental screening	Dental health is often poor

often necessary. Malathion (Ovide) is available by prescription only, and is effective with a single application. Although it is an organophosphate, neurologic toxicity has not been described. Malathion lotion is flammable, so hair dryers or electric hair-curling devices should be avoided. A systematic review found no evidence that any one of these pediculicides was superior to another.[42] However, in certain regions where resistance has emerged to one or more agents, there may be variable efficacy. Resistance is not thought to be widespread in the United States, but formal surveillance is not done.

Many experts recommend using a fine-toothed comb to remove nits for several days after the application of the topical agent. However, nits are difficult to remove, and there is no evidence that combing increases the cure rate.

For refractory cases, some recommend the use of oral ivermectin,[43] but it is not approved for this use, and comparative data are lacking. The use of combination therapy with topical permethrin 1% and oral trimethoprim-sulfamethoxazole has also been advocated for refractory cases[44] but has not been studied adequately.[45]

Lindane (Kwell) is available by prescription, has lower efficacy than the topical agents mentioned above, and can cause seizures if applied excessively. It should rarely be used. There are no data regarding the use of petrolatum, mayonnaise, or other home remedies used to "suffocate" the lice. Head shaving is an unnecessary and excessive measure for a benign condition.

Reinfestation is a common reason for "treatment failure," as is misdiagnosis. The child may have nits but no lice, or they may have hair casts (pseudonits) or even dandruff, both of which can be removed much more easily than the oval nits.[46]

School Exclusion Issues

A survey of 382 school nurses found that 60% supported a "no-nit" rule of forced absenteeism for any children with nits in their hair.[47] However, nits can persist for several weeks, even after effective treatment of lice. Even in children without recent treatment, most nits do not develop into lice. Of 50 school children with newly diagnosed nits, only 9 (18%) developed lice in the ensuing 2 weeks. Lice were especially unlikely to develop if all the nits were greater than $\frac{1}{4}$ inch from the scalp.[48] Many

TABLE 21-9. MANAGEMENT OF EXPOSURES TO SELECTED DISEASES

DISEASE	PROPHYLAXIS
Chickenpox	
1. Exposed susceptible immunosuppressed child 2. Newborn of mother with onset of rash within 5 days before or 48 hours after delivery 3. Susceptible pregnant woman 4. Premature infant (≥28 weeks' gestation) with no maternal history of chickenpox 5. Premature infant (<28 weeks' gestation or ≤1,000 g), regardless of maternal history of chickenpox	Varicella-zoster immune globulin (VZIG) within 96 hours of exposure; 125 units per 10 kg of body weight intramuscularly (minimum dose: 125 units; maximum dose: 625 units)
Exposed, healthy household contacts (≥12 months old, no history of varicella vaccination, no history of natural varicella disease, and not immunocompromised)	Vaccinate with varicella vaccine if within 72 hours of exposure[101]
H. influenzae	
1. Child <4 years of age in the household who is incompletely immunized or a child <12 months old in the household regardless of immunization status or an immunocompromised child in the household, regardless of age and immunization status	1. Rifampin 20 mg/kg once daily (maximum 600 mg per day) for 4 days to all nonpregnant household contacts[a]
2. Child care or nursery school contacts (some withhold prophylaxis unless 2 or more cases of invasive disease in 60 days)	2. Rifampin, as above, to all child care contacts,[a] nonpregnant adults and children, regardless of age
3. Index case	3. Rifampin, as above, if invasive disease is treated with a regimen other than cefotaxime or ceftriaxone
Meningococcus	
1. Household contact,[b] especially young children 2. Child care or nursery school contact[b] 3. Direct exposure to index patient's secretions through kissing or sharing toothbrushes or eating utensils[b] 4. Mouth-to-mouth resuscitation, unprotected contact during endotracheal intubation[b]	Rifampin 10 mg/kg per dose (maximum 600 mg) orally b.i.d. for 2 days (if ≤1 month old, 5 mg/kg per dose orally b.i.d. for 2 days) Or Ceftriaxone (125 mg intramuscularly [IM] once if ≤12 years, 250 mg IM once if >12 years); preferred in pregnancy Or Ciprofloxacin (500 mg orally once in nonpregnant adults ≥18 years old)
Measles	
1. Exposed susceptible contact born after 1956 (except pregnant women and immunocompromised persons)	1. Live attenuated measles vaccine[c] (within 72 hours of exposure) *and* immune globulin[d] **0.25 mL/kg** IM (within 6 days of exposure), maximum 15 mL
2. Exposed susceptible pregnant women	2. Immune globulin **0.25 mL/kg** IM (within 6 days of exposure), maximum 15 mL
3. Exposed susceptible immunocompromised persons	3. Immune globulin **0.5 mL/kg** IM (within 6 days of exposure), maximum 15 mL

[a] For *H. influenzae*, a contact is defined as a person residing with the index patient or a nonresident who spent 4 or more hours with the index case for at least 5 of the 7 days preceding the day of hospital admission of the index case.

[b] During the 7 days before onset of disease in the index case.

[c] Children as young as 6 months may receive measles vaccination during an outbreak or if exposed to a case of measles; however, they should be revaccinated at age 12–15 months and at 4–6 years.

[d] Immune globulin is not indicated for household contacts who have received 1 dose of vaccine at 12 months of age or older unless they are immunocompromised.

Source: Adapted from American Academy of Pediatrics. Bite wounds. In: Pickering LK, ed. *2000 Red Book*: Report of the Committee on Infectious Diseases. Elk Grove Village, IL: American Academy of Pediatrics 2000: 155–159, with permission.

children are excluded from school based on a misdiagnosis of head lice; in fact, noninfested children are quarantined at least as often as infested ones.[40] Not surprisingly, "no-nit" policies are not effective in controlling head lice. They do, however, result in millions of missed school days in U.S. children each year—a classic case of the cure being worse than the disease.[39,47]

■ REFERENCES

1. Sloand EM, Pitt E, Klein HG. Safety of the blood supply. JAMA 1995;274:1368–73.
2. Bresee JS, Mast EE, Coleman PJ, et al. Hepatitis C virus infection associated with administration of intravenous immune globulin. A cohort study. JAMA 1996;276:1563–7.
3. Bos OJ, Sunye DG, Nieuweboer CE, et al. Virus validation of pH 4-treated human immunoglobulin products produced by the Cohn fractionation process. Biologicals 1998; 26:267–76.
4. Morrison G. Zoonotic infections from pets. Understanding the risks and treatment. Postgrad Med 2001;110:24–26, 29–30, 5–6 passim.
5. Tan JS. Human zoonotic infections transmitted by dogs and cats. Arch Intern Med 1997;157:1933–43.
6. Glaser C, Lewis P, Wong S. Pet-, animal-, and vector-borne infections. Pediatr Rev 2000;21:219–32.
7. Weiss HB, Friedman DI, Coben JH. Incidence of dog bite injuries treated in emergency departments. JAMA 1998; 279:51–3.
8. Brogan TV, Bratton SL, Dowd MD, Hegenbarth MA. Severe dog bites in children. Pediatrics 1995;96:947–50.
9. Jones N, Khoosal M. Infected dog and cat bites. N Engl J Med 1999;340:1841.
10. Talan DA, Citron DM, Abrahamian FM, et al. Bacteriologic analysis of infected dog and cat bites. Emergency Medicine Animal Bite Infection Study Group. N Engl J Med 1999; 340:85–92.
11. Lion C, Escande F, Burdin JC. *Capnocytophaga canimorsus* infections in human: review of the literature and cases report. Eur J Epidemiol 1996;12:521–533.
12. Hovenga S, Tulleken JE, Moller LV, et al. Dog-bite induced sepsis: a report of four cases. Intensive Care Med 1997; 23:1179–80.
13. Raffi F, Barrier J, Baron D, et al. *Pasteurella multocida* bacteremia: report of thirteen cases over twelve years and review of the literature. Scand J Infect Dis 1987;19:385–93.
14. Callaham M. Prophylactic antibiotics in common dog bite wounds: a controlled study. Ann Emerg Med 1980;9: 410–4.
15. American Academy of Pediatrics. Bite wounds. In: Pickering LK, ed. 2000 Red Book: report of the Committee on Infectious Diseases. Elk Grove Village, IL: American Academy of Pediatrics, 2000:155–9.
16. Medeiros I, Saconato H. Antibiotic prophylaxis for mammalian bites. Cochrane Database Syst Rev. 2001: CD001738.
17. Cornwell JM. Dog bite prevention: responsible pet ownership and animal safety. J Amer Vet Med Assoc 1997;210: 1147–8.
18. Griego RD, Rosen T, Orengo IF, et al. Dog, cat, and human bites: a review. J Am Acad Dermatol 1995;33:1019–29.
19. Bunzli WF, Wright DH, Hoang AT, et al. Current management of human bites. Pharmacother 1998;18:227–34.
20. Baker MD, Moore SE. Human bites in children. A six-year experience. Am J Dis Child 1987;141:1285–90.
21. De Smet L, Stoffelen D. Clenched fist injury: a pitfall for patients and surgeons. Acta Orthop Belg 1997;63:113–7.
22. Kelly IP, Cunney RJ, Smyth EG, et al. The management of human bite injuries of the hand. Injury 1996;27:481–4.
23. Gonzalez MH, Papierski P, Hall RF. Osteomyelitis of the hand after a human bite. J Hand Surg [Am] 1993;18: 520–2.
24. Zubowicz VN, Gravier M. Management of early human bites of the hand: a prospective randomized study. Plast Reconstr Surg 1991;88:111–4.
25. Brook I. Microbiology of human and animal bite wounds in children. Pediatr Infect Dis J 1987;6:29–32.
26. Goldstein EJ. Bite wounds and infection. Clin Infect Dis 1992;14:633–8.
27. Goldstein EJ, Citron DM. Comparative activities of cefuroxime, amoxicillin-clavulanic acid, ciprofloxacin, enoxacin, and ofloxacin against aerobic and anaerobic bacteria isolated from bite wounds. Antimicrob Agents Chemother 1988;32:1143–8.
28. Pretty IA, Anderson GS, Sweet DJ. Human bites and the risk of human immunodeficiency virus transmission. Am J Forensic Med Pathol 1999;20:232–9.
29. Dominguez KL. Management of HIV-infected children in the home and institutional settings. Care of children and infections control in schools, day care, hospital settings, home, foster care, and adoption. Pediatr Clin North Am 2000;47:203–39.
30. Ho DD, Byington RE, Schooley RT, et al. Infrequency of isolation of HTLV-III virus from saliva in AIDS. N Engl J Med 1985;313:1606.
31. Cancio-Bello TP, de Medina M, Shorey J, et al. An institutional outbreak of hepatitis B related to a human biting carrier. J Infect Dis 1982;146:652–6.
32. Figueiredo JF, Borges AS, Martinez R, et al. Transmission of hepatitis C virus but not human immunodeficiency virus type 1 by a human bite. Clin Infect Dis 1994;19: 546–7.
33. Gerberding JL. Management of occupational exposures to blood-borne viruses. N Engl J Med 1995;332:444–51.
34. Lauer GM, Walker BD. Hepatitis C virus infection. N Engl J Med 2001;345:41–52.
35. Centers for Disease Control and Prevention. Updated U.S. public health service guidelines for the management of occupational exposures to HBV, HCV, and HIV and recommendations for postexposure prophylaxis. MMWR Morb Mort Wkly Rep 2001;50:20–2.
36. Cardo DM, Culver DH, Ciesielski CA, et al. A case-control study of HIV seroconversion in health care workers after percutaneous exposure. Centers for Disease Control and Prevention Needlestick Surveillance Group. N Engl J Med 1997;337:1485–90.
37. Garcia-Algar O, Vall O. Hepatitis B virus infection from a needle stick. Pediatr Infect Dis J 1997;16:1099.
38. Jenista JA. The immigrant, refugee, or internationally adopted child. Pediatr Rev 2001;22:419–9.
39. Roberts RJ. Head lice. N Engl J Med 2002;346:1645–50.

40. Pollack RJ, Kiszewski AE, Spielman A. Overdiagnosis and consequent mismanagement of head louse infestations in North America. Pediatr Infect Dis J 2000;19:689–93; discussion 694.

41. Mumcuoglu KY, Friger M, Ioffe-Uspensky I, et al. Louse comb versus direct visual examination for the diagnosis of head louse infestations. Pediatr Dermatol 2001;18:9–12.

42. Dodd CS. Interventions for treating head lice. Cochrane Database Syst Rev. 2001:CD001165.

43. Bell TA. Treatment of Pediculus humanus var. capitis infestation in Cowlitz County, Washington, with ivermectin and the LiceMeister comb. Pediatr Infect Dis J 1998;17: 923–4.

44. Hipolito RB, Mallorca FG, Zuniga-Macaraig ZO, et al. Head lice infestation: single drug versus combination therapy with one percent permethrin and trimethoprim/sulfamethoxazole. Pediatrics 2001;107:E30.

45. Pollack RJ. Head lice infestation: single drug versus combination therapy. Pediatrics 2001;108:1393.

46. Lam M, Crutchfield CE 3rd, Lewis EJ. Hair casts: a case of pseudonits. Cutis 1997;60:251–2.

47. Price JH, Burkhart CN, Burkhart CG, et al. School nurses' perceptions of and experiences with head lice. J Sch Health 1999;69:153–8.

48. Williams LK, Reichert A, MacKenzie WR, et al. Lice, nits, and school policy. Pediatrics 2001;107:1011–5.

49. Cano MV, Hajjeh RA. The epidemiology of histoplasmosis: a review. Semin Respir Infec 2001;16:109–18.

50. Werner SB, Pappagianis D, Heindl I, et al. An epidemic of coccidioidomycosis among archeology students in northern California. N Engl J Med 1972;286:507–12.

51. Schneider E, Hajjeh RA, Spiegel RA, et al. A coccidioidomycosis outbreak following the Northridge, Calif., earthquake. JAMA 1997;277:904–8.

52. Baumgardner DJ, Buggy BP, Mattson BJ, et al. Epidemiology of blastomycosis in a region of high endemicity in north central Wisconsin. Clin Infect Dis 1992;15:629–35.

53. Dodge HJ, Ajello L, Engelke OK. The association of a bird-roosting site with infection of school children by Histoplasma capsulatum. Am J Pub Health 1965;55:1203–11.

54. Kapoor A, Flechner SM, O'Malley K, et al. Cryptococcal meningitis in renal transplant patients associated with environmental exposure. Transplant Infect Dis 1999;1: 213–7.

55. Kauffman CA. Sporotrichosis. Clin Infect Dis 1999;29: 231–6.

56. Gregory DW, Schaffner W. Pseudomonas infections associated with hot tubs and other environments. Infect Dis Clin North Am 1987;1:635–48.

57. Samples JR, Binder PS, Luibel FJ, et al. Acanthamoeba keratitis possibly acquired from a hot tub. Arch Ophthalmol 1984;102:707–10.

58. Luttichau HR, Vinther C, Uldum SA, Moller J, Faber M, Jensen JS. An outbreak of Pontiac fever among children following use of a whirlpool. Clin Infect Dis. 1998;26: 1374-8.

59. Khoor A, Leslie KO, Tazelaar HD, et al. Diffuse pulmonary disease caused by nontuberculous mycobacteria in immunocompetent people (hot tub lung). Am J Clin Pathol 2001;115:755–62.

60. Fiorillo L, Zucker M, Sawyer D, et al. The pseudomonas hot-foot syndrome. N Engl J Med 2001;345:335–338.

61. Kee F, McElroy G, Stewart D, et al. A community outbreak of echovirus infection associated with an outdoor swimming pool. J Public Health Med 1994;16:145–8.

62. Harley D, Harrower B, Lyon M, et al. A primary school outbreak of pharyngoconjunctival fever caused by adenovirus type 3. Commun Dis Intell 2001;25:9–12.

63. Friedman MS, Roels T, Koehler JE, et al. Escherichia coli O157:H7 outbreak associated with an improperly chlorinated swimming pool. Clin Infect Dis 1999;29:298–303.

64. Anonymous. Shigellosis outbreak associated with an unchlorinated fill-and-drain wading pool—Iowa, 2001. MMWR Morb Mort Wkly Rep 2001;50:797–800.

65. MacKenzie WR, Kazmierczak JJ, Davis JP. An outbreak of cryptosporidiosis associated with a resort swimming pool. Epidemiol Infect 1995;115:545–53.

66. Greensmith CT, Stanwick RS, Elliot BE, et al. Giardiasis associated with the use of a water slide. Pediatr Infect Dis J 1988;7:91–4.

67. Blair JE, Woo-Ming MA, McGuire PK. Aeromonas hydrophila bacteremia acquired from an infected swimming pool. Clin Infect Dis 1999;28:1336–7.

68. Choong KY, Roberts LJ. Molluscum contagiosum, swimming and bathing: a clinical analysis. Aust J of Dermatol 1999;40:89–92.

69. Kamihama T, Kimura T, Hosokawa JI, et al. Tinea pedis outbreak in swimming pools in Japan. Public Health 1997; 111:249–53.

70. Jernigan JA, Farr BM. Incubation period and sources of exposure for cutaneous Mycobacterium marinum infection: case report and review of the literature. Clin Infect Dis 2000;31:439–43.

71. Hoeffler DF. "Swimmers' itch" (cercarial dermatitis). Cutis 1977;19:461–5, 467.

72. Ross AGP, Bartley PB, Sleigh AC, et al. Schistosomiasis. N Engl J Med 2002;346:1212–20.

73. Centers for Disease Control and Prevention. Update: Leptospirosis and unexplained acute febrile illness among athletes participating in triathlons—Illinois and Wisconsin, 1998. JAMA 1998;280:1474–5.

74. Janda JM, Abbott SL. Infections associated with the genus Edwardsiella: the role of Edwardsiella tarda in human disease. Clin Infect Dis 1993;17:742–48.

75. Gold WL, Salit IE. Aeromonas hydrophila infections of skin and soft tissue: report of 11 cases and review. Clin Infect Dis 1993;16:69–74.

76. DeNapoli TS, Rutman JY, Robinson JR, et al. Primary amoebic meningoencephalitis after swimming in the Rio Grande. Texas Medicine 1996;92:59–63.

77. Lehane L, Rawlin GT. Topically acquired bacterial zoonoses from fish: a review. Med J Aust 2000;173:256–9.

78. Jackson LA, Kaufmann AF, Adams WG, et al. Outbreak of leptospirosis associated with swimming. Pediatr Infect Dis J 1993;12:48–54.

79. Moreno-Ancillol A, Dominguez-Noche C, Gil-Adrados AC, Cosmes PM. Hypersensitivity pneumonitis due to occupational inhalation of fungi-contaminated corn dust. J Investig Allergol Immunol 2004;14:165–7.

80. Sullivan PA, Bang KM, Hearl FJ, et al. Respiratory disease risks in the construction industry. Occup Med 1995;10: 313–34.

81. Frontera JA, Gradon JD. Right-side endocarditis in injec-

tion drug users: review of proposed mechanisms of pathogenesis. Clin Infect Dis 2000;30:374–9.

82. Fox IM, Brady K. Acute hematogenous osteomyelitis in intravenous drug users. J Foot Ankle Surg 1997;36:301–5.

83. Werner SB, Passaro D, McGee J, et al. Wound botulism in California, 1951-1998: recent epidemic in heroin injectors. Clin Infect Dis 2000;31:1018–24.

84. Centers for Disease Control and Prevention. Update: yersinia enterocolitica bacteremia and endotoxin shock associated with red blood cell transfusions—United States, 1991. MMWR Morb Mortal Wkly Rep 1991;40:176–-8.

85. Foreman NK, Wang WC, Cullen EJ Jr, Endotoxic shock after transfusion of contaminated red blood cells in a child with sickle cell disease. Pediatr Infect Dis J 1991;10: 624–6.

86. Goodnough LT, Brecher ME, Kanter MH, et al. Transfusion medicine. First of two parts—blood transfusion. N Engl J Med 1999;340:438–47.

87. Mungai M, Tegtmeier G, Chamberland M, et al. Transfusion-transmitted malaria in the United States from 1963 through 1999. N Engl J Med 2001;344:1973–8.

88. Gerber MA, Shapiro ED, Krause PJ, et al. The risk of acquiring Lyme disease or babesiosis from a blood transfusion. J Infect Dis 1994;170:231–4.

89. Schmunis GA. *Trypanosoma* cruzi, the etiologic agent of Chagas' disease: status in the blood supply in endemic and nonendemic countries. Transfusion 1991;31:547–57.

90. Wells GM, Woodward TE, Fiset P, et al. Rocky Mountain spotted fever caused by blood transfusion. JAMA 1978; 239:2763–5.

91. De Schryver A, Meheus A. Syphilis and blood transfusion: a global perspective. Transfusion. 1990;30:844-7.

92. Schreiber GB, Busch MP, Kleinman SH, et al. The risk of transfusion-transmitted viral infections. The Retrovirus Epidemiology Donor Study. N Engl J Med 1996;334: 1685–90.

93. Chang HJ, Miller HL, Watkins N, et al. An epidemic of Malassezia pachydermatis in an intensive care nursery associated with colonization of health care workers' pet dogs. N Engl J Med 1998;338:706–11.

94. Duchin JS, Koster FT, Peters CJ, et al. Hantavirus pulmonary syndrome: a clinical description of 17 patients with a newly recognized disease. The Hantavirus Study Group. N Engl J Med 1994;330:949–55.

95. Ostrowski SR, Leslie MJ, Parrott T, et al. B-virus from pet macaque monkeys: an emerging threat in the United States? Emerg Infect Dis 1998;4:117–21.

96. Centers for Disease Control and Prevention. Raccoon roundworm encephalitis—Chicago, Illinois, and Los Angeles, California, 2000. JAMA 2002;287:580–1.

97. Capitini CM, Herrero IA, Patel R, et al. Wound infection with Neisseria weaveri and a novel subspecies of *Pasteurella multocida* in a child who sustained a tiger bite. Clin Infect Dis 2002;34:e74–6.

98. Barbour AG, Maupin GO, Teltow GJ, et al. Identification of an uncultivable *Borrelia* species in the hard tick *Amblyomma americanum*: possible agent of a Lyme disease-like illness. J Infect Dis 1996;173:403–9.

99. Miller LC, Comfort K, Kely N. Immunization status of internationally adopted children. Pediatrics 2001;108: 1050–1.

100. Hostetter MK, Iverson S, Thomas W, et al. Medical evaluation of internationally adopted children. N Engl J Med 1991;325:479–85.

101. American Academy of Pediatrics. Committee on Infectious Diseases. Varicella vaccine update. Pediatrics 2000;105: 136–41.

CHAPTER 22

Infections Complicating Chronic Diseases

Certain chronic diseases of children are associated with a higher than expected frequency of infectious complications. Some of these patients are immunocompromised hosts (ICH) and their unusual infecting organisms are referred to as opportunistic pathogens, because the microorganism may be normal flora or may only rarely produce disease in healthy children. Other patients may have a normal immune system, but the presence of an anatomic abnormality predisposes them to particular infections. Often, a combination of these factors exists.

This chapter classifies infections by the abnormal organ system or the disease rather than by the infecting agent or the physiologic defect of the host (Table 22-1). Infections in transplant recipients are included here. The approach to the child with a possible but unknown immune deficiency is covered in Chapter 23, as is the management of the child with a known primary immune disorder. HIV infection is covered in Chapter 20.

Several other infections in children with chronic illness are discussed elsewhere in this book where it seems more logical. The problem of fever in patients with heart disease is discussed in the section on endocarditis in Chapter 18. Intravascular device infections are covered in Chapter 10, neurosurgical shunt infections in Chapter 9, and postoperative wound infections in Chapter 17.

■ SPLENIC ABSENCE OR DYSFUNCTION

Individuals who are born without a spleen (congenital asplenia), who have been splenectomized for any reason, or whose splenic function is impaired by disease, such as sickle cell anemia, are at a significantly increased risk for fatal septicemia. In many cases, the infection is fulminating and is typically caused by encapsulated bacteria, usually *Streptococcus pneumoniae* or, less commonly, *Haemophilus influenzae* type b. In infants younger than 6 months with congenital asplenia, the organism is more likely to be an encapsulated strain of *Klebsiella* or *E. coli*.[1] Other infections to which asplenic patients are especially susceptible include meningococcemia, malaria, babesiosis, and *Capnocytophaga canimorsus* infection, which is associated with dog bites.

Functions of the Spleen

The frequency of encapsulated organisms in bacteremia in the asplenic patient provides strong evidence that the spleen aids in phagocytosis, both by the filtering effect of macrophages and production of specific Ig (immunoglobulin) M antibodies to opsonize bacteria.[2] Heavily encapsulated bacteria, such as the pneumococcus, are poorly opsonized by complement. The patient without capsular-specific antibodies from prior infection or from immunization relies on splenic macrophages to recognize and remove the bacteria before overwhelming sepsis ensues. The importance of the spleen is much greater during the first 2 years of life, possibly because other organs can later take over part of its function. Other protective roles of the spleen include synthesis of tuftsin (a stimulator of phagocytes), production of a platelet humoral factor and possibly production of other humoral factors related to immunity, and clearance of intraerythrocytic parasites, such as that of malaria. The spleen is believed to be necessary for normal thymic maturation during the neonatal period and to be involved in B-cell and T-cell interactions.

Howell-Jolly Bodies

These are very small, round, dark blue inclusions within red blood cells and are made up of nuclear debris. The spleen usually removes red cells containing these inclusions, and thus their presence is suggestive of hyposplenism. If the possibility of asplenia is suspected, a manual review of the

TABLE 22-1. CONTENTS OF THIS CHAPTER

ORGAN SYSTEM	DISEASES
Splenic absence or dysfunction	Sickle cell anemia, other hemoglobinopathies, postsplenectomy, congenital asplenia, functional asplenia
Collagen disease	Systemic lupus erythematosus, others
Lung disease	Cystic fibrosis, Down syndrome
Endocrine disease	Diabetes mellitus, polyendocrinopathies
Heart disease	Congenital heart disease, velocardiofacial syndrome
Kidney disease	Nephrotic syndrome, uremia, peritoneal dialysis, hemodialysis
Liver disease	Cirrhosis, others
Neoplastic disease	Hematologic malignancies, solid tumors
Hematopoietic stem cell transplant	
Solid organ transplant	

peripheral smear should be requested. Howell-Jolly bodies may be found in the peripheral smear in normal neonates, but are uncommon later in life. Interference phase-contrast microscopy can be used to detect red cells that are "pocked," which has slightly greater sensitivity[3] and specificity[4] for asplenia than does the presence of Howell-Jolly bodies.

If Howell-Jolly bodies are discovered incidentally, a history should be obtained, both regarding previous episodes of sepsis as well as the looking for causes of asplenia and hyposplenia. An abdominal ultrasound should be performed, looking for the spleen. If the spleen is present, a technicium-99m liver-spleen scan should be performed. If there is no uptake of the radioactive tracer by the spleen, a diagnosis of functional hyposplenism can be made.[5]

Clinical Manifestations

Overwhelming postsplenectomy infection often begins with a nonspecific influenza-like prodrome with fever, chills, malaise, myalgia, and headache. In addition, gastrointestinal symptoms such as vomiting, diarrhea, and abdominal pain may be prominent, distracting the physician from the diagnosis and resulting in delayed treatment.[6] The prodrome, which may last a few days or only a few hours, is followed by rapid progression to septic shock, with hypotension and disseminated intravascular coagulation. Symmetric peripheral gangrene may result. The mortality is greater than 50%. In contrast, if bacteremia is recognized and treated

prior to the development of clinical sepsis, the mortality rate is less than 10%.[5]

Specific Conditions

Congenital Asplenia

This may occur as an isolated finding but is most commonly associated with complex congenital cardiac defects, especially atrioventricular canal, transposition of the great arteries, pulmonary stenosis or atresia, and total anomalous pulmonary venous return. Children with these defects should have an abdominal ultrasound looking for the presence of a spleen. After the first month of life, such children are at greater risk of dying of sepsis than from their cardiac defect; thus, antibacterial prophylaxis is warranted.[1] Some of these children have accessory splenic tissue in the peritoneal cavity (polysplenia). However, the degree of protection offered by accessory spleens is variable, and antibacterial prophylaxis is probably warranted.[5] Heterotaxy syndromes are usually associated with asplenia or polysplenia. In addition to cardiac defects, patients may have primary ciliary dyskinesia, biliary atresia, intestinal malrotation, and multiple other anomalies.[7,8]

Postsplenectomy

Removal of the spleen may be necessary because of splenic trauma, malignancy, or hypersplenism (such as occurs in immune thrombocytopenic purpura). Children are at a higher risk of postsplenectomy sepsis than adults, and the risk is greater in persons undergoing splenectomy because of malignancy or thalassemia than for trauma.[9] This may be because of the frequent presence of splenic implants (splenosis) in patients who undergo splenectomy for trauma, which is sometimes (but not predictably) protective.[10]

The highest risk for infection is during the first 2 years after splenectomy. However, a third of infections occur up to 5 years later, and cases of fulminant infection have been reported more than 20 years postsplenectomy. The increased risk of dying of serious infection, although not quantifiable, is clinically significant and almost certainly lifelong.[11]

Functional Asplenism

In addition to the hemoglobinopathies, splenic dysfunction has been linked to a variety of conditions, including celiac disease, ulcerative colitis, portal hypertension, systemic lupus erythematosus, Graves' disease, polyarteritis nodosa, sarcoidosis, and HIV infection.[5] An important category of patients with functional hyposplenism are those who have received splenic irradiation for cancer or those who have undergone a stem cell transplant and develop graft-versus-host disease.[12,13]

Sickle Cell Anemia

Due to autoinfarction of the spleen, children with sickle cell anemia are at substantially increased risk for sepsis. In the first 5 years of life, the risk for pneumococcal sepsis is approximately 400 times that of the general population.[14] Patients with other hemoglobinopathies, such as sickle-C disease, are at intermediate risk.[15] The greatest risk is in young children with high fever and elevated white blood cell (WBC) count.[16] However, some children will present in a more subtle fashion. Bacteremia should be considered in all children with sickle cell anemia and fever (T greater than 38°C) especially in the first 5 years of life. In such children, blood cultures should be obtained and empiric treatment with ceftriaxone given. Children at higher risk (less than 2 years old, temperature greater than 40°C, WBC less than 5000/mcL or greater than 30,000/mcL, those who are ill-appearing or have pulmonary infiltrates or another focus of infection) should be admitted to the hospital for intravenous antibiotics. Well-appearing children at lower risk are often treated as outpatients, with careful follow-up and a second dose of ceftriaxone intramuscularly until the initial culture is negative at 48 hours.[17]

In addition to sepsis with encapsulated bacteria, patients with sickle cell anemia are also at risk for other infectious complications. As described in Chapter 11, infection with parvovirus B19, the agent of erythema infectiosum, can precipitate severe hypoplastic crisis in patients with sickle cell disease. The increased risk of osteomyelitis (especially due to *Salmonella* spp.), and the difficulty in distinguishing this condition from the more common bone infarction, is discussed in Chapter 16.

The *acute chest syndrome* is the leading cause of death among patients with sickle cell disease. It can be defined as a new pulmonary infiltrate involving at least one complete lung segment and one or more of the following findings: temperature greater than 38.5°C (seen in 80% of patients), cough (62%), chest pain (44%), or wheezing (26%).[18] The lower lobes are typically involved, and effusions develop in about half of cases. Acute chest syndrome is most commonly caused by infection; infarction and fat embolism are also frequent causes. In a prospective multicenter study of 671 episodes among 538 patients (all of whom underwent bronchoalveolar lavage), an infectious cause was found in 249 (37%).[18] Of the 249 episodes triggered by infection, *Chlamydia pneumoniae* was the most frequently identified organism, found in 71 (29%). Other frequent causes were *Mycoplasma pneumoniae* (20%), respiratory syncytial virus (10%), and *Staphylococcus aureus*, *S. pneumoniae*, *Mycoplasma hominis*, and parvovirus (4% each). Eighteen (3%) of the 528 patients died, and infection was a factor in 10 deaths. *S. pneumoniae*, *E. coli*, *H. influenzae*, legionella, cytomegalovirus, *S. aureus*, and chlamydia were implicated in fatal cases. Appropriate management of the acute chest syndrome includes a third-generation cephalosporin and a macrolide, as well as oxygen, bronchodilator therapy, and often, red cell transfusion.

Prevention

Effective prevention of invasive disease in patients with an absent or dysfunctional spleen requires a three-pronged approach of education, vaccination, and prophylactic antibiotics.[5]

Education

In one survey, of 63 patients who had undergone a splenectomy in the previous few years, only 10 (16%) were aware of any health precautions.[19] Asplenic patients should be aware of the need to notify their physician or seek immediate medical care in the event of any acute febrile illness. Patients should be encouraged to wear a Medi-Alert bracelet indicating their asplenic status.[11] They should be counseled regarding the risk of *C. canimorsus* sepsis after dog bites.

Expert travel advice is especially important. Travel to areas where malaria is endemic should be discouraged.[11] If travel to such areas is necessary, patients should be made aware of their increased risk of severe falciparum malaria and the need for strict adherence to effective antimalarial prophylaxis as well as protective measures, such as the use of DEET-containing insect repellent and mosquito netting. Patients traveling to sub-Saharan Africa should receive quadrivalent meningococcal vaccine if they have not already done so.

Pneumococcal Vaccination

Patients with an absent or dysfunctional spleen should definitely be vaccinated against *S. pneumoniae*. Unfortunately, 30–60% of eligible patients never receive the pneumococcal vaccine.[19,20] In the case of elective splenectomy, the vaccine should be given at least 2 weeks before surgery since asplenic individuals have impaired antibody production.

The recent introduction of the seven-valent conjugated pneumococcal vaccine (PCV7) represents a significant advance in the prevention of invasive pneumococcal disease. In contrast to the 23-valent polysaccharide pneumococcal vaccine (PPV23), the conjugate vaccine is immunogenic in young infants and induces immunologic memory both in healthy children[21] and in children with sickle cell diesase.[22] Children should receive the primary series of PCV7 as described in Table 22-2. Children 2 years old or more who have been primed with PCV7 have a significant booster response to PPV23.[21,22] Thus, in order to receive protection against the additional serotypes contained in the 23-valent vaccine, high-risk children who have received PCV7 should also receive PPV23, according to the schedule in Table 22-3.

Children at high risk for invasive pneumococcal disease who have already received PPV23 (but who have not received PCV7) should receive 2 doses of PCV7, 2 months apart. Although the vaccine is only FDA approved for children up to age 9 years, it has been shown to be immunogenic in persons aged 4–30 years with sickle cell disease,[23] and administering PCV7 to older children with high-risk conditions is not contraindicated.[24]

In children with functional or anatomic asplenia, the parents and patients should understand the risk of fulminant pneumococcal disease and that vaccination does not guarantee protection.[25] Prompt medical attention is required for febrile illnesses. Immediate expectant antimicrobial treatment should be given for suspected bacteremia, the initial signs and symptoms of which may be subtle.

H. influenzae Type b Vaccine

Children with an absent or dysfunctional spleen should have their immunization history reviewed. Most children in the United States will have re-

---

TABLE 22-2. RECOMMENDED SCHEDULE FOR USE OF 7-VALENT PNEUMOCOCCAL CONJUGATE VACCINE (PCV7)

AGE AT FIRST DOSE (MOS)	PRIMARY SERIES	ADDITIONAL DOSE
2–6	3 doses, 2 mos apart	1 dose at 12–15 mos
7–11	2 doses, 2 mos apart	1 dose at 12–15 mos
12–23	2 doses, 2 mos apart	–
≥24		
Healthy children 24–59 mos old	1 dose	–
High-risk children[a,b]	2 doses, 2 mos apart	–

[a] Sickle cell disease, asplenia, HIV infection, chronic illness, immunocompromising condition.
[b] PCV7 is only FDA approved for children up to age 9 years; however, its use is not contraindicated in older children with high-risk conditions.
Source: Adapted from: Preventing pneumococcal disease among infants and young children. Recommendations of the Advisory Committee on Immunization Practices (ACIP). MMWR Recomm Rep 2000;49:1–35, with permission.

TABLE 22-3. SCHEDULE FOR VACCINATION USING 23-VALENT POLYSACCHARIDE VACCINE (PPV23) FOR CHILDREN AGED 2 YEARS OR MORE WHO HAVE PREVIOUSLY RECEIVED THE 7-VALENT CONJUGATE VACCINE (PCV7)

POPULATION	SCHEDULE FOR PPV23	REVACCINATION WITH PPV23
Healthy children	None	No
Children with sickle cell disease or asplenia, HIV infection, or other immunocompromising condition	1 dose of PPV23 given at age ≥2 yrs (and ≥2 months after last dose of PCV7)	Yes (one revaccination 3–5 years after previous PPV23 dose)[a]
Other chronic illness	1 dose of PPV23 given at age ≥2 yrs (and ≥2 mos after last dose of PCV7)	Not recommended

[a] Some experts recommend that patients with HIV infection receive PPV23 every 5 years.
Source: Adapted from: Preventing pneumococcal disease among infants and young children. Recommendations of the Advisory Committee on Immunization Practices (ACIP). MMWR Recomm Rep 2000;49:1–35, with permission.

ceived conjugate *H. influenzae* type b vaccination. Children who have not completed the primary series and booster at 12–15 months of age should be vaccinated. Asplenic children older than 5 years who have not previously been vaccinated should receive 2 doses, 2 months apart.[26] The vaccine has been shown to be immunogenic in children with sickle cell disease.[27]

N. meningitidis Vaccine

Quadrivalent meningococcal vaccine contains purified polysaccharides of serogroups A, C, Y, and W135 and is poorly immunogenic in young children. No vaccine is available for the prevention of serogroup B disease. Meningococcal vaccine should be given to all children with functional or anatomic asplenia at 2 years of age or older. The need for additional doses is unclear, but reimmunization does not elicit a booster response to serogroup C.[28] A meningococcal group C conjugate vaccine was introduced into routine use for infant immunization in the United Kingdom in 1999, but is not currently available in the United States.[29]

Influenza Vaccine

Influenza vaccination is effective in reducing the risk of secondary bacterial infection thus, children with hyposplenia and their household contacts should receive annual influenza immunization.[30] Despite this recommendation, immunization rates in such high-risk patients younger than 65 years are typically low (30–40%).[31] Influenza vaccine has been shown to be reasonably immunogenic in pre-

school and school-aged children with sickle cell disease.[32]

Prophylactic Antibiotics

Daily oral penicillin has been shown to decrease the risk of serious bacterial infection by 84% in young children with sickle cell disease.[33] Prophylaxis should begin as soon as the child is found to have sickle cell disease and preferably by 2 months of age. Most experts recommend penicillin V 125 mg b.i.d. for children younger than 5 years and 250 mg b.i.d. for those aged 5 years or older (alternatively, amoxicillin 20 mg/kg daily may be given). For the penicillin-allergic child, options are limited. Trimethoprim-sulfamethoxazole or erythromycin may be given, but the rates of pneumococcal resistance to these organisms are higher than to the penicillins.

Penicillin prophylaxis generally results in an overall decrease in the nasopharyngeal carriage rate of *S. pneumoniae*.[34] An increase in the proportion of penicillin-resistant pneumococci colonizing the nasopharynx of children taking penicillin prophylaxis has been reported in some studies[34,35] but not in others.[36,37] Despite the concern about increasing resistance rates, penicillin's safety profile, low cost, and lack of a suitable alternative oral agent argues for its continued status as the prophylactic drug of choice.

The optimal duration of therapy is not known. A multicenter study compared continuing penicillin prophylaxis with placebo after the age of 5 years in 400 children with sickle cell anemia.[38] Four (2%) of placebo recipients developed systemic infection with *S. pneumoniae* as compared with 2 (1%) of those receiving penicillin prophylaxis, a result that was not statistically significant. The authors concluded that children with sickle cell anemia who have not had a prior severe pneumococcal infection or a splenectomy and are receiving comprehensive care may safely stop prophylactic penicillin at 5 years of age. However, the confidence limits around their estimates were wide, and it is possible that a larger trial would have demonstrated a statistically significant result. Many experts continue penicillin prophylaxis indefinitely.

The duration of prophylaxis in persons with anatomic or functional asplenia of another cause has not been studied. The *Red Book* states only that prophylaxis be strongly considered for all asplenic children younger than 5 years of age and for at least 1 year after splenectomy (in patients of any age).[39] However, a British working group stated that lifelong prophylaxis should be offered in all cases. They especially recommend prophylaxis in patients who meet any of the following criteria: patients in the first two years after splenectomy, patients younger than 16 years old, and patients who have underlying impaired immune function.

Whether the asplenic patient is on prophylactic antibiotics or not, patients and parents need to be made aware of the importance of seeking prompt medical care if the patient develops a fever. This is preferable to self-administration of antibiotics when patients develop fever, although this may be considered in unusual circumstances when the patient does not have quick access to a hospital or clinic.

■ COLLAGEN DISEASE

Children with chronic collagen diseases often have fever or complications that are not infectious. Sometimes, corticosteroids or other immunosuppressive drugs are used, resulting in the same kinds of opportunistic infections found in children with transplants.

Systemic Lupus Erythematosus

Infection is a leading cause of morbidity and mortality in systemic lupus erythematosus (SLE).[40] In a prospective study of 200 patients with SLE, 65 (32%) developed infection over a 2-year period.[41] Disease activity was the only variable independently associated with infection.

Most patients with SLE do not have specific complement defects. However, the diagnosis of SLE in a young male patient should alert the clinician to the possibility of complement deficiency (especially C1q, C2, and C4),[42] with the consequent predisposition to severe infection with encapsulated bacteria (Chapter 23).[43,44] Some patients with SLE have a mutation in the gene for mannose-binding lectin, which is associated with both higher disease activity and increased risk of infection.[45]

In a review of 63 hospitalized adults with SLE and fever, about 60% of the fevers were caused by the disease itself and about 23% were caused by infections.[46] Shaking chills, leukocytosis, neutrophilia, and normal levels of anti-DNA antibodies were observed more frequently in infectious episodes, whereas leukopenia was more likely to indicate a noninfectious process. Some studies report that an elevated C-reactive protein in a febrile patient with SLE is suggestive of infection,[47,48] whereas other studies show it to be of poor predictive value.[49,50]

Granulocyte colony stimulating factor has been used to increase neutrophil counts in patients with SLE-associated neutropenia. Unfortunately, in one study 3 (33%) of 9 patients experienced serious adverse effects (exacerbation of CNS [central nervous system] symptoms in two and leukocytoclastic vasculitis in one).[51]

Juvenile Rheumatoid Arthritis (JRA)

Sometimes, septic arthritis occurs in adults with rheumatoid arthritis, but it is extremely rare in children. Platelet dysfunction, renal papillary necrosis, and, rarely, Reye syndrome may be related to aspirin therapy. Pericarditis and myocarditis occur, but are usually not of infectious origin.

Hemophagocytic lymphohistiocytosis (HLH), also referred to as hemophagocytic syndrome or macrophage activation syndrome,[52,53] is a rare but potentially lethal complication of systemic onset JRA. Although HLH is not an infectious process per se, it appears that certain infectious agents (e.g., Epstein-Barr virus) may trigger it in susceptible hosts.[54] In children with JRA, the presentation is dramatic, with acute onset of fever, lymphadenopathy, and hepatosplenomegaly.[53] One or more cell lines are depressed, liver enzymes are elevated, and clotting abnormalities may occur. The ferritin level is usually extremely high, and the ESR (erythrocyte sedimentation rate) is often unexpectedly low. The diagnosis is made by bone marrow examination, which demonstrates phagocytosis of various cells by macrophages. Initial treatment is with high dose corticosteroids, but some patients do not respond. Consultation with a pediatric rheumatologist or hematologist is critical.

Mixed Connective Tissue Disease (MCTD)

This disease resembles a mixture of SLE, systemic sclerosis, rheumatoid arthritis, and dermatomyositis, and produces a high titer of speckled antinuclear antibody. An immune response to ribonuclear protein (RNP) is the defining serologic feature of MCTD.[55] The disease often presents with Raynaud's phenomenon, followed by fever and arthralgia.[56] Lymphadenopathy and parotid gland enlargement also can give it the appearance of an infectious disease. Patients may have hypergammaglobulinemia and a positive rheumatoid factor.[56] Severe thrombocytopenia can occur, and fatal meningococcemia has been reported.[57]

In a review of 224 children reported in the literature over a 25-year period, common long-term problems included loss of joint function, restrictive lung disease, scleroderma-like skin changes, renal involvement, and esophageal dysmotility. Cardiovascular problems included cardiomyopathy, myopericarditis, and pulmonary hypertension. Seventeen (8%) of the 224 patients died. Infection (usually sepsis) was the most common cause of death and was implicated in seven patients.[58]

Reye Syndrome

Children receiving maintenance aspirin are at increased risk of encephalopathy from Reye syndrome (Chapter 9).[59] Hepatotoxicity without encephalopathy can also occur secondary to salicylate therapy. Children receiving long-term aspirin should be immunized against influenza and varicella.

■ CYSTIC FIBROSIS

Cystic fibrosis is common, affecting approximately 30,000 persons in the United States. Mutations in the cystic fibrosis transmembrane conductance regulator (CFTR) gene result in defective chloride transport in the epithelial cells of the respiratory, hepatobiliary, gastrointestinal, and reproductive tracts, as well as the pancreas.[60] Multiple different mutations have been identified, and severity of the disease varies greatly among patients.[61] The primary causes of morbidity and mortality are airway inflammation, bronchiectasis, and obstructive pulmonary disease, which occur as a direct result of persistent endobronchial bacterial infection.

Pathogenesis and Microbiology

In the lung, decreased transport of chloride, sodium, and water results in dehydrated, viscous secretions that cause airway obstruction and create a favorable environment for persistent bacterial colonization. Initially, the airways are colonized with *S. aureus*, and non-typable *H. influenzae*. However, by the end of the first decade, *Pseudomonas aeruginosa* gradually becomes the predominant pathogen. During the transition from intermittent infection to permanent colonization, *P. aeruginosa* transforms from a motile, nonmucoid phenotype to a nonmotile, highly mucoid phenotype.[62] The mucoid *P. aeruginosa* forms a biofilm that makes it highly resistant to antibiotics. This chronic bacterial endobronchitis is associated with an intense neutrophilic inflammatory response that damages the airway and impairs local host-defense mechanisms. Other bacteria sometimes causing pulmonary infections in patients with cystic fibrosis include *Burkholderia cepacia*, *Serratia marcescens*, and *Stenotrophomonas maltophilia*. Fungi (especially *Aspergillus* spp.) and non-tuberculous mycobacteria also can contribute to disease.[63,64]

Clinical Manifestations and Therapy

Intermittent exacerbations of chronic lung infection are frequent in patients with cystic fibrosis. Such exacerbations are usually heralded by increased cough and sputum production. Physical examination may show an increased respiratory rate and new or increased crackles or wheezes. Chest radiography will often show a new or progressive infiltrate, and spirometry will demonstrate a decline in pulmonary function. Chronic sinusitis (with or without nasal polyposis) is common in children with cystic fibrosis and may require endoscopic sinus surgery in addition to antibiotics.[65]

The therapy of exacerbations should be based on the results of sputum culture and sensitivity. Although a relatively insensitive predictor of lower airway pathogens, throat culture testing is often used for children too young to produce sputum. Combination intravenous therapy with' an antipseudomonal beta-lactam agent (such as ceftazidime or cefepime) and an aminoglycoside is usually given for approximately 14 days. For milder exacerbations, an oral fluoroquinolone, such as ciprofloxacin, is sometimes given. Although not approved for use in children, fluoroquinolones are generally well-tolerated in children with cystic fibrosis,[66] and the benefits of their use appear to outweigh the risks in this population.[67] An inhaled antibiotic, such as tobramycin or colistin may also be used; however, they have not been studied in the setting of acute exacerbations.[68] Recombinant human DNase can be given by inhalation to reduce the viscosity of the sputum[69] and some variation of chest physiotherapy is performed to enhance clearance of pulmonary secretions.[70] This aggressive approach to pulmonary exacerbations is believed to be a major reason for the increased life expectancy among patients with cystic fibrosis during the past few decades.

Chronic antibiotic therapy to prevent pulmonary exacerbations is controversial but should probably be avoided. A multicenter study of 119 children with newly diagnosed cystic fibrosis was conducted to determine if continuous therapy with cephalexin was superior to placebo. After 7 years, there were no significant differences between the two groups in pulmonary function, frequency of exacerbations, nutritional status, or chest radiography scores. Although children in the cephalexin group were less likely to be colonized with *S. aureus*, they were twice as likely to be colonized with *P. aeruginosa*.[71] A retrospective study of 639 German children with cystic fibrosis also showed an increased risk of colonization with *P. aeruginosa* among those who had received antistaphylococcal prophylaxis.[72]

Intermittent inhaled tobramycin was recently studied in a placebo-controlled trial.[73] A total of 520 patients were randomly assigned to receive either 300 mg of inhaled tobramycin or placebo twice daily for 4 weeks, followed by 4 weeks with no study drug. Patients received treatment or placebo in three on-off cycles for a total of 24 weeks. At the end of the study period, patients receiving tobramycin had improved pulmonary function, decreased density of colonization with *P. aeruginosa*, and a 26% lower rate of hospitalization for pulmonary exacerbation. The drug was well tolerated. However, several important questions remain. The drug is expensive, and it is possible that once-daily administration would be as effective. In addition, whether long-term intermittent use will increase the development of drug-resistant strains of *P. aeruginosa* is unknown. Because of this concern, some centers reserve its use for exacerbations, when one or more systemic antibiotics are given simultaneously.

Viral infections are a common predisposing factor for exacerbations of cystic fibrosis. Patients and their household contacts should receive the influenza vaccine yearly. Although *S. pneumoniae* is not a common cause of infection in patients with cystic fibrosis, it is reasonable to administer the pneumococcal vaccine as well.

Allergic Bronchopulmonary Aspergillosis (ABPA)

This condition is a hypersensitivity lung disease caused by bronchial colonization with *Aspergillus fumigatus*. The presence of colonization with *A. fumigatus* in patients with cystic fibrosis can be has high as 50%;[74] however, less than 10% of patients develop ABPA.[75,76] Standard diagnostic criteria were recently proposed by a consensus group.[76] They require the presence of two of three major criteria (immediate skin test reactivity to *A. fumigatus*, precipitating antibodies to *A. fumigatus*, and total serum IgE greater than 1,000 IU/mL), and two of six minor criteria (*A. fumigatus* in sputum, bronchoconstriction, peripheral eosinophil count more than 1,000/mcL, pulmonary infiltrates, elevated serum IgE or IgG to *A. fumigatus*, and response to corticosteroids).

If untreated, irreversible bronchiectasis may result. Conventional therapy has consisted mainly of systemic corticosteroids that, although effective, have numerous side-effects (such as growth failure, diabetes mellitus, and osteoporosis). Although randomized trials are lacking, anecdotal reports suggest that itraconazole treatment is associated with fewer episodes of ABPA and allows for decreased steroid use.[77] Aerosolized amphotericin B has also been used in this setting, but no data are available regarding its effectiveness.

Nontuberculous Mycobacteria

These organisms (especially *M. avium* complex *and M. chelonae*) are isolated from sputum cultures in 3–30% of patients with cystic fibrosis.[64] A pathogenic role has not been established, but some patients appear to improve clinically after a course of antimycobacterial therapy. Such therapy should be considered for the patient with repeatedly positive sputum cultures, persistent symptoms, and declining pulmonary function despite routine antibacterial—and in some cases, antifungal—treatment.

Extrapulmonary Manifestations

As expected from the pathophysiology, multiple other organ systems are involved in cystic fibrosis. Pancreatic exocrine deficiency occurs in about 80% of patients, diabetes mellitus in up to 20%, and obstructive biliary tract disease in 15–20% of patients.[60] Recurrent arthritis occurs in some patients, occasionally accompanied by erythema nodosum.[78]

Outcome

The median life expectancy is now greater than 30 years, and it is projected that for newborn infants it will become more than 40 years.[61] Lung transplantation is an option for some patients to further increase survival but is limited by the availability of donor organs. The 5-year survival rate for lung transplant recipients with cystic fibrosis is about 50%.[79] Gene transfer therapy for cystic fibrosis is currently under investigation, but multiple hurdles to its successful implementation still remain.[80]

■ DOWN SYNDROME

Children with Down syndrome have well-documented immunological alterations, including a lower number of B cells, lower numbers of IgG2 and IgG4 subclasses, inverted CD4/CD8 ratio, and decreased T-cell proliferative responses to mitogens.[81,82] Although not well studied, it is apparent that children with Down syndrome have an increased incidence of viral and bacterial respiratory infections, especially pneumonia and otitis media. In one series of 100 children with Down syndrome who underwent surgical correction of their heart defects, 38% had postoperative pneumonia.[83]

Part of the predisposition to infections relates to anatomic abnormalities, such as pulmonary hypoplasia and collapsed eustachian tubes.[84,85] Children with Down syndrome also frequently have stenotic ear canals, leading to difficulty visualizing the tympanic membrane and underdiagnosis and undertreatment of otitis media.[86] When these children undergo frequent ear examinations by an otolaryngologist, as many as 80% will be found to have chronic otitis media.[85] Although hearing loss in children with Down syndrome is common, recent studies suggest that it is largely preventable with

early and aggressive management of chronic otitis media.[85] Most children with Down syndrome will require placement of tympanostomy tubes in the first 2 years of life.

■ ENDOCRINE DISEASE

Diabetes Mellitus

In patients with diabetes, acute infections lead to difficulty in controlling blood glucose levels and are the most common precipitant of ketoacidosis.[87,88] Adult patients with diabetes have an increased susceptibility to certain infections,[89] but whether this is true for children with diabetes is less clear. Adult diabetic patients have an increased frequency of candidiasis (especially vaginal), staphylococcal infections (especially boils), infected decubitus ulcers, rhinocerebral mucormycosis, and malignant otitis externa.[89] These infections rarely occur in children with diabetes.

Neutrophils from patients with diabetes demonstrate decreased chemotaxis, phagocytosis, and killing,[87] and this decreased neutrophil function is more pronounced in patients whose diabetes is poorly controlled.[88] In addition, some organisms (such as *Candida albicans* and *E. coli*) are more virulent in a high-glucose environment.[87]

Polyendocrinopathies

Autoimmune polyendocrinopathy syndrome (APS) type 1 (also referred to as autoimmune polyendocrinopathy-candidiasis-ectodermal dystrophy or APECED) is an autosomal recessive disorder characterized by chronic mucocutaneous candidiasis, hypoparathyroidism, Addison's disease and sometimes other features such as insulin-dependent diabetes mellitus (IDDM).[90,91] Some patients have severe cell-mediated immune dysfunction, whereas others have few problems with infections. Symptoms usually begin in childhood. It is discussed in more detail in Chapter 23. APS type 2 is an association of Addison's disease with autoimmune thyroid disease, IDDM, or both.

A rare X-linked syndrome called IPEX (immunodysregulation, polyendocrinopathy, enteropathy, X-linked) has recently been elucidated.[92] Boys present early in life with variable combinations of IDDM, diarrhea, eczema, anemia, thrombocytopenia, lymphadenopathy, and hypothyroidism.[93] It is usually lethal in infancy or childhood. No specific immune abnormality has been detected, but patients are at high risk for infections, and sepsis is a common cause of death. Some patients respond to chronic immune suppressive therapy, and a few patients have undergone successful bone marrow transplanation.[92]

■ HEART DISEASE

Congenital Heart Disease

Children with congenital heart disease (CHD) are at increased risk for pneumonia, particularly if the defect is associated with chronic pulmonary congestion. Children with CHD have a rate of hospitalization for RSV infection that is three-fold to five-fold higher than age-matched controls.[94] Once hospitalized, they more frequently require mechanical ventilation (20%) and have a higher mortality rate (3%) than children without heart disease.[95] A recent multicenter study compared monthly palivizumab during RSV season with placebo in 1,287 children younger than 2 years of age with CHD.[96] The intervention was safe and effective. Among placebo recipients, the rate of RSV hospitalization was 10%; the rate among children receiving palivizumab was 5%. Children with CHD most likely to benefit from palivizumab are those who are less than 12 months old[94] and who have congestive heart failure, pulmonary hypertension, or cyanotic heart disease.

22q11.2 Deletion Syndrome (Velocardiofacial Syndrome)

Between 10% and 30% of children with various conotruncal cardiac anomalies will be found to have 22q11.2 deletion syndrome (velocardiofacial syndrome). The syndrome has previously been referred to as DiGeorge syndrome or Catch 22. In addition to the heart defect, patients usually have hypotonia, palatal anomalies, and mild developmental delay. Anomalies of other organ systems may occur as well, including thymic hypoplasia. These children frequently have impairment in T cell production and function,[97] which tends to improve over time (Chapter 23).[98] Children with impaired T cell function or with low CD4 counts (Chapter 20 for levels based on age) should receive trimethoprim-sulfamethoxazole (TMP-SMX) for PCP (*Pneumocystis jiroveci*) prophylaxis.

Fever in a patient with congenital or rheumatic heart disease is discussed in the section on endocarditis (Chapter 18). Infections in cardiac transplant recipients are discussed later in this chapter.

■ KIDNEY DISEASE

This section reviews the infectious complications of nephrotic syndrome, uremia, hemodialysis, and peritoneal dialysis.

Nephrotic Syndrome

Nephrotic syndrome is characterized by edema, hypoalbuminemia, proteinuria, and hyperlipidemia. Viral respiratory infections appear to be a common trigger for exacerbations of nephrosis.[99] Children with nephrotic syndrome are at increased risk of infection for several reasons. Partly due to protein loss in the urine, they have decreased serum levels of immunoglobulins.[100] They also have decreased serum complement concentration,[101] impaired lymphocyte blastogenesis,[102] and splenic hypofunction.[103] In addition, patients with nephrotic syndrome are frequently on corticosteroids or other immunosuppressive agents.

Peritonitis

The classic infection in children with nephrotic syndrome is spontaneous bacterial peritonitis (SBP) caused by *S. pneumoniae*. However, other gram-positive organisms such as *Enterococcus* and viridans streptococci are occasionally seen, as are gram-negative organisms (especially *E. coli*).[104,105] Sepsis in patients with peritonitis is not uncommon and is occasionally fatal.[104] Patients with one episode of peritonitis are at increased risk for a second episode.

Children with SBP usually present with the acute onset of fever and abdominal pain, although occasionally the onset is subacute and the symptoms are subtle. Abdominal tenderness is apparent in an older child but may be difficult to discern in an infant. If SBP is suspected, cultures of blood and peritoneal fluid should be obtained. The peritoneal fluid usually contains more than 250 neutrophils per mcL. Empiric broad-spectrum antibiotics should be given to cover the pneumococcus and gram-negative organisms. The combination of vancomycin and a third- or fourth-generation cephalosporin is reasonable initial coverage. In the severely ill patient, an aminoglycoside should probably be added. Antibiotics are tailored to susceptibility testing and are given for 10–14 days.

Other Infections

In addition to peritonitis and sepsis, cellulitis is more common in children with nephrotic syndrome.[106] During therapy with corticosteroids or other immunosuppressive agents, the child with nephrotic syndrome is at risk for many of the infections described in the sections on leukemia and transplantation.

Prevention

Children with nephrotic syndrome should receive pneumococcal vaccination (Tables 22-2 and 22-3). Whether prophylactic penicillin is of benefit is unclear. In one study, there was no increase in pneumococcal peritonitis for the 7 years after the policy of penicillin prophylaxis was discontinued.[105] Consideration should be given to the use of TMP-SMX for PCP prophylaxis in children receiving prolonged courses (more than 14 days) of high-dose prednisone (more than 20 mg per day or more than 2 mg/kg per day).[107,108]

Uremia

Patients with uremia are at increased risk for infections, which are a common cause of death in this population.[109] Such patients have impaired neutrophil function secondary to excessive parathyroid hormone and elevated intracellular calcium.[110] Use of calcium-channel blockers has been shown to improve neutrophil phagocytosis in uremic patients.[110] However, whether this translates into decreased incidence of infection is unknown. Other mechanisms such as iron overload contribute to the increased risk of infection in patients with chronic renal failure.[111] As discussed in the next section, the use of dialysis brings additional infectious risk.

In addition to the routine childhood vaccines, children with chronic renal failure should receive pneumococcal vaccination (Table 22-3) as well as yearly influenza vaccination.[112]

Peritoneal Dialysis

Peritonitis

Peritonitis is a common complication of peritoneal dialysis. In two studies of children on peritoneal dialysis, the rate of peritonitis varied from one episode per 5.6 patient-months[113] to one episode per 13.2 patient-months.[114] Infection can occur with any contaminating organism, particularly *S. aureus*

and *S. epidermidis*.[115] If a nephrectomy has been performed, gram-negative enteric rods are more common.[116] Fungi, particularly *Candida albicans*, are less common.

The diagnosis of peritonitis is usually suspected when the effluent is cloudy, a much more reliable finding than fever or peripheral leukocytosis.[117] Abdominal pain is common but not universal. Routine screening cultures of the dialysate are not useful.[117] The skin sites rarely look infected. In general, the diagnosis of peritonitis requires the presence of at least two of the following three criteria: (i) organisms on gram stain or culture of peritoneal dialysis fluid; (ii) cloudy fluid (more than 100 white cells per mcL with more than 50% neutrophils); and (iii) symptoms of peritoneal irritation.[118] False-negative gram stains are common. In about 20% of cases, the culture is negative as well, particularly if there has been prior antimicrobial therapy.[119] Optimally, 50–100 mL of effluent should be centrifuged and gram stained. The concentrate should then be injected into blood culture bottles.[120]

For patients without systemic toxicity, intraperitoneal administration of antibiotics is usually sufficient and can usually be accomplished as an outpatient. If the patient is toxic appearing, intravenous antibiotics are administered with the doses adjusted for renal failure. The International Society for Peritoneal Dialysis has published detailed guidelines for the treatment of peritonitis in children receiving peritoneal dialysis.[121] Initial empiric therapy should usually be with intraperitoneal cefazolin and ceftazidime. For continuous antibiotic therapy, which is preferred, both are given as a loading dose of 250 mg of the antibiotic in the first liter of dialysate, followed by 125 mg of antibiotic in each subsequent liter of dialysate. The peritoneal dialysis exchange containing the loading dose should dwell in the abdomen for 4–6 hours. For intermittent therapy, both are dosed at 15 mg/kg in a single peritoneal dialysis exchange every 24 hours.

The antibiotic regimen can be tailored to culture and susceptibility results. Isolates requiring vancomycin therapy can be treated intraperitoneally with a loading dose of 500 mg per liter of dialysate followed by a maintenance dose of 30 mg per liter of dialysate. For intermittent therapy, 30 mg/kg is given intraperitoneally; subsequent doses are given when the serum level is less than 10 μg/mL, usually 5 to 7 days later. For patients with culture-negative peritonitis who improve clinically with cefazolin and ceftazidime, these agents are continued for 2 weeks. Most culture-positive infections are treated for 2 weeks as well. Exceptions include infections due to *S. aureus, Pseudomonas, Stenotrophomonas,* anaerobes, and polymicrobial infections, which are treated for 3 weeks, and may often necessitate removal of the peritoneal dialysis catheter. Lack of clinical response to appropriate antibiotics for 3 days is an additional indication for catheter removal. Approximately 20% of patients will still have positive peritoneal fluid cultures 3 days into therapy; this is not necessarily an indication for catheter removal or changing antibiotics.[122]

Successful treatment of fungal peritonitis usually requires removal of the catheter.[123] Treatment is with amphotericin B or fluconazole for a minimum of 2 weeks after catheter removal. For infections that require catheter removal, a new peritoneal catheter can usually be placed 2–3 weeks later.[121]

Adjunctive therapies sometimes used for patients with peritonitis include decreasing the fill volume in patients with significant abdominal pain, low-dose intraperitoneal heparin to maintain catheter patency, and intravenous immune globulin for children with documented hypogammaglobulinemia.[121] Some physicians use antifungal prophylaxis with oral nystatin or fluconazole during prolonged antibacterial therapy, and there is some evidence that this decreases the incidence of secondary *Candida* peritonitis.[124,125]

Exit Site and Tunnel Infections

In a large multicenter study of children on peritoneal dialysis, 11% of patients had an exit site or tunnel infection within 30 days of catheter placement; by 12 months, the number rose to 30%.[114] Patients with these local infections were twice as likely to develop peritonitis or to need access revision, and were three times more likely to be hospitalized than patients without these local infections. When infected, the exit site is elevated and erythematous, and there may be purulent or serous drainage. Tunnel infections occur deeper along the cannula tract. Any exudate from the site should be cultured. Exit site infections are usually treated with a combination of topical and systemic antibiotics for 2–4 weeks. Tunnel infections generally require catheter removal for cure.

Prevention

Rates of peritonitis are lowest with the use of a double-cuffed catheter, with a downward directed tunnel, placed by an experienced surgeon.[126] The use of a perioperative antibiotic administered intravenously decreases the incidence of postoperative peritonitis.[127] A single dose of cefazolin is recommended unless the patient is known to be colonized with methicillin-resistant *S. aureus*, in which case vancomycin can be used.[121] The use of mupirocin ointment applied to the nares[128] or to the catheter exit site[129] has been demonstrated to decrease the incidence of exit-site infections and peritonitis caused by *S. aureus*. Unfortunately, emergence of mupirocin-resistant *S. aureus* has recently been reported in patients receiving continuous prophylaxis for 4 years.[130]

Hemodialysis

Hemodialysis may be done using several different types of access. Native arteriovenous fistulas carry the lowest risk of infection, followed by prosthetic arteriovenous grafts, tunneled central venous catheters, and nontunneled central catheters, which carry the highest risk of infection.[131,132] *S. aureus* and coagulase-negative staphylococci are the most common causes. Hemodialysis patients with fever should have blood cultures drawn both peripherally and from their access site if possible. Indium white cell scans can be particularly useful in localizing the site of infection in a clotted, nonfunctional access site.[132] Patients with symptoms of severe sepsis should generally receive intravenous vancomycin, gentamicin, and a third-generation cephalosporin pending culture results. Well-appearing patients without known colonization with MRSA can be treated initially with cefazolin (with or without gentamicin).[132] If the bacteremia is cleared promptly, the catheter can be left in place and antibiotics given for a minimum of 3 weeks; infections due to *S. aureus* are treated for at least 4 weeks. For patients with persistent bacteremia, the catheter should be removed and the possibility of endocarditis entertained.[133]

Patients on hemodialysis are at increased risk for both hepatitis B virus (HBV) and hepatitis C virus (HCV) infection (Chapter 13). Strict attention to infection-control practices in hemodialysis units is necessary to prevent transmission of these viruses.[134] All patients on hemodialysis should receive the HBV vaccine series and have immunity documented. The dose of HBV vaccine used in dialysis patients is higher than in healthy persons.[135] Hemodialysis recipients should also have baseline

ALT (alanine aminotransferase) and anti-HCV testing. Anti-HCV-negative patients should be retested every 6 months.[136] HIV transmission has not been documented in dialysis centers in the United States, and routine testing for HIV infection is not recommended.

Prevention

Guidelines for preventing fistula-, graft-, and catheter-associated infections in this population have been published.[137] Nasal mupirocin is used to eradicate nasal carriage of *S. aureus*. In one study, its use resulted in a four-fold decrease in the incidence of *S. aureus* bacteremia, compared with historical controls.[138] Treatment is given twice daily for 5 days, then weekly to prevent recolonization. It may be most cost-effective to treat all patients on hemodialysis, regardless of their carriage status. For patients with catheters, applying mupirocin to the exit site as part of daily site care is also appropriate.[139]

■ LIVER DISEASE

Liver disease in children may be chronic, such as cirrhosis secondary to galactosemia or biliary atresia, or acute, such as that caused by hepatitis A or B virus. The complications of hepatitis are discussed in the chapter on hepatitis syndromes (Chapter 13). Children with chronic liver disease have an increased frequency of severe infections, which may be due in part to defective neutrophil motility[140] and decreased levels of complement.[141]

Cirrhosis

Patients with cirrhosis and ascites are at particular risk for spontaneous bacterial peritonitis (SBP). In this setting, SBP can be defined as ascitic fluid with 250 neutrophils/mcL or more, and a positive culture.[142] Fever and abdominal pain occur in approximately two-thirds of patients. Gram-negative enteric bacteria (such as *E. coli* and *Klebsiella pneumoniae*) are most frequently implicated, but gram-positive cocci (especially *S. pneumoniae*) are a relatively common cause in children.[141]

Cefotaxime has been shown to be superior to the combination of ampicillin and tobramycin;[143] it is usually used empirically until culture results are available. Duration of therapy depends on presence of bacteremia and initial response, but is usually 7–14 days. Culture-negative SBP in patients with 250 neutrophils/mcL or more, should be treated the same as culture-positive cases. Patients with fewer than 250 neutrophils/mcL but with growth of a single organism are treated if they have symptoms consistent with SBP.[142] Patients with polymicrobial infection should undergo abdominal CT (computed tomography) and surgical evaluation for the possibility of an intraabdominal source of infection.

Patients with cirrhosis and acute gastrointestinal bleeding are at increased risk for bacterial infections, probably because shock increases bacterial translocation. Norfloxacin given orally for 7 days significantly decreases the risk of infection in adult cirrhotics with a gastrointestinal bleed.[144] It is also effective for adults with a chronically increased risk of SBP (such as those with ascitic fluid protein levels less than 1 g/dL).[145] However, the long-term use of norfloxacin selects for colonization with quinolone-resistant organisms (such as enterococci), which may be a limitation of this strategy.[146] Regimens using ciprofloxacin or TMP-SMX are likely to result in a similar trade-off.[147,148]

Prolonged Total Parenteral Nutrition (TPN)

Children with short bowel syndrome and certain other disorders require prolonged nutritional therapy via the intravenous route for survival. As a result of bacterial translocation across the intestinal wall,[149] such patients are at particularly high risk for bacteremia. In one study, children with short gut syndrome experienced catheter-related infections 6 times more frequently than children without short gut syndrome.[149] Whereas skin flora are the predominant organisms causing catheter-related infections in other populations, enteric organisms are responsible for about two-thirds of infections in children with short bowel syndrome.[149] Yeasts are also relatively more common. The approach to prevention and treatment of catheter-related infections in this population is similar to that of other patients (Chapter 10).[150]

Malnutrition

Malnutrition with resultant immune deficiency and infection is the leading cause of infant and childhood death worldwide.[151] Those infectious diseases that are more frequent or more severe in the malnourished include measles, malaria, tuberculosis, infectious diarrhea, pneumonia, and HIV infection.

The interplay between malnutrition and infection is complex—infection predisposes to malnutrition and malnutrition predisposes to infection.[152] Profound immune deficiency, particularly reduced T-cell function, is found in children with both forms of protein-energy malnutrition (marasmus and kwashiorkor).[153] In addition, increasing evidence points to the independent effect of micronutrient deficiencies in the risk of infection in the developing world.[154,155] In general, the immune deficiency is related to the duration and degree of malnutrition and is reversible with adequate nutrition.

Hepatic Portoenterostomy

Children with biliary atresia are at risk for cholangitis even after a corrective portoenterostomy (Kasai procedure).[156] In one series of 75 children with fever after hepatic portoenterostomy, cholangitis was the most common cause of fever in the first 3 months, and pneumonia was a more common cause thereafter.[157] However, late cases of cholangitis are not uncommon.[158] Children with fever after portoenterostomy should have blood cultures obtained and should receive empiric therapy to cover *S. pneumoniae*, enteric organisms, and *Pseudomonas aeruginosa*. Cefepime or piperacillin are reasonable choices. An aminoglycoside is added if the patient is ill-appearing.

■ NEOPLASTIC DISEASE

It is useful to distinguish between the infections that complicate hematologic malignancies such as leukemia, lymphoma, and Hodgkin's disease, and those complicating nonhematologic malignancies such as neuroblastoma and Wilms' tumor. Infection is the cause of death in about 10–30% of children dying with nonhematologic neoplasms.[159] Many of the principles involving infections of leukemia and other hematologic malignancies are applicable to aplastic anemia, transplantation, and nonhematologic malignancies. Leukemia is the prototype example in terms of frequency and number of problems.

Mechanisms

Leukemia usually is associated with an acquired immunodeficiency secondary to chemotherapy and to prevention of proliferation of normal cells by malignant cells. Corticosteroid therapy acts by inhibiting the inflammatory process and by altering lympho-cyte function. Anticancer drugs cause marrow suppression as well as diminution of antibody-mediated and cell-mediated immunity. They also cause ulcerations of mucosal surfaces, which allow invasion by colonizing flora.

Neutropenia

Neutropenia, defined as an absolute neutrophil count (ANC) less than 500 per mm^3, is the most important risk factor for development of infection in the child on chemotherapy. The likelihood of infection is directly related to both the severity and the duration of the neutropenia. In the absence of empiric antibiotic therapy, virtually 100% of children with prolonged (more than 3 weeks), severe (ANC less than 100 per mm^3) neutropenia will develop an invasive bacterial infection.[160] Even with empiric therapy, the incidence of infection in this subgroup of patients is quite high. Because of the low leukocyte count, the classic signs of inflammation (swelling, redness, and warmth) may be absent. Pain is often preserved and should not be lightly dismissed. Similarly, symptoms of respiratory infection (tachypnea, hypoxia) may precede the appearance of an infiltrate on chest x-ray.

The neutropenic patient is at risk for infections with various infectious agents that may involve multiple different organ systems. These will be discussed under the categories of prophylaxis, management when fever occurs, and diagnosis and management of focal infections. Fever associated with intravascular devices is common and is discussed in Chapter 10.

Prophylaxis

Some specific infections can be prevented in neutropenic patients during induction chemotherapy using relatively nontoxic antimicrobial agents. Although it also reduces the frequency of fever and bacterial infections,[161] the main use of prophylactic TMP-SMX is to prevent PCP.[162] Patients with leukemia, lymphoma, or Hodgkin's disease should receive PCP prophylaxis for the duration of their chemotherapy. Because of its superior efficacy, TMP-SMX should be used unless the patient is allergic to sulfa medications. The dose is usually 5 mg/kg per day of the trimethoprim component in two divided doses, 3 days per week. Second-line agents, all of which are less effective than TMP-SMX, include dapsone, atovaquone, and aerosolized pentamidine. Most children with solid tumors undergoing routine cyclic chemotherapy do not require PCP prophylaxis. However, patients with brain tumors receiving corticosteroids are at risk for PCP and should receive prophylaxis.[163]

The use of broader spectrum antibiotics to prevent infections in afebrile neutropenic patients is controversial. Fluoroquinolones are sometimes used for this purpose in adults. Although they decrease the incidence of gram-negative infections, they do not alter infection-related morbidity or overall mortality.[164] Because of the risk of emergence of resistant isolates, this practice is generally discouraged.[165]

Similarly, routine prophylactic use of antifungal agents is not warranted, but may be considered in certain circumstances. An example may be the child receiving intensive induction chemotherapy for acute myelocytic leukemia who is expected to be profoundly neutropenic for 6 or more weeks.[166]

There is usually no indication for the empirical use of antiviral drugs in the treatment of febrile neutropenic patients without evidence of viral disease.[167]

Colony stimulating factors (G-CSF and GM-CSF) have been shown to shorten the duration of neutropenia, but their effect on decreasing morbidity is modest.[168] Although they may be considered in certain circumstances, current guidelines from the American Society of Clinical Oncology do not recommend their routine use.[169]

Fever

Fever in this setting can be defined as a single oral temperature of 38.3°C or more, or a temperature of 38.0°C for more than 1 hour.[167] Fever in the neutropenic patient should be considered a medical emergency, as up to half of these patients may have invasive bacterial infection as the cause of their fever, and it is difficult to discriminate those with bacterial infection from those without. A set of clinical and laboratory findings independently predictive of a high risk of bacterial infection has been constructed[170] and prospectively validated.[171] Five predictors of high risk were identified (listed in order of significance): (i) C-reactive protein greater than 9.0 mg/dL, (ii) hypotension, (iii) relapse of leukemia as the cancer type, (iv) platelet count greater than 50,000/dL, and receipt of chemotherapy within 7 days of the febrile episode.[170] While the presence of one or more of these factors por-

tends a higher risk of bacterial infection, their absence, unfortunately, cannot rule out serious infection.

For all patients with neutropenic fever, a history should be obtained and a physical examination performed. Two blood cultures should be collected, and intravenous antibiotic therapy should be started promptly. This requires verbal communication between the physician, pharmacist, and nurse. Single-drug therapy with an antipseudomonal cephalosporin is usually appropriate. Cefepime is favored over ceftazidime because of its superior coverage of viridans streptococci and pneumococci. Cefepime is also more likely to retain activity against organisms that possess extended spectrum beta-lactamases or type 1 inducible beta-lactamases.

The addition of vancomycin should be considered in the following situations: (a) clinically suspected catheter-related infections, (b) known colonization with penicillin-resistant pneumococci or methicillin-resistant *S. aureus*, and (c) hypotension.[167] Vancomycin is also frequently given empirically in centers with a high incidence of cephalosporin-resistant viridans streptococci. If vancomycin is started, it should be discontinued if the cultures are negative at 48 hours. In the septic-appearing patient, an aminoglycoside is added to the two-drug regimen above. An agent active against gram-negative organisms should be continued for the duration of the neutropenia, even if the cultures remain negative.[172] In some centers, children with negative cultures at low risk for serious infection are switched to an oral antibiotic such as cefixime.[173] In adults, a fluoroquinolone plus amoxicillin-clavulanate is sometimes used. This practice should usually be reserved for patients who defervesce promptly or who have low-grade fever, who appear well clinically, and whose expected duration of neutropenia is short (less than 10 days).

For patients who remain febrile for 5–7 days after initiation of a course of broad-spectrum antibiotics, empiric antifungal therapy with amphotericin B is indicated.[167] Alternatively, one of the lipid formulations of amphotericin B can be used.[174] These drugs are substantially less nephrotoxic. However, their effectiveness is similar to that of conventional amphotericin, and they are significantly more expensive. Voriconazole is a new triazole with activity against *Aspergillus* spp. that may have a role in the empiric treatment of persistently febrile and neutropenic patients.[175] Unlike amphotericin, which must be given intravenously, it is also available in an oral form. One disadvantage of voriconazole is a high incidence of transient visual side-effects. Hepatotoxicity also occurs.[176]

Focal Infections

Pneumonia

The lungs are a common site of focal infection in the child with cancer.[177,178] Noninfectious causes of pulmonary infiltrates must also be kept in mind.[179] These include pulmonary edema or hemorrhage, leukemic or lymphomatous infiltrates, metastases (e.g., osteogenic sarcoma), radiation pneumonitis, drug toxicity (e.g., methotrexate), atelectasis, and adult respiratory distress syndrome.

The likely causes and diagnostic approach depend on the radiographic pattern. Focal pneumonias are more likely to be bacterial or fungal but can be caused by viruses or *Pneumocystis*.[178] Diffuse interstitial infiltrates are most commonly caused by viral infections, *Pneumocystis*, or atypical bacteria. Single or multiple nodular infiltrates are worrisome for fungal infection (especially *Aspergillus*) or *Nocardia*. The nodules may only be detected by chest CT.

Tuberculosis is a difficult diagnostic problem, because patients are often anergic, with a negative tuberculin test. A careful exposure history is critical. The endemic mycoses (cryptococcosis, blastomycosis, histoplasmosis, and coccidioidomycosis) are occasional causes of pneumonia in leukemia.[180,181] *Legionella* is a rare cause of focal pneumonia.[182] Dermatophytes occasionally cause disseminated diseases in these children.[183]

Blood cultures are obtained and antibacterial therapy is begun empirically. Depending on disease severity, tempo of progression, and response to initial therapy, invasive diagnostic procedures may be indicated. The risk of such procedures should be viewed in light of the potential value of the result. In general, an attempt to make an etiologic diagnosis is important, because the list of possible causes is long. Bronchoalveolar lavage (BAL) is often useful in diagnosing the cause of diffuse infiltrates, such as PCP or viruses. The diagnostic yield is much lower for focal infiltrates.[179] Unfortunately, transbronchial biopsy is relatively insensitive in detecting fungal infection, and open lung biopsy may be required.[184] With any of these procedures, communication with the microbiology laboratory is essential to ensure that appropriate studies are done for common and opportunistic pathogens.[185]

Pneumocystis jiroveci (carinii) Pneumonia (PCP)

This is rare when TMP-SMX is used prophylactically but the possibility should still be considered. Subacute onset of fever, marked tachypnea, hypoxia, and bilateral diffuse alveolar or interstitial densities are characteristically found, but virtually any radiologic pattern can occur. Hypoxemia is secondary to an alveolar-capillary diffusion block. Symptoms often begin at the time that corticosteroids are being tapered.[163] The diagnosis is best confirmed by observing the organism in specially stained smears obtained from tracheal aspirates, BAL, or open lung biopsy. The treatment of choice is TMP-SMX 15–20 mg/kg day divided every 6 to 8 hours for 2–3 weeks, initially given intravenously. Children with severe hypoxemia (PaO2 less than 70 mm Hg) are given methylprednisolone 2 mg/kg day initially and then tapering doses.[186]

Skin Infections

Skin infections can be caused by viral, bacterial, or fungal pathogens and may represent local infection or a manifestation of systemic disease. In addition, skin lesions may be from a noninfectious source, such as leukemic infiltrate or one of the neutrophilic dermatoses (pyoderma gangrenosum or Sweet syndrome).[187] Ecthyma gangrenosum is characterized by one or more tender subcutaneous nodules with central necrosis. It is classically caused by systemic infection with *P. aeruginosa* but can also be caused by multiple other agents, including gram-negative enteric organisms, *Aeromonas*, *Stenotrophomonas*, *S. aureus*, Group A streptococcus, herpes simplex virus, *Candida*, *Aspergillus*, *Fusarium*, and the agents of mucormycosis.[188–201] Patients with fever, neutropenia, and a focal skin lesion should undergo skin biopsy, which results in a specific diagnosis in approximately 50% of cases.[202]

Gastrointestinal Tract Infections

Infections involving the gastrointestinal tract are common in neutropenic patients, as the chemotherapy can cause mucosal damage at any point from the mouth to the anus. Oral mucositis predisposes the patient to bacteremia with oral flora, including viridans streptococci and anaerobes. Thus, empiric antibiotics in the patient with fever, neutropenia, and severe mucositis should include an agent with anaerobic activity. This can be accomplished by adding metronidazole to the regimen or by using piperacillin/tazobactam or ticarcillin/clavulanate instead of ceftazidime or cefepime.

Esophagitis is most commonly caused by *Candida*, but HSV and CMV are other possible causes. Definitive diagnosis requires esophagoscopy with biopsy and culture. Patients are usually treated empirically with fluconazole and endoscopy reserved for those who fail to respond clinically.

Diarrhea is common in children undergoing chemotherapy and often no cause is found. The most common infectious cause is antibiotic-associated colitis due to *Clostridium difficile*.[203] Occasionally, typical enteric bacteria, viruses, or parasites are implicated (Chapter 12).[204]

Neutropenic enterocolitis (also referred to as typhlitis) is a life-threatening complication of chemotherapy (especially Ara-C) in patients with hematologic or solid tumors. It is characterized by necrotizing inflammation of the cecum and ascending colon.[205] Patients usually present with fever, diarrhea (often bloody), and severe abdominal pain, which may be diffuse or localized (usually right lower quadrant). Diagnosis is usually confirmed by the finding of cecal wall thickening on ultrasound or CT. Blood cultures are positive in a little less than 50% of patients.[205] Management includes bowel rest, nasogastric suction, and broad spectrum antibiotics, including coverage for gut anaerobes and enterococci.[205,206] Serial plain films are done to look for evidence of bowel perforation. Most cases are managed medically, but perforation, obstruction, massive hemorrhage, and abscess formation are indications for surgery.[206] The mortality rate is approximately 20%.[205]

Disseminated *Candida* infections often involve the liver and spleen and are commonly referred to as hepatosplenic candidiasis (HSC). The typical presentation is that of unexplained fever that persists once the neutropenia resolves. Abdominal pain and hepatosplenomegaly are variable. Early on, laboratory and imaging studies are normal, but over several days the alkaline phosphatase level becomes elevated and multiple low attenuation lesions are visible by CT. MRI (magnetic resonance imaging) is slightly more sensitive, and ultrasound less sensitive than CT in detecting the lesions.[207] The lesions are not specific for *Candida*, and biopsy may be indicated to establish the diagnosis. Initial treatment is with amphotericin B (or a lipid formulation) for 1–2 weeks. Oral fluconazole is then given until calcification or resolution of lesions (usually 3–4 months).[208,209] Chemotherapy need not be withheld during therapy for HSC.[210]

Ear and Sinus Infections

Otitis media is a common infection in children with and without malignancy. The typical organisms are implicated, but resistance may be more common in the child on chemotherapy because of frequent antibiotic use. Occasionally, *Pseudomonas* or other gram-negative organisms are the cause. Sinus infections are also common in children with malignancy. Fever and face pain are the usual presenting features, sometimes accompanied by subtle erythema or swelling over the paranasal sinuses. Nasopharyngeal cultures do not predict the cause of the sinus infection.[211] Sinus CT is done to document infection and look for evidence of bony destruction. Broad-spectrum coverage (including anaerobes) is indicated. If there is no clinical response after 48 hours of therapy, a surgeon should be consulted and biopsies performed to rule out the possibility of fungal sinusitis.[211] In the neutropenic patient, fungal infection of the sinuses requires aggressive medical and surgical management to prevent extension to the brain.

■ HEMATOPOIETIC STEM CELL TRANSPLANT (HSCT)

The term HSCT encompasses bone marrow transplant (BMT) as well as transplantation of peripheral blood stem cells and umbilical cord blood stem cells. HSCT is increasingly being used to treat a variety of malignancies as well as certain nonmalignant hematologic, immunologic, and metabolic conditions.[212] Most of the concepts discussed in the previous section on infections in children with neoplastic disease are directly applicable to HSCT recipients. However, certain infections are more common and/or more severe in HSCT recipients and, in general, more aggressive strategies for prophylaxis are indicated. This is particularly true for allogeneic HSCT recipients. Patients undergoing autologous transplants are at a somewhat lower risk for infections. The type of allogeneic transplant also affects the risk of infection. Patients undergoing HLA (histocompatibility locus antigen)-matched sibling transplant are at lower risk than those undergoing a matched unrelated donor transplant. Patients receiving a T-cell depleted graft from a partially matched donor are at highest risk.[213] Comprehensive guidelines for preventing infections in HSCT recipients have been developed and should be consulted for details.[214]

Pretransplant Evaluation

A detailed history of past infections, unusual exposures, and allergies should be taken, and a thorough physical examination performed. In addition to a tuberculin skin test, the following serologic testing is performed on both the HSCT candidate and the donor: herpes group viruses (CMV, EBV, HSV, VZV[varicella zoster virus]), hepatitis viruses (A, B, and C), HIV, HTLV (human T-cell lymphotropic virus), and syphilis serology. Other serologic testing (such as for endemic mycoses or toxoplasmosis) varies by center. In addition, some centers perform surveillance cultures on HSCT candidates from various sites (e.g., nasopharynx and rectum) for bacteria, viruses, and fungi. Obtaining a baseline chest x-ray on the HSCT candidate is appropriate.

Mechanisms and Timing

After the conditioning regimen and until marrow engraftment occurs (usually by 3–4 weeks), the HSCT recipient is profoundly neutropenic. Bacterial and fungal infections are most common during the first month posttransplant, as is infection with herpes simplex virus. Fever and neutropenia is nearly universal during the first month posttransplant, necessitating the use of broad-spectrum antibiotics and placing the patient at risk for *C. difficile* colitis. The most common cause of diarrhea, however, is acute graft-versus-host disease (GVHD).[215]

HSCT recipients have profound cell-mediated and humoral immunodeficiencies as well. This is particularly true if the patient has received a graft that has been depleted of T-cells. Immunosuppressants (such as prednisone and cyclosporine) used to prevent GVHD further impair the cell-mediated immune system. Thus, infections occurring during the first 3 months postengraftment are often caused by viruses, such as CMV, or by *Pneumocystis jiroveci*. Some HSCT recipients (particularly those with chronic GVHD or delayed T-cell engraftment) continue to be at high risk for infection even during the late posttransplantation period (more than 100 days posttransplant). Infection due to VZV and encapsulated bacteria predominate during this period.[216]

Although a myriad of organisms may cause in-fection in the HSCT recipient, those that are particularly important and can be targeted for prevention will be highlighted here.

Bacterial Infections

In general, the approach is similar to that discussed in the section on patients with cancer. One possible exception is that some experts recommend against the use of monotherapy in the transplant recipient with fever and neutropenia.[217] An antipseudomonal cephalosporin plus vancomycin is appropriate in this setting. Routine use of prophylactic antibiotics in the absence of fever is not generally recommended,[214] but many centers employ them nonetheless. The use of IVIG should probably be limited to those patients with documented hypogammaglobulinemia.

Fungal Infections

The most common fungi causing infections in HSCT recipients are *Candida* spp. and *Aspergillus* spp. Syndromes associated with *Candida* infection include thrush, esophagitis, fungemia, and disseminated infection (especially hepatosplenic candidiasis). The incidence of each of these manifestations has been dramatically reduced by the routine use of fluconazole prophylaxis from the time of conditioning until engraftment (sometimes longer).[218] Although this has been associated with an increase in infections with *C. krusei* and *C. glabrata* (which are frequently resistant to fluconazole) in some centers,[219] it has not been a significant problem in most centers.

Fluconazole does not have activity against *Aspergillus* spp. (or other filamentous fungi) and these have become the most common cause of fungal infection in HSCT patients in some centers.[220] Patients who receive matched unrelated donor marrow or undergo unrelated cord blood transplantation are at higher risk than those who have autologous or matched sibling transplants. Patients with severe GVHD are eight-fold more likely to develop aspergillosis.[221] The most common clinical syndromes associated with *Aspergillus* infection are focal pneumonia, sinusitis, and CNS disease. Positive blood cultures are rare. Patients with proven or suspected pulmonary aspergillosis should have a head CT scan performed to rule out CNS involvement. The treatment for aspergillosis is conventional amphotericin B or a lipid formulation, often using higher than usual doses. The role of caspofungin in pediatric patients with invasive aspergillosis is still undefined. Variconazole is promising in this setting. Surgical drainage of sinus infection and resection of localized lung disease are generally advised. Despite therapy, the mortality for invasive aspergillosis remains high. This has led some centers to attempt to prevent infection in the highest risk settings (e.g., allogeneic matched unrelated donor or T-cell depleted grafts). Aerosolized amphotericin B has been instilled into the airways,[222] but there are no studies with comparison controls. Other approaches include the use of low-dose or alternate-day amphotericin B (conventional or lipid formulation) given intravenously,[223] but data with concurrent controls are lacking. A randomized trial of voriconazole prophylaxis in prophylaxis is ongoing.

Pneumocystis jiroveci Pneumonia (PCP)

As in patients with hematologic malignancies, PCP is an important and readily preventable infection in the HSCT recipient. TMP-SMX should be used for prophylaxis from the time of engraftment until at least 6 months posttransplant (and longer if there is GVHD or lymphopenia).[214] Other regimens are inferior, particularly aerosolized pentamidine.[224] Marrow suppression with TMP-SMX is uncommon when used on a three-times-a-week schedule.

Community-acquired Viruses

Children undergoing HSCT are at particular risk for severe disease caused by common respiratory viruses. Of 281 stem cell transplants performed at St. Jude Children's Research Hospital over a 4-year period, 32 (11%) were complicated by respiratory virus infection within the first year posttransplant.[225] The most commonly implicated virus was parainfluenza virus (PIV), followed by adenovirus, influenza, and RSV. Risk factors for infection were allogeneic transplant and severe GVHD. If lower respiratory tract disease develops, the mortality is high; thus, prevention is paramount. Patients should be cared for in positive-pressure isolation rooms. Patients, their families, and all care-providers should receive influenza vaccination. Viral cultures should be performed in patients at the first sign of respiratory symptoms. Some centers use monthly prophylaxis with RSV-Ig (Respigam) during the RSV season. Although published data are lacking, this is a reasonable approach. The use of

humanized monoclonal antibody to RSV (palivizumab) can also be used but, unlike RSV-Ig, it does not offer protection against other respiratory viruses, such as parainfluenza virus.

Early detection and prompt treatment of infections is likely to lead to improved outcome compared with attempting treatment once lower respiratory tract disease is apparent. In a compassionate use study of pediatric HSCT recipients with RSV infection, early treatment with a combination of aerosolized ribavirin and high-dose RSV-Ig resulted in improved outcome compared with historical controls.[226] Ribavirin has activity against PIV,[227] and RSV-Ig contains neutralizing antibodies to PIV-3,[228] so this regimen is reasonable for HSCT recipients with parainfluenza virus infection as well.

In addition to respiratory tract disease, adenovirus causes hemorrhagic cystitis, hepatitis, and gastroenteritis in the HSCT recipient.[229] Cidofovir, a nucleoside analogue of cytosine has *in vitro* activity against adenovirus. Although comparative trials are lacking, anecdotal reports suggest that this agent is effective against adenovirus in the setting of HSCT.[230–232] Nephrotoxicity is seen commonly at the usual dose (5 mg/kg per week) and can be lessened by the concomitant use of probenecid. In our experience, lower doses of 1–3 mg/kg per week are still effective but much less nephrotoxic.

As with the other viruses mentioned above, illness caused by influenza can be fatal in this population.[225] Prior to transplant, HSCT candidates and their household contacts should receive the influenza vaccine. HSCT recipients are unlikely to make an antibody response in the first 6 months after transplant, and vaccination is not recommended during this period.[233] If a community outbreak of influenza occurs during this period and the patient is not in isolation, prophylaxis with rimantadine (influenza A) or oseltamivir (influenza A or B) should be considered. These agents should also be used for treatment of documented infection in this population as discussed in Chapter 7.

Cytomegalovirus (CMV)

It is useful to distinguish between CMV infection (detection of the virus, viral proteins, or nucleic acid) and CMV disease (symptoms referable to a particular organ along with detection of the virus in tissue samples).[234] Prior to the routine use of CMV prophylaxis or monitoring, CMV was a common cause of pneumonia in HSCT recipients and was frequently fatal. CMV pneumonia presents in a nonspecific manner with fever, cough, hypoxemia, and diffuse interstitial infiltrates on chest x-ray. Treatment is with ganciclovir, but prevention is greatly preferred. CMV can also cause disease of the gastrointestinal tract; esophagitis and colitis are common syndromes and require biopsy for definitive diagnosis.

Among HSCT recipients, those at highest risk for infection (and disease) are those who are CMV seropositive prior to transplant. CMV seronegative recipients of marrow from a CMV-positive donor are at intermediate risk. If both recipient and donor are CMV negative, the risk is negligible as long as CMV negative (or leukocyte-filtered) blood products are used.[235] For patients at risk for CMV disease (i.e., seropositive donor or recipient), one of two strategies should be employed: prophylaxis or preemptive therapy.

Prophylaxis involves administering ganciclovir intravenously (or valganciclovir orally) during the high-risk time period for CMV infection (engraftment until approximately 100 days posttransplant). This strategy is highly effective, but is limited by ganciclovir-induced neutropenia, which occurs in about one-third of patients.[236] In addition, late-onset CMV disease may occur after prophylaxis has been discontinued.[237] Some centers use CMV-Ig in addition to ganciclovir prophylaxis, but the effect of this combination compared with ganciclovir alone has not been studied. Prophylaxis is probably the best option for the highest risk patients, such as those receiving T-cell depleted stem cells.[238]

Preemptive therapy involves screening the blood of at-risk patients weekly for the presence of CMV by pp65 antigen detection or PCR.[214] Patients testing positive are then given ganciclovir until the test is negative and for a minimum of 3 weeks (some centers continue therapy till 100 days posttransplant). If screening tests are available, this approach is preferred for patients at lower risk for CMV disease, such as autologous HSCT recipients. Patients at high risk for late CMV disease (such those with GVHD or chronically low CD4 counts) should probably continue to be monitored even after day 100.

Varicella-zoster virus (VZV)

Primary varicella (chickenpox) and to a lesser extent reactivation of latent varicella (zoster) are potentially fatal complications in HSCT recipients.[239,240] With primary varicella, skin lesions are numerous, severe and may be hemorrhagic. In addition, about half of patients will develop organ involvement, especially pneumonitis and hepatitis. Zoster in HSCT recipients is usually dermatomal but can cause disseminated infection.[241] Prompt recognition of VZV infection and institution of intravenous acyclovir (at a dose of 1,500 mg/m^2 per day divided every 8 hours) dramatically reduces the mortality and morbidity of these infections in the ICH.[242,243] Patients are treated for 10–14 days and until all lesions are crusted over. Although not well studied, oral valacyclovir can probably be used once the patient has had a clinical response. HSCT recipients who are seronegative for VZV should receive VZIG within 96 hours of exposure to a person with varicella. They should be observed closely for the development of skin lesions as the efficacy of VZIG in this population is relatively low.[242] All household and other close contacts of HSCT recipients who do not have a history of chickenpox should receive the varicella vaccine.[214]

Herpes Simplex Virus (HSV)

HSV infection is usually caused by reactivation of latent virus in a seropositive HSCT recipient. In the absence of prophylaxis, 75% of HSV seropositive patients (and up to 15% of seronegative patients) will develop symptomatic HSV disease, usually 2–3 weeks after transplant.[244–246] The most common presentation is severe ulcerative mucositis, which may be difficult to distinguish from that caused by the conditioning regimen. Thus, oral lesions should generally be tested for HSV by culture or PCR. Esophagitis, pneumonitis, hepatitis, and disseminated disease can also occur. All HSCT recipients who are HSV seropositive should receive acyclovir prophylaxis,[214] which decreases the incidence of infection to less than 5%.[247] Some centers provide prophylaxis for HSV-seronegative recipients as well. The schedule varies among centers, but a reasonable approach is to begin intravenous acyclovir during the conditioning regimen, continue it until the time of engraftment, and then switch to oral acyclovir until 6 months posttransplant.[247] Valacyclovir has been associated with the development of thrombotic thrombocytopenic purpura in HSCT recipients and should be used with caution in this population.[248] Patients receiving ganciclovir or valganciclovir for CMV prophylaxis need not receive acyclovir.

Epstein-Barr Virus (EBV)

In contrast to the situation in solid organ transplant recipients, EBV-induced posttransplant lymphoproliferative disorder (PTLD) is relatively uncommon among HSCT recipients. The incidence is highest in those receiving an allogeneic HLA-mismatched transplant from an EBV seropositive donor, especially if the graft is T-cell depleted.[249] In one study of 18 children with PTLD after bone marrow transplant, the median onset of symptoms was 137 days (range, 48–617 days) posttransplant.[250] Fever and adenopathy are the usual initial manifestations, but multiple organs may be affected. Uncommonly, symptoms may mimic GVHD.[251] The disease is the result of uncontrolled proliferation of EBV-infected and transformed B cells, which in the normal host are kept in check by the T-cell immune response. Definitive diagnosis requires biopsy of affected tissue with histologic confirmation. Treatment consists of decreasing immunosuppression, if possible. No antiviral agent has demonstrated efficacy. In HSCT recipients with PTLD, the EBV-infected B cells are of donor origin.

Thus, a promising approach to treatment and prevention in this group of patients involves the infusion of EBV-specific cytotoxic T lymphocytes prepared from donor leukocytes.[252]

Immunization of the HSCT Recipient

Most HSCT recipients lose immunity to vaccine preventable diseases after transplantation.[253] Thus, it is appropriate to revaccinate them after their transplant. However, they do not respond to immunization in the immediate posttransplant period; thus, immunizations are generally deferred until 12 months posttransplant (Table 22-4).[214] Although not studied in this population, the use of conjugated pneumococcal vaccine at 12 months followed by boosting with polysaccharide pneumococcal vaccine at 24 months may provide a better antibody response.[21] Although varicella vaccine is contraindicated in the HSCT recipient, vaccination of household and other close contacts is important to decrease the patient's risk of exposure to wild-type virus.

TABLE 22-4. RECOMMENDED VACCINATIONS FOR HSCT RECIPIENTS[a]

VACCINE	TIME AFTER HSCT		
	12 MONTHS	14 MONTHS	24 MONTHS
Inactivated vaccine			
Diphtheria, tetanus, pertussis			
<7 years	DTaP	DTaP	DTaP
≥7 years	Td	Td	Td
Hib conjugate	Hib conjugate	Hib conjugate	Hib conjugate
Hepatitis B (HBV)	HBV	HBV	HBV
PPV23	PPV23	–	PPV23
Hepatitis A (HAV)	Not routinely indicated		
Influenza	Lifelong, seasonal administration, beginning before HSCT and resuming ≥6 months after HSCT		
Meningococcal	Not routinely indicated; administer if functionally asplenic		
Inactivated polio (IPV)	IPV	IPV	IPV
Live-attenuated vaccines			
Measles, mumps, rubella	–	–	MMR[a]
Varicella	Not recommended for HSCT patients until further data available		

Abbreviations: HSCT, hematopoietic stem cell transplant; GVHD, graft-versus-host disease; Hib, *Haemophilus influenzae* type b; PPV23, 23-valent pneumococcal polysaccharide vaccine.
[a] Administer only if HSCT recipient is not on immunosuppressive therapy and does not have GVHD.
Source: Adapted from: Preventing pneumococcal disease among infants and young children. Recommendations of the Advisory Committee on Immunization Practices (ACIP). MMWR Recomm Rep 2000;49:1–35, with permission.

■ SOLID ORGAN TRANSPLANT (SOT)

Like the HSCT recipient, SOT recipients are at increased risk for a variety of common and opportunistic infections. However, many of the issues relating to infectious risk are quite different between the two groups. Unlike HSCT recipients, SOT recipients are not usually immunocompromised prior to the transplant, they do not undergo a conditioning regimen that makes them profoundly neutropenic, they do not generally require a long-term central venous catheter, and they are not at risk for GVHD. On the other hand, the induction regimen at the time of transplant induces profound impairment of the cellular immune system, and they must remain on a combination of immunosuppressive agents for life to prevent rejection of the allograft. Thus, from an infectious disease standpoint, recipients of various solid organs have more in common with each other than with HSCT recipients.

There are several infection-related aspects of SOT that vary based on the particular organ being transplanted. Some donor organs are more likely to carry (and transmit) a particular pathogen than others (Table 22-5). In general, for these organisms, the highest risk situation is when the donor is seropositive and the recipient is seronegative prior to transplant. Many of the infections in the immediate posttransplant period are unique to the anatomic area of the grafted organ (Table 22-5).

The following solid organ transplants will be discussed in this section: kidney, liver, intestine, heart, and lung. Sometimes, more than one organ is transplanted simultaneously (e.g., heart-lung or liver-intestine), but for simplicity we will consider only single-organ transplants. Pancreas transplantation is uncommon in children and will not be discussed.[254]

Pretransplant Evaluation

This evaluation generally consists of a detailed exposure history, an assessment of remote and recent infections, a review of the vaccination history and drug allergies, and a physical examination.[257] A tuberculin skin test is performed on all SOT candidates and donors. Serologic testing for the following organisms is performed on both donor and recipient: herpes group viruses (CMV, EBV, HSV, VZV), hepatitis viruses (HAV, HBV, HCV), HIV, HTLV, syphilis, and measles. For heart transplants, toxoplasma serology should be obtained as well. For patients from the southwestern United States, serology for *Coccidioides immitis* is obtained. A sputum culture should be obtained in the lung transplant candidate. Immunizations should be given to bring the child up to date. This includes live-attenuated vaccines, unless there are other contraindications to their use (e.g., the patient is receiving more than 2mg/kg per day of prednisone). Live vaccines should be given at least 2 weeks (and preferably 4 weeks) prior to the date of transplant.

Timing of Infections

The timetable of infections after SOT is organized into 3 segments: the first month, 1–6 months, and

TABLE 22-5. COMMON INFECTIONS IN SOLID ORGAN TRANSPLANTS BASED ON ORGAN TRANSPLANTED[a]

ORGAN	INFECTIONS TRANSMITTED BY THE DONOR ORGAN	INFECTIONS SPECIFIC TO THE ANATOMIC AREA
Kidney	CMV, EBV, BK virus[255]	Urinary tract infection, especially pyelonephritis (GPC, GNB, *Candida*)
Liver	CMV, EBV	Intraabdominal abscess, cholangitis (GNB, enterococcis, *Candida*, *Aspergillus*)
Intestine	CMV, EBV	Bacteremia (gut flora), intraabdominal abscess (GNB, enterococcis, *Candida*)
Heart	CMV, EBV, toxoplasmosis[256]	Mediastinitis (*S. aureus*)
Lung	CMV, EBV	Mediastinitis, pneumonia, lung abscess (*S. aureus*, GNB, *Aspergillus*)

Abbreviations: GPC, gram positive cocci; GNB, gram negative bacilli; CMV, cytomegalovirus; EBV, Epstein-Barr virus.
[a] Bacteremia and wound infections are relatively common in all patients posttransplant.

more than 6 months after transplantation.[258] During the first month posttransplant, most infections are nosocomially acquired or related to surgical complications. These include bacterial and candidal bloodstream and wound infections, as well as organ-specific infections (Table 22-5). As in the HSCT recipient, HSV reactivation is also common during the first month. The second through the sixth month is when the patient is at greatest risk for opportunistic infections, such as CMV, PCP, and aspergillosis. After 6 months posttransplant, community-acquired infections and VZV reactivation are most common.

Prophylaxis for Bacterial And Fungal Pathogens

Intravenous perioperative antibiotics are indicated at the time of transplant and are usually given until 48–72 hours posttransplant. The exact regimen used depends on the type of transplant and the patient's history of recent infections. Kidney and heart transplant recipients often receive cefazolin. Liver and intestine transplant recipients commonly receive ampicillin and cefotaxime. Depending on sputum culture results, cefepime is reasonable coverage for the lung transplant recipient. TMP-SMX, which is used for PCP prophylaxis, has the added benefit of providing coverage against many common bacteria, as well as *Nocardia*.[259] It also provides effective prophylaxis against toxoplasmosis,[260] which is a concern in heart transplant recipients. The use of oral selective bowel decontamination prior to liver transplant is controversial; some studies have suggested a benefit,[261] whereas others have not.[262]

The issue of antifungal prophylaxis in the SOT recipient is complex. Many centers use an oral nonabsorbable agent such as nystatin; however, its efficacy is questionable.[263] Some centers give fluconazole for 4 weeks after transplant to prevent candidal infection. The literature regarding the efficacy of this approach is conflicting.[264,265] In addition, fluconazole does not have activity against *Aspergillus*, which is a particular concern among liver and lung transplant recipients. Itraconazole and voriconazole are options for orally administered agents, but, like fluconazole, they cause significant increases in cyclosporine and tacrolimus levels. Because the risk of fungal infections among liver transplant recipients is primarily in the first month posttransplant, it may be reasonable to give one of these agents (or

even amphotericin) during this period to selected high-risk patients.[263,266] The risk period for fungal infections among lung transplant recipients is longer, and many centers give itraconazole for at least 6 months posttransplant.[266]

Pneumocystis jiroveci Pneumonia (PCP)

PCP presents in a similar fashion to that in cancer patients described above. Low-dose, three times per week TMP-SMX is highly effective in preventing this potentially severe illness. Although the peak incidence is between 2 and 6 months posttransplant, as many as one-third of cases occur more than 1 year after transplant.[267] TMP-SMX should be started as soon after transplant as the patient is able to take oral medications. If tolerated, it should be continued indefinitely.[268]

Community-acquired Viruses

If acquired during a period of maximal immunosuppression (i.e., immediately posttransplant or during treatment for allograft rejection), these infections may be severe, as discussed above for the HSCT recipient, especially in young children.[269,270] Accordingly, for children less than 2 years old, it may be reasonable to use monthly RSV-Ig (or palivizumab) as prophylaxis during the first winter posttransplant.

Adenovirus infection is a particular concern. In one series, 49 (10%) of 484 pediatric liver transplant recipients developed adenovirus infection. The most common sites of involvement were the liver, lung, and gastrointestinal tract.[271] Anecdotal reports suggest benefit of low-dose cidofovir (1 mg/kg, 3 days per week).[272] Among pediatric heart transplant recipients, identification of adenoviral genome by PCR in myocardial biopsies is associated with significantly decreased graft survival.[273]

Cytomegalovirus (CMV)

Unlike the case of HSCT recipients, in which recipient serostatus is the best predictor of CMV disease, the SOT patient at highest risk for CMV disease is one who is CMV-seronegative and who receives an organ from a CMV-seropositive donor (D+/R-). The group with the next highest risk includes those in whom both donor and recipient are CMV-seropositive (D+/R+), followed by the group in which only the recipient is seropositive (D-/R+). Patients receiving anti T-cell antibodies to prevent rejection are at particularly increased risk for CMV disease, whether it is the donor or the recipient who is CMV seropositive.[274] In general, if both donor and recipient are seronegative, the risk of CMV disease is negligible.

Whether ganciclovir should be used prophylactically or preemptively with monitoring is controversial.[275] Prophylaxis is probably best for the highest risk patients (D+/R- or those receiving anti T-cell therapy for rejection). Other patients can be monitored weekly by pp65 antigen or PCR and treated only if the test becomes positive. Treatment is generally for 3 weeks and until the test is negative. The duration of prophylaxis varies between centers, but 3 months is typical. Oral valganciclovir is highly bioavailable and is an option for patients old enough to swallow pills.[276] A liquid formulation is being studied.

Varicella zoster virus (VZV)

VZV infection can be severe in SOT recipients.[277] The approach to prevention, postexposure prophylaxis, and treatment is similar to that discussed for the HSCT recipient above.

Herpes Simplex Virus (HSV)

HSV infection can be severe in the SOT recipient,[278] and acyclovir is safe and effective in preventing HSV disease.[279] If either the recipient or donor is HSV seropositive, acyclovir is generally given orally 5 mg/kg b.i.d. for the first 4–6 weeks posttransplant. It should also be considered in the patient being treated for an episode of acute allograft rejection, as we have seen severe HSV pneumonia in this circumstance. Acyclovir prophylaxis is unnecessary if the patient is already on ganciclovir.

Epstein-Barr Virus (EBV)

EBV-associated posttransplant lymphoproliferative disorder (PTLD) is a potentially fatal complication of SOT. It is a particularly frequent problem in children, who are more likely to be EBV seronegative prior to transplant. The risk of PTLD is approximately 20–25% in children who are EBV seronegative, and 5% in those who are seropositive prior to liver transplant.[280,281] Seronegative patients who receive an EBV-seropositive organ are at greatest risk in the first year after transplant. Seronegative patients who receive an EBV-seronegative organ may develop community-acquired infection at any time after transplant, sometimes many years later (with risk of late-onset PTLD). Other risk factors relate to the type, duration, and intensity of immunosuppressive agents used.[281]

EBV infection in transplant recipients may result in several different syndromes: (i) asymptomatic infection or nonspecific viral syndrome, (ii) classical infectious mononucleosis, and (iii) PTLD. PTLD can further be broken down into categories based on histology and genetic markers (polyclonal plasmacytic hyperplasia, monoclonal polymorphic PTLD, and malignant lymphoma).[282] These syndromes are a continuum, and benign manifestations may evolve into more serious syndromes.[283] Fever and adenopathy are common presenting symptoms, but multiple organs can be involved, including the allograft, gastrointestinal tract, liver, and brain. Tissue biopsy is necessary to establish the diagnosis of PTLD.[284] Early detection is critical, but unfortunately PCR testing for EBV has proven to be neither highly sensitive nor specific for PTLD. In our experience, there is no cutoff level that predicts the development of PTLD. The mainstay of therapy consists of decreasing immunosuppression.[283] Other therapies include anti-CD20 monoclonal antibodies and conventional chemotherapy. Antiviral agents (such as ganciclovir) and passive antibody (such as CMV-Ig) are often used but have not been proven beneficial in the prevention or treatment of PTLD. Cell-based therapy is more problematic in the setting of SOT because the infected B-lymphocytes are of recipient (not donor) origin, and because patients are usually EBV-seronegative prior to transplant. Thus, they do not possess EBV-specific cytotoxic T-lymphocytes that could be expanded *ex vivo*.[284]

Immunization of SOT Recipients

It is a paradox of modern medicine that as many as two-thirds of children have not received their full complement of immunizations at the time of transplantation.[285,286]

Live-attenuated Vaccines

Most SOT candidates are not immunocompromised prior to transplant and should receive both inactivated and live-attenuated vaccines. Ideally, live vaccines should be given at least 2 weeks prior to transplant.[287] Live vaccines are not generally administered posttransplant. Although some centers use them in certain patients after immunosuppression has been reduced,[288] larger studies of the safety of this approach are needed.

Inactivated Vaccines

If a child receives a transplant before the primary series is completed, immunizations should usually be resumed starting 6–12 months posttransplant (and at least 3 months after completing therapy for an episode of allograft rejection). An exception is influenza vaccine, which should be given to all SOT recipients older than 6 months and their household contacts as soon as it becomes available each fall. For most vaccine-preventable illnesses, serological correlates of immunity are not available. Thus, serologic testing to confirm immunity is generally not done, except for hepatitis A and B viruses, where it may be considered.[287] Although not well studied in this population, a reasonable approach to pneumococcal vaccination involves the sequential use of conjugated vaccine and polysaccharide vaccine, as outlined in Tables 22-2 and 22-3.

■ REFERENCES

1. Waldman JD, Rosenthal A, Smith AL, et al. Sepsis and congenital asplenia. J Pediatr 1977;90:555–9.
2. Ellis EF, Smith RT. The role of the spleen in immunity. With special reference to the post-splenectomy problem in infants. Pediatrics 1966;37:111–9.
3. Corazza GR, Ginaldi L, Zoli G, et al. Howell-Jolly body counting as a measure of splenic function. A reassessment. Clin Lab Haematol 1990;12:269–5.
4. Feder HM Jr, Pearson HA. Assessment of splenic function in familial asplenia. N Engl J Med 1999;341:210–2.
5. Brigden ML, Pattullo AL. Prevention and management of overwhelming postsplenectomy infection—an update. Crit Care Med 1999;27:836–42.
6. Lynch AM, Kapila R. Overwhelming postsplenectomy infection. Infect Dis Clin North Am 1996;10:693–707.
7. Ticho BS, Goldstein AM, Van Praagh R. Extracardiac anomalies in the heterotaxy syndromes with focus on anomalies of midline-associated structures. Am J Cardiol 2000;85:729–34.
8. Lin AE, Ticho BS, Houde K, et al. Heterotaxy: associated conditions and hospital-based prevalence in newborns. Genet Med 2000;2:157–72.
9. Dickerman JD. Splenectomy and sepsis: a warning. Pediatrics 1979;63:938–41.
10. Moore GE, Stevens RE, Moore EE, et al. Failure of splenic implants to protect against fatal postsplenectomy infection. Am J Surg 1983;146:413–4.
11. Guidelines for the prevention and treatment of infection in patients with an absent or dysfunctional spleen. Working Party of the British Committee for Standards in Haematology Clinical Haematology Task Force. Br Med J 1996; 312:430–34.
12. Coleman CN, McDougall IR, Dailey MO, et al. Functional hyposplenia after splenic irradiation for Hodgkin's disease. Ann Intern Med 1982;96:44–7.
13. Kalhs P, Panzer S, Kletter K, et al. Functional asplenia after bone marrow transplantation. A late complication related to extensive chronic graft-versus-host disease. Ann Intern Med 1988;109:461–4.
14. Zarkowsky HS, Gallagher D, Gill FM, et al. Bacteremia in sickle hemoglobinopathies. J Pediatr 1986;109:579–85.
15. Topley JM, Cupidore L, Vaidya S, et al. Pneumococcal and other infections in children with sickle-cell hemoglobin C (SC) disease. J Pediatr 1982;101:176–9.
16. Kravis E, Fleisher G, Ludwig S. Fever in children with sickle cell hemoglobinopathies. Am J Dis Child 1982; 136:1075–78.
17. Wilimas JA, Flynn PM, Harris S, et al. A randomized study of outpatient treatment with ceftriaxone for selected febrile children with sickle cell disease. N Engl J Med 1993;329:472–6.
18. Vichinsky EP, Neumayr LD, Earles AN, et al. Causes and outcomes of the acute chest syndrome in sickle cell disease. National Acute Chest Syndrome Study Group. N Engl J Med 2000;342:1855–65.
19. White KS, Covington D, Churchill P, et al. Patient awareness of health precautions after splenectomy. Am J Infect Control 1991;19:36–41.
20. Kinnersley P, Wilkinson CE, Srinivasan J. Pneumococcal vaccination after splenectomy: survey of hospital and primary care records. Br Med J 1993;307:1398–9.
21. O'Brien KL, Steinhoff MC, Edwards K, et al. Immunologic priming of young children by pneumococcal glycoprotein conjugate, but not polysaccharide, vaccines. Pediatr Infect Dis J 1996;15:425–30.
22. O'Brien KL, Swift AJ, Winkelstein JA, et al. Safety and immunogenicity of heptavalent pneumococcal vaccine conjugated to CRM(197) among infants with sickle cell disease. Pneumococcal Conjugate Vaccine Study Group. Pediatrics 2000;106:965–72.
23. Vernacchio L, Neufeld EJ, MacDonald K, et al. Combined schedule of 7-valent pneumococcal conjugate vaccine followed by 23-valent pneumococcal vaccine in children and young adults with sickle cell disease. J Pediatr 1998; 133:275–8.
24. Preventing pneumococcal disease among infants and young children. Recommendations of the Advisory Committee on Immunization Practices (ACIP). MMWR Recomm Rep 2000;49:1–35.
25. Buchanan GR, Smith SJ. Pneumococcal septicemia despite pneumococcal vaccine and prescription of penicillin prophylaxis in children with sickle cell anemia. Am J Dis Child 1986;140:428–32.
26. American Academy of Pediatrics. Haemophilus influenzae infections. In: Pickering LK, ed. 2000 Red Book: Report of the Committee on Infectious Diseases. Elk Grove Village, IL: American Academy of Pediatrics, 2000:262–72.
27. Rubin LG, Voulalas D, Carmody L. Immunogenicity of Haemophilus influenzae type b conjugate vaccine in children with sickle cell disease. Am J Dis Child 1992;146: 340–2.
28. Granoff DM, Gupta RK, Belshe RB, et al. Induction of immunologic refractoriness in adults by meningococcal C polysaccharide vaccination. J Infect Dis 1998;178:870–4.
29. Jodar L, Feavers IM, Salisbury D, et al. Development of

vaccines against meningococcal disease. Lancet 2002; 359:1499–508.

30. Prevention and control of influenza: recommendations of the Advisory Committee on Immunization Practices (ACIP). MMWR Recomm Rep 1999;48:1–28.

31. Neuzil KM, Griffin MR, Schaffner W. Influenza vaccine: issues and opportunities. Infect Dis Clin North Am 2001; 15:123–41, ix.

32. Glezen WP, Glezen LS, Alcorn R. Trivalent, inactivated influenza virus vaccine in children with sickle cell disease. Am J Dis Child 1983;137:1095–7.

33. Gaston MH, Verter JI, Woods G, et al. Prophylaxis with oral penicillin in children with sickle cell anemia. A randomized trial. N Engl J Med 1986;314:1593–9.

34. Steele RW, Warrier R, Unkel PJ, et al. Colonization with antibiotic-resistant *Streptococcus pneumoniae* in children with sickle cell disease. J Pediatr 1996;128:531–5.

35. Sakhalkar VS, Sarnaik SA, Asmar BI, et al. Prevalence of penicillin-nonsusceptible *Streptococcus pneumoniae* in nasopharyngeal cultures from patients with sickle cell disease. South Med J 2001;94:401–4.

36. Woods GM, Jorgensen JH, Waclawiw MA, et al. Influence of penicillin prophylaxis on antimicrobial resistance in nasopharyngeal *S. pneumoniae* among children with sickle cell anemia. The Ancillary Nasopharyngeal Culture Study of Prophylactic Penicillin Study II. J Pediatr Hematol Oncol 1997;19:327–33.

37. Norris CF, Mahannah SR, Smith-Whitley K, et al. Pneumococcal colonization in children with sickle cell disease [see comment]. J Pediatr 1996;129:821–7.

38. Falletta JM, Woods GM, Verter JI, et al. Discontinuing penicillin prophylaxis in children with sickle cell anemia. Prophylactic Penicillin Study II. J Pediatr 1995;127: 685–90.

39. American Academy of Pediatrics. Asplenic children. In: Pickering LK, ed. 2000 Red Book: Report of the Committee on Infectious Diseases. Elk Grove Village, IL: American Academy of Pediatrics, 2000:66–7.

40. Iliopoulos AG, Tsokos GC. Immunopathogenesis and spectrum of infections in systemic lupus erythematosus. Semin Arthritis Rheum 1996;25:318–36.

41. Zonana-Nacach A, Camargo-Coronel A, Yanez P, et al. Infections in outpatients with systemic lupus erythematosus: a prospective study. Lupus 2001;10:505–10.

42. Hohler T, Buschenfelde KH. Systemic lupus erythematosus. N Engl J Med 1994;331:1235.

43. Densen P. Complement deficiencies and infection. In: Valanakis JE, Frank MM, eds. The Human Complement System in Health and Disease. New York: Marcel Dekker Inc, 1998:409–21.

44. Bansal AS. Predispositions to meningococcemia. N Engl J Med 1997;337:204.

45. Garred P, Voss A, Madsen HO, Junker P. Association of mannose-binding lectin gene variation with disease severity and infections in a population-based cohort of systemic lupus erythematosus patients. Genes Immunity 2001;2:442–50.

46. Stahl NI, Klippel JH, Decker JL. Fever in systemic lupus erythematosus. Am J Med 1979;67:935–940.

47. Hind CR, Ng SC, Feng PH, et al. Serum C-reactive protein measurement in the detection of intercurrent infection in Oriental patients with systemic lupus erythematosus. Ann Rheum Dis 1985;44:260–1.

48. Becker GJ, Waldburger M, Hughes GR, et al. Value of serum C-reactive protein measurement in the investigation of fever in systemic lupus erythematosus. Ann Rheum Dis 1980;39:50–2.

49. Maury CP, Helve T, Sjoblom C. Serum beta 2-microglobulin, sialic acid, and C-reactive protein in systemic lupus erythematosus. Rheumatol Int 1982;2:145–9.

50. Zein N, Ganuza C, Kushner I. Significance of serum C-reactive protein elevation in patients with systemic lupus erythematosus. Arthritis Rheum 1979;22:7–12.

51. Euler HH, Harten P, Zeuner RA, et al. Recombinant human granulocyte colony stimulating factor in patients with systemic lupus erythematosus associated neutropenia and refractory infections. J Rheumatol 1997;24: 2153–7.

52. Palazzi DL, McClain KL, Kaplan SL. Hemophagocytic syndrome in children: an important diagnostic consideration in fever of unknown origin. Clin Infect Dis 2003; 36:306–12.

53. Sawhney S, Woo P, Murray KJ. Macrophage activation syndrome: a potentially fatal complication of rheumatic disorders. Arch Dis Child 2001;85:421–6.

54. Okano M, Gross TG. Epstein-Barr virus-associated hemophagocytic syndrome and fatal infectious mononucleosis. Am J Hematol 1996;53:111–5.

55. Hoffman RW, Greidinger EL. Mixed connective tissue disease. Curr Opin Rheumatol 2000;12:386–90.

56. Yokota S. Mixed connective tissue disease in childhood. Acta Paediatr Jpn 1993;35:472–9.

57. Singsen BH, Bernstein BH, Kornreich HK, et al. Mixed connective tissue disease in childhood: a clinical and serologic survey. J Pediatr 1977;90:893–900.

58. Michels H. Course of mixed connective tissue disease in children. Ann Med 1997;29:359–64.

59. Rennebohm RM, Heubi JE, Daugherty CC, et al. Reye syndrome in children receiving salicylate therapy for connective tissue disease. J Pediatr 1985;107:877–80.

60. Ramsey BW. Management of pulmonary disease in patients with cystic fibrosis. N Engl J Med 1996;335: 179–88.

61. Doull IJ. Recent advances in cystic fibrosis. Arch Dis Child 2001;85:62–6.

62. Brennan AL, Geddes DM. Cystic fibrosis. Curr Opin Infect Dis 2002;15:175–82.

63. Milla CE, Wielinski CL, Regelmann WE. Clinical significance of the recovery of *Aspergillus* species from the respiratory secretions of cystic fibrosis patients. Pediatr Pulmonol 1996;21:6–10.

64. Oliver A, Maiz L, Canton R, et al. Nontuberculous mycobacteria in patients with cystic fibrosis. Clin Infect Dis 2001;32:1298–303.

65. Gentile VG, Isaacson G. Patterns of sinusitis in cystic fibrosis. Laryngoscope 1996;106:1005–9.

66. Hampel B, Hullmann R, Schmidt H. Ciprofloxacin in pediatrics: worldwide clinical experience based on compassionate use—safety report. Pediatr Infect Dis J 1997;16: 127–9; discussion 160–22.

67. Richard DA, Nousia-Arvanitakis S, Sollich V, et al. Oral ciprofloxacin vs. intravenous ceftazidime plus tobramycin in pediatric cystic fibrosis patients: comparison of

antipseudomonas efficacy and assessment of safety with ultrasonography and magnetic resonance imaging. Cystic Fibrosis Study Group. Pediatr Infect Dis J 1997;16: 572–8.

68. Campbell PW, 3rd, Saiman L. Use of aerosolized antibiotics in patients with cystic fibrosis. Chest 1999;116: 775–88.

69. Fuchs HJ, Borowitz DS, Christiansen DH, et al. Effect of aerosolized recombinant human DNase on exacerbations of respiratory symptoms and on pulmonary function in patients with cystic fibrosis. The Pulmozyme Study Group. N Engl J Med 1994;331:637–42.

70. Thomas J, Cook DJ, Brooks D. Chest physical therapy management of patients with cystic fibrosis. A meta-analysis. Am J Respir Crit Care Med 1995;151:846–50.

71. Stutman HR, Lieberman JM, Nussbaum E, et al. Antibiotic prophylaxis in infants and young children with cystic fibrosis: a randomized controlled trial. J Pediatr 2002; 140:299–305.

72. Ratjen F, Comes G, Paul K, et al. Effect of continuous antistaphylococcal therapy on the rate of P. aeruginosa acquisition in patients with cystic fibrosis. Pediatr Pulmonol 2001;31:13–6.

73. Ramsey BW, Pepe MS, Quan JM, et al. Intermittent administration of inhaled tobramycin in patients with cystic fibrosis. Cystic Fibrosis Inhaled Tobramycin Study Group. N Engl J Med 1999;340:23–30.

74. Nelson LA, Callerame ML, Schwartz RH. Aspergillosis and atopy in cystic fibrosis. Am Rev Respir Dis 1979; 120:863–73.

75. Laufer P, Fink JN, Bruns WT, et al. Allergic bronchopulmonary aspergillosis in cystic fibrosis. J Allergy Clin Immunol 1984;73:44–8.

76. Geller DE, Kaplowitz H, Light MJ, et al. Allergic bronchopulmonary aspergillosis in cystic fibrosis: reported prevalence, regional distribution, and patient characteristics. Scientific Advisory Group, Investigators, and Coordinators of the Epidemiologic Study of Cystic Fibrosis. Chest 1999;116:639–46.

77. Nepomuceno IB, Esrig S, Moss RB. Allergic bronchopulmonary aspergillosis in cystic fibrosis: role of atopy and response to itraconazole. Chest 1999;115:364–70.

78. Newman AJ, Ansell BM. Episodic arthritis in children with cystic fibrosis. J Pediatr 1979;94:594–6.

79. Yankaskas JR, Mallory GB Jr. Lung transplantation in cystic fibrosis: consensus conference statement. Chest 1998; 113:217–26.

80. Flotte TR, Laube BL. Gene therapy in cystic fibrosis. Chest 2001;120:124S–31S.

81. Spina CA, Smith D, Korn E, et al. Altered cellular immune functions in patients with Down's syndrome. Am J Dis Child 1981;135:251–5.

82. Cuadrado E, Barrena MJ. Immune dysfunction in Down's syndrome: primary immune deficiency or early senescence of the immune system? Clin Immunol Immunopathol 1996;78:209–14.

83. Malec E, Mroczek T, Pajak J, et al. Results of surgical treatment of congenital heart defects in children with Down's syndrome. Pediatr Cardiol 1999;20:351–4.

84. Cooney TP, Thurlbeck WM. Pulmonary hypoplasia in Down's syndrome. N Engl J Med 1982;307:1170–3.

85. Shott SR, Joseph A, Heithaus D. Hearing loss in children

with Down syndrome. Int J Pediatr Otorhinolaryngol 2001;61:199–205.

86. Roizen NJ, Martich V, Ben-Ami T, et al. Sclerosis of the mastoid air cells as an indicator of undiagnosed otitis media in children with Down's syndrome. Clin Pediatr 1994;33:439–43.

87. Geerlings SE, Hoepelman AI. Immune dysfunction in patients with diabetes mellitus (DM). FEMS Immunol Med Microbiol 1999;26:259–65.

88. Rayfield EJ, Ault MJ, Keusch GT, et al. Infection and diabetes: the case for glucose control. Am J Med 1982; 72:439–50.

89. Joshi N, Caputo GM, Weitekamp MR, et al. Infections in patients with diabetes mellitus. N Engl J Med 1999;341: 1906–12.

90. Baker JR Jr. Autoimmune endocrine disease. JAMA 1997; 278:1931–7.

91. Peterson P, Nagamine K, Scott H, et al. APECED: a monogenic autoimmune disease providing new clues to self-tolerance. Immunol Today 1998;19:384–6.

92. Wildin RS, Smyk-Pearson S, Filipovich AH. Clinical and molecular features of the immunodysregulation, polyendocrinopathy, enteropathy, X linked (IPEX) syndrome. J Med Genetics 2002;39:537–45.

93. Powell BR, Buist NR, Stenzel P. An X-linked syndrome of diarrhea, polyendocrinopathy, and fatal infection in infancy. J Pediatr 1982;100:731–7.

94. Boyce TG, Mellen BG, Mitchel EF Jr, et al. Rates of hospitalization for respiratory syncytial virus infection among children in Medicaid. J Pediatr 2000;137:865–70.

95. Navas L, Wang E, de Carvalho V, et al. Improved outcome of respiratory syncytial virus infection in a high-risk hospitalized population of Canadian children. Pediatric Investigators Collaborative Network on Infections in Canada. J Pediatr 1992;121:348–54.

96. Feltes TF, Cabalka AK, Meissner HC, et al. Palivizumab prophylaxis reduces hospitalization due to respiratory syncytial virus in young children with hemodynamically significant congenital heart disease. J Pediatr 2003;1432: 532–40.

97. Sullivan KE, Jawad AF, Randall P, et al. Lack of correlation between impaired T cell production, immunodeficiency, and other phenotypic features in chromosome 22q11.2 deletion syndromes. Clin Immunol Immunopathol 1998;86:141–6.

98. Pierdominici M, Marziali M, Giovannetti A, et al. T cell receptor repertoire and function in patients with DiGeorge syndrome and velocardiofacial syndrome. Clin Exp Immunol 2000;121:127–32.

99. MacDonald NE, Wolfish N, McLaine P, et al. Role of respiratory viruses in exacerbations of primary nephrotic syndrome. J Pediatr 1986;108:378–82.

100. Kemper MJ, Altrogge H, Ganschow R, et al. Serum levels of immunoglobulins and IgG subclasses in steroid sensitive nephrotic syndrome. Pediatr Nephrol 2002;17: 413–17.

101. Strife CF, Jackson EC, Forristal J, et al. Effect of the nephrotic syndrome on the concentration of serum complement components. Am J Kidney Dis 1986;8:37–42.

102. Moorthy AV, Zimmerman SW, Burkholder PM. Inhibition of lymphocyte blastogenesis by plasma of patients

with minimal-change nephrotic syndrome. Lancet 1976; 1:1160–2.

103. McVicar MI, Chandra M, Margouleff D, et al. Splenic hypofunction in the nephrotic syndrome of childhood. Am J Kidney Dis 1986;7:395–401.

104. Tain YL, Lin G, Cher TW. Microbiological spectrum of septicemia and peritonitis in nephrotic children. Pediatr Nephrol 1999;13:835–37.

105. Krensky AM, Ingelfinger JR, Grupe WE. Peritonitis in childhood nephrotic syndrome: 1970-1980. Am J Dis Child 1982;136:732–6.

106. Sickler SJ, Edwards MS. Group B streptococcal cellulitis in a child with steroid-responsive nephrotic syndrome. Pediatr Infect Dis J 2001;20:1007–9.

107. Murphy JL, Kano HL, Chenaille PJ, et al. Fatal *Pneumocystis* pneumonia in a child treated for focal segmental glomerulosclerosis. Pediatr Nephrol 1993;7:444–5.

108. American Academy of Pediatrics. Corticosteroids. In: Pickering LK, ed. 2000 Red Book: Report of the Committee on Infectious Diseases. Elk Grove Village, IL: American Academy of Pediatrics, 2000:61–2.

109. Vanholder R, Van Biesen W. Incidence of infectious morbidity and mortality in dialysis patients. Blood Purif 2002; 20:477–80.

110. Massry S, Smogorzewski M. Dysfunction of polymorphonuclear leukocytes in uremia: role of parathyroid hormone. Kidney Int 2001;78:S195–6.

111. Vanholder R, Ringoir S. Infectious morbidity and defects of phagocytic function in end-stage renal disease: a review. J Am Soc Nephrol 1993;3:1541–54.

112. Laube GF, Berger C, Goetschel P, et al. Immunization in children with chronic renal failure. Pediatr Nephrol 2002;17:638–42.

113. Ariza M, Lopez M, Quesada T. Complications of CAPD in children: six years experience in Caracas, Venezuela. Adv Peritoneal Dial 1991;7:269–71.

114. Furth SL, Donaldson LA, Sullivan EK, et al. Peritoneal dialysis catheter infections and peritonitis in children: a report of the North American Pediatric Renal Transplant Cooperative Study. Pediatr Nephrol 2000;15:179–82.

115. Powell D, Luis ES, Calvin S, et al. Peritonitis in children undergoing continuous ambulatory peritoneal dialysis. Am J Dis Child 1985;139:29–32.

116. Warady BA, Campoy SF, Gross SP, et al. Peritonitis with continuous ambulatory peritoneal dialysis and continuous cycling peritoneal dialysis. J Pediatr 1984;105: 726–30.

117. McClung MR. Peritonitis in children receiving continuous ambulatory peritoneal dialysis. Pediatr Infect Dis 1983;2:328–32.

118. Vas S, Oreopoulos DG. Infections in patients undergoing peritoneal dialysis. Infect Dis Clin North Am 2001;15: 743–74.

119. von Graevenitz A, Amsterdam D. Microbiological aspects of peritonitis associated with continuous ambulatory peritoneal dialysis. Clin Microbiol Rev 1992;5:36–48.

120. Sewell DL, Golper TA, Hulman PB, et al. Comparison of large volume culture to other methods for isolation of microorganisms from dialysate. Perit Dial Int 1990;10: 49–52.

121. Warady BA, Schaefer F, Holloway M, et al. Consensus guidelines for the treatment of peritonitis in pediatric patients receiving peritoneal dialysis. Perit Dial Int 2000; 20:610–24.

122. Schaefer F, Klaus G, Muller-Wiefel DE, et al. Intermittent versus continuous intraperitoneal glycopeptide/ceftazidime treatment in children with peritoneal dialysis-associated peritonitis. The Mid-European Pediatric Peritoneal Dialysis Study Group (MEPPS). J Am Soc Nephrol 1999; 10:136–45.

123. Warady BA, Bashir M, Donaldson LA. Fungal peritonitis in children receiving peritoneal dialysis: a report of the NAPRTCS. Kidney Int 2000;58:384–9.

124. Lo WK, Chan CY, Cheng SW, et al. A prospective randomized control study of oral nystatin prophylaxis for *Candida* peritonitis complicating continuous ambulatory peritoneal dialysis. Am J Kidney Dis 1996;28:549–52.

125. Robitaille P, Merouani A, Clermont MJ, et al. Successful antifungal prophylaxis in chronic peritoneal dialysis: a pediatric experience. Perit Dial Int 1995;15:77–9.

126. Verrina E, Honda M, Warady BA, et al. Prevention of peritonitis in children on peritoneal dialysis. Peri Dial Int 2000;20:625–30.

127. Sardegna KM, Beck AM, Strife CF. Evaluation of perioperative antibiotics at the time of dialysis catheter placement. Pediatr Nephrol 1998;12:149–52.

128. Anonymous. Nasal mupirocin prevents *Staphylococcus aureus* exit-site infection during peritoneal dialysis. Mupirocin Study Group. J Am Soc Nephrol 1996;7:2403–8.

129. Thodis E, Bhaskaran S, Pasadakis P, Bargman JM, et al. Decrease in *Staphylococcus aureus* exit-site infections and peritonitis in CAPD patients by local application of mupirocin ointment at the catheter exit site. Perit Dial Int 1998;18:261–70.

130. Annigeri R, Conly J, Vas S, et al. Emergence of mupirocin-resistant *Staphylococcus aureus* in chronic peritoneal dialysis patients using mupirocin prophylaxis to prevent exit-site infection. Perit Dial Int 2001;21:554–9.

131. Lew SQ, Kaveh K. Dialysis access related infections. ASAIO J 2000;46:S6–12.

132. Nassar GM, Ayus JC. Infectious complications of the hemodialysis access. Kidney Int 2001;60:1–13.

133. McCarthy JT, Steckelberg JM. Infective endocarditis in patients receiving long-term hemodialysis. Mayo Clin Proc 2000;75:1008–14.

134. Tokars JI, Arduino MJ, Alter MJ. Infection control in hemodialysis units. Infect Dis Clin North Am 2001;15: 797–812, viii.

135. Hepatitis B virus: A comprehensive strategy for eliminating transmission in the United States through universal childhood vaccination. Recommendations of the Immunization Practices Advisory Committee (ACIP). MMWR Recomm Rep 1991;40:1–25.

136. Recommendations for preventing transmission of infections among chronic hemodialysis patients. MMWR Recomm Rep 2001;50:1–43.

137. NKF-DOQI clinical practice guidelines for vascular access. National Kidney Foundation-Dialysis Outcomes Quality Initiative. Am J Kidney Dis 1997;30:S150–91.

138. Boelaert JR, Van Landuyt HW, Godard CA, et al. Nasal mupirocin ointment decreases the incidence of *Staphylococcus aureus* bacteraemias in haemodialysis patients. Nephrol Dial Transplant 1993;8:235–9.

139. Piraino B. *Staphylococcus aureus* infections in dialysis patients: focus on prevention. ASAIO J 2000;46:S13–7.

140. Maggiore G, De Giacomo C, Marconi M, et al. Defective neutrophil motility in children with chronic liver disease. Am J Dis Child 1983;137:768–70.

141. Larcher VF, Manolaki N, Vegnente A, et al. Spontaneous bacterial peritonitis in children with chronic liver disease: clinical features and etiologic factors. J Pediatr 1985;106: 907–12.

142. Such J, Runyon BA. Spontaneous bacterial peritonitis. Clin Infect Dis 1998;27:669–74;quiz 675–6.

143. Felisart J, Rimola A, Arroyo V, et al. Cefotaxime is more effective than is ampicillin-tobramycin in cirrhotics with severe infections. Hepatology 1985;5:457–62.

144. Soriano G, Guarner C, Tomas A, et al. Norfloxacin prevents bacterial infection in cirrhotics with gastrointestinal hemorrhage. Gastroenterology 1992;103:1267–72.

145. Grange JD, Roulot D, Pelletier G, et al. Norfloxacin primary prophylaxis of bacterial infections in cirrhotic patients with ascites: a double-blind randomized trial. J Hepatology 1998;29:430–6.

146. Dupeyron C, Mangeney N, Sedrati L, et al. Rapid emergence of quinolone resistance in cirrhotic patients treated with norfloxacin to prevent spontaneous bacterial peritonitis. Antimicrob Agents Chemother 1994;38:340–4.

147. Singh N, Gayowski T, Yu VL, et al. Trimethoprim-sulfamethoxazole for the prevention of spontaneous bacterial peritonitis in cirrhosis: a randomized trial. Ann Intern Med 1995;122:595–8.

148. Rolachon A, Cordier L, Bacq Y, et al. Ciprofloxacin and long-term prevention of spontaneous bacterial peritonitis: results of a prospective controlled trial. Hepatology 1995;22:1171–4.

149. Kurkchubasche AG, Smith SD, Rowe MI. Catheter sepsis in short-bowel syndrome. Arch Surg 1992;127:21–4; discussion 24–5.

150. Buchman AL. Complications of long-term home total parenteral nutrition: their identification, prevention and treatment. Dig Dis Sci 2001;46:1–18.

151. De Onis M, Monteiro C, Akre J, et al. The worldwide magnitude of protein-energy malnutrition: an overview from the WHO Global Database on Child Growth. Bull World Health Organ 1993;71:703–12.

152. Campbell H, Gove S. Integrated management of childhood infections and malnutrition: a global initiative. Arch Dis Child 1996;75:468–71.

153. Chandra RK. Golan memorial lecture. Nutritional regulation of immunity and infection: from epidemiology to phenomenology to clinical practice. J Pediatr GastroenterolNutr 1986;5:844–52.

154. Guerrant RL, Lima AA, Davidson F. Micronutrients and infection: interactions and implications with enteric and other infections and future priorities. J Infect Dis 2000; 182:S134–8.

155. Tomkins A. Malnutrition, morbidity and mortality in children and their mothers. Pro Nutr Soc 2000;59: 135–46.

156. Gottrand F, Bernard O, Hadchouel M, et al. Late cholangitis after successful surgical repair of biliary atresia. Am J Dis Child 1991;145:213–5.

157. Kuhls TL, Jackson MA. Diagnosis and treatment of the febrile child following hepatic portoenterostomy. Pediatr Infect Dis 1985;4:487–90.

158. Ecoffey C, Rothman E, Bernard O, et al. Bacterial cholangitis after surgery for biliary atresia. J Pediatr 1987;111: 824–9.

159. Hughes WT. Early side effects in treatment of childhood cancer. Pediatr Clin North Am 1976;23:225–32.

160. Bodey GP, Buckley M, Sathe YS, et al. Quantitative relationships between circulating leukocytes and infection in patients with acute leukemia. Ann Intern Med 1966;64: 328–40.

161. Goorin AM, Hershey BJ, Levin MJ, et al. Use of trimethoprim-sulfamethoxazole to prevent bacterial infections in children with acute lymphoblastic leukemia. Pediatr Infect Dis 1985;4:265–9.

162. Hughes WT, Rivera GK, Schell MJ, et al. Successful intermittent chemoprophylaxis for *Pneumocystis carinii* pneumonitis. N Engl J Med 1987;316:1627–32.

163. Sepkowitz KA, Brown AE, Telzak EE, et al. *Pneumocystis carinii* pneumonia among patients without AIDS at a cancer hospital. JAMA 1992;267:832–7.

164. Cruciani M, Rampazzo R, Malena M, et al. Prophylaxis with fluoroquinolones for bacterial infections in neutropenic patients: a meta-analysis. Clin Infect Dis 1996;23: 795–805.

165. Murphy M, Brown AE, Sepkowitz KA, et al. Fluoroquinolone prophylaxis for the prevention of bacterial infections in patients with cancer—is it justified? Clin Infect Dis 1997;25:346–8.

166. Bow EJ, Laverdiere M, Lussier N, et al. Antifungal prophylaxis for severely neutropenic chemotherapy recipients: a meta analysis of randomized-controlled clinical trials. Cancer 2002;94:3230–46.

167. Hughes WT, Armstrong D, Bodey GP, et al. 2002 guidelines for the use of antimicrobial agents in neutropenic patients with cancer. Clin Infect Dis 2002;34:730–51.

168. Mitchell PL, Morland B, Stevens MC, et al. Granulocyte colony-stimulating factor in established febrile neutropenia: a randomized study of pediatric patients. J Clin Oncol 1997;15:1163–70.

169. Ozer H, Armitage JO, Bennett CL, et al. 2000 update of recommendations for the use of hematopoietic colony-stimulating factors: evidence-based, clinical practice guidelines. American Society of Clinical Oncology Growth Factors Expert Panel. J Clin Oncol 2000;18: 3558–85.

170. Santolaya ME, Alvarez AM, Becker A, et al. Prospective, multicenter evaluation of risk factors associated with invasive bacterial infection in children with cancer, neutropenia, and fever. J Clin Oncol 2001;19:3415–21.

171. Santolaya ME, Alvarez AM, Aviles CL, et al. Prospective evaluation of a model of prediction of invasive bacterial infection risk among children with cancer, fever, and neutropenia. Clin Infect Dis 2002;35:678–83.

172. Pizzo PA. Management of fever in patients with cancer and treatment-induced neutropenia. N Engl J Med 1993; 328:1323–32.

173. Shenep JL, Flynn PM, Baker DK, et al. Oral cefixime is similar to continued intravenous antibiotics in the empirical treatment of febrile neutropenic children with cancer. Clin Infect Dis 2001;32:36–43.

174. Walsh TJ, Finberg RW, Arndt C, et al. Liposomal ampho-

tericin B for empirical therapy in patients with persistent fever and neutropenia. National Institute of Allergy and Infectious Diseases Mycoses Study Group. N Engl J Med 1999;340:764–71.

175. Walsh TJ, Pappas P, Winston DJ, et al. Voriconazole compared with liposomal amphotericin B for empirical antifungal therapy in patients with neutropenia and persistent fever. N Engl J Med 2002;346:225–34.

176. Anonymous. Voriconazole. Med Lett Drugs Ther 2002; 44:63–5.

177. Pizzo PA, Robichaud KJ, Wesley R, et al. Fever in the pediatric and young adult patient with cancer. A prospective study of 1001 episodes. Medicine (Baltimore) 1982; 61:153–65.

178. Siegel SE, Nesbit ME, Baehner R, et al. Pneumonia during therapy for childhood acute lymphoblastic leukemia. Am J Dis Child 1980;134:28–34.

179. Wilson GJ, Dermody TS. Respiratory infections in immunocompromised children. Semin Pediatr Infect Dis 1995; 6:156–65.

180. Cox F, Hughes WT. Disseminated histoplasmosis and childhood leukemia. Cancer 1974;33:1127–33.

181. MacDonald N, Steinhoff MC, Powell KR. Review of coccidioidomycosis in immunocompromised children. Am J Dis Child 1981;135:553–56.

182. Kovatch AL, Jardine DS, Dowling JN, et al. Legionellosis in children with leukemia in relapse. Pediatrics 1984;73: 811–15.

183. Apaliski SJ, Moore MD, Reiner BJ, et al. Disseminated Trichosporon beigelii in an immunocompromised child. Pediatr Infect Dis 1984;3:451–4.

184. Levine SJ. An approach to the diagnosis of pulmonary infections in immunosuppressed patients. Semin Respir Infect 1992;7:81–95.

185. Shelhamer JH, Gill VJ, Quinn TC, et al. The laboratory evaluation of opportunistic pulmonary infections. Ann Intern Med 1996;124:585–99.

186. Barone SR, Aiuto LT, Krilov LR. Increased survival of young infants with Pneumocystis carinii pneumonia and acute respiratory failure with early steroid administration. Clin Infect Dis 1994;19:212–3.

187. Lear JT, Atherton MT, Byrne JP. Neutrophilic dermatoses: pyoderma gangrenosum and Sweet's syndrome. Postgrad Med J 1997;73:65–8.

188. Fergie JE, Huang DB, Purcell K, et al. Successful treatment of Fusarium solani ecthyma gangrenosum in a child with acute lymphoblastic leukemia in relapse. Pediatr Infect Dis J 2000;19:579–81.

189. Kimyai-Asadi A, Tausk FA, Nousari HC. Ecthyma secondary to herpes simplex virus infection. Clin Infect Dis 1999;29:454–5.

190. Wirth F, Perry R, Eskenazi A, et al. Cutaneous mucormycosis with subsequent visceral dissemination in a child with neutropenia: a case report and review of the pediatric literature. J Am Acad Dermatol 1997;36:336–41.

191. Rodot S, Lacour JP, van Elslande L, et al. Ecthyma gangrenosum caused by Klebsiella pneumoniae. Int J Dermatol 1995;34:216–7.

192. Vartivarian SE, Papadakis KA, Palacios JA, et al. Mucocutaneous and soft tissue infections caused by Xanthomonas maltophilia. A new spectrum. Ann Intern Med 1994;121: 969–73.

193. Fergie JE, Patrick CC, Lott L. Pseudomonas aeruginosa cellulitis and ecthyma gangrenosum in immunocompromised children. Pediatr Infect Dis J 1991;10:496–500.

194. Hewitt WD, Farrar WE. Bacteremia and ecthyma caused by Streptococcus pyogenes in a patient with acquired immunodeficiency syndrome. Am J Med Sci 1988;295: 52–4.

195. Rajan RK. Spontaneous bacterial peritonitis with ecthyma gangrenosum due to Escherichia coli. J Clin Gastroenterol 1982;4:145–8.

196. Fine JD, Miller JA, Harrist TJ, et al. Cutaneous lesions in disseminated candidiasis mimicking ecthyma gangrenosum. Am J Med 1981;70:1133–5.

197. Turnbull D, Parry MF. Ecthyma-like skin lesions caused by Staphylococcus aureus. Arch Intern Med 1981;141:689.

198. Panke TW, McManus AT, Spebar MJ. Infection of a burn wound by Aspergillus niger. Gross appearance simulating ecthyma gangrenosa. Am J Clin Pathol 1979;72:230–2.

199. Moyer CD, Sykes PA, Rayner JM. Aeromonas hydrophila septicaemia producing ecthyma gangrenosum in a child with leukaemia. Scand J Infect Dis 1977;9:151–3.

200. Shackelford PG, Ratzan SA, Shearer WT. Ecthyma gangrenosum produced by Aeromonas hydrophilia. J Pediatr 1973;83:100–1.

201. Del Pozo J, Garcia-Silva J, Almagro M, et al. Ecthyma gangrenosum-like eruption associated with Morganella morganii infection. Br J Dermatol 1998;139:520–1.

202. Allen U, Smith CR, Prober CG. The value of skin biopsies in febrile, neutropenic, immunocompromised children. Am J Dis Child 1986;140:459–61.

203. Bartlett JG. Clinical practice. Antibiotic-associated diarrhea. N Engl J Med 2002;346:334–9.

204. Miller RA, Holmberg RE Jr, Clausen CR. Life-threatening diarrhea caused by Cryptosporidium in a child undergoing therapy for acute lymphocytic leukemia. J Pediatr 1983; 103:256–9.

205. Gomez L, Martino R, Rolston KV. Neutropenic enterocolitis: spectrum of the disease and comparison of definite and possible cases. Clin Infect Dis 1998;27:695–9.

206. Moir CR, Scudamore CH, Benny WB. Typhlitis: Selective surgical management. Am J Surg 1986;151:563–6.

206a. Slavin MA, Grigg AP, Schwarer AP. Fatal anaerobic bacteremia after hematppoietic stem cell transplant. Leuk Lymphoma 2004;45:143–5.

207. Kontoyiannis DP, Luna MA, Samuels BI, et al. Hepatosplenic candidiasis. A manifestation of chronic disseminated candidiasis. Infect Dis Clin North Am 2000;14: 721–39.

208. Rex JH, Walsh TJ, Sobel JD, et al. Practice guidelines for the treatment of candidiasis. Infectious Diseases Society of America. Clin Infect Dis 2000;30:662–78.

209. Sallah S, Semelka RC, Wehbie R, et al. Hepatosplenic candidiasis in patients with acute leukaemia. Br J Haematol 1999;106:697–701.

210. Walsh TJ, Whitcomb PO, Revankar SG, et al. Successful treatment of hepatosplenic candidiasis through repeated cycles of chemotherapy and neutropenia. Cancer 1995; 76:2357–62.

211. Kavanagh KT, Hughes WT, Parham DM, et al. Fungal sinusitis in immunocompromised children with neoplasms. Ann Otol Rhinol Laryngol 1991;100:331–6.

212. Armitage JO. Bone marrow transplantation. N Engl J Med 1994;330:827–38.

213. Skinner J, Finlay JL, Sondel PM, et al. Infectious complications in pediatric patients undergoing transplantation with T lymphocyte-depleted bone marrow. Pediatr Infect Dis 1986;5:319–24.

214. Guidelines for preventing opportunistic infections among hematopoietic stem cell transplant recipients. MMWR Recomm Rep 2000;49:1–125, CE121–128.

215. Cox GJ, Matsui SM, Lo RS, et al. Etiology and outcome of diarrhea after marrow transplantation: a prospective study. Gastroenterology 1994;107:1398–407.

216. Sable CA, Donowitz GR. Infections in bone marrow transplant recipients. Clin Infect Dis 1994;18:273–81; quiz 282–4.

217. Serody JS. Fever in immunocompromised patients. N Engl J Med 2000;342:217–8.

218. Goodman JL, Winston DJ, Greenfield RA, et al. A controlled trial of fluconazole to prevent fungal infections in patients undergoing bone marrow transplantation. N Engl J Med 1992;326:845–51.

219. Wingard JR, Merz WG, Rinaldi MG, et al. Increase in *Candida krusei* infection among patients with bone marrow transplantation and neutropenia treated prophylactically with fluconazole. N Engl J Med 1991;325:1274–7.

220. Pannuti C, Gingrich R, Pfaller MA, et al. Nosocomial pneumonia in patients having bone marrow transplant. Attributable mortality and risk factors. Cancer 1992;69: 2653–62.

221. Benjamin DK Jr, Miller WC, Bayliff S, et al. Infections diagnosed in the first year after pediatric stem cell transplantation. Pediatr Infect Dis J 2002;21:227–34.

222. Conneally E, Cafferkey MT, Daly PA, et al. Nebulized amphotericin B as prophylaxis against invasive aspergillosis in granulocytopenic patients. Bone Marrow Transplant 1990;5:403–6.

223. O'Donnell MR, Schmidt GM, Tegtmeier BR, et al. Prediction of systemic fungal infection in allogeneic marrow recipients: impact of amphotericin prophylaxis in high-risk patients. J Clin Oncol 1994;12:827–34.

224. Vasconcelles MJ, Bernardo MV, King C, et al. Aerosolized pentamidine as pneumocystis prophylaxis after bone marrow transplantation is inferior to other regimens and is associated with decreased survival and an increased risk of other infections. Biol Blood Marrow Transplantation 2000;6:35–43.

225. Lujan-Zilbermann J, Benaim E, Tong X, et al. Respiratory virus infections in pediatric hematopoietic stem cell transplantation. Clin Infect Dis 2001;33:962–8.

226. DeVincenzo JP, Hirsch RL, Fuentes RJ, et al. Respiratory syncytial virus immune globulin treatment of lower respiratory tract infection in pediatric patients undergoing bone marrow transplantation - a compassionate use experience. Bone Marrow Transplant 2000;25:161–5.

227. Wendt CH, Hertz MI. Respiratory syncytial virus and parainfluenza virus infections in the immunocompromised host. Semin Respir Infect 1995;10:224–31.

228. Englund JA. Diagnosis and epidemiology of community-acquired respiratory virus infections in the immunocompromised host. Biol Blood Marrow Transplant 2001;7: 2S–4S.

229. Hale GA, Heslop HE, Krance RA, et al. Adenovirus infection after pediatric bone marrow transplantation. Bone Marrow Transplant 1999;23:277–82.

230. Ribaud P, Scieux C, Freymuth F, et al. Successful treatment of adenovirus disease with intravenous cidofovir in an unrelated stem-cell transplant recipient. Clin Infect Dis 1999;28:690–1.

231. Bordigoni P, Carret AS, Venard V, et al. Treatment of adenovirus infections in patients undergoing allogeneic hematopoietic stem cell transplantation. Clin Infect Dis 2001;32:1290–7.

232. Legrand F, Berrebi D, Houhou N, et al. Early diagnosis of adenovirus infection and treatment with cidofovir after bone marrow transplantation in children. Bone Marrow Transplantation 2001;27:621–6.

233. Engelhard D, Nagler A, Hardan I, et al. Antibody response to a two-dose regimen of influenza vaccine in allogeneic T cell-depleted and autologous BMT recipients. Bone Marrow Transplant 1993;11:1–5.

234. Ljungman P, Griffiths P, Paya C. Definitions of cytomegalovirus infection and disease in transplant recipients. Clin Infect Dis 2002;34:1094–7.

235. Bowden RA, Slichter SJ, Sayers M, et al. A comparison of filtered leukocyte-reduced and cytomegalovirus (CMV) seronegative blood products for the prevention of transfusion-associated CMV infection after marrow transplant. Blood 1995;86:3598–3603.

236. Goodrich JM, Bowden RA, Fisher L, et al. Ganciclovir prophylaxis to prevent cytomegalovirus disease after allogeneic marrow transplant. Ann Intern Med 1993;118: 173–8.

237. Boeckh M, Gooley TA, Myerson D, et al. Cytomegalovirus pp65 antigenemia-guided early treatment with ganciclovir versus ganciclovir at engraftment after allogeneic marrow transplantation: a randomized double-blind study. Blood 1996;88:4063–71.

238. Zaia JA. Prevention of cytomegalovirus disease in hematopoietic stem cell transplantation. Clin Infect Dis 2002; 35:999–1004.

239. Morgan ER, Smalley LA. Varicella in immunocompromised children. Incidence of abdominal pain and organ involvement. Am J Dis Child 1983;137:883–5.

240. Feldman S, Hughes WT, Daniel CB. Varicella in children with cancer: seventy-seven cases. Pediatrics 1975;56: 388–97.

241. Atkinson K, Meyers JD, Storb R, et al. Varicella-zoster virus infection after marrow transplantation for aplastic anemia or leukemia. Transplantation 1980;29:47–50.

242. Feldman S, Lott L. Varicella in children with cancer: impact of antiviral therapy and prophylaxis. Pediatrics 1987;80:465–72.

243. Prober CG, Kirk LE, Keeney RE. Acyclovir therapy of chickenpox in immunosuppressed children—a collaborative study. J Pediatr 1982;101:622–5.

244. Saral R, Burns WH, Laskin OL, et al. Acyclovir prophylaxis of herpes-simplex-virus infections. N Engl J Med 1981;305:63–7.

245. Engelhard D, Marks MI, Good RA. Infections in bone marrow transplant recipients. J Pediatr 1986;108: 335–46.

246. Wade JC, Day LM, Crowley JJ, et al. Recurrent infection with herpes simplex virus after marrow transplantation:

role of the specific immune response and acyclovir treatment. J Infect Dis 1984;149:750–6.

247. Lundgren G, Wilczek H, Lonnqvist B, et al. Acyclovir prophylaxis in bone marrow transplant recipients. Scand J Infect Dis Suppl 1985;47:137–44.

247a. Danve-Szatanek C, Aymard M, Thouvenot D, et al. Surveillance network for herpes simplex virus resistance to anti-viral drugs: 3-year follow-up. J Clin Microbiol 2004; 42:242–9.

248. Chulay JD, Bell AR, Miller GB. Longterm safety of vala-cyclovir for suppression of herpes simplex virus infections, Infectious Diseases Society of America Program and Abstracts, 34th Annual Meeting, New Orleans, LA, September 18-20, 1996.

249. Gerritsen EJ, Stam ED, Hermans J, et al. Risk factors for developing EBV-related B cell lymphoproliferative disorders (BLPD) after non-HLA-identical BMT in children. Bone Marrow Transplant 1996;18:377–82.

250. Chiang KY, Hazlett LJ, Godder KT, et al. Epstein-Barr virus-associated B cell lymphoproliferative disorder following mismatched related T cell-depleted bone marrow transplantation. Bone Marrow Transplant. 2001;28: 1117–23.

251. Claviez A, Tiemann M, Wagner HJ, et al. Epstein-Barr virus-associated post-transplant lymphoproliferative disease after bone marrow transplantation mimicking graft-versus-host disease. Pediatric Transplantation 2000;4: 151–5.

252. Rooney CM, Smith CA, Ng CY, et al. Infusion of cytotoxic T cells for the prevention and treatment of Epstein-Barr virus-induced lymphoma in allogeneic transplant recipients. Blood 1998;92:1549–55.

253. Singhal S, Mehta J. Reimmunization after blood or marrow stem cell transplantation. Bone Marrow Transplant 1999;23:637–46.

254. Sutherland DE, Gruessner RW, Dunn DL, et al. Lessons learned from more than 1,000 pancreas transplants at a single institution. Ann Surg 2001;233:463–501.

255. Lin PL, Vats AN, Green M. BK virus infection in renal transplant recipients. Pediatr Transplant 2001;5: 398–405.

256. Michaels MG, Wald ER, Fricker FJ, et al. Toxoplasmosis in pediatric recipients of heart transplants. Clin Infect Dis 1992;14:847–51.

257. Avery RK. Recipient screening prior to solid-organ transplantation. Clin Infect Dis 2002;35:1513–19.

258. Fishman JA, Rubin RH. Infection in organ-transplant recipients. N Engl J Med 1998;338:1741–51.

259. Fox BC, Sollinger HW, Belzer FO, et al. A prospective, randomized, double-blind study of trimethoprim-sulfamethoxazole for prophylaxis of infection in renal transplantation: clinical efficacy, absorption of trimethoprim-sulfamethoxazole, effects on the microflora, and the cost-benefit of prophylaxis. Am J Med 1990;89:255–74.

260. Carr A, Tindall B, Brew BJ, et al. Low-dose trimethoprim-sulfamethoxazole prophylaxis for toxoplasmic encephalitis in patients with AIDS. Ann Intern Med 1992;117: 106–11.

261. Arnow PM, Carandang GC, Zabner R, et al. Randomized controlled trial of selective bowel decontamination for prevention of infections following liver transplantation. Clin Infect Dis 1996;22:997–1003.

262. Hellinger WC, Yao JD, Alvarez S, et al. A randomized, prospective, double-blinded evaluation of selective bowel decontamination in liver transplantation. Transplantation 2002;73:1904–9.

263. Collins LA, Samore MH, Roberts MS, et al. Risk factors for invasive fungal infections complicating orthotopic liver transplantation. J Infect Dis 1994;170:644–52.

264. Winston DJ, Pakrasi A, Busuttil RW. Prophylactic fluconazole in liver transplant recipients. A randomized, double-blind, placebo-controlled trial. Ann Intern Med 1999; 131:729–37.

265. Lumbreras C, Cuervas-Mons V, Jara P, et al. Randomized trial of fluconazole versus nystatin for the prophylaxis of Candida infection following liver transplantation. J Infect Dis 1996;174:583–8.

266. Singh N. Antifungal prophylaxis for solid organ transplant recipients: seeking clarity amidst controversy. Clin Infect Dis 2000;31:545–53.

267. Gordon SM, LaRosa SP, Kalmadi S, et al. Should prophylaxis for *Pneumocystis carinii* pneumonia in solid organ transplant recipients ever be discontinued? [see comments]. Clin Infect Dis 1999;28:240–6.

268. Arend SM, van't Wout JW. Editorial response: prophylaxis for *Pneumocystis carinii* pneumonia in solid organ transplant recipients—as long as the pros outweigh the cons. Clin Infect Dis 1999;28:247–9.

269. Pohl C, Green M, Wald ER, et al. Respiratory syncytial virus infections in pediatric liver transplant recipients. J Infect Dis 1992;165:166–9.

270. Apalsch AM, Green M, Ledesma-Medina J, et al. Parainfluenza and influenza virus infections in pediatric organ transplant recipients. Clin Infect Dis 1995;20:394–9.

271. Michaels MG, Green M, Wald ER, et al. Adenovirus infection in pediatric liver transplant recipients. J Infect Dis 1992;165:170–4.

272. Carter BA, Karpen SJ, Quiros-Tejeira RE, et al. Intravenous cidofovir therapy for disseminated adenovirus in a pediatric liver transplant recipient. Transplantation 2002; 74:1050–2.

273. Shirali GS, Ni J, Chinnock RE, et al. Association of viral genome with graft loss in children after cardiac transplantation. N Engl J Med 2001;344:1498–503.

274. Paya CV. Role of immunoglobulins and new antivirals in treatment of cytomegalovirus infection. Transplant Proc 1995;27:28–30.

275. Green M, Michaels M. Preemptive therapy of cytomegalovirus disease in pediatric transplant recipients. Pediatr Infect Dis J 2000;19:875–7.

276. Pescovitz MD, Rabkin J, Merion RM, et al. Valganciclovir results in improved oral absorption of ganciclovir in liver transplant recipients. Antimicrob Agents Chemother 2000;44:2811–5.

277. Feldhoff CM, Balfour HH Jr, Simmons RL, et al. Varicella in children with renal transplants. J Pediatr 1981;98: 25–31.

278. Kusne S, Dummer JS, Singh N, et al. Infections after liver transplantation. An analysis of 101 consecutive cases. Medicine (Baltimore) 1988;67:132–43.

279. Paya CV, Hermans PE, Washington JA 2nd, et al. Incidence, distribution, and outcome of episodes of infection in 100 orthotopic liver transplantations. Mayo Clin Proc 1989;64:555–64.

280. Newell KA, Alonso EM, Whitington PF, et al. Posttransplant lymphoproliferative disease in pediatric liver transplantation. Interplay between primary Epstein-Barr virus infection and immunosuppression. Transplantation 1996;62:370–5.

281. Younes BS, McDiarmid SV, Martin MG, et al. The effect of immunosuppression on posttransplant lymphoproliferative disease in pediatric liver transplant patients. Transplantation 2000;70:94–9.

282. Chadburn A, Chen JM, Hsu DT, et al. The morphologic and molecular genetic categories of posttransplantation lymphoproliferative disorders are clinically relevant. Cancer 1998;82:1978–87.

283. Green M, Michaels MG, Webber SA, et al. The management of Epstein-Barr virus associated post-transplant lymphoproliferative disorders in pediatric solid-organ transplant recipients. Pediatr Transplant 1999;3: 271–81.

284. Paya CV, Fung JJ, Nalesnik MA, et al. Epstein-Barr virus-induced posttransplant lymphoproliferative disorders. ASTS/ASTP EBV-PTLD Task Force and The Mayo Clinic Organized International Consensus Development Meeting. Transplantation 1999;68:1517–25.

285. Ginsburg CM, Andrews W. Orthotopic hepatic transplantation for unimmunized children: A paradox of contemporary medical care. Pediatr Infect Dis J 1987;6: 764–5.

286. Thall TV, Rosh JR, Schwersenz AH, et al. Primary immunization status in infants referred for liver transplantation. Transplant Proc 1994;26:191.

287. Burroughs M, Moscona A. Immunization of pediatric solid organ transplant candidates and recipients. Clin Infect Dis 2000;30:857–69.

288. Zamora I, Simon JM, Da Silva ME, et al. Attenuated varicella virus vaccine in children with renal transplants. Pediatr Nephrol 1994;8:190–2.

CHAPTER 23

The Child with Frequent, Severe, or Unusual Infections: Congenital Immunodeficiency Syndromes

■ OVERVIEW

It is impossible to pass through life without acquiring a large number of infections. Most of these infections occur during early childhood, a time when there is considerable immunologic naiveté. The child's immune system begins to build up defenses against infection by being exposed to various pathogens.

Not so long ago, children stayed at home throughout their toddler years. When these children attended kindergarten, they began to develop frequent respiratory infections. Absenteeism was high. These days, many children are in day care centers from infancy; thus, the time of frequent infection has been switched from early school age to infancy and the toddler years. Pediatricians offices are bombarded with many children who are experiencing yet another in a long series of infections.

■ FREQUENCY OF INFECTION

The important question is: How many infections is too many? Dr. Wald and colleagues performed an observational study that looked at the number of respiratory infections acquired by otherwise normal children in day care and preschool situations.[1] They found that the average child experienced 4 or 5 respiratory infections a year, and that some children experienced as many as 12 per year. When you consider that a common cold lasts approximately 10–14 days in a child of this age, and that most of these infections are clustered in the winter months, it becomes clear why some parents state that their child is "always sick."

Differentiation Between Normal and Immunodeficiency States

Given that even a child with a normal immune system can frequently be ill, how does one differentiate between a normal child who has a naive immune system and frequent exposure to infectious agents, and a child who has a faulty immune response to infection? In general, the normal child with frequent infections has normal growth and development, no family history of immune deficiency states or early childhood death, and appears well between episodes of sickness. It is rare to find a severe immunodeficiency in a child who is normally grown and developed and who has an entirely normal physical examination apart from the signs of the current disease. Children with primary immunodeficiency states, on the other hand, are more likely to have: (a) growth failure, (b) abnormal development, (c) severe or invasive infections, (d) family history of immune deficiency or early childhood demise, and (e) infections with opportunistic or unusual organisms (i.e., pathogens not normally considered virulent).

The history and physical examination is often enough, therefore, to determine which children should receive evaluation of immune system function, and what laboratory tests should be ordered.

■ FREQUENT RESPIRATORY TRACT INFECTIONS

The type and severity of infections should be carefully documented. Chest radiographs should be reviewed to verify the diagnosis of pneumonia and to determine whether single or multiple lobes have been involved. Foreign body aspiration is a common cause of recurrent unilobar pneumonia.

The child's risk for recurrent respiratory infection should also be explored. Children who attend day care or group child-care settings have a higher incidence of respiratory infections.[1,2] Exposure to environmental tobacco smoke in the first 2 years of life has been shown in several studies to increase the rate of respiratory illness by one-and-a half- to two-fold.[2,3] Otherwise healthy infants with frequent infections are also more likely to be bottle-fed than breast-fed.[4]

Children with normal immune function usually acquire common cold-like illnesses, whose duration is usually less than 2 weeks and from which recovery is complete. Acute otitis media (AOM) may frequently accompany viral respiratory tract infections even in the normal host, because of the fact that the pathogenesis of AOM is often related to eustachian tube dysfunction and other anatomic realities of early childhood (Chapter 2). Normal children may have frequent AOM but individual episodes usually respond to appropriate antimicrobial therapy. Because true bacterial sinusitis is less common than AOM, multiple episodes of properly diagnosed sinusitis is more suggestive of either immune deficiency or problems of mucociliary clearance such as cystic fibrosis (Chapter 22) or primary ciliary dyskinesia. Unfortunately, bacterial sinusitis can be difficult to diagnose (Chapter 5).

An isolated episode of pneumonia, either with a clinical history suggestive of viral infection or an atypical pneumonia pathogen, or with a confirmed common cause of pneumonia such as *Streptococcus pneumoniae* is not suspicious for immune deficiency. In addition, keep in mind that some parents will report that their child has had "recurrent pneumonia," when in fact the history is more compatible with multiple episodes of reactive airways disease. However, multiple episodes of radiographically documented pneumonia, pneumonia requiring hospitalization on more than one occasion, or pneumonia in concert with frequent sinusitis or episodes of otitis media should raise "red flags" in the clinician's mind. A combination of that type of history, and growth failure or developmental delay is highly suggestive of immune deficiency.

Diagnostic Possibilities in the Child with Frequent Respiratory Tract Infections

Normal Child

As previously discussed, many immunologically normal children experience frequent, transient, nonsevere respiratory tract infections, occasionally in tandem with AOM. Although there are no scientific data to buttress this claim, our practice experience suggests that many of these children are fair-skinned, blue-eyed, and blond. If the child has had

no invasive infections, is well between episodes, has a history suggestive of frequent exposure to infectious agents, is exposed to tobacco smoke in the home, has normal growth and development, has a normal physical examination, and/or has never been hospitalized for infection, the parents may be reassured that the child does not have an immune deficiency. Frequency of infections may be decreased by common sense behaviors such as frequent handwashing, decreasing exposure to environmental tobacco smoke, and removal from day care or placement in a day care with fewer children. As these children grow, their immune system strengthens and the frequency of infection naturally decreases. In general, infection and illness are less frequent in the summer months.

In addition to the modifiable factors listed above, bad luck is frequently the stated explanation for why some children experience "more than their share" of respiratory infections. However, it is likely that certain genetic polymorphisms play a role in the risk for infection. For example, mannose binding lectin (MBL) is an acute phase protein that is secreted by hepatocytes. Part of the innate immune system, it is able to activate complement via the classic pathway. Several mutant alleles in the MBL gene have been described, and about 5% of the population is homozygous for these mutant alleles; thus, they have very low levels of MBL in serum.[5] A population-based, prospective cohort study from Greenland showed that among children aged 6–17 months, MBL-insufficient children experienced 2.9 times more acute respiratory infections (95% CI, 1.8–4.8) than MBL-sufficient children.[6] There was no effect among children aged 18–23 months, suggesting that once the adaptive immune system matures, the presence of MBL is less important.

Polymorphisms in other genes that encode proteins involved in immune function are also relatively common. Examples include the 4th component of complement (C4) and the Fcγ receptor on phagocytic cells (a receptor necessary for bacteria opsonized with Ig [immunoglobulin] G to be ingested by phagocytes). Patients with either of these defects (partial C4 deficiency or the presence of an Fcγ receptor with decreased affinity for IgG-coated bacteria) appear to be at increased risk for various infections.[7]

Cystic Fibrosis (CF)

Children with CF often present in the first few years of life with a history of frequent respiratory infections and poor growth. They may have a history of slow passage of meconium in the newborn period. Parents may also state that kissing the child leaves a salty taste in the mouth. Because CF is common (prevalence ~1 in 2,500), easily diagnosed, and requires complex medical care, a sweat test for this condition should be ordered whenever the diagnosis is considered (Chapter 22).

Primary Ciliary Dyskinesia (PCD)

This is the preferred term for a group of disorders characterized by abnormal ciliary structure or function. About 50% of patients with PCD have situs inversus, in which case the term Kartagener syndrome is used. Like CF, PCD is usually transmitted in an autosomal recessive fashion. It is much less common than CF; the estimated prevalence is 1 in 20,000. However, symptoms are milder than in patients with CF, and it is probably underdiagnosed.[8] In one series of 55 children with PCD, 37 (67%) had a history of neonatal respiratory distress, 38 (69%) had situs inversus, and 42 (76%) had a history of early-onset persistent rhinorrhea. The mean age at diagnosis was 4.4 years, which is considerably younger than in most series.[9] Bronchiectasis and nasal polyps are common but do not usually manifest until the second decade of life. One group has proposed the following criteria for investigating the possibility of PCD: (a) patients with chronic otitis, rhinosinusitis, and bronchitis in whom other entities have been excluded (CF, allergy, immunologic disorders, and α_1-antitrypsin deficiency); (b) term infants with neonatal respiratory distress syndrome of unknown cause; and (c) patients with situs inversus and recurrent airway infections.[10]

The diagnosis is usually made by epithelial cell brushing from the nasal turbinates or bronchi. Ciliary beat frequency is evaluated by phase-contrast microscopy and ultrastructural changes are detected by electron microscopy. Concurrent bacterial infection can cause secondary ciliary dyskinesia, so ciliary brushings should be obtained at least 4–6 weeks after resolution of a respiratory infection.

Structural Abnormalities of the Lung

A child who has recurrent pneumonia, especially if all episodes occur in the same lobe, may have a structural abnormality that predisposes to the development of infection, such as congenital cystic adenomatoid malformation or pulmonary seques-

tration (Chapter 8). These conditions are best diagnosed by fine cut computed tomography.

Transient Hypogammaglobulinemia of Infancy (Transient Hypogammaglobulinemia of Early Childhood)[11]

Perhaps the most common of the usually symptomatic humoral immune deficiency syndromes, transient hypogammaglobulinemia of infancy may be just an exaggeration and prolongation of the physiologic gamma globulin nadir that all infants experience.[12] These children are typically well during the first 3–6 months of life, when passive antibody from their mothers provides protection against most common pathogens. As this pool of passive antibody disappears, however, these patients begin to experience recurrent respiratory tract infections. Common cold syndrome and AOM are the most common syndromes, but sinusitis, bronchiolitis, and pneumonia may also occur. Recurrent gastroenteritis or "formula intolerance" has also been described.[12] Generally, babies with this syndrome do not become infected with atypical pathogens, nor do they experience severe or life-threatening infections. In contrast to patients with X-linked agammaglobulinemia (discussed in the following text), patients with transient hypogammaglobulinemia of infancy have normal levels of circulating B cells and mount normal responses to diphtheria and tetanus immunizations.[13] Although IgG is the principal antibody isotype affected, levels of other antibodies may also be decreased. In one series of 40 patients, IgG levels were low in 30 (75%), IgA levels were low in 17 (43%), and IgM levels were low in 10 (25%). Physical examination should reveal the presence of lymphoid tissue, without lymphadenopathy. Immunoglobulin levels eventually normalize; occasionally, patients will require IVIG therapy for a few months to a year.[12,14] In most patients, immunoglobulin levels are normal by age 3 years, but in some they may be subnormal until 5 years.[14] In a few, transient hypogammaglobulinemia of infancy is a precursor of a persistent immunoglobulin problem, usually IgA deficiency.[11]

X-Linked Agammaglobulinemia (XLA, Bruton's Disease)

XLA is due to a B-cell maturational defect.[15] It is caused by a mutation in the gene encoding Bruton tyrosine kinase (BTK), a cytoplasmic protein required for the growth and development of B-cell precursors. Without it, B-cells never become antibody-secreting cells; therefore, antibody is scant to absent. Circulating B cells in the blood are similarly missing. This disorder presents similarly to transient hypogammaglobulinemia of infancy, previously described, in that the first few months of life are uneventful, attributable to passive maternal antibody. Thereafter, the child develops frequent sinopulmonary infections, mostly due to encapsulated gram-positive organisms, especially *S. pneumoniae*. Most of these bacterial infections can be readily treated with antibiotics; their frequency, however, can lead to destructive processes in the lungs and sinuses. Patients with agammaglobulinemia are also subject to severe or prolonged infections with nonenveloped viruses, especially the enteroviruses. Chronic enteroviral meningitis is an especially interesting syndrome seen almost exclusively in patients with XLA.[16] Progressive viremia and paralytic poliomyelitis secondary to live attenuated oral polio vaccine (no longer available in the United States) has also been described in these patients. T-cell function is normal or nearly so. Therefore, patients with this disorder do not suffer from fungal infections or prolonged infection with enveloped viruses, such as respiratory syncytial virus (RSV) or influenza virus. The gene defect for XLA has been located to the X chromosome at position Xq21.2-22. Carrier females are immunologically normal. Physical examination of these children is generally unremarkable except that lymphoid tissue is scant. If a patient with a compatible clinical history has no visible tonsils and no palpable lymph node enlargement, the diagnosis of XLA should be strongly considered.

Common Variable Immunodeficiency (CVID)

CVID is a complex and heterogeneous immune dysregulation syndrome characterized by hypogammaglobulinemia, recurrent bacterial infections, and a variety of immunological abnormalities. In addition to recurrent infections (primarily upper and lower respiratory infections), patients with this syndrome are also at increased risk for autoimmune disease and malignancy.[17] The incidence is approximately 1 in 100,000. The exact genetic defect is unknown, and it is likely that several different defects can result in the CVID phenotype. CVID can occur at any age; in most patients the disease does

not become clinically apparent until the second or third decade of life. Its presentation can mimic that of cystic fibrosis. Most cases are sporadic but sometimes there is a family history of CVID (or of selective IgA deficiency). Unlike patients with XLA, circulating numbers of B cells are usually normal. However, IgG, IgM, and IgA levels are all usually decreased. In at least some cases of CVID, the fundamental immunologic abnormality is probably due to a defect in T cell help.[18]

Like patients with XLA, patients with CVID experience recurrent infections (especially sinusitis, otitis media, and pneumonia) with encapsulated organisms. Diarrhea, particularly due to *Giardia*, is common. Persistent enteroviral meningitis has also been described but is less common than in patients with XLA.[19] Some patients with CVID also develop infections typical of patients with T-cell defects, such as *Pneumocystis* pneumonia.

About 20% of patients with CVID develop an autoimmune disease. Hemolytic anemia and immune thrombocytopenic purpura are the two conditions most commonly seen. Lymphoproliferation occurs in about 30% of patients and is manifested by adenopathy and splenomegaly. Some patients develop malignant lymphoma.

Hyper-IgM Syndrome

Two boys with a clinical syndrome resembling that of X-linked agammaglobulinemia who had grossly elevated levels of IgM and low to absent IgG and IgA were the first case reports of the syndrome now called Hyper-IgM syndrome. Subsequently, female cases were also reported. The phenotype is similar to that of XLA, except that patients with Hyper-IgM syndrome are also prone to some opportunistic infections, especially *Pneumocystis jiroveci* pneumonia. Patients with this syndrome also have a high incidence of autoimmune hematologic problems, including hemolytic anemia, thrombocytopenic purpura, and, especially, neutropenia. The disorder is caused by the inability to "class switch." Resting B cells express IgM; antigenic stimulation, therefore, produces IgM first. In order to produce IgG or IgA, class switching must take place. In the absence of the ability to class switch, IgM levels become elevated. Although most patients have very elevated total IgM levels (more than 1,000 mg/dL), some patients have levels in the normal range. IgG levels are usually less than 150 mg/dL and IgA is not detectable. Class switching requires two signals, one of which is the interaction of CD40 (expressed on B cells) and CD154 (CD40 ligand, expressed on T cells). Patients with the X-linked form of Hyper-IgM syndrome are incapable of producing functional CD154. This defect can be detected in utero.[20] Patients with the less common autosomal recessive variant have a different genotype. In these patients, class switching does not take place, despite appropriate cross-linking of CD40, suggesting a downstream signaling defect.[21]

Selective IgA Deficiency

IgA is the most plentiful immunoglobulin in the body. Much of it is locally produced and secreted, and the presence of specific IgA on mucosal surfaces has been shown to be protective against a variety of infections that begin with replication at those sites. These two facts, taken together, would suggest that IgA deficiency would predispose to frequent and severe infections of the respiratory and gastrointestinal tracts. However, most people with IgA deficiency do not know they are IgA deficient, as they are entirely asymptomatic.[22] It has been estimated that from 1 in 300 to 1 in 700 individuals lacks appreciable IgA, which makes IgA deficiency the most common immunoglobulin deficiency.

IgG subclass Deficiency

IgG can be divided into four different subclasses. Some people have a deficiency of one or more of these subclasses, sometimes even in the face of a normal total IgG. There is considerable controversy regarding the role of IgG subclass deficiency in patients with frequent sinopulmonary infections. Patients with frequent, nonsevere infections who have deficiencies of one or more of the IgG subclasses have certainly been described. However, subclass deficiencies can also be found in healthy control subjects, particularly children in the first 4 years of life.

The fundamental question is whether there is a difference in the function of the different IgG subclasses; if there is not, then as long as total IgG levels are normal, subclass deficiency would not be expected to cause any problems. When subclass deficiencies were first described, there were reports that IgG2 was more important in the response to polysaccharide antigens. A failure to respond well to polysaccharide antigens would certainly predispose one to the type of infections generally seen in antibody-deficient patients. However, this was an in vitro finding, and it was not supported by subsequent in vivo experiments. Many papers describing frequent and severe infections in patients who have a combination of IgA deficiency and IgG subclass deficiency have been published.[23,24] Despite this, it is not clear how much of the problem stems from the IgA deficiency, and how much, if any, is attributable to the associated IgG subclass deficiency. It is probably fair to say that IgG subclass deficiency by itself is rarely a cause of significant recurrent infectious problems. A small percentage of patients with IgG subclass deficiency later go on to develop common variable immunodeficiency. In addition, in some families, one individual will have selective IgA deficiency, another will have IgG subclass deficiency, and yet another will develop CVID. Thus, these conditions may represent a spectrum of abnormalities of B-cell maturation.

One expert has suggested the following criteria for diagnosis of clinically significant IgG subclass deficiency: (a) a history of recurrent bacterial infections, primarily respiratory; (b) impaired response to immunization with protein and/or polysaccharide antigens; (c) significant reductions in serum concentrations of one or more IgG subclasses; and (d) age 4 years or older.[25]

Failure to Respond to Polysaccharide Antigens

Antibodies to protein antigens and antibodies to polysaccharide antigens are made through different pathways. Antibodies to polysaccharides are made by thymus-independent (T-independent) pathways. These pathways are generally not well developed in children until about the age 2 years. This explains why babies do not make good responses to polysaccharide vaccines (like the 23-valent polysaccharide pneumococcal vaccine or the quadrivalent meningococcal vaccine). Some patients never really fully develop the ability to mount responses to polysaccharide antigens.[26] These patients may be plagued by recurrent infections with encapsulated bacteria, especially *S. pneumoniae*. Their immunoglobulin levels may be normal, and IgG subclasses may also be normal, although low levels of IgG2 are not uncommon.

Human Immunodeficiency Virus infection (HIV)

Although recurrent respiratory tract infections is not the usual presentation of children with untreated HIV infection, the mother's HIV status should be ascertained in all children with frequent infections, and the child should be tested for HIV antibody if the mother's status is unknown.

Early Complement Component Deficiency

Complement deficiencies are considerably less common than immunoglobulin deficiencies. Deficiency of one of the early components (especially C1q), however, closely resembles immunoglobulin deficiency. These patients generally suffer recurrent sinopulmonary infections with encapsulated bacteria (*S. pneumoniae* is the most common pathogen).[27] As a secondary effect, serum IgG may be decreased; IgG2 and IgG4 are almost always low.[28]

Patients with C3 deficiency are generally more severely affected and suffer more frequent recurrences of infection. They are also more likely to have systemic infections such as bacteremia or meningitis. About 80% of these children also develop autoimmune disorders.[27]

■ EVALUATION

Evaluation of the immune system should be undertaken when the child exceeds the expected number, type, or severity of infections. Often, the history and physical examination alone will strongly suggest that the child's immune system is normal; in that case, reassurance should be provided. The following are elements that may be included when a work-up seems indicated.

Evaluation Elements

Complete Blood Count (CBC)

Though nonspecific, much useful information can be obtained from the CBC, including the presence or absence of anemia, neutropenia, neutrophilia, eosinophilia, and lymphopenia.

Peripheral Blood Smear

The presence of Howell-Jolly bodies suggests functional or anatomic asplenia.

Immunoglobulin Levels

Most laboratories are able to provide total immunoglobulin levels in a reasonable amount of time. Generally, IgG, IgA, and IgM levels are reported unless others are specified. When hyper-IgE syndrome (discussed later) is suspected, it is advisable to ask for IgE levels as well. It is not necessary to ask for IgG subclass levels on a routine basis. Immunoglobulin levels do not provide information about the production of specific immunity, but this is still a reasonable first screening test.

Specific Antibody Titers

It is often useful to know whether the patient is able to mount an antibody response to an antigen to which he or she is known to be exposed. Most patients have had some immunizations; therefore, antibody levels against one or more of these immunogens can be obtained. Antitetanus and antidiphtheria antibody titers are commercially available. These antibodies are of the T-dependent type. To test T-independent responses, one can administer the 23-valent polysaccharide pneumococcal vaccine and measure the type-specific antibody response 1 month later. Ideally, prevaccination and postvaccination titers are measured simultaneously. If the child has previously received the 7-valent conjugated pneumococcal vaccine, one cannot ascribe a response to those 7 serotypes (4, 6, 9, 14, 18, 19, and 23) as indicative of a functional response to polysaccharide antigens. Also, recall that children younger than about 2 years are expected to have a very poor immune response to polysaccharide antigens, no matter how they are tested.

If the child has a protective antibody titer to tetanus but a low titer to diphtheria, the child should be given a booster vaccine, and the level rechecked in 2–3 weeks. If it boosts into the normal range, the patient is able to mount appropriate T-dependent antibody responses.

HIV Antibody

Unless it can be specifically proven that the child could not possibly have HIV infection, HIV antibody titer should be obtained as part of the workup of any child with frequent, recurrent, or recalcitrant infections. Infection with an opportunistic pathogen is even more suggestive of the possibility of HIV infection.

Sweat Chloride Measurement

A sweat chloride is a simple screening test for cystic fibrosis. The test results are reliable when it is performed at a site with considerable experience.

Patients with suspected CF should be referred to such a site to obtain the test.

Examination of Ciliary Structure and Function

If more common causes of recurrent respiratory infections have been ruled out, an ENT (ear, nose and throat) physician can be consulted to perform a ciliary biopsy.

Lung Imaging

A chest radiograph should be obtained to look for evidence of chronic lung disease or bronchiectasis. If the patient has a suspected anatomic abnormality or foreign body, a fine-cut chest CT (computed tomography) should be obtained.

CH50 (Total Hemolytic Complement)

A CH50 is a reasonable screening test for patients in whom early complement component deficiency is suspected.

Asthma and Allergy Testing

If suspected based on history and physical examination, pulmonary function testing in children more than 6 years old or a trial of bronchodilator therapy (children younger than 6 years) should be considered. Referral to an allergist for skin testing may be indicated if the child has symptoms suggestive of allergies (such as sneezing, itching, or a prominent seasonal component).

■ MANAGEMENT

Because the infections are not severe, patients with transient hypogammaglobulinemia of infancy usually do not require intravenous immunoglobulin replacement therapy (IVIG). They can be followed every 3–6 months for serial evaluation of their immunoglobulin status. Recovery of serum levels to normal usually occurs spontaneously sometime before the second birthday. The prognosis is excellent.

As patients with XLA are incapable of mounting antibody responses, standard vaccines need not be given. Lifetime replacement with IVIG is required. With IVIG replacement, many patients are able to lead essentially normal lives.

Unlike XLA, not all patients with CVID require monthly IVIG infusions. The decision to treat patients with IVIG should be based on measurement of the patient's functional antibody response and on the frequency and severity of recurrent infections. For patients in whom IVIG is indicated, 200–400 mg/kg is given every 3–4 weeks to maintain trough serum levels of IgG greater than 400 mg/dL.[29]

Treatment of Hyper-IgM syndrome with IVIG corrects the immune deficiency and usually also corrects neutropenia, if it is present. Some patients may require G-CSF as well.

One must be careful about the use of IVIG as a "diagnostic trial" in the patient with recurrent infections and IgG subclass deficiency. IVIG provides very effective passive immunity to many of the pathogens normally encountered in the first few years of life. For example, boys with XLA who are placed on monthly IVIG in the first few months of life have far fewer than the 6–8 colds per year that the normal child experiences.[25] This same benefit is obtained in healthy children, for whom this intervention is obviously not indicated.

IVIG is contraindicated in patients with selective IgA deficiency. These patients have IgE antibodies to IgA. Thus, minor amounts of IgA in IVIG can lead to fatal anaphylaxis.[30]

In most instances, prophylactic antibiotics are not indicated for these conditions. However, diagnosis of infections should be pursued aggressively, including the identification of the responsible organism. For severe immunodeficiency syndromes in this category (e.g., XLA, hyper-IgM syndrome), treatment often requires administration of intravenous antibiotics, at least initially. In addition, infections should generally be treated longer than in immunocompetent hosts.

■ RECURRENT ABSCESSES, FURUNCLES, BOILS, OR LYMPHADENITIS

Some children present for medical care because of superficial skin abscesses. Most of these are caused by *S. aureus* infection. It is not uncommon for a child with a normal immune system to develop a staphylococcal skin or lymph node infection. If these respond to drainage and antibiotic therapy and do not return, no further evaluation is necessary. However, some patients develop abscesses on a recurrent basis, deep-seated or solid organ abscesses, or develop abscesses that are recalcitrant to therapy. This may raise some concern about immune function.

Diagnostic Possibilities in Children with Recurrent Abscesses

Normal Child

Occasionally, a normal child will be plagued with recurrent furunculosis. Most of the time, these patients are preschoolers or teenagers. Abscesses may develop at any location, but they are always fairly superficial. They may occur in crops or singly. When the abscesses are drained and cultured, they are always staphylococcal. The isolates may be either methicillin sensitive or methicillin resistant. They always respond to drainage and antibiotic therapy. The period of time between recurrences varies. The physical examination is entirely normal except for the abscess(es).

Children with recurrent furunculosis are almost always nasal carriers of staphylococci. The pathogenesis involves recurrent self-inoculation with the organisms that reside in the nasopharynx. Therapy consists of an attempt to break the cycle of recurrences by (i) eradicating the nasal carriage of staphylococci, and (ii) keeping the skin and fingers as clean as possible.

Most patients who present with recurrent furunculosis are immunologically normal. In the absence of any other finding, treating the patient with drugs that eradicate carriage and providing education about the pathophysiology of the abscesses is enough to eradicate the condition (Chapter 17).

Hyper IgE Syndrome (Job Syndrome, Job-Buckley Syndrome)

Hyper IgE syndrome is now known to be a systemic disease, of which immune deficiency is one manifestation. Affected patients typically suffer from moderate to severe atopic dermatitis and recurrent staphylococcal skin abscesses. The facies is often described as coarse. They may also develop pneumonia with pneumatocele or abscess formation. Serum immunoglobulin E levels are extremely elevated (usually greater than 2,000 IU/mL), but tend to decrease over time.

In one series of 30 patients with hyper IgE syndrome, all patients over the age of 8 years had systemic manifestations, principally of the teeth and bones.[31] Three-quarters had failure or delay of primary tooth shedding, presumably due to lack of root resorption. More than half had recurrent long-bone fractures, about 70% had hyperextensible joints, and by the age of 16 years, 75% had scoliosis.

The syndrome is inherited in an autosomal dominant fashion with variable penetrance.[31] The gene has been linked to the proximal part of chromosome 4q.[32] The actual immunologic defect is decreased neutrophil chemotaxis, and probably a TH1/TH2 imbalance due to impaired production of interferon-gamma.[33] Some patients develop T-cell lymphomas.[34] Cases of fungal lung abscess and cryptococcal meningitis in patients with Hyper-IgE have been reported.[35,36] Treatment is with antistaphylococcal antibiotics and sometimes with intravenous immune globulin.[37] Bone marrow transplant is not helpful.[38]

Chronic Granulomatous Disease (CGD)

CGD is a rare disorder in which leukocytes are able to ingest microbes but not are not able to adequately kill them once they are ingested. The problem stems from defects in any of the four subunits of NADPH oxidase, pivotal in forming reactive oxygen species used for killing. About 70% of affected individuals have the X-linked form, which tends to be the most severe. The remaining forms are autosomal recessive.

Patients with CGD tend to have recurrent and recalcitrant infections with catalase-positive organisms. Specifically, infections with S. aureus, Serratia marcescens, Burkholderia cepacia, Aspergillus spp, and Nocardia spp are troublesome. Abscesses of the liver, lungs, or other organs often occur, and must be approached aggressively with prompt surgical drainage and intravenous antibiotics. Bone infections in patients with CGD tend to be caused by Serratia marcescens. Signs and symptoms of serious infections may be subtle or appear late, so vigilance is required. In one series of 61 hepatic abscesses in 22 patients, 29 (48%) of them were recurrent, and 20 (33%) were persistent. Fever was the predominant presenting complaint. The erythrocyte sedimentation rate was increased in almost all.[39] Although the surgical complication rate was 56%, surgery plus antibiotic therapy eradicated all the infections. Eighty-eight percent of surgical aspirates grew S. aureus in culture.[39] Patients may develop granulomas in the gastrointestinal or genitourinary tracts, leading to symptoms of obstruction. The diagnosis is suspected in patients who present with frequent severe infection or with specific infections that would be rare in those without CGD, namely, staphylococcal abscesses of organs or soft tissues at an early age, *Serratia* osteomyelitis at any age, pulmonary or disseminated nocardiosis, or invasive aspergillus infection. The nitroblue tetrazolium (NBT) test is used to screen for CGD and flow cytometry is used for confirmation.

Daily trimethoprim-sulfamethoxazole (TMP-SMX) reduces the incidence of severe bacterial infection without altering the risk for fungal infection.[40] Fungal infections can be reduced by giving itraconazole.[41] Liquid formulations are better absorbed than the pill form. Most experts also feel that interferon-gamma helps to reduce the number of invasive bacterial infections.[42]

Bone marrow transplant has been fraught with difficulty and bad outcomes. Some have reported good success rates using myeloablative bone marrow transplant with haploidentical sibling donors;[43] others have used nonmyeloablative transplants using T-cell depleted allografts.[44] Gene therapy has been only transiently successful in the research setting and is not used.

Hyper-IgM Syndrome

This syndrome, previously discussed, is sometimes accompanied by frequent abscess formation.

Evaluation of the Child with Recurrent Abscesses

Serum Immunoglobulins

Patients with hyper IgE syndrome usually have extremely elevated levels of IgE, almost always greater than 2,000 IU/mL. Most patients with hyper IgM syndrome have elevated levels of IgM and depressed levels of IgA and IgG.

Nitroblue Tetrazolium Test

This test is performed by placing a yellow dye in contact with the patient's phagocytic cells in the laboratory. In normal persons, the presence of oxygen radicals turns the dye blue, whereas cells from patients with CGD are unable to reduce the dye. Results are reported as percent activity, as some patients with CGD retain some activity. Female carriers of the disease have approximately 50% of normal activity, but are not clinically symptomatic. Although a useful screening test, both false positives and false negatives occur. If the NBT test is negative

and CGD is strongly suspected, a direct test of neutrophil oxidative burst using flow cytometric methods should be performed.[45]

Management

The management of the immunologically normal child with recurrent furunculosis is discussed in the previous text, and in more detail in Chapter 17. Patients with hyper-IgE syndrome or CGD should be referred to subspecialists in infectious diseases and immunology, as their care is complex. Those with hyper-IgE syndrome need monthly immunoglobulin therapy. Those with CGD may receive TMP-SMX, itraconazole, and possibly injections of interferon gamma.

Infection with Fungi or Other Opportunistic Pathogens

Patients who develop infections with organisms that possess little inherent virulence almost always have some disorder of the immune system. In patients with severe immunodeficiency states, eradication of these infections can be difficult. People with T-cell defects (cellular immune deficiencies) have difficulty eradicating viral infections, especially those caused by enveloped viruses (RSV, influenza, parainfluenza, herpes group viruses, and the like). They also have problems controlling fungal infections, and may present with persistent or aggressive thrush, or skin or pulmonary fungal infections. There are several patterns of infection that can be seen. These will be discussed separately although there may be considerable overlap in how patients present.

Early-onset Fulminant *Pneumocystis jiroveci (formerly carinii)* Pneumonia (PCP)

Pneumocystis jiroveci is everywhere in the environment. Typically, infection with PCP does not cause any symptoms because it is rapidly eliminated by the immune system. Patients with severe immune deficiency states may become very sick from PCP during the first few months of life. They present to the hospital hypoxic and in florid respiratory distress. Many require mechanical ventilation and aggressive supportive care.

Diagnostic Possibilities in the Child with Early-Onset Fulminant PCP

Severe Combined Immunodeficiency (SCID)

SCID is the appellation given to a genetically heterogenous group of disorders that have in common severe impairment of both the cellular and humoral arms of the immune system. The incidence is estimated to range from 1 in 50,000 to 1 in 500,000 births.[46] The most common cause in the United States is deficiency of the common gamma chain of the interleukin-2 receptor. This results from a mutation in the gene for the common gamma chain, which is located on the X chromosome, and accounts for almost half of all cases.[46] The protein in question is called the "common gamma chain" because it is common to cell-surface receptors of five different interleukin molecules, explaining why its functional absence results is severe deficiency in B cells, T cells, and natural killer cells.[47] The next most common form is autosomal recessive SCID, seen in about a fifth of patients. Adenosine deaminase (ADA) deficiency, one of the earliest described causes of the syndrome, accounts for about 15%.

Despite the variety of causes, all share in common a profound inability to fight off infections. The absolute lymphocyte count is low in nearly all cases. Levels of serum immunoglobulins are low (due to placental transfer) or absent. Lymph nodes, tonsils, and thymic tissue are scant or absent. Patients often have a history of poor growth and/or persistent diarrhea before presenting with fulminant PCP. In addition to PCP, babies with SCID can suffer life-threatening infections with varicella, RSV, adenovirus, parainfluenza viruses, CMV (cytomegalovirus), EBV (Epstein-Barr virus), or fungi. Babies from other countries may have disseminated infection with BCG (the live-attenuated tuberculosis vaccine). The mean age at diagnosis is 6 months.[46] SCID is uniformly fatal during infancy or early childhood if not treated with bone marrow transplant.

AIDS

Early-onset fulminant PCP was once a fairly common way for a baby infected with HIV to come to medical attention. Fortunately, this presentation is becoming quite scarce, thanks to the institution of universal screening of pregnant women for antibody to HIV and careful follow-up of their babies. Those who are found to be HIV infected are placed on TMP-SMX until the age of 1 year, regardless of CD4 cell count, because in babies the CD4 cell count is not predictive of who is at-risk for severe PCP. Occasionally, a woman without prenatal care will deliver a baby who develops fulminant PCP.

■ EVALUATION

Methods

Complete Blood Count

Most babies with SCID have a decreased absolute lymphocyte count (ALC). Lymphopenia in an infant should never be ignored, even if it is detected incidentally. The mean ALC in a 6-month-old is 6,500/mcL and the lower limit of normal is 4,000/mcL. For a 2-month-old, the corresponding values are 6,000/mcL and 3,000/mcL, respectively.[48]

About 5% of infants with SCID have normal or elevated lymphocyte counts, presumably from transplacental passage and subsequent expansion.[46]

HIV Antibody

HIV should be ruled out in any patient with early-onset PCP, as HIV infection is many times more common than SCID.

Serum Immunoglobulins

Serum immunoglobulins will be low in babies with SCID. However, most infants will have some passively acquired IgG if tested in the first 6 months of life.

■ TREATMENT

The patient should be admitted to an intensive care unit, and if PCP is suspected, therapy with intravenous TMP-SMX be started. An intensivist, an infectious disease specialist, and an immunologist should be involved in the child's care. Getting the baby through the acute episode is the primary concern, and then making a diagnosis. If SCID is strongly suspected by the presentation and laboratory values, arrangements for transfer to a center experienced in pediatric bone marrow transplant should be made. A pediatric infectious diseases specialist can manage the child with AIDS. In either case, prophylactic TMP-SMX should be given. The child with SCID will probably require IVIG prior to transfer. Patients with SCID should not receiveany vaccines (they will not respond to inactivated vaccines and they can develop fatal infections from live-attenuated ones).

■ CANDIDIASIS (PERSISTENT THRUSH; ESOPHAGEAL OR TRACHEOBRONCHIAL CANDIDIASIS; PERSISTENT SKIN AND MUCOUS MEMBRANE CANDIDIASIS)

Infants less than 6 months of age often suffer from oral candidiasis (thrush), and it may be difficult to eradicate, even in the absence of immune deficiency. These babies may be frequently reinoculated with the organism via bottles, pacifiers, or even the breast-feeding mother's nipples. Thrush after the age of 6 months is uncommon and should make the clinician suspect immunodeficiency. Candidiasis of the esophagus or tracheobronchial tree is suggestive of severe T-cell immunodeficiency at any age. Chronic fungal infection of the nails does not necessarily imply immunodeficiency, but when multiple nails, the skin, and the mucous membranes are involved it is suggestive of chronic mucocutaneous candidiasis, discussed in the following text.

Diagnostic Possibilities in the Child with Candidiasis

Severe Combined Immunodeficiency (SCID)

Discussed earlier.

22q11.2 Deletion Syndrome (DiGeorge Syndrome, Velocardiofacial Syndrome, Conotruncal Anomaly Face Syndrome [Takao Syndrome])

Microdeletion of a portion of the 22q11.2 gene produces a variety of abnormalities of tissues derived from the third and fourth pharyngeal pouch tissues, including the cardiac outflow tract, thymus, and parathyroid gland. These abnormalities are now referred to as 22q11 deletion syndrome. Complete DiGeorge syndrome is the most serious in terms of immunologic deficits, as these patients lack T-cell activity. Despite the serious nature of the immune problem, patients usually present with other problems associated with this phenotype, such as with seizures or tetany from hypocalcemia, or in florid congestive heart failure from an interrupted aortic

arch. The complete DiGeorge syndrome also includes a typical facies, with short palpebral fissures, a short philtrum and small mouth, and sometimes micrognathia. Cleft or high-arched palate may also be seen. Learning and speech delays, feeding problems with growth failure, and musculoskeletal defects are common but lesser known; long-term neurological problems are rare but have been described.[49] Growth is usually poor in the first years of life, but obesity is common in those who survive to adolescence.[50]

The degree of impairment of cellular immunity varies greatly. In some cases, although decreased T-cell counts are usually found in the peripheral blood, functional cellular immunity is preserved.[51] Additionally, T-cell immunity usually improves over time.[52]

Although classically thought of as a pure cellular immunodeficiency, some patients may have concomitant humoral shortcomings. In one cohort of 32 patients with 22q11 deletion syndrome, 26 (81%) had recurrent infections, and of those, half had abnormal serum immunoglobulin levels and just over half had blunted humoral response to pneumococcal polysaccharide vaccination.[53] The phenotype of 22q11 deletion syndrome varies widely, even in patients with identical genotypes. Monozygotic twins may be variously affected, for example.[54] The genetic abnormality may arise de novo, or the genotype (but not phenotype) may be inherited in an autosomal dominant fashion.[55] Asymptomatic close relatives may also harbor the genetic aberration.[56]

The diagnosis should be suspected in any patient with dysmorphic features, cardiac outflow tract defect, and recurrent infections. The diagnosis is established by fluorescent in situ hybridization (FISH). Treatment of the immune defect is primarily supportive. Patients with less than 15% CD4 cells/mcL and those with functional T-cell abnormalities should receive *Pneumocystis* prophylaxis with TMP-SMX.[57]

One group of researchers restored T-cell function by transplanting thymic tissue into the muscles of the thigh.[58] This technique is still experimental at this time.

HIV/AIDS

Discussed above, and in chapter 20.

Hyper-IgE Syndrome

In one review, 25 (83%) of 30 patients with hyper-IgE syndrome (previously described) also had chronic candidiasis of the mucous membranes and nails.[31]

Chronic Mucocutaneous Candidiasis (CMC).

CMC is the name given to a heterogeneous group of disorders that share in common the predilection toward chronic, recurrent, or recalcitrant candidiasis of the mucous membranes, skin, and/or nails. Invasive candidiasis is rare. There are at least five clinically distinct forms of importance in pediatrics: (a) chronic oral candidiasis; (b) familial chronic mucocutaneous candidiasis, which has its onset by age 2 years and is seen mostly in families with consanguinity; (c) autoimmune polyendocrinopathy-candidiasis-ectodermal dystrophy, discussed in the following text; (d) chronic localized candidiasis, in which patients develop exuberant lesions commonly called "candidal granulomas" or "cutaneous horns;" and (e) candidiasis with chronic keratitis, which is autosomal dominantly inherited and often associated with alopecia areata or totalis.[59] A sixth form, called CMC with thymoma, is only seen in older adults. The autoimmune polyendocrinopathy form deserves special mention. It is an autosomal recessive disease and has been linked to chromosome 21.[60] Most patients eventually develop disorders of two or more endocrine glands, the most commonly affected being the parathyroid, the adrenal, and the ovaries.[61] The usual presenting symptoms are recalcitrant thrush and candidal diaper dermatitis, and the endocrinopathy may not develop until adulthood. Therefore, yearly endocrine evaluations are recommended for patients with CMC. These patients may also develop alopecia.

Accompanying disorders are seen in many patients with CMC. Approximately two-thirds of patients have enamel dysplasia, 50% have dystrophy of the nails, 25% have alopecia, 20% have malabsorption, and 10% have autoimmune hepatitis, keratoconjunctivitis, or vitiligo.[59] For most patients, the immune defect is specific for species of candida. In the typical case, their T-cells are unable either to proliferate properly or to produce appropriate cytokines in response to stimulation with candidal antigens.[59] Some patients have features overlapping with common variable immunodeficiency. TH1-type cytokine responses (especially interleukin-2) are most likely to be aberrant;[62] these cytokines are critical to cytotoxic T-cell responses, so important in immunity to fungi.

The diagnosis is clinical. The patient's T-cell responses to common mitogens and to candidal antigens can be tested at some referral laboratories. Treatment is with antifungal agents. Because antifungals do not correct the underlying immune defect, recurrence of the clinical problem after cessation of therapy is common.

Myeloperoxidase Deficiency

Myeloperoxidase is the principal component of azurophilic granules. Its deficiency is the most common genetic disorder of neutrophils.[63] Thankfully, most people with myeloperoxidase deficiency are entirely asymptomatic. The exception is when patients with myeloperoxidase deficiency also have other chronic conditions, most commonly diabetes mellitus. These patients are prone to disseminated candidiasis.[64] The diagnosis of myeloperoxidase deficiency should be considered in patients with diabetes mellitus who develop invasive candidiasis. The diagnosis is established by peroxidase staining on peripheral blood.

Evaluation of the Child with Invasive or Persistent Candidiasis

Careful history and physical examination must be performed, with special attention to associated features of the above disorders, as described. The patient should be tested for antibody to HIV by ELISA. Other testing depends upon the specifics of the clinical situation, as described in the individual sections.

Treatment

Oral or intravenous fluconazole, or intravenous amphotericin B may be indicated, depending upon the severity and distribution of the candidal infection. Fungal cultures and susceptibility testing are indicated. Treatment aimed at eliminating or abrogating the underlying cause may be required, depending upon the predisposing condition. Consultation with an expert in pediatric infectious diseases or an immunologist is usually advisable.

■ RECURRENT INVASIVE NEISSERIAL INFECTION

More than one episode of invasive neisserial infection (whether meningococcal or gonococcal) is highly suspicious for the presence of either a late component complement defect (LCCD) (especially

C6, C7, or C8 deficiency) or an alternative component defect (virtually always properdin deficiency). Patients with late complement deficiencies cannot form the membrane attack complex (MAC) needed to lyse *Neisseria* spp. Two-thirds of all patients with late complement component deficiencies suffer at least one meningococcal infection, and about half have recurrent disease. Recurrent infection is less common with C9 or properdin deficiencies.

There are several features of meningococcal disease that differ between patients with and without late complement component defects. In the normal host, the average age at the time of infection is 3 years, and more than 50% of all infections occur prior to age 5 years. In the patient with LCCD, the average age at time of first infection is between 14 and 17 years. Patients with LCCD tend to be infected with less common serogroups such as Y and W-135. They sometimes develop invasive infection with "nonpathogenic" species of *Neisseria*, such as *N. lactamica* and *N. subflava*. Both recurrence and relapse (defined as recurrent symptoms within 1 month caused by the same serotype) are much more common in those with LCCD. Interestingly, patients with LCCD tend to be less sick during meningococcal infection than do immune competent hosts, and the mortality rate is 10 times lower. (reference)

Assaying for complement deficiency with CH50 is a low-yield, but relatively cheap and important intervention in patients with invasive meningococcal or gonococcal disease. Certainly, older patients with unusual serogroups merit the test. Some experts advise testing all patients. Patients proven to have complement deficiency can have the risk of repeat meningococcal disease decreased considerably by meningococcal vaccination.[65]

■ IMMUNODEFICIENCY SYNDROMES IN WHICH ASSOCIATED FINDINGS MAY DOMINATE THE CLINICAL PICTURE

22q11.2 Deletion Ssyndrome

Described in detail above, in the section on opportunistic infections.

Wiskott-Aldrich Syndrome (WAS)

WAS is an X-linked disorder marked by moderate to severe eczema, thrombocytopenia, and variable immunodeficiency. It is caused by mutations in the gene encoding the Wiskott-Aldrich Syndrome Protein (WASP). WASP is important to actin polymerization and thus to the cytoskeleton of hematopoietic cells. Immunologic events depend on actin reorganization in response to signals that come from the cell surface through the T-cell receptor and Fc-gamma receptors.[66] The genotype is variable. Carrier females are almost never affected. The phenotype of WAS varies as well; cases that were originally called X-linked thrombocytopenia have been reclassified as WAS based on information from molecular diagnostic tests.[67] In addition to immunodeficiency, patients with WAS are prone to having autoimmune conditions or IgA nephropathy.[68] They also have an increased incidence of hematopoietic cancers.[68]

The diagnosis of WAS should be entertained in male patients with refractory thrombocytopenia, with or without eczema and recurrent infection. The diagnosis can be established by protein techniques (immunoblots) or by flow cytometry. Prenatal diagnosis by PCR (polymerase chain reaction) is now possible.[69] Treatment is with bone marrow transplantation. Obtaining marrow from a haploidentical sibling produces the best results, although unrelated donor marrow leads to approximately the same outcome provided the transplant is performed prior to age 5 years.[70] Small series of patients with severe T-cell defects treated with umbilical cord blood stem cells have shown promising results.[71] In vitro, transfection of cell lines by a retrovirus that expresses the WASP gene fully restores function,[72] suggesting a possible future role for gene therapy.

Ataxia-Telangiectasia

As the name implies, this disorder causes ataxia and conjunctival telangiectasias, along with a variable degree of immunodeficiency, usually manifest as recurrent sinopulmonary infections. The disease is due to an autosomal recessive defect in the Ataxia-Telangiectasia Mutant (ATM) gene, which is important in repairing oxidative and irradiative damage to DNA.[73,74] For this reason, patients with ataxia-telangiectasia are also subject to an increased risk of cancers, especially breast cancer in females.[75,76] Cases of unusual tumors, including EBV-driven leiomyosarcomas, such as those seen in children with HIV, have been reported.[77] Immunologic testing in these patients shows a decreased number of naïve CD4 and CD8 T-lymphocytes,[78] reflecting restricted diversity of both the B- and T-cell repertoires.[79]

B-cell receptor signaling is normal,[80] and terminal differentiation into effector cells is likewise normal. About 50–80% have selective IgA deficiency.[79]

The diagnosis is made clinically. Patients may have elevated serum alpha-fetoprotein levels.[81] In vitro colony survival assay in response to irradiation can be helpful in establishing the diagnosis. Less than 21% of the cells from patients with ataxia-telangiectasia survive irradiation, versus greater than 36% of cells from unaffected controls.[82]

Chediak-Higashi Syndrome

This is a rare autosomal recessive disorder in which malfunction of secretory lysosomes results in partial oculocutaneous albinism, hematologic abnormalities, immune suppression, and, often, a progressive debilitating peripheral neuropathy caused by axonal dysfunction. The genetic cause is a mutation of the LYST gene, which is important in lysosomal trafficking. Patients usually suffer recurrent bacterial infections. Immunologic defects include impaired chemotaxis and decreased natural killer cell function.[83] In vitro, cells from patients with Chediak-Higashi syndrome do not produce as much myeloperoxidase as do control cells,[84] which suggests decreased white blood cell killing. There appear to be multiple forms of the disease, all with differing severities; genotype predicts phenotype.[85] The majority of affected patients, however, have the severe form, which may follow a biphasic course because many patients enter into an "accelerated phase," caused by nonmalignant lymphohistiocytic infiltration of multiple organs,[86] leading to repeated infections and bleeding complications, often ending in death.[87] Bone marrow transplantation restores immune function, but, unfortunately, does not seem to change the neurological outcome.[88]

Leukocyte Adhesion Deficiency (LAD)

LAD (type I) is an autosomal recessive disorder caused by mutations in the CD18 gene, which encodes the beta subunit of a number of different cell surface integrins.[89] Integrins are adhesion molecules on white blood cells that enable them to adhere to endothelial cell surfaces, which they must do in order to leave the circulation and migrate to sites of infection. This inability of the white blood cells to travel to sites of trauma or infection leads to several predictable clinical features of the disease: (i) delayed umbilical cord separation with or without omphalitis; (ii) poor wound healing; (iii) decreased pus formation; (iv) elevated peripheral blood white cell counts; and (v) recurrent bacterial and fungal infections of skin and mucous membranes.[90] Varying severities have been described. In some cases, deeper infections such as pneumonia, sinusitis, or mastoiditis occur. Other patients suffer from recurrent ulcerative lesions of the skin. Patients with LAD have high white blood cell counts even when they are well, and they can be extremely high (greater than 50,000/dL) during illnesses.

The diagnosis is established by assaying for the presence of CD11/CD18 by flow cytometry. Although retroviral gene transfer has reestablished expression of CD18 in vitro,[91] successful treatment of LAD still requires bone marrow transplantation.[92]

A separate autosomal recessive condition termed LAD type II is associated with severe mental retardation, seizures, growth failure, and microcephaly. As with LAD type I, there is defective pus formation and a failure of neutrophil recruitment to sites of inflammation. The leukocyte defect is caused by a lack of fucosylated cell-surface proteins on neutrophils.[93]

Cyclic Neutropenia

In this condition, defects in the neutrophil elastase gene[94] cause patients to have profound neutropenia on a cyclic basis, generally every 21 days. Periods of neutropenia last 3–6 days. Neutropenic episodes are usually accompanied by fever; thus, periodic fever accompanied by mild malaise may dominate the clinical picture (Chapter 10). Oral ulcerations, gingivitis, or periodontal disease is also common. During periods of neutropenia, these patients are prone to infection. Most patients suffer only minor skin or respiratory tract infections.[95] However, patients with cyclic neutropenia are at risk for severe opportunistic infections. Some have contracted life-threatening diseases such as *Clostridium septicum* septicemia, normally only seen in patients with hematologic malignancies.[96] Careful attention to dental hygiene may thwart the progression of periodontal disease.[97] Definitive treatment is with granulocyte colony-stimulating factor (G-CSF).[95]

Other Genetic Syndromes

Multiple genetic syndromes are associated with various immune defects. In addition to those previously discussed, others include ICF (immuno-deficiency, centromeric instability, facial anomaly) syndrome; Nijmegen breakage syndrome; Bloom syndrome; cartilage-hair hypoplasia; Griscelli syndrome; and Schimke immunoosseus dysplasia.[98]

Other genetic syndromes in which immune dysfunction is an occasional feature are short-limb skeletal dysplasia, Omenn syndrome, hypohidrotic and anhidrotic ectodermal dysplasia, Cohen syndrome, Kabuki syndrome, Roifman syndrome, deletion of chromosome 10p14-p13, partial deletion of chromosome 4p, and CHARGE association.[98]

The reader is referred to the review by Ming and colleagues for a detailed description of the genetic syndromes and their associated immune defects.[98]

■ REFERENCES

1. Wald ER, Dashefsky B, Byers C, et al. Frequency and severity of infections in day care. J Pediatr 1998;112(4):540–6.
2. Fleming DW, Cochi SL, Hightower AW, et al. Childhood upper respiratory tract infections: to what degree is incidence affected by day-care attendance? Pediatrics 1987;79(1):55–60.
3. Li JS, Peat JK, Xuan W, et al. Meta-analysis on the association between environmental tobacco smoke (ETS) exposure and the prevalence of lower respiratory tract infection in early childhood. Pediatr Pulmonol 1999;27:5–13.
4. Oddy WH, Sly PD, de Klerk NH, et al. Breast feeding and respiratory morbidity in infancy: a birth cohort study. Arch Dis Child 2003;88:224–8.
5. Babovic-Vuksanovic D, Snow K, Ten RM. Mannose-binding lectin (MBL) deficiency. Variant alleles in a midwestern population of the United States. Ann Allergy Asthma Immunol 1999;82:134–43.
6. Koch A, Melbye M, Sorensen P, et al. Acute respiratory tract infections and mannose-binding lectin insufficiency during early childhood. JAMA 2001;285:1316–21.
7. Winkelstein JA, Childs B. Why do some individuals have more infections than others? JAMA 2001;285:1348–9.
8. Meeks M, Bush A. Primary ciliary dyskinesia (PCD). Pediatr Pulmonol 2000;29:307–16.
9. Coren ME, Meeks M, Morrison I, et al. Primary ciliary dyskinesia: age at diagnosis and symptom history. Acta Paediatr 2002;91:667–9.
10. Holzmann D, Ott PM, Felix H. Diagnostic approach to primary ciliary dyskinesia: a review. Eur J Pediatr 2000;159:95-8.
11. McGeady SJ. Transient hypogammaglobulinemia of infancy: need to reconsider name and definition. J Pediatr 1987;110:47–50.
12. Cano F, Mayo DR, Ballow M. Absent specific viral antibodies in patients with transient hypogammaglobulinemia of infancy. J Allergy Clin Immunol 1990;85:510–3.
13. Dressler F, Peter HH, Muller W, et al. Transient hypogammaglobulinemia of infancy: five new cases, review of the literature and redefinition. Acta Paediatr Scand 1989;78:767–84.

14. Kilic SS, Tezcan I, Sanal O, et al. Transient hypogammaglobulinemia of infancy: clinical and immunologic features of 40 new cases. Pediatr Int 2000;42:647–50.
15. de Weers M, Verschuren MCM, Kraakman MEM, et al. The Bruton's tyrosine kinase gene is expressed throughout B cell differentiation, from early precursor B cell stages preceding immunoglobulin gene rearrangement up to mature B cell stages. Eur J Immunol 1993;23:3109–14.
16. McKinney RE Jr, Katz SL, Wilfert CM. Chronic enteroviral meningoencephalitis in agammaglobulinemic patients. Rev Infect Dis 1987;9:334–56.
17. Sneller MC. Common variable immunodeficiency. Am J Med Sci 2001;321:42–8.
18. Wright JJ, Wagner DK, Blaese RM, et al. Characterization of common variable immunodeficiency: identification of a subset of patients with distinctive immunophenotypic and clinical features. Blood 1990;76:2046–51.
19. Rotbart HA, Webster AD, Pleconaril Treatment Registry Group. Treatment of potentially life-threatening enterovirus infections with pleconaril. Clin Infect Dis 2001;32:228–35.
20. DiSanto JP, Markiewicz S, Gauchat J-F, et al. Prenatal diagnosis of X-linked hyper-IgM syndrome. N Engl J Med 1994;330:969–73.
21. Revy P, Muto T, Levy Y, et al. Activation-induced cytidine deaminasae (AID) deficiency causes the autosomal recessive form of the hyper-IgM syndrome. Cell 2000;102:565–75.
22. Weber-Mzell D, Kotanko P, Hauer AL, et al. Gender, age, and seasonal effects on IgA deficiency: a study of 7293 Caucasians. Eur J Clin Invest 2004;34:224–8.
23. Oxelius VA, Laurell AB, Lindquist B, et al. IgG subclasses in selective IgA deficiency: importance of IgG2-IgA deficiency. N Engl J Med 1981;304:1476–7.
24. Ugazio AG, Out TA, Plebani A, et al. Recurrent infections in children with "selective" IgA deficiency: association with IgG2 and IgG4 deficiency. Birth Defects 1983;19:169–72.
25. Lawton AR. IgG subclass deficiency and the day-care generation. Pediatr Infect Dis J 1999;18:462–6.
26. Gigliotti F, Herro HG, Kalwinsky DK, et al. Immunodeficiency associated with recurrent infections and an isolated in vivo inability to respond to bacterial polysaccharides. Pediatr Infect Dis J 1988;7:417–20.
27. Densen P. Chapter 19. Complement Deficiencies and Infection. In: Volanakis JE, Frank MM, eds. The human complement system in health and disease. New York: Marcel Dekker Inc., 1998:409–21.
28. Bird P, Lachmann PJ. The regulation of IgG subclass production in man: low serum IgG4 in inherited deficiencies of the classical pathway of C3 activation. Eur J Immunol 1988;18:1217–22.
29. Sneller MC. Common variable immunodeficiency. [Review] Am J Med Sci 2001;321:42–8.
30. Burks AW, Sampson HA, Buckley RH. Anaphylactic reactions after gamma globulin administration in patients with hypogammaglobulinemia. Detection of IgE antibodies to IgA. N Engl J Med 1986;314:560–4.
31. Grimbacher B, Holland SM, Gallin JI, et al. Hyper-IgE syndrome with recurrent infections—an autosomal dominant multisystem disorder. N Engl J Med 1999;340:692–702.
32. Grimbacher B, Schaffer AA, Holland SM, et al. Genetic

linkage of hyper IgE syndrome to chromosome 4. Am J Hum Genet 1999;65:735–44.

33. Borges WG, Augustine NH, Hill HR. Defective interleukin-12/interferon-gamma pathway in patients with hyperimmunoglobulinemia E syndrome. J Pediatr 2000;136:176–80.

34. Chang SE, Huh J, Choi JH, et al. A case of hyper-IgE syndrome complicated by cutaneous, nodal, and liver peripheral T cell lymphomas. J Dermatol 2002;29:320–2.

35. Santambrogio L, Nosotti M, Pavoni G, et al. Pneumatocele complicated by fungal lung abscess in Job's syndrome. Successful lobectomy with the aid of videothoracoscopy. Scand Cardiovasc J 1997;31:177–9.

36. Garty BZ, Wolach B, Ashkenazi S, et al. Cryptococcal meningitis in a child with hyperimmunoglobulin E syndrome. Pediatr Allergy Immunol 1995;6:175–7.

37. Bilora F, Petrobelli F, Boccioletti V, et al. Moderate-dose intravenous immunoglobulin treatment of Job's syndrome. Case report. Minerva Med 2000;91:113–6.

38. Gennery AR, Flood TJ, Abinun M, et al. Bone marrow transplantation does not correct the hyper IgE syndrome. Bone Marrow Transplant 2000;25:1303–5.

39. Lublin M, Bartlett DL, Danforth DN, et al. Hepatic abscess in patients with chronic granulomatous disease. Ann Surg 2002;235:383–91.

40. Margolis DH, Melnick DA, Alling DW, et al. Trimethoprim-sulfamethoxazole prophylaxis in the management of chronic granulomatous disease. J Infect Dis 1990;162:723–6.

41. Gallin JI, Alling DW, Malech HL, et al. Itraconazole to prevent fungal infections in chronic granulomatous disease. N Engl J Med 2003;348:2416–22.

42. The International Chronic Granulomatous Disease Cooperative Study Group. A controlled trial of interferon gamma to prevent infection in chronic granulomatous disease. N Engl J Med 1991;324:509–16.

43. Seger RA, Gungor T, Belohradsky BH, et al. Treatment of chronic granulomatous disease with myeloablative conditioning and an unmodified hematopoietic allograft: a survey of the European experience 1985-2000. Blood 2002;100:4344–50.

44. Horwitz ME, Barrett AJ, Brown MR, et al. Treatment of chronic granulomatous disease with nonmyeloablative conditioning and a T-cell depleted hematopoietic allograft. N Engl J Med 2001;22:881–8.

45. O'Gorman MR, Corrochano V. Rapid whole-blood flow cytometry assay for diagnosis of chronic granulomatous disease. Clin Diagn Lab Immunol 1995;2:227–32.

46. Buckley RH, Schiff RI, Schiff SE, et al. Human severe combined immunodeficiency: genetic, phenotypic, and functional diversity in one hundred eight infants. J Pediatr 1997;130:378–87.

47. Buckley RH. Primary immunodeficient diseases due to defects in lymphocytes. N Engl J Med 2000;343:1313–24.

48. Gossage DL, Buckley RH. Prevalence of lymphocytopenia in severe combined immunodeficiency.[comment]. N Engl J Med 1990;323:1422–3.

49. Roubertie A, Semprino M, Chaze AM, et al. Neurological presentation of three patients with 22q11 deletion (CATCH 22 syndrome). Brain Dev 2001;23:810–4.

50. Diglio MC, Marino B, Cappa M, et al. Auxological evaluation in patients with DiGeorge/velocardiofacial syndrome (deletion 22q11.2 syndrome. Genet Med 2001;3:30–3.

51. Martin Mateos MA, Perez Duenas BP, Iriondo M, et al. Clinical and immunological spectrum of partial DiGeorge syndrome. J Investig Allerg Clin Immunol 2000;10:352–60.

52. Pierdominici M, Marziali M, Giovannetti A, et al. T cell receptor repertoire and function in patients with DiGeorge syndrome and velocardiofacial syndrome. Clin Exp Immunol 2000;121:127–32.

53. Gennery AR, Barge D, O'Sullivan JJ, et al. Antibody deficiency and autoimmunity in 22q11.2 deletion syndrome. Arch Dis Child 2002;86:422–5.

54. Goodship J, Cross I, Scambler P, et al. Monozygotic twins with chromosome 2q11 deletion and discordant phenotype. J Med Genet 1995;32:746–8.

55. Cuneo BF. 22q11.2 deletion syndrome: DiGeorge, velocardiofacial, and conotruncal anomaly face syndromes. Curr Opin Pediatr 2001;13:465–72.

56. McDonald-McGinn DM, Tonnesen MK, Laufer-Cahana A, et al. Phenotype of the 22q11.2 deletion in individuals identified through an affected relative: cast a wide FISHing net! Gent Med 2001;3:23–9.

57. Sullivan KE, Jawad AF, Randall P, et al. Lack of correlation between impaired T cell production, immunodeficiency, and other phenotypic features in chromosome 22q11.2 deletion syndromes. Clin Immunol Immunopathol 1998;86:141–6.

58. Markert ML, Boeck A, Hale LP, et al. Transplantation of thymic tissue in complete DiGeorge syndrome. N Engl J Med 1999;341:1180–9.

59. Kirkpatrick CH. Chronic mucocutaneous candidiasis. Pediatr Infect Dis J 2001;20:197–206.

60. Nagamine K, Peterson P, Scott HS, et al. Positional cloning of the APECED gene. Nat Genet 1997;17:393–8.

61. Ahonen P, Myllarniemi S, Sipila I, et al. Clinical variation of autoimmune polyendocrinopathy-candidiasis-ectodermal dystrophy (APECED) in a series of 68 patients. N Engl J Med 1990;322:1829–36.

62. Lilic D. New perspectives on the immunology of chronic mucocutaneous candidiasis. Curr Opin Infect Dis 2002;15:143–7.

63. Nauseef WM. Insights into myeloperoxidase biosynthesis from its inherited deficiency. J Mol Med 1998;76:661–8.

64. Lanza F. Clinical manifestation of myeloperoxidase deficiency. J Mol Med 1998;76:676–81.

65. Densen P, Weiler JM, Griffiss JM, et al. Familial properdin deficiency and fatal meningococcemia. Correction of the bactericidal defect by vaccination. N Engl J Med 1987;316:922–6.

66. Thrasher AJ. WASp in immune-system organization and function. Nat Rev Immunol 2002;2:635–46.

67. Lawson SE, Thompson L, Williams MD. Wiskott Aldrich syndrome presenting as congenital thrombocytopenia. Clin Lab Haematol 1999;21:397–9.

68. Nonoyama S, Ochs HD. Wiskott-Aldrich syndrome. Curr Allergy Asthma Rep 2001;1:430–7.

69. Ariga T, Iwamura M, Miyakawa T, et al. Prenatal diagnosis of the Wiskott-Aldrich syndrome by PCR-based methods. Pediatr Int 2001;43:716–19.

70. Filipovich AH, Stone JV, Tomany SC, et al. Impact of donor type on outcome of bone marrow transplantation for

Wiskott-Aldrich syndrome: collaborative study of the International Bone Marrow Transplant Registry and the National Marrow Donor Program. Blood 2001;15:1598–603.

71. Knutsen AP, Wall DA. Umbilical cord blood transplantation in severe T-cell immunodeficiency disorders: two-year experience. J Clin Immunol 2000;20:466–76.

72. Wada T, Jagadeesh GJ, Nelson DL, et al. Retrovirus-mediated WASP gene transfer corrects Wiskott-Aldrich syndrome T-cell dysfunction. Hum Gene Ther 2002;13: 1039–46.

73. Reichenbach J, Schubert R, Schindler D, et al. Elevated oxidative stress in patients with ataxia telangiectasia. Antioxid Redox Signal 2002;4:465–9.

74. Khanna KK, Lavin MF, Jackson SP, et al. ATM, a central controller of cellular responses to DNA damage. Cell Death Differ 2001;8:1052–65.

75. Spring K, Ahangari F, Scott SP, et al. Mice heterogenous for mutation in ATM, the gene involved in ataxia-telangiectasia, have heightened susceptibility to cancer. Nat Genet 2002;32:185–90.

76. Geoffroy-Perez B, Janin N, Ossian K, et al. Cancer risk in heterozygotes for ataxia-telangiectasia. Int J Cancer 2001; 15:288–93.

77. Reyes C, Abuzaitoun O, De Jong A, et al. Epstein-Barr virus-associated smooth muscle tumors in ataxia-telangiectasia: a case report and review. Hum Pathol 2002;33: 133–6.

78. Schubert R, Reichenbach J, Zielen S. Deficiencies in CD4 + and CD8 + T cell subsets in ataxia telangiectasia. Clin Exp Immunol 2002;129:125–32.

79. Giovannetti A, Mazzetta F, Caprini E, et al. Skewed T cell receptor repertoire, decreased thymic output, and predominance of terminally differentiated T cells in ataxia-telangiectasia. Blood 2002;100:4082–9.

80. Speck P, Ikeda M, Ikeda A, et al. Signal transduction through the B cell antigen receptor is normal in ataxia-telangiectasia B lymphocytes. J Biol Chem 2002;277: 4123–7.

80a. Rosen FS, Cooper MD, Wedgwood RJP. The primary immunodeficiencies. N Engl J Med 1984;311:235–309.

81. Huang KY, Shyur SD, Wang CY, et al. Ataxia telangiectasia: report of two cases. J Microbiol Immunol Infect 2001;34: 71–5.

82. Sun X, Becker-Catania SG, Chun HH, et al. Early diagnosis of ataxia-telangiectasia using radiosensitivity testing. J Pediatr 2002;140:724–31.

83. Shiflett SL, Kaplan J, Ward DM. Chediak-Higashi syndrome: a rare disorder of lysosomes and lysosome related organelles. Pigment Cell Res 2002;15:251–7.

84. Kjeldsen L, Calafat J, Borregaard N. Giant granules of neutrophils in Chediak-Higashi syndrome are derived from azurophil granules but not from specific and gelatinase granules. J Leukoc Biol 1998;64:72–7.

85. Karim MA, Suzuki K, Fukai K, et al. Apparent genotype-phenotype correlation in childhood, adolescent, and adult Chediak-Higashi syndrome. Am J Med Genet 2002;108: 16–22.

86. Introne W, Boissy RE, Gahl WA. Clinical, molecular, and cell biological aspects of Chediak-Higashi syndrome. Mol Genet Metab 1999;68:283–303.

87. Liang JS, Lu MY, Tsai MJ, et al. Bone marrow transplantation from an HLA-matched unrelated donor for treatment of Chediak-Higashi syndrome. J Formos Med Assoc 2000; 99:499–502.

88. Ward DM, Shiflett SL, Kaplan J. Chediak-Higashi syndrome: a clinical and molecular view of a rare lysosomal storage disorder. Curr Mol Med 2002;2:469–77.

89. Shaw JM, Al-Shamkhani A, Boxer LA, et al. Characterization of four CD18 mutants in leucocyte adhesion deficient (LAD) patients with differential capacities to support expression and function of the CD11/CD18 integrins LFA-1, Mac-1 and p150,95. Clin Exp Immunol 2001;126: 311–8.

90. Akbari H, Zadeh MM. Leukocyte adhesion deficiency. Indian J Pediatr 2001;68:77–9.

91. Wilson JM, Ping AJ, Krauss JC, et al. Correction of CD18-deficient lymphocytes by retrovirus-mediated gene transfer. Science 1990;248:1413–6.

92. Mancias C, Infante AJ, Kamani NR. Matched unrelated donor bone marrow transplantation in leukocyte adhesion deficiency. Bone Marrow Transplant 1999;24:1261–3.

93. Price TH, Ochs HD, Gershoni-Baruch R, et al. In vivo neutrophil and lymphocyte function studies in a patient with leukocyte adhesion deficiency type II. Blood 1994; 84:1635–9.

94. Horwitz M, Benson KF, Person RE, et al. Mutations in ELA2, encoding neutrophil elastase, define a 21-day biological clock in cyclic haematopoiesis. Nat Genet 1999; 23:433–6.

95. Lubitz PA, Dower N, Krol AL. Cyclic neutropenia: an unusual disorder of granulopoiesis effectively treated with recombinant granulocyte colony-stimulating factor. Pediatr Dermatol 2001;18:426–32.

96. Bar-Joseph G, Halberthal M, Sweed Y, et al. Clostridium septicum infection in children with cyclic neutropenia. J Pediatr 1997;131:317–9.

97. Pernu HE, Pajari UH, Lanning M. The importance of regular dental treatment in patients with cyclic neutropenia. Follow-up of two cases. J Periodontol 1996;67:454–9.

98. Ming JE, Stiehm ER, Graham JM. Genetic syndromes associated with immunodeficiency. Immunol Allergy Clin North Am 2002;22:261–78.

Index

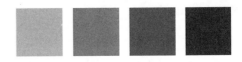

Page numbers followed by "t" indicate tables. Page numbers in *italics* indicate figures.